Fifth Edition

Exploring the Dimensions of Human Sexuality

Jerrold S. Greenberg, EdD, FASHA, FAAHE
Professor Emeritus
University of Maryland

Clint E. Bruess, EdD, CHES, FASHA, FAAHE
Dean Emeritus
University of Alabama at Birmingham
Professor Emeritus
Birmingham-Southern College

Sara B. Oswalt, MPH, PhD, CSE
Associate Professor
University of Texas at San Antonio

JONES & BARTLETT
LEARNING

World Headquarters
Jones & Bartlett Learning
5 Wall Street
Burlington, MA 01803
978-443-5000
info@jblearning.com
www.jblearning.com

Jones & Bartlett Learning books and products are available through most bookstores and online booksellers. To contact Jones & Bartlett Learning directly, call 800-832-0034, fax 978-443-8000, or visit our website, www.jblearning.com.

Substantial discounts on bulk quantities of Jones & Bartlett Learning publications are available to corporations, professional associations, and other qualified organizations. For details and specific discount information, contact the special sales department at Jones & Bartlett Learning via the above contact information or send an email to specialsales@jblearning.com.

Production Credits

Publisher: William Brottmiller
Executive Editor: Shoshanna Goldberg
Editorial Assistant: Sean Coombs
Production Manager: Julie Champagne Bolduc
Production Assistant: Stephanie Rineman
Marketing Manager: Grace Richards
VP, Manufacturing and Inventory Control: Therese Connell

Composition: diacriTech
Cover Design: Michael O'Donnell
Rights & Photo Research Associate: Amy Rathburn
Cover Image: © Kenny Yeoh/ShutterStock, Inc.
Printing and Binding: Courier Companies
Cover Printing: Courier Companies

To order this product, use ISBN: 978-1-4496-9801-0

Library of Congress Cataloging-in-Publication Data
Greenberg, Jerrold S.
  Exploring the dimensions of human sexuality / by Jerrold S. Greenberg, Clint E. Bruess, and Sara B. Oswalt.—5th ed.
    p. cm.
  Includes bibliographical references and index.
  ISBN 978-1-4496-4851-0
  ISBN 1-4496-4851-7
  1. Sex (Psychology) 2. Hygiene, Sexual. 3. Interpersonal relations. 4. Sexual ethics. I. Bruess, Clint E. II. Oswalt, Sara B. III. Title.
  HQ21.G67118 2014
  306.7—dc23

2012032815

6048

Printed in the United States of America
17 16 15 14 13   10 9 8 7 6 5 4 3 2 1

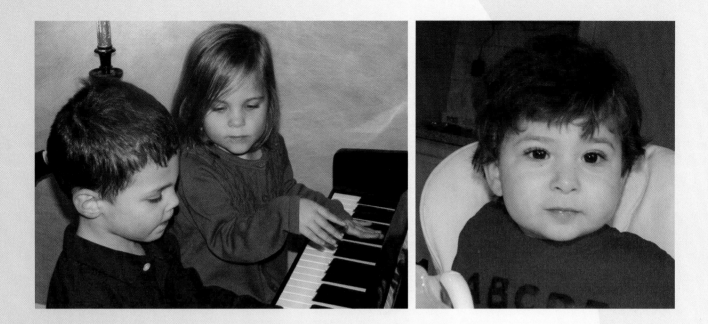

This book is dedicated to three of the cutest grandchildren possible: Jonah, Zoe, and Garrett.
The joy they bring is unsurpassed.

— *Jerrold S. Greenberg*

To Susan J. Laing with appreciation for her part in a wonderful relationship.

— *Clint E. Bruess*

To Martijn Middelplaats for his unwavering support and unconditional love.

— *Sara B. Oswalt*

Brief Contents

Contents

Features

Gender Dimensions

Ethical Dimensions

Human sexuality is an important component of a healthy lifestyle. It is not a topic to be hidden or avoided, as this can lead to serious consequences for one's health and overall life satisfaction. Conversely, when human sexuality is understood, the result is a healthier lifestyle and an increased ability to achieve consistency between one's actions and moral principles. The authors of this text have seen the effects of both approaches to human sexuality in their own families.

The benefit of perceiving sexuality as a topic of discussion and understanding can be seen in one example of a telephone call from one of the author's daughters. She said that her 14-year-old daughter asked about noises she sometimes heard coming from her parents' bedroom. Her mother explained that the noises were her mom and dad enjoying physical contact as part of showing love for each other. Fortunately, she had previously talked with her daughter about sexuality and reproduction, so she was able to refer back to that conversation. She asked her father for advice regarding how she handled the situation and what she should do further. He responded that she should be pleased that her daughter felt comfortable enough to talk with her about the noises, and that it was very positive that she had explained sexuality and reproduction to her daughter so she had accurate information that was appropriate for her age. Beyond that, the author simply said that his daughter was on the right track related to the sexuality education of her daughter, and the best thing to do moving forward was continue to keep the lines of communication open.

On the other hand, an example of how human sexuality is inappropriately conceptualized occurred when the son of a different author was entering fifth grade. School personnel organized a committee of parents to review instructional materials for the sexuality education course. As luck would have it, the author was selected to serve on this committee. At the first committee meeting, he was surprised to learn that the program focused exclusively on reproductive anatomy and physiology, and asked, with an inquiring tone, "How will you help students process their feelings pertaining to sexuality?" The answer was that the reproductive system would be taught just as any other body system would, with no plans to include a discussion of feelings associated with sexuality. At that point the author volunteered to resign from the parent review committee and asked to join the "Digestive System Parent Review Committee." Of course, there was none. That allowed the author to point out that there really is a distinction between education regarding sexuality and education pertaining to other health issues, and that this distinction needs to be addressed with students. We do that in this book by exploring the varied dimensions of human sexuality.

In fact, we have known students who would have liked to enroll in our human sexuality courses but did not due to their discomfort regarding sexuality. Some were embarrassed to have their friends or relatives find out that they did not know *everything* about sex. Others felt uncomfortable discussing sexuality in a class with their peers. And still others believed they knew more than they really did, although in reality it was not enough to live a sexually healthy life. Consequently, in *Exploring the Dimensions of Human Sexuality, Fifth Edition* we make a special effort to engage students in a nonjudgmental manner and make the content interesting, resulting in enhanced learning.

The Dimensions of Human Sexuality

In many regards, human sexuality today does not differ from that of our ancestors' times. Biologically, human reproduction occurs the same way. As in the past, religion and culture have a significant impact on our sexuality; as does public policy. As longtime sexuality educators, we know that no single aspect of sexuality can be separated from the others, and no single aspect is more important than the others. Therefore, we have chosen to write a text that presents all aspects of sexuality as interconnected and significant. Throughout this text you will find an emphasis on health and well-being based on the assumption that we are all sexual beings and that sexuality should be viewed in its totality—with biological, psychological, and sociocultural dimensions.

The dimensions discussed in the book can be broken down into biological, psychological, and sociocultural categories. Some examples are described here.

Biological Dimensions
Physiology
The basis of understanding sexuality is knowledge about the physiology of how our bodies work. Factual information lays the foundation of critical thinking—without the facts, you cannot begin to think critically about your sexuality. The greater your knowledge, the more likely you are to take responsibility for your sexual health.

Gender

The physiological differences between genders create the foundation for the development of psychological and social wellness and strongly influence our perceptions of sexual wellness. Gender Dimensions receive a full chapter and boxed treatment in every chapter.

Psychological Dimensions

Psychology

Developing a positive image of self and sexuality is critical to developing sexual wellness. For example, a positive body image lends itself to your overall wellness; a negative self-image can lead to drug abuse (steroids or diet pills) or psychological disorders (anorexia, bulimia, binge eating disorder, or muscle dysmorphia). Body image is so important that we devote a minichapter ("In Focus") to the topic—the most comprehensive coverage in the market!

Spirituality

Religious and spiritual beliefs influence feelings about sexual behavior, premarital sexual activity, adultery, divorce, contraception, abortion—even masturbation. Spiritual issues are discussed in Multicultural Dimensions boxes and in the opening chapter.

Sociocultural Dimensions

Multicultural

Cultures within the United States and around the world differ in their views of sexuality. From semi-nude beaches in the south of France to Middle Eastern Muslim communities where women are covered from head to hand to foot, ours is a world of diversity. Sometimes these diverse behaviors are a part of the culture, and other times they are given legal sanction. A good example of this is the many ways in which abortion is viewed. Such views range from strict prohibition, including strong laws, to simply viewing abortion as a method of birth control, such that it is common for women to have as many as four or five abortions. Your ability to respect your sexual partner's cultural beliefs and feelings will result in a higher level of satisfaction for both of you. To help students better understand sexual diversity, each chapter contains one boxed example pertaining to a culture within the United States and another example pertaining to a culture from elsewhere in the world.

Ethics

Ethical decision-making takes on legal and moral implications concerning sexuality. The law and courts become involved in such far-flung areas as access to abortion clinics, workplace sexual harassment, and ownership of frozen embryos. Moral implications of ethical decisions include sexual coercion and underscore the importance of taking responsibility for your sexual wellness. Ethical Dimensions boxes appear in every chapter, and Chapter 18 (Sexual Ethics, Morality, and the Law) covers these issues more in-depth.

Public Policy

Public policy also affects our sexual behavior. For example, the Healthy People 2020 national health objectives promote sexual health awareness pertaining to acquired immune deficiency syndrome (AIDS) and sexually transmitted infections (STIs), unwanted teenage pregnancies, and prenatal care. Furthermore, public policy on free speech continues to allow the uncontrolled distribution of pornographic material on the Internet. Unfortunately, as a result of public policy, access to proper health care, birth control, and other influences on sexual health are often unavailable for the poor.

Integration

Integrated Theme

With so many factors influencing our sexual behavior, we have created a striking full-page feature: *Exploring the Dimensions of Human Sexuality,* an integrated approach that ties all these strands together. This feature assists students in understanding how many different aspects affect their sexual health and influence their sexual behavior. Our intent is to help students envision the convergence of the many aspects of sexuality and help them make sexual decisions that lead to a lifetime of positive sexual health and wellness.

Integrated Website

Exploring the Dimensions of Human Sexuality also links to the Jones & Bartlett Learning website (go. jblearning.com/dimensions5e), where each dimension is presented in greater depth. Students can click on a particular chapter and find self-assessments, exercises, research links, and information that will allow them to explore further their own dimensions of human sexuality. Integrating the book and website actively engages the students in the learning process. *See the Visual Walkthrough on page xx for an example of this feature.*

Pedagogy

Because we realize that learning best occurs when students are actively involved, we have created a text that goes beyond merely presenting factual knowledge about the varied dimensions of human sexuality. For example, we provide numerous ways for students to explore the dimensions of human sexuality and determine how each affects their *personal* sexuality. This exploration is facilitated through the pedagogical features described below. In addition, *Exploring the Dimensions of Human Sexuality, Fifth Edition* presents accurate, up-to-date, state-of-the-art content by regularly updating the text. This updating occurred in the 2002 edition, the 2004 edition, the 2007 edition, the 2011 edition, and in this 2014 edition.

There are numerous pedagogical features employed in *Exploring the Dimensions of Human Sexuality* to enhance student learning.

In Focus: Body Image

We offer a comprehensive look at the concept of body image in a minichapter. It is rare to find so much detail on this subject. Together in one place we discuss how body image affects self-esteem and sexuality, how the quest for a perfect body creates problems ranging from eating disorders to cosmetic surgery and steroid abuse, and how body image affects both genders. There are also three other In Focus chapters: Unexpected Pregnancy Outcomes, HIV and AIDS, and Alternative Sexual Behaviors.

The Dimensions of Human Sexuality Boxed Features

A carefully designed program reinforces the dimensions theme of the textbook with five distinct types of boxes in each chapter: Multicultural Dimensions, Global Dimensions, Gender Dimensions, Communication Dimensions, and Ethical Dimensions. *Please refer to page xx of the Visual Walkthrough for detailed descriptions of these features.*

Critical Thinking

Exploring the Dimensions of Human Sexuality, Fifth Edition requires students to think critically about how the multifaceted dimensions relate to them. To that end, we have embedded critical thinking questions within the text to help students reflect on the subject matter and understand its implications for their sexual health. Critical thinking questions are found in boxes, in photo captions, and in the end-of-chapter section—including application questions related to the chapter-opening story, critical thinking questions about material, and a critical thinking minicase. Critical thinking questions help students recall information and synthesize new material with existing knowledge and stimulate students to make informed judgments about the information provided.

Myth vs. Fact and Did You Know. . . Boxes

Students' sexual health and wellness are also influenced by sexual myths and folklore. Many of our brief sidebars are designed to set students straight on such myths. "Did You Know..." boxes add whimsical and high-interest information to engage the student further.

Chapter-Opening Story

Each chapter opens with an engaging real-life story that explores the concepts to be discussed in the chapter. Students are drawn into the chapter material with a high-interest case and introduced to the topics that will be discussed. At the end of the chapter, students are asked to relate the chapter's information to application questions about the opening story.

Reviewing the Dimensions of Human Sexuality

Each chapter ends with an interactive feature designed to help students take responsibility for their sexual health and wellness. This section includes an interactive self-assessment designed to help students understand and clarify their own feelings about sexuality issues presented in that chapter. It also includes discussion questions, application questions pertaining to the opening story, critical thinking questions, a critical thinking minicase, and a self-assessment.

Updates to the Fifth Edition

Throughout this new edition, extensive updates have been made to focus on information and statistics about recent developments. Information from hundreds of new references has been added—almost all of these references were published in the last few years. Suggested readings at the end of each chapter were updated, as was the Web Resources section at the end of each chapter. Some sections within chapters have been moved to improve organization, others have been deleted, and new sections have been added to reflect changes related to human sexuality. New and more appropriate photos and illustrations have replaced older ones as needed. Examples of changes and updates within selected chapters include the following:

- Chapter 1 offers additional global and multicultural examples, including a box about the Islamic culture.

- Chapter 2 includes the latest research related to sexuality. There are 15 new references in that chapter alone.

- Chapter 3 examines the newer electronic modes of communication related to sexuality.

- Chapter 4 includes the latest research on the G spot, female ejaculation, and speculation regarding the existence of a female prostate. Table 4.2 includes the latest information from the National Women's Health Center on premenstrual symptoms.

- The latest PSA screening recommendation of the U.S. Preventive Services Task Force was added in Chapter 5. In addition, a new Gender Dimensions box focused on testicular self-exam is presented.

- In Chapter 6 a table was added depicting the age of first intercourse globally and in 41 countries including the United States *(When You First Had Sex)*. Also, a new Did You Know box discusses controversial research that concluded that women who experience vaginal orgasms can be identified by how they walk.

- Chapter 7 now includes an updated discussion about different options for emergency contraception.

- In Chapter 8, new research and references related to the use and effect of drugs during pregnancy were included. There is also revised information on water births and associated risks, additional information on disorders of sexual development, and an expanded section on assisted reproductive technologies.

- In Focus: Unexpected Pregnancy Outcomes includes updated information about medical abortion in the United States. There is also a recent summary of state laws regarding abortion availability and restrictions. An extensive rewrite was done related to domestic and international adoption practices and challenges.

- In Chapter 9, information about the first federal report since 1963 on the welfare of women was included. New features include a Did You Know box about the effects "checking out" someone of the other gender can have on students' performance, and a Multicultural Dimensions box on the women's movement in France, along with updated information throughout the chapter.

- In Focus: Body Image has new information on eating disorders and an overview of literature related to muscle dysmorphia.

- Chapter 10 includes new information about pansexuality and asexuality. A new Ethical Dimensions box related to teaching about gay history is also included, in addition to a new Did You Know box about the National Institute of Medicine's assessment of the health status of the LGBT population.

- In Chapter 11 there is new information about gender during the early years. Comparisons between comprehensive sexuality education programs and abstinence-only-until-marriage programs are summarized based on current research.

- In Chapter 12, there is a new Global Dimensions box about young people, unprotected sexual activity, and trustworthy information. Another new Global Dimensions box contains information about single-parent households in various countries. New information about various family styles is also included, and the chapter has 36 new references.

- In Focus: Alternative Sexual Behaviors contains a new Multicultural Dimensions box on paraphilias across cultures along with updated information about paraphilias in general.

- In Chapter 13, research about gay and straight men's most arousing sexual fantasies was added as was the latest data pertaining to male and female college students' viewing of Internet pornography. A new Did You Know box about sexual activity among older adults and a new table (Table 13.3) on median age of first intercourse by country and gender were also added.

- Chapter 14 contains a new Multicultural Dimensions box on sexual violence in various cultures. A new Did You Know box on stalking was also added along with six new suggested readings and 20 new references.

- Chapter 15 now includes discussion about expedited partner therapy. In addition to an expanded and more thorough discussion of HPV and its related complications, there are updated prevalence rates and treatment recommendations for all STIs.

- In Focus: HIV and AIDS includes updated statistics about prevalence and rate of HIV in the United States and internationally, information about antiviral medication as a prophylactic medication, and recent vaccine developments. An expanded discussion about risk of contracting HIV through organ donation, a revised discussion about new testing mechanisms, and an extensively updated section on prevention strategies also have been added.

- In Chapter 16, discussion about the potential medicalization of sexual function and dysfunction is included. Terminology is streamlined and updated; a review of hypersexuality (commonly referred to as sex addiction) and new strategies in sex therapy are also included.

- In Chapter 17, there is new information about dating and relationships on reality TV shows, as well as on videos and video games. There is also a new Global Dimensions box on international differences related to prostitution.

- Chapter 18 includes an expanded discussion of stem cell research. The issue of polygamy is also discussed and its morality explored.

When appropriate, boxed material has been changed and updated throughout the fifth edition of this book. Statistics have also been updated throughout the book. For example, the most current statistics regarding STIs, adoptions, abortions, birth rates, marriage and divorce rates, prevalence of sexual behaviors, and many other categories are presented.

Writing this book has been a service-learning activity for us. We did abundant and thorough research to identify state-of-the-art knowledge and attitudes pertaining to sexuality and learned a great deal in doing so. That was the "learning" part of the service-learning equation. The "service" part relates to our interest in helping to enhance the sexual health and wellness of our readers. As such, we hope you find the information we included, the issues we raised and discussed, and the myths we debunked useful as you live, express your sexuality, and make decisions related to your sexuality. If that is the case, the time, effort, and energy we have devoted to writing this text will have been well worth that investment.

About the Authors

Jerrold S. Greenberg, EdD, FASHA, FAAHE

Dr. Jerrold S. Greenberg is Professor Emeritus in the School of Public Health at the University of Maryland. Dr. Greenberg earned his baccalaureate and master's degrees from The City College of New York and then continued his education at Syracuse University where he earned his doctorate. Dr. Greenberg has taught at Syracuse University, Boston University, and the State University of New York at Buffalo before accepting a professorship at the University of Maryland in 1979. Dr. Greenberg has written more than 50 books on such topics as elder care, health, stress management, physical fitness, sexuality, and methods of health education. In addition, he has published more than 80 articles in professional journals and in lay magazines. Among Dr. Greenberg's honors are: the University of Maryland Service–Learning Advocate of the Year award for 2003–2004; the American School Health Association's Distinguished Service Award; selection as Alliance Scholar by the American Alliance for Health, Physical Education, Recreation, and Dance; the Presidential Citation, the Certificate of Appreciation, and the Scholar Award of the American Association for Health Education; selection for inclusion in Who's Who in America, Outstanding Young Men of America, and Who's Who in World Jewry. Dr. Greenberg has also served on the editorial boards of the professional journals *Health Education* and *The Journal of School Health;* and as a reviewer for other professional journals. In addition, Dr. Greenberg has conducted stress management workshops for professional, business, and lay organizations throughout the United States.

Clint E. Bruess, EdD, CHES, FASHA, FAAHE

Dr. Clint E. Bruess is Dean Emeritus of the School of Education and Professor Emeritus of Health Education at the University of Alabama at Birmingham. He is also Professor Emeritus at Birmingham-Southern College. He earned his baccalaureate degree at Macalester College, his master's at the University of Maryland, and his doctorate at Temple University.

Dr. Bruess was a professor at West Chester University, Towson University (also department chair), and The University of Alabama at Birmingham (also department chair and later Dean of the School of Education), before becoming Division Chair and Professor at Birmingham-Southern College. He also directed the School Health Education Project for the National Center for Health Education for 3 years.

Dr. Bruess has coauthored more than 15 textbooks in the areas of human sexuality, sexuality education, personal health, and school health programs. In addition, he has published numerous articles in professional journals and served in elected and appointed positions for the American School Health Association (also a Fellow), American Association for Health Education (also a Fellow), and Society of Public Health Educators. Dr. Bruess continues to review professional articles for *Health Education, The Journal of School Health, The International Journal of Health Education, The American Journal of Health Behavior,* and serves on the editorial board of the *American Journal of Sexuality Education.*

Sara B. Oswalt, MPH, PhD, CSE

Sara B. Oswalt is an Associate Professor in the Department of Health and Kinesiology at the University of Texas at San Antonio. She attended Pennsylvania State University for her undergraduate degree, Indiana University for her master's degree, and the University of Georgia for her doctorate degree. She worked as a college health educator for 8 years, spending 6 of those years as the sexual health coordinator for the University of Georgia.

Dr. Oswalt has authored more than 25 journal articles. Her research interests are directed at college students, assessing their health status and the evaluation of college and university efforts to address those health issues. She has a special interest in sexual health issues for the college population. She regularly teaches sexuality courses for undergraduate students and is also an AASECT (American Association of Sexuality Educators, Counselors, and Therapists) Certified Sexuality Educator (CSE).

Acknowledgments

We would like to thank Dr. Sue Tendy, EdD of the U.S. Military Academy at West Point for her contributions to the material on sexual harassment in the military. Our sincere thanks and appreciation goes to the Jones & Bartlett Learning Health Science team: Shoshanna Goldberg, Executive Editor; Sean Coombs, Editorial Assistant; Julie Bolduc, Production Manager; Stephanie Rineman, Production Assistant; and Jennifer Stiles, Marketing Manager. We would like to acknowledge the dedication and hard work of these individuals, for without them this project would never have been realized. Finally, we would like to thank the many reviewers who guided us throughout the various stages of this project. Their voices, criticism, and support have truly made this a better text.

Robert E. Braun, MPH, CHES
The University of Toledo

Dr. Charles Chase
West Texas A&M University
Sports and Exercise Sciences

Dr. Kirsten Lupinski
Health, Physical Education, and Recreation
Albany State University

Deneen Long-White, MS, CHES
Howard University

Dr. Maureen McHarey
Dean, Health and Rehabilitation Services
Community College of Rhode Island
Visiting Lecturer
Providence College
School of Continuing Education

Molly A. McKinney
University of Toledo

A Visual Walkthrough

Exploring the Dimensions of Human Sexuality, Fifth Edition is designed around the central theme that our feelings, attitudes, and beliefs regarding sexuality are continually influenced by our internal and external environments. All aspects of sexuality—biological, spiritual, psychological, and sociocultural—are interconnected and significant. The boxed feature program, additional pedagogy, and ancillaries of this new textbook have been designed around these core concepts.

BOXED FEATURES

Communication Dimensions
These boxes discuss communication issues that arise around sexuality between the genders, partners from different ethnic groups, and others.

Multicultural Dimensions
To better appreciate how various people view sexuality we offer a multicultural boxed feature. These boxes deal exclusively with diversity issues within the United States.

Global Dimensions
Sexuality is viewed very differently outside of the United States. Issues such as divorce in China and international differences in discussing sexuality are discussed in the Global Dimensions boxes.

Gender Dimensions
Issues arising from gender are integrated throughout the text, discussed in detail in the Gender Dimensions chapter, and featured in the Gender Dimensions boxes found in each chapter. Topics covered in these boxes include communication breakdown between genders, responsibility for contraception, and many others.

Ethical Dimensions
The importance of ethics in sexuality is underscored in the Ethical Dimensions box features. This is where topics such as abstinence-only education and the ethics surrounding technological advances are discussed.

Pedagogical Design

Chapter-Opening Pedagogy Each chapter-opening spread gives the reader a glimpse of the content with chapter objectives, a list of the Dimensions of Human Sexuality boxed features that will follow, and a list of topics also explored on the companion website. In addition, a high interest and engaging real-life story draws students into the chapter material and introduces them to the topics that will be discussed. This opening story is revisited at the end of the chapter in the application questions.

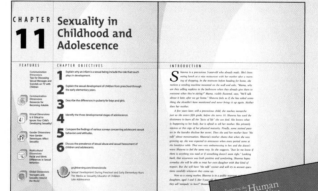

Exploring the Dimensions of Human Sexuality This feature organizes the multifaceted issues in each chapter into biological, psychological, and sociocultural factors. This visual element is integrated with the companion website where instructors and students can further explore these dimensions.

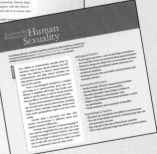

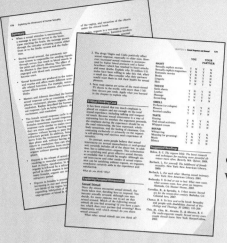

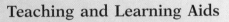

Reviewing the Dimensions of Human Sexuality This end-of-chapter activity gives students the opportunity to review and apply key chapter concepts. Items in this section include discussion questions, critical thinking questions, and application questions that relate to the chapter-opening story. The Exploring Personal Dimensions section directs students to focus on personal choices and take responsibility for their sexual health and well-being.

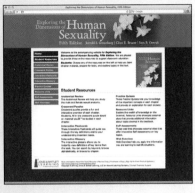

Teaching and Learning Aids

Exploring the Dimensions of Human Sexuality Online

go.jblearning.com/dimensions5

The companion website is integrated with the *Exploring the Dimensions of Human Sexuality* feature found in each main chapter of the text and offers four central components:

- ■ Resource links give the instructor the ability to integrate the Web into the curriculum.

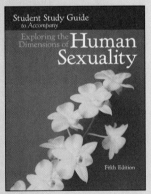

- ■ Instructor resources such as PowerPoint lecture presentations, a TestBank, and an instructor's manual assist in classroom preparation.
- ■ Student activities such as web exercises and self-assessments involve students in the dimensions of human sexuality in a structured online environment.
- ■ Student study tools like an anatomical review, animated flashcards, crossword puzzles, and practice quizzes offer students the opportunity to review chapter concepts and prepare for exams.

An Interactive Online Workbook allows students to review chapter topics and assess their own sexuality behaviors in relation to these topics. Exercises and activities include Chapter Summary, Fill in the Blanks, Review the Dimensions, Focus on the Facts, Quick Questions, and Test Your Knowledge.

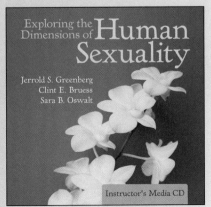

Instructor's Media CD

offers the instructor maximum flexibility in preparing for class, designing and presenting lectures, and generating tests. The Media CD features PowerPoint lecture outlines and an image and table bank. Content can be implemented into many of the common distance learning programs. (Available for both PC and Macintosh.)

SPECIAL FEATURES

Myth vs Fact Students' sexual health and wellness are influenced by sexual myths and folklore. Myth vs Fact features common myths associated with the material presented in each chapter along with the fact to dispel each myth.

Brief Did You Know… sidebars add whimsical and high-interest information to further engage the student.

In Focus Minichapters The authors have included focused minichapters that delve into topics that affect students' lives. These take a fully comprehensive look at subjects such as body image, unexpected pregnancy, HIV and AIDS, and alternative sexual behaviors. The concentrated chapters offer today's students a deeper understanding of issues about which they should be informed.

Service–Learning Appendix Although we are all rightfully concerned with our own sexual health and well-being, the authors encourage readers to also recognize the responsibility to contribute to the sexual health of the communities in which they reside. An *Introduction to Service–Learning* appendix, available on the companion website, gives an overview of the concept of service–learning and suggests specific activities through which readers can contribute to sexual health in their communities. These activities employ a service–learning methodology; that is, students provide service while learning chapter content at the same time.

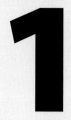

CHAPTER 1

Introducing the Dimensions of Human Sexuality

CHAPTER OBJECTIVES

 1 Identify and discuss the dimensions of human sexuality, including biological, psychological, and sociocultural factors.

 2 Discuss the historical aspects of human sexuality, including the sexual revolution, the role of gender, and the role of culture.

 3 Apply critical thinking methods to human sexuality.

 4 Outline the reasons to study human sexuality, including the steps of the decision-making process.

go.jblearning.com/dimensions5e

Global Dimensions: Male Genital Mutilation
and Circumcision Practices
Prostate Cancer
Care from Organizations and Available Publications

INTRODUCTION

*L*et us begin our exploration of the many dimensions of human sexuality by examining how they affect the life of one person: Lisa, an 18-year-old college freshman, involved in her first serious—and sexual—relationship. After several months of dating, Lisa experiences the scare of her life: Her period is late. After a few days she purchases a home-pregnancy kit. As she waits until the morning to take the test, she begins to think about the role of sexuality in her life.

Like most people who grow up in the United States today, Lisa received basic sexuality education in public school. But that brief overview—which Lisa and her friends giggled through—touched only on the physical aspects of reproduction. Nothing prepared her for the emotions she felt during her current relationship, or how her social and cultural upbringing would affect her sexual behavior.

Lisa is a Korean American, a member of a family who respect heritage and tradition. Her parents, a university professor and a homemaker, were born in Korea and had an arranged marriage. The traditional Korean view of sexuality is conservative, and virginity is highly prized for marriage. Although Lisa holds on to many traditional views, she also struggles with the permissive attitude toward sexuality that prevails in the U.S. culture today—an attitude that her boyfriend shares (Brennan, 1999).

An unexpected pregnancy for Lisa would be a major tragedy in her family. Pregnancy outside marriage would shame not only the individual (and make her an "unperson") but also the entire family. Her family could choose to exile her.

Korean Americans tend not to tolerate secrecy by children and exert strict parental control. The Korean culture discourages open discussion of feelings and seeking out of psychological counseling. Thus Lisa is in a *crisis because she feels she cannot tell her parents, but she also cannot tell anyone else (who may in turn tell her parents). In fact, Lisa has yet to tell her boyfriend what is upsetting her.*

Religion plays a major role in many people's sexuality. For Lisa's parents, whose cultural traditions in Korea can be traced to Confucianism, abortion may be a possibility (as a means of saving face for the family). But many Korean American immigrants are members of fundamentalist Christian groups, who often prohibit abortion. Lisa wonders what she will do if, in fact, she is really pregnant.

Lisa is lucky: She is not pregnant. But Lisa has realized that she has to start taking greater responsibility for her sexual behavior. How can she incorporate the many dimensions affecting her sexuality into her personal sexuality?

This chapter begins our exploration of the many dimensions of sexuality and how they affect our lives.

The Dimensions of Human Sexuality

When you think about human sexuality, what do you think of? Some form of physical contact? Human reproduction? Feelings when you see an attractive person? Human sexuality is all that and more. **Human sexuality** is a part of your total personality. It involves the interrelationship of biological, psychological, and sociocultural dimensions.

human sexuality
A part of your total personality. It involves the interrelationship of biological, psychological, and sociocultural dimensions.

The Sexuality Information and Education Council of the United States (SIECUS) defines human sexuality as encompassing the sexual knowledge, beliefs, attitudes, values, and behaviors of individuals. Its various dimensions include the anatomy, physiology, and biochemistry of the sexual response system; identity, orientation, roles, and personality; and thoughts, feelings, and relationships. The expression of sexuality is influenced by ethical, spiritual, cultural, and moral concerns (SIECUS, 2012).

The Alberta Society for the Promotion of Sexual Health (ASPSH) indicates that sexuality means many things: feelings about ourselves, roles we play in society, and reproduction. It is not limited to how we behave sexually. It is the total of our physical, emotional, and spiritual responses, thoughts, and feelings. Sexuality is more about who we are than about what we do (ASPSH, 2011).

Sexuality is a natural part of life. The concepts of human sexuality are learned. From our viewpoint, human sexuality involves at least three dimensions—biological, psychological, and sociocultural. Each dimension has many subdimensions. The interactive relationship of these dimensions describes an individual's total sexuality.

The Interactive Nature of Sexual Dimensions

A complex set of biological, psychological, and sociocultural variables plays a role in all our sexual interactions. The decision to be sexually active is a result of many factors. Sexual arousal is a physiological function. Psychologically, our body image and feelings of self-worth may inhibit getting involved ("I'm not good enough for her"; "I'm not attractive enough for him"). A lack of self-worth may also inhibit arousal. Our culture helps us develop a sense of what is attractive—height, weight, hair style, skin tone. In addition, religious beliefs affect our sexual undertakings, as do legal and ethical considerations. Role models set by family and friends influence us as well.

All these dimensions constantly interact and influence our sexuality. Although we discuss them separately for clarity, remember that almost all sexuality-related decisions we make are influenced by more than one dimension.

Biological Dimension

The basis of understanding sexuality is physiological knowledge about how our bodies work. Factual information lays the foundation of decision making—without the facts, you cannot begin to think critically about your sexuality. The greater your knowledge, the more likely you are to take responsibility for your sexual health.

Until relatively recently, most of the research into human sexuality focused on physiology. For example, a model of the human sexual response cycle, published by the well-known researchers Masters and Johnson in 1966, focused mainly on physiology.

Fisher (1992) emphasizes the genetic aspects of behavior. In her view, humans have a common nature, a set of unconscious tendencies that are encoded in our genes. She believes that although we are not aware of these predispositions, they still motivate our actions. Although she recognizes that culture plays a role in one's sexuality, she also seems to support **essentialism**, the belief that the essence of sexuality is biological.

> **essentialism**
> Belief that once the cultural and historical aspects are taken away, the essence of sexuality is biological.

The biological dimension of our sexuality involves our physical appearance, especially the development of physical sexual characteristics; our responses to sexual stimulation; our ability to reproduce or to control fertility; and our growth and development in general. Although human reproductive function does not begin until puberty, human sexual–erotic functioning begins immediately after birth and lasts a lifetime. It is important to realize that biological functioning, as it relates to sexuality, is a part of the natural functioning of human beings. These biological aspects also relate to the other dimensions of sexuality, and all the dimensions work together to produce an individual's total sexuality—which, in turn, is part of the total personality (Bruess & Schroeder, 2014).

The physiological differences between the sexes help to lay the groundwork for the development of psychological and social wellness, and our gender strongly influences our perceptions of sexual wellness. For example, the sexual double standard, in which men are expected to be promiscuous and women are not, is a belief held by many people in the United States. In our human sexuality classes we always ask students to complete the sentences "A man who carries a condom in his wallet is _____" and "A woman who carries a condom in her purse is _____." The man is routinely described as "responsible," the woman as "a slut."

Gender DIMENSIONS

The Multifaceted Dimension of Gender

The first words our parents heard after we emerged from the womb declared our biological gender: "It's a boy!" or "It's a girl!" Our parents bought crib sheets and clothes that were pink or blue to match our gender.

We soon learned the sociocultural meanings of gender: Boys and girls are socialized to play in different styles and usually learn to prefer different sets of toys. Our moms and/or dads tended to do gender-specific chores. Teenage boys are somehow allowed to be sexually active, whereas girls are discouraged from such activities (a concept known as the "double standard").

Psychologically, girls are encouraged to show their emotions, whereas boys learn to suppress emotions. This leads to differing communication styles as well: Females are generally more expressive verbally than males. (Of course, there are many expressive men and inexpressive females. Remember that Lisa in our opening story has been culturally socialized to suppress open discussion of feelings.)

One couple announced the birth of their baby, Storm, but decided not to share the baby's gender. They felt that their decision gave Storm the freedom to choose who he or she wanted to be. They said that kids receive messages from society that encourage them to fit into existing boxes, including those with regard to gender. To other people they simply said, "Please, can you just let Storm discover for him/herself what s(he) wants to be?" (Roth, 2011).

Socially, there are many gender inequalities that will be covered in detail throughout this text. In the workplace, a woman often earns less than a man earns (a concept known as the "wage gap") and often faces a tougher time getting promoted into upper management (a concept known as the "glass ceiling"). After a woman goes home from work, she usually does more household chores (known as the "second shift") than her spouse.

Why are such topics covered in a human sexuality course? Because our gender—who we are as men and women and how we experience ourselves as male and female—is an essential component of our sexuality.

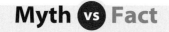

Myth: Human sexuality relates mainly to biological functioning.
Fact: Human sexuality includes a biological dimension but also includes psychological and socio-cultural dimensions.

Myth: Most people are well informed about human sexuality.
Fact: Unfortunately, most people still have relatively poor knowl-

edge of sexuality. Therefore, many myths about human sexuality still exist.

Myth: Sexual "normality" is similar among various cultures.
Fact: Sexual attitudes and behaviors differ greatly among cultural groups. There is no set standard for "normality."

Psychological Dimensions

Although sexual activity is definitely physical, it also involves psychology—our sense of being. The noted sexual therapist Dr. Ruth Westheimer has a favorite saying, that sexual behavior "is all between the ears."

A major psychological factor that affects our sexual wellness is body image. A positive body image lends itself to a feeling of overall wellness; a negative self-image can lead to drug abuse (use of steroids or diet pills) or psychological disorders (anorexia, bulimia, binge eating disorder, or muscle dysmorphia).

The psychological dimension of sexuality is probably the clearest example of learned aspects of sexuality. Our attitudes and feelings toward ourselves and other people begin to develop very early in life. From the time we are born, we get signals from all around us telling us how to think and act. We learn that some words are "wrong" or "dirty" and that certain parts of our body are "unmentionable." We even learn to be careful about what conversational topics we enter into with certain people. If we feel one way about ourselves but think others would find these feelings unacceptable, we learn to hide our true feelings and to pretend. After all, thinking or talking about sexuality is not a good idea anyway (or so we have learned). Some of us are lucky enough to grow up with a more positive set of experiences. Regardless of whether our experiences are positive or negative, however, our learned responses to them become integral to our sexuality.

Sociocultural Dimensions

The biological and psychological components of sexuality are affected by society and culture. The sociocultural dimension of sexuality is the sum of the cultural and social influences that affect our thoughts and actions.

In contrast to a perception of sexuality's being controlled mainly by biological or genetic characteristics,

Tiefer (1995) promotes the idea of **social constructionism**, which proposes that sexual identities and experiences are acquired from and influenced and modified by an ever-changing social environment. According to social constructionists, people acquire and assemble meanings, skills, and values from the people around them. This dimension of sexuality is the sum of the cultural influences that affect our thoughts and actions, both historical and contemporary. For example, historical influences become evident when one considers roles of males and females as well as certain customs.

> **social constructionism**
> The belief that sexual identities are acquired from and influenced and modified by an ever-changing social environment.

Indeed, we are surrounded by social influences on our sexuality. Among the sources of influence are religion, multiculturalism, socioeconomic status, ethics, the media, and politics. We will look at each influence here briefly and will revisit them throughout the text.

Religious Influences

Religious and spiritual beliefs influence feelings about morality, sexual behavior, premarital sexual behavior, adultery, divorce, contraception, abortion, and masturbation.

It is hard to know for sure what influences the attitudes of college students toward many controversial issues, but religion is certainly one of the important influences. It is interesting to note the findings of the UCLA Higher Education Research Institute. Since 1966, this group has done a comprehensive survey of college freshmen.

In 1999 only 40% of freshmen agreed that it is OK for two people who like each other to have sexual intercourse, even if they have known each other for only a short time. In 2001, this percentage increased only slightly, to 41.8%, and in 2002 it was 42.2%. In 2005 it increased a little more, to 46.2%. This represents lower support for casual sexual behavior among the entering class than the all-time high of 52% in 1987. Interestingly, in 2002 this idea was supported by 55.2% of males and 31.7% of females. In 2005 it was supported by 59.8% of males and 35.1% of females. Only half of 1999's freshman class backed efforts to keep abortion legal. This was after a record low figure after 6 years of decline, but in 2001 the proportion increased to 53.9% and in 2002 it was 55%—about equal for males and females. In 2005 it was 53.9%—again about equal for males and females. In 2007 it was 56.9%, and in 2009 it was 58.2%; in both instances it remained about equal for males and females. In 2012 support for legal abortion rose to 60.7%. Support for laws protecting abortion peaked

Romance reality shows have been successful with television viewers. With so many people looking for love, networks have no shortage of candidates, but it remains to be seen whether real romance can blossom in front of the camera. Do you watch romance reality shows? Why do you think society has embraced them? Do you think it's healthy to make a game out of love?

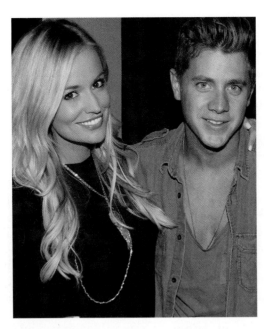

in 1990 at 65% (Characteristics of freshmen, 2001; The nation: Attitudes and characteristics of freshmen at 4-year colleges, 2002; This year's freshmen at 4-year colleges: A statistical profile, 2005; The American freshman: National norms for fall 2007, 2008; This year's freshmen at 4-year colleges: A statistical profile, 2009; Survey Tracks Changes in Political Views of Freshmen, 2012).

The percentage of freshmen supporting the legal right of gay couples to marry was 57.9% in 2002, 59.3% in 2003, 56.7% in 2005, 63.5% in 2007, 66.2%

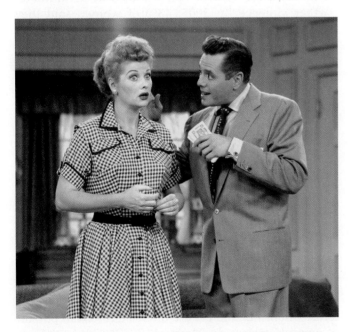

In its infancy, television was reluctant to show a biracial couple. When Lucille Ball and Desi Arnaz proposed the *I Love Lucy* show in the early 1950s, television executives wanted a white actor to play opposite Lucy, fearing problems of showing a white-and-Latino couple. Lucy and Desi were forced to put up $5,000 of their own money to create a pilot, which was, of course, a success.

in 2009, and 71.3% in 2012. Interestingly, in 2007 this position was supported by 55.3% of males as compared to 70.3% of females. In 2009 it was supported by 58.8% of males and 72.4% of females. In 2003, 24.8% said they supported laws prohibiting gay relationships; in 2005, 21.5% believed this; and in 2007, 24.3% did (Rooney, 2003; This year's freshmen at 4-year colleges: A statistical profile, 2005; The American freshman: National norms for fall 2007, 2008; This year's freshmen at 4-year colleges: A statistical profile, 2009; Survey tracks changes in political views of Freshmen, 2012).

In 2011 it was reported that two-thirds of entering first-year students supported legal marital status for same-gender couples. Slightly more than three-fourths of entering students (76.5%) agreed with the statement that "Gays and lesbians should have the legal right to adopt a child," with 48% agreeing strongly and 28.5% agreeing somewhat. Women supported the rights of gays and lesbians to adopt more than men, regardless of political orientation (The American freshman, 2011).

The percentage who believed married women should confine their activities to the home and family reached a 15-year low of 21.5% in 2002 and was 21% in 2005 (Rooney, 2003; This year's freshmen at 4-year colleges: A statistical profile, 2005; The American freshman: National norms for fall 2007, 2008; This year's freshmen at 4-year colleges: A statistical profile, 2009).

Religion plays a major role in many people's sexuality, including Lisa from the opening story. For Lisa's parents, whose cultural traditions in Korea can be traced to Confucianism, abortion might have been a possibility (as a means of saving face for the family).

Religion can also play a role in use or nonuse of medical services related to sexuality. It can even influence the availability of such services when policies allow service providers to refuse to provide services that are against their personal beliefs. For example, a pharmacist might refuse to sell contraceptives because he does not believe in their use, or a doctor might refuse to perform an abortion because she does not believe abortions are morally appropriate.

Through the years, religiosity (an intense religious belief) has been found to influence the number of sexual partners, the frequency of various forms of sexual behavior, the age at first sexual intercourse, types of sexual behaviors, standards related to sexual activity before marriage, and even marital satisfaction. Religiosity also seems to influence the sexual behaviors of college students. A study conducted at a southeastern university showed that both males and females who reported less frequent worship attendance and weaker religious feelings were more likely to participate in sexual behaviors than those with more frequent worship attendance and stronger religious feelings (Penhollow, Young, & Denny, 2005).

Multicultural Influences

Cultures within the United States differ in their views of sexuality. Your ability to respect your sexual partner's cultural beliefs and feelings will result in a higher level of satisfaction for both of you.

First we must distinguish between ethnic background and ethnicity. A person's ethnic background is usually determined by birth and is related to country of origin, native language, race, and religion. **Ethnicity** refers to the degree of identification an individual feels with a particular ethnic group (Harrell & Frazier, 1999).

ethnicity
The degree of identification an individual feels with a particular ethnic group.

Our opening story underscores this concept. Had Lisa been pregnant, she would have found herself torn between her parents' strong ethnicity and the individual cultural beliefs and practices that she

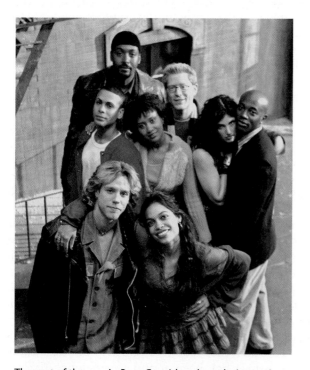

The cast of the movie *Rent*. Considered revolutionary in the mid-1990s, the story dealt frankly with HIV/AIDS and gay relationships. Such sensitivity has become commonplace in almost all media today.

learned in school and college. Such difficult cultural conflicts might place some people in a position like Lisa's at high risk for potential serious problems.

Cultural influences from citizens of other countries also play a dramatic role in U.S. culture. This is especially important for college students in the United States, because 1 in 10 students is from another country. These students' local cultural understandings of the body, health, and morality shape their use of contraceptive methods and abortion. For example, in the United States, abortion is not viewed as a method of contraception. In some other countries, however, abortion is viewed as a primary method of birth control. Some women from these countries might have as many as four or five abortions. Two other examples of multicultural influences related to Brazil and China follow.

In Brazil, compared with members of evangelical religions, other men are significantly more likely to report having had an extramarital partner and unprotected extramarital sexual intercourse in the last 12 months. Region of residence is also strongly associated with extramarital sexual activity. Compared with men in southern or central Brazil, those in the north are three times more likely to have had extramarital sexual intercourse and unprotected sexual intercourse in the last year (Hill et al., 2004).

Chinese women whose beliefs and experiences reflect traditional norms limiting gender equality may be at increased risk of being subjected to intimate-partner violence. In 2005, 43% of women said they had been physically or sexually abused by a partner, with 26% experiencing such events during the past year. Several factors suggesting adherence to traditional gender roles were associated with the likelihood of reporting intimate-partner violence. For example, women who had turned down a job because of their partner, women who thought that wife-beating is sometimes justified, and women who believed that a wife has a duty to have intercourse with her husband had elevated odds of having been abused (Xu et al., 2005).

A third multicultural example deals with the topic of gendercide. In some cultures, women are aborted, killed, and neglected to death. In China and northern India, 120 males are born for every 100 females. The destruction of baby girls is a product of three forces: the ancient preference for sons, a modern desire for smaller families, and ultrasound scanning and other technologies that identify the gender of a fetus. Unborn daughters are often sacrificed in pursuit of a son (Gendercide, March 6, 2010).

Socioeconomic Influences

Socioeconomic status and education also influence sexual attitudes and behaviors, at least within the same ethnic group. Examples of this influence include low-income individuals often thinking and acting differently than middle-class individuals, being more likely to engage in sexual intercourse at an earlier age, and having children outside of marriage.

Educational levels also seem to influence sexual behavior. Examples include people with more education masturbating more and people with at least some college education having more sexual partners than those who did not attend college.

Socioeconomic status influences more than just sexual activities. The poor have less access to proper health care, birth control, care during pregnancy, day care for children, and positive sexual role models.

Lisa, from our opening story, is affected by her family's high socioeconomic status. The prevailing indicator of success among second-generation Korean Americans is high academic achievement at prestigious universities, followed by pursuit of professional careers. Lisa's academic performance to this point has reflected this cultural value. An unexpected and unwanted pregnancy would create a major obstacle to achieving the expected success and thus create an added intergenerational cultural conflict.

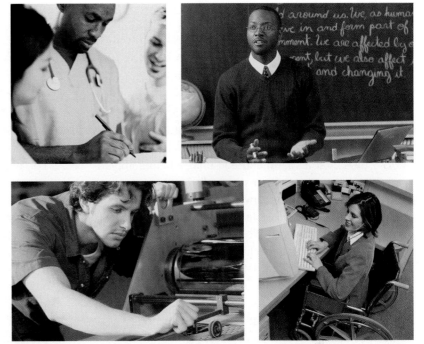

All people are sexual beings, and our experiences influence our thinking about sexuality.

Ethical Influences

The ethics of sexuality involves questioning the way we treat ourselves and other people. Examples of sexually oriented ethical dilemmas include the following:

- Should I or should I not participate in a certain sexual behavior?

- Is it ethical to use a prostitute?

- Is it ethical not to disclose my full sexual history to a new partner?

- Is it ethical to engage in sexual behaviors with a person who is underage?

- Is it ethical to use a position of power to obtain sexual partners?

Ethical issues are not necessarily the same as legal concerns. For example, prostitution is illegal in the United States except in a few counties in Nevada. However, the ethical question of prostitution would look at the morality of hiring a prostitute—who may be selling her body as a last resort to survive. Also, the age of maturity in your state (the age at which you are deemed legally of age to engage in sexual activity) is probably 16 or 17 years old. Thus, it would be illegal to have a sexual partner younger than that age. However, in Tokyo, Japan, the legal age for girls is 12 years. Is it ethical for you to have a sexual partner who is of age in the country you are visiting, even if she is very young?

How we consider such questions and ultimately decide what is right and wrong profoundly shapes our sexuality. Ethical decision making underscores the importance of taking responsibility for your sexual wellness.

Media Influences

It has long been recognized that the media help shape public attitudes on many topics—especially sexuality, gender roles, and sexual behaviors. The depictions of sexuality we encounter in the media are there mainly to entertain and sell products. Consequently, the media do not provide us with realistic depictions.

Television shows are filled with portrayals of sexual activity and "double-meaning" comments. The music industry has countless sexual images. Listen to the words of many currently popular songs and you will hear the sexual content. Magazines, tabloids, and books contribute to the many sexual themes that bombard us. Next time you are in the checkout line at the supermarket, take a look at the number of magazine covers that relate to sexuality. Numerous advertisements also use sexual themes to sell products. We are told that if we buy the right soap, toothpaste, clothes, or cars we will look sexier and be more attractive.

Some people have argued that, if they would so choose, the media could promote sexual health by

¿? Ethical DIMENSIONS

Should Human Embryos Be Used for Stem Cell Research?

In 2005 the National Academies released guidelines for embryonic stem cell research. They were amended in 2007, 2008, and 2010. Stem cells are harvested 3 to 5 days after a sperm and egg unite—before implantation in the uterus. Such stem cells have the capacity to develop into almost any type of tissue in the body. Although it is also possible to extract "adult" stem cells from bone marrow, skin, blood, and other types of tissue, adult stem cells have more limited applications than stem cells from embryos. The National Academies developed guidelines because such research is controversial.

Supporters of stem cell research point out that stem cells can be used to treat many human conditions—such as diabetes, Parkinson's disease, and multiple sclerosis. Someday stem cells might even be used to grow spare body parts. Supporters believe researchers should press on to find "cures" for such conditions because the results could be helpful to so many people. Opponents are strongly against research in which embryos are destroyed. Pro-life groups and others believe government funding should not be provided for such research and that it should not be done at all.

For many years stem cell research has been an important political and ethical issue. Many issues, such as whether a woman should become pregnant to produce stem cells to be used for research, have been heavily debated. Others argue about whether stem cell research results in the taking of a human life.

The guidelines of the National Academies prohibit not only the cloning of human beings, but also payments to egg donors and use of eggs without the donor's informed consent. Debates about stem cell research are likely to continue for years to come.

Source: Data from Stem cells at the National Academies. Washington, DC: National Academies, 2011. Available: http://dels-old.nas.edu/bls/stemcells.

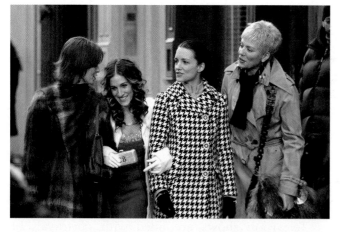

On the surface, *Sex and The City* presented four successful, single women living, loving, and having it all in New York City. Beneath the shoes, clothes, and beautiful faces in beautiful places, some saw the show as an insightful commentary on loss, loneliness, and the failure of sexual liberation.

communicating accurate information and portraying realistic situations. For example, they might show effective communication about sexuality and relationships, interactions as verbally and physically respectful, more examples of responsible sexual activity, more instances where healthy sexual encounters are anticipated and not last-minute responses to the heat of passion, and the importance of having good

information and using contraceptives and condoms to prevent unwanted pregnancies and diseases.

Political Influences

Even public policy affects our sexual behavior. For example, the U.S. government's *Healthy People 2010* and *2020* projects attempt to use health promotion to establish AIDS and sexually transmitted infection (STI) awareness, decrease unwanted teenage pregnancies, and increase the number of women who receive prenatal care. Also, the U.S. constitutional right to free speech allows the uncontrolled distribution of some pornographic material on the Internet.

Even political elections—including choosing elected officials and voting on ballot initiatives—can have a profound effect on policies and on thinking about human sexuality. Consider the political ramifications of election results.

As a result of the 2002 elections, for the first time in decades the same political party (in this case, the Republicans) that occupied the White House also controlled the U.S. House and the Senate. This provided an opportunity for that political party to strongly influence various policy issues, including those related to sexuality. The Republican Party has openly supported limiting the right of women to get abortions. It also has clearly desired to emphasize abstinence from sexual activity as the major way to

Global DIMENSIONS

The Islamic Influence

Islam is the world's fast-growing religion, and its followers are called Muslims. Islam is very common in the Middle East, but it also exists in many other parts of the world. One-fifth of the world's population is Muslim, and 2 to 8 million Muslims live in the United States.

As with other religions, Muslims have differing beliefs on many aspects of sexuality. However, generally Muslims oppose intercourse before marriage, but value it highly within marriage. Both genders are considered to have high interest in sexual behavior and get great satisfaction from it. Both males and females are encouraged to show modesty in public by wearing loose-fitting, body-covering clothing.

Controversy sometimes occurs among Muslims over traditions, such as, women wearing headscarves. Trying to support secularism, the Muslim country of Turkey for decades banned women from wearing headscarves in universities. In early 2008, Turkey's parliament lifted the ban, allowing university women to wear headscarves. However, the issue remains controversial. People opposed to women wearing headscarves protested at some campuses, while some university leaders continued to enforce the ban that parliament had removed.

Sources: Data from Hodge, D., & Nadir, A. Moving toward culturally competent practice with Muslims: modifying cognitive therapy with Islamic tenets. *Social Work, 53* (2008), 31–41; Martin, C. A head scarf is not just a scarf. *Christian Science Monitor* (February 25, 2008) 9–11.

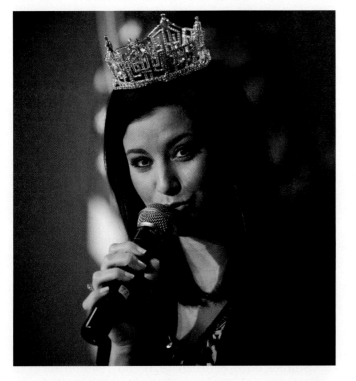

Even Miss America can be involved in politics related to sexuality.

control pregnancies and STIs among young people. It has gone so far as to provide federal funding for certain types of educational programs only if they emphasize abstinence. It also has not been very supportive of rights for homosexuals.

Many issues in the 2008 elections related to sexuality. There was the first female major party candidate for president. It was announced that the teenage daughter of the female candidate for Vice-President of the United States was pregnant and not married. During the presidential campaign, platforms and debates included discussions about the legality of abortion, rights for homosexuals (including marriage and adoption), stem cell research, and abstinence-only versus comprehensive sexuality education. After Barack Obama was inaugurated as president in 2009, these issues, along with many others, continued to influence politics. Political issues, in turn, continued to influence human sexuality in many ways.

It remains common for political candidates to be questioned about their views on a number of issues related to sexuality. Abortion, homosexual rights, and some medical advances (e.g., genetic engineering, stem cell research, and variations of artificial insemination) are often the most common sexuality topics discussed in political circles. However, the context and focus of such discussions change periodically. For example, a discussion about health insurance might focus on whether abortion services should be covered. A discussion about homosexual rights might focus on tax issues or the future of homosexuals in the military. We can be confident that politics will continue to influence thinking about human sexuality, and vice versa.

Historical–Cultural Influences on Sexuality

Just as many sociocultural influences have affected human sexuality, so have some interesting historical–cultural influences. Because we cannot consider all of

? Did You Know ...

During the first seven to eight decades of the 1900s, there was a steady increase in the rates of premarital sexual intercourse for 15- to 19-year-old students. In 1991, 54.1% had ever engaged in sexual intercourse. The rates then gradually declined, reaching 45.6% in 2001. Then they again increased to 47.8% in 2007 (49.8% of males and 45.9% of females).

In 2007, the number of teens who have had sexual intercourse increased dramatically with grade level: from 32.8% of ninth graders, to 43.8% of tenth graders, to 55.5% of eleventh graders, to 64.6% of twelfth graders. Nationwide, 7.1% of students had sexual intercourse for the first time before 13 years of age. Overall, the proportion of students who had ever had sexual intercourse was higher among black (66.5%) and Hispanic (52.0%) students than among white (43.7%) students.

However, as reported in 2010, the numbers of each group who participated in sexual intercourse again went down. Overall, the number having ever had sexual intercourse was 31.6% for ninth graders, 40.9% for tenth graders, 53% for eleventh graders, and 62.3% for twelfth graders. Nationwide, 5.9% of students had had sexual intercourse for the first time before age 13 years. Overall, the population of students who ever had sexual intercourse was higher among black (65.2%) and Hispanic (49.1%) students than among white (42%) students.

Note that in each case the numbers were *smaller* in 2010 than in 2007. This is mentioned because many people think that these numbers keep going up, and that is not necessarily the case.

Source: Data from Youth risk behavior surveillance—United States, 2007. *Morbidity and Mortality Weekly Report, 57, no. SS-4* (June 6, 2008), 21–23; Youth risk behavior surveillance—United States, 2009. *Morbidity and Mortality Weekly Report, 59, no. SS-5* (June 4, 2010), A–142.

Myth vs Fact
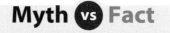

Myth: Rates of premarital intercourse increased rapidly in the first 60–70 years of the 20th century.
Fact: There was a rather steady rate of premarital sexual intercourse during the first six to seven decades of the 20th century.

Myth: We have long known that early childhood experiences are important to sexual development.
Fact: It was not until at least the middle of the 20th century that it was recognized that early childhood experiences are important to a child's healthy development.

them, and because most of these topics are covered in greater depth elsewhere in this text, we briefly focus on some from a historical standpoint—namely, the sexual revolution, control of sexual behavior, conception, contraception, and gender roles. As you read about these historical–cultural influences, think about how you and people you know may have been affected by them.

The Sexual Revolution

No doubt you have heard references to the sexual revolution. The meaning of this term varies according to the speaker; however, it is clear that many changes related to sexuality have occurred in the past 80 to 100 years. Whether there has been an actual revolution—or perhaps an evolution—is for you to decide after considering some facts and observations.

Many people talk about a sexual revolution in reference to rates of sexual intercourse before marriage. Many of our history books would lead us to believe that in the past, Americans were sexually chaste before marriage. If we read between the lines, however, we find that this is not necessarily true. Reiss (1973) informs us that in the late 1700s in Massachusetts, one of three women in a particular church confessed fornication to her minister (the actual number was probably higher yet). The U.S. western frontier society relied heavily on prostitution. The women's liberation movement of the 1870s revealed numerous sexual affairs. And the first vulcanized rubber condom was displayed at the Philadelphia World's Fair in 1876. These are not isolated events, and they should make us question what we think about the sexual purity and innocence of our forebears (Bruess & Schroeder, 2014).

Studies done between 1920 and 1945 do seem to indicate that the greatest increases in rates of premarital sexual intercourse occurred in the early 1900s (Bell, 1966). This means that the so-called sexual revolution began early in the 20th century and not in more recent years. Many older people who seem so concerned about changes in sexual behavior were in the middle of the sexual revolution themselves. Our best research tells us that approximately 35% to 45% of females and 55% to 65% of males participated in sexual intercourse before marriage during most of the first six to seven decades of the 20th century (Bruess & Schroeder, 2014).

? Did You Know . . .

During the Middle Ages, some people believed in witches, whom they accused of having sexual relations with the devil. Because that was not generally acceptable behavior, something had to be done about it. Some women who were sexually "loose" were simply ignored, but others were labeled as witches, and witch hunts were common. Women were put on trial, and, if they were found guilty of witchcraft, attempts were made to free them from the devil. This was done by a "laying on of hands" by an appropriate religious leader. If these attempts failed, it was sometimes thought better to kill the witch than to let her live.

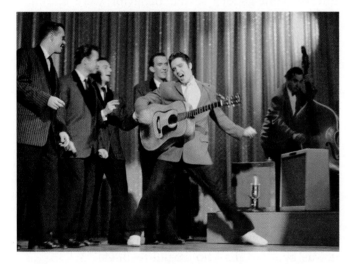

Some people thought this performance by Elvis Presley was obscene.

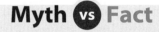

Myth: Contraceptive methods were not available until the 20th century.

Fact: Methods used to prevent pregnancy are as old as recorded history.

Many changes that influence our thinking about sexuality occurred in the first six to seven decades of the 20th century. For example, as traditional moral viewpoints were questioned, people began to wonder about whether any one standard of morality could apply universally. Social scientists talked about people defining their own morality, while religious leaders often saw morality as determined by an order higher than mere humans.

Several events also occurred during this period that contributed to a trend toward more receptivity to the topic of sexuality. For example, wars exposed many people to other cultures, and the uncertainty of survival contributed to a philosophy of "Live tonight, for tomorrow we may die." The result was a change in the concept of sexual morality. In addition, there was a rise in the status of women as they became better educated, a more significant part of the workforce, more aggressive, and more active partners in sexual activity.

Rapid improvements in communication and transportation also had a tremendous effect on sexuality. First the telephone became a convenient way to promote interpersonal relationships, and today the Internet provides a means for people to meet, send quick love messages, and stay in touch. Magazines, TV, and films continued to have many sexual themes, and the car became a "bedroom on wheels," providing a way to have private sexual activity.

It became accepted that early childhood experiences are important to the development of young children—including their sexual development. This understanding has had ramifications for sexuality education programs for children of all ages.

Important events that influenced sexuality include the research of Alfred Kinsey in the 1940s and 1950s related to sexual behavior, the first nationwide appearance of Elvis Presley in 1956 (considered obscene by many), and the introduction of the bikini swimsuit in 1959. The lyrics of popular songs became more sexually suggestive, and record smashing by opponents of these songs occurred in an attempt to censor the music.

The 1960s work of William Masters and Virginia Johnson on human sexual response also greatly contributed to our knowledge of how we function sexually and how and why we sometimes do not function. In addition to basic information about sexual functioning, their research provided the foundation for sexual counseling and methods for dealing with human sexual inadequacy.

Increasingly reliable contraceptives, especially the pill (introduced in the United States in 1960), were developed and accepted by large numbers of people. Today many reliable and relatively safe contraceptive methods are available, and the vast majority of married couples use contraception.

In the late 20th century and early 21st century, books, classes, and radio and television programs about sexuality, as well as numerous websites related to sexuality, became common. The press reports the findings of virtually every new study, and discussions about sexuality in American society are out of the closet and into public forums.

Control of Sexual Behavior

Throughout the history of Western culture, there have been many attempts to control sexual behavior. Most of these are found in moral and legal codes of the time. For example, early Christian moralists taught that because sexual activity outside marriage had a purpose other than **procreation**, it was a sin. Even within marriage, sexual union was lawful only if it was performed for the purpose of begetting children. Almost all medieval theologians emphasized that it was a mortal sin to embrace one's spouse solely for pleasure (Aries & Bejin, 1985, 115).

> **procreation**
> Sexual intercourse for the purpose of reproduction.

There were many other religious influences and restrictions. For example, intercourse was objectionable on all fast or feast days, during the days a female was menstruating, for 40 days after childbirth, during pregnancy, and during breastfeeding. Also, intercourse between husband and wife was supposed to take place in the "natural" position, with the wife on her back and the husband on top. All other positions were considered "unnatural."

Many religious people thought that only the lowest type of people engaged in oral–genital sexual activity or anal intercourse. Homosexuality was considered an abomination and punishable by death.

A belief in witchcraft was another means of controlling sexual behavior. Strong feelings, especially lust and passion, were believed to arise from evil spirits, and because women (and not men) inspired lust, some religious leaders saw women as witches or agents of the devil. Witches were tortured, ostensibly to drive the devil out of them, or killed. Bewitchment was said to account for the mysterious and overwhelming emotional effects that women had on men, sometimes driving them to irrational acts. Witch trials were held throughout the Middle Ages,

particularly during the 15th century (Sadock, Kaplan, & Freedman, 1973).

In 17th-century England, the Puritan influence was responsible for legislation to prevent amusements such as dancing, singing, and the theater. Women were treated as prostitutes if they wore long hair or makeup. On Sundays any activities not related to worship were banned.

By the end of the 18th century, sexual behavior was subdued and spontaneity inhibited. People conducted their lives very discreetly. Harsh negative attitudes toward same-gender sexual behavior were common during this time, and many people who practiced that behavior were reportedly put to death. So strong were fears and feelings during the period that people who asked for leniency for those convicted of sodomy (which includes almost any sexual behavior one wishes to prohibit) were themselves in danger of persecution. Eighteenth-century studies of sexuality emphasized physiology and generally concluded that excessive sexual activity—specifically, expelling of semen to excess—had debilitating physical consequences.

In the 19th century, during Victorian times, sexual drives were generally repressed. Though it was believed that men had natural and spontaneous sexual desires, women supposedly had dormant sex drives unless subjected to undue excitation. Children, it was believed, had no sexual feelings.

Much was done to protect the people of Victorian times from sexual arousal. Sexual references in literature and general conversation were suppressed, as were most sexual feelings. Masturbation, a particularly repudiated activity, was called the "secret sin," "self-pollution," and the "solitary vice." Devices were even developed to place around the male's penis at night to prevent **spermatorrhea** (more commonly called **nocturnal emissions** or **wet dreams**) (Figure 1.1).

> **spermatorrhea (wet dreams, or nocturnal emissions)**
> Emission of semen during sleep.

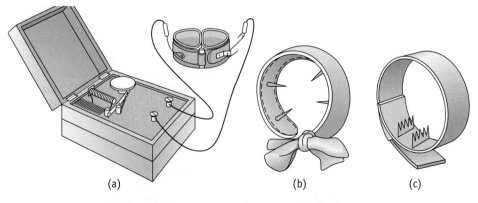

(a)   (b)   (c)

FIGURE **1.1** Devices designed to prevent wet dreams. One device caused a bell to ring when erection occurred (a). For some devices, no bell was needed (b and c).

In the early 20th century, as conservative morality about sexuality diminished and people argued that sexual expression was natural and normal, some secular attempts were made to legislate sexual morality. This resulted in censorship, prohibition, and the revival of old statutes against certain sexual behaviors, such as homosexuality, oral–genital relations, and sodomy.

Theoretically, in the United States there is a separation of church and state, but legal debates about such subjects as abortion, access to sexual information and services, homosexuality, and sexual behaviors have prompted some people to wonder about that separation.

Conception

Much of our information about prehistoric people is obtained by analyzing the remains of their art. In addition, we can make inferences about primitive cultures from the art that exists today. Prehistoric cave paintings indicate that more than 30,000 years ago sexuality was an important part of culture. Some of these stone engravings suggest human intercourse, and some show women and men with exaggerated body parts.

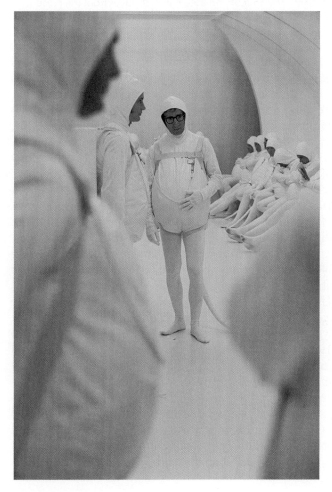

Despite the attention to sexuality in their art and perhaps their religion, prehistoric people apparently did not understand its role in reproduction. Consequently, theorists believe that a number of explanations for childbirth existed. One notion may have been that children were sent by ancestral deities; sexual intercourse was reserved solely for pleasure. Or a woman became pregnant by sitting over a fire on which she had roasted a fish received from the prospective father. An Australian tribe believed that a woman conceived by eating human flesh. Some cultures thought it was possible for a man to become pregnant (Tannahill, 1980). Some of these theories might seem humorous, but they are really no more peculiar, or at least no more wrong, than such modern superstitions as "You can't get pregnant if you do it only once." By the time of the first written records, however, it appears that humans were aware that they played some part in reproduction, even if they did not know how.

Throughout recorded history, many theories and myths about conception existed. For example, Aristotle theorized that the human fetus resulted from the mixture of menstrual blood and seminal fluid. One hundred years before Aristotle, the Greek poet Aeschylus believed that a child was conceived by a male alone (Where do babies come from?, 1987).

The microscope allowed scientists to see sperm for the first time. In 1677, the Dutch naturalist Anton van Leeuwenhoek described the human sperm discovered by one of his students. Many scientists, however, refused to accept that sperm could be responsible for creating human life. Other scientists claimed they had seen tiny humans inside sperm. This thinking led to the belief that a tiny, fully formed person would not grow until he or she reached the female "nest." At the same time other scientists, known as **ovists**, claimed that the preformed baby was contained in the female and the sperm served only to activate its development. It was not until 1875 that it was demonstrated that the sperm penetrates and combines with the egg (Where do babies come from?, 1987).

ovist
Adherent to the 17th-century belief that the preformed baby was contained within the female body and that the male's sperm simply activated its development.

Woody Allen's farcical treatment of sperm cells in *Everything You Always Wanted to Know about Sex ...* reflects what was once thought true. When sperm cells were discovered by a magnifying glass in 1677, scientists believed that they saw tiny men (called *animalcules*) inside sperm cells. Other scientists even claimed to see microscopic horses in horse sperm!

It is impossible to know the overall effect of the accurate understanding of conception; however, it would seem that such knowledge was useful to both males and females. The understanding that sexual intercourse could result in conception must have influenced sexual behavior and made it possible to have at least some control over whether or not to procreate. The control of reproduction is possible today; throughout most of history it was not.

Contraception

Although the process of reproduction was not understood until relatively recently, **contraception**—methods employed to prevent pregnancy—is as old as recorded history. More than 4,000 years ago Egyptian women used medicated tampons as contraceptives. Lint, moistened in a mixture of acacia tips ground with honey, was placed into the vagina. Many other practices, some of them dangerous, were used in the centuries that followed (*The ecology of birth control*, 1971). Among these were inserting spongy or absorbent fabrics into the vagina or mixing crocodile dung with a paste and inserting the mixture into the vagina. It is said that Persian women placed lemon-soaked sponges in the vagina to prevent pregnancy. It is interesting to note that these methods have some merit. Most of them attempted to form a barrier or alter the acid–base relationship within the vagina. In fact, many of today's contraceptive methods are based on these same principles.

> **contraception**
> Means of preventing pregnancy in spite of sexual intercourse.

The first modern contraceptive device, which was eventually called the condom, appeared in the mid-16th century. It was designed to protect the wearer against the plague of syphilis then spreading throughout Europe. The condom was first made of fine linen, then of animal intestine, and finally of rubber. Even though its original use was for protection from disease, its potential as a contraceptive was quickly noticed (*The ecology of birth control*, 1971).

In the middle of the 19th century, the German physician Mensinga perfected the rubber diaphragm. He believed that women should have equal rights with men and that their lives would be improved by controlling the number of children they conceived. In the United States, the diaphragm was generally unknown until after World War I. Although condoms were not as effective as diaphragms, and although they depended on the male's willingness to use them, they were manufactured in great quantities at the end of the 19th century and thus became cheaper and more available (Bullough, 1976a, 651). Today, 5.5 billion condoms are manufactured in the United States each year.

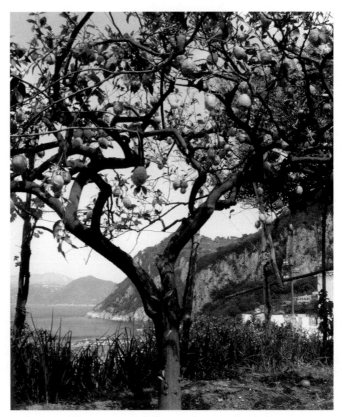

Humans have sought and used contraceptives from the present day to ancient times, when ingredients ranged from lemons to crocodile dung.

The idea of the intrauterine device (IUD) was borrowed from an ancient practice of camel drivers, who put a round stone (or an apricot pit, according to some accounts) into the uterus of a female camel to prevent pregnancy on long trips. During the 1920s, a German gynecologist modernized the idea by substituting a ring of surgical silk or silver (The ecology of birth control, 1971). It was not until experiments with IUDs were performed in Israel and Japan in 1959, however, that their use became widespread.

A number of effective spermicides appeared on the market at the end of the 19th century. The early ones, marketed in a suppository form, probably worked by blocking the cervix with an oily film. Numerous other chemicals soon appeared on the market (Bullough, 1976a, 651). Foams and jellies were introduced in the early 20th century. Research on an oral contraceptive was widespread in the 1950s, but it was not until 1960 that the first oral contraceptive was approved for public use. It can probably be said that this event marked the beginning of the modern era of contraception.

It was 30 years later, in 1990, that the U.S. Food and Drug Administration approved levonorgestrel (Norplant). This hormonal contraceptive implant system was six capsules 34 mm long, inserted beneath the skin of a woman's upper arm. Its release marked

Communication
DIMENSIONS

The CERTS Model Wendy Maltz developed the CERTS model for healthy sexuality. The letters stand for Consent, Equality, Respect, Trust, and Safety. Consent means you can freely and comfortably choose whether or not to engage in sexual activity. Equality means your sense of personal power is on an equal level with your partner. Respect means you have positive regard for yourself and for your partner. Trust means you trust your partner on physical and emotional levels. Safety means you feel secure and safe within the sexual setting.

Maltz suggests that spending time together and engaging in lots of honest, open communication are good ways to make sure that the CERTS conditions are operating in your relationship. Meeting the CERTS conditions does not guarantee that everything will be perfect, but it can help you feel secure knowing that you've minimized the possibility of something bad resulting from your sexual experiences.

Source: Data from *The CERTS model for healthy sex.* 2011. Available: http://www.healthysex.com/page/certs-model.

the first time long-term (in this case, up to 5 years) hormonal control of conception was available in the United States (FDA OKs hormonal implant, 1990).

Not necessarily considered a form of contraception, abortion is a means of controlling births. Abortion early in pregnancy was legal in ancient China and Europe. In the 13th century the Roman Catholic church indicated that the soul developed 40 days after conception in males and 90 days after conception in females, and abortion was allowed within those intervals. In the late 1860s the Catholic church declared that life begins at conception; that doctrine led to its abortion ban (O'Keefe, 1995).

Early American law allowed abortion until the woman felt fetal movement, but during the 1860s abortion became illegal in the United States except to save the woman's life. In addition to the religious beliefs of some people, reasons for this included health problems related to crude abortion procedures, the belief that population growth was needed for economic reasons, and maybe a male-dominated political system's response to more women seeking independence and equality (Sheeran, 1987). It was not until 1973 that the U.S. Supreme Court in its famous *Roe* v. *Wade* decision legalized a woman's right to decide to terminate her pregnancy before the fetus could survive independently of the woman's body. Debates about this issue continue.

Gender Roles

"The paramount destiny and mission of women are to fulfill the noble and benign offices of wife and mother. This is the law of the Creator." Words of a time long past? Not quite. This is actually an excerpt from a Supreme Court opinion rendered in the first case tried under the Fourteenth Amendment in 1873. The court's decision upheld the denial of the right of

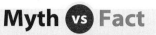
Myth vs Fact

Myth: Open discussion about sexuality will have negative results—people will be more likely to be sexually permissive.
Fact: Healthy communication about sexuality will help people develop into sexually healthy adults—open discussions do not have negative results.

Myth: The relatively open attitudes in thinking about sexuality in Sweden have resulted in higher rates of teen pregnancy and sexually transmitted infections.
Fact: Swedish attitudes and practices related to sexuality have resulted in lower rates of teen pregnancy and sexually transmitted infections.

Myth: Abortion has been illegal throughout most of the history of the United States.
Fact: Early American law allowed abortion until a woman felt fetal movement. In the 1860s abortion became illegal in the United States, but in 1973 the Supreme Court legalized a woman's right to terminate her pregnancy.

Myth: What is sexually arousing to people is very much the same regardless of the culture.
Fact: In different cultures the idea of what is sexually arousing varies a great deal.

women to practice law (Bardes, Shelley, & Schmidt, 1998).

Historically, the role of the woman as a sexual partner has been to satisfy male needs. In India, for example, women were viewed as nothing without men. In the West, women who enjoyed sexual activity dared not speak of it publicly because of the severe penalties for doing so. Throughout the ages women were viewed as property of men (Spielvogel, 1997). In most societies, if a woman committed adultery, was raped, or lost her virginity, she was considered damaged property. A woman's father or husband could expect to gain compensation for this damage, or, in the case of adultery, he might even kill her and her partner if they were caught (Bullough, 1976b, 677–679).

In many societies men enjoyed a status vastly superior to that of women. This status can probably be accounted for by (1) men's greater physical strength, (2) women's repeated pregnancies in the absence of reliable contraceptive methods, and (3) the ideology that disparity in male and female roles was divinely ordained. Men used their greater physical strength to trap animals and handle livestock, to defend themselves, and to intimidate women. Because women were often pregnant and spent much of their time caring for children, little time was left to alter their inferior status. Those who felt male and female

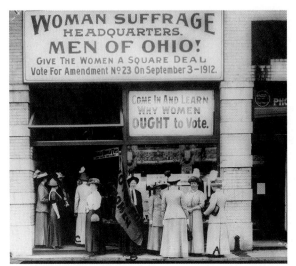

Women did not get the right to vote in the United States until 1920.

roles had a divine origin saw any attempts to change these roles as antireligious (Murstein, 1974, 566).

The ancient Greeks believed that men were primarily mental and spiritual in their makeup and that women were primarily physical and earthy. Because the Greeks believed the mind and body were separate entities, this meant men had a higher nature and deserved greater privileges. Several centuries later, however, Jesus insisted on the basic equality of the sexes. He opposed Jewish divorce law, which allowed women to be disposed of as property (Nelson, 1978).

Throughout medieval times, women were thought to be inferior to men. Their motives were suspect, they were thought to be sinful, and their female functions were belittled. Some still believed Aristotle's earlier claim that the female was little more than an incomplete male. Both religious and scientific thinking seemed to support these ideas (Bullough, 1976b).

In the early 1800s there were more male children than female children in the western states and territories of the United States. Some researchers have thought this was because nutrition and health of young females were neglected because their labor was not as economically valued. Others have indicated that this imbalance simply occurred because more boys were born in, survived childhood in, or moved to western regions (Courtwright, 1990). This presents another example in which it is difficult to determine the real reasons for the situation.

However, the mid- to late 1800s and the early 1900s witnessed many advances in the status of women in the United States. After the first major organized meeting on the rights of women in 1848, there was a sort of legal emancipation, an opening of work opportunities, and an ideological acceptance of the equality of the sexes. Actual changes in behavior,

however, did not keep pace with this verbal acceptance. The average woman was probably more interested in receiving greater respect and consideration, and in receiving the right to vote, than in having equal professional rights. Most articles advocating the causes important to women today were written by highly educated men and women, and probably the majority of Americans were not even aware of these new ideas (Murstein, 1974, 379). Nonetheless, the seeds of the women's rights movement were planted.

The women's suffrage movement began in the late 19th century with the goal of obtaining the right to vote for women. The passage in 1920 of the Nineteenth Amendment to the U.S. Constitution guaranteed women the right to vote. World War II created an environment for increased gender equality. As men were required to leave home for military duty, thousands of women left their traditional roles in the home and took paying jobs for the first time. It was not until the 1960s, however, after many postwar marriages, the baby boom, and continued disappointment about women's roles, that a new movement for gender equality became evident.

Some people had thought that the ratification of the Nineteenth Amendment would end the struggle for women's rights, but this had not happened. In 1963 the Equal Pay Act, which stated that women must receive pay equal to that of men if they perform the same work, was enacted. In 1964 women were included in the protections of the Civil Rights Act. This made it clear that equality of opportunity for women was endorsed by the federal government (Degler, 1980, 442). Still, women today earn an average of less than 90 cents for every dollar men earn.

In 1963 Betty Friedan published *The Feminine Mystique*, which helped create a widespread movement for women's rights. She urged women to make a life for themselves in addition to their homes and families. The case for women's equality was also championed in a number of other books. In 1966 Friedan organized the National Organization for Women (NOW), which has consistently advocated women's rights. By 1970 a number of other organizations that pushed for women's equality were formed, including the Women's Equity Action League and

Multicultural DIMENSIONS

Pregnancy and Health

When speaking of culture, sociologists generally refer to the "learned values, beliefs, norms, behaviors, and even material objects that are passed from one generation to the next." Within the culture of the United States, however, are many subcultures—groups of people with shared values within the overall culture. Each subculture has a distinctive way of looking at life that sets it off from the prevalent culture. In the United States, these groups may be defined by ethnicity, age, religion, sexuality, geographical location, and national origin. The Multicultural Dimensions boxes look at varied subcultures within the United States.

The first multicultural issue we explore relates to teen pregnancy in developing countries. In January 2009, UNICEF released its annual report entitled *The State of the World's Children, 2009*. The report pointed out that women in the world's least developed countries are 300 times more likely to die in childbirth or from pregnancy-related complications than are women in developed countries. Put another way, women in developing countries have a 1 in 76 chance of dying from pregnancy or childbirth-related complications, compared with a 1 in 8,000 chance for women in developed countries. A child born in a developing country is almost 14 times more likely to die during the first month of life than a child born in a developed one. Approximately 70,000 young women ages 15 to 19 die in childbirth annually.

It is obvious that better medical intervention is a key to improving the health of mothers and their children. But more than just medical intervention is required: There also needs to be a change in how women are viewed and how things get done to really make a difference. For example, it is essential to have a stable environment that empowers women and respects their rights. Educating girls and women is one of the most fundamental ways to improve maternal and newborn health and benefits both families and societies. Essential interventions will be guaranteed only within the context of improved education and the abolition of discrimination.

Source: Data from *The state of the world's children, 2009.* New York: UNICEF, 2009.

---

the Women's Political Caucus. So successful was the women's movement that it has been considered "possibly the most lasting legacy of the ... period of protests" (Degler, 1980, 446).

In recent years many issues related to women's roles have been raised. Women now work in a variety of jobs previously thought to be only for males, and there are more women in positions of authority. Discrimination against pregnant women in the workplace has lessened, many women delay having children to pursue other interests, and there is an increased acceptance of child care while women work. Varied opinions about women's roles continue. Studies about gender and leadership style, gender differences in work, family conflict, gender and the influence of achievement evaluations, gender in the college classroom, among others, continue to provide reams of information about women and their roles and status. But whether we have achieved equality between the sexes is still a matter of debate.

Thinking Critically About Human Sexuality

You have probably observed that, when it comes to many topics related to health and sexuality, there are "experts" everywhere. The concept of critical thinking is important to being able to judge the accuracy of what these people say as well as lots of other information you hear related to sexuality. In this case, the word *critical* does not mean being negative or criticizing people or things. It means being careful and somewhat analytical.

In essence, then, **critical thinking** is thinking that prevents blindly accepting conclusions or arguments (or headlines) and instead closely examines all assumptions. This includes carefully evaluating existing evidence and cautiously assessing all conclusions (Baron, 1998).

> **critical thinking**
> Thinking that avoids blind acceptance of conclusions or arguments and closely examines all assumptions.

Critical thinking is like the scientific methods you may have used in other classes. In practice, it involves guidelines such as these (Baron, 1998):

1. Never jump to conclusions; gather as much information as you can before making up your mind about any issue.

2. Keep an open mind; do not let your existing views blind you to information or new conclusions.

3. Always ask "How?" as in "How was this evidence gathered?"

4. Be skeptical; always wonder about *why* someone is making an argument, offering a conclusion, or trying to persuade you.

5. Never be stampeded into accepting some view or position by your own emotions—or by arguments and appeals designed to play on your emotions.

Not every guideline will apply in every situation, but the important goal is to develop a style of thinking using as many of the guidelines as seems appropriate in a given situation.

Correlation Versus Causation

A research study found that for people 60 years and older, the 62% who drank coffee still enjoyed active sex lives, compared with only 37% of those who were not coffee drinkers (Plotnik, 1993). Does coffee lead to a better sex life for seniors? Or are the two events just coincidental? The study shows a **correlation**, a relationship between two events. But it does not show a **causation**, a relationship in which one event causes the other.

correlation
A relationship between two events.

causation
A relationship in which one event causes another event to occur.

It is easy to show that a correlation exists, but correlations do not show cause and effect. There is a high correlation between the winning conference of the Super Bowl and the stock market: When the NFC wins, the stock market goes up in most years; when the AFC wins, the market goes down in most years. In fact, from 1972 to 1985 there was a perfect correlation. However, no scientific study is needed to understand that the Super Bowl does not cause the stock market to go up or down.

Returning to the coffee example, perhaps people older than 60 years old who are in good health enjoy both coffee and sexual activity. However, there does not appear to be a causal link between caffeine use and sexual activity. In contrast, a study showing a correlation between the drug Viagra and an active sex life would appear to have a causal link. So, correlations can sometimes help predict behavior and point to possible causes of behavior. Further studies can help validate the causation.

Being a Good Consumer of Sexual Information

We are bombarded with information—and misinformation—about sexuality issues. In fact, most best-selling newsstand periodicals lure readers with information about "new" sexual techniques or sex

surveys. It is important to keep the principles of the scientific method in mind when reading popular literature.

Consider a study that garnered a great deal of media attention: The medical anthropologists Soma Grismaijer and Sidney Ross Singer (2002) surveyed 4,700 women and concluded that their odds of having breast cancer increased the longer women wore bras. Their hypothesis was that the cinching effect of a bra suppresses the lymphatic system below a woman's armpit, blocking an internal network of vessels that are intended to flush toxic wastes from the body. Over time, these toxins accumulate in the breast tissue and create an environment in which cells can turn cancerous.

The results of the survey appear to confirm their hypothesis: Of women who wore bras 24 hours a day, in three of four breast cancer developed; of women who wore bras less than 12 hours a day, in one in seven breast cancer developed; of women who rarely wore bras, in only 1 in 168 did breast cancer develop (Joseph, 1998).

The study appears to have found a *correlation* between length of bra-wearing time and breast cancer. However, few medical scientists would agree that a *causation* exists; many would even question the correlation. First, consider the design of the survey on which the conclusion was based: Participants were not randomly selected, following accepted statistical guidelines. For example, women who have had breast cancer might be more willing to participate in a breast-cancer study. Nor were participants questioned about preexisting breast-cancer risks. In addition, participants answered only 12 questions regarding their bra-wearing habits.

A scientific approach to the correlation of bra use and breast cancer would be to find a large, randomly selected sample of women who wear bras for specific lengths of time each day. The women would need to be prescreened for breast-cancer risk and would need to undergo medical exams before participating. Family history of cancer, age, race, body mass, weight, diet, exercise, alcohol or drug consumption, and other factors would have to be controlled in some manner. A matching control group (not selected by bra-wearing time) would add further validity. The study could follow the women across a long period, perhaps 15 to 25 years.

Thus a critical review of the study quickly calls into doubt the causal factor between bra use and breast cancer. Even the correlation appears to be contrived. However, it does open the door for further studies.

A final point about the scientific method should be made here: When this study first appeared in popular print media, the information provided varied by the source. News media presented the story as provocative and quirky but with powerful opposition voiced by medical doctors and cancer specialists. But one popular "health" magazine reported the study in a way that suggested a causal link—and placed an ad on the opposite page for a "health drug" claiming to lower risk of breast cancer. Always remember to think about why someone is publishing the study. In this case, it was clearly done to help sell a product.

■ Why Study Sexuality?

There are many reasons for studying human sexuality, including obtaining accurate sexual knowledge, clarifying personal values, improving sexual decision making, learning the relationship between human sexuality and personal well-being, and exploring how the varied dimensions of human sexuality influence one's sexuality.

Sexual Knowledge

A major reason for studying human sexuality is to acquire a sound foundation of sexual knowledge. Only knowledge can dispel sexual myths, superstitions, and misinformation that block understanding, inhibit communication, and create confusion. Correct information lays the groundwork for sexual decision making. The greater your knowledge, the more likely you are to take responsibility for your sexual health. Studies have found that college students want specific factual information (probably pertaining to a sexual encounter), as well as the answer to the age-old question, "Am I normal?" (Caron & Bertran, 1988).

The issue of sexual and physical normality underscores the psychological dimensions of human sexuality. It is normal to wonder whether your appearance and/or sexual desires are normal. Many men worry about the size and shape of their penis, and women often worry about the size and shape of their breasts. Learning about the wide variety in appearances may help you feel better about yourself. Learning more about sexuality can often increase your sense of personal worth, or **self-esteem**.

self-esteem
Sense of personal worth.

Factual knowledge can also help you interpret sociocultural traditions or myths. History is filled with examples of myths about the biological nature of sexuality. Aristotle, for example, thought that menstrual fluid was the substance from which the embryo was formed, a belief held for centuries. Leonardo da Vinci's anatomical drawings show a tube running from the uterus to the breasts of a woman, depicting the common belief that the menstrual fluid that did not flow during pregnancy was diverted to the breasts to make milk—this in spite of the fact that he had dissected female cadavers and certainly never saw such a tube! The U.S. culture is by no means free of sexual myths, as you will discover throughout this text.

A major issue relating to sexual knowledge involves how to engage in "safer sex." Which activities can lead to the transmission of STIs and HIV? Is your partner, for example, in a high-risk group? What can be done to lower the risk of transmitting STIs and HIV? Does your partner share your knowledge—and concern—about such issues? If not, should you be willing to engage in sexual activity with that person?

Personal Values

A second reason for studying sexuality is to clarify personal sexual **values**, those beliefs to which we attach the most worth. By exploring your own dimensions of human sexuality, you may come to understand the origins and nature of your sexual values, as well as the values of others.

values
Those beliefs to which we attach the most worth.

Remember Lisa from our opening story. She began to understand how sexuality fit into her personal values, especially those involving her family. The values that her family and culture held were very important to Lisa, and she fretted over the prospect of becoming an "unmember" of her family, were she to become pregnant outside marriage.

Responsible Sexual Decision Making

A third reason for studying sexuality is to improve your sexual decision-making skills. Most people have had some sexual experience. A large majority of college students have had sexual intercourse, and almost all have participated in some form of sexual activity. But experience alone does not necessarily provide wisdom or skill in sexual decision making. The study of sexuality provides a sound foundation of sexual information, promotes an understanding of sexual attitudes, and examines a broad range of sexual issues.

For example, assume you were dating Lisa in the opening story. Without an understanding of the many social and cultural factors that influence her sexuality, you would find it hard to understand her feelings. Her communication style is restricted by her cultural background, which discourages openly discussing feelings and seeking psychological

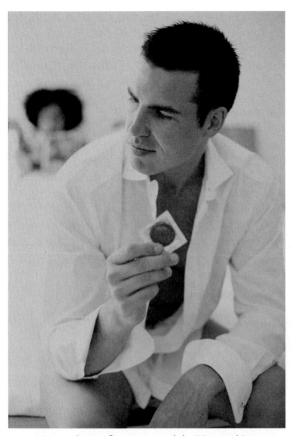
Many values influence sexual decision making.

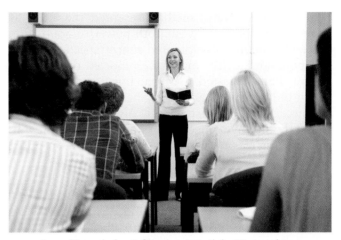
Sound knowledge influences sexual decision making.

counseling. Lack of understanding of why Lisa holds in her feelings could lead to a deterioration of your relationship.

Dr. Drew, the dry-witted host of *Loveline,* a radio and TV talk show that answers viewers' sexuality questions, often suggests that listeners think about their actions before they get involved in sexual situations. A frequently occurring situation on the show is that of having sexual activity with a roommate's lover, which callers often claim "just happened." Dr. Drew responds that, in most cases, it does not just happen—the two parties consciously flirt, possibly dress enticingly, and in the end must find a time and place to be alone. Dr. Drew suggests that had the parties stopped to think about the actions they were taking, they could have made the sexually responsible decision not to engage in sexual activity.

A Decision-Making Model

A simple but formal model of the decision-making process consists of the following steps (Bruess & Richardson, 1995).

1. *Recognition.* Only with the recognition of an issue can a decision be made. For example, a couple who consider engaging in sexual intercourse need to recognize the risk of pregnancy, transmission of STIs or HIV, and overstepping of a partner's personal dimensions.

The best decision making requires defining the issue as precisely as possible: For example, which forms of contraception are acceptable? Which forms are unacceptable? What can be done to promote safer sexual activity? How does my partner feel about this? Which physiological or cultural dimensions might influence my partner's decisions?

2. *Evaluation.* Having recognized a need to make decisions, it is time to gather relevant information, analyze the possible choices, and decide on the best alternative. For example, the latex condom might be a choice for contraception and lowering of the possibility of STI transmission. But the condom also has a lower rate of contraception effectiveness than some other methods. Another choice might be using a contraceptive method with a higher effectiveness rate—such as the pill—combined with a latex condom for STI protection. Further consideration might be necessary if one person is unwilling to use contraceptives because of religious beliefs. Or perhaps one partner has an allergy to latex condoms (in which case polyurethane condoms could be substituted). The decision to remain abstinent could also be discussed.

3. *Implementation.* When a decision has been reached, the plan needs to be put into action. A decision to combine the pill with latex condoms is not effective unless you can delay intercourse until the woman has received a prescription for the pill and taken it for about a month and the man has purchased latex condoms (and learned how to use them).

Communication
DIMENSIONS

Talking About Your Human Sexuality Class

Expect to find a great deal of interest when you tell people you are taking a class in human sexuality. Inevitably, many of your friends, colleagues, neighbors, and family members will ask, "What are you learning?" How you answer that question says a great deal about your tactfulness, how people perceive your knowledge, and how interestingly and humorously you can present delicate information. We have dealt with this question for years, and here are some suggestions:

- Be careful talking about sexual information at work. One *Seinfeld* episode revolved around Jerry being unable to remember a new girlfriend's name—except that it rhymed with a female body part. Eventually, he remembers her name is Dolores—which rhymes (sort of) with clitoris. One man embarrassed a sexually inhibited female colleague by describing the episode at work. The woman, who did not know the term *clitoris,* was further embarrassed when the man showed her the definition in a dictionary (in front of several colleagues). She complained to human resources, and he was fired. He sued the company and won a settlement, which is currently in the appeals process. Do not give people sexual information they do not want to hear! As illustrated in the *Seinfeld* case, it is best to change subjects—or even apologize—if someone is uncomfortable with what you are saying. Watch for nonverbal cues as well. Pressing a point may cost you friends.

- Do not go into detail. Use the KISS method (Keep It Simple and Sincere). If you find the human sexual response cycle interesting, discuss it in general terms: "I was surprised to learn that males and females have the same physiological response to sexual activity." If asked further questions, simply arrange for the person to borrow your book.

- Do not gross people out. In general, people do not want to hear sordid stories relating to sexuality. Information on atypical sexual behaviors, female genital mutilation, or sexual slavery is not usually dinnertime conversation. Recognize diversity. In fact, many people will be highly offended by hearing such information.

- Do not be afraid to say something in a straightforward manner. Show comfort with the subject matter by using sexual terminology in a polite, accurate manner. No one will be offended by the use of the word *penis* or *vagina* if used in context—especially if you are answering someone's question.

- Do not lecture. No matter how hard you try (or how sincere you are), you simply will not change friends' sexual behavior by telling them what they are doing wrong.

4. *Review.* After putting the decision into practice, there should be a periodic review. Are the desired results being achieved, or should another alternative be tried? Perhaps after making the decision, something new is learned about the issues that raises questions about the choice. For example, Lisa's pregnancy scare would likely make her seek out a more effective contraceptive method. If so, the decision-making process can be started again. In fact, you will find yourself renewing the decision-making process throughout your life, according to how your circumstances change.

Sexual Health and Wellness

Finally, sexual education can contribute to safer sexual behavior. Given that some sexual behaviors can result in pregnancies and/or the spread of STIs (including HIV), it is important for people of all ages to understand which practices can result in safer sexual behavior and to incorporate such practices into personal relationships.

Note that although we use the term *safer sex,* no sexual activity can be deemed *perfectly* safe. Although knowing a partner's sexual history, using latex condoms consistently, and avoiding certain sexual behaviors can *reduce* your risk of STIs and HIV, they do not *eliminate* the risk. Condoms can break or be improperly used. Your partner may not wish to disclose a complete sexual history (especially embarrassing or abusive situations). Alcohol can also get in the way of judgment.

Following safer sexual practices does not end with youth. The number of older Americans with HIV/AIDS is rising steadily. As of 2011, 28% of those diagnosed with HIV were 45 years and older (Centers for Disease Control and Prevention, 2011).

Practicing safer sexual behavior can promote sexual health and wellness, as well as improve self-esteem. The failure to practice safer sexual behavior can result in physiological, psychological, and social trauma. Although many STIs are "curable," some (such as genital herpes) can only be controlled. Knowing that you have herpes or genital warts may lead to lower self-esteem and a reluctance to seek out partners. Contracting HIV would mean a lifetime of treatment to prevent contracting AIDS. An unwanted pregnancy can have devastating results for both the parents and the child. For Lisa, pregnancy outside marriage could have resulted in losing her family.

So how do we know if someone is sexually healthy? The Alberta (Canada) Society for the Promotion of Sexual Health lists 17 criteria for sexually healthy individuals. Among the criteria are: appreciate their own bodies, avoid exploitative relationships, interact with both genders in appropriate and respectful ways, demonstrate tolerance for people with different values, decide what is personally "right" and act upon these values, talk with a partner about sexual activity before it occurs, and seek further information about sexuality as needed.

Service–Learning Projects in Your Community

While we focus on how you can develop a healthy and sexually responsible lifestyle, we recognize that all of us also have a responsibility to contribute to the health of our communities. We live in a college community, and in a city, town, or village. We live in a state and in this country. And, of course, we are part of a global community as well. With the knowledge you learn in your sexuality course and by reading this book, you have a unique opportunity to contribute to the sexual health of the communities with which you are associated. One of the best ways to do that is through service–learning. **Service–learning** is an educational method that involves students applying what they learn in their coursework in the community so as to contribute to the welfare of that community. For example, after studying the effects of gangster rap music on the sexual attitudes of young people, you might choose to write to local government representatives advocating that warnings be provided with music of this nature. Or you might volunteer at a rape crisis center. As a result of our commitment to you, and to help you organize to meet your commitment to your communities, we provide suggestions for sexuality-related service–learning activities on the website for this text.

service–learning
Educational method that involves students applying what they learn in their coursework in the community to contribute to that community's welfare.

Exploring the Dimensions of Human Sexuality

Our feelings, attitudes, and beliefs regarding sexuality are influenced by our internal and external environments. Go to go.jblearning.com/dimensions5e to learn more about the biological, psychological, and sociological factors that affect your sexuality.

Case Study

Many factors influence our sexuality. For example, consider your physical appearance. At first glance, it appears to be a biological factor, set by genetics. But your body image, or self-concept of your appearance, is psychological. Sociocultural factors also come into play—your perception is influenced by the culture in which you live and conveyed by the media that surround you.

Biological Factors

- Gender
- Genetics
- Reproduction
- Fertility control
- Sexual arousal and response
- Physiological cycles and changes
- Physical appearance
- Growth and development

Sociocultural Factors

- Socioeconomic status
- Laws
- Religion
- Culture
- Ethnic heritage
- Media and ad information
- Family, neighbors, and friends
- Ethics

Psychological Factors

- Emotions
- Experience
- Self-concept
- Motivation
- Expressiveness
- Learned attitudes and behaviors
- Body image

Summary

- Sexuality is part of our personality, and it involves the interrelationship of biological, psychological, and sociocultural dimensions.

- Sociocultural influences include religious influences, multicultural influences, ethical influences, and political influences.

- The sexual revolution had many influences on present thinking about human sexuality.

- Throughout history there have been many attempts to control sexual behavior. Most of these efforts can be seen in the moral and legal codes of the time.

- Throughout recorded history, many theories and myths about conception have existed. It was not until 1875 that it was demonstrated that the sperm penetrates and combines with the egg.

- Methods employed to prevent pregnancy have been used for thousands of years. The condom first appeared in the mid-16th century.

- Abortion in early pregnancy was legal in ancient China and Europe. In 1973 the U.S. Supreme Court legalized a woman's right to decide to terminate her pregnancy.

- There have been changes in gender roles throughout the centuries. In recent years many issues related to women's roles continue to be raised.

- It is important to use sound critical thinking skills when making decisions related to human sexuality.

- Studying human sexuality is important to obtain accurate sexual knowledge, clarify personal values, improve sexual decision making, understand the relationship between human sexuality and personal well-being, and explore how the varied dimensions of human sexuality influence one's sexuality.

Discussion Questions

1. List the three main dimensions of sexuality and their subdivisions, and give examples of each.

2. Trace the historical aspects of human sexuality, including the sexual revolution and the changing roles of gender and culture.

3. Explain a method for critical thinking, and differentiate between correlation and causation. Give examples to back up your answer.

4. Explain the main reasons for studying human sexuality.

Application Questions

Reread the chapter-opening story and answer the following questions.

1. If Lisa were pregnant, what advice would you give her? Consider Lisa's sexual dimensions, including the reaction of her family, her religion, and her communication style.

2. If you were Lisa's lover, how might you respond to the situation? To answer this question, you need to reconcile your sexual dimensions with Lisa's.

3. Do all Korean Americans have the same set of sexual dimensions? How might such dimensions differ, depending on age? Length of time in the United States? Geographic location? Socioeconomic status?

Critical Thinking Questions

1. Consider your own sexuality. Write about how each of the three dimensions affects you. Which has the greatest effect on you? The least? Explain your answers.

2. Use the decision-making model to decide whether to engage in a sexual activity that you have not yet done. Having thought the issue through, would you proceed? Which precautions might you take to promote safer sexual behavior?

Critical Thinking Case

Should an Artificial Womb Be Used?

People often need to focus on ethical questions related to conception. For example, an article in the *New York Times Magazine* by Perri Klass (September 29, 1996, 117–119) reports that Japanese researchers developed a technique called *extrauterine fetal incubation* (EUFI). They took goat fetuses, supplied them with oxygenated blood, and suspended them in incubators that contained artificial amniotic fluid (the fluid that surrounds a fetus in a pregnant woman's uterus) heated to body temperature. So far, the researchers have been able to keep goat fetuses alive for 3 weeks, but they are confident they can extend the length of time and ultimately be able to apply this technique to humans. When they do, we will have an artificial womb. This will allow us to have more control over conception and birth than ever before.

If it were ever possible, should an artificial womb be used for human pregnancies? Which circumstances would warrant the use of an artificial womb for human births? Consider the case in which a woman had fertile eggs but had had her uterus removed as a result of cancer. Should she be able to use EUFI to have a baby? What about the female executive who wants a family but worries that a pregnancy (and postpartum leave) will sideline her career? What about the couple who would otherwise use a human surrogate womb?

Consider further social consequences: Should insurance companies pay for the cost of using the artificial womb? Should the government allot Medicaid money for the socioeconomically deprived who wish to use such a service? Or should such a service be available only to the wealthy?

Exploring Personal Dimensions

Sexuality and Human Relations

A number of internal and external forces in your life influence the decisions you make regarding sexual behavior. What you do may be in harmony with some of these forces and in conflict with others.

Directions

Give a value to the following forces in your life as they pertain to your sexual behavior (i.e., what makes you choose to be sexually active or what makes you refrain from sexual activity). If you are married, apply this tool to a specific sexual behavior such as your degree of fidelity to your spouse or your degree of sexual activity with your spouse.

a = a major force influencing my sexual behavior

b = a moderate force influencing my sexual behavior

c = an insignificant force influencing my sexual behavior

1. Religious influence   a   b   c
2. Family influence   a   b   c
3. How it feels when we kiss and hug   a   b   c
4. My own self-image (how I think I   a   b   c
   look to others)
5. My sense of right or wrong   a   b   c
6. Radio, television, or movies   a   b   c
7. How it feels to touch someone   a   b   c
8. How I learned to act   a   b   c
9. The way I feel inside   a   b   c
10. Literature (books, magazines)   a   b   c
    or music
11. Pleasure   a   b   c
12. My judgment   a   b   c
13. My sense of what I should and   a   b   c
    should not do
14. Friends' influence   a   b   c
15. Physical stimulation   a   b   c
16. Introversion or extroversion   a   b   c
    (how outgoing I am)
17. My morals or values   a   b   c
18. The expectations/relationship   a   b   c
    I have with boyfriend/girlfriend
    (for marrieds, consider friends
    other than spouse)
19. Fear of, or anticipation of,   a   b   c
    pregnancy
20. Desire to feel good about myself   a   b   c

Scoring

a = 3   b = 2   c = 1

Total values as follows from top to bottom of the four columns.

Column A	Column B	Column C	Column D
1. _____	2. _____	3. _____	4. _____
5. _____	6. _____	7. _____	8. _____
9. _____	10. _____	11. _____	12. _____
13. _____	14. _____	15. _____	16. _____
17. _____	18. _____	19. _____	20. _____
Totals _____	_____	_____	_____

Interpretation

Column A represents the degree to which your morals and values or beliefs influence your sexual behavior and decisions.

Column B represents the degree to which social forces influence your sexual behavior.

Column C represents the degree to which biological factors influence your sexual behavior and decisions.

Column D represents the degree to which psychological forces influence your sexual behavior and decisions.

The relative influences can be compared directly with each other to see which area is the strongest or whether they are equal. You may interpret the results as follows:

11–15	major influence
6–10	moderate influence
1–5	insignificant influence

Suggested Readings

Alberta Society for the Promotion of Sexual Health. *Definitions of sexual health*, 2011. Available: http://www.aspsh.ca/definitions_of_sexual _health.

Bruess, C. E. Sexuality education, in *Battleground schools*, Mathison, S., & Ross, W. eds, Westport, CT: Greenwood/Praeger, 2008.

Bruess, C. E., & Schroeder, E. *Sexuality education: Theory and practice*, 6th edition. Boston, MA: Jones and Bartlett, 2014.

Edwards, W. M., & Coleman, E. Defining sexual health: A descriptive overview. *Archives of Sexual Behavior, 33, no. 3* (June 2004), 189–195.

Lefkowitz, E. S., Shearer, C. L., & Boone, T. L. Religiosity, sexual behaviors, and sexual attitudes during emerging adulthood. *Journal of Sex Research, 41, no. 2* (January 2004), 150–159.

Levine, J. Promoting pleasure: What's the problem? *SIECUS Report 30, no. 4* (April/May 2002), 19–22.

Report of the Task Force on the Sexualization of Girls. Washington, DC: American Psychological Association, 2007.

Rice, S. What does it mean to be healthy? *American Journal of Sexuality Education, 1, no. 2* (2006), 75–82.

Taverner, W. J. Sexual health in prime time. *American Journal of Sexuality Education, 1, no. 4* (2006), 71–82.

Web Resources

For links to the websites below, visit *go.jblearning. com/dimensions5e* and click on Resource Links.

Sexuality Information and Education Council of the United States
www.siecus.org

Source for the Consensus Statement on Adolescent Sexual Health and other information related to healthy sexuality.

Alberta Society for the Promotion of Sexual Health
www.aspsh.ca

Source for an excellent definition of sexuality.

Sex & Sexuality
www.plannedparenthood.org/health-topics/ sexuality-4323.htm

Information from Planned Parenthood about how understanding our sexuality can help us enjoy our lives more.

Sexual Health Network
www.sexualhealth.com/aboutus.php

A network dedicated to providing easy access to sexuality information, education, support, and other resources.

Teens Health
http://kidshealth.org/teen/sexual_health

Designed to help both males and females learn the facts about sexual health.

References

The American freshman. *Research Brief*, Higher Education Research Institute, UCLA, January 2011.

The American freshman: National norms for fall 2007. *Chronicle of Higher Education, 54*, 24 (February 1, 2008), A34.

Aries, P., & Bejin, A. *Western sexuality.* New York: Basil Blackwell, 1985.

ASPSH. *Definitions of sexual health*, 2011. Available: http://aspsh .ca/definitions_of_sexual_health.

Bardes, B. A., Shelley II, M. C., & Schmidt, S. W. *American government and politics today: The essentials.* Belmont, CA: West/Wadsworth, 1998.

Baron, R. A. *Psychology*, 4th ed. Needham Heights, MA: Allyn & Bacon, 1998.

Bell, R. R. *Premarital sex in a changing society.* Englewood Cliffs, NJ: Prentice-Hall, 1966.

Brennan, J. Reconciling immigrant values, in *Case studies in cultural diversity*, Ferguson, V. D., ed. Sudbury, MA: Jones and Bartlett, 1999, 185–189.

Bruess, C. E., & Richardson, G. *Decisions for health.* Dubuque, IA: Brown & Benchmark, 1995, 1.14–1.16.

Bruess, C. E., & Schroeder, E. *Sexuality education: Theory and practice*, 6th ed. Boston: Jones & Bartlett, 2014.

Bullough, V. L. *Sex, society & history.* New York: Science History Publications, 1976a.

Bullough, V. L. *Sexual variance in society and history*, New York: John Wiley & Sons, 1976b.

Caron, S. L., & Bertram, R. M. What college students want to know about sex. *Medical Aspects of Human Sexuality, 22* (April 1988), 18–20.

Centers for Disease Control and Prevention. *Basic statistics.* Atlanta, GA: Centers for Disease Control and Prevention,

2011. Available: http://www.cdc.gov/hiv/topics/surveillance/basic.htm#hivaidsage.

Characteristics of freshmen, 2001. *Chronicle of Higher Education, 68, no. 1* (August 31, 2001), 22–23.

Courtwright, D. T. The neglect of female children and childhood: Sex ratios in nineteenth century America: A review of the evidence. *Journal of Family History, 15* (1990), 313–323.

Degler, C. N. *At odds: Women and the family in America from the revolution to the present.* New York: Oxford University Press, 1980.

The ecology of birth control. Chicago: G. D. Searle, 1971.

FDA OKs hormonal implant. *Family Planning Perspectives, 20, no. 6* (November/December 1990), 1–4.

Fisher, H. E. *Anatomy of love.* New York: W. W. Norton, 1992.

Gendercide. *The Economist* (March 6, 2010), 13.

Grismaijer, S., & Singer, S.R. *Dressed to kill.* Pahoa, HI: ISCD Press, 2002.

Harrell, G. D., & Frazier, G. L. *Marketing: Connecting with customers.* Upper Saddle River, NJ: Prentice Hall, 1999, 26.

Hill, Z. E., Cleland, J., & Ali, M. M. Religious affiliation and extramarital sex among men in Brazil. *International Family Planning Perspectives, 30, no. 1* (2004), 20–26.

Joseph, J. Singing the push-up blues, *ABCNews.com* (September 7, 1998).

Murstein, B. L. *Love, sex, and marriage.* New York: Springer, 1974.

The nation: Attitudes and characteristics of freshmen. *Chronicle of Higher Education, 49, no. 1* (August 30, 2002), 26.

Nelson, J. B. *Embodiment: An approach to sexuality and Christian theology.* Minneapolis: Augsburg, 1978.

O'Keefe, M. The times are trying politicians' souls. *The Oregonian* (April 20, 1995), A1.

Penhollow, T. M., Young, M., & Denny, G. Predictors of quality of life, sexual intercourse, and sexual satisfaction among active older adults. *American Journal of Health Education, 40, 1* (January/February 2009), 14–22.

Plotnik, R. *Introduction to psychology,* 3rd ed. Pacific Grove: CA: Brooks/Cole, 1993, 27–28.

Reiss, I. L. Changing trends, attitudes and values on premarital sexual behavior in the U.S., in *Human sexuality and the mentally retarded,* de la Cruz, F. F., & La Vock, G. D., eds. New York: Brunner/Mazel, 1973, 286–289.

Rooney, M. Freshmen show rising political awareness and changing social views. *The Chronicle of Higher Education, 49, no. 21* (January 31, 2003), A35–A38.

Roth, Z. Parents keep child's gender under wraps. Yahoo! News, May 26, 2011. Available: http://news.yahoo.com/blogs/lookout/parents-keep-child-gender-under-wraps-170824245.html.

Sadock, B. J., Kaplan, H. I., & Freedman, A. M. *The sexual experience.* Baltimore: Williams & Wilkins, 1973.

Sheeran, P. *Women, society, the state and abortion: A structuralist analysis.* New York: Prager, 1987.

SIECUS position statements on human sexuality, 2012. Available: http://siecus.org/index.cfm.

Spielvogel, J. J. *Western civilization,* 3rd ed. St. Paul, MN: West, 1997.

Survey Tracks Changes in Political Views of Freshmen. *Chronicle of Higher Education, 58, no. 22* (February 3, 2012), A11.

Tannahill, R. *Sex in history.* New York: Stein & Day, 1980.

This year's freshmen at 4-year colleges: A statistical profile. *Chronicle of Higher Education, 51, no. 22* (February 4, 2005), A34.

This year's freshmen at 4-year colleges: A statistical profile. *Chronicle of Higher Education, 55, 21* (January 30, 2009), A19.

Tiefer, L. *Sex is not a natural act.* Boulder, CO: Westview Press, 1995.

Where do babies come from? *Family Life Educator* (Winter 1987), 5–7.

Xu, X, Zhu, F., O'Campo, P. Koenig, M. A., Mock, V., & Campbell, J. Prevalence of and risk factors for intimate partner violence in China. *American Journal of Public Health 95, no. 1* (2005), 78–85.

CHAPTER

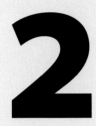

2

Sexuality Research

FEATURES

Ethical Dimensions
Permission to
Do Research on
Sexual Behavior

**Multicultural
Dimensions**
The Wyatt Surveys on
African American and
White Women in
Los Angeles

Global Dimensions
The Liu Report:
Sexual Behavior in
Modern China

Gender Dimensions
Differences in
Research Results

**Communication
Dimensions**
Talking About
Sexuality Research
Results

CHAPTER OBJECTIVES

1 Describe the various methods used in sexuality research, including the steps in the scientific process.

2 Identify the ethical issues involved in sexuality research.

3 Describe the work of early sexuality researchers, including how they set the stage for modern research.

4 Summarize the contributions of major modern sexuality researchers.

go.jblearning.com/dimensions5e

Ethical Dimensions: Permission to Do Research
on Sexual Behavior
Alfred Kinsey
William Masters and Virginia Johnson
Youth Risk Behavior Surveillance System

INTRODUCTION

You have probably heard the joke, "My mind is made up; don't confuse me with the facts." Unfortunately, when it comes to sexuality research, this attitude too often prevails. For example, a few years ago one of our students mentioned that one of his parents had asked him how his courses were going that term. When he mentioned he was learning about research on human sexuality, there were a few seconds of silence.

He explained that he had been raised in a home where sexuality was not discussed. He asked his parent about the silence, and the answer came back that it was a little difficult to think about research on such a topic. What did the researchers do? How did they do it? Why would they even want to do research on sexuality?

Our student explained that for a few minutes he felt he was the parent while he tried to answer these questions. Fortunately, he had already read information on this topic, so he thought he did a pretty good job.

This is not an isolated instance of lack of understanding, or even of repression, when it comes to sexuality research. For instance, in many places in this chapter you will find references to the National Health and Social Life Survey (NHSLS). In 1988, a team of researchers at the University of Chicago won a federal government grant competition to conduct an extensive research study on sexual behavior. In 1989, however, conservative members of Congress attacked its research for a number of reasons (Laumann, Michael, & Gagnon, 1994). They said it was a plot by homosexuals to legitimate the normality of gay and lesbian lifestyles; it was an unwarranted intrusion by the government in private matters; it was not needed; it should not be supported with taxpayers' money; and the project staff had an antifamily agenda.

During a federal governmental review, facts about the research were widely misrepresented. It was also claimed that the researchers had published statements that they had not, and statements were taken out of context in an attempt to show that the researchers should not be doing the research. As a result, the previously approved government grant was cancelled. The research was then completed with private funding. Since the study of human sexuality still prompts anxiety and even fear in some people, as well as a hesitancy to talk about the subject with other people, sexuality research can be difficult.

In this chapter we present some of the major 20th- and 21st-century research on sexuality to show you how knowledge about human sexuality is obtained and to discuss some of the findings that researchers believe can aid individuals in accepting and understanding the sexual parts of their personalities. We turn to the findings after identifying some of the methodology used in sexuality research.

■ Research Methods

Research is undertaken to expand our knowledge about specific factors in our environment. Our current knowledge of human sexuality is based on relatively few studies. Perhaps by reading about issues and techniques related to research in general, you will better understand and evaluate the studies we discuss, as well as ask yourself how valid the findings are.

The first task of any researcher, regardless of the subject, is to ask an explicit question. The next is to design a way of gathering the relevant information. In sexuality research the most common methods used are surveys, case studies, and experimental research. Less common is the method of direct observation, a method used more in sexual research clinics but also used extensively in the research of Masters and Johnson (discussed shortly). Each method of research has its advantages and disadvantages, some of which are discussed here.

A good researcher chooses a method according to the particular problem and population being studied. For example, a survey would be used when a large number of responses are desired, as in a study of adolescent behavior. Observation might be desirable when a small number of subjects are involved, as in measuring responses of people who are engaging in a sexual behavior while being electrically monitored.

The Scientific Method

Sexology is the study of sexuality. To study sexuality appropriately, it is necessary to use the **scientific method**—that is, research conducted in an atmosphere free from bias—because it is the most objective way to establish new knowledge in any field. Scientists must always approach research studies without preconceived ideas of what their studies will show. In addition, they cannot have preconceived agendas to show what sexual behavior *should* be. Researchers do not set out to "prove" something but instead conduct research scientifically to discover what *is*—not necessarily just what they want it to be. Researchers follow proper procedures and discover information through research that can then be generalized to the real world outside the study.

> **sexology**
> The study of sexuality.
>
> **scientific method**
> Research conducted in an atmosphere free from bias.

As we will explain, the scientific method involves the following steps:

1. *Identifying a research question* (which could be based on personal interest or experience, on social concerns, or on the interests of those funding the research, such as government agencies or private industry)

2. *Reviewing the literature*

3. *Formulating a hypothesis (or two or more hypotheses)*

4. *Operationalizing variables*

5. *Collecting data*

6. *Analyzing the data to test the hypotheses*

The scientific method first involves identifying a research question. Not all questions about sexuality lend themselves to scientific research, because many involve subjective values, morals, and philosophical questions. (However, scientific research can provide information that can help us address even these types of questions.)

Second, to inform themselves adequately, researchers must review literature related to the research question. Thus the researchers learn what is already known about the topic, think of ways to conduct the desired research, and possibly even come up with new research questions.

Third, a hypothesis is formulated. A **hypothesis** is a tentative proposal or an educated guess about the results of a research study. It often deals with the relationship between two variables. A **variable** is a measurable event that varies or is subject to change (such as frequency of sexual behavior, use of contraceptives, or amount of alcohol ingested).

hypothesis
A tentative proposal or an educated guess about the results of a research study.

variable
A measurable event that varies or is subject to change.

Fourth, operationalizing the variables means specifying how they are going to be measured. For example, some variables, such as gender or income level, are easy to measure. Others, such as sexual desire or satisfaction in a relationship, are not. There are many ways to measure these variables, and the research has to state clearly how this will be done.

Fifth, collecting the data involves using methods such as survey research, case studies, experimental research, and direct observation. Each of these is explained in greater detail shortly.

Sixth, the data are analyzed to test the hypotheses. Data can be analyzed to describe situations, to show a relationship between variables, or to show that one situation causes another. Each of these methods of analysis demands the use of appropriate statistical methods.

Various forms of bias can be problematic. For example, in addition to possible bias of researchers, there could be bias of research subjects. If all subjects are college educated, they will probably be biased. Or, if some subjects are really not willing to participate or

to be honest even if they agree to participate, they will also be biased. This type of bias is referred to as **volunteer bias**—characteristics of volunteers that are likely to influence research results.

One of the goals of the scientific method is to find information that can be generalized to the real world outside the study. Obviously, when researchers are trying to learn more about human sexuality, they cannot get information from *all* human beings. Therefore, they must study a relatively small group of people from which the results may be generalized to a larger population. **Generalization**, the ability to conclude that the same results would be obtained outside the study, can occur only if all aspects of the scientific method are properly planned, carried out, and controlled as much as possible.

The **population** is the group being studied in a research project. Usually only a **sample** (a segment of the larger population) participates, because the total

volunteer bias
Characteristics of volunteers that are likely to influence research results.
generalization
The ability to conclude that the same results would be obtained outside the study.

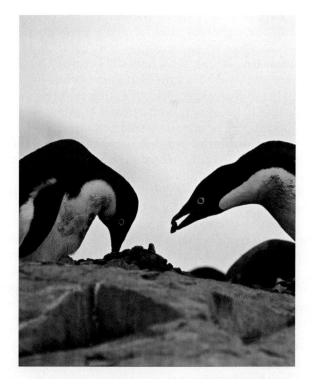

Researchers on Antarctica's Ross Island have noted that female penguins, desperate for stones for their real nest, were willing to engage in "courtship" with an unpaired male penguin in exchange for stones. The penguin expert Eric Bennett decided to try an experiment at the Baltimore Zoo: He dressed up as a penguin and surrounded himself with lots of rocks. Within minutes, female penguins began presenting themselves for courtship. Does Bennett's experiment reflect the scientific method?

population
The group being studied in a research project.

sample
A segment of the larger population.

random sample
A sample that represents the larger population and that is chosen without bias, so that every member of the larger population has an equal chance to be selected.

population would be too large and unwieldy. A **random sample** represents the larger population and is chosen in a way that eliminates bias. If the sample is selected properly, the researcher can generalize findings to the larger population.

Survey Research

Much information about human sexuality has been obtained by **surveys** asking people about sexual attitudes and experiences. This kind of data can be obtained orally (face-to-face interviews) or in written form (pencil-and-paper questionnaires). Researchers use surveys when information from a large number of people is desired. For example, they might use a survey to find out how people feel about condom advertisements on television.

The **interview** allows the interviewer to explain the purpose and value of the survey, to clarify and explain the questions, and to report answers clearly. However, some individuals may not report their sexual experiences and views honestly because they may be embarrassed to admit particular behaviors and thoughts to a stranger. Also, the subjects being interviewed may be equally embarrassed to admit they do not participate in certain sexual activities.

Questionnaires are less expensive than interviews, which require many people to conduct the interviews. A questionnaire that the subject can fill out at his or her convenience makes many people feel more relaxed and reinforces anonymity; the privacy may also ensure more honest answering. In addition, the questionnaire eliminates the subject's being influenced by the interviewer's facial or bodily gestures.

The major concern with any **self-report data** is that subjects may include inaccuracies. Accuracy is obviously necessary for reliable research. For instance, people often have difficulty recalling past events, and events can become highly embellished or minimized the longer the time between experience and reporting. Recall

survey
Research in which people complete questionnaires or are personally interviewed.

interview
Oral research method designed to gather information.

questionnaire
Written instrument designed to gather information.

self-report data
The respondents' descriptions of something.

involves estimating **frequency** and/or **duration** of behaviors, and many people have problems remembering numbers.

frequency
How often something occurs or has occurred.

duration
How long something occurs or has occurred.

Case Studies

Case studies are in-depth studies of individuals or small, select groups of individuals. Those under study are generally followed over a period of months or years. Case studies provide a chance to look at specific behaviors or characteristics in great depth. Also, because case studies generally cover a relatively long period, the researcher is able to explore cause-and-effect relationships in detail. For example, much information about sex offenders and people with sexual-response difficulties has been obtained through case studies.

case study
In-depth study of individual(s) or small groups.

With case studies, however, there is no way to use proper sampling techniques, making it difficult to generalize case-study results to the rest of the population. For instance, how do we know that sex offenders or those receiving treatment for sexual-response problems are like the rest of the population?

Experimental Research

In an **experiment**, behavior can be studied under controlled conditions. A common experimental design is one in which two groups are matched and compared. The groups are identical but for one important difference—the **experimental group** is subjected to a particular event or condition, whereas the **control group** is not. Both groups are observed, and the results are compared to determine whether the experimental condition had an effect. For example, a researcher could compare the responses of different groups of people (perhaps grouped by gender or age) to erotic materials.

Experimental research allows control over variables thought to influence responses or behavior. At the same time, the somewhat artificial setting may influence behavior or response. Merely

experiment
Observation of behavior (or effects) under controlled conditions.

experimental group
In an experiment, the group subjected to a particular event or condition.

control group
In an experiment, the group not subjected to a particular event or condition.

knowing you are in a study or being in a laboratory might alter your reaction.

Ethical DIMENSIONS

Permission to Do Research on Sexual Behavior

A faculty member at Mercer University in Macon, Georgia, was told by the president of the university that he could not conduct research in the form of a survey of sexual behavior of undergraduate students at Mercer (Wilson, 2002). The president said the project simply was not appropriate at a Baptist institution.

The president was concerned that the survey's explicit questions might offend students and their parents. Even though a 13-member campus review board unanimously approved the survey, top university administrators said that the survey was also subject to their approval. This procedural step had never before been invoked. One of the vice presidents said that such a survey could have negative impacts on admissions and parents' attitudes about the school.

Taking the opposite position, the researchers involved in the study said that better safe-sex programs were needed for Mercer undergraduates, and that a well-done survey about sexual behavior would be a good place to start. The faculty and students working together on the project hoped to publish the results in a scholarly journal. They indicated that preventing them from conducting the survey denied them academic freedom. They were upset that the result was an apparently arbitrary decision of senior administrators.

What do you think? Was it ethical for the researchers to conduct the survey? Was it ethical for the president to tell them they could not conduct the survey? Should the senior administrators have allowed the survey to be conducted even if they did not like the idea of the survey's being done on their campus?

Source: Data from Wilson, R. An ill-fated sex survey, *The Chronicle of Higher Education, 48, no. 47* (August 2, 2002), A10–A12.

Direct Observation

Observation is a method in which subjects are watched in a laboratory, a class, a natural setting, or the workplace. It can be an accurate way to collect sexual information—particularly if the researcher controls the setting. A prime example of observational research has been the human sexual-response research of Masters and Johnson.

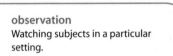

observation
Watching subjects in a particular setting.

The major drawback of direct observation is the required expenditure of time and money. In addition, people are likely to be reluctant to perform sexual activity in a laboratory where they are being observed. Some people also question the ethics of participating in observational research either as the researcher or as the subject. When people do feel relatively comfortable and volunteer for observational research related to sexuality, one must always ask whether their sexual responses in such a setting replicate those obtained in the privacy of their normal environment. Another important question is whether people who are comfortable doing this are similar to the majority of people who aren't: Put another way, can the findings be generalized?

Focus Groups

A **focus group** is a form of research where a group of approximately 6 to 10 people are asked about their feelings or attitudes toward a topic and then discuss related issues. For example, the participants might be asked what they think about equal rights

focus group
A form of research where a group of 6 to 10 people are asked about a topic and then discuss related issues.

for homosexuals and heterosexuals. The leader usually has a focus-group script that guides the discussion (it includes questions, follow-up questions, and other instructions). A typical focus-group session might last for 1–2 hours. It is important to have extensive interchange among the participants to get as many thoughts and ideas as possible from the group. Focus-group members sometimes talk among themselves in reaction to a topic or question from the focus-group leader—with the leader listening and taking notes for analysis later.

There are arguments both for and against focus groups. Some experts believe they are valuable ways to get important information from a group of people in a relatively inexpensive way. Other experts think they can be very time-consuming, the group cannot possibly be large enough to be a representative sample of the population, and the group can be unduly influenced by the researcher. Traditionally, most focus groups meet in person, but today there are also teleconference focus groups and online focus groups.

Interpreting Statistics

In many kinds of sexuality research, statistics related to the results will be presented. When we hear about statistical results, we have to differentiate between correlation and causation. **Correlation** is a statistical measure that shows how variables are naturally related in the real world. For example, studies might show that youth who watch more television also participate in more sexual behavior. That is interesting information, but it tells us nothing about *why* that relationship exists; it only tells us that the relationship *does* exist.

> **correlation**
> A statistical measure that shows how variables are naturally related to each other.

How do we know if the results of a study are accurate? Perhaps the findings just happened to occur in this study, but wouldn't occur in other similar studies. We can use statistics to help us determine how likely it is that the results will also occur in other studies. A number of statistical methods can be used to determine statistical significance. **Statistical significance** refers to the likelihood that a study's results are due to chance. If the results are significant at the .05 level, for example, there is only a 5% chance those results are due to chance. If it has been reported that people who don't use condoms develop HIV to a greater extent than those who do use condoms, and that finding is significant at the .05 level, we can be confident that the difference is attributable to not using condoms rather than to chance. In other words, not using condoms "caused" more people to develop HIV as compared to the rate found among people who did use condoms.

> **statistical significance**
> The likelihood that a study's results are due to the relationship uncovered between the study's variables as opposed to chance.

How can you use this information to contribute to your sexual health? When you are deciding whether to engage in a sexual behavior, you can read studies to see if there are statistically significant differences between those who engage in that behavior and those who do not. This will give you confidence that these differences are a result of that behavior, and that you can expect similar results if you decide to engage in that sexual behavior.

Issues in Sexuality Research

Despite the care and planning that go into implementing a research project, the success of a project depends on the cooperation of the subjects. The most difficult task in studying humans is finding a large group who will stay with the project to completion. When mail questionnaires are used, for example, the response rate is generally less than 40% of the total number distributed—and often close to 20%. Interviews are expensive, but the response rate can be high, depending on the interviewer's expertise and awareness. The interviewer must establish rapport with the subjects so that they are not embarrassed, intimidated, or totally unresponsive.

When asked to be surveyed about sexual behavior, many people will refuse, but others will participate. Therefore, those who do participate may be more or less sexually experienced and liberated than those who choose not to take part. This volunteer bias may allow us to draw conclusions from the study results about how some people view sexual matters, but it does not allow us to conclude that people in general behave or believe that way. When people answer surveys or consent to be interviewed, there are always problems of reporting accuracy, ability to recall past experiences as they really occurred, and willingness to be truthful, particularly about sexual matters, when facing an interviewer. Consider, for example, that reporting and evaluating how we feel now are easier than reporting how we felt sometime in the past. In recalling how and where we learned about sexuality or what sexual activities we were involved in as children, we are easily influenced by events that took place in intervening years, by changes in behavior socially defined as normal (or at least permissible), and by our own maturity. Even if subjects want and intend to give honest responses, they may feel reluctant to share the intimate details of their activities with a stranger, worry about the researcher's attitude toward their sexual behavior—particularly in an interview—or be afraid that their responses are not genuinely confidential.

Research on sexuality faces some additional problems. Many conditions affect our sexuality, including broad cultural and social definitions of sexuality roles and proper sexual behavior, as well as characteristics such as ethnic origin, religion, personal experience, and education. Such conditions and their effects may be too complex to measure or control. Also, cooperative subjects may be hard to find, because in our culture people feel anxiety, self-consciousness, and a

Multicultural DIMENSIONS

The Wyatt Surveys on African American and White Women in Los Angeles

You will sometimes see research findings indicating differences in sexual behaviors and attitudes between people of different races. Care is needed when interpreting such findings, because it is often hard to differentiate between what may be a result of racial culture, what may be a result of socioeconomic differences, and what may be random or coincidental. A good example of this is provided by the Wyatt surveys.

Wyatt and her colleagues used Kinsey-style face-to-face interviews to examine the sexual behavior of 122 white and 126 African American 18- to 36-year-old women in Los Angeles. The two samples were balanced in relation to demographic characteristics such as age, education, number of children, and marital status.

Wyatt reported that by age 20, 98% of the people in her study (both white and African American) had experienced premarital sexual intercourse. When social class differences were considered, the ages of first intercourse for African American and white women were similar.

To control for demographic differences between white and African American women, Wyatt limited the subjects to demographically similar (age, education, social class) women. Her sample of African American women then matched the demographic characteristics of the larger African American Los Angeles population. However, because of Wyatt's efforts to use demographically similar groups, the white sample did not match the demographic characteristics of the larger white Los Angeles population because it contained a greater proportion of white women from lower-income families. This is an example of a trade-off in research. Wyatt wanted to be sure her two groups were demographically similar but in doing so ended up with one group that was not demographically similar to its larger population. This is not necessarily bad; however, it illustrates that we must understand what the researchers have done to interpret the results accurately.

Sources: Data from Wyatt, G. E. The sexual abuse of Afro-American and white American women in childhood, *Child Abuse and Neglect, 9* (1985), 5, 7, 19; Wyatt, G. E., Peters, S. D., & Guthrie, D. Kinsey revisited, Part I: Comparisons of the sexual socialization and sexual behavior of white women over 33 years, *Archives of Sexual Behavior, 17* (3, 1988a), 201–209; Wyatt, G. E., Peters, S. C., & Guthrie, D. Kinsey revisited, Part II: Comparisons of the sexual socialization and sexual behavior of black women over 33 years, *Archives of Sexual Behavior, 17* (4, 1988b), 289–332.

---

reluctance to share private thoughts, experiences, and memories about sexuality. For example, many people would not want to talk about their experiences with forcible sexual behavior. Even talking about whether one masturbates and, if so, how frequently, is not something most people are eager to do.

There can also be some limitations in sexuality research. For example, nonresponse (refusal to participate) can make it difficult to get responses from the desired subjects. Also, self-selection volunteer bias may be a problem. Volunteers for sexuality research may be more sexually experienced and hold more positive attitudes toward sexuality than nonvolunteers. Finally, there may be a demographic bias. As seen in Kinsey's work and even today, it is often easier to get subjects for sexuality research who are white, middle-class, white-collar workers and college students.

Adding to the difficulty of gathering accurate information is the influence of the researcher's own values and biases. The researcher may have very strong opinions about issues in the study and may—perhaps unintentionally—phrase questions in favor of his or her views, emphasize certain words in a face-to-face interview, and/or have certain racial, ethnic, or cultural views that affect rapport with the subjects in the study. Interviewers and writers of questionnaires may have perceptions about the group they are surveying, which can also influence how questions are asked or phrased. When the information is collected and interpreted, the researcher must consciously prevent personal feelings and attitudes from affecting analysis and reporting. For example, a researcher who might be either strongly for or strongly against abortion would need to be very careful when asking questions about abortion and recording the answers of a research subject. It would be wise to have several researchers with different views work together to check questionnaires and procedures to be sure there is as much **objectivity** as

objectivity
Being sure the results are the same no matter who asks the questions or records the answers.

possible—that is, be sure the results are the same no matter who asks the questions or records the answers.

Ethical Issues in Sexuality Research

Recently there has been increased attention to the need to protect the people participating in any form of human research. Because of the intimate nature of sexual research, the ethical issues involved in this field are particularly important.

An ethical issue of particular concern is obtaining the **informed consent** of participants; subjects of research studies must agree in writing to participate *after* the purposes, risks, and benefits of the study have been explained to them. Consent is obtained to ensure that subjects both understand what the project entails and agree to undergo the experience as described. This requirement protects subjects against physical and psychological abuse by irresponsible researchers and protects researchers against claims that subjects were taken advantage of. Investigators are now required by law to obtain an individual's consent to be subjected to the project as described; those testing minors must also obtain parental or guardian permission.

Researchers do not have the right to coerce people to participate in a study, and they must be honest when presenting information about the research. They also have a responsibility to protect the confidentiality of their participants. They must be sure that personal facts can never be connected to a given

informed consent
Document required to participate in a research study after the purposes, risks, and benefits of the study have been explained.

individual. It is obvious that participants must also be protected from physical and psychological harm. Many methods must be used to guarantee the anonymity of participants and to be sure confidential information is never released.

Human-research review committees commonly exist in government agencies and in universities. These committees must review and approve any research designs and procedures that will use human subjects. Such committees consider the value of the research and compare it to any potential risks to the participants. It can be difficult for committees to decide whether to allow a researcher to carry out a particular study—especially if children are involved. This is one reason why we do not have better information about the sexual thoughts and experiences of young people.

Additional ethical questions arise in studies of the sexual behaviors and attitudes of various racial groups. Some people argue that such research is important to better understanding of diverse feelings and practices. In contrast, others believe that describing sexual behaviors and attitudes according to racial groups contributes to stereotypical thinking.

vaginal plethysmography
Insertion of a probe into a woman's vagina to measure changes in blood volume.

penile strain gauge
A wire or cuff placed around the penis to measure physiological changes over time.

plethysmograph
A laboratory measuring device that charts physiological changes over time.

Another interesting ethical issue arises from the ways that have been developed to measure physiological changes in the vagina or the penis due to sexual stimulation. **Vaginal plethysmography** involves inserting a probe into a woman's vagina to measure increased blood volume, an indication of sexual arousal. Changes in blood volume over time can be charted with this device. Similarly, a **penile strain gauge** can be used. This is a wire or cuff placed around the penis that is attached to a **plethysmograph**, a laboratory measuring device that charts physiological changes over time and records changes in the girth of the penis as it responds to sexual arousal or loss of arousal.

Plethysmography has been used to see whether a person has certain sorts of sexual interests, such as a sexual interest in children. For example, if it were suspected that a person were sexually attracted to children, the device might provide additional information that could lead to a referral for possible treatment. Following treatment, the device could be used again to see whether the degree of sexual interest in children has decreased. However,

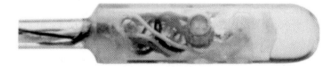

The vaginal plethysmograph is used to measure sexual response by detecting changes in the amount of blood in the vaginal walls. The device is used in sexuality research.

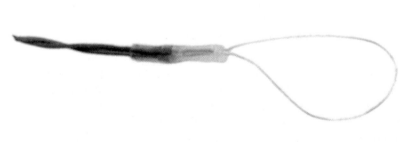

The penile strain gauge is used to measure erectile response by detecting changes in the circumference of the penis. The device is used in sexuality research.

because people can sometimes learn to control their physiological responses, this is not a foolproof test. Also, it would be a mistake to base too many assumptions about a person's future sexual behaviors on one measure of physiological response. Use of penile and vaginal plethysmography is likely to be debated for years to come.

Finally, it is crucial to be sure a test has **validity**—that is, that it tests what it is supposed to test. For example, a sexual-knowledge test must be a good representation of overall sexual knowledge. This might be shown by a comparison to a known good test or by expert ratings.

validity, validation
Demonstration that tests measure what they are designed to measure.

Most research on sexual feelings, attitudes, responses, and behavior depends on participants' reporting about themselves. Some people believe that sexuality research is useless and meaningless because subjects can lie about their sexual behavior, exaggerate their experiences, or feel too embarrassed to discuss personal sexual matters openly and honestly. Others believe that we need information about sexual matters and must encourage research, even while acknowledging its limitations. Although it is difficult to validate information that people include on a questionnaire or divulge in an interview, validation is frequently done by asking for the same information in another part of the survey or in conversation and cross-checking whether the information given is the same in both instances.

Given the variety of attitudes toward sexuality in our society, the many different opinions concerning moral and ethical issues related to sexuality, and even the disagreement as to whether sexuality should be researched at all, researchers have a difficult job. They must design a scientifically sound study, create confidence in that study, and guarantee their subjects' privacy.

Evaluating Sexuality Information on the Internet

Anyone who uses a search engine to look for information about "sex" or "sexuality" finds so many hits that it is not humanly possible to review all of the sites mentioned. In addition, although accurate and reliable information about sexuality can be found on the Internet, so can a preponderance of information about sexuality that is incorrect or misleading. How can you determine whether information about sexuality found on the Internet is accurate? Here are some suggestions (National Center for Complementary and Alternative Medicine, 2011):

1. *Who runs the site?* Any good website related to sexuality should make it easy for you to learn who is responsible for the site and its information.

2. *Who pays for the site?* The source of a site's funding should be readily apparent. The funding source can affect what content is presented, how the content is presented, and what the site owners want to accomplish on the site.

3. *What is the purpose of the site?* An "About This Site" link appears on many sites; if it's there, use it. The purpose of the site should be clearly stated and help you evaluate the trustworthiness of the information.

4. *Where does the information come from?* If the person or organization in charge of the site did not create the information, the original source should be clearly labeled. This identification allows others to easily find original sources of information.

5. *What is the basis of the information?* The site should describe the evidence on which the material is based. Facts and figures from valid research should have references. Also, opinions or advice should be clearly set apart from information that is based on research results.

6. *How is the information selected?* Is there an editorial board? Do people with excellent professional and scientific qualifications review the material before it is posted?

7. *How current is the information?* Websites should be reviewed and updated on a regular basis, and the most recent update or review date should be clearly posted. Even if the information is still accurate, you want to know whether the site owners have reviewed it recently to ensure that it is still valid.

8. *How does the site choose links to other sites?* What is the policy of the website owner about how links to other sites are established? What are the criteria for the sites that are linked to the website?

9. *What information about you does the site collect, and why?* Any credible website should tell you exactly what it will and will not do with personal data gathered about you. Many commercial sites sell data about their users to other companies. Don't sign up for anything you don't fully understand.

10. *How does the site manage interactions with visitors?* There should be a way for you to contact the site owners with problems, feedback, and questions. Information about the terms for using any site services should be readily available as well.

Early Sexuality Researchers

We have some information about sexual practices throughout human history. Although not all of the information was gathered in a systematic way, in Western civilization attempts to study human sexual behavior systematically date back at least to the ancient Greeks. Physicians, such as Hippocrates, and philosophers, such as Plato and Aristotle, are the forefathers of sexuality research. They made extensive observations and offered the first elaborate theories regarding sexual responses and dysfunctions, reproduction and contraception, abortion, legislation related to sexuality, and sexual ethics (The Kinsey Institute, 1998).

In Rome, Greek physicians such as Soranus and Galen further advanced sexual knowledge. Their work prompted later Islamic scholars to spend much time on sexual questions. These studies, together with the Greek and Roman manuscripts, became standard texts at medical schools and stimulated a rebirth of anatomical research in the 16th, 17th, and 18th centuries. In the 19th century, new concerns about overpopulation and sexual psychology intensified efforts to study the topic of sexuality. Finally, at the turn of the 20th century, the investigation of sexuality became a legitimate endeavor in its own right (The Kinsey Institute, 1998).

Richard von Krafft-Ebing

Richard von Krafft-Ebing (1840–1902) wrote during a period when Victorian standards strongly suppressed thinking about human sexuality. Because he was a product of this period, and because he was a physician who worked primarily with sexually disturbed people, von Krafft-Ebing's writings (1902) indicated that sexual activity is something to fear.

He supported what we now know as the double standard, whereby men have sexual freedoms that women do not. He may have supported this perspective because of his apparent discomfort with the sexuality of women.

Von Krafft-Ebing's writings had a tremendous influence on many physicians as well as the public. Even though he seemed to be biased and made some false

assumptions, his writings convinced some physicians and researchers that the study of sexuality was legitimate. This helped prepare the way for Ellis and Freud.

Henry Havelock Ellis

Henry Havelock Ellis (1859–1939), an English psychologist and physician who studied human sexuality, grew up in fear of what he had been told about the danger of nocturnal emissions. He was also concerned about his general ignorance of human sexuality. Between 1896 and 1910 Ellis published a six-volume series entitled *Studies in the Psychology of Sex,* which included the following beliefs:

1. Masturbation is common for both sexes.

2. Orgasm in males and females is very much the same.

3. Homosexuality and heterosexuality are a matter of degree.

4. Women do have sexual desire, contrary to Victorian thought.

5. There is no one norm for human sexuality. Thoughts and acts vary among individuals and cultures.

6. There should be sexuality education for both sexes starting at early ages.

7. There should not be laws against contraception or private sexual behavior.

It is clear that Ellis's ideas were controversial and ahead of their time, particularly his support of sexuality education. In fact, some people today still have difficulty accepting his beliefs. Ellis's work influenced the later pursuits of many sexuality researchers and writers.

Sigmund Freud

Sigmund Freud (1856–1939), a psychological researcher, developed theories about human development, personality, and psychopathology that have influenced our thinking today. To develop into a well-adjusted person, according to Freud, one had to progress successfully through a number of psychosexual stages.

Freud viewed sexuality and sexual pleasure as a central part of human life and felt that people naturally sought to have as much pleasure and as little pain as possible. He indicated that sexual activity was natural and that procreation was secondary to pleasure, and he cautioned against severe restrictions on sexual instincts. People, he maintained, could become neurotic if denied natural expression of their sexual instincts.

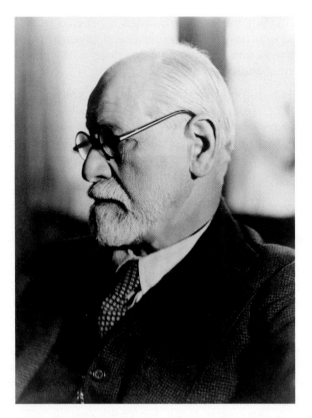

Freud's theories have influenced thinking about sexuality for more than 100 years.

One of Freud's important contributions was his suggestion that early childhood experiences had strong consequences for adult functioning. Largely because of Freud's work, sexual thoughts and behaviors are still considered to be major influences on contemporary life in general.

Magnus Hirschfeld

Magnus Hirschfeld (1868–1935) was a German physician who started his career in medicine and was soon drawn to the study of human sexuality. He was a transvestite (he coined the word "transvestism") in addition to being a homosexual. He believed that sexual orientation was a naturally occurring trait worthy of scientific study rather than social hostility. He urged homosexuals from all walks of life to come out and get involved in a growing campaign for emancipation. He promoted the idea that sexual honesty was necessary for healthy living.

Hirschfeld produced many books and papers concerning sexuality and succeeded in bringing the discussion of homosexuality into the halls of government as well as the homes of everyday people. As German fascists gained power in the 1920s, however, he was physically attacked at least twice and there were political attempts to suppress his work.

By 1930 he was forced into exile and made his home in France.

Katherine Davis

Katherine Davis (1860–1935) was born in Buffalo, New York, and educated in the United States. She taught high school science for 10 years, then went on to earn a Ph.D. degree in economics in 1900. In 1901 she began working in the field of corrections, and in 1914 became the commissioner of corrections for New York City.

She quickly moved to improve conditions in the penal institutions, then became interested in topics related to the well-being of women. From 1918 to 1928 she was general secretary of the New York Bureau of Social Hygiene board of directors, where she directed research on many topics related to public health. In 1929 she published *Factors in the Sex Life of Twenty-Two Hundred Women*. In addition, she was the author of many articles in professional and popular journals (Women in American history, 2005).

Her survey of married Caucasian women of above-average intelligence, education, and social position revealed some interesting results (History of sex surveys: Factors in the sex life of 2200 women, 2005). For example, contraception (then called "voluntary parenthood") was approved in principle by almost 90% of the respondents and practiced by 73%. Of those who claimed to have "happy" marriages, only one out of four worked outside the home. Based on this fact, the researchers concluded that working was not conducive to marital happiness.

Ninety percent of the married women considered their husband's sex drives to be as strong as or stronger than their own. A little over 3% believed their sex drives were stronger. Masturbation was admitted to by 65% of the unmarried women and 40% of the married women, but 2 out of 3 of these women considered the habit "morally degrading." Slightly more than 50% of the single women said they had experienced "intense emotional reactions" with other women, and over 25% admitted that the relationship involved overt homosexual expression.

Dr. Davis's research included some opinion questions. She found that 39% of the women thought sexual intercourse was necessary for complete physical and mental health, 19% thought a young woman was justified in having intercourse before marriage, 21% thought a young man was justified in having intercourse before marriage, 85% thought married people were justified in having intercourse for reasons other than having children, 63% thought information regarding birth control methods should be available for unmarried people, and 72% felt that it was acceptable for an abortion to be performed.

Clelia Mosher

Clelia Mosher (1863–1940) was born in Albany, New York. She was educated at Stanford University, where in her master's thesis she debunked a widespread myth of that time: the belief that women breathed differently than men, and were therefore unfit for exercise. Mosher found that this difference was caused by women being laced into tight-fitting corsets, and that there was no reason that they could not otherwise participate in strenuous exercise.

Mosher completed medical school at Johns Hopkins in 1899. In 1923 she wrote a book entitled *Women's Physical Freedom*. She explained her views on women's health, menstruation, and breast care. She promoted a positive view of women's potential and argued against many Victorian attitudes.

Over a period of 30 years, she surveyed Victorian women, most of whom were born about the time of the Civil War, about their sexual lives. This was probably the first known survey of sexual attitudes and behaviors. She gave her nine-page survey to a total of 47 women. Therefore, the sample size was small and the women were not representative of Victorian women in general. Most were faculty wives at universities and also well educated for that era. Even though it was a biased sample, it is noteworthy because it is the only known survey of Victorian women. This was a period when women were not supposed to be sexual. Interestingly, her findings were not published until 1980. Here are some of them:

- Although Victorian women were not supposed to feel sexual desire, 35 of the 47 women indicated that they liked sexual intercourse.

- Thirty-four of the women had experienced orgasms.

- Many of the women indicated that it could be a problem because it took them longer to reach orgasm than their male partner. They said there was a need for men to know about this.

- More than two-thirds of the women used some kind of birth control. Douching was the most common, followed by withdrawal and "timing." Obviously, we do not consider these methods very reliable today. Some husbands used a "male sheath" (a condom), and two women used a "rubber cap over the uterus" (either a diaphragm or a cervical cap). One woman said she used "cocoa butter," but she did not explain why or how.

- Three of the women said that their ideal would be to never have sexual intercourse at all. But most of the women expressed their sexual desires and experienced orgasms. Most seemed to enjoy sexual relations with their husbands.

It is impressive that Mosher was able to accomplish her research at the height of the Victorian era. It seems that she was a talented woman who tried hard to improve the status of women at the same time she was doing groundbreaking research.

20th-Century Sexuality Researchers

The 19th-century model of sexuality and sexual behavior was a medical one. Individuals who differed from the accepted norms were considered ill or, in scientific terms, deviant or pathological; however, little was known about sexual attitudes, behaviors, and activities. There was a dearth of knowledge about human sexuality from the psychological, psychosocial, and physiological perspectives. Research into sexual attitudes and behaviors lacked respectability, and many institutions would not fund or support it. In the 1930s changes in public attitudes in the United States, desire for contraception (both for child spacing and for

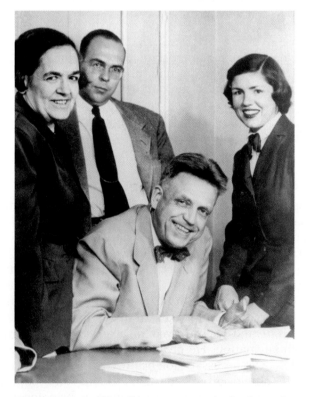

Alfred Kinsey and his colleagues were at the forefront of using scientific methodology to study human sexuality. His research, begun in 1938, was revolutionary in that it covered a wide range of sexual activities and applied statistical methods to sexuality research.

population control), and a more open interest in the scope of sexual behavior led to greater acceptance of human sexuality as a legitimate field for research.

What follows is an overview of the more prominent research in human sexual behavior during the 20th century. Although some of this work was done in the late 1930s, you will find that many of the issues are not very different from those you are concerned with and possibly are experiencing now.

Our overview covers two categories—scientific literature and popular literature. In most instances it is obvious which category applies, but admittedly in a few cases the point is arguable. We hope that a review of these studies will not only add to your sum of information but also help you to expand and develop your sexuality and interpersonal relationships.

Scientific Literature

Alfred C. Kinsey: Establishing Scientific Sex Research

Alfred Kinsey, a biologist and zoologist, joined the faculty of Indiana University in 1920. He gained academic recognition early in his career through his writings in biology. In 1937 Kinsey became the teacher of a newly introduced course in marriage and sexuality education. As his interest in the subject grew, he began to amass information concerning sexual activities and beliefs about sexuality. Dr. Kinsey's scientific background led him to gather facts and statistical data. Kinsey eventually gathered the largest amount of information on human sexuality ever collected.

The interviews conducted by Kinsey and his colleagues covered six ways in which males and females achieve orgasm in our culture: masturbation, nocturnal sex dreams and emissions, heterosexual petting, heterosexual premarital intercourse, homosexual intercourse, and sexual contact with animals. The questions focused on nine major areas: social and economic data, marital history, sexuality education, physical and physiological data, nocturnal sex dreams, masturbation, heterosexual history, homosexual history, and animal contacts. Using these highly specific interviews, Kinsey and his associates collected data from only white males and females. They represented rural and urban areas in each state and a range of ages, marital statuses, educational levels, occupations, and religions. The sample contained a disproportionately high number of better-educated people living in cities. All subjects were volunteers. Kinsey's studies may be the best-known example of survey research related to sexuality, but his sample cannot be viewed as representative of the U.S. population. *Sexual Behavior in the Human Male* (1948) is based on interviews with 5,300 males; *Sexual Behavior in the Human Female* (1953) on interviews with 5,900 females.

Americans had little knowledge about sexual behavior in this culture until Kinsey presented his findings. His conclusions generated a great deal of public reaction. Kinsey concluded that there was a relationship between sexual behaviors and attitudes on the one hand and education and socioeconomic characteristics on the other hand. In males, the lower the educational level, the higher the premarital activity. For women, the findings were the opposite—the higher the educational level, the more likely the premarital activity. He found that those women who had experienced premarital orgasm were more likely to experience marital orgasm. Most of the married females reported orgasm response through coital and noncoital sexual behavior. Only about 2% of women reported a complete lack of sexual arousal. A great many of Kinsey's subjects reported childhood sexual experiences, which reinforced Freud's belief that sexual expression is experienced in childhood. Kinsey concluded from all the data that people are sexual from early childhood through adulthood. Despite its limitations, Kinsey's work was hailed as the first large-scale study of sexual behavior. Some of Kinsey's major findings are described in the following paragraphs.

Masturbation Close to 92% of males in Kinsey's sample stated that they had masturbated at some point in their lives, with the highest incidence reported between 16 and 20 years of age; about 62% of all females reported that they had masturbated. The higher the educational level, the greater the incidence of masturbation in both men and women. In both males and females, the stronger the religious adherence, the lower the incidence of masturbation.

Nocturnal Dreams About Sex Dreams about sex were experienced by both sexes. From the data Kinsey concluded that 70% of females had dreams about sex. About 90% of the females who reported sex dreams had heterosexual dreams with sexual partners they could not identify. About 37% of 45-year-old women had experienced dreams that led to orgasm. The highest incidence of nocturnal emissions was reported by 71% of single males aged 21 to 25 years.

Premarital Intercourse With regard to heterosexual premarital intercourse, Kinsey found that 22% of all adolescent males had experienced intercourse. Among college males 67% had experienced premarital intercourse. Males of lower social class reported greater frequency of premarital intercourse than those of higher social class. Nearly 50% of the females reported premarital intercourse. About two-thirds of the married females reported sexual orgasm before marriage through any one of five

Global DIMENSIONS

The Liu Report: Sexual Behavior in Modern China

Dalin Liu and associates (1997) interviewed 23,000 Chinese people over a period of 18 months. The nationwide survey about sexual attitudes and behavior, a Chinese "Kinsey Report," was the first conducted in China. Liu reported the following:

1. For high school students, the mean age of first ejaculation was 14.4 years.
2. College students were highest in their masturbation rates (59% for males and 17% for females) as compared to high school students (13% for males and 5% for females), city married subjects (33% for males and 12% for females), and village married subjects (9% for males and 11% for females).
3. Thirteen percent of the college student males and 6% of the college student females had experienced premarital sexual activity. This compared with 22% of the city married men and 16% of the city married women, and 35% of the village married men and 15% of the village married women.
4. Among all groups, college students had the highest proportion of those who had homosexual behavior (8%) as compared to less than 1% of city married

subjects and just over 2% of village married subjects.
5. Sexual satisfaction was reported by 55% of married males and 67% of married females.
6. Ninety-five percent of the college students and 67% of the married subjects felt positively about the female's initiating sexual activity. Four percent of the college students and 11% of the married subjects felt negatively about this idea.
7. Fifty-six percent of college students, as compared to 10% of married subjects, approved of extramarital sexual activity. Thirty-nine percent of the college students and 79% of the married subjects felt very negative about extramarital sexual activity.
8. Most Chinese couples engage in little or no foreplay before initiating intercourse. Many wives report some discomfort during intercourse as a result of insufficient vaginal lubrication.
9. Women are more likely than men to initiate divorce proceedings (three of five divorces are requested by women).

Source: Data from Liu, D., Man Lun Ng, Li Ping Zhou, & Haeberle, E. J. *Sexual behavior in modern China.* New York: Continuum, 1997.

---

techniques: masturbation, nocturnal dreams, heterosexual petting, heterosexual coitus, and homosexual contacts. At all social levels, males and females who were devoutly religious reported much less premarital intercourse than nondevout subjects. Kinsey also found that people who married earlier had experienced premarital intercourse at a younger age, and those who married later had begun premarital intercourse at a later age.

Homosexual Activity Kinsey found homosexual incidence highest in high school males. About 37% of all males had some homosexual experience between adolescence and old age. Twenty-five percent of females aged 30 years and over had been erotically aroused by other females, and 17% had experienced sexual contact with other females. Female homosexual contact was greatest in the college and graduate school groups.

The Kinsey Institute is still operating. It is called the Kinsey Institute for Research in Sex, Gender, and Reproduction and is located at Indiana University. In 2004 Kinsey's life was the subject of a popular movie.

William Masters and Virginia Johnson: The Physiology of Sexual Response

The research efforts and studies of Masters and Johnson are probably the most widely known and cited of all sex-related data. These researchers were the first to observe people's sexual behaviors in a laboratory setting and to identify physiological changes during sexual arousal. William Masters was a gynecologist and Virginia Johnson a psychologist. Together they were the directors of what was the Reproductive Biology Research Foundation in St. Louis and is now the Masters and Johnson Institute. In 1966 they published their data in *Human Sexual Response*, and in 1970 they published *Human Sexual Inadequacy*.

Once the two started their research, they informed university contacts and professionals that they were in search of volunteer study subjects. Of the 1,273 volunteers who initially applied, Masters and Johnson selected 694—276 married couples, 106 unmarried women, and 36 unmarried men. Ninety-eight of the single people had been married previously.

The investigators obtained social and sexual histories for all their subjects, gave them information to explain the studies, and introduced them to the laboratory setting. For experiments involving sexual intercourse, married couples were used as subjects; in studies other than intercourse (such as masturbation and controlled vaginal tests with an artificial phallus), unmarried subjects participated.

Through direct observation, filming, and monitoring with instruments, Masters and Johnson recorded a variety of changes in the physiology of the body in general and in the genitals and reproductive organs in particular. Most of their findings related to physiological responses to sexual arousal that had never before been measured or documented. Their major finding, generally accepted as true since the results were published, was the existence of a cycle of physiological events in response to sexual stimulation. The whole cycle, known as the *human sexual response*, occurs in

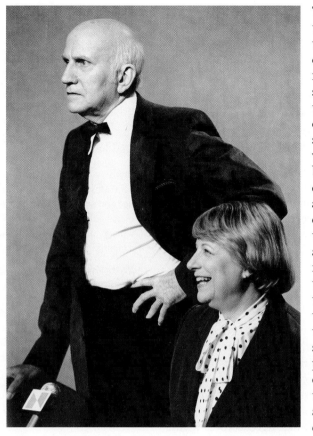

William Masters and Virginia Johnson were the first sexuality researchers to observe people's sexual behaviors in a laboratory setting. Among their many contributions to sexuality research is the human sexual response cycle.

This study of sexual dysfunction put the relationship of the physiology and the psychology of sexual response in sharper focus. Causes of sexual dysfunction, the relationship of the partners who experienced dysfunction, and sexual interaction in general were the concerns of this book. Masters and Johnson defined *sexual dysfunction* as an inability to respond emotionally and physically to sexual arousal. They were able to give a range of dysfunctions, defining six basic types—three for women and three for men. The dysfunctions were also defined in terms of the phases of the sexual response cycle. The physiological, psychological, and emotional (or situational) causes were suggested and defined, with treatment developed to deal with the causes and symptoms presented. Their research has provided a great deal of knowledge of physiological changes that occur in the

both sexes in four phases, always in order: excitement, plateau, orgasm, and resolution. This research showed that males and females have many similar responses, as well as responses specific to the physiology of each sex. The research of Masters and Johnson now serves as the basis for modern therapy, education, and counseling; cross-disciplinary research; and general information about sexual functioning.

As well developed as it is, Masters and Johnson's research is not without criticism. Some professionals believe that their model of human sexual response ignores psychological and cognitive aspects of arousal. One can only speculate because Masters and Johnson are no longer here to defend themselves. However, it could also be argued that their original model was intended to only demonstrate what happens biologically and that other factors could be considered later. We will never know for sure, but you should realize that criticisms of their work do exist. It is interesting, however, that their second study was expanded to consider a broader range of factors related to human sexual response.

The second major Masters and Johnson study, *Human Sexual Inadequacy,* was published in 1970.

body during sexual activities.

In 1979 Masters and Johnson published *Homosexuality in Perspective.* This study of the sexual response of homosexuals added much information to the human sexuality literature. The data were gathered by studying the sexual response cycles of 38 lesbian couples and 42 male homosexual couples between 1957 and 1970. The researchers reported that there was little difference between homosexuals and heterosexuals in sexual functioning and response to sexual stimulation. However, homosexuals appeared to communicate with partners more effectively during sexual activity than did heterosexuals. The broadest conclusion reported in this publication was that homosexuality is not a disease and that homosexuals, like heterosexuals, are individuals who have sexual concerns.

Masters and Johnson and You The work of Masters and Johnson affects your sexual life in many ways. Both you and your partner can now better understand your bodies' responses to sexual stimulation. Knowing that you proceed through several identifiable phases during your sexual response cycle will make you and/

Myth vs Fact

Myth: Most women prefer a sexual partner who has a large penis.
Fact: Surveys indicate this is not true. Plus, we know that a female's vagina can adjust to different size penises and that there is far less difference in the sizes of erect penises than of soft penises.

Myth: Sexual activity usually ends soon after age 60.
Fact: Most people older than 60 years in relatively good health continue to participate in many forms of sexual activity.

Myth: Masturbation is physically harmful.
Fact: Masturbation does not harm the body in any way.

Myth: Anal intercourse between uninfected people can transmit human immunodeficiency virus (HIV).
Fact: If there is no infection, there will be no HIV transmission. To contract acquired immunodeficiency syndrome (AIDS), a person must first be infected with HIV.

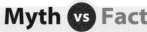

Myth vs Fact

Myth: Most husbands have extramarital affairs.
Fact: The rates may vary in different studies, but the National Health and Social Life Survey reported that 25% of men and 15% of women had extramarital affairs.

Myth: Few women masturbate.
Fact: Most men and women, married and unmarried, occasionally masturbate. About 50% to 68% of females masturbate at least once a month.

Myth: Most normal women have orgasms from penile thrusting alone.
Fact: Different women prefer different kinds of stimulation. Many do not reach orgasm from penile thrusting alone.

Myth: A man cannot have an orgasm without an erection.
Fact: He can have an orgasm even if he does not have an erection.

Myth: Erectile dysfunction (sometimes referred to as "impotence" by the layperson) usually cannot be treated successfully.
Fact: With counseling, medical treatments, surgical treatments, and better sexual knowledge alone or in combination, most instances of erectile dysfunction can be treated.

June Reinisch and Ruth Beasley found these nine myths to be commonly believed. More information about these myths can be found in later chapters in this book and in their book The Kinsey Institute New Report on Sex (1991). New York: St. Martin's.

or any sexual partner more willing to proceed at a sexual pace in synchrony with your physiology. The results will be greater sexual satisfaction and less sexual dysfunction. Because of the work of Masters and Johnson and that of others motivated by Masters and Johnson's studies, a person experiencing problems with sexual functioning has access to a whole warehouse of effective sexual therapy modalities. As with the work of Kinsey, the studies of Masters and Johnson not only broke ground for sexual research as a profession, but also produced some very useful information for the general public.

The National Health and Social Life Survey

A University of Chicago research team conducted the first comprehensive survey of adult sexual behavior since Kinsey's research (Laumann et al., 1994). The National Health and Social Life Survey (NHSLS) was designed to assess the incidence and prevalence of a broad range of sexual practices and attitudes within the U.S. population.

When the AIDS epidemic began in the 1980s, experts were not well informed about contemporary sexual practices. Believing that such data might help prevent the spread of HIV, in 1987 an agency within the U.S. Department of Health and Human Services asked for proposals to study adult sexual attitudes and practices. The research team from the University of Chicago was awarded a grant in 1988 to support a survey of 20,000 people.

As mentioned earlier, after 2 years of planning, federal funds for the project were withdrawn. In 1991, because conservative members of Congress were offended by the idea of using government funds for research on sexual behavior, legislation was passed to eliminate federal funding for such studies.

The research team then obtained funding from several private foundations. They were able to proceed, but with a much smaller sample. After sampling techniques were used to select a representative sample of 4,369 18- to 59-year-old Americans, 79% of the sample agreed to participate. This gave them a sample size of 3,432.

Although they did have a high participation rate, they had been forced to limit their sample size. This resulted in a population that was representative of white Americans, black Americans, and Hispanic Americans; however, there were too few representatives of other groups to provide useful information about them.

The research team trained 220 professional interviewers, and all 3,432 subjects were interviewed face-to-face. The interviewers made sure the respondents understood all questions. The questionnaire also had internal checks to measure consistency of answers and to validate the responses.

Here are a few examples of their findings: (1) Of married persons, 93.7% had had only one sexual partner in the last year as compared with 38% of those never married and not cohabitating; (2) married people were much more likely than singles to report being extremely or very happy; (3) 9.1% of men and 4.3% of women reported engaging in any same-sex activity since puberty (for nearly half of these men the behavior occurred only before the age

Gender DIMENSIONS

Differences in Research Results

When reviewing research results, researchers have historically commonly found relatively large differences between genders in the amount of heterosexual sexual behavior. Even when comparing the amounts for males and females of the same age, it is common to see much higher rates for males than females. The reasons for this are not known, but this situation makes for interesting discussion because one must wonder who the males are having heterosexual behavior with if the numbers are much smaller for females.

Gender differences also often exist when it comes to reasons for first sexual intercourse (Laumann et al., 1994). For example, among those females who wanted their first vaginal intercourse to happen when it did, just over half the males were motivated by a curiosity about sexual behavior, but a little less than one-quarter of the females were. However, about one-quarter of the males had intercourse because of affection for their partner, whereas 47.5% of the females did it for this reason. Only about 3% of the females said that physical pleasure was their main reason, compared to about four times as many men (12%) who said this.

However, Alexander and Fisher (2003) reported on the differences in self-reported sexual behaviors between males and females. They pointed out that at least some of these differences may be because women don't always answer such surveys honestly, but give answers that they believe are expected of them. Women's sensitivity to social expectations for their sexual behavior might cause them to be less than honest when asked about their sexual behavior. It might also be that men claim more sexual behavior than they actually had because they feel that is expected of them. In their study, men and women were asked about their sexual behavior when they believed they were connected to a lie detector machine. Although there were still some gender differences, women's answers were much closer to men's under these circumstances.

Watch for these kinds of comparisons as you consider research on sexual behavior and think about reasons why gender differences might exist.

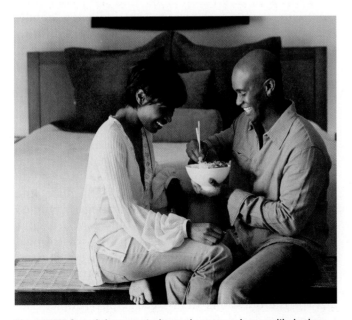

The NHSLS found that married people are much more likely than singles to report being very happy.

of 18 years). About 1.4% of the women and 2.8% of the men reported a homosexual identity.

Popular Literature

Shere Hite: Women's Sexuality, Men's Sexuality, and Women and Love

Between 1972 and 1976, when her findings were published in *The Hite Report*, Shere Hite mailed more than 100,000 60-item essay-type questionnaires to such women's groups as the National Organization for Women, university women's organizations, and women's newsletters. She also placed notices in *The Village Voice, Mademoiselle, Brides, Ms.,* and *Oui* magazines asking women to send for questionnaires. Hite received completed questionnaires from 3,109 women, who expressed their personal feelings about masturbation, orgasm, intercourse, clitoral stimulation, lesbianism, sexual slavery (satisfying males' needs during sexual activity and ignoring their own needs), and the sexual revolution. Many women reported

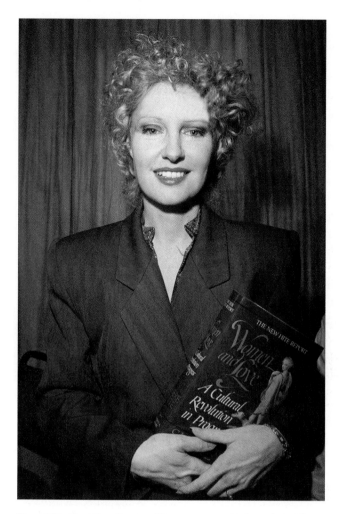

Shere Hite completed several important research projects about sexual behavior.

that they experienced orgasm more frequently from clitoral stimulation than from coitus and that they achieved deep orgasm from masturbation. Furthermore, they described a history of orgasm in general. Of the sample, 8% preferred sexual activity with other women, 53% said that they preferred sexual activity with themselves, and 17% preferred no sexual activity at all. Although the question was not directly asked, many women offered the information that they were curious about and might be interested in a sexual encounter with another woman. The majority of older women said that sexual pleasure increased with age, but many respondents older than 45 years reported difficulty in finding new sexual partners.

The findings published in *The Hite Report* were of great interest, for despite the fact that only a relatively small portion of the total female population was reached, no study had previously afforded such large numbers of women the opportunity to express their preferences and desires in matters of sexuality. However, remember that Hite recruited her subjects by inserting a notice in magazines such as

Oui, The Village Voice, Ms., and *Mademoiselle.* Rather than being representative of all women, this small, select group of women is considered to be what is called a biased sample. Hite did not statistically analyze her data; rather, she used what are described as anecdotal reports—essays written by individuals describing their sexual activities and the feelings they experienced.

In 1981 Hite published *The Hite Report on Male Sexuality* using the same anecdotal analysis, this time presenting the views of 7,200 men. Men preferred intercourse to masturbation or oral–genital sexual activity. They were generally unaware that women could achieve orgasm by means other than intercourse. They expressed ignorance of when a female orgasm occurs and expressed anxious feelings about not knowing. Some of the males expressed anger over always being the initiators of sexual activity yet volunteered that sexually aggressive women were difficult for them to deal with. Many men stated that they grew up not being allowed to express themselves emotionally, for the culture demanded that men be strong and showing emotion was not defined as indicating strength. Again, because the Hite study of males was anecdotal, it is not considered to be of statistical note.

In 1987 Hite published *Women and Love: A Cultural Revolution in Progress.* After spending 7 years analyzing surveys from 4,500 women, she concluded that women are fed up with men. Despite women's liberation and the sexual revolution, Hite reported that women remain oppressed, and even abused, by men. Four of five women in her study said they still had to fight for their rights within relationships, 87% said that men became more emotionally dependent than women, 92% complained that men communicate with women in language that indicates "condescending, judgmental attitudes," 95% reported forms of "emotional and psychological harassment," 79% said they seriously question whether they should put so much energy into love relationships, 98% wished for more verbal closeness with male partners, 70% of the women married 5 years or more said they had extramarital affairs more often for emotional closeness than for sexual activity, and 87% of the married women said they have their deepest emotional relationship with a woman friend.

Many respectable researchers, both male and female, questioned Hite's findings. Criticisms pointed to a highly self-selected sample—only a 4.5% return from more than 100,000 questionnaires distributed to a variety of women's groups in 43 states—and a likely disproportion of unhappy people, because unhappy people were probably more willing to answer the questions than were happy people. Hite indicated a desire for men to see what women feel works in relationships, but others feared that Hite's

Remember that the main purpose of sexual themes in newspapers, in magazines, and on radio and TV may be to sell newspapers and magazines and raise ratings of the programs. Also, there is a motivation to entertain people. It may be possible to get some sound information about sexuality through these sources; however, caution is needed if you are going to be a wise consumer. It is probably healthy to be skeptical until you have a chance to verify the information in accepted professional journals.

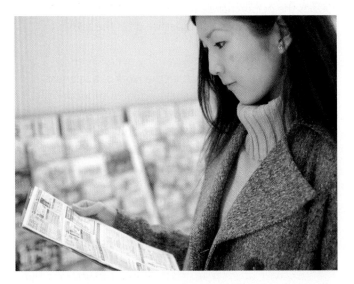

Readers must carefully evaluate information about human sexuality found in popular literature.

book encouraged women to take the easy way out and blame everything on men.

Lorna Sarrel and Philip Sarrel: The Redbook Report on Sexual Relationships

In 1980 *Redbook* magazine published a sexuality questionnaire to which approximately 20,000 women and 6,000 men responded. The questionnaire was primarily concerned with the quality of relationships and the interpersonal communication of couples. More than half of the men (60%) and less than half of the women said that sharing feelings was very important to their relationships. Seventy-five percent of those who answered the questionnaire rated their current sexual relationships as being good or excellent. Fifteen percent reported sexual dysfunction, and these people said that they spoke very little about sexuality with their partner. Of particular interest is the fact that 40% of men and women who were parents said that lack of privacy interfered in some way with their enjoyment of sexual activity. Many individuals accepted sexual activity to satisfy a partner even if they did not want to make love at the time, and half of those who did said they "end up enjoying it."

This study is not indicative of sexual relationships of the population in general, because the readership of *Redbook* in 1980 tended to be youthful, married, better educated, and financially more secure than the general population. However, these people do represent a very large group of our population and they certainly do show an interest in sexual matters, are comfortable with the subject, and possess a willingness to discuss sexuality and interpersonal relationships. It is fair to believe that they did represent many couples in the society (Sarrel & Sarrel, 1980).

June Reinisch and Ruth Beasley: The Kinsey Institute New Report on Sex

The inclusion of a 1991 book within our popular literature section may be debatable, but it is indeed written for the general public. In fact, one of its authors said, "It's a great book to have in the bathroom, when you have time to read bits and pieces. It is designed to be a 'friendly encyclopedia,' telling readers in question-and-answer format almost everything they wanted to know about sexuality" (Dolan, 1990).

Research from the Kinsey Institute and the results of a Roper poll of 2,000 adults show that knowledge about sexuality is still at a very low level. For example, half of the adults tested did not know that a lubricant such as Vaseline or baby oil can cause microscopic holes in a condom or a diaphragm in as little as 60 seconds. This lack of understanding hardly contributes to safer sex practices.

Of women aged 30 to 44 years, only 55% received a passing grade on the test, and 52% of men in the same age group did. Men answered correctly more often on matters of sexual practices, and women knew more about their own sexual health. People living in the Midwest had the highest scores, and those in the South and the Northeast had the lowest.

Seventeen Magazine and The Kaiser Family Foundation: SexSmarts Survey on Teen Sexual Behavior

The latest in a series of surveys of teens aged 15–17 years found that only 1 in 10 teens who have had

Communication
DIMENSIONS

Talking About Sexuality Research Results

It is not easy to analyze findings of sexual research, and it is common to hear others talking about some "new findings" they just heard about. What if someone tells you about some sexual "research" and some interesting findings? What can you suggest to help the person (and you) analyze whether the research seems sound? Here are some possibilities for questions and conversational points.

- Was the scientific method used? This method does not rely just on testimonials or someone's opinion. It requires proper sampling techniques, accurate measurement and observation, and appropriate statistical analysis of the findings to reach valid conclusions.
- Is the study replicable? One study, taken alone, seldom proves anything. To be valid, one researcher's findings must be repeatable by others.
- Have the research findings been properly used? For example, conclusions based on data from one population may not apply to another population, and the

results from animal studies cannot be applied with certainty to humans.
- Were the proper statistics used and were they used correctly? Many people tend to accept statistical data without question, although statistical errors do occur.
- What is the competency of the author or researcher? Does the person have a record of excellent previous research? What kinds of expertise does the author or researcher have?
- Has the research been reviewed by peers? Peer review is the process in which the work of a scientist is reviewed by others who have equal or superior knowledge. It may be done while the study is being developed or afterward, as when results of the study are being considered for publication in a scientific journal.

Even these questions will not guarantee appropriate judgments about the accuracy of sexual research, but it can be very helpful to see whether there are good answers to them. They may also inspire some very interesting conversation.

sexual intercourse discussed his or her sexual plans with parents ahead of time, and more than a third did not tell their parents about their sexual history at all. Forty-eight percent of all survey respondents and 56% of sexually active respondents never talked with a parent about "how to know when you are ready to have sex." Eighty percent of respondents said teens do not discuss sexual issues with their parents because they worry that their parents will disapprove or will assume that they are already participating in sexual behavior if they discuss the subject with them (Kaiser Family Foundation and *Seventeen* magazine release latest SexSmarts Survey on teen sexual behavior, 2002).

Eighty-four percent of all respondents said they had never talked with a healthcare provider about how to know when one is prepared for sexual behavior. More than two-thirds had not discussed contraception, HIV and AIDS, condoms, or STIs with a health care provider. Nearly two-thirds had spoken with a sexual partner about "what they are comfortable doing sexually." Fifty-eight percent had never discussed STIs with a partner, 56% had never discussed HIV and AIDS with a partner, and 53% of all respondents and 28% of sexually active teens had never discussed contraception with a partner. Most cited lack of knowledge about sexual issues, fear

of what a partner might think, and embarrassment as reasons they do not discuss sexual issues with partners.

NBC News and People Magazine: National Survey of Young Teens Sexual Attitudes and Behavior

NBC News and *People Magazine* had the Princeton Survey Research Associates International conduct a survey of 1,000 young teenagers (ages 13–16) and their parents. The results were reported in 2004 and updated in 2005 (Nearly 3 in 10 young teens sexually active, 2005). Teens were asked about their sexual health, behavior, and attitudes, and parents were asked for their views on the sexual lives of today's teens.

The survey showed that parents and teens have somewhat different opinions on the pressure teens face and their attitudes. For example, 85% of parents strongly or somewhat agreed that "there is a lot of pressure on teenagers to have sex by a certain age," compared with 66% of the teens. Forty-seven percent of parents strongly or somewhat agreed with the statement, "for teens oral sex is not as big a deal as sexual intercourse," compared with 75% of teens.

The survey confirmed that teens engage in a wide range of sexual behavior, from kissing to sexual

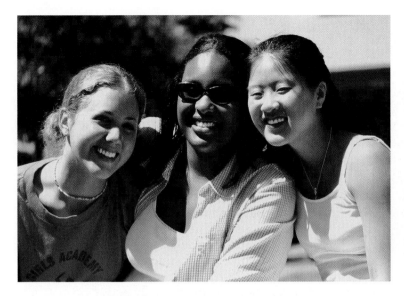

By the time they finish high school, the percentage of females who have had sexual intercourse is about 62%, with about 38% who have not.

intercourse. For example, 58% of all teens (ages 13–16) reported having "kissed someone romantically," 27% reported having "been with someone in an intimate or romantic way," 21% reported having "touched someone's genitals or private parts," 13% reported having engaged in sexual intercourse, and 12% reported having engaged in oral sex. Among the 12% of all teens who reported having had oral sex, 1% first had oral sex at age 11, 8% at age 12, 19% at age 13, 22% at age 14, 29% at age 15, and 16% at age 16.

As might be expected, older teens (ages 15–16) reported higher rates of sexual behavior. Seventy-two percent had "kissed someone romantically," 41% had "been with someone in an intimate or romantic way," 37% had "touched someone's genitals or private parts," 21% had engaged in sexual intercourse, and 19% had engaged in oral sex.

Parents seemed to underestimate whether their teens had engaged in sexual behavior. When asked about their own child, 83% believed he or she had not engaged in sexual activity beyond kissing.

According to the study, many teens were not protecting themselves from pregnancy or STIs. Thirty percent who had oral sex reported "always" using "protection such as a condom" during oral sex, 14% reported using protection "most of the time," 13% "some of the time," and 42% reported "never" using protection during oral sex.

Thirty-six percent of teens who had sexual intercourse used birth control every time, 6% used it "almost every time," 8% used it "most of the time," 7% used it "only sometimes," 1% "hardly ever," and 40% never used birth control.

The survey showed that many factors, from parent's reactions to curiosity to sexual desire,

play a role in teens' decisions about sexual behavior. Eighty-two percent of teens who had engaged in sexual intercourse cited having met the right person as a major or minor reason for their decision, 71% cited curiosity, 68% cited sexual desire, 56% cited a hope that it would make their relationship even closer, 34% cited pressure from their partner, and 18% cited a desire "to be more popular and accepted" as a major or minor reason for their decision.

For those who had never engaged in sexual intercourse, 89% cited feeling they were too young as a major or minor reason for their decision, 88% cited "a conscious decision to wait," 86% cited worries about STIs, 85% cited worries about pregnancy, 84% cited worries about what their parents would think, 75% cited not having met the right person yet, 63% cited religious or moral beliefs, 54% cited worries about what their friends would think, and 49% cited not having had the opportunity as a major or minor reason for their decision.

Among those who had engaged in oral sex, 76% cited "the other person wanted to" as a major or minor reason for their decision, 71% cited having met the right person, 69% cited the belief that "you are still a virgin if you have oral sex," 68% cited not having to worry about pregnancy, 64% cited curiosity, 40% cited wanting to avoid sexual intercourse, 35% cited the belief you can't get STIs from oral sex, 24% cited wanting to avoid being touched or undress, and 21% cited "wanting to be more popular and accepted" as a major or minor reason for their decision.

■ Examples of Research in the 21st Century

It is almost impossible to count the many research studies related to human sexuality done in recent years. And until these studies stand the test of time, it is difficult to tell which, if any, might become classics. The following is a chronological summary of selected, more recent, research studies.

Studies on Premarital Sexual Attitudes and Behavior
Dailard (2001) reported on the findings of the National Longitudinal Study of Adolescent Health (more commonly called the "Add Health Survey"). She indicated that teens' reports of ever having had sexual intercourse increase dramatically with grade level, from 16% among 7th and 8th graders to 60% among 11th graders. Teenagers who are African

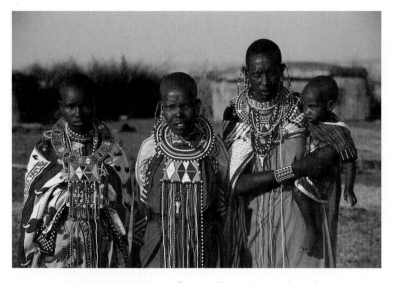

Sexual standards are influenced by culture and gender.

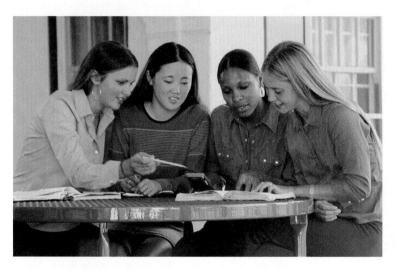

Rates of sexual activity vary with differences in ethnicity.

American or in low-income or single-parent families are more likely to have had sexual intercourse than their peers. In addition, the Add Health Survey strongly indicates that whether a teenager has ever had sexual intercourse is largely explained by that individual's own sexual history and his or her perceptions about the costs and benefits of having sexual intercourse. In sharp contrast, the data indicate that other major risk behaviors—such as cigarette smoking, drug and alcohol use, weapons-related violence, and suicidal thoughts and attempts—are shaped more by factors such as problems with school or work or the number of friends who regularly smoke or drink.

Dennison and Russell (2005) pointed out that more than 1,000 published reports employed data from the Add Health Study. Findings from these reports indicate that adolescents at the upper and lower ends of the intelligence distribution were less likely to have engaged in intercourse, religiosity reduced the risk of coital debut in both males and females, youth from intact families were less likely to have engaged in intercourse, greater parental involvement was related to a lower likelihood of sex initiation, and most teens had their first sexual experience within the context of a romantic relationship. The average waiting time before engaging in sexual intercourse within these romantic relationships was 5 months. In addition, students who felt connected at school reported later ages at sexual initiation, girls participating in sports tended to delay sexual activity, and students who took abstinence pledges were less likely than nonpledgers to practice safe sex once they became sexually active.

In 2002 the Kaiser Family Foundation reported the results of a national survey of 1,200 adolescents and young adults 13–24 years old (Substance use and risky sexual behavior, 2002). It concluded that for many teens and young adults, alcohol use and drug use are closely linked to sexual decision making and risk taking. Nearly 90% said their peers used alcohol or drugs before having sexual intercourse at least some of the time, and many young people reported that condoms are often not used when people are drinking or using drugs. More than a third of sexually active young people reported that alcohol or drugs had influenced their decisions about sex. Almost as many had "done more" sexually than they had planned while under their influence. As a result, they reported they worried about STIs and pregnancy.

It is interesting that most sexually active teenagers had sexual intercourse for the first time in their parents' homes, late at night (Most sexually active teens first had sex at home, 2002). On the basis of a national survey that had tracked 8,000 children aged 12–16 years since 1997, the study found that 56% of those who had been sexually active said they first had sexual intercourse at their family's home or at the family home of a partner, 12% said at a friend's house, 4% said in a vehicle, 3% said at an outdoor location, 3% said at a hotel or motel, and 10% said at another location. In addition, 42% said they first had sexual intercourse between 10 P.M. and 7 A.M. and 28% said between 6 P.M. and 10 P.M. Only 15% of respondents said they had intercourse for the first time between 3 P.M. and 6 P.M. This study dispels the myth that teens most often have sexual intercourse after school, when parents are at work.

? Did You Know . . .

Many studies of sexual behavior have examined only whether a person reports ever having had sexual intercourse. When investigating the safety of sexual behavior, it is also helpful to know how often people have participated in sexual intercourse in a recent time, with whom, and which types of sexual practices have been used. For example, we know that teenagers and nonwhite women are at greater risk of contracting HIV than are older women, but teenagers are less consistently sexually active than are older women (Klitsch, 1990). Similarly, nonwhite women are statistically more likely to contract sexually transmitted infections than white women; however, they are less consistently sexually active than white women. Again, researchers need to consider the type of behavior or practice, not just the amount, to determine the degree to which safe sexual behavior is practiced.

TABLE 2.1 Youth Risk Behavior Surveillance (YRBS) Results, 2004 and 2010

Sexual Behavior	2004	2010
Percent of high school students (grades 9–12) who had sexual intercourse	47%	46%
Percent of sexually active students who used a condom at last sexual intercourse	63%	61%
Incidence of intercourse for African American males	74%	72%
Incidence of intercourse for Hispanic males	57%	53%
Incidence of intercourse for white males	41%	40%
Incidence of intercourse for African American females	61%	54%
Incidence of intercourse for Hispanic females	46%	45%
Incidence of intercourse for white females	42%	45%
Incidence of intercourse for 9th grade students	33%	34%
Incidence of intercourse for 10th grade students	44%	41%
Incidence of intercourse for 11th grade students	53%	53%
Incidence of intercourse for 12th grade students	62%	62%
Had first intercourse before age 13 years	7%	6%
Had sexual intercourse during their lifetime with four or more partners	14%	14%

Sources: Data from Grunbaum, J., Kann, L., Kinchen, S., Ross, J., Hawkins, J., Lowry, R., Harris, W. A., McManus, T., Chyen, D., & Collins, J. Youth risk behavior surveillance—United States, 2003. In: *Surveillance Summaries, Morbidity and Mortality Weekly Report, 53, no. SS-2* (2004), 1–20; Eaton, D. K., Kann, L., Kinchen, S., Shanklin, S. Ross, J., Hawkins, J., Harris, W. A., Lowry, R., McManus, T., Chyen, D., Lim, C., Whittle, L., Brener, N. D., & Wechsler, H. Youth risk behavior surveillance—United States, 2009. In: *Surveillance Summaries, Morbidity and Mortality Weekly Report, 59, no. SS-5* (2010), 1–143.

Changes in sexual risk behavior among U.S. high school students (grades 9–12) over a 10-year period were reported in 2002 (Trends in sexual risk behaviors among high school students, 2002). The percentage who reported ever having had sexual intercourse decreased by 16%. In 1991, 56% had participated, but in 2001 only 46% had done so. Also, the overall proportion who had had four or more partners dropped by 24%—from 19% in 1991 to 14% in 2001.

The overall prevalence of "current sexual activity"—defined as having intercourse at any point during the 3 months preceding the survey—did not change between 1991 and 2001. It was reported by about one-third of the respondents. Condom use rose between 1991 and 1999 but had "leveled off" since then. In 2001 about 58% of sexually active teens used condoms, compared to about 46% in 1991. The percentage of sexually active students who had used drugs or alcohol before their most recent intercourse increased 18% between 1991 and 2002.

For a number of years the U.S. Centers for Disease Control has periodically conducted a Youth Risk Behavior Surveillance (YRBS). A portion of the questions within the survey of health behaviors of students in grades 9–12 relate to sexual behavior. Some of the YRBS results reported in 2004 and 2010 are shown in Table 2.1.

In 2005 Halpern-Felsher et al. reported that ethnically diverse 9th-grade adolescents evaluated oral sexual activity as significantly less risky than vaginal intercourse on health, social, and emotional consequences. They also believed that oral activity is more acceptable than vaginal intercourse for adolescents their own age in both dating and nondating situations, oral sexual activity is less of a threat to their values and beliefs, and more of their peers will have oral sexual activity than vaginal intercourse in the near future. More study participants reported having had oral sexual activity (20%) than vaginal intercourse (14%), and more intended to have oral sexual activity in the next 6 months (32%) than vaginal intercourse (26%).

In 2005, South et al. studied the effect of residential mobility on the timing of first premarital sexual intercourse. They found that adolescents who had recently moved were about one-third more likely than nonmobile adolescents to experience first premarital intercourse. They further found that much of the difference between adolescents who moved and those who didn't in the onset of sexual activity was attributable to the greater propensity for delinquency and weaker academic performance among members of movers' school-based friendship networks.

In 2008, Lescano et al. studied factors associated with anal intercourse among adolescents and young adults. Recent heterosexual anal intercourse was reported by 16% of the 1,348 respondents. Females who engaged in anal intercourse were more likely to be living with a sexual partner, to have had two or more partners, and to have experienced coerced intercourse. For males, only a sexual orientation other than heterosexual was a significant predictor of engaging in heterosexual anal intercourse.

In 2011, Lehmiller et al. reported on gender differences in approaching friends with benefits (FWB) relationships. They defined FWB relationships as consisting of friends who are sexually, but not romantically, involved. They engage in sexual activity on occasion, but otherwise have a basic friendship. Their results indicated many similarities in terms of how males and females approached FWB relationships, but several important differences emerged. Sexual activity was a more common motivation for men to begin such relationships, whereas emotional connection was a more common motivation for women. Also, men were more likely to hope that the relationship stayed the same over time, whereas women expressed more desire for it to change into either a full-fledged romance or a basic friendship. Both men and women were more committed to the friendship than to the sexual aspect of the relationship. The researchers felt their findings were largely consistent with the notion that traditional gender role expectations and the sexual double standard may influence how men and women approach FWB relationships.

Studies on Ethnic Differences in Sexual Attitudes and Behavior

Only relatively recently have researchers looked at the influence of ethnic differences in sexual attitudes and behavior. Examples of such studies are given in the following discussion.

Ford and coworkers (2001) reported that the sexual partners of white and black adolescents are likely to be similar to them. In contrast, the sexual partners of Latino adolescents and of adolescents of "other" race or ethnicity are more likely to be of a different racial or ethnic group. As adolescents get older, their partners become more heterogeneous.

Cavanagh (2004) studied the sexual debut of girls in early adolescence. She found that among white girls, those who matured early were more likely to have sexual intercourse in early adolescence, and this was partially due to the friendship groups of which they were a part. Early puberty seemed to draw white girls into larger friendship groups characterized by riskier behavior and lower academic achievement. Hispanic girls were similar to white girls in key ways, but different in others. For them, as for whites, both early puberty and friendship group characteristics were closely related to sexual debut, but unlike whites, friendship group characteristics did not mediate the association between early pubertal timing and sexual debut. Early pubertal timing mattered for Hispanics in other ways not captured in the model used in the study. There was also another factor uniquely characterizing Hispanics—the presence of older boys. Interestingly, among African American girls, there were no meaningful associations among early pubertal timing, the friendship group, and sexual debut.

Other studies have shown a variety of ethnic differences related to sexuality. For example, Connell et al. (2004) found that African American groups are more aware of STIs and HIV than either white or Hispanic groups. However, African Americans tend to have a higher percentage of people testing positive for HIV/AIDS (Johnson & Jackson, 2004). The prevalence rate of HIV has been found to be 16% for African Americans, 7% for Hispanics, and 3% for whites (Harawa et al., 2004). Also, Hispanic youth seem to be at a greater risk for experiencing early intercourse than white youth (Adam et al., 2005).

Regarding birth control, use of injectable contraceptives is high among African American women, but not as high among Asian Indian or white women (Burgard, 2004). Knowledge disparities can also be seen when comparing ethnic groups. For example, 41% of Hispanic women and 75% of African American women have heard of emergency contraception as compared to 99% of white women (Chuang & Freund, 2005).

Studies on the Use of Contraception

Ford and colleagues (2001) reported that the less similar adolescents and their sexual partners are to one another—whether because of a difference in age, grade, or school—the less likely they are to use condoms and other contraceptive methods. The likelihood of having sexual relations with adolescents with different characteristics increases as adolescents get older.

Oncalem and King (2001) reported that many college students either have tried to talk their sexual partners out of using a condom or have had a partner try to dissuade them from condom use. Nearly 14% of women and nearly 17% of men who had engaged in sexual intercourse admitted to having actively tried to dissuade a partner from the couple's using condoms. Thirty percent of men and 41% of women said that a sexual partner had tried to dissuade them. The most frequent reasons cited were (1) that sexual intercourse feels better without a condom, (2) that the woman will not get pregnant, and (3) that the person will not get a sexually transmitted infection.

While it may seem obvious, Bruckner et al. (2004) reported that the factor most strongly associated with the risk of pregnancy among young women is contraceptive use, with nonusers being significantly more likely than inconsistent and consistent users to become pregnant. However, these researchers also indicated that adolescents who become pregnant do not sufficiently appreciate the negative consequences, and that prevention programs should target participants' attitudes toward pregnancy. If more positive attitudes toward contraception can be developed, this will help shape effective contraceptive use.

While there are many reasons for close involvement between parents and adolescents, Frisco (2005) pointed out an interesting relationship to contraceptive use. Her research showed that parental involvement in education shapes teenagers' attitudes about school and work by encouraging achievement and by providing a home environment that values education. Such parental involvement also increases the odds that young women will use contraception, especially increasing the likelihood of using specific reliable birth control methods.

Manlove et al. (2008) examined a sample of sexually experienced 15- to 19-year-old males to identify factors associated with condom use. They found that Hispanic males and those who did not receive formal sexuality education had lower odds of condom use and/or consistency. African American males and those with more positive attitudes about condoms had greater odds of both using condoms and using them

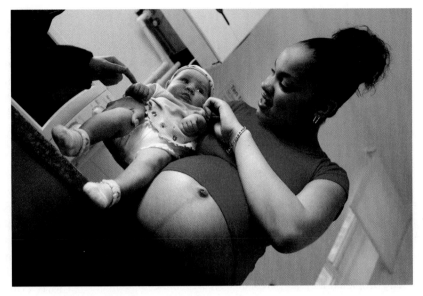

Adolescents give many reasons why they did not use contraception.

consistently. Males who were older at most recent sexual intercourse, who had an older sexual partner or a casual sexual partner, who were in longer relationships, or who engaged in more frequent sexual intercourse had reduced odds of contraceptive use.

In 2010, the Guttmacher Institute (Facts on contraceptive use in the United States, 2010) reported that of the 43 million fertile, sexually active women who do not want to become pregnant, 89% use a method of contraception. Sixty-three percent of reproductive-age women who practice contraception use nonpermanent methods, including hormonal methods (such as the pill, patch, implant, injectable, and vaginal ring), the IUD, and condoms. The remaining women rely on female or male sterilization. For women younger than age 30, the most common method is the pill. Among women aged 30 and older, more rely on sterilization. Overall, pills are used by 28% of users, tubal sterilization by 27%, male condoms by 16%, a vasectomy by 10%, an IUD by 6%, withdrawal by 5%, an injectable by 3%, a vaginal ring by 2%, an implant by 1%, and periodic abstinence (calendar method) by a little less than 1%.

Related to control of births, in 2011 it was reported (Facts on induced abortion in the United States, 2011) that the overall U.S. abortion rate declined after 1981. The abortion rate among U.S. women of childbearing age declined from about 29.3 per 1,000 women in 1981 to about 19 in 2011. Sixty-one percent of abortions are obtained by women who have one or more children; 18% are obtained by teenagers. Women in their twenties account for more than half of all abortions, and women who have never married and are not cohabiting account for 45% of all abortions.

Among the 34.2% of currently sexually active high school students (grades 9–12) in the United

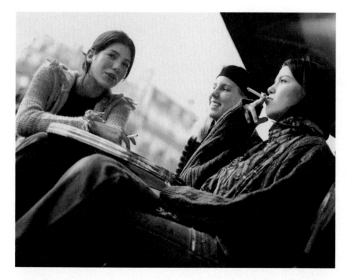

Young people say they get a lot of their sexual information from their peers.

States, 61% reported that either they or their partner used a condom during the last sexual intercourse, 20% used birth control pills, 3% used Depo-Provera, 23% used either birth control pills or Depo-Provera, and 9% used both a condom and birth control pills or Depo-Provera (Eaton et al., 2010).

Other Representative Studies

The Guttmacher Institute (Facts on American teens' sexual and reproductive health, 2011) reported that each year almost 750,000 U.S. women ages 15–19 become pregnant. Two-thirds of all teen pregnancies are among 18- and 19-year-olds. The peak rate of teen pregnancies was 117 per 1,000 women ages 15–19, which occurred in 1990. Since then, there has been a steady decline to about 70 per 1,000. However, the U.S. teen pregnancy rate continues to be one of the highest in the developed world—more than twice as high as rates in Canada (28 per 1,000) or Sweden (31 per 1,000). About 59% of U.S. teen pregnancies end in birth, 27% in abortion, and 14% in miscarriage.

In 2011, Pazol et al. reported that approximately 410,000 teens ages 15–19 gave birth in 2009. The national teen birth rate was 39.1 per 1,000 females, a 37% decrease since 1991, and the lowest rate ever recorded. State-specific teen birth rates varied from 16.4 to 64.2 births per 1,000 females and were highest among southern states. Birth rates for black and Hispanic teens were 59.0 and 70.1 births per 1,000 females, respectively, compared with 25.6 for white teens.

In 2011, Torian et al. reported that sharp increases were reported from 1981 to 1995 in the number of new AIDS cases and deaths in the United States, reaching highs of over 75,400 in 1992 and 50,600 in 1995, respectively. However, with the introduction of highly active antiretroviral therapy, AIDS diagnoses and deaths declined substantially from 1995 to 1998 and remained stable from 1998 to 2008, at an average of just over 38,200 AIDS diagnoses and 17,400 deaths per year, respectively. Despite the decline in AIDS cases and deaths, at the end of 2008 an estimated 1,178,350 persons were living with HIV, including 236,000 (20.1%) whose infection was undiagnosed. Most (75%) persons living with HIV were male, and 65.7% of the males were men who have sexual activity with men. HIV prevalence rates for blacks or African Americans (1,819 per 100,000 population) and Hispanics or Latinos (593) were approximately eight times and two and a half times the rate among whites (238), respectively.

Daniel and Balog (2009) reported that the age of female puberty seems to have decreased in the United States and western countries as child health and nutrition have improved and obesity has become more common. Environmental contaminants, particularly endocrine disruptors, may also play a role in lowering the age of puberty. Puberty at an early age increases the risk of stress, poor school performance, teen pregnancy, eating disorders, substance abuse, and a variety of health issues that may appear later in life, including breast cancer and heart disease. The age of first breast development is dropping faster than that of first menstrual period (menarche). While the age of menarche dropped from a mean of 17.5 years in the middle of the 19th century to 12.5 years by the middle of the 20th century, girls begin menstruating only a few months earlier today than girls 40 years ago.

Biro et al. (2010) indicated that 15% of U.S. girls have breast development, an early sign of puberty, by age 7. Black girls are more likely to have early breast development, with 23% starting by age 7 compared to almost 15% of Hispanic girls. They found that 10% of white girls began developing breasts by age 7, which is twice the rate of a 1997 study.

Examinations of associations between religiosity and sexual behaviors and attitudes have shown interesting results. In 2004 Lefkowitz et al. found relationships between religiosity (group affiliation, attendance at religious services, attitudes, perceptions of negative sanctions, and adherence to sanctions) and sexuality. They reported that religious behavior was the strongest predictor of sexual behavior. In 2005 research by Penhollow et al. indicated that religiosity variables, especially frequency of religious attendance and religious feelings, were significant predictors of sexual behavior.

Interestingly, in 2011 McFarland et al. reported that among older married adults religion is largely unrelated with frequency of sexual behavior and satisfaction, although religious integration in daily life shares a weak, but positive, association with pleasure from sexual activity.

In 2004 Vlassoff et al. assessed the costs and benefits of sexual and reproductive health interventions. Their study showed that poor sexual and reproductive health account for a substantial share of the global burden of disease. Their research indicated that the benefits of sexual and reproductive health interventions are far-reaching. For example, in addition to medical benefits, maternal health care lowers death and disability due to pregnancy-related causes, helps families remain intact, enables higher household savings and investment, and encourages higher productivity. Prevention and treatment for STIs and treatments for medical conditions also help reduce social stigma and help parents remain healthy so they are better able to care for and invest in their children. Contraceptives, together with maternal health services, minimize the adverse health effects of unintended pregnancy and high-risk births, including unsafe abortion, hemorrhage, infection, anemia, low birth weight, and malnutrition. These researchers concluded that sexual and reproductive health interventions are a good investment.

In 2005 Mosher et al. reported data from the National Survey of Family Growth. They indicated that, among adults 25–44 years of age, 97% of men and 98% of women had had vaginal intercourse; 90% of men and 88% of women had had oral sexual activity with an opposite-sex partner; and 40% of men and 35% of women had had anal sexual activity with an opposite-sex partner. About 6.5% of men had had oral or anal sex with another man. Eleven percent of women reported having had a sexual experience of any kind with another female.

Koch (2006) reported on women's bodies being a "puzzle" for college men. She found that college men believed women and their bodies are complex "puzzles" that are difficult to understand. The college men also felt ignorance about women's bodies, particularly their genital/reproductive anatomy and menstruation. Confusion over how to deal with women's body image was another major theme. The men believed that women are too concerned about their body image. Most felt that having better knowledge of women's bodies and the experiences they go through would improve their relationships with women.

As electronic devices have played much larger roles in the lives of college students, some issues related to electronic devices and sexuality have arisen. For example, the National Campaign to Prevent Teen and Unplanned Pregnancy and CosmoGirl.com commissioned a survey of teens and young adults to explore electronic activity (Sex and Tech, 2008). The key findings showed that a significant number of teens have electronically sent, or posted online, nude or semi-nude pictures or videos of themselves. Sexually suggestive messages were even more prevalent than sexually suggestive images. Most respondents knew that it was potentially dangerous to post sexually suggestive content, but did it anyway. Many of the teens and young adults said they were pressured by friends to send or post sexual content. Most said it was a "fun and flirtatious" activity.

The National Survey of Sexual Health and Behavior (NSSHB) (2010) included data from the largest nationally representative study of sexual-health behaviors ever fielded. It included information about sexual experiences and condom-use behaviors of 5,865 adolescents and adults ages 14–94. This survey generated so much information that the initial findings were presented in nine separate research articles in a special issue of *The Journal of Sexual Medicine* published on October 1, 2010. According to the study's findings, 1 in 4 acts of vaginal intercourse in the United States are condom protected (1 in 3 among singles). Information was obtained on the percentage of Americans (by age group) performing certain sexual behaviors in the past year. Behaviors included masturbated alone, masturbated with partner, received oral from woman, received oral from man, gave oral to woman, gave oral to man, vaginal intercourse, received penis in anus, and inserted penis in anus. As one example, percentages for vaginal intercourse by age group were as follows: 14–15 (9% for males and 11% for females); 16–17 (30% for males and 30% for females); 18–19 (53% for males and 62% for females); 20–24 (63% for males and 80% for females); 25–29 (86% for males and 87% for females); 30–39 (85% for males and 74% for females); 40–49 (74% for males and 70% for females); 50–59 (58% for males and 51% for females); 60–69 (54% for males and 42% for females); and 70+ (43% for males and 22% for females).

Here is a sampling of other findings from the NSSHB:

- Condoms are used twice as often with casual sexual partners as with relationship partners.

- The sexual repertoires of U.S. adults are extremely variable, with more than 40 combinations of sexual activity described at adults' most recent sexual event.

- Many older adults continue to have pleasurable sex lives, reporting a range of different behaviors and partner types.

- About 85% of men report that their partner had an orgasm at the most recent sexual event; this compares to 64% of women who report having had an orgasm at their most recent sexual event. (A difference that is too large to be accounted for by some of the men having had male partners at their most recent event.)

- Men are more likely to have an orgasm when sexual activity includes vaginal intercourse; women are more likely to have an orgasm when they engage in a variety of sexual acts and when oral sexual activity or vaginal intercourse is included.

- Whereas about 7% of adult women and 8% of men identify as gay, lesbian, or bisexual, the proportion of individuals in the United States who have had same-gender sexual interactions at some point in their lives is higher.

- At any given time, most U.S. adolescents are not engaging in partnered sexual behavior. While 40% of 17-year-old males reported vaginal intercourse in the past year, only 27% reported the same in the past 90 days.

- Adults using a condom for intercourse were just as likely to rate the sexual event positively in terms of arousal, pleasure, and orgasm than when having intercourse without one.

Research on Sexuality Education

Research has been done to evaluate the effect of sexuality education programs. For example Kirby (2001) reported that some sexuality and HIV education programs can delay the onset of intercourse, reduce the number of partners, reduce the frequency of sexual intercourse, increase condom or contraceptive use, and thereby decrease sexual risk taking. Also, some programs that have addressed nonsexual risk or protective factors (such as attachment to family, parental monitoring, and attachment to school) have reduced sexual risk taking. Characteristics of effective programs include the following: (1) They focus on reducing one or more behaviors that lead to unintended pregnancy or STIs; (2) they provide basic, accurate information about the risks of teen sexual activity and about ways to avoid intercourse or use methods of protection against pregnancy and STIs; (3) they provide examples of practice with communication, negotiation, and refusal skills; (4) they continue for a sufficient length of time; and (5) they employ teaching methods designed to involve the participants and induce them to personalize the information.

In 2004 Albert reported on a poll that showed a divide among parents and teenagers on whether comprehensive sexuality education encourages young people to engage in sexual activity. Forty-four percent of the parents said that messages beyond abstinence-only education might encourage sexual activity, but

68% of the teens said that "more information does not automatically translate into more sex." The survey also showed that teenagers most often seek information about sexuality from their parents, but most parents don't believe their kids listen to them. Ninety percent of the parents said they do not know how to discuss sexuality with their children.

Unfortunately, evaluations of comprehensive sexuality education have tended to focus mainly on whether the programs have helped young people delay sexual activity and prevent unwanted pregnancy and disease (Haffner & Goldfarb, 1998). Other goals, such as helping young people develop an appreciation of their bodies or communicate effectively with peers and partners, are often overlooked. Evaluations of sexuality education need to be improved so they reflect broad program goals. In the meantime, many evaluations have found that high-quality sexuality education programs increase knowledge, clarify values, increase parent–child communication, help young people delay the initiation of sexual intercourse, increase the use of contraception and condoms, do not encourage young people to begin intercourse, and do not increase the frequency of sexual intercourse.

Kohler et al. (2008) found that young people who received comprehensive sexuality education were significantly less likely to report a teen pregnancy compared to those who received no sexuality education. Abstinence-only programs were not significantly associated with a risk reduction for teen pregnancy when compared with no sexuality education. In comparing abstinence-only programs with comprehensive sexuality education, comprehensive programs were associated with a 50% lower risk of teen pregnancy. Also, teaching about contraception was not associated with an increased risk of adolescent sexual activity or an STI.

Kirby (2008) found that most abstinence programs did not delay initiation of sexual activity and that only 3 of 9 had any significant positive effects on any sexual behavior. In contrast, two-thirds of comprehensive programs showed strong evidence that they positively affected young people's sexual behavior, including both delaying initiation of sexual activity and increasing condom and contraceptive use for those who decided to become sexually active. He concluded that abstinence programs have little evidence to warrant their widespread replication; conversely, strong evidence suggests that some comprehensive programs should be disseminated widely.

In their publication *Comprehensive Sex Education: Research and Results* (2009), Advocates for Youth summarized what the research indicates. They stated that evaluations of comprehensive sexuality education programs show that such programs can help youth delay onset of sexual activity, reduce the frequency of sexual activity, reduce the number of sexual partners, and increase condom and contraceptive use. Also, those who receive comprehensive sexuality education are "NOT more likely to become sexually active, increase sexual activity, or experience negative sexual health outcomes." Conversely, they also indicated that there is little, if any, evidence to show that abstinence-only programs are effective— even at achieving abstinence among teens.

Related to sexuality education, some professionals have promoted virginity pledges. Rosenbaum (2009) found that 5 years after giving pledges, 82% of pledgers denied having ever pledged. Pledgers and nonpledgers did not differ in premarital sexuality activity, sexually transmitted diseases, and anal and oral sex variables. Pledgers were less likely to protect themselves from pregnancy and disease before marriage.

The Future of Sexuality Research

More sexuality research is definitely needed. Not only do we need to have more information on sexual behavior itself, but we also need to explore how we make decisions to engage in sexual activity, how the quality of relationships can be improved, and which factors will be important in helping people achieve sexual satisfaction throughout the life cycle. A variety of cultural and societal factors (age, religion, education) have always affected sexual decision making, but recently a change in societal attitudes toward marriage, divorce, childbearing, and sexual relationships has become evident. The stresses these new attitudes bring to bear on personal relationships need to be explored in the near future.

There are real challenges related to sexuality research. Tiefer (1994), in her presidential address to the International Academy of Sex Research, emphasized three crises facing sexology. First, the media are inundating the public with sexual topics. Second, many people in academic circles still hesitate to accept sexuality research as being as legitimate as other forms of research. Finally, there is a tendency for sexuality research to focus only on medical topics and not on the comprehensive nature of people and society. We have learned a great deal through sexuality research; however, even better research methods are needed to fit together the psychological, the biological, and the sociological aspects of sexuality research.

In closing, Tables 2.2 and 2.3 summarize the sexuality research of selected researchers.

TABLE 2.2 Selected Sexuality Researchers and Their Studies (Grouped by Type of Method)

Author(s)	Date	Title
Interview survey		
Scientific literature		
Kinsey, Pomeroy, & Martin	1948	*Sexual behavior in the human male*
	1953	*Sexual behavior in the human female*
Laumann, Gagnon, Michael, & Michaels	1994	*The social organization of sexuality*
Carolina Population Center	2001	National longitudinal study of adolescent health (The "Add Health Survey")
Karofsky	2001	Parent–teen communication and the initiations of sexual intercourse
Bancroft et al.	2004	Sexual activity and risk taking in young heterosexual men: The relevance of sexual arousability, mood, and sensation seeking
Burgard	2004	Factors associated with contraceptive use in late and post apartheid South Africa
Bruckner & Bearman	2004	Ambivalence and pregnancy: Adolescents' attitudes, contraceptive use and pregnancy
Cavanagh	2004	The sexual debut of girls in early adolescence: The intersection of race, pubertal timing, and friendship group characteristics
Connell & Freund	2004	Investigating ethnic differences in sexual health: Focus groups with young people
Harawa et al.	2004	Associations of race/ethnicity with HIV prevalence and HIV related behaviors
Johnson & Jackson	2004	What is the significance of black–white differences in risky sexual behavior?

Continued

TABLE 2.2 **Selected Sexuality Researchers and Their Studies (Grouped by Type of Method)—cont'd**

Author(s)	Date	Title
Interview survey		
Scientific literature		
U.S. Centers for Disease Control and Prevention (Grunbaum et al.)	2004	Youth risk behavior surveillance system
Adam et al.	2005	Acculturation as a predictor of the onset of sexual intercourse among hispanic and white teens
Chuang & Freund	2005	Emergency contraception knowledge among women in a Boston community
Frisco	2005	Parental involvement and young women's contraceptive use
Halpern Fisher et al.	2005	Oral versus vaginal sex among adolescents: Perceptions, attitudes, and behavior
South et al.	2005	Residential mobility and the onset of adolescent sexual activity
Popular literature		
Hite	1976	*The Hite report*
	1981	*The Hite report on male sexuality*
	1987	*Women and love: A cultural revolution in progress*
Sarrel & Sarrel	1980	The *Redbook* report on sexual relationships
Reinisch & Beasley	1991	*The Kinsey Institute new report on sex*
Kaiser Family Foundation and *Seventeen* magazine	2002	SexSmarts survey on teen sexual behavior
NBC News and *People Magazine*	2004	National Survey of Young Teens Sexual Attitudes and Behavior
Direct observation		
Scientific literature		
Masters & Johnson	1966	*Human sexual response*
	1970	*Human sexual inadequacy*
	1979	*Homosexuality in perspective*

TABLE 2.3 **Examples of Additional Research**

Author(s)	Date	Title
Oncalem & King	2001	Comparison of men's and women's attempts to dissuade sexual partners from the couple using condoms
Kirby	2001	Emerging answers: Research findings on programs to reduce sexual risk taking and teen pregnancy
Ford et al.	2001	Characteristics of adolescents' sexual partners and their association with use of condoms and other contraceptive methods
Kaiser Family Foundation	2002	Substance use and risky sexual behavior: Attitudes and practices among adolescents and young adults
Child Trends	2002	National longitudinal survey of youth (Most sexually active teens first had sex at home, late at night, survey shows)
Greenbaum et al.	2004	Youth Risk Behavior Surveillance—United States, 2003
Lefkowitz et al.	2004	Religiosity, sexual behaviors, and sexual attitudes during emerging adulthood
Vlassoff et al.	2004	Assessing costs and benefits of sexual and reproductive health interventions
Penhollow et al.	2005	The impact of religiosity on the sexual behaviors of college students

TABLE 2.3 **Examples of Additional Research—cont'd**

Author(s)	Date	Title
Moshser et al.	2005	Sexual behavior and selected measures: Men and women 15–44 years of age, United States, 2002
Koch	2006	Women's bodies as a "puzzle" for college men: Grounded theory research
Kirby	2008	Impact of sexuality education programs on adolescent sexual behavior
Kohler et al.	2008	Sexuality education and the initiation of sexual activity
Lescano et al.	2008	Correlates of heterosexual anal intercourse among at-risk adolescents and young adults
Manlove et al.	2008	Condom use and consistency among male adolescents in the United States
Sex and Tech	2008	Results from a survey of teens and young adults
Daniel & Balog	2009	Early female puberty
Rosenbaum	2009	Patient teenagers? A comparison of the sexual behavior of virginity pledgers and matched nonpledgers
Biro et al.	2010	Pubertal assessment and characteristics
Eaton et al.	2010	Youth Risk Behavior Surveillance—United States, 2009
Guttmacher Institute	2010	Facts on contraceptive use in the United States
National Survey of Sexual Health and Behavior (NSSHB)	2010	Research about sexual-health behaviors
Guttmacher Institute	2011	Facts on induced abortion in the United States
Guttmacher Institute	2011	Facts on American teens' sexual health
Lehmiller et al.	2011	Friends with benefits relationships
McFarland et al.	2011	Role of religion on sexual behavior and satisfaction
Pazol et al.	2011	U.S. teen pregnancy statistics
Torian et al.	2011	U.S. HIV statistics

Exploring the Dimensions of Human Sexuality

Our feelings, attitudes, and beliefs regarding sexuality are influenced by our internal and external environments. Go to go.jblearning.com/dimensions5e to learn more about the biological, psychological, and sociological factors that affect your sexuality.

It's amazing how many factors are involved in even basic research on sexuality. Political forces have banned the use of government money for research dealing with sexuality, so monies must be provided by private foundations or companies, which may have a political or financial agenda of their own.

Learned behaviors prompt many people to answer questions as they think they should be answered, instead of with the truth, and that tendency can create survey bias. The limited number of people willing to respond to a sexuality survey, especially in lower socioeconomic classes, also hinders researchers.

Finally, cultural, ethnic, and religious biases may hinder researchers from getting the data needed. For example, a survey of sexual behavior based on religious affiliation would do poorly, because many Muslim (the number-two religion in the United States) women would not allow interviews or would do so only with their husband present.

Biological Factors

- The medical model was the focus of sexuality research in the 19th century.
- The sexual response cycle was discovered by the researchers Masters and Johnson.
- Physiological changes in the vagina or penis can be monitored by the vaginal plethysmograph and penile strain gauge, respectively.

Sociocultural Factors

- The gender "double standard" research goes back to the 19th century, when discomfort with women's sexuality prompted such beliefs.
- Education leads to both a later age of first intercourse and a higher likelihood of using contraception at first intercourse.
- Religious adolescents are less likely to participate in sexual intercourse; when they do, they are less likely to use reliable contraceptives.
- Ethical considerations abound in sexuality research.

Psychological Factors

- The NHSLS data found that married people were much more likely than single people to report being extremely or very happy.
- Behaviors and practices, as well as frequency of sexual activity, need to be accounted for in sexuality research.
- Motivation to respond to a sexual research survey may create a bias in the sample.
- Learned attitudes and behaviors may influence answers given on sexuality surveys.

Summary

- The scientific method involves identifying a research question, reviewing literature, formulating a hypothesis, operationalizing the variables, collecting data, and analyzing the data to test the hypothesis.

- Research in sexuality can involve surveys, case studies, experimental research, and direct observation.

- Ethical issues in sexuality research include informed consent, confidentiality, anonymity, and protection of subjects.

- Evaluating information about sexuality found on the Internet is often difficult. We need to ask ourselves important questions, such as the purpose of the site or the source of the information, to better evaluate Internet sexuality content.

- Early sexuality researchers included Richard von Krafft-Ebing, Henry Havelock Ellis, Sigmund Freud, Magnus Hirschfeld, Katherine Davis, and Clelia Mosher.

- In the mid-20th century, Alfred Kinsey did extensive research on sexual attitudes and behavior of males and females.

- The research of Masters and Johnson gave us a great deal of information about human sexual response.

- Many studies have been done to help us know more about premarital sexual attitudes and behavior, teen pregnancy, ethnic differences in sexual attitudes and behaviors, use of contraception, changes in selected statistical relationships, and the effects of sexuality education.

- More sexuality research is definitely needed. Needs include knowing more about how we make decisions about sexual behavior, how to improve the quality of relationships, and which factors will help achieve sexual satisfaction throughout the life cycle.

Discussion Questions

1. Compare and contrast the varied methods of sexuality research.

2. Describe the ethical issues involved in sexuality research, citing examples of each.

3. Who were the early sexuality researchers, and what did they figure out? Is their research still considered valid?

4. List the major modern sexuality researchers and describe their contributions. How has their research changed sexuality?

Application Questions

Reread the story that opens the chapter and answer the following questions.

1. Imagine your parents asked you to explain what sexuality researchers do—and why. Prepare a brief response to their query.

2. Explain which dimensions of human sexuality would influence congressional funding for a study on sexuality. Would representatives from some states be more willing to support sexuality research? Explain your answer.

3. For over a year, allegations of sexual relations between former President Clinton and White House intern Monica Lewinsky rocked the news. Evaluate why, in light of a sexual scandal, the president's approval ratings continued to climb.

Critical Thinking Questions

1. What motivates a person to take the time and effort to respond to a human sexuality research questionnaire? Could that motivation lead to a sample bias?

2. Masters and Johnson were not the only team to discover a human sexual response cycle. How is it possible that different research groups obtained different results regarding a physiological response?

3. In 1991, the U.S. federal government pulled support from the NHSLS research project and passed legislation prohibiting the spending of federal funds on sexuality research. Although this was clearly a political move, it raises the question, Why should the government support such research? Put another way, how does sexuality research help the American people?

4. Imagine that you and/or your lover read a popular magazine sex survey that showed that a large percentage of people were doing a sexual activity that you had never tried. Would that motivate you to try something new? Would you encourage your lover to try it? How would you feel if your lover asked you to try it?

Critical Thinking Case

Years ago it was widely reported that Russian track and field athletes were encouraged to have sexual relations the night before a major meet. In fact, reports claimed that those who did so performed better (closer to their potential). Imagine that the coach of your college's track team has just learned this information. He has asked you to design a sexuality research project, using scientific methodology, to prove or disprove the hypothesis that sexual activity leads to improved athletic performance.

> Which method(s) of research would give you the best results? Explain why. Is it possible to prove the validity of such a hypothesis? Which other factors might be involved? Which ethical issues might you encounter? How could those issues be overcome?

Exploring Personal Dimensions

Sexuality Research
Mark each of the following statements "true" or "false."

_____ 1. All research completed as part of the National Health and Social Life Survey was financially supported by the U.S. federal government.

_____ 2. The first step in the scientific method is identifying a research question.

_____ 3. A hypothesis is a statement based on research results.

_____ 4. Kinsey's research is an example of survey research.

_____ 5. The research of Masters and Johnson is an example of experimental research.

_____ 6. A plethysmograph is used in the laboratory to measure and chart physiological changes over time.

_____ 7. Most normal women have orgasms from penile thrusting alone.

_____ 8. The Sex and Tech study in 2008 showed that a significant number of teens have electronically sent, or posted online, nude or semi-nude pictures or videos of themselves.

_____ 9. The Liu Report can be correctly referred to as a Chinese National Health and Social Life Survey.

_____10. More than half the U.S. students in grades 9–12 have participated in sexual intercourse.

_____11. Both the proportion of adolescent females in the United States who have experienced sexual intercourse and their likelihood of pregnancy have increased in recent years.

_____12. Good sexuality education programs do not hasten the onset of sexual intercourse and may increase the use of contraception—particularly condoms.

Interpretation
All of the even-numbered statements are true and all of the odd-numbered statements are false. If you were correct on at least 10 statements, you did well. If you were not correct on at least 10 statements, find the correct answers in the chapter. All of the correct answers are in this chapter on sexuality research.

Suggested Readings

Brecher, E. *The sex researchers*. New York: Signet Books, 1969.

Chandrda, A., Mosher, W.D., Copen, C, & Sionean, C. Sexual behavior, sexual attraction, and sexual identity in the United States: Data from the 2006–2008 National Survey of Family Growth. National *Health Statistics Report, 36* (March, 2011),1–36. Available: *http://www.cdc.gov/nchs/data/nhsr/nhsr036.pdf*.

Dodge, B., Reece, M., Herbenick, D., Schick, V., Sanders, S., & Fortenberry, J.D. Sexual health among U.S. black and Hispanic men and women. A national representative study. *The Journal of Sexual Medicine, 7, Issue Supplement a5* (October 2010), 330–345.

Harbenick, D., Reece, M., Schick, V., Sanders, S.A., Dodge, B., & Fortenberry, J.D. Sexual behavior in the United States: Results from a national probability sample of men and women ages 14–94. *The Journal of Sexual Medicine, 7, Issue Supplement a5* (October 2010), 255–265.

Pomeroy, W. *Dr. Kinsey and the Institute for Sex Research*. New York: Harper & Row, 1972.

Wang, B., Hertog, S., Meier, A., Lou, C., & Gao, E. The potential of comprehensive sex education in China: Findings from suburban Shanghai. *International Family Planning Perspectives 31, no. 2* (June 2005), 63–72.

U.S. Department of Commerce and the Executive Office of the President. *Women in America: Indicators of social and economic well-being*. March 2011. Available: http://www.whitehouse.gov/sites/default/files/rss_viewer/Women_in_America.pdf.

Web Resources

For links to the websites below, visit go.jblearning .com/dimensions5e and click on Resource Links.

Information on Marie Stopes, an early sexuality researcher
www.encyclopedia.com/topic/Marie_Carmichael_ Stopes.aspx

Contains additional information about an early sexuality researcher.

Society for the Scientific Study of Sexuality: Annual Review of Sex Research
www.sexscience.org

Provides updated information on various sexuality research topics.

The Kinsey Institute Research Program
www.kinseyinstitute.org/research/surveylinks.html

Information about many present and past sexuality research studies.

The Alan Guttmacher Institute: New Research and Analysis
www.agi-usa.org

With emphasis on research related to pregnancy and to abortion, the Guttmacher Institute has information on many sexuality research topics.

Sexuality Information and Education Council of the United States
www.siecus.org

Information and publications on numerous sexuality topics are available from the Sexuality Information and Education Council of the United States (SIECUS).

References

Advocates for Youth. *Comprehensive sex education: Research and results*, 2009. Available: http://www.advocatesforyouth.org/ publications-a-z/1487-publications.

Albert, Bill. *With one voice 2004: America's adults and teens sound off about teen pregnancy.* Washington, D.C.: National Campaign to Prevent Teen Pregnancy, December 2004.

Biro, F. M., Galvez, M. P., Greenspan, L. C., Succop, P. A., Van-geepuram, N., Pinney, S. M., Teitelbaum, S., Windham, G. C., Kushi, L. H., & Wolff, M. S. Pubertal assessment method and baseline characteristics in a mixed longitudinal study of girls. *Pediatrics, 126, no. 3* (September 1, 2010), e583–e590.

Bruckner, H., Martin, A., & Bearman, P. S. Ambivalence and pregnancy: Adolescents' attitudes, contraceptive use and pregnancy. *Perspect Sex Reprod Health, 36, no. 6* (November/December 2004), 248–257.

Burgard, S. Factors associated with contraceptive use in late- and post-apartheid South Africa. *Studies in Family Planning, 35, no. 2* (June 2004), 91–104.

Cavanagh, S. E. The sexual debut of girls in early adolescence: The intersection of race, pubertal timing, and friendship group characteristics. *Journal of Research on Adolescence, 14, no. 3* (September 2004), 285–312.

Chuang, C. H., & Freund, K. M. Emergency contraception knowledge among women in a Boston community. *Contraception, 71, no. 2* (Feb. 2005), 157–160.

Connell, P., McKevitt, C., & Low, N. Investigating ethnic differences in sexual health: Focus groups with young people. *Sexually Transmitted Infections, 80, no. 4* (August 2004), 300–305.

Dailard, C. Recent findings from the "Add Health" survey: Teens and sexual activity. *The Guttmacher Report, 4, no. 4* (August 2001), 1–3, 2–4.

Daniel, E., & Balog, L. F. Early female puberty: A review of research on etiology and implications. *The Health Educator, 41, no. 2* (Fall 2009), 47–53.

Dennison, R. P., & Russell, S. T. Positive perspectives on adolescent sexuality: Contributions of the National Longitudinal Study of Adolescent Health. *Sexuality Research & Social Policy, 2, 4* (December 2005), 54–59.

Dolan, B. No sex please, we're ignorant. *Time* (September 17, 1990), 71.

Eaton, D. K., Kann, L., Kinchen, S., Shanklin, S., Ross, J., Hawkins, J. Harris, W. A., Lowry, R., McManus, T. Cheyen, D., Lim, C., Whittle, L., Brener, N. D., & Wechsler, H. Youth risk behavior surveillance—United States, 2009. In: *Surveillance Summaries,* June 4, 2010, *Morbidity and Mortality Weekly Report, 59, no. SS-5* (2010), 1–143.

Facts on American teens' sexual and reproductive health. Guttmacher Institute, January 2011. Available: http://www. guttmacher.org/pubs/FB-ATSRH.html.

Facts on contraceptive use in the United States. Guttmacher Institute, May 2011. Available: http://www.guttmacher.org/ pubs/fb_contr_use.html.

Facts on induced abortion in the United States. Guttmacher Institute, June 2010. Available: http://www.guttmacher.org/ pubs/fb_induced_abortion.html.

Ford, K., Woosung, S., & Lepowski, J. Characteristics of adolescents' sexual partners and their association with use of condoms and other contraceptive methods. *Family Planning Perspectives, 33, no. 3* (May/June 2001), 100–105, 132.

Frisco, M. Parental involvement and young women's contraceptive use. *Journal of Marriage and Family, 67, no. 1* (February 2005), 110–121.

Haffner, D. W., & Goldfarb, E. S. *But, does it work? Improving evaluations of sexuality education.* Sexuality Information and Education Council of the United States, 1988.

Halpern-Felsher, B. L., Cornell, J. L., Kropp, R. Y., & Tschann, J. M. Oral versus vaginal sex among adolescents: Perceptions, attitudes, and behavior. *Pediatrics, 115, no. 4* (April 2005), 845–851.

Harawa, N. T., et al., Associations of race/ethnicity with HIV prevalence and HIV-related behaviors. *Journal of Acquired Immune Deficiency Syndrome, 35, no. 5* (March 2004), 526–536.

History of sex surveys: Factors in the sex life of 2200 women. Trivia-Library.com (2005). Available: www.trivia-library.com.

Hite, S. *The Hite report.* New York: Macmillan, 1976.

Hite, S. *The Hite report on male sexuality.* New York: Alfred Knopf, 1981.

Hite, S. *Women and love: A cultural revolution in progress.* New York: Alfred Knopf, 1987.

Johnson, E. H., & Jackson, L. A. What is the significance of black–white differences in risky sexual behavior? *Journal of the National Medical Association, 86, no. 10* (October 2004), 745–759.

Kaiser Family Foundation and *Seventeen* magazine release latest SexSmarts survey on teen sexual behavior. Kaiser Family Foundation (July 9, 2002). Available: www.kaisernetwork .org/daily_reports.

Kinsey, A. C., Pomeroy, W. B., & Martin, C. E. *Sexual behavior in the human female.* Philadelphia: Saunders, 1953.

Kinsey, A. C., Pomeroy, W. B., & Martin, C. E. *Sexual behavior in the human male.* Philadelphia: Saunders, 1948.

The Kinsey Institute. *The history and concept of sexology,* 1998.

Kirby, D. *Emerging answers: Research findings on programs to reduce sexual risk-taking and teen pregnancy.* Washington, DC: National Campaign to Prevent Teen Pregnancy, 2001.

Kirby, D. H. The impact of abstinence and comprehensive sex and STD/HIV education programs on adolescent sexual behavior. *Sexuality Research Social Policy, 5, no. 3* (September 2008), 18–27.

Klitsch, M. Subgroups of U.S. women differ widely on exposure to sexual intercourse. *Family Planning Perspectives, 22* (1990), 94–95.

Koch, P. B. Women's bodies as a "puzzle" for college men: Grounded theory research. *American Journal of Sexuality Education, 1, 3* (2006), 51–72.

Kohler, P. K., Manhart, L. E., & Lafferty, W. E. Abstinence-only and comprehensive sex education and the initiation of sexual activity and teen pregnancy. *Journal of Adolescent Health, 42, no. 4* (April 2009), 344–351.

Laumann, E. O., Michael, R. T., & Gagnon, J. H. A political history of the National Sex Survey of Adults. *Family Planning Perspectives, 26, no. 1* (1994).

Lefkowitz, E. S., Gillen, M. M., Shearer, C. L., & Boone, T. L. Religiosity, sexual behaviors, and sexual attitudes during emerging childhood. *Journal of Sex Research, 41, no. 2* (May 2004), 150–159.

Lehmiller, J. J., VanderDrift, L. E., & Kelly, J. R. Sex differences in approaching friends with benefits relationships. *Journal of Sex Research, 48, no. 2–3* (March 2011), 275–284.

Lescano, C. M., Houck, C. D., Brown, L. K., Doherty, G., DiClemente, R. J., Fernandez, M. I., Pugatch, D., Schlenger, W. E., & Silver, B. J. Correlates of heterosexual anal intercourse among at-risk adolescents and young adults. *American Journal of Public Health, 99* (2009), 1131–1136.

Manlove, J., Ikramullah, E., & Terry-Humen, E. Condom use and consistency among male adolescents in the United States. *Journal of Adolescent Health, 43, 4* (October 2008), 325–333.

Masters, W. H., & Johnson, V. E. *Homosexuality in perspective.* Boston: Little, Brown, 1979.

Masters, W. H., & Johnson, V. E. *Human sexual inadequacy.* Boston: Little, Brown, 1970.

Masters, W. H., & Johnson, V. E. *Human sexual response.* Boston: Little, Brown, 1966.

McFarland, M. J., Uecher, J. E., & Regerus, M. D. The role of religion in shaping sexual frequency and satisfaction: Evidence from married and unmarried older adults. *Journal of Sex Research, 48, no. 2 & 3* (March 2011), 297–308.

Mosher, W. D., Chandra, A., & Jones, J. Sexual behavior and selected health measures: Men and women 15–44 years of age, United States, 2002. *Advance Data from Vital and Health Statistics, 362* (September 15, 2005), 1–17.

National Center for Complementary and Alternative Medicine. *10 things to know about evaluating medical resources on the Web,* 2011. Available: http://nccam.nih.gov/health /webresources/.

National Survey of Sexual Health and Behavior. Center for Sexual Health Promotion, Indiana University, 2010. Available: http://www.nationalsexstudy.indiana.edu.

Nearly 3 in 10 young teens sexually active: NBC News, *People* magazine commission landmark national poll. *NBC News* (January 19, 2004, updated January 31, 2005). Available: http://www.msnbc.msn.com/id/6839072.

Oncalem, R. & King, B. Comparison of men's and women's attempts to dissuade sexual partners from the couple using condoms. *Archives of Sexual Behavior, 30, no. 4* (August 2001), 379–391.

Pazol, K., Warner, L., Gavin, L., Callaghan, W. M., Spitz, A. M., Anderson, J. E., Barfield, W. D., & Kann, L. Vital signs: Teen pregnancy—United States, 1991–2009. *Morbidity and Mortality Weekly Report, 60, no. 13* (April 8, 2011), 414–420.

Penhollow, T., Young, M., & Denny, G. The impact of religiosity on the sexual behaviors of college students. *American Journal of Health Education, 36, no. 2* (March/April 2005), 75–83.

Rosenbaum, J. E. Patient teenagers? A comparison of the sexual behavior of virginity pledgers and matched nonpledgers. *Pediatrics, 123, 1* (January 2009), e110–e120.

Sarrel, P., & Sarrel, L. The *Redbook* report on sexual relationships, part I. *Redbook* (October 1980), 73–80.

Sex and Tech. Washington, DC: *National Campaign to Prevent Teen and Unplanned Pregnancy,* 2008. Available: http://www .thenationalcampaign.org/sextech/PDF/SexTech_Summary.pdf.

South, S. J., Haynie, D. L., & Bose, S. Residential mobility and the onset of adolescent sexual activity. *Journal of Marriage and Family, 67, no. 2* (May 2005), 499–514.

Substance use and risky sexual behavior: Attitudes and practices among adolescents and young adults. *American Journal of Health Education, 33, no. 5* (September/October 2002), 278–281.

Tiefer, L. Three crises facing sexology. *Archives of Sexual Behavior, 23, no. 4* (1994), 361–373.

Torian, L., Chen, M., Rhodes, P., & Hall, H. I. HIV surveillance—United States, 1991–2008. *Morbidity and Mortality Weekly Report, 60, no. 21* (June 3, 2011), 689–693.

Trends in sexual risk behaviors among high school students—United States, 1991–2001. *Morbidity and Mortality Weekly Report, 51, no. 38* (September 27, 2002), 856–859.

Vlassoff, M., Singh, S., Darroch, J. E., Carbone, E., & Bernstein, S. *Assessing costs and benefits of sexual and reproductive health interventions.* New York: Guttmacher Institute, 2004.

von Krafft-Ebing, R. *Psychopathia sexualis.* Stuttgart, Germany, 1902.

Women in American history. *Britannica Online.* Available: http://www.britannica.com.

CHAPTER 3

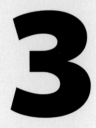

Sexual Communication

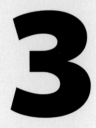

CHAPTER OBJECTIVES

1 Describe the process of sexual communication, including nonverbal communication.

2 Identify barriers to sexual communication, including gender differences, attitudes about sexuality, and sexual language.

3 Discuss techniques for improving sexual communication.

go.jblearning.com/dimensions5e

Attitudes About Sexuality
Learning Assertiveness
Global Dimensions: International Differences in
    Discussing Sexuality

INTRODUCTION

*T*wo for the Road (1967) is a movie starring Audrey Hepburn as Joanna and Albert Finney as Mark. When they first meet on the road in Europe, Joanna is in a touring girls' choir and Mark is a struggling architect. The film follows their life together—through courtship and marriage, infidelity, and parenthood—all on the road in a variety of cars (hence the title), through a score of time-shifting vignettes.

The film presents a lovely portrayal of a young couple growing in—and eventually out of—love. It not only shows the life cycle of a 12-year relationship, but also brilliantly portrays how communication changes during that life cycle.

As the couple meets and falls in love at a dizzying pace, conversation flows. It seems there is nothing that Joanna and Mark cannot talk about. They openly share their worlds together, delighting in the pleasure of each other. They communicate with touch, holding hands, kissing, making love (although in a 1967 family movie the lovemaking is only implied).

In one blissful scene, the young lovers are shown to their table in a French restaurant. Joanna and Mark hold hands, giggle, smile, make eye contact while walking across the restaurant. But they notice an older married couple who are eating their dinner. The couple is simply eating—no conversation, no touching, no eye contact. Mark turns to Joanna and suggests, "I guess married people don't talk."

But as their relationship and life change, so does their communication style. In time, Joanna and Mark have experienced life together, and they do not talk about it as much as they used to talk about their lives before they met. The mistakes they made as youths disappear into their sophisticated adulthood. There are no silly mistakes to giggle about anymore.

*In time, they begin to know each other so well that each can antici-
pate what the other is going to say or wants to do. Verbal expression
becomes infrequent, because it no longer seems very important.*

*And their lives change, too: They become parents, and Mark becomes
a well-known architect. Children and work decrease the amount of time
they have for each other. Again, life changes alter communication styles.*

*Eventually, Joanna and Mark are back in the same French res-
taurant, but this time as a married couple—no talk, no touch, no eye
contact. A young couple, holding hands and giggling, looks at them; he
whispers something in her ear. Joanna and Mark have come full circle—
they are the married couple who do not talk!*

*Of course, one of the pleasures of being in a long-term relationship
is that there is such a high level of comfort that sometimes you do not
have to talk. Yet the very essence of a relationship is communication.
Over time, if you rely on your assumptions about what the other person wants, needs, or thinks, the relationship begins to break down—and
knowing what your partner wants all the time can become old hat. As
people do in real life, Joanna and Mark fail to bridge the gap between not
needing to talk constantly and not communicating.*

*Joanna and Mark's relationship deteriorates. They meet new people, have
affairs—all in an effort to relive those days of carefree expression, of newness
and excitement. Eventually the marriage ends; the full cycle of the relationship
has been portrayed in less time than it may take you to read this chapter!*

*Many of you who have had long-term relationships can probably
relate to the story of Joanna and Mark. When partners fail to communicate freely about sexuality or other topics, their relationship is bound to be
limited—in scope and time. You have a great opportunity to enrich your
relationships and sexual experiences when you can communicate with
your partner about arousing mind and body experiences, your feelings
about each other, and the other's preferences in life and in sexuality.*

■ The Process of Communicating Sexually

Effective communication begins with an understanding of how communication works. The basic communication model (Figure 3.1) illustrates the five
steps of the communication process. Let us consider
how the basic communication model might work in
a relationship in which partners are participating in
some sexual activity.

First, the sender has an idea. Partner A (the
sender) does not want to have sexual intercourse.
The nature of the idea is influenced by many factors,
such as the context of the situation and the sender's
mood, background, culture, and frame of reference.
For example, Partner A may be too tired or upset,
perhaps it is already too late at night, or perhaps
Partner A does not know enough about Partner B.
Whatever the reasons, Partner A does not want to
participate.

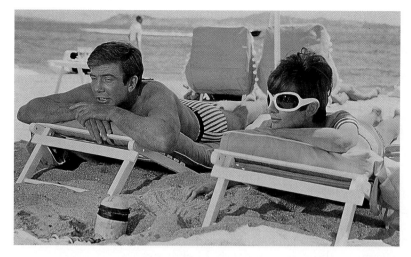

The movie *Two for the Road* (1967) explores the life cycle of a relationship, as well as the way communication changes through the cycle. From your own personal experience, does communication change in a relationship over the long term?

Second, the sender encodes the idea in a message. **Encoding** means converting the idea into words or gestures to convey meaning. Partner A says, "I do not want to have sexual intercourse." A potential problem is that words have different meanings for different people. If misunderstandings result from missed meanings, that process is called **bypassing**. For example, Partner B may think all forms of sexual behavior except sexual intercourse are acceptable to Partner A. It may also be possible that Partner B thinks Partner A is just "saying" this and does not really mean it.

Third, the message travels over a channel. Channels include speech, telephones, fax machines, computers, and written correspondence. In this case, the channel contains speech and gestures. Partner A's voice tones, inflections, and gestures are part of the channel.

Fourth, the receiver (Partner B) decodes the message. **Decoding** means translating the message from its symbol form into meaning. Communication can be successful only when decoding is accurate. Various forms of "noise," however, can distort the message. In its simplest sense, the noise of a crowded room makes hearing difficult. Noise can also be represented by misinterpretation of words, voice tones, or gestures; emotional reactions; or the use of alcohol or other drugs. In our

example, after having several drinks, Partner B hears, "Come and convince me."

Fifth, the receiver responds verbally or nonverbally—this is called **feedback**. Feedback helps the sender know whether the message was received and understood. In view of what Partner B heard, feedback is sent in the form of further sexual advances, because "noise" disturbed the transmission of Partner A's message.

Note that in Figure 3.1 the model provides for continual sending, receiving, and feedback. In our example, it is likely that the feedback provided by Partner B will result in additional communication from Partner A, and so the process continues.

Nonverbal Communication

Nonverbal communication includes all unwritten and unspoken messages. These may be sent intentionally or unintentionally. These silent signals exert a strong influence on the receiver in our basic communication model, but interpreting them can be difficult. For example, does the fact that Person A is looking down indicate modesty or just fatigue? Do crossed arms indicate that a person is unwilling to communicate or that a person feels cold?

The vast majority of message meaning (some experts say

encoding
Converting an idea into words or gestures to convey meaning.

bypassing
When misunderstandings result from missed meanings.

decoding
Translating the message from its symbol form into meaning.

feedback
When the receiver responds verbally or nonverbally.

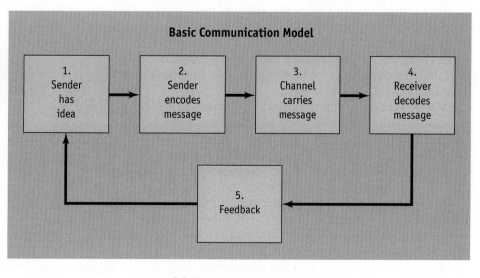

FIGURE **3.1** The basic communication model.

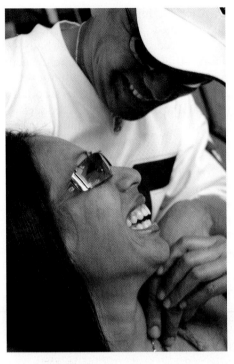

You can show interest in your partner with nonverbal communication. Gazing into each other's eyes, leaning in toward each other, smiling, and touching are all ways of conveying interest in one another.

as much as 93%) (Guffey, 1999) is sent nonverbally. Messages can be difficult to decipher when verbal and nonverbal messages seem to contradict each other. For example, if Person A says it is acceptable to participate in sexual intercourse but then is not very responsive, Person B may have a problem knowing what Person A is really communicating.

When verbal and nonverbal messages conflict, receivers often have more faith in the nonverbal cues than what is said. It is important to recognize the significance of nonverbal communication, but it is unwise to attach a specific meaning to each gesture in every situation.

Note the body posture of your classmates. During an interesting class activity, most of them will probably be leaning or looking toward the lecturer or the center of the group, indicating that they are involved in what is happening. During a boring class, they will probably be leaning away from the lecturer or group. We call this physical behavior *body language*. Communicating by body posture often conveys as much as, or more than, the spoken word. When people feel uncomfortable about expressing their thoughts or feelings verbally, body language may be the only form of communication in which they participate.

We all recognize the importance of communicating nonverbally: We smile when we say hello, scratch our heads when perplexed, and hug a friend to show affection. (We also have an array of body terms to describe our nonverbal behavior: "Keep a stiff upper lip," "I can't stomach him," "She has no backbone," "I'm tongue-tied," "He caught her eye," "I have two left feet," "That was spine-tingling.") We show appreciation and affection, revulsion and indifference with expressions and gestures. We tell people we are interested in them by merely making eye contact and, as the male peacock displays his feathers, we display

our sexuality by the ways we dress and walk and even by the way we stand.

Unfortunately, the nonverbal expression of feelings and thoughts is easy to misinterpret. College students often indicate that they think there are differences in male and female nonverbal communication. Many males and females say that women are more expressive and better at sending and receiving nonverbal messages. This might include smiling, having an expressive face, using hands to communicate, and having an expressive voice. In contrast, men might be louder, more likely to interrupt, and be more uneasy about the use of nonverbal behaviors.

Consequently, to depend on nonverbal communication alone to express yourself sexually is to risk being misunderstood. Furthermore, if your partner is depending on nonverbal communication to express feelings to you, it is up to you to find out—verbally—whether you are getting the right message. Without such a reality check, your partner, although totally failing to connect, might assume that he or she is communicating effectively. For example, imagine that a man and woman on their first date begin hugging, kissing, and caressing each other after a movie. The woman's breathing speeds up, and the man, taking this as a sign of sexual arousal and interest, presses onward. When the woman suddenly pushes free and complains that the man is too impatient, he is confused. The problem here is one of interpretation rather than incompatibility: The rapid breathing that the man took as a sign of arousal was really a sign of nervousness. If these people had been more effective verbal communicators, they would have been able to clarify the situation in the beginning. Instead they reached a silent impasse, with him confused and

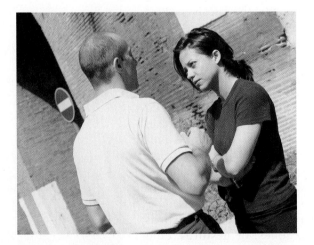

Misinterpretation of your partner's body language can often lead to conflict in a relationship.

Multicultural DIMENSIONS

Female and Male Subcultures?

Male–female communication is related to gender issues. In the business world males and females seem to be members of different subcultures: Even though meetings in the executive suite increasingly are coed gatherings, there are often real differences in the behavior of females and males.

It could be called the "bad-boy/good-girl" clash. Men seated around conference tables often start acting like adolescents—putting on a show of bravado while trading "witty" put-downs to protect themselves from the pain of criticism. As a prerequisite to success, their culture has taught them to be both self-effacing and self-promoting.

Women, by contrast, have learned from their culture to be earnest perfectionists, eager to show they have done all their homework by explaining every point; yet they are quick to admit mistakes. A woman executive reported seeing this at a meeting where a female colleague began her presentation with many apologies. She told the group that all the information she needed was not available, that she had been rushed, that her slides probably contained typos. She said she was sorry several times but then went on to give a flawless presentation with perfect slides. The man who followed her launched right into his presentation with no apologies whatsoever—and his slides were much less well put together.

On average, men talk more at meetings than women, and so their ideas typically are adopted more often. Men also are more comfortable making up things, so if someone asks about a particular financial figure, for example, they may offer one. A woman is more likely to say, "I'm not sure about that." Women give the impression that they do not know what they are talking about, whereas many men seem confident whether they know a little or a lot.

However, it is probably possible to change behaviors and expectations in different cultures. For example,

at Eddie Bauer & Co. in Seattle, where half of all managers are women, female executives report a "comfort level" about speaking freely at meetings that they did not feel working at other places. Style differences seem to relate more to job categories than to gender.

Of course, we cannot assume that all males or females will behave exactly as those described do. We also have to remember that possible communication differences are not always a result of being a male or a female. For example, the differences might be related to status rather than gender. The point is that we need to be aware of possible subcultural differences in our personal relationships as well as in our business relationships. Understanding these possible differences can be helpful in improving communication in all relationships.

On a very different note related to possible female and male subcultures, it is known that many women pretend, or "fake," orgasm, but is this also true for men? Among 180 male and 101 female college students, it was found that both men and women pretended orgasm (28% and 67%, respectively). Most pretended during penile–vaginal intercourse, but some pretended during oral sexual activity, manual stimulation, and phone sex. Frequently reported reasons for faking were that orgasm was unlikely, they wanted the sexual activity to end, and they wanted to avoid negative consequences (for example, hurting their partner's feelings) and to obtain positive consequences (for example, pleasing their partner). Results also suggest a sexual script in which women should orgasm before men and that men are responsible for women's orgasms.

Note the implications in this study related to communication between sexual partners before and during sexual activity.

Source: Data from Hymowitz, C. Men, women fall into kids' roles in meetings, *The Birmingham News* (December 20, 1998), D1–D2; Muehlenhard, C. L., & Shippee, S. K. Men's and women's reports of pretending orgasm. *Journal of Sex Research, 47, no. 6* (Nov.–Dec. 2010), 552–567.

---

her resentful. It can work the other way around, too; both people may want to touch each other but feel too awkward to show it and thus are disappointed.

There are many forms of nonverbal communication. Segal (2008) listed eye contact, facial expression, tone of voice, posture, touch, intensity, timing and pace, and sounds that convey understanding (such as "ahhh," "ummm," and "ohhh") as the most

important nonverbal clues. Probably three of the most important forms of nonverbal communication are proximity, eye contact, and touching.

Another name for proximity is *nearness*. Even in our example of students' leaning in the direction of the speaker if they are interested, they are showing nearness. Most often, however, proximity refers to the face-to-face distances between people. Although

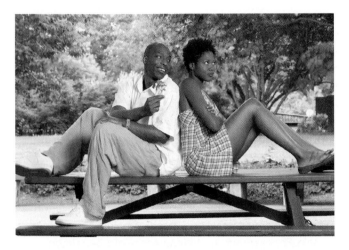

Body position can be a barrier to effective communication.

there are differences, in most cultures moving closer indicates increased interest or intimacy, and moving farther away indicates the opposite.

Making eye contact with another person shows interest. This can be true when one is simply listening to another person; however, making eye contact with another person for a little longer than usual can also be a signal of interest in a relationship.

Touching can be very important in a relationship, and it can show interest, intimacy, and emotional closeness. It can range from a slight touch to show concern or connection to the intimate touching associated with sexual relationships. Touch must be used with caution. For example, if someone you do not know very well touches you, that action could be offensive to you. Also, in social and work situations it is important to be careful in using touch to prevent appearing overly intimate and to avoid giving any suggestion of sexual harassment.

Van Wagner (2009) provides some nonverbal communication tips. Here are a few of them:

1. Pay attention to nonverbal signals. This will help improve communication for both the sender and the receiver.

2. Look for incongruent behaviors. When words don't match up with nonverbal signals, people tend to ignore what is said and

focus instead on nonverbal expressions of moods, thoughts, and emotions.

3. Use good eye contact. Do not stare fixedly into someone's eyes—but note that failing to look others in the eye makes it seem like there is something to hide.

4. Ask questions about nonverbal signals. If there is confusion about a person's nonverbal signals, it can help to ask questions.

5. Be aware that signals can be misread. A person's overall demeanor tells a lot more than a single gesture.

■ Barriers to Effective Sexual Communication

The basic communication model is successful only when the receiver understands the message as intended by the sender. In real life, that is hard to accomplish. Consider all the times that you thought you had delivered a clear message, only to be misunderstood. Most messages reach their destination but are disrupted by communication barriers. The most common barriers to successful communication are bypassing, frame of reference, and lack of language and listening skills (Guffey, 1999). To this list we add mind-altering drugs (which include alcohol). Figure 3.2 summarizes ways that barriers play a part in sexual miscommunication.

Barriers to Communication

Sender has idea	Sender encodes message	Channel carries message	Receiver decodes message
Girl does not want to engage in sexual activities	Girl says, "I don't think we're ready to have sex"	Barriers distort message	Boy hears, "Come on and convince me"

Common Barriers to Sexual Communication

Frame of reference	Male was more sexually experienced.
Language skills	Female may fear situation and not speak directly.
Listening skills	Male heard only what he wanted to hear; he did not listen to the tone of her voice or look for nonverbal communication.
Emotional interference	Ego prompted him to believe that the girl wanted him.
Mind-altering drugs	Alcohol or drugs were likely involved.

FIGURE **3.2** Common barriers to communication.

- *Bypassing:* We all attach meanings to words, but individuals may attach different meanings. Consider the confusion that results if your partner does not want to engage in "sexual relations." You may back off all physical contact. Yet some people—including the former President Bill Clinton—consider sexual relations to refer only to penile–vaginal intercourse. So it is important to understand what meaning your partner attaches to a word.

- *Frame of reference:* Your frame of reference is your unique set of experiences. Your sociocultural upbringing strongly influences your style of communication. A belief in the sexual double standard, in which men pursue women and women "give in" to men, affects the male's frame of reference in our example. For example, the Korean culture often discourages open discussion of feelings and seeking out of psychological counseling. Therefore, a Korean woman might not be comfortable telling her boyfriend that she was afraid she might be pregnant.

- *Lack of language skills:* In a new situation, you may not be prepared to communicate effectively. For example, one partner may fear the situation and not know how to communicate effectively that the other's sexual pursuit is unwelcome.

- *Lack of listening skills:* We often listen selectively and interpret messages to our advantage. In our example, the male heard only what he wanted to hear ("Come on and convince me"). He failed to listen to the tone of his partner's voice or look for nonverbal cues.

- *Mind-altering drugs:* Use of alcohol and drugs creates a powerful barrier to communication. More than half of all date rapes involve alcohol. As your inhibitions and ability to communicate clearly fade, so does your ability to control the situation.

Gender Communication Issues

In a popular magazine, Scheidlower (1997) indicated that communication difficulties between the sexes are related to a lack of vocabulary. Men and women are unable to reach a mutual understanding of certain concepts because they cannot describe them to each other. He compares the reality of situations with the words women use in their language ("she-speak").

Here are two examples (*the authors recognize that these examples are quite sexist, but we include them because many people, unfortunately, believe in these stereotypes*):

- "He-speak": A new car has "331 horsepower, five-speed transmission, V-8, four valves per cylinder, dual overhead cam, and a twin turbocharger." "She-speak": "It's red."

- "He-speak": A new amplifier has "twin mono-blocks, low THD, only 40 watts per channel, but it's a small room, so the low-impedance speakers will still work; it'll be expensive if we blow any Gold Aero KT-88 output tubes." "She-speak": "That thing is not going in *my* living room."

Scheidlower's point is that if we want to have high-quality relationships, we have to make an effort. Whether there is really a difference in vocabulary between the genders is for each of us to decide, but we can also do our part to reduce the possibility of a problem of miscommunication.

Gender roles can strongly shape our communication patterns. Because men have traditionally focused on their place in the hierarchy, they tend to be good at public speaking. Women, who have traditionally focused on nurturing relationships, tend to be better at speaking in private. On the emotional level, women tend to be good at verbalizing thoughts and feelings in close relationships. Men, in contrast, tend to be good at dismissing their feelings or keeping them to themselves. For men, expressing feelings does not help determine their status or help them compete in the outside world. It can be helpful to be aware of the context and the power of gender roles to influence what we hear, what we say, and what is the purpose of our communication (Worden & Worden, 1998).

Do males and females naturally communicate differently, or are their communication behaviors learned just as other behaviors are? Some people believe that males are socialized to be more assertive and direct, in both verbal and nonverbal communication. Eye contact, body placement, and rough physical contact by males can communicate intention, superiority, and territoriality. Historically, women have generally been socialized to have a less pronounced presence. They tend, for example, to listen empathetically, communicate and elicit emotions, and process conflict. As a result, a familiar complaint of women in heterosexual relationships is that male partners "never want to talk about things," "aren't sensitive to their needs," and "just don't understand." Conversely, males often wonder how a seemingly innocuous comment could cause their female partner's sudden silence or desire

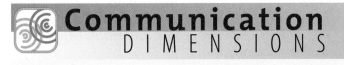

Communication
DIMENSIONS

Adult Sexting In recent years there have been a number of examples of adult sexting—even some that involved prominent politicians, sports stars, and other celebrities. Is adult sexting just a new form of pornography? When is it a harmless way to communicate, and when is it damaging or even dangerous? Is it different for people in their 20s as opposed to older adults? Six experts gave their opinions on some of these questions.

Pepper Schwartz, professor of sociology at the University of Washington, said that adult sexting is a form of flirtation. It is a dangerous flirtation if pictures are being sent that you might not want 200 million people to see, but it can be sexy and playful among mutually consenting adults. If sexting is not performed in the context of a mutually collaborative and intimate relationship, it can feel like an act of sexual aggression. People should have the right to block unwanted pictures and gross messages.

Michelle Drouin, assistant professor of psychology at Indiana University-Purdue University Fort Wayne, indicated that her research with 745 U.S. college students showed that sexting is a popular means of sexual communication within both committed romantic relationships and casual sexual relationships. For those with insecure attachments, sexting may help fulfill relationship needs and demands. This may be especially true for emotionally distant men, who were less likely to call, text, or engage in face-to-face sexual conversations with a partner.

S. Craig Watkins, professor at the University of Texas at Austin, said that he is not convinced that the raunchy behavior online is equivalent to porn. However, sexting certainly reveals how our sexual norms and the expression of our sexual selves are evolving in ways that make all of us vulnerable.

Susan Lipkins, a psychologist in Port Washington, New York, said that for most people sexting is a form of flirting. For some, it is a form of gossip; for others a form of harassment. For those born around 1987 or later, sexting is simply a form of communication. However, for those a little older sexting may have different implications. Adults who sext may be doing so to assert their power within a group or toward a particular person, to increase their popularity, to use their status and enhance it, or to display their aggression. In general, sexters view sexting as harmless and fun, whereas nonsexters see it as dangerous.

Finally, K. Jason Krafsky and Kelli Krafsky, coauthors of *Facebook and Your Marriage*, indicated that there is a double standard that applies to the virtual world and real world, with two different sets of rules, acceptable behavior, and consequences. Making unwanted sexual advances virtually is called "cyberflirting," but in the real world it is sexual harassment. Being sexually active with multiple partners on the Internet is called "virtual sex," but in the real world it is engaging in high-risk and irresponsible behavior. Sending lewd pictures of your private parts online is called "sexting," but in the real world it is a crime called indecent exposure. They point out that we should not buy the lie that we can have dual citizenship in both worlds, breaking the rules in one without consequence in the other.

What do you agree with or disagree with that these six experts have said? What does all of this have to do with communication about sexuality?

Source: Data from Room for debate: A running commentary on the news. What's wrong with adult sexting? *The New York Times* (June 9, 2011). Available: http://www.nytimes.com/roomfordebate/2011/06/09/whats-wrong-with-adult-sexting?nl=todaysheadlines&emc=thab1.

to talk about where the relationship is going. People internalize the values attached to gendered communication to the point that men become used to living within conflict and women prefer the roles of peacemaker and relationship builder. Some people argue that looking at gender exclusively as the source of different communication styles is a mistake and that such elements as upbringing, socioeconomic status, culture, and ethnicity must be considered within this context (Do women and men communicate differently?, 2003).

Reeder (2005) pointed out that research findings regarding communication differences related to gender are simply contradictory. For example, some studies show men to be more assertive, while others find women to be as assertive or even more assertive than men. When it comes to most communication behaviors, such as leadership style, sociability, or displays of power in intimate relationships, Reeder indicated that academic research reveals little to no difference between genders. Mehl et al. (2007) reported further evidence that there may not

Ethical
DIMENSIONS

Ethics, Communication, and Date Rape

One example of potential communication difficulties is sexual behavior on a date. Keeping our basic communication model in mind, let us consider some ethical issues related to communication and date rape.

It has been found that 69% of men and 54% of women believe that some women like to be talked into having sexual intercourse. Because bypassing (misunderstanding that results from a mixed message) can occur if a male believes this, there can be an ethical responsibility for the male or the female to be sure certain messages are accurately interpreted.

Some cultural images of romantic interaction in sexual situations may lead to many ethical questions about date rape. For example, is it part of a dating ritual for a woman to resist a man's initial sexual advances? What is her ethical responsibility to be sure she is sending accurate—and not misleading—messages?

If a woman is drunk or has used other chemical substances that can influence judgment, what is the ethical responsibility of the male in regard to his actions? Should the female have considered the ethics of putting herself (and the male) in that situation in the first place? If she is under the influence of chemical substances, she may send (encode) a message in a way she does not intend.

If a male is drunk or has used other chemical substances that can influence his judgment, the "noise" (see the communication model in Figure 3.2) can interfere with his ability to decode the message being sent accurately. What is his ethical responsibility for accurate communication in this situation?

The feedback being sent is an important part of our communication model. If a woman goes to a man's apartment or invites the man to her apartment for a drink and then participates in heavy petting, do her actions suggest consent? Is it ethical for her to do these things if she has no intent of participating in sexual intercourse? How should she provide accurate feedback so there is accurate communication?

How about if a woman is dressed in revealing clothing? Is it ethical for her to do this if she is not interested in sexual activity? Is it ethical for a man to interpret the wearing of revealing clothing as an invitation for sexual activity?

Date rape may be a result of miscommunication. Following the steps of our basic communication model (sender having an idea, sender encoding the message, message traveling over a channel, receiver decoding the message, and feedback traveling to the sender) and considering how bypassing can occur and how noise can interfere with accurate communication give us many ethical issues related to communication and date rape to consider. Clear communication is needed to help prevent date rape.

Relatedly, what is the prevalence of implied versus verbal consent at first intercourse among U.S. college students? Higgins et al. (2010) found that among those with consensual first intercourse experiences, 49% provided nonverbal consent. Respondents who used condoms at first intercourse were more likely to provide verbal consent, suggesting that condoms may prompt sexual discussion (or vice versa). In contrast, those who provided nonverbal consent were less likely to have used contraception. It seems, then, that college students who do not discuss whether to engage in vaginal intercourse for the first time are less likely to use contraception.

Source: Data from Is there a date rape crisis in society? In *Taking sides: Clashing views on controversial issues in family and personal relationships,* 4th ed., Vail, A., ed. Guilford, CT: Dushkin/McGraw-Hill, 1999; Higgins, J. A., Trussell, J., Moore, N. B., & Davidson, J. K. Sr. The language of love?—Verbal versus implied consent at first heterosexual intercourse: Implications for contraceptive use. *American Journal of Health Education,* 44, no. 4 (July/August 2010), 218–230.

be the gender differences previously thought. They had 396 participants wear voice recorders for several days. It was found that women and men both spoke about 16,000 words per day. Overall, communication research suggests that male–female differences are actually quite small. Gender seems to account for only 1% of the variation in communication behaviors. Other factors play a more significant role, such as the type of relationship and the context within which the communication takes place.

Attitudes About Sexuality

Some people are prevented from communicating openly by attitudes learned at home. Some parents "protect" young children from references to sexuality.

Gender DIMENSIONS

Sexual Behavior in Marriage

Listen to this couple in their mid to late 20s, married 9 years:

Wife: I don't understand him. He's ready to go any time. It's always been a big problem with us right from the beginning. If we've hardly seen each other for two or three days and hardly talked to each other, I can't just jump into bed. If we have a fight, I can't just turn it off. He has a hard time understanding that. I feel like that's all he wants sometimes. I have to know I'm needed and wanted for more than just jumping into bed.

Husband: She complains that all I want from her is sex, and I try to make her understand that it's an expression of love. I'll want to make up with her by making love, but she's as cold as the inside of the fridge. I get mad when that happens. Why shouldn't I? Here I'm trying to make up and make love, and she's holding out for something—I don't know what.

Wife: He keeps saying he wants to make love, but it just doesn't feel like love to me. Sometimes I feel bad that I feel that way, but I just can't help it.

Husband: I don't understand. She says it doesn't feel like love. What does that mean, anyway? What does she think love is?

Wife: I want him to talk to me, to tell me what he's thinking. If we have a fight, I want to talk about it so we could maybe understand it. I don't want to jump in bed and just pretend it didn't happen.

Husband: Talk! Talk! What's there to talk about? I want to make love to her and she says she wants to talk. How's talking going to convince her I'm loving her?

In sexual behavior, as in other matters, the barriers to effective communication are high and the language people use only further confuses and mystifies them. He says he wants to make love, but she says, "It doesn't feel like love." Neither quite knows what the other is talking about; both feel vaguely guilty and uncomfortable, aware only that somehow they're not connecting. He believes that he has already given her a profound declaration of love: He married her and they share a home.

Yet she says, "Just once, I'd like him to love me without it ending up in sex. But when I tell him that, he thinks I'm crazy."

For him, perhaps, it does seem crazy. Sexual activity may be the one way in which he can allow himself the expression of deep feeling. His wife, however, finds it difficult to be comfortable with her feelings in the same area. She keeps asking for something that she can understand and is comfortable with—a demonstration of his feelings in nonsexual ways. He keeps giving her the one thing he can understand and is comfortable with—his feelings wrapped up in a blanket of sex. Thus some husbands and wives find themselves in an impossibly difficult bind, one that stems from the cultural context in which girls and boys grow to adulthood.

We are suggesting that the man's ever-present sexual readiness is not simply an expression of urgent sexual need but is also a complex response to a socialization process that restricts the development of the emotional side of his personality. Conversely, the woman's insistent plea for a nonsexual emotional statement is a response to a process that encourages the development of the emotional side of her personality.

When as teenagers these children are exposed to talk about sexuality—on the street or at school—they often feel guilty for participating in or eavesdropping on such forbidden conversations. When parents fail to acknowledge our sexuality as children, we should not be surprised if suppressed feelings permeate our adult sexual lives.

Some writers suggest that men often do not communicate well with women because they have a "fear of intimacy" that is really a fear of rejection. One way to deal with this is for men to learn to talk about their lives more openly, as women have learned to do. Developing their own friendships with other men can help men acquire personal skills that will also improve their relationships with women (Dickson, 2000).

Parent–Teen Communication

An excellent example of the importance of good communication is that between parents and their children—especially their adolescent children. Karofsky (2001) reported a correlation between the level of adolescent–parent communication, as perceived by the teenager, and abstinence from initiation of sexual intercourse. High levels of communication with mothers were most closely associated with abstinence. The amount of parent–teen communication declined as the teen got older. The authors suggest two possibilities: (1) As communication declined at home, teenagers sought a replacement for intimacy with their parents and then participated in sexual

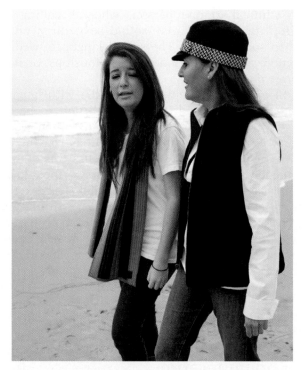

Many teens would welcome communication with their parents about sexuality.

intercourse; or (2) as teenagers became sexually active, they were reluctant to discuss these and other personal issues with their parents, and therefore communication declined.

Dailard (2001) reported that teenagers who feel their parents are warm, caring, and supportive are more likely to delay sexual activity than their peers. Teens who feel highly satisfied with their relationship with their mother are more likely to use contraception and to delay sexual activity and are less likely to have an unplanned pregnancy.

When it comes to communicating with their children about sexuality, many parents consider the task a daunting one, for which they feel ill equipped. Parents often do not have meaningful conversations with sons and daughters because they do not know what to say or how to begin, fearing that talking to children about sexuality may either scare children or encourage them in sexual behaviors at a young age. Most parent–child discussions about sexuality are limited, indirect, and uncomfortable. Yet, parents' failure to provide adolescents with appropriate information and decision-making skills may place teens at risk for negative outcomes such as pregnancy or STI. Only about 15% of adolescents have had conversations about sexuality with their parents. Mothers are more likely than fathers to discuss birth control, adolescent pregnancy, and sexual morality with both sons and daughters (Filomeno, 2002).

Parents and teens also seem to have different estimations of how often they have discussed sexuality (Grunbaum et al., 2004). Forty-two percent of parents said they talked to their teenagers about sexuality and sexual relationships "very often," 43% said they talked "somewhat often," 12% said "not too often," and 2% said "never." In contrast, 11% of teens of those same parents said they talked to their parents about sexuality and sexual relationships "very often," 30% said they talked "somewhat often," 40% said "not too often," and 18% said "never."

Albert (2004) reported that 90% of parents said they did not know how to discuss sexuality with their children. He also pointed out that parents are selling themselves way too short, and that they need to have conversations about sexuality with their children at earlier ages. In fact, 91% of adults and 87% of teens think it would be easier for young people to delay sexual activity and avoid unwanted pregnancy if they could discuss sexuality with their parents.

There are many reasons for good parent–child communication about sexuality. However, the association between parent–child communication and adolescent pregnancy risk remains unclear (Sample lesson plan using JSR, 2005). One difficulty in studying this relationship is that there is little or no agreement between what parents and teens perceive to have communicated between them. Measures of communication content, as well as the frequency, timing, and quality of communication, vary so much across studies that it is hard to establish a pattern of findings.

El-Shaieb and Wurtele (2009) surveyed 214 parents of young children about their plans for sexual discussions with their children. Parents reported being educated mostly by their mothers and rated both of their parents as ineffective educators. Compared to a similar survey of parents conducted over 25 years earlier, these parents intended to discuss sexual abuse at an earlier age, but to delay discussing genital differences, birth, and reproduction. Compared to fathers, mothers intended to discuss sexuality at earlier ages and anticipated this to be more effective. Parents' intentions to discuss varied between sons and daughters for certain topics, and there were two topics (masturbation and nocturnal emissions) many parents did not intend to discuss with their children.

Because many college students eventually decide to become parents, here are some tips about talking with kids about sexuality (Silverberg, 2008). Perhaps the most important one is to make talking with your children about sexuality a lifelong conversation. Instead of just having a "big sex talk," recognize that many small moments of learning and teaching about sexuality happen throughout a child's development. El-Shaieb and Wurtele (2009) indicated that parents need guidance about when and how best to discuss sexual issues with their children. To help them get ready, parents need to: (a) learn about healthy sexual development, (b) consider the influence of their own experiences learning about sexuality, (c) understand the impact of ineffective sexuality education in one generation leading to poor sexuality education in the next, (d) understand the role of demographic influences on their communication styles, and (e) discuss with other parents various dilemmas confronting them in their sexuality education efforts. Also, it is important to be comfortable when it comes to talking about sexuality. Many things, such as reading this book and taking a sexuality class, can greatly help to increase your comfort level with this topic. It is also good to make it OK for your kids to ask about sexuality. All children have such questions, and it helps to create an environment where they feel comfortable asking them. Finally, it is important to use age-appropriate information. A number of excellent resources, such as many of those mentioned throughout this text, are available that can help people understand more about age-appropriate sexuality information.

Sexual Language

One of us was invited to speak with a group of elderly people about sexuality. Proceeding with undaunted courage, he began the session with exercises designed to neutralize the emotional impact of sexual words. He showed slides containing one or two words and instructed the participants to shout in unison the word appearing on the slide. The first slide was shown and the audience shouted *love* with much enthusiasm. Buoyed up by the group's cooperation and interest, he projected the next slide—*hug*. The audience again shook the room with their shouts. From that point on, however, it was all downhill. With each successive word, the decibel level of the voices lowered—no small wonder, considering the remaining words: *kiss, caress, pet, sexual intercourse, oral sex, penis,* and *vagina.* The point was made. Many people are uncomfortable with sexual language. How can sexual communication be effective if we cannot even speak the language?

When discussing sexual topics, people often find that the words themselves prevent rational, thoughtful, comfortable interaction. Some words evoke such strong emotions—embarrassment, guilt, shame, or anger—that they interfere with thoughtful discourse. Generally, the greater the emotion, the greater the interference.

For example, it may be that the term used influences what a partner hears: "Penis," "dick," and "cock" may all have different connotations for different people. Calling a vagina a "vagina" may sound very clinical to one person, whereas calling it a "pussy" or a "cunt" may sound sexy, dirty, or just fine to someone else. The sexual language used can promote communication and relationships, or it can inhibit them.

In addition to being comfortable with language related to sexuality, it is also important to be sure we are talking about the same thing when we use sexual terms. For example, what does "having sex" mean? It can be interesting to discuss this question with college students. Does "having sex" include only penile–vaginal intercourse? Does anal sexual activity count? How about oral sexual activity? Mutual masturbation? Does intense petting and body contact constitute having sex? It is common to hear college students as well as other people refer to "having sex." But to be sure we are communicating clearly we have to be sure we have the same definitions for the terms we are using.

◼ Techniques for Improving Sexual Communication

As we have discussed, there are many reasons for good sexual communication. One of these includes a need to communicate about desires related to sexual activity. Miller and Byers (2004) interviewed 153 heterosexual couples about their actual and ideal duration of foreplay and intercourse, as well as their partners' desired duration of foreplay and intercourse. Both men's and women's perceptions of their partners' ideal duration of foreplay and intercourse were found to be more strongly related to their own sexual stereotypes than to their partners' self-reported sexual desires. This suggested that people rely on sexual stereotypes when estimating their partners' ideal sexual scripts. Improving communication about sexuality could help eliminate such misperceptions. There are no magical methods for attaining free, open, and comfortable communication about sexual topics, but we do have some suggestions.

First, Owen (2008) provides some suggestions to improve the overall atmosphere for communication. She indicates that it is important to realize that one does not know everything. This leads to asking good questions. Also, it helps to ask the right questions. For example, "Is this what you like?" can be a great question that also shows concern about the other person. Being open-minded and nonjudgmental is helpful as well. Maintaining care and trust also leads to better communication. One person is much more likely to open up to another if there is confidence that the information will not be shared with others. Other suggestions for improving communication are found in the following pages.

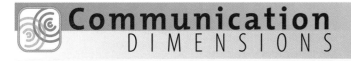
Communication
DIMENSIONS

Clarity in Sexual Communication

In the communication process, the idea sent and the message actually received are ideally the same. But as you likely know from experience, matters do not always work that way. Often, the words chosen, the tone of voice, the body language, or the context in which the message is delivered blurs the true intent of the sender. When you add the ambiguity of sexual language, communicating clearly becomes even more difficult.

Consider former President Bill Clinton and his now-infamous words in a press conference on January 26, 1998: "I did not have sexual relations with that woman—Miss Lewinsky." To President Clinton, "sexual relations" specifically referred to penile–vaginal intercourse, sexual activity in which he and Monica Lewinsky did not participate.

In his own parlance, Clinton was telling the truth. Yet few would agree with him. One reason was the context of the comment—a formal press conference in the White House. Also, the delivery of the comment—with strong body language and tersely delivered words—made it appear that there was no relationship at all between Clinton and Lewinsky.

Now consider how such language ambiguity might affect a newer relationship.

Let us say that you suggest beginning a more "serious relationship" with someone. Your partner responds that the relationship is not ready for "sexual relations." At this point, it is not clear what either party has said. A "serious relationship" could imply having sexual activity, but it could also imply seeing each other more often or not seeing other people. The "sexual relations" comment in the context of an intimate conversation could be construed to refer to any sexual activity.

Thus it is important to be clear in communicating about sexuality with a partner. If you or your partner cannot talk about sexuality, that may be a sign that you are not ready to be involved in a sexual relationship.

A good way to start a conversation is to talk about sexual histories. By starting the conversation and opening it up for participation, you will make it more comfortable for your partner. Talk about sexual activities that you have enjoyed and would like to share with your partner.

Before entering into a sexual relationship, you should talk about any STIs that you or a partner may have had, and any STI and/or HIV testing you have had (and why you had it done). In addition, you should discuss using latex condoms to prevent STI transmission as well as using a contraceptive method to prevent pregnancy.

Planning

One common barrier to good sexual communication is the complete avoidance of the subject by both partners. We suggest that partners set aside time to discuss sexuality as they would any other topic of mutual interest and of significance to their relationship. In setting up a time for such a discussion, it is wise to make the following plans.

1. Make sure you have plenty of time for your discussion. Do not be cut short when one of you has to run off somewhere.

2. Do not allow others to interrupt your discussion by calling you or by barging in on you.

3. Accept all feelings and the right to express these feelings verbally. For example, it is just as appropriate to say, "I feel angry when …" as it is to say, "I feel terrific when …"

4. Take a risk—really describe your thoughts and needs. Do not expect your partner to guess what they are.

5. Approach the discussion with both people understanding that the goal is to improve your relationship rather than to see who can shock whom.

6. Expect changes but not miracles. Sexual communication requires continued dialogue. You might want to seek the help of other family members, friends, peer counselors, members of the clergy, psychologists, sexuality counselors, or others who can contribute to your ability to communicate sexually.

Working to improve your sexual communication will help you and your partner develop a deeper trust, a greater sense of intimacy, and a feeling of adventure about your relationship.

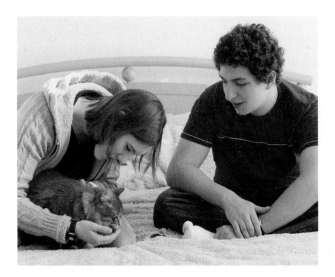

It can take work to have good sexual communication.

Flooding

A technique for learning to use and become comfortable with sexual language is called **flooding**. In one use of this technique, people stand in front of a mirror, look themselves in the eye, and repeat over and over again the words they feel uncomfortable using.

> **flooding**
> Experiencing something so frequently that you no longer are aroused by it. This is a technique used to become more comfortable with sexual terminology.

We are not necessarily referring to profanity. We are talking about sexual language. Learning to feel comfortable with these words and being able to use them should be your goals.

Learning Assertiveness

Some people just have a tough time communicating—period. Inevitably they have trouble communicating sexually. When this is the case, working to improve only the sexual side of communication is a mistake. Therefore, we turn now to a topic that concerns one's ability to express oneself with confidence in all areas—the quality of assertiveness and the means to develop it.

The first step toward grasping what it means to be assertive is to distinguish assertive, aggressive, and nonassertive behaviors. **Assertiveness** means standing up for your basic rights *without violating* anyone else's. **Aggressiveness** means standing up for your basic

> **assertiveness**
> Standing up for one's basic rights without violating anyone else's rights.
>
> **aggressiveness**
> Standing up for one's basic rights, but at the expense of someone else's basic rights.

rights (or more) *at the expense* of someone else's rights. **Nonassertiveness** means *giving up* your basic rights so that other people can achieve theirs.

> **nonassertiveness**
> Giving up one's basic rights so others may achieve theirs.

For example, an assertive style of verbal sexual communication would be one in which you stand up for your own sexual rights and needs by expressing your wishes, while allowing your partner the same freedom.

Body language, too, can be aggressive, nonassertive, or assertive. Aggressive body language includes a pointing finger, leaning toward the other person, glaring, and using a loud, angry tone of voice. Nonassertive body language is characterized by slumped posture, a lack of eye contact, handwringing, hesitant speech, nervous whining or laughing, and not saying or doing what you want to. Assertive behavior, by contrast, entails sitting or standing tall, looking directly at the person you are talking to, speaking in explicit statements with a steady voice, and using the gestures or physical contact that is right for you.

As a first step toward learning to be assertive, consider this formula, developed by Bower and Bower (1976), for organizing assertive verbal responses. The formula, which they call DESC, involves

1. **D**escribing the other person's behavior or the situation as objectively as possible (as in sentences taking the form "When you...")

2. **E**xpressing your feelings about the other person's behavior or the situation that you just described (as in statements beginning with "I feel...")

3. **S**pecifying changes you would like to see made ("I would like..." or "My preference is...")

4. **C**hoosing the consequences you are prepared to accept (a) if the situation changes to your satisfaction and (b) if it does not ("If you..., I will..." or "If you don't..., I will...")

Using the DESC form, then, let us look at an example of assertive sexual communication: "When you expect me to become sexually aroused in two minutes of foreplay (Describe), I feel as though I'm being used (Express). I would like us to spend more time touching, kissing, and hugging (Specify). If you agree to devote more time to foreplay, I will relax and pay special attention to your sexual needs. If you don't agree to devote more time to foreplay, I won't have intercourse with you (Choose)." Note that our imaginary speaker describes the situation from a personal point of view, expressing his or her own feelings and preferences, as well as the consequences of the listener's choice.

The form of the DESC message just described suggests the philosophical basis of the assertion theory: We are in control of ourselves alone; we have no right to tell others how to behave; we need not tolerate the other person's behavior when it is contrary to our own desires. The basis of assertive behavior is the combination of self-respect with respect for others. One could find no better formula for effective sexual communication.

Expressing Yourself Nonverbally

Words are important, but they do not say it all. Do not be afraid to smile, wink, hug, touch, kiss, or in other ways communicate your affection for another. As we said earlier, in the way you walk, sit, gesture, and so on, you are "talking" to your partner, whether you intend to or not. But you can also consciously use those gestures to help get your message across.

Seeking Information (Listening)

Verify your interpretation of the other person's verbal, and especially nonverbal, communication. Listen actively, and ask whether your understanding of your partner's feelings and intentions is accurate. Listening is often hard and takes real skill. If you want to hear what others say effectively, make sure you are not a

- *Mind reader:* You hear little or nothing as you think, "What is this person really thinking or feeling?"

- *Rehearser:* Your mental tryouts for "Here's what I'll say next" tune out the speaker.

- *Filterer:* Some call this selective listening—hearing only what you want to hear.

- *Dreamer:* Drifting off during a face-to-face conversation can lead to an embarrassing "What did you say?" or "Could you repeat that?"

- *Identifier:* If you refer everything you hear to your experience, you probably did not hear what was said.

- *Comparer:* When you get side-tracked assessing the messenger, you are sure to miss the message.

- *Derailer:* Changing the subject too quickly tells others you are not interested in anything they have to say.

- *Sparrer:* You hear what is said but quickly belittle it or discount it. That puts you in the same class as the derailer.

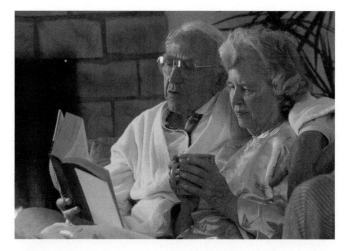

Sitting close together, touching, and smiling are all ways to show you care. Nonverbal communication is important; expressing feelings in words is also vital.

- *Placater:* Agreeing with everything you hear just to be nice or to prevent conflict does not make you a good listener (Why don't we hear others?, 2005).

The leadership expert Stephen Covey speaks of "attentive" and "empathetic" listening—not the fake or manipulative kind but rather "listening with the intent to understand." Covey speaks and writes about situations related to business; however, the basics of good listening skills apply to intimate relationships as well. Good listeners are rare; most of us have to squelch our natural inclination to talk.

The characteristics of good listeners are as follows:

1. The most visible characteristic is body language—nodding encouragingly, perhaps leaning into the conversation, not glancing around the room or looking for something.

2. Good listeners demonstrate that they are mentally engaged in what the speaker is saying by making brief comments from time to time and asking focused questions—patiently waiting for the answer before providing one.

3. They listen with the "third ear," seeking to understand those thoughts that are not expressed.

4. They try to understand, rather than first being understood. They try to see the topic of conversation from the speaker's standpoint first. Good listeners push back the urge to express personal opinions until they are asked or until the time is appropriate.

5. Good listeners have to be trusted. They never repeat confidences and personal problems without consent of the party involved (Listening to understand, 1998).

Global
DIMENSIONS

International Differences in Discussing Sexuality

International differences exist related to the topic of human sexuality. One way to gain an understanding of these differences is to consider how sexuality education is viewed in some countries. Here are some examples.

1. In Mexico, it is the government's policy to stabilize growth. Family planning is supposed to be implemented by means of education and public services. At the same time, the conservative Catholic church opposes sexuality education.

2. In Chile, sexuality is not a subject that is talked about by family members or in schools.

3. In China, there is virtually no institutional sexuality education. People rely on folklore, sexually explicit materials, and approved marriage manuals for sexuality information.

4. In Denmark, sexuality and social-life education has been a compulsory subject in schools since 1970, and it was a tradition long before then.

5. In Egypt, discussion of sexuality is socially unacceptable. Egypt uses an approach that emphasizes repression rather than education.

6. In Greece, sexuality education does not exist in the school curriculum. Greece is one of the few European countries without sexuality education.

7. In India, sexuality education is not offered in schools because society believes it would "spoil the minds" of children.

8. In Iran, to get a marriage license, couples must take a segregated course in family planning.

9. In Japan, sexuality education in schools (typically focused on reproductive issues) is mandated, beginning at age 10 or 11 years. The Ministry of Education believes that teachers should teach HIV and AIDS prevention to students without mentioning sexual intercourse.

10. In Kenya, the government opposes sexuality education in schools. Young people turn to their peers for sexuality information.

11. In Romania, sexuality education was removed from the schools in the early 1980s. The major sources of contraception and sexuality information are friends, mass media, and healthcare providers.

12. In Singapore, women are highly ignorant about their bodies, including being unable to locate the vagina. Women complain also of pain during intercourse because of lack of foreplay. Some women who believe they are barren actually turn out to be virgins.

13. In Sweden, sexuality education has been a compulsory subject in schools since 1955. It is well integrated into the school curriculum. In addition, Swedish children receive their first sexuality education at home, from their parents.

14. In Thailand, there are strong taboos surrounding the discussion of sexuality and disease. HIV/AIDS education has been stifled, and many do not know how the disease is spread.

15. In the United Kingdom, sexuality education has been required in secondary schools since 1993. In Northern Ireland, it is not mandated, but it is encouraged in the teaching of health education. In Scotland, jurisdiction over the provision of sexuality education lies with the local education authority. In general, teens report that they believe their parents should be their main source of sexuality information; however, in practice they are more likely to turn to their friends for information.

Although it is difficult to draw definite conclusions from this information, it appears that there can be real differences in the ability of people from various countries to engage in effective communication about human sexuality. For example, think about the differences that are likely to exist between people from Sweden and those from Thailand or from Egypt. Of course, we cannot generalize about all people from any country, because many differences are possible within countries. But these differences can strongly influence communication about sexuality.

Source: Data from Carson, S. L. *Cross-cultural perspectives on human sexuality.* Boston: Allyn & Bacon, 1998.

Hostile settings and other communication hindrances can defeat even the best listeners. Here are a few steps to avoid those pitfalls:

1. Choose the physical environment. Find a quiet, nonthreatening place to talk if you want to ensure true understanding.

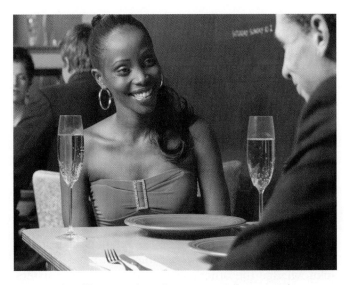

Good listeners show they are mentally engaged.

2. Cut the interruptions. It can be difficult to communicate if the phone rings or if a person pops in at the door.

3. Recognize differences. People communicate best in different ways. Some of us are primarily auditory, whereas others are visual or "hands-on."

4. Persist. Refuse to believe that you cannot understand another person's message.

Steps Toward Change

Counselors often work with couples to help them improve their communication skills. In summary, the counselor (1) encourages **active listening**; (2) elicits feedback from each partner by asking each to summarize what he or she just heard; (3) facilitates the expression of feelings and thoughts directly and succinctly; (4) requests the use of **"I" statements** (beginning each sentence with "I" to express personal feelings better and avoid blaming the other partner) instead of questions; and (5) prohibits interruptions and blaming (Worden & Worden, 1998). These techniques will help all of us communicate much more effectively.

> **active listening**
> Paraphrasing what someone has said to demonstrate interest and understanding.
>
> **"I" statement**
> Statement that begins with an "I" to express personal feelings.

Resolving Conflicts

In relationships—even the best of relationships—conflicts arise. Too often poor communication skills (such as improper listening), a combative or offensive stance geared toward winning rather than communicating, an inability to acknowledge another's point, or a refusal to consider alternative solutions interferes with the healthy resolution of these conflicts. As a result, conflicts threaten the continuation of the relationship and, at the least, tear little pieces from it, potentially leaving the relationship bankrupt. To gain a sense of how these poor communication skills impair effective conflict resolution, consider the following dialogue.

> Paul: *Well, Barbara, as you know, I really care for you, and I hope we can continue to develop our relationship. We can't go any further tonight, though, because I'd like you to be tested for HIV.*
> Barbara: *Now you ask—right in the middle of this romantic time! Why didn't you say something about this before?*
> Paul: *You've got some nerve. You should have realized this is something we need to consider.*
> Barbara: *I should have realized? How was I supposed to know you were concerned about HIV status? You never said anything about it.*
> Paul: *Why should I take the chance of getting HIV? You're pretty selfish, aren't you?*
> Barbara: *I've had it! Either we're going to trust each other and move ahead in our relationship or you can say good-bye right now.*
> Paul: *In that case, GOOD-BYE!*

In this example, both Paul and Barbara are trying to win: Paul wants Barbara to have an HIV test, and Barbara wants Paul to have faith and move ahead with their relationship. Neither Paul nor Barbara can possibly win this battle, although they are probably unaware of this. If they proceed with their relationship (including sexual intercourse and other intimate behaviors), Paul will be uneasy because of his concern about HIV. He will probably feel his concerns are not very important to Barbara, will resent her lack of concern, and will have a difficult time participating freely in the relationship.

However, if Barbara agrees to the HIV test, she will feel that Paul did not trust her and "forced" her to take the test. She may also feel he waited to spring the idea on her and wonder why it did not arise earlier.

It becomes evident, then, that regardless of which way they go, one or the other will be resentful. This resentment will probably result in a weakening, or possibly a dissolution, of their relationship. So, no matter who wins, both really lose.

This situation is not totally hopeless, though. Consider the effect on resolving their conflict if Paul and Barbara had communicated as follows:

Paul: *Well, Barbara, as you know, I really care for you, and I hope we can continue to develop our relationship. We can't go any further tonight, though, because I'd like you to be tested for HIV.*

Barbara: *Now you ask—right in the middle of this romantic time! Why didn't you say something about this before?*

Paul: *You feel we should have discussed this earlier?*

Barbara: *Yes, and HIV status is something we both need to be concerned about.*

Paul: *You have a concern about my HIV status, too?*

Barbara: *You bet! And I think it is only fair that we treat ourselves and each other equally in this situation.*

Paul: *You think that it would be a problem if you got the HIV test and I didn't?*

Barbara: *Yes.*

Paul: *Would you be embarrassed if other people knew you had taken the test?*

Barbara: *Yes, I guess I would.*

Paul: *It sounds like my request might have hurt you at least a little?*

Barbara: *Yes, I guess it did.*

Paul: *I'm glad that you also care about our relationship. But HIV is really a serious health problem today, and I am worried about it. And I'm bothered that you didn't understand my concern.*

Barbara: *I guess you do have a reason to be concerned. I'm sorry.*

Paul: *Well, let's see what alternatives we have.*

Barbara: *Maybe I should just go ahead and be tested.*

Paul: *Or perhaps we should both be tested.*

Barbara: *How about agreeing that we will honestly share the results with each other but also that the results are private and not anyone else's business?*

Paul: *That's fine with me. In fact, we don't even need to tell anyone else we took the tests. That is our private matter.*

Barbara: *Would it make sense to agree to take the tests as soon as possible so we both know the results as soon as we can?*

Paul: *That seems sensible, and since your schedule in the next couple of weeks is so busy, I'll be happy to work around your schedule.*

Barbara: *Okay. Remember, though, the next time either of us has concerns or suggestions we need to bring them up as early as possible.*

In this example, Paul took the initiative in resolving his interpersonal conflict with Barbara. He began by employing a technique known as *active listening,* or *reflective listening.* The key to this technique is that the listener paraphrases the words of the speaker to indicate that he or she comprehends the meaning of the speaker's message. The listener tries to pick up on hidden messages and feelings not actually verbalized and paraphrases those as well. For example, Paul understood that Barbara would be embarrassed if other people knew she had taken the test, even though she never explicitly stated that. When Paul was able to understand and listen so well to Barbara—well enough to identify feelings she had not verbalized—Barbara was convinced that Paul cared enough to understand her needs. *Then* Barbara was ready to hear about Paul's needs and became more receptive to his viewpoint. Paul next expressed his opinion and the reasons for his feelings. The point of reflective listening is to enable each participant to acknowledge the other's view and to be less insistent in arguing for his or her own.

The next step in this technique is to propose as many alternative solutions as possible through brainstorming. The result is a win–win, rather than a no–win, situation, reached through a mutual agreement that it is possible to agree. Paul agrees that they both will be tested and that they will treat the testing and the results confidentially. He also shows respect for Barbara's busy schedule and says he is willing to work around it.

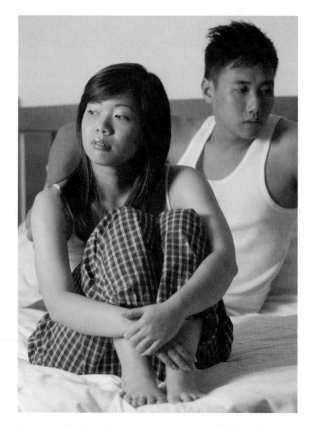

Communication about HIV status can be difficult, but it is very important.

Myth vs Fact

Myth: For most people, good communication comes naturally.
Fact: Although some people may seem to be naturally better than others at communication, good communication is a lot of work for almost everyone.

Myth: Because sexuality is such an open topic today, most people can discuss it rather easily.
Fact: Even though sexuality seems more open, many people still experience much difficulty in talking about sexual topics and personal relationships.

Myth: Communication skills are basically the same in all cultures.
Fact: Although most skills may be quite similar, communicating with people from another culture can be challenging. Even though the language may be the same, communication methods and meanings may greatly differ.

Myth: Because men and women now have the same rights and are equal, they communicate in the same ways.

Fact: Conditions can be slow to change. Even though men and women have equal rights, we still need to be sensitive to differences in learning and motivation related to communication.

Myth: The most important part of communication is the meaning of the words we use.
Fact: It has often been said that "actions speak louder than words." It is also true that nonverbal communication is often more important, and revealing, than words used.

Myth: It is a bad idea to take a risk when trying to communicate with another person. The technique may backfire.
Fact: There are risks in most things we do, and developing and using good communication skills can involve disclosing personal feelings and desires. In a trusting relationship, this should not be too risky.

In addition, Paul and Barbara have improved their relationship *because* of this conflict. The conflict instigates a discussion about their needs and, therefore, provides the opportunity for them to demonstrate their feelings for each other by organizing to satisfy those needs. Instead of threatening the relationship, the conflict has actually improved it.

To reiterate, the steps in this conflict resolution process are as follows:

1. *Active listening:* Reflecting to the other person his or her own words and feelings.

2. *Identifying your position:* Stating your own thoughts and feelings about the situation, and explaining why you feel this way.

3. *Proposing and exploring alternative solutions:* First brainstorming and then evaluating the possibilities.

Although you may feel awkward using this technique initially, and your conversations may seem stilted, with practice it will become a part of your style and will be very effective. The payoffs are huge; do not give up on it.

A similar way to resolve conflict involves four steps (Resolve conflict in four steps, 1995): (1) *Identify the interests* of each person. Ask each person, "What do you want?" Then listen carefully to the answers. (2) *Identify higher levels of interest* by asking, "What does having that do for you?" It is important to understand what each of us really wants. (3) *Create an agreement frame* by asking, "If I could show you how to get X, would you do Y?" X is the person's real interest, and Y is what you want from the person. (4) *Brainstorm for solutions.* Do not just give a solution and expect the other person to accept it. Commitment results from being involved in finding a solution. The solutions must satisfy the interests of all parties.

Giving and Receiving Criticism

Imagine a "sex critic" planned to evaluate your sexual functioning as a movie critic critiques movies! All of us would probably feel threatened, and because of that, our abilities to function normally would most likely be compromised. Well, in a very real sense, our sexual partners are our sex critics. They evaluate what we do in terms of how pleasing it is for both them and us. It would be nice if we could receive our "sex critique" without feeling threatened by it, without feeling that it denigrated our self-esteem. It would also be nice if we were open enough both to give and to receive feedback about our sexual functioning in a way that enhanced our sexual lives and those of our partners. Well, we can learn both to receive and to give criticism in a way that is truly constructive. Here are a few hints:

1. Find a private, relaxing place to discuss thoughts and feelings about your sexual relationship. You do not want to feel uncomfortable in your environment while discussing such a sensitive topic. Feeling uncomfortable will not be conducive to either receiving or giving feedback on such a sensitive issue.

2. Devote sufficient time to such a discussion. It would be unfortunate if you were beginning to communicate well on significant matters just as one of you had to leave.

3. Limit distractions so that your attention is focused on the conversation. Rather than wondering who might overhear you or who might inadvertently hit you in the head with a Frisbee, find a quiet, private place for your discussion.

4. It is probably not wise to do these things just before or just after a sexual encounter. Plan a relaxed time for this discussion.

Communication
D I M E N S I O N S

Guidelines for Healthy Sexual Communication

A great source of information about sexual communication is Healthy Sex.com. Wendy and Larry Maltz provide insights related to many aspects of sexuality. They provide 15 communication guidelines for healthy sexual communication. In addition to the points already mentioned in this chapter, they include the following points directly related to sexuality:

- Both partners need to make a commitment to engage in a discussion about intimate concerns.
- When discussing sexual intimacy concerns, keep in mind that partners are apt to feel scared, embarrassed, or hurt. Emphasize what you like and what works well before making a new request or discussing something that bothers you.
- See intimate problems as a normal and natural part of a relationship. Turn them into opportunities to learn and grow as a couple.
- Seek professional help when needed. Don't allow unresolved sexual issues to fester and erode your positive feelings for each other.

Source: Data from Maltz, W., & Maltz, M. Communication guidelines for healthy sex. Healthy Sex.com. Available: http://www.healthysex.com/page/communication-guidelines/.

In addition to these general suggestions, when *giving criticism* try to remember to

1. Begin your comments on a positive note. "You know, when you kiss me I really feel great." Then move to the behavior you would like to change. "I enjoy your touches so much that it would be terrific if you could ...."

2. Be specific regarding the change you are recommending. Rather than announcing, "You don't hold me enough," suggest, "When we watch television, I'd really like it if you would put your arm around me."

3. Be aware of the limitations of your partner. Do not expect more than your partner is able to give. To critique something that cannot or will not be changed may harm the relationship. If your partner is slow to arouse, asking him or her to speed up is unrealistic and, we might add, unfair. It is criticism given for no useful purpose.

When *receiving criticism* try to remember to

1. Separate your partner's suggestions and recommendations from your self-worth. You are no less of a person because you might need to adjust some of your sexual behavior. In fact, if you were not open to suggestion, then you might suspect you have a problem.

2. Assume a nondefensive attitude. Rather than attempting to justify your present actions, ask questions to understand the criticism better. Then, if you disagree, you will know why you disagree.

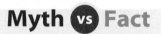

Myth vs Fact

Myth: Being assertive means standing up for your basic rights at the expense of someone else's rights.
Fact: Being aggressive is standing up for your basic rights at the expense of someone else's. Being assertive means standing up for your basic rights without violating anyone else's.

Myth: Conflicts will always get in the way of good relationships.
Fact: It is true that conflicts are a part of life, but if we learn how to deal with them effectively they can help us grow and have better relationships.

3. If the criticism is too general, ask for specific suggestions to help you make the recommended change. In addition, inquire as to how your partner can help make this change more likely to occur. Ask your partner to participate in remedying the situation or action being criticized.

4. Whether or not you agree with the criticism, thank your partner for being honest enough to express the concern to you. Acknowledge that it is not easy to discuss such matters and you appreciate the opportunity to consider something you have been doing or not been doing that is causing a problem. Encourage future suggestions that have the potential to improve your relationship.

With these recommendations for giving and receiving criticism, your relationship should improve. That is because not only will the specific suggestions lead to actual changes, but the practice of opening up your relationship to discussions of problems will, in itself, help foster a style of communicating that will serve you well in all aspects of your relationship. It will then be easier to discuss matters that bother you, and it will be easier to express emotions such as love, caring, and wonderment. The relationship will improve with this style of communication.

When trying to communicate effectively, it can be helpful to have some ground rules. Silverberg (2009) suggests that talking with a partner about these rules can help in developing your own set of rules. Here are some examples:

1. Check in and check out. At the beginning of the conversation, spend a minute talking about your day and how you are feeling so you know what each person is bringing into the conversation. It can also help to take a minute at the end of the conversation to say how it went.

2. Define safety for yourselves and to each other. Discuss what is needed to feel safe so partners can talk honestly and openly.

3. Listen without interrupting. This can be a hard rule to follow, but it is a very important one.

4. Respect differences in interests and desires. If one person exposes personal information, the other person should consider that a compliment, even if the desire is not something he or she is interested in doing.

5. Bring a sense of goodwill to the conversation. Neither partner should be trying to intentionally hurt the other or be mean to the other.

6. Anyone can call time-out at any time. To have a safe conversation, partners need to feel they can stop the conversation at any time. This doesn't mean that one partner should storm out in the middle of a sentence, but rather that either partner can ask for a time-out to end the conversation at that time with the agreement to pick it up at a later point.

Final Thoughts on Sexual Communication

In this chapter we have discussed the importance of word meanings, nonverbal communication, cultural and personal backgrounds, and attitudes toward communication about sexuality. We have also seen that there are many ways to improve our ability to communicate significantly but that doing so usually takes a great deal of effort.

At the same time, however, to be effective, communication must be truthful. In practice, this is often not the case. For example, lying is common in relationships involving college students (Saxe, 1991). The majority of these lies (41%) were about relations with other partners. In another study, respondents said they did not regard their lies as serious, did not plan them, and did not worry about getting caught. They averaged about two lies each day (DePaulo et al., 1996).

Communication difficulties may even increase the level of risk—especially for females. Rickert and associates (2002) reported that about 20% of women believe they never have the right to stop foreplay, including at the point of intercourse; refuse to have sexual intercourse, even if they have had intercourse with that partner before; make their own decisions about contraception, regardless of their partner's wishes; ask their partner whether he has been examined for STIs; or tell their partner that they want to make love differently or that he is being too rough. Moreover, more than 40% of young women believe that they never have or only sometimes have the right to tell a relative they are not comfortable with being hugged or kissed in certain ways. These findings show that some young women may be unable to communicate their sexual beliefs and desires clearly and are therefore at risk for undesired outcomes.

Finally, it is interesting to note what a number of leading sexologists have said about communication. They were asked to relate the most important information they had learned about sexuality over the years. Here are some of the ideas they expressed about communication (Haffner & Schwartz, 1998):

1. It is hard to be honest about past sexual experiences with a new partner.

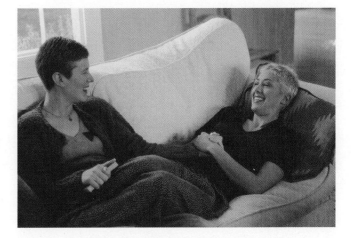

Appropriately giving and receiving criticism will enhance communication in a relationship.

2. Some sexual secrets—unless they pose a health threat—are better left unshared.

3. Nonverbal communication often works better than words in bed.

4. Talking during sexual activity—sharing fantasies, using forbidden words—can be very sexy.

5. Couples who have nothing to say to each other in restaurants are usually married—and they may be in trouble.

6. Open, honest communication is the most important foundation for a relationship.

7. You cannot underestimate the value of humor.

8. After humor, consideration is the second most important ingredient in a sexual relationship. Most people appreciate a sensitive and thoughtful partner.

9. Most people are not comfortable talking about sexual issues.

10. Consent requires communication.

11. It is better to talk about sexual feelings, desires, and boundaries in relationships.

12. Talking about scenes in movies or books can sometimes be a good way to communicate what you like in sexual behavior and relationships.

Exploring the Dimensions of Human Sexuality

Our feelings, attitudes, and beliefs regarding sexuality are influenced by our internal and external environments. Go to go.jblearning.com/dimensions5e to learn more about the biological, psychological, and sociological factors that affect your sexuality.

Case Study

Your ability to communicate sexually plays an important role in your sexual wellness and self-image. Your capacity to discuss sexual histories, contraceptives, and safer sexual activities can help prevent unwanted pregnancy and transmission of STIs and HIV.

From a psychological standpoint, a positive self-image as a communicator gives you confidence. A negative self-image may hinder your ability to ask for dates, to ask for sexual activities that you like, or to ask for safer sexual activities.

Sexual communication is influenced by virtually all social and cultural phenomena, including religion, ethnic heritage, language, family traditions, peers, geographical region, and even mass media.

Gender plays a pervasive role: Men and women communicate in different styles and express emotions differently.

Consider the confusion of sexual language: If your partner suggested that you were not close enough to engage in "sexual relations," you might back off any type of physical contact. It is important to talk with your partner to make sure each of you understands what the other wants.

Biological Factors

- Physiological reactions—such as blushing or erections—are nonverbal means of communicating sexual attraction.
- Alcohol or drugs can distort the communication process.
- Physical touching can indicate interest, intimacy, and emotional closeness.
- Hearing loss over time can inhibit communication and frustrate a partner.

Sociocultural Factors

- Media strongly influence sexual communication.
- Gender affects style of communication.
- Sexuality education may increase confidence.
- Cultures influence communication style.
- Religion may influence the sexual activities in which one participates.
- Family and peers set an example of sexuality.

Psychological Factors

- Emotions can overwhelm the ability to communicate.
- The role of the double standard in thinking may alter the communication process.
- Ego may get in the way of listening to a partner.
- Self-image and body image may distort communication.

Summary

- The process of communication consists of having an idea, the sender encoding a message, sending the message over a channel, the receiver decoding a message, and the receiver providing feedback.

- Nonverbal communication includes all unwritten and unspoken messages. It is a very important part of effective communication, but it can also be easy to misinterpret.

- Barriers to communication include bypassing, the frame of reference, lack of language skills, lack of listening skills, and use of mind-altering drugs.

- There are many things that parents can do to improve communication about sexuality with their children, including making conversations about sexuality ongoing, knowing individual comfort levels, and making it acceptable for children to ask about sexuality.

- Communication can be improved by planning, using flooding, learning assertiveness, using effective nonverbal communication, and using good listening skills.

- Counselors often help people improve their communication skills by encouraging active listening, eliciting feedback from each partner, facilitating the expression of thoughts directly, using "I" statements, and not allowing interruptions and blaming.

- It can be helpful to establish ground rules to help promote good sexual communication. Examples include listening without interruption and respecting differences in desires and interests.

Discussion Questions

1. Describe the steps of the communication process. Explain how they would work in discussing specific relationship or sexuality issues.

2. What are the barriers to effective sexual communication? How can they be overcome?

3. How can you improve your communication abilities? Which techniques would work best for you? Which would not work for you? Explain why.

Application Questions

Reread the chapter-opening story and answer the following questions.

1. If you were teaching this course, and Joanna and Mark were students, what information would you want them to leave with from your course?

2. The changes in communication style across the life cycle of the relationship can enhance or harm it. For example, anticipating what your partner wants can lead to a strengthened relationship, but it can also lead to deterioration of communication. What could Joanna and Mark have done to maintain interest in their relationship? (You may want to think about what successful couples you know do to stay happy.)

Critical Thinking Questions

1. Should sexual partners communicate all they think and feel so that they can better respond to each other's needs? Or should sexual partners be selective in relating their innermost thoughts and feelings? Explain why or why not. Would your opinion change from situation to situation?

2. You are excited about an upcoming first date when you overhear a conversation describing your date as someone who has had many sexual partners in the past. You have no idea whether the information is correct. Later, on your date, your partner implies a willingness to engage in sexual activity. Although you like the person and are sexually attracted, you are unable to forget what you overheard. How can you open the discussion of sexual histories without offending your date?

3. On the last episode of MTV's *Road Rules Latin America*, all five of the campers (three males and two females) climb naked into a Jacuzzi as a final "gathering of friends." In real life, if you climbed naked into a Jacuzzi with some "close friends," what kind of sexual message might that be sending? What if you climbed into the Jacuzzi with just one other person whom you wanted to get to know better?

Critical Thinking Case

The following is a true date-rape case that occurred at Georgetown University years ago. Kim and Mark (names changed) decided to go to the senior black-tie dance together. Both had agreed beforehand that it would not be a "real date." But during the long evening of drinking and dancing, their plans changed.

They met at 8:30 and went to two parties, the dance, and a bar before returning to Mark's apartment at about 4:00 A.M. Kim had lost her key and had agreed to go back to his apartment. "I decided I wouldn't mind kissing him." They kissed, undressed, and climbed into his bed. Kim said later that she had frequently shared a bed with her previous boyfriend without having sexual intercourse and assumed she could do the same with Mark. When Mark asked whether he should get a condom, Kim said they did not know each other well enough to have sex. At that point, the stories diverge.

Kim said she told Mark, "I've never had sex before, and I don't want to have it on a whim." Then, "all of a sudden, he was on top of me, forcing himself into [me].... I kept trying to push him off with my hands and squirming around, and I kept saying I didn't want to have sex."

Mark said in an affidavit that she was "kissing me and thrusting her pelvis against me.... At no time during our sexual activity did I use any kind of physical force against Kim. Nor did I threaten Kim verbally."

How could communication have gone so awry? Consider the dimensions of human sexuality as you explain what went wrong. Then describe what could have been done to prevent the incident.

Exploring Personal Dimensions

Measure Your Assertiveness
Indicate how characteristic or descriptive each of the following statements is of you by using the code given.

+3 very characteristic of me, extremely descriptive

+2 rather characteristic of me, quite descriptive

+1 somewhat characteristic of me, slightly descriptive

–1 somewhat uncharacteristic of me, slightly nondescriptive

–2 rather uncharacteristic of me, quite nondescriptive

–3 very uncharacteristic of me, extremely nondescriptive

_____ 1. Most people seem to be more aggressive and assertive than I am.

_____ 2. I have hesitated to make or accept dates because of "shyness."

_____ 3. When the food served at a restaurant is not done to my satisfaction, I complain about it to the waiter or waitress.

_____ 4. I am careful to avoid hurting other people's feelings, even when I feel that I have been injured.

_____ 5. If a salesperson has gone to considerable trouble to show me merchandise that is not quite suitable, I have a difficult time saying no.

_____ 6. When I am asked to do something, I insist upon knowing why.

_____ 7. There are times when I look for a good, vigorous argument.

_____ 8. I strive to get ahead as well as most people do.

_____ 9. To be honest, people often take advantage of me.

_____10. I enjoy starting conversations with new acquaintances and strangers.

_____11. I often don't know what to say to attractive persons of the opposite sex.

_____12. I will hesitate to make phone calls to business establishments and institutions.

_____13. I would rather apply for a job or for admission to a college by writing letters than by going through personal interviews.

_____14. I find it embarrassing to return merchandise.

_____15. If a close and respected relative were annoying me, I would smother my feelings rather than express my annoyance.

_____16. I have avoided asking questions for fear of sounding stupid.

_____17. During an argument I am sometimes afraid that I will get so upset that I will shake all over.

_____18. If a famed and respected lecturer makes a statement that I think is incorrect, I will have the audience hear my point of view as well.

_____19. I avoid arguing over prices with clerks and salespeople.

_____20. When I have done something important or worthwhile, I manage to let others know about it.

_____21. I am open and frank about my feelings.

_____22. If someone has been spreading false and bad stories about me, I see him or her as soon as possible to "have a talk" about it.

_____23. I often have a hard time saying "no."

_____24. I tend to bottle up my emotions rather than make a scene.

_____25. I complain about poor service in a restaurant and elsewhere.

_____26. When I am given a compliment, I sometimes just don't know what to say.

_____27. If a couple near me in a theater or at a lecture were conversing rather loudly, I would ask them to be quiet or to take their conversation elsewhere.

_____28. Anyone attempting to push ahead of me in a line is in for a good battle.

_____29. I am quick to express an opinion.

_____30. There are times when I just can't say anything.

Scoring

To score this scale, first change the signs (+ or –) to the opposite for items 1, 2, 4, 5, 9, 11, 12, 13, 14, 15, 16, 17, 19, 23, 24, 26, and 30. Next, total the plus (+) items, then total the minus (–) items, and, last, subtract the minus total from the plus total to obtain your score. This score can range from –90 through 0 to +90. The higher the score (closer to 190), the more assertively you usually behave. The lower the score (closer to +90), the more nonassertive is your typical behavior. This particular scale does not measure aggressiveness.

> Source: Rathus, S. A. A 30-item schedule for assessing assertive behavior, *Behavior Therapy*, 4 (1973), 398, 406. Copyright © 1973 Academic Press, Orlando, FL.

Suggested Readings

Baxter, L. A. Family communication environments and rule-based social control of adolescents' healthy lifestyle choices. *Journal of Family Communication, 5, no. 3* (July 2005), 209–214.

Cherry, K. Top 10 nonverbal communication tips. About.com Psychology, 2011. Available: http://psychology.about.com/od/nonverbal-communication/tp/nonverbaltips.htm.

DeVore, E. R., & Ginsburg, K. R. The protective effects of good parenting on adolescents. *Current Opinions in Pediatrics, 17, no. 4* (August 2005), 460–465.

Guilamo-Ramos, V., & Bouris, A. Working with parents to promote healthy adolescent sexual development. *The Prevention Researcher, 16, no. 4* (November 2009), 7–11.

Hinchliff, S., Gott, M., & Galena, E. "I daresay I might find it embarrassing": General practitioners' perspectives on discussing sexual health issues with lesbian and gay patients. *Health & Social Care in the Community, 13, no. 4* (July 2005), 345–353.

Owen, C. The importance of sexual communication. suite101.com, July 2008. Available: http://improving-relationships.suite101.com.

Rosenfeld, S. M. Psychosocial correlates of sexual communication. *Dissertation Abstracts International: Section B: The Sciences & Engineering, 65, no. 9-B* (2005), 4849.

Savitsky, D., Keysar, B., Epley, N. Carter, T., & Swanson, A. The closeness-communication bias: Increased egocentrism among friends versus strangers. *Journal of Experimental Social Psychology, 47* (2011), 269–273.

Segal, J. Nonverbal communication. *Helpguide Newsletter* (October 2008). Available: http://www.helpguide.org/mental/eq6_nonverbal_communication.htm.

Silverberg, C. How to talk with your kids about sex. About.com Sexuality, December 2009. Available: http://sexuality.about.com/od/talkingwithyourkids/a/talk_to_you_kids_about_sex.htm.

Silverberg, C. Sexual communication ground rules. About.com Sexuality, January 2009. Available: http://sexuality.about.com/od/improvingsexcommunication/a/ground_rules.htm.

Somers, C. The sexual communication scale: A measure of frequency of sexual communication between parents and adolescents. *Adolescence, 38, no. 149* (Spring 2003), 43–56.

Tannen, D. *You just don't understand*. New York: Morrow, 1990 (also available in paperback from Ballantine, 1991).

Web Resources

For links to the websites below, visit go.jblearning.com/dimensions5e and click on Resource Links.

Planned Parenthood: Educator's Update
www.plannedparenthood.org

Gives ideas that can help communication between parents and their children.

Double Your Dating: Sexual Communication Workbook
www.freewebs.com/maestro_mr/SCW.pdf

Gives hints about many aspects of sexual communication within relationships.

MindTools: Communication Skills
www.mindtools.com/page8.html

Contains numerous articles related to communication skills in many different situations.

Queendom: The Land of Tests

www.queendom.com/tests/access_page/index
.htm?idRegTest=2288

You can find out how your interpersonal skills rate
by taking a Communication Skills Test.

Sexual Communication & Relationships: About
.com Sexuality

*http://sexuality.about.com/od/communication/Sexual_*
Communication_Relationships.htm

Gives suggestions related to talking about sexuality
with kids and teens, talking with partners, talking
with medical personnel, communication in alternative relationships, and communication quick tips.

Sexual Communication: Health 24

www.health24.com/sex/Tips_techniques/1253-1254,
32463.asp

Provides an overview of ways to help improve
communication about sexuality with a partner.

References

Albert, Bill. *With one voice 2004: America's adults and teens
sound off about teen pregnancy.* Washington, D.C.: National
Campaign to Prevent Teen Pregnancy, December 2004.

Bower, S. A., & Brower, G. *Asserting yourself: A practical guide
for positive change.* Reading, MA: Perseus Books, 1976.

Dailard, C. Recent findings from the "Add Health" survey:
Teens and sexual activity. *The Guttmacher Report, 4, no. 4*
(August 2001), 1–3, 2–4.

DePaulo, B. M., Kirkendol, S. E., Kashy, S. E., Wyer, M. M., &
Epstein, J. A. Lying in everyday life. *Journal of Personality
and Social Psychology, 70, no. 5* (1996), 979–997.

Dickson, A. Men friends. *Time, 155, no. 4* (January 17, 2000), 89.

Do women and men communicate differently? In *Taking sides:
Issues in family and personal relationships,* Schroeder, E.,
ed. Guilford, CT: McGraw-Hill/Dushkin, 2003.

El-Shaieb, M., & Wurtele, S. K. Parents' plans to discuss sexuality
with their children. *American Journal of Sexuality Education, no. 4* (April–June 2009), 103–115.

Filomeno, A. H. Promoting parent–adolescent communication
to facilitate healthy sexual socialization of youth. *Health
Education Monograph Series, 19, no. 2* (2002),17–21.

Grunbaum, J., Kann, L., Kinchen, S., Ross, J., Hawkins, J.,
Lowry, R., Harris, W. A., McManus, T., Chyen, D., &
Collins, J. Youth risk behavior surveillance—United States,
2003. In: *Surveillance Summaries,* May 21, 2004. *Morbidity
and Mortality Weekly Report, 53, no. SS-2* (2004), 1–20.

Guffey, M. E. *Business communication: Process and product,* 3rd
ed. Belmont, CA: Wadsworth, 1999.

Haffner, D. W., & Schwartz, P. *What I've learned about sex.* New
York: Perigee Books, 1998.

Karofsky, P. F. Relationship between adolescent–parental communication and initiation of first intercourse by adolescents.
Journal of Adolescent Health, 28, no. 1 (January 2001),
41–45.

Listening to understand. *The Pryor Report Success Workshop,* a
supplement to *The Pryor Report Management Newsletter*
(August 1998).

Miller, S. A., & Byers, E. S. Actual and desired duration of foreplay and intercourse: Discordance and misperceptions
within heterosexual couples. *Journal of Sex Research, 41,
no. 3* (August 2004), 301–309.

Owen, C. The importance of sexual communication. *suite101.
com,* July 2008. Available: http://improving-relationships
.suite101.com.

Reeder, H. M. Exploring male–female communication: Three lessons on gender. *Journal of School Health, 75, no. 3* (March
2005), 115–117.

Rickert, V. I., Sanghvi, R., & Wiemann, C. M. Is lack of sexual
assertiveness among adolescent and young adult women a
cause for concern? *Perspectives on Sexual and Reproductive
Health, 34, no. 4* (July/August 2002), 16–28.

Sample lesson plan using JSR. Allentown, PA: Society for the
Scientific Study of Sexuality, 2005. Available: http://www
.sexscience.org/publications.

Saxe, L. Lying: Thoughts of an applied social psychologist.
American Psychologist, 46, no. 4 (1991), 409–415.

Scheidlower, J. Sex talk, *Esquire,* 127 (January 1997), 29.

Segal, J. Nonverbal communication. *Helpguide Newsletter,*
October 2008. Available: http://www.helpguide.org/mental/
eq6_nonverbal_communication.htm.

Silverberg, C. How to talk with your kids about sex. *About.com
Sexuality,* March 2008. Available: http://sexuality.about.
com/od/sexeducationforparent1/a/talk_sex_kids.htm?p=1.

Silverberg, C. Sexual communication ground rules. *About.com
Sexuality,* January 2009. Available: http://sexuality.about
.com/od/improvingsexcommunication/a/ground_rules.htm.

Van Wagner, K. Top 10 nonverbal communication tips. *About.
com Psychology,* 2009. Available: http://psychology.about.
com/od/nonverbalcommunication/tp/nonverbaltips.htm.

Why don't we hear others? *Communication Briefings, 22, no. 1*
(July 2005), 1.

Worden, M., & Worden, B. D. *The gender dance in couples
therapy.* Pacific Grove, CA: Brooks/Cole, 1998.

CHAPTER 4

Female Sexual Anatomy and Physiology

CHAPTER OBJECTIVES

 1 Name and describe the parts of the female reproductive system, to include external and internal genitalia.

 2 Discuss the role of breasts in sexual arousal and response, as well as in the reproductive function of lactation.

 3 Explain the role of hormones as they pertain to sexuality.

 4 Describe what occurs during menstruation, to include menarche, the menstrual cycle, and problems associated with each.

 5 Cite various diseases that can affect the female reproductive system and the self-care procedures, as well as medical treatments, associated with these diseases.

go.jblearning.com/dimensions5e

Global Dimensions: Female Genital Mutilation
Amenorrhea
Breast Cancer

INTRODUCTION

O *ne of the authors of this text was sitting at his desk preparing
for an upcoming class. On the desk were diagrams of the female
and male reproductive systems, colored pictures with various
parts differentiated from others by different pastel colors and shading.
Before long, a colleague walked into the office. The visitor was a professor
of educational administration and the proud recipient of a baccalaureate
degree in mathematics, a master's degree in counseling, and a doctorate
in educational administration. In short, this was an educated man, one
on whom students and family relied and whose opinions were accorded
the respect someone of his stature deserves. As he entered the office, he
glanced at the desk and was fascinated with the reproductive system diagrams. When he inquired as to their purpose, he was told that they were
to be used in a sexuality education class to help students learn about
their sexual organs. It was then that he sheepishly admitted his own ignorance about the structure and function of the reproductive system. For the
next 20 minutes, he and his colleague proceeded to discuss the reproductive systems of females and males, referring to the diagrams on the desk.*

*The only surprising aspect of this incident was the openness with
which this educated man admitted his ignorance. In general, people
know less about themselves, both physically and psychologically, than
they know about cars or ecology or sports or politics or contemporary
musicians or any of the hundreds of topics people care about or find fas-
cinating. The less we know about our bodies, the less well equipped we
are to keep them healthy. The more we know, the more choices we have
and the better decisions we can make. Appropriate health maintenance
should be valued similarly by males and females, and both genders need
to adopt certain behaviors, such as periodic medical screenings, to*

maintain their health. However, men's and women's reproductive health issues are not the same.

The purpose of this chapter is to describe the anatomy of the female reproductive system as a step toward creating a comprehensive picture of human sexuality.

■ The Female Reproductive System

Both females and males have external and internal genitals, or reproductive organs. We begin with the external female genitals and progress inward.

The External Genitals

The external female genitals are the mons pubis, labia majora, labia minora, clitoris, vestibule, and urethral opening (Figure 4.1). All of these organs together are called the **vulva**.

The Mons Veneris
The **mons pubis** (also called the **mons veneris**, or **mount of Venus**) is the rounded, soft area above the pubic bone that becomes covered with hair at puberty. Since the mons contains numerous nerve endings, it can be sexually stimulated.

> **vulva**
> The female external genitalia.
>
> **mons pubis (mons veneris, mount of Venus)**
> The rounded, soft area above the vaginal opening that becomes covered with hair at puberty.

The Labia Majora
The **labia majora** (major lips) are two large folds of skin whose main function is to protect the external genitalia. Unless the labia majora are spread apart, the other external genitalia are not visible. The outer surfaces of the labia majora also grow hair after puberty, and the inner surfaces remain smooth. Within the tissue of the labia majora are smooth muscle fibers, nerves, and vessels for blood and lymph.

The Labia Minora
The **labia minora** (minor lips) are two folds of skin lying inside the labia majora. Loaded with blood vessels and nerve receptors, the labia minora and their upper part, the clitoris, are very sensitive to stimulation. During sexual arousal, blood fills the labia minora, causing them to spread, making the vagina more

> **labia majora**
> Two large folds of skin whose main function is to protect the external genitalia and the opening of the vestibule (defined later).
>
> **labia minora**
> Two folds of skin lying inside the labia majora, which contain numerous blood vessels and nerve receptors.

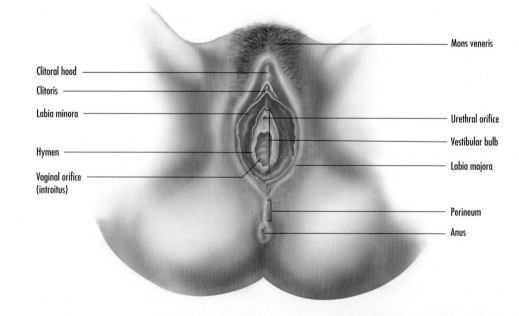

Clitoral hood
Clitoris
Labia minora
Hymen
Vaginal orifice (introitus)

Mons veneris
Urethral orifice
Vestibular bulb
Labia majora
Perineum
Anus

FIGURE **4.1** Female external reproductive organs.

Female Genital Mutilation in Various Parts of the World

Female genital mutilation has been used throughout the world as a means of diminishing sexual stimulation. The result, the argument goes, is that fewer women participate in sexual intercourse outside marriage and fewer women engage in masturbation. Female mutilation can take several different forms. The most simple form is *circumcision*, whereby the clitoral hood is removed. In a *clitoridectomy*, the clitoris itself is surgically removed. Genital *infibulation* is the most complex procedure: The clitoris and the labia minora are removed, and both sides of the vulva are scraped raw and then stitched together. When the tissue grows together, only a small opening remains through which urine and the menstrual flow pass. During these procedures, it is unusual for sterile instruments to be used. Most of the time razor blades or broken glass is used to do the cutting, without the benefit of pain-reducing medications or disinfectants. Therefore, as you might imagine, aside from causing psychological trauma, female mutilation can result in serious medical complications. The combination of infections, bleeding, and pain can cause shock, gangrene, and even death.

Female mutilation is common in some African, Middle Eastern, and Asian countries. The United Nations estimates that 70 million girls and women have been subjected to female genital mutilation in Africa and Yemen. Mutilated women are also increasingly found in Europe, Australia, Canada, and the United States, primarily among immigrants from Africa and southwestern Asia (UNICEF, 2011a)—this in spite of the World Health Organization (WHO) and the United Nations Children's Fund (UNICEF) 1980 joint plan to lobby leaders of countries in which female mutilation is common to work toward eliminating this practice. A new statement, with wider United Nations support, was then issued in February 2008 (World Health Organization, 2008). Numerous other organizations and governments have publicly opposed female genital mutilation, even though the tendency is to avoid interference in cultural practices of sovereign countries. Grass-roots organizations, such as the Kenyan women's organization Maendeleo ya Wanawake, and Tostan in Senegal, have also sprung up around the world with the goal of eliminating female genital mutilation. These groups conduct educational campaigns encouraging women to break the generational cycle of female genital mutilation by preventing their daughters from experiencing it. The prevalence of female genital mutilation is declining. It is measurably less common among younger women than older ones, and among daughters compared with their mothers. But progress is slow, and millions of girls remain threatened by the practice (UNICEF, 2011b).

accessible. Within the labia minora lie **Bartholin's glands**. The glands slightly lubricate the labia during coitus (intercourse).

The Clitoris

The **clitoris** is the most sensitive structure in the female body. This small organ contains two spongy bodies, the **corpora cavernosa**, that have the capacity to fill with blood during arousal. (The penis, a similar organ, contains spongy bodies that react to arousal in a similar way.) During sexual stimulation, the corpora cavernosa fill with blood, causing the clitoris to become erect. Popular knowledge about the sensitivity of the clitoris has led males to seek out and stimulate it to arouse their female sexual partners. Here is a case in which knowledge can have either a positive or a negative effect on sexual relationships. Men who carefully and delicately stimulate the clitoris may sexually arouse their partner, but those who rub incessantly will only irritate the clitoris and thereby irritate their partner.

The clitoris is covered by the **clitoral hood**. As can be seen in Figure 4.1, the hood is attached to the labia minora. One function of the clitoral hood is to protect the glans of the clitoris. When we discuss the male reproductive organs, we will observe that the foreskin of the penis protects the glans penis in a similar way.

Knowing about the anatomy of the reproductive system offers guidance for sexual functioning,

Bartholin's glands
Small glands located within the labia minora that secrete a few drops of fluid during sexual arousal.

clitoris
The structure located at the upper part of the labia minora that is homologous to the penis and is very sensitive to stimulation.

corpora cavernosa
A cavernous structure located within the clitoris and the penis that fills with blood during sexual excitement, causing erection.

clitoral hood
The skin covering the clitoris.

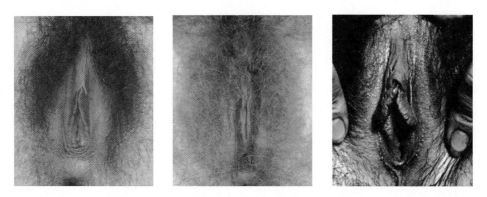

Many variations exist in the female external genitals.

and the relationship of the clitoris, the clitoral hood, and the labia minora provides a case in point. During sexual excitement, the clitoris retracts under the clitoral hood. Therefore, stimulating the clitoris requires pulling back the clitoral hood, pulling the labia majora upward, or putting pressure on the hood or clitoris itself. For example, during sexual intercourse, the clitoris can be stimulated if the penis is positioned correctly. One position that will stimulate the clitoris is called "riding high." With the female lying on her back, the male places his penis into the vagina so that its upper shaft rubs on the clitoris. Another option is for the penis to be pressed, thrusting downward, on the lower part of the labia minora so as to create downward movement of the hood and its contact with the clitoris. Many women, however, require additional manual stimulation of the clitoris to cause orgasm during intercourse.

The Vestibule
When the clitoris is erect and the labia minora spread, the urethral and vaginal openings (called the **vestibule**) become visible.

The Urethral Opening
The urethral opening, where urine is excreted, is not generally considered a part of the reproductive system in females, although there is some evidence that women who do experience something akin to ejaculation do so through the urethra.

The Hymen
The **hymen**, a thin connective tissue containing a relatively large number of blood vessels, covers the opening of the vagina in women who have an intact hymen. The function of this tissue is unknown. Hymens vary in shape and size: A hymen may surround the vaginal opening (an **annular** hymen), bridge it (a **septate** hymen), or form a sievelike covering (a **cribriform** hymen) (Figure 4.2).

Normally all forms of hymens have openings that are large enough to permit menstrual flow or the insertion of a tampon or a finger, but that are usually too small to permit an erect penis to enter without

vestibule
The area containing the vaginal and urethral openings.

hymen
A thin connective tissue covering the opening of the vagina.

annular
Type of hymen that surrounds the vaginal opening.

septate
Type of hymen that bridges the vaginal opening.

cribriform
Type of hymen that creates a sievelike covering for the vaginal opening.

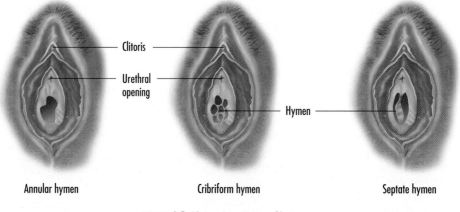

Annular hymen   Cribriform hymen   Septate hymen

FIGURE **4.2** The various types of hymens.

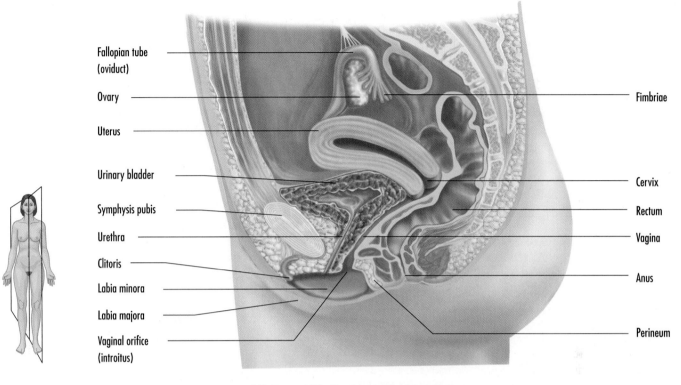

Fallopian tube
(oviduct)

Ovary

Uterus

Urinary bladder

Symphysis pubis

Urethra

Clitoris

Labia minora

Labia majora

Vaginal orifice
(introitus)

Fimbriae

Cervix

Rectum

Vagina

Anus

Perineum

FIGURE **4.3** Organs of the female reproductive system.

the hymen tearing. Historically the presence of an intact hymen was considered proof that a woman had never had intercourse. But the hymen can be ruptured by accident or by normal exercise, as well as by intercourse, so a tear in the tissue is not a reliable indication that a woman is no longer a virgin. The rupturing of the hymen during first intercourse generally does not result in a great deal of pain and bleeding, although some people expect it to do so. Pain is usually related to muscular tension due to anxiety or to entry of the penis into the vagina before the vagina is sufficiently lubricated; care and attention can ordinarily prevent it. A few drops of blood may be noticeable.

The Internal Genitals

The female internal genitals consist of such structures as the vagina, uterus, fallopian tubes, and ovaries. These structures of the female internal genitalia, as well as relevant surrounding structures, are depicted in Figures 4.3 and 4.4.

The Vagina
The **vagina** is a hollow, tunnel-like structure, about 4.5 inches (11.4 centimeters) long, that opens outward to the vestibule and at the opposite end into the uterus. The vagina has several reproductive functions: It surrounds the penis and receives its ejaculate during intercourse, serves as the route of exit for the newborn, and provides an exit for menstrual flow. When the vagina is empty, its lips and walls are in contact, but during childbirth the vagina can expand wide enough for the baby to pass through, and during intercourse it can both expand and close tightly enough on a penis to provide sexual satisfaction. Soft transverse folds in the vaginal wall enable the vagina to expand, and muscle fibers within the walls enable it to contract, as they do in orgasm. No muscles surround the vaginal entrance (the **introitus**); however, the **pubococcygeal** and **bulbocavernosus muscles** that support the vagina can be voluntarily contracted so as to intensify sexual responsiveness by forcing the vaginal walls to close on the penis. Exercises to help women develop greater control of these muscles (called **Kegel exercises** after their proponent) are frequently recommended by

vagina
A hollow, tunnel-like structure of the female internal genitalia whose reproductive functions are to receive the penis and its ejaculate, serve as a route of exit for the newborn, and provide an exit for menstrual flow.

introitus
The vaginal entrance.

pubococcygeal muscle
A muscle that encircles the vagina and supports it.

bulbocavernosus muscle
A muscle that encircles and supports the vagina.

Kegel exercises
Exercises to help women develop greater control of muscles supporting the genitalia.

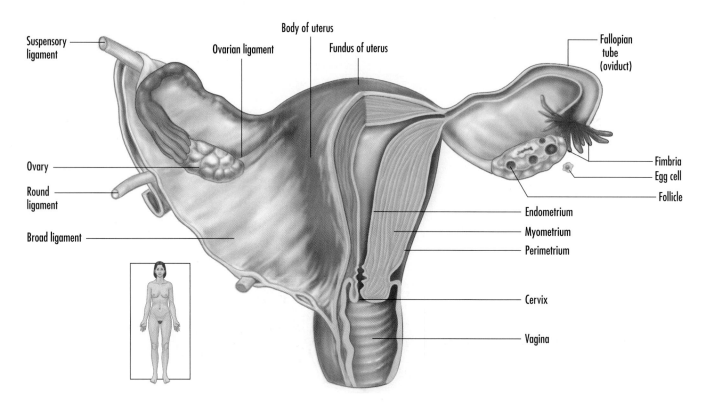

FIGURE **4.4** An anterior view of the female reproductive organs showing the relationships of the ovaries, fallopian tubes, uterus, cervix, and vagina.

sexual counselors (Kegel, 1952). To learn to control the pubococcygeal muscles, try the following:

1. Insert a finger into the vagina and contract muscles in that area until you feel the vagina squeeze the finger.

2. Practice squeezing and then relaxing these muscles—first slowly, then rapidly.

3. Practice the preceding exercise about three times daily until you feel you have voluntary control of the pubococcygeal muscles.

The Grafenberg Spot

One would think that after centuries of studying the human body and its sexual nature there would be little room for disagreement regarding its function. Not so. The existence and the effect of the **Grafenberg spot (G spot)** provide a case in point.

The stimulation of an area along the anterior (front) wall of the vagina, several inches into the vaginal canal and just below the bladder, appears to be sexually exciting for many females. This area is known as the Grafenberg spot, named after Ernest Grafenberg, the gynecologist who first noted its erotic potential (Figure 4.5) (Grafenberg, 1950). The presence of glands in this area has been known for some time (Skene, 1980), and it is these glands—called **Skene's glands**—through which a type of ejaculate

is expelled in some women when they experience orgasm by stimulation of the G spot (Grafenberg, 1950; Sevely & Bennett, 1978; Addiego et al., 1981; Belzer, 1981; Perry & Whipple, 1981; Zaviacic et al., 1988).

Others maintain that there is no one particular spot in the vagina that is more sensitive than others to stimulation. For example, the noted sexual therapist Helen Singer Kaplan believes there are many spots within the vagina that are sexually arousing, and the G spot is merely one of those (Kaplan, 1983). Masters and Johnson agree with Kaplan; they report that only 10% of the women they studied "had an area of heightened sensitivity in the front wall of the vagina or a tissue mass that fit the various descriptions of this area" (Masters, Johnson, & Kolodny, 1985). Although some women reported sensitivity in the front wall of the vagina, a study by Alzate and Londono (1984) could not locate a specific spot such as that described by Grafenberg. Heath (1984) found an area of erotic sensitivity and concluded that it is larger than

Grafenberg spot (G spot)
An area located along the anterior wall of the vagina, several inches into the vaginal canal, that when stimulated in some women may result in sexual excitement and/or orgasm.

Skene's glands
Glands located along the walls of the vagina that are thought to be analogous to the male prostate gland and the site from which some women eject a fluid during orgasm.

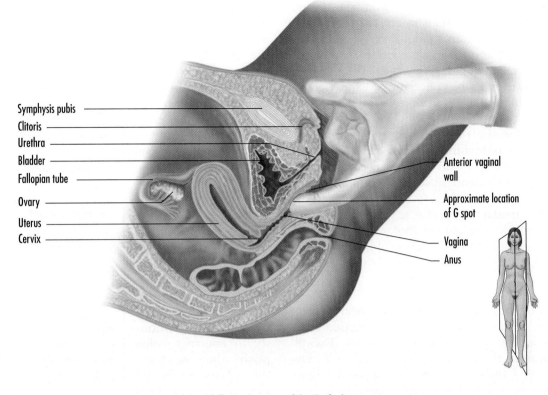

Symphysis pubis
Clitoris
Urethra
Bladder
Fallopian tube
Ovary
Uterus
Cervix

Anterior vaginal wall
Approximate location of G spot
Vagina
Anus

FIGURE **4.5** The location of the Grafenberg spot.

previously described: about the width of the middle two fingers and at least two-thirds the length.

In a more recent study of female twins, 56% of the women studied reported having a G spot, even though there was determined to be no genetic basis for its existence (Burri, Cherkas, & Spector, 2010). However, there still remain skeptics. For example, some researchers explain the sensation on the anterior wall of the vagina as pressure and movement of the clitoris during vaginal penetration and not a distinct G spot area (Foldes & Buisson, 2009). At the 2009 meeting of the International Society for the Study of Women's Sexual Health Congress, the *Journal of Sexual Medicine* held a debate among experts regarding the existence of the G spot. The conclusion was that more research is needed to determine whether the G spot actually exists (Jannini et al., 2010).

The Female Prostate

The existence of a female prostate and ejaculate, although controversial, was first described centuries ago. In the 4th century, several Chinese Taoist texts mentioned female ejaculation. In the 7th century, the Indian *Kamasutra* mentioned it, as did Aristotle (in 300 B.C.) and Galen (in the 2nd century) (Korda, Goldstein, & Sommer, 2010).

That glandular tissue exists in the area of the G spot is not debatable. The pathologist Robert Mallon (1984)

conducted autopsies on women and found evidence of this glandular tissue, as did Heath (1984). Both of these researchers found prostatelike glandular tissue in the front wall of the vagina. When the substances within these glands were analyzed, they were found to contain fluids similar to those found in the male prostate. Hence, some sexuality experts have concluded that there are a female prostate (the Skene's glands) and a female ejaculate. Further evidence for a female ejaculate is offered by Addiego and colleagues (1981), who analyzed the fluid expelled by females at the time of orgasm and found it to contain an enzyme (prostatic acid phosphatase, or PAP) characteristic of semen. However, when Goldberg and associates (1983) studied this ejaculate, they concluded that it was similar to urine. Alzate and Hoch (1986) also found ejaculate secreted through the urethra. To complicate matters further, a study conducted by Belzer and associates (1984) concluded that the ejaculate obtained from women contained significantly more prostatic acid phosphatase than did their urine. More recently, researchers using ultrasound and biochemical analysis concluded that there is glandular tissue surrounding the length of the female urethra containing a duct that secretes fluid during orgasm. Upon analysis, that fluid was more similar to prostate secretions than urine (Wimpissinger et al., 2007). Obviously, further study is needed to confirm the existence of a female ejaculate beyond any doubt.

That some women expel a fluid from the vagina during orgasm has been demonstrated. The prevalence of this phenomenon remains unknown. Whether this fluid is similar to that of the male prostate is a matter of much research and debate. What is not discussed or researched, however, is the concern first expressed by the Boston Women's Health Collective (1998) regarding the possibility that the G spot orgasm will become a new "ideal" for the sexually liberated woman. It would indeed be unfortunate if this new ideal created pressure on women who do not experience erotic feelings when the Grafenberg spot is stimulated and, therefore, perceive themselves to be inadequate sexually. When the media popularize sexual information, as they did with the Grafenberg spot, often education is needed to remind the public about the many paths to sexual fulfillment. This is particularly true today.

The Uterus

At the top of the vagina lies the **uterus**, a pear-shaped hollow organ with muscular walls. Its function is to nurture the developing embryo and fetus. Except during pregnancy, the uterus is about 3 inches (8 centimeters) long, 3 inches wide at the top, and 1 inch (2.5 centimeters) thick. The uterus extends into the vagina at its **cervix**; the actual opening to the uterus in the cervix is called the **os**. The upper two-thirds of this cavity is called the **corpus**, and the top end is called the **fundus**. Most uteruses tilt forward (that is, they are *anteflexed*) over the bladder; approximately 20% tilt backward (*retroflexed*) (Figure 4.6). Women with retroflexed uteruses are more likely to experience discomfort during menstruation and may have more

difficulty in inserting a diaphragm as a result of the angle of the cervix. Contrary to widespread belief, however, the ability to conceive is in no way affected by the position of the uterus.

The uterus consists of three layers. The outermost layer, the **perimetrium**, is very elastic, enabling the uterus to accommodate a growing embryo during pregnancy. The middle layer, the **myometrium**, consists of smooth muscles, whose ability to contract helps push the newborn through the cervix and into the vagina (which during childbirth acts as the birth canal). The innermost layer of the uterus is the **endometrium**. This layer is loaded with blood vessels and can therefore provide the nourishment necessary to sustain a developing fetus. It

uterus
A pear-shaped hollow structure of the female genitalia in which the embryo and fetus develop before birth.

cervix
The mouth of the uterus, through which the vagina extends.

os
The opening to the uterus.

corpus
The upper two-thirds of the uterus.

fundus
The upper end of the uterus, closest to the opening of the fallopian tubes.

perimetrium
The outermost layer of the uterus, sometimes termed the *serosa*, a very elastic layer that allows the uterus to accommodate a growing embryo and fetus.

myometrium
The middle layer of the uterus, consisting of smooth muscle that aids in the pushing of the newborn through the cervix.

endometrium
The innermost layer of the uterus, to which the fertilized egg attaches and by which it is nourished as it develops before birth, which is partly discharged (if pregnancy does not occur) with the menstrual flow.

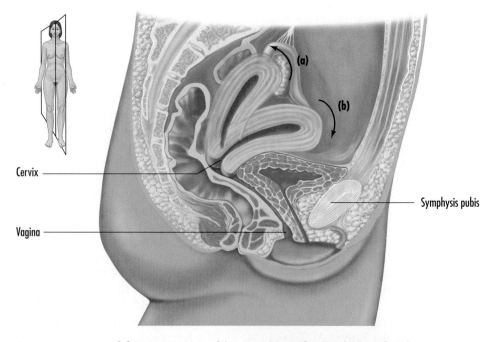

Cervix

Vagina

Symphysis pubis

FIGURE **4.6** Various positions of the uterus: (a) retroflexed and (b) anteflexed.

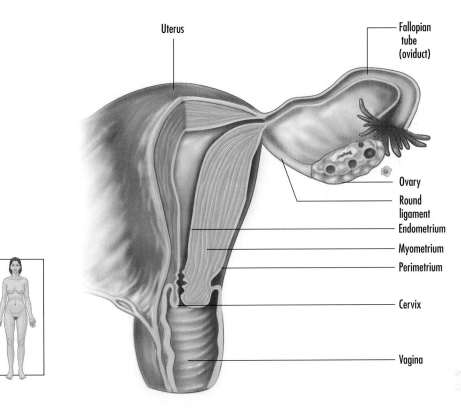

FIGURE **4.7** Layers of the uterine wall.

fallopian tubes (oviduct)
The routes through which eggs leave the ovaries on their way to the uterus, in which fertilization normally occurs.

ovary
A structure of the female genitalia that houses ova before their maturation and discharge and that produces estrogen and progesterone.

Graafian follicle
A part of the ovary from which a mature egg ruptures, allowing the corpus luteum to develop in the location where the egg was released.

corpus luteum
A yellowish structure that develops in the Graafian follicle at the discharge of an ovum and that produces progesterone and estrogen.

progesterone
A hormone secreted by the corpus luteum signaling the endometrium to develop in preparation for a zygote.

estrogen
A hormone produced by the ovaries whose level in the blood helps control the menstrual cycle.

fimbriae
The fingerlike ends of the fallopian tubes that catch the ova when they are discharged from the ovaries.

builds up and partly sloughs off as the menstrual flow in every menstrual cycle, unless fertilization takes place. Figure 4.7 depicts the anatomical relationships of the three layers of the uterus.

The Fallopian Tubes and the Ovaries
At the fundus, the uterus opens into the two **fallopian tubes** (we will use this more common name, although **oviduct** might be more appropriate). At the other end of each tube is an **ovary**, the organ that produces and stores the *ova*, or eggs. When a female is born, each of her ovaries contains approximately 40,000 to 400,000 eggs. Every egg has the potential to be fertilized by a sperm to become an embryo. After the girl reaches puberty, one of these eggs is usually discharged through the wall of one of her ovaries during each menstrual cycle.

The egg develops inside a capsule called a **Graafian follicle** and is discharged when it has matured. The discharged egg, now matured and freed from its capsule and the ovary, is ready to be fertilized by a male's sperm. When the follicle ruptures to discharge its egg, the empty follicle, now a yellowish structure called the **corpus luteum**, secretes a hormone (**progesterone**) that signals the endometrium to prepare for a fertilized egg. Progesterone and **estrogen**, another hormone produced by the ovaries, play significant roles in menstruation, birth, growth, and aging.

When the ovum is discharged from the ovary, it is directed into the fallopian tubes. As shown in Figure 4.4, these tubes serve as routes for ova to reach the uterus. The newly released ovum is caught by the fingerlike end of the fallopian tube, called a **fimbria**, and is guided into the cone-shaped open end of the tube. If fertilization takes place, it usually takes place there.

cilia
Hairlike structures that guide objects, such as ova, moving past them.

ectopic pregnancy
The attachment and development of the zygote in a location other than in the uterus.

mammary glands
Milk-secreting glands located in the female breast.

prolactin
A pituitary hormone that stimulates the production of milk from the mammary glands.

areola
The darkened part of the breast immediately surrounding the nipple.

Whether fertilized or not, the ovum continues on its journey through the tube, moved along in a sweeping motion by tiny hairlike structures called **cilia**. The destination of the fertilized ovum is the endometrium in the uterus, where it becomes attached and continues its development. An unfertilized ovum also travels to the endometrium, then disintegrates, and eventually is expelled through the vagina, along with some of the endometrium, in the process called *menstruation*. (Once an ovum is expelled, the menstrual cycle is completed. Soon an ovary will discharge another mature egg and the process will begin again.)

It should be noted that occasionally a woman may produce more than one egg per cycle, thereby becoming prone to multiple births. Fertility drugs, which may result in multiple births, are suspected of causing the maturation of several eggs per cycle. Sometimes the fertilized egg may attach in the abdominal cavity or the fallopian tube rather than in the uterus. This is termed an **ectopic pregnancy**.

■ The Breasts

Although the female breasts are not reproductive organs, they do have significance in sexual arousal and response, and they serve an important reproductive function in providing milk for the newborn infant. Each breast contains about 15 to 20 clusters of milk-secreting structures called **mammary glands** (Figure 4.8). Each of these mammary gland clusters

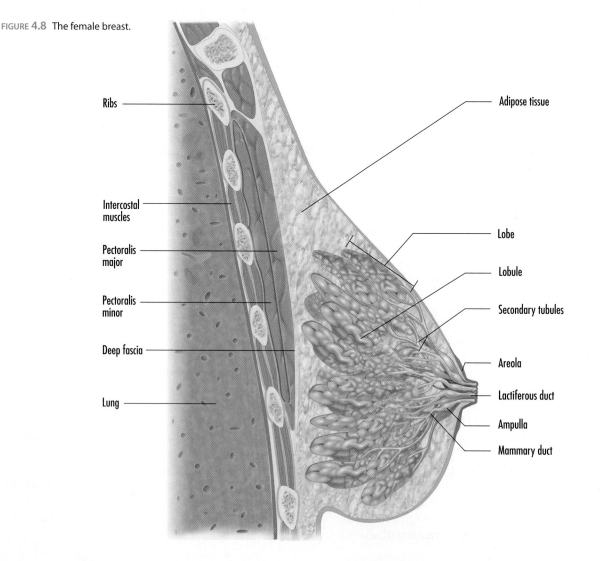

FIGURE **4.8** The female breast.

Ribs

Intercostal muscles

Pectoralis major

Pectoralis minor

Deep fascia

Lung

Adipose tissue

Lobe

Lobule

Secondary tubules

Areola

Lactiferous duct

Ampulla

Mammary duct

has an opening to the nipple, where the milk ducts open. The stimulation of the newborn's sucking on the nipple causes the pituitary gland to secrete a hormone called **prolactin**, which in turn stimulates the production of breast milk.

Most of the breast is fat and connective tissue. Except for small muscles in the area of the nipple and **areola** (the darkened skin around the nipple), there are no muscles in the breast. Because the breast is muscle-free, exercises to increase breast size are ineffective. Over the years the breasts may hang lower than normal if the ligaments are stretched by lack of support or by jostling (for example, not wearing a bra while jogging).

The nipples—of men as well as women—are richly supplied with nerve endings that respond with pleasurable sexual feelings when stimulated. During sexual arousal the nipples become erect. The size of the breasts or their shape is not related to sensitivity. Women with either small or large breasts may be equally sexually stimulated by the fondling of the breasts. Though some have characterized our society as making a fetish of large breasts, preferences in breast size and shape vary from individual to individual. It should be noted, however, that although breast size varies, extent of glandular tissue is comparable in all women's breasts. Because the amount of glandular tissue is the same, women with small breasts produce the same amount of breast milk after childbirth as women with larger breasts and are therefore as successful breastfeeding their babies as are women with larger breasts.

Our society has so emphasized breast size that many women have their breasts reconstructed. In the past, liquid silicone was injected to enlarge the breast, but approximately 60% of women experienced problems such as infection, deformity, or exceptional hardness of the breast. More recently, silicone pouches containing saline solution have been implanted to reshape the breast. However, in 1992, in response to reported breakage of the pouches, the Dow Chemical Company, the largest manufacturer of silicone pouches, stopped manufacturing them and agreed to pay for their removal for women who so desired. The most recent research, however, indicates that silicone implants are not the health issue previously thought. In a study of the research related to silicone breast implants, the Institute of Medicine (a subgroup of

the National Academy of Sciences) found no convincing evidence that chronic disease was more likely to develop in women with silicone breast implants than women without implants (Reuters, 1999). Furthermore, during a lawsuit against breast implant manufacturers, a federal judge appointed a panel of scientists to study the issue and report their findings to the court. The court-appointed panel found no convincing evidence that silicone breast implants cause disease of the immune system as alleged in the lawsuit. The Food and Drug Administration also approved silicone-gel implants for breast enhancement in 2003. Silicone pouch implants are still regularly used in breast reconstruction for women who have had a radical mastectomy due to cancer of the breast.

We also need to be concerned about other health issues regarding the breast, such as cancer of the breast. (We discuss this in greater detail later in the chapter.) Suffice it to say here that women need to obtain periodic medical checkups by a health professional to make sure that any abnormalities are identified early, thereby increasing the likelihood that treatment will be successful and as noninvasive as possible.

Table 4.1 reviews the functions of the female reproductive organs.

■ The Hormones

What happens at the sight of an attractive person in a skimpy bathing suit? If the stimulus is sufficiently interesting, it can result in the first stages of sexual response—for example, increased heart rate, vaginal lubrication, and erection of the penis or clitoris. How does the visual image result in these physical changes? The chain of events is rather complex. It starts with the **hypothalamus**, a structure in the brain that, either through direct nerve pathways or through chemicals called **releasing factors**, can instruct

hypothalamus
A structure in the brain that controls the pituitary gland and is directly connected by nerve pathways to various organs of the body.

releasing factors
Chemicals released from the hypothalamus that affect the function of various body parts.

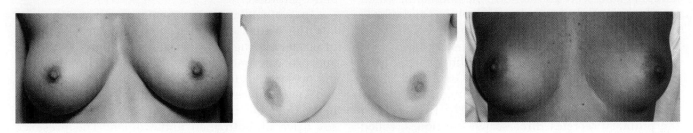

The size and shape of breasts vary among women.

TABLE 4.1 Functions of the Female Reproductive Organs

Organ	Function
Ovary	Production of egg cells and female sex hormones
Fallopian tube	Conveying of egg cell toward uterus; site of fertilization; transport developing zygote to uterus
Uterus	Protection and sustaining of life of embryo and fetus during pregnancy
Vagina	Conveying of uterine secretions to the outside of body; receiving of erect penis during sexual intercourse; transport of fetus during birth process
Labia majora	Enclosing and protection of other external reproductive organs
Labia minora	Formation of margins of vestibule; protection of openings of vagina and urethra
Clitoris	Organ richly supplied with sensory nerve endings associated with feeling of pleasure during sexual stimulation
Vestibule	Space between labia minora that includes vaginal and urethral openings
Vestibular glands	Secretion of fluid that moistens and lubricates vestibule

various body parts to function. The hypothalamus might be said to serve as a bridge between external stimuli and physiological responses. But let us go back to the bathing suit. Two things happen: (1) When the individual perceives the external stimulus as sexually exciting, the hypothalamus "tells" the pituitary gland to secrete its hormones, and (2) these chemicals stimulate the adrenal gland to secrete its hormones and the testes and ovaries to secrete their hormones. These secretions change the blood flow (producing vasocongestion), the heart rate, breathing, vaginal moistness, and so on.

These powerfully acting **hormones** are chemical substances that influence organs and tissues. They are produced by **endocrine glands**, glands that secrete their products into the bloodstream. The thyroid, for example, secretes a hormone that travels to the heart and increases the heart rate. The adrenal gland secretes the hormone adrenalin, which travels to the bronchial tubes of the lungs and dilates them. As we have just seen, the secretions of several glands are involved in sexual response.

The **pituitary**, a pea-shaped gland located at the base of the brain, serves as a sort of master gland to the others in the system. It stimulates the other glands to release their hormones. The front part of the pituitary secretes three sexual hormones, called **gonadotropins**, which act on or stimulate the **gonads**

(the testes and ovaries). The gonads are also endocrine glands, and they produce their own hormones. The three gonadotropins are **follicle-stimulating hormone (FSH)**; **luteinizing hormone (LH)**, often called the **interstitial-cell-stimulating hormone (ICSH)** in males; and prolactin (produced only during pregnancy and breastfeeding). Once stimulated by these gonadotropic hormones, the gonads produce their own hormones: estrogens, progesterones, and androgens. The adrenal gland also secretes androgen directly.

In women, estrogens and progesterones regulate the menstrual cycle, with estrogens important in producing vaginal lubrication. Although estrogens and progesterones have no known function in men, the presence of too much estrogen in the male body can lower interest in sexual activity and may result in enlargement of the breasts. **Androgens** affect the sex drive of both men and women: The presence of too much causes excessive sexual appetite, the

hormone
A chemical substance secreted by a ductless gland, which is carried to an organ or tissue where it has a specific effect.

endocrine glands
Glands that secrete their products into the bloodstream.

pituitary
The "master gland," an endocrine gland located at the base of the brain that stimulates the other endocrine glands to produce their hormones.

gonadotropins
Sexual hormones secreted by the pituitary that stimulate the gonads to produce their hormones.

gonads
The male testes and the female ovaries, which produce gonadotropin hormones responsible for the development of secondary sexual characteristics.

follicle-stimulating hormone (FSH)
A hormone, secreted by the anterior portion of the pituitary gland, that "instructs" the ovaries to prepare an egg to be released from a follicle.

luteinizing hormone (LH)
A hormone, secreted by the anterior portion of the pituitary gland, that stimulates ovulation.

interstitial-cell-stimulating hormone (ICSH)
A hormone, secreted by the anterior portion of the pituitary gland in males, that stimulates the production of sperm.

androgens
Male sex hormones.

spermatocytes
Cells that develop through several stages to form sperm.

testosterone
The male sex hormone produced in the testes that is responsible for the development of male secondary sexual characteristics.

menarche
The time when a female begins her first menstrual cycle, usually at 8 to 16 years of age.

menstruation
The cyclical emission of the blood-enriched endometrium when pregnancy does not occur.

presence of too little androgen decreases sexual interest. FSH stimulates cells in the seminiferous tubules (called **spermatocytes**) to produce sperm.

Despite the fact that hormones account for and influence sexual differences, males and females produce the same hormones. Estrogens and progesterones are considered female hormones and androgens male hormones, but both males and females produce all three. They do differ in the amounts they produce, however. For example, males have levels of the strongest androgen (**testosterone**) 10 times those of females, and females have significantly more estrogens than males. Obviously, too, males and females differ in the organs activated by the hormones. Long before we begin to think about hormones and our sexuality, hormones have already had significant effects.

Menstruation

At some time during puberty, a girl reaches **menarche**; that is, she has her first menstrual cycle. Then, and cyclically thereafter unless she is pregnant, blood (actually the blood-enriched endometrium) is discharged (or flows) from her uterus through her vagina for several days. The Latin origin of the word **menstruation** is *mensis*, meaning "month," because the menses, or periods, supposedly occur monthly. Actually they are not so predictable. Between menarche and menopause, when menstruation ceases, a woman's menstrual cycle may stabilize in a 28- to 30-day pattern (20- to 40-day cycles are also quite normal), or it may never stabilize. Cycles may vary in length from period to period, or they may be stable for a long time, fluctuate, and become stable again. Menstruation has been called the "curse," the "monthly sickness," and worse, but it is a normal physiological response to hormonal activity.

Menarche

The reason menstruation begins when it does is not exactly known. One hypothesis relates to the increase in body fat at puberty as a result of

hormonal secretions. Evidence for this hypothesis can be found in long-distance runners. Many women who jog long distances lose considerable weight and body fat. It is not uncommon for such women to experience secondary **amenorrhea**; that is, they no longer menstruate regularly. In fact, some experts estimate that as many as 50% of women runners experience a cessation of menstruation (Barrack et al., 2010). In addition, women suffering from anorexia nervosa—a condition in which the woman is so preoccupied with being thin that she eats very little and loses a great deal of body weight and fat—often lose their periods. In truth, though, no one really knows why women joggers or anorexics cease to menstruate, and, at least for the joggers, there appears to be more going on than just a loss of body fat. Other studies have found that many thin female joggers continue to menstruate, and many heavier ones do not.

amenorrhea
The absence of menstruation in a woman who should be menstruating.

Menstrual Physiology

The menstrual cycle begins when the pituitary gland secretes two hormones: FSH, which stimulates the growth, or "ripening," of follicles in the ovary; and LH, which stimulates the ovary to release one egg, that is, to *ovulate*. Once the egg is released, the area from which it was released (the Graafian follicle) becomes a yellow body (corpus luteum). The Graafian follicle secretes the hormone estrogen, and the yellow body secretes progesterone and estrogen. Progesterone causes the lining of the uterus to thicken and store nutrients in preparation to receive, implant, and nourish a fertilized egg, called a **zygote**. If the egg is not fertilized, the yellow body degenerates and thus becomes unable to secrete progesterone any longer. The lack of progesterone is a signal to expel the unneeded endometrium. This tissue, which is gradually shed over the course of a few days, is the menstrual flow. The cycle is then ready to begin anew.

zygote
A fertilized egg.

proliferative phase
The first part of the menstrual cycle, during which FSH production is increased and the follicles are maturing.

Phases of the Menstrual Cycle

Figures 4.9 and 4.10 depict the roles of hormones in the menstrual cycle and its phases. The first phase is termed the **proliferative phase**. It is during this

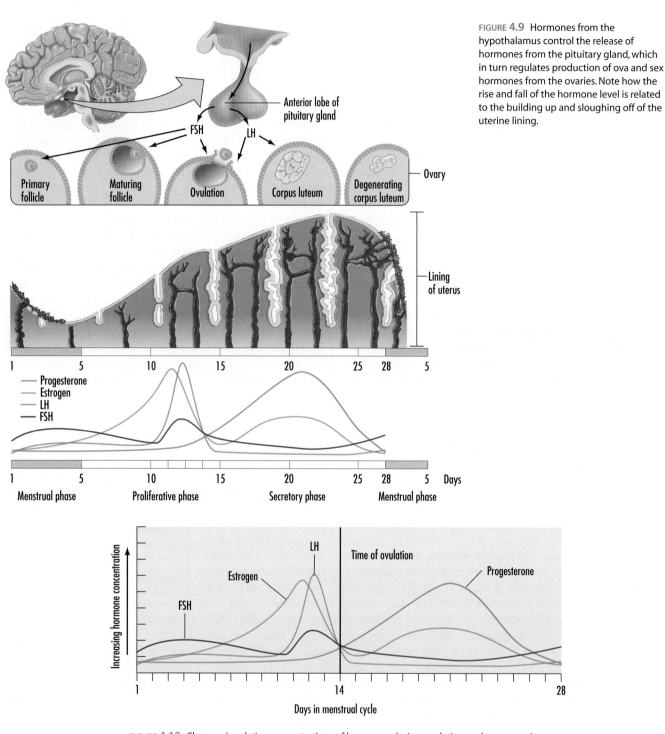

FIGURE **4.9** Hormones from the hypothalamus control the release of hormones from the pituitary gland, which in turn regulates production of ova and sex hormones from the ovaries. Note how the rise and fall of the hormone level is related to the building up and sloughing off of the uterine lining.

FIGURE **4.10** Changes in relative concentrations of hormones during ovulation and menstruation.

phase that FSH production is increased by the pituitary gland, which in turn stimulates the follicles in the ovaries to mature. The follicles then can produce estrogen, which causes the endometrial lining of the uterus to thicken and prepare for the implantation of the

secretory phase
The second part of the menstrual cycle, during which ovulation occurs and the production of LH stimulates the development of the corpus luteum.

zygote. The pituitary then increases production of LH in response to the elevated levels of estrogen in the bloodstream, causing one follicle to prepare to expel an ovum (the Graafian follicle), and the proliferative phase proceeds until ovulation.

The **secretory phase** of the menstrual cycle begins once ovulation occurs and entails continued secretions of LH, which stimulate the development of the corpus luteum. The corpus luteum secretes progesterone, causing further thickening and engorgement of blood of the endometrium. If implantation does not occur, the pituitary shuts down production of FSH and LH, causing degeneration of the corpus luteum. The result is a decrease in the secretions of estrogen and progesterone.

menstrual phase
The part of the menstrual cycle during which the endometrial lining is sloughed off as the menstrual flow.

follicular phase
The part of the menstrual cycle during which menstruation occurs and the pituitary increases the production of FSH so the follicles mature: a combination of the menstrual and proliferative phases.

ovulation
The part of the menstrual cycle when the ovum is discharged from the ovary.

luteal phase
The same phase of the menstrual cycle as the secretory phase, which includes ovulation and the production of LH from the corpus luteum.

The next phase of the menstrual cycle is the **menstrual phase**, in which the endometrial lining of the uterus is sloughed off as the menstrual flow.

Some sexuality experts divide the menstrual cycle into three different phases: the **follicular phase**, **ovulation**, and the **luteal phase**. The follicular phase coincides with the menstrual and proliferative phases, ovulation is marked by the discharge of the ovum from the Graafian follicle, and the luteal phase is the same as the secretory phase. This categorization pertains to changes in the ovaries, whereas the previous categorization refers to changes in the uterus.

As noted in Figure 4.10, in a 28-day cycle ovulation occurs on day 14, with the menstrual flow lasting for 4 days. The great variation in the menstrual cycle—among women and even in any one woman—should be emphasized. The 28-day cycle, although often spoken of as *the* cycle, is not very common. Furthermore, in spite of menstrual cycles' differing in length, there is little difference in the luteal phase of these cycles. That is, regardless of the length of the menstrual cycle, once ovulation occurs, it basically takes 14 days until menstruation begins. For example, if a woman's cycle is 42 days long, she will ovulate on day 28, and 14 days later she will menstruate; if her cycle is 30 days long, she will ovulate on day 16 and will still menstruate 14 days later.

Effects of Menstruation on the Body and Mind

Menstruation can have several physical and emotional effects, which vary greatly from woman to woman and from one cycle to another. Eighty-five percent of women of reproductive age experience physical or emotional changes associated with their menstrual cycle, and approximately 40% of women are bothered by menstrual cycle–related conditions such

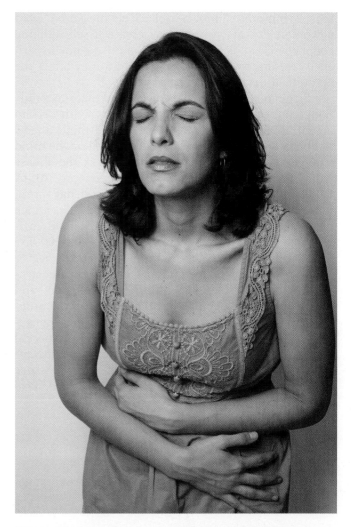

Menstruation can affect a woman's body and mind. Cramps and backaches can occur, as well as feelings of nervousness or depression. Different women are affected differently by menstruation—some women have minor symptoms whereas others have symptoms that are more severe.

as premenstrual syndrome or premenstrual dysphoric disorder (Ballagh & Heyl, 2008). It is estimated that 2.5 million women are affected by menstrual disorders each year (Clayton, 2008). There is evidence that some 10% of women take time off from work, school, or other activities because of menstrual discomfort (Patterson, 1990). Some women report cramps, backaches, and pimples; others report none of these symptoms. Some women report feeling depressed, bloated, nervous, or weak, and others do not.

Whether a woman experiences any of these effects—be they physical or emotional—may be a function of what she expects to experience. Evidence for this hypothesis does exist. For example, when researchers conducting studies of menstruating women inform the women of what the study is about, women report more of these symptoms than when they do not know what is being studied (Brooks, Ruble, & Clark, 1977; Ruble & Brooks-Gunn, 1979). Because many of these symptoms cannot be objectively measured, what a woman expects to feel may create a self-fulfilling prophecy. That is not to say women do not experience real discomfort; rather, the mind may affect the amount of discomfort experienced.

Stress researchers have determined that the mind–body connection is a real one. That is, with certain actual illnesses and diseases, either the mind affects the body so as to prepare it to become ill or the mind changes the body in a way that makes the illness worse than it might otherwise be (Greenberg, 2011). Other factors that might influence menstrual symptoms include diets too high in saturated fats, a lack of regular exercise, and work in extremely cold environments (Greenwood, 1986; Barnard et al., 2000).

The preceding discussion is not meant to negate the real physical and emotional effects of menstruation. For example, depending on one's age, and whether one has given birth to a child or not, cramping associated with menstruation can vary. Teenagers and perimenopausal women—those in the period between the beginning of menopause and the complete cessation of a woman's period—report worse cramping than is usual, whereas women who have given birth to a child report less cramping.

Menstrual Problems

Several conditions associated with menstruation require special attention. Among these conditions are dysmenorrhea, amenorrhea, and premenstrual syndrome.

Dysmenorrhea

Painful menstruation is termed **dysmenorrhea**. Many women experience some discomfort and pain during some menstrual cycles, and other women experience discomfort and pain regularly. It has been estimated that 70% to 90% of menstruating women have some degree of menstrual problems on a regular basis (Sommerfield, n.d.). Women may experience severe abdominal cramping, a bloated feeling, headaches, backaches, and nausea. An estimated 10% to 15% of women experience menstrual pain each month severe enough to prevent normal daily function at school, work, or home (Smith, 2012).

The cause of **primary dysmenorrhea**—that is, pain during menstruation—is not specifically known. Many health practitioners identify the cause as **prostaglandins**, substances produced by body tissues that act as hormones. Prostaglandins, which are found in unusually high amounts in women with dysmenorrhea, cause the muscles in the uterus to contract. This contraction causes pain and cuts off some of the blood supply (with its oxygen) to the uterus, thereby causing more discomfort.

To treat primary dysmenorrhea, physicians sometimes prescribe antiprostaglandin medications such as naproxen (Aleve), Anaprox, or Ponstel. These medicines inhibit the production of prostaglandins and relieve pain, dizziness, headache, nausea, vomiting, and irritability in many women. Many women who do not use prescription drugs find aspirin or ibuprofen helpful in relieving pain (these also somewhat inhibit prostaglandin production). Other remedies proposed for dysmenorrhea include eating more fish and vegetables and less animal fats and taking calcium, vitamin B, and magnesium supplements. Drinking plenty of fluids has also been recommended, because it seems that when the body is dehydrated, the hormone vasopressin is secreted. Vasopressin conserves body fluids, an effect that is not what a woman feeling bloated needs. Oral contraceptives can also help relieve menstrual pain by eliminating ovulation and thereby decreasing the amount of prostaglandin produced (American College of Obstetricians and Gynocologists, 2009). In addition, placing a heating pad on the abdomen, lightly massaging the abdomen with the fingertips (effleurage), drinking warm beverages, taking a warm shower, doing waist-bending exercises, having an orgasm, and walking may alleviate some menstrual pain.

Secondary dysmenorrhea is painful menstruation caused by some other identifiable condition. For example, **endometriosis** (a condition in which endometrial cells attach and develop on some body tissue other than the uterus) can cause secondary dysmenorrhea, as can pelvic inflammatory disease, uterine tumors, and blockages of the opening to the uterus (the os). In these cases, treatment consists of finding and removing the cause of the menstrual pain, which may require surgery or medication.

dysmenorrhea
Painful menstruation.

primary dysmenorrhea
Painful menstruation, the cause of which is unknown.

prostaglandins
Hormonelike substances produced by body tissue that may cause dysmenorrhea.

secondary dysmenorrhea
Painful menstruation caused by some identifiable condition such as endometriosis.

endometriosis
The growth of the endometrium uterine lining at a location other than in the uterus.

primary amenorrhea
A condition in which a woman of age 18 years or older has never menstruated.

secondary amenorrhea
A condition in which a woman has ceased menstruating after menarche.

Amenorrhea

Amenorrhea is the absence of menstrual flow. If a woman has never menstruated and is 18 years or older, her condition is called **primary amenorrhea**. If menstruation ceases after menarche, the condition is called **secondary amenorrhea**. Amenorrhea may be caused by pregnancy, malfunctioning of the ovaries, cysts or tumors, disease, hormonal imbalance, poor nutrition, or emotional distress. It may also be caused by strenuous exercise of the sort done by runners and young dancers (Koutedakis & Jamurtas, 2004; Torstveit & Sundgot-Borgen, 2005). The causes of amenorrhea in physically active women are not known. Some experts hypothesize that exercising women experience a decrease in body fat that may contribute to the cessation of their periods, as it does in anorexic women. Lower body fat may interfere with production of the amount of estrogen needed to menstruate. Among female athletes, amenorrhea is quite common (Mayo Clinic, 2007a), and it is suspected the cause is a combination of low body fat, the stress upon the body as a result of strenuous physical exercise, and the psychological stress associated with competition. Although the actual cause of amenorrhea in female athletes is difficult to determine, it does not follow that some physical condition does not exist in any one woman—athlete or not—that can be identified as the cause of her menstrual problem. It is advised that women whose menses cease consult their physicians to discuss any conditions or illnesses that are treatable.

The fear of pregnancy also has been known to create enough anguish and anxiety in sexually active women to cause a cessation of menses. Fearing pregnancy, many couples wait with bated breath for the evidence that the woman is not pregnant—menstruation. A slight delay in her period (not unusual) makes the woman anxious about the possibility of an unwanted pregnancy. Her anxiety can then further delay menstruation or create amenorrhea. Thus a vicious cycle develops that only a pregnancy test or the menstrual flow can break. Any woman who has been sexually active and has missed more than one period should have a pregnancy test.

Premenstrual Syndrome

Some women experience mood changes and other physical and emotional discomforts just before their menstrual periods. This condition is referred to as **premenstrual syndrome (PMS)**. In fact, more than 150 disorders have been associated with premenstrual syndrome; some of the more common ones are depression, tension, anxiety, mood swings, irritability or anger, difficulty in concentrating, lethargy, weight gain, fluid retention, bloating, breast soreness, joint or muscle pain, nausea, vomiting, and headaches (Mayo Clinic, 1998). It has been estimated that at some time during their reproductive years 75% of women experience PMS (Mayo Clinic, 2007b).

> **premenstrual syndrome (PMS)**
> Marked mood fluctuation during the week before menstruation, accompanied by physical symptoms.

Premenstrual syndrome was described by Katharina Dalton, a leading researcher in the treatment of PMS, in *Once a Month* (1979): "Once a month with monotonous regularity, chaos is inflicted on American homes as premenstrual tension and other menstrual problems recur time and again with demoralizing repetition." Reading this, many women found solace in the fact that other women had similar experiences each menstrual cycle. It is undeniable that many women do experience something akin to PMS fairly regularly (see Table 4.2).

There is no laboratory test or other sure way to diagnose premenstrual syndrome. Doctors rely on the woman's menstrual history, often requesting that patients keep a diary of the onset, duration, and the nature and severity of symptoms for at least two menstrual cycles. If symptoms such as those cited are present in the week before a woman's period, subside as her period starts, and are absent the week

TABLE 4.2 Premenstrual Symptoms

The Office of Women's Health of the U.S. Department of Health and Human Services lists the following symptoms of PMS:

• Acne	• Swollen or tender breasts
• Feeling tired	• Trouble sleeping
• Upset stomach	• Bloating
• Constipation	• Anxiety
• Diarrhea	• Headache or backache
• Appetite changes or food cravings	• Joint or muscle pain
• Trouble with concentration or memory	• Tension, irritability, mood swings, crying spells
• Depression	

Source: Reproduced from the National Women's Health Center. *Premenstrual Syndrome.* 2010. Available: http://www.womenshealth.gov/faq/premenstrual-syndrome.cfm.

after her period, she is diagnosed as having PMS. This diagnosis is important not only to determine the treatment to recommend but also to help screen out other conditions commonly confused with PMS, such as contraceptive side effects, dysmenorrhea, eating disorders, substance abuse, depression, and other psychiatric disorders.

There have been numerous theories about the causes of PMS. These are described in the following list, along with the recommended treatment based on the theory of causation.

1. *Prostaglandins.* As a woman's uterine lining begins to shed during the menstrual cycle, prostaglandins (hormones) are released into her bloodstream. As the prostaglandins build up, they cause the uterine walls to become tense and to contract, resulting in cramping. As with dysmenorrhea, antiprostaglandin medications are recommended, such as aspirin, acetaminophen (for example, Tylenol or Datril), naproxen (Aleve), or ibuprofen (Motrin, Advil, or Nuprin).

2. *Progesterone.* Progesterone builds up during the menstrual cycle, causing PMS symptoms. Antiprogesterone medications are recommended to alter the menstrual cycle (speeding or delaying the onset of bleeding).

3. *Natural opiates.* Women experience a drop in the level of the neurotransmitter beta-endorphin, which is manufactured in the brain the week before the menstrual flow. This neurotransmitter has been described as the body's natural opiate in that it alleviates pain and generally makes you feel good. Treatment involves administering the drug naloxone, which maintains high levels of beta-endorphins.

late luteal phase dysphoric disorder (LLPDD)
A type of premenstrual syndrome in which mental and emotional symptoms occur the week before menstruation. This is the name given to that condition by the American Psychiatric Association.

4. *State of mind.* The symptoms of PMS are the result of brain activity—that is, the mind. Moods, perceptions, thoughts, ideas, self-confidence, and self-image are "choreographed" by the brain premenstrually. Treatment, therefore, entails counseling and other means to help women change their states of mind.

Other treatments include the following:

1. Birth control pills to stop ovulation.

2. Medications such as injectable medroxyprogesterone acetate (Depo-Provera) to stop ovulation and menstruation temporarily in severe cases.

3. Antidepressants in lower dosages than usually prescribed for depression, such as fluoxetine hydrochloride (Prozac), sertaline hydrochloride (Zoloft), paroxetine hydrochloride (Paxil), and venlafaxine hydrochloride (Effexor), if symptoms are mainly emotional.

4. A vegetarian diet.

5. Naturopathic medicine that includes lifestyle and dietary changes and may consist of nutritional supplements, botanical medicines, homeopathy, Chinese medicine, acupuncture, hydrotherapy, manipulation, physical therapy, or minor surgery (Phalen, 2000).

In addition, the following is recommended (Mayo Clinic, 2007b):

1. Maintain a healthy body weight.

2. Lower the intake of salt and salty foods, especially before the period, to reduce fluid retention and bloating.

3. Avoid alcohol before the period to minimize depression and mood swings.

4. Avoid caffeine, such as in coffee, cola, and tea, to reduce moodiness, tension, and breast tenderness.

5. Increase the intake of carbohydrates such as breads, potatoes, cereals, vegetables, and rice.

? Did You Know . . .

When the American Psychiatric Association included PMS in its *Diagnostic and Statistical Manual of Mental Disorders IV* as an illness, terming it **late luteal phase dysphoric disorder (LLPDD)**, some people objected to the potential negative economic and social impact for all women. They believed it promoted a view of women as unreliable and unstable. However, others were grateful that women could then collect health insurance for treating PMS and that research would be focused on the condition.

6. Exercise regularly to enhance the sense of well-being.

7. Reduce stress by getting plenty of sleep, practicing a relaxation technique regularly, and trying yoga or massage.

Premenstrual Dysphoric Disorder

As many as 10% of women experience premenstrual symptoms so severe they cannot maintain their daily routines (Mayo Clinic, 2008). Some experts believe this is a result of a condition they term *premenstrual dysphoric disorder* (PMDD). PMDD has been described as a supercharged PMS, and is cited in the *Diagnostic and Statistical Manual of Mental Disorders, Fourth Edition.* PMDD's symptoms include

• A marked depressive mood

• A decreased interest in usual activities

• Lethargy, fatigability, or lack of energy

• Hypersomnia (falling asleep when not wanting to) or insomnia (difficulty falling asleep)

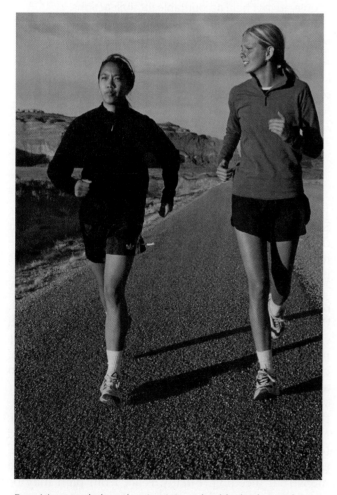

Exercising regularly and maintaining a healthy body weight are two strategies that are recommended to help women limit the severity of their menstrual and premenstrual symptoms.

There is disagreement among women's health specialists about whether PMDD should be categorized as a "mental disorder." Some believe that classifying menstrual problems as a mental disorder stigmatizes women. As one psychologist argued: "It's a label that can be used by a sexist society that wants to believe that women go crazy once a month" (Daw, 2002). Others believe a PMDD classification acknowledges women's feelings and focuses researchers' attention on developing medications to help premenstrual women. The medications now used to treat PMDD include ibuprofen (Advil, Motrin, Midol Cramp), ketoprofen (Orudis KT), naproxen (Aleve), or aspirin (National Women's Health Center, 2010).

Endometriosis

Sometimes tissue resembling the inner lining of the uterus (the endometrium) is found outside the uterus. This condition is known as *endometriosis*. Endometriosis is found most often on the lining of the pelvic cavity, the ovaries, the rectum, and the colon, and in the uterus and on the bladder. Sometimes it is also found on the small intestine, liver, spleen, and lymph nodes. Endometriosis is, unfortunately, not an uncommon occurrence. In fact, it affects 63 million women and girls in the United States, 1 million in Canada, and millions more worldwide (Endometriosis Association, 2010). Although it can affect all women, endometriosis is most common among 25- to 30-year-olds, and it has also occurred in girls as young as 11 years of age.

The causes of endometriosis are not known, although there are several theories. One theory holds that pieces of the endometrium somehow find themselves in the fallopian tubes and are transported into the pelvic cavity. This is called *retrograde menstruation*. The endometrium pieces then adhere to one another to form adhesions, which cause pain. Another theory is based on the realization that in the early stages of fetal development there are but a few cells present and that these cells eventually differentiate into different tissue. This theory posits that perhaps cells outside the uterus, for some unknown reason, take on the function of cells in the endometrium. Still another theory argues that endometrial cells are transported through the bloodstream or through the lymph system to sites elsewhere in the body. Finally, some researchers believe that endometriosis is caused by a breakdown in the function of the immune system, resulting in an inability to destroy endometrium cells that manage to leave the uterus.

Women who acquire endometriosis usually experience a great deal of pelvic pain. This pain most often occurs just before or during menstrual bleeding, and usually abates after bleeding ceases. Pain may also

¿? Ethical DIMENSIONS

Should PMS Be Used as an Excuse for Socially Unacceptable Behaviors?

In 1980 and 1981, in two separate trials, British courts set free two women who admitted to murder because they were judged to suffer from PMS. In the first case, a barmaid, Sandie Smith, stabbed another barmaid during a fight. Testimony proved Smith had a history of violent outbursts that, when subsequently treated, were controlled with injections of progesterone. In the other case, Christine English purposely drove her car into her lover after an argument. English, too, was able to prove that she suffered from PMS and that she had menstruated a few hours after the murder. Both women were judged to have "diminished responsibility" and had their charges reduced to manslaughter. They were then released contingently on their getting treatment for their PMS.

Some people believe that PMS is so unsettling a condition that the physical discomfort and the emotional changes can understandably make a woman irritable, angry, hostile, and prone to do things she might not otherwise do. Given an incident to provoke such a reaction, even violent acts can be performed without the woman's really being responsible for them. These women should be encouraged to seek treatment for their illness rather than be regarded as criminals. They should be treated with compassion rather than imprisoned. Advocates of this position would contend that these women are not in control of their decisions and should, therefore, be excused for their actions.

Others argue that murder is never excusable. If women are allowed to offer PMS as a defense, then any ill person can use a similar defense. That would allow antisocial behavior to occur without any punishment or societal sanctions. Anarchy would result. Women, or other sick people, could (short of committing murder) sign contracts and not be held responsible for them, could steal items from stores and not be prosecuted for that theft, and could even sexually abuse children without fear of reprisal. Opponents of this PMS defense conceive of an unmanageable situation if PMS sufferers, or any other group of ill people, are not held accountable for their actions.

If you were a judge, would you rule that "diminished responsibility" was a justifiable defense for women who experienced PMS? What other behaviors would you allow to be excused by PMS? What other physical or emotional conditions would you allow to be similarly used to explain people's actions?

---

be experienced in the lower back or lower abdomen and may be associated with urination. Fatigue and/or bloated feelings may occur, there may be blood in the urine and/or heavy menstrual bleeding, and diarrhea or constipation may result. In addition to causing these uncomfortable symptoms, endometriosis can lead to serious health consequences. For example, scar tissue can form and result in infertility. Or, adhesions can connect organs such as the uterus, fallopian tubes, ovaries, and intestines.

Endometriosis is treated in several ways, depending on the severity of the symptoms and the location of the tissue. Laparoscopic surgery—in which two small incisions are made in the abdomen through which is inserted a viewing instrument to perform the surgical cut—can be helpful in identifying the existence of endometrial tissue outside the uterus and determining its location. Then the tissue can be surgically removed before the procedure is completed.

Sometimes the tissue has spread so extensively that the surgeon needs to open the abdomen to remove it rather than merely inserting a laparoscope. This procedure is called a *laparotomy*.

In addition to surgery, there are medications that result in lower levels of estrogen than normal and, therefore, alleviate much of the pain associated with endometriosis. Some of these drugs are synthetic hormones that stop the ovaries from producing estrogen, causing cessation of menstruation. These are known as *gonadotropin-releasing hormone analogues (GnRH analogues)*. Another drug sometimes used is a synthetic hormone derived from testosterone (Danazol). More frequently, oral contraceptives are prescribed to prevent ovulation and reduce (when estrogen and progestin are used in combination) or eliminate menstrual bleeding. Finally, relief from pain may be obtained temporarily with ibuprofen or other analgesics (pain relievers).

Myth (vs) Fact

Myth: The menstrual cycle is 28 days long and does not fluctuate in length for any one woman.
Fact: The most prevalent menstrual cycle happens to be 30 days long. Even so, the cycle varies greatly from woman to woman and even for any one woman.

Myth: Women are usually emotionally "low" premenstrually and emotionally "high" at ovulation.
Fact: This has not been conclusively determined. There are conflicting research findings and criticism of the methodology researchers have employed to answer this question.

Myth: Women's work activity needs to be adjusted during their periods.
Fact: Though this myth has been used to support job discrimination practices against women, there is no evidence that women cannot function normally in their jobs when menstruating.

Myth: Women should not swim or exercise as usual during their periods.
Fact: With the usual hygienic practices used by women, there are no known physical reasons for not exercising as usual. For some women, iron supplementation may be necessitated by the iron lost in the menstrual blood, but that precaution is a simple one.

Myth: Women's sexual desire is at a peak just before and just after menstruation.
Fact: For some women and for some cycles this may be true. However, sexual desire involves more than one's physical condition—the nature of the relationship, the setting, one's comfort with sexuality, one's health, and so on—so that expecting sexual desire to be determined solely by the menstrual cycle is unrealistic.

The Menstrual Cycle and Sex

Many researchers have searched for a relationship between sexual interest and the time of the menstrual cycle. Findings of these studies have, for the most part, been contradictory (Bullivant et al., 2004). Some researchers report that women are more interested in sex just *before* menstruation (AskMen, 2011), and others find them most interested *during* menstruation (Friedman et al., 1980). Still others report the *middle* of the menstrual cycle to be the most sexually active (Adams, Gold, & Burt, 1978) or the time just

after the menses to be when most sexual fantasizing occurs (Matteo & Rissman, 1984). Several other studies have not found the midcycle related in any way to heightened sexual arousal (Slob et al., 1991; van Goozen et al., 1997).

When are women most sexually aroused? The answer to this question probably varies from one woman to another and, in addition to menstrual physiology, depends on such factors as one's lover, the setting, and numerous psychosocial factors such as the woman's comfort with her body, her level of self-esteem, and her religious and cultural beliefs regarding menstruation. The bottom line is that women can be sexually aroused at any time during their menstrual cycle (menstruation.com.au, 2008).

Although there are no medical reasons to refrain from coitus during menstruation (if one or both partners are HIV-negative, see the Did You Know box on this page), many couples do so. At least one study found over half the men and women surveyed believed couples should not engage in sexual intercourse when the woman is menstruating (Research Forecasts, 1981). According to a 1996 study, 16 percent of women 20 to 37 years of age reported that they had had sexual intercourse during their last menstrual period (Tanfer & Aral, 1996). Some people refrain from coitus during menstruation because of religious taboos. For example, in Orthodox Judaism menstruating women are considered unclean and are supposed to sleep in a separate bed. When they are through menstruating, Jewish women are supposed to cleanse themselves in a ritual bath called a *mikvah*. Others refrain from sexual intercourse during menstruation because of the potential messiness. Still others refrain because of the physical discomfort they feel—bloating, cramping, or fatigue. And, finally, there are women who are ashamed of their menstrual flow and prefer to keep it a private matter not shared with anyone. A couple who refrains from sexual intercourse during menstruation should be comfortable with their decision, whatever the reason; likewise, a

(?) Did You Know . . .

If a couple decides to engage in sexual intercourse when the woman is menstruating, they should realize that transmission of HIV is probably more likely at this time of the menstrual cycle than at any other. That is because of the blood present and the probability that some of that blood will have contact with an opening (albeit microscopic) into the body. If HIV is in that blood, it can infect the sexual partner. The "safer sex"

practice of refraining from sexual intercourse while a woman is menstruating is usually overlooked. From the woman's perspective, participating in coitus while menstruating can facilitate HIV entry into her body.

couple who decides to engage in coitus during this time should be comfortable with their decision.

A couple who decide to engage in sexual intercourse during the menstrual period can take several actions to make that experience as enjoyable as possible. First, they should discuss any concerns they may have—for example, the potential messiness or any religious inhibitions. Second, the woman can wear a diaphragm or cervical cap to hold back the menstrual flow. Because the menstrual fluid can sometimes irritate the penis, the man should wear a condom (a good idea anytime coitus occurs). With these simple actions, coitus during menstruation can be a positive and rewarding experience.

Menopause

Usually between the ages of 40 and 55 years, women produce progressively less estrogen and progesterone, as an effect of aging on the ovaries. Whereas the pituitary continues to produce FSH and LH, the ovaries can no longer respond to these pituitary hormones as they once could. This decrease in estrogen and progesterone occurs over approximately a 5- to 10-year period and results in a cessation of menstruation. The period when these changes take place is called the **perimenopause**, or the **climacteric**; when menstruation has not occurred for a year, we call that **menopause**.

perimenopause (climacteric)
The period just before menopause when the production of estrogen and progesterone is decreasing, usually a 5- to 10-year period.

menopause
The time when a woman's menstrual cycle ceases, usually between 40 and 55 years of age.

Sexually Related Diseases: Self-Care and Prevention

Some diseases are not transmitted by sexual activity but do affect sexual organs. These are termed sexually related diseases (SRDs). Advances in chemical and surgical treatment of diseases of the sex organs have improved 5- and 10-year survival rates and made restoration of function more attainable than ever before. Maintaining reproductive health means following safer sexual practices, paying attention to your body, monitoring it for certain signs, using the specialized health services available, and seeking information—from organizations and publications—on issues related to reproductive health. Successful treatment of SRDs generally depends on early diagnosis of potential problems.

The Female Reproductive System

Self-care and disease prevention activities for the female involve many of the sexual organs, including the breasts, cervix, uterus, ovaries, and vagina.

The Breasts

The most common breast disorders are cancer, cystic mastitis (mammary dysplasia), fibroadenoma, nipple discharge, and breast abscess. Most of these disorders occur only in women, but men are susceptible to breast cancer, too.

Breast Cancer The breast is the leading site of cancer in American women and the second major cause of cancer death (the first is lung cancer). At the time of this writing, it is estimated that 207,080 new cases of **breast cancer** will have been diagnosed in women in 2010, and 1,970 cases will have been diagnosed in men (American Cancer Society, 2010a). After increasing about 4% per year in the 1980s, breast cancer incidence rates have dropped slightly. Still, 39,840 women and 390 men will probably have died of breast cancer in 2010. And yet, death rates from breast cancer continue to decline, especially among younger women. The 5-year survival rate for localized breast cancer increased from 72% in the 1940s to 98% in 2010. If the cancer has spread regionally, however, the 5-year survival rate drops to 84%, and, if the cancer has spread to distant locations (metastasized), the survival rate drops to 23%. Eighty-two percent of women diagnosed with breast cancer survive 10 years, and 90% survive 5 years.

breast cancer
The most common type of cancer in women.

No specific cause of breast cancer is known, but epidemiological studies have identified certain risk factors that predispose women to breast cancer. One of these risk factors is age. As women get older, the risk increases. The risk is also higher in women who have a family history of breast cancer, who experienced an early menarche or a late menopause, who recently used oral contraceptives or postmenopausal estrogens, and who never had children or had the first live birth at a late age. Other suspected risk factors are a diet high in fat, although a large-scale 1999 study calls this relationship into question (Holmes et al., 1999); exposure to pesticides and other selected chemicals; alcohol consumption; weight gain; and physical inactivity. In addition, two new genes that appear to make women susceptible to breast cancer have been discovered, BRCA1 and BRCA2. However, only 5% to 10% of breast cancers are thought to be inherited, and only 5% of breast cancer patients were found to have the gene BRCA1 or BRCA2. One study found that 75% of women in whom breast cancer develops have no identifiable risk factor other than gender and age (Hortobagyi, McLelland, & Reed, 1990). This makes it especially important for all women to learn breast self-examination and to have regular breast examinations by a physician.

Breast self-examination (BSE) is a self-care procedure women can adopt. Although medical specialists actively check for breast cancer in routine examinations, some experts believe that checking one's own breasts every menstrual cycle increases the chances of early detection. The

> **breast self-examination (BSE)**
> A periodic self-care procedure that involves feeling the breast for any abnormalities. The test is performed once every menstrual cycle or every month after menopause.

technique is simple. If cancer is present, the earlier it is diagnosed, the better the chance for survival.

In April 1987 a committee of the United States Public Health Service (which had been established to recommend those medical procedures with demonstrated effectiveness and those without) caused concern among cancer prevention specialists by citing BSE as a procedure whose value had not been clearly shown. The committee was charged with reviewing the scientific evidence for many medical screenings and examination procedures and eliminating those that contributed to the increasing cost of health care. As such they decided that BSE was not employed by enough women and cancers not found in enough quantity to warrant public health campaigns to encourage women to perform the examination. Other cancer experts, who argued that BSE does not cost a woman any money and that it can uncover early treatable cancers, recommended that women ignore the committee's finding and continue doing monthly BSEs. Canadians have also weighed in on this issue. The Canadian Task Force on Preventive Health Care (Baxter, 2001) studied the benefits and harms associated with breast self-examinations and found no evidence of effectiveness and evidence of harm. The harm included an increase in the number of physician visits for the evaluation of benign breast lesions and significantly higher rates of benign breast biopsy findings. As a result, the Canadian Task Force recommended that women not perform breast self-examinations. The American Cancer Society (2007a) takes a neutral stance, stating in their guidelines that breast self-exam is an option for women starting in their 20s. More recently, after conducting an extensive review of the research literature, the U.S. Preventive Services Task Force (2009) concluded there were more risks than benefits associated with breast self-exams and, therefore, recommended against teaching women how to perform breast self-examination.

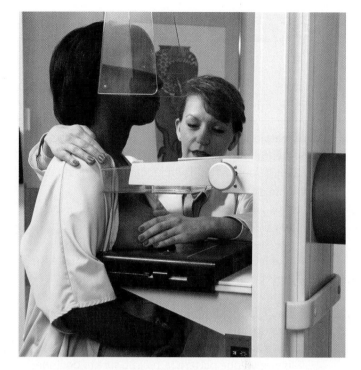

It is recommended by several organizations that women older than age 40 get a mammogram annually. Younger women should have annual clinical breast exams every 3 years.

If choosing to perform BSE, for best results, perform the exam when the skin is wet or moist—after showering or after applying body lotion. Menstruating women should perform this test 1 week after their period; postmenopausal women should check their breasts at least once a month. All women should check their breasts visually in the mirror and by means of this exam. Consult a gynecologist if you find a lump, a thickening, or any other unusual feature. These symptoms may include pain in the breast, discharge from the nipple, a change in the character of the nipple itself, or changes in the character of the breast.

In addition, the American Cancer Society, the American Medical Association, and the National Comprehensive Cancer Network recommend that women have regular breast examinations by a physician. These examinations include both **clinical breast exams** and **mammography** screening, depending on a woman's age and medical history.

> **clinical breast exam**
> A breast examination conducted by a physician to detect any abnormalities.
>
> **mammography**
> An X ray of the breasts to detect any abnormality before it is visible or palpable.

A clinical breast exam is similar to BSE, except that it is conducted by a physician trained to detect any

Gender
DIMENSIONS

Breast Self-Examination
By regularly examining her own breasts, a woman may notice any changes that occur. The best time for breast self-examination (BSE) is about a week after your period ends, when your breasts are not tender or swollen. If you are not having regular periods, do BSE on the same day every month.

1. Lie down with a pillow under your right shoulder and place your right arm behind your head.
2. Use the finger pads of the three middle fingers on your left hand to feel for lumps in the right breast.
3. Press firmly enough to know how your breast feels. A firm ridge in the lower curve of each breast is normal. If you are not sure how hard to press, talk with your doctor or nurse.
4. Move around the breast in a circular, up-and-down line, or wedge pattern (a, b, c). Be sure to do it the

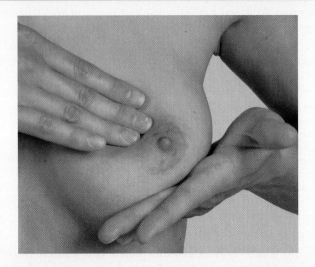

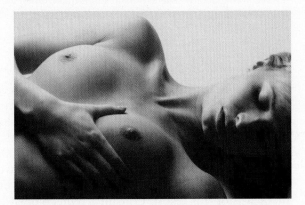

same way every time, check the entire breast area, and remember how your breast feels from month to month.
5. Repeat the exam on your left breast, using the finger pads of the right hand. (Move the pillow to below your left shoulder.)

6. If you find any changes, see your doctor right away.
7. Repeat the examination of both breasts while standing, with one arm behind your head. The upright position makes it easier to check the upper and outer part of the breasts (toward your armpit). This is where about half of breast cancers are found. You may want to do the standing part of the BSE while you are in the shower. Some breast changes can be felt more easily when your skin is wet and soapy.

For added safety, you can check your breasts for any dimpling of the skin, changes in the nipple, redness, or swelling while standing in front of a mirror right after your BSE each month.

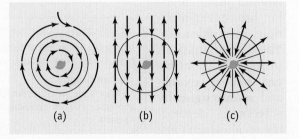

(a)   (b)   (c)

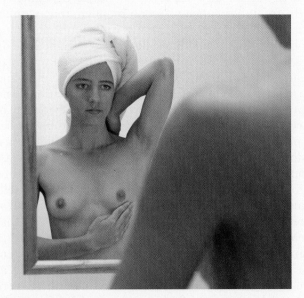

abnormalities. It is suggested that women aged 20 years and older have a clinical breast examination regularly, preferably every 3 years between ages 20 and 40 years and annually thereafter. However, the U.S. Preventive Services Task Force also questioned the value of clinical breast exams (2009).

Mammography is also recommended. A mammogram is an X ray of the breast that often allows physicians to detect breast lumps before they would be palpable by a physician (see Figure 4.11). Some organizations argue that women older than age 40 years should have a mammogram annually. However, whether women in their 40s or women over 74 years old receive benefit from mammograms has been called into question by the U.S. Preventive Services Task Force (2009). (See Table 4.3.) The Centers for Disease Control and Prevention (2008) reported that in 2008, 76% of women aged 40 years and older had had a mammogram within the previous 2 years. Obviously, we have a long way to go in educating women about the need to get mammograms and the benefits they can expect.

There is increasing interest in using breast magnetic resonance imaging (MRI) as a screening test for breast cancer. The use of MRI to detect breast cancer is being studied at the time of this writing. Some studies have shown that MRI is associated with higher false-positive rates. Thus women who are screened with MRI may have more unnecessary surgical biopsies. At the present time, it is still undetermined whether the increase in cancer detection achieved with MRI, in conjunction with the as-yet-undemonstrated decrease in death rates as a result, conveys enough of a benefit to warrant recommendations for wider use of this technology, given the large increase in false-positive rates and the possibility of overdiagnosis (National Cancer Institute, 2008a).

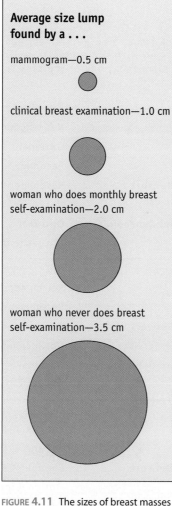

Average size lump found by a . . .

mammogram—0.5 cm

clinical breast examination—1.0 cm

woman who does monthly breast self-examination—2.0 cm

woman who never does breast self-examination—3.5 cm

FIGURE **4.11** The sizes of breast masses detectable by mammography, physical examination, and self-examination illustrate the importance of screening mammography in the early detection of breast cancer.

When breast cancer is suspected, a **biopsy** is performed. In a **needle biopsy** a fine needle is inserted into the tumor and fluid or cells are withdrawn. If the lump dissipates as soon as fluid is obtained, the lump is confirmed as a cyst and generally no further procedure is needed. An **open biopsy** is a minor surgical procedure during which tissue of the tumor is removed and examined for possible cancer (**carcinoma**).

Patients who have breast cancer are classified in terms of stages. These stages are determined by the characteristics of the tumor and the lymph nodes and whether **metastasis**—spread of the cancer to other body sites—has occurred. Treatment naturally depends on the stage of the cancer. The treatment of breast cancer may involve **lumpectomy**, in which only the breast lump and lymph nodes under the arm are removed, usually followed by radiation therapy; **mastectomy**, in which the breast and lymph nodes under the arm are removed; **chemotherapy**, treatment with drugs; **radiation therapy**; and **hormone therapy**. There are three kinds of mastectomy: *simple mastectomy*, in which the whole breast is removed, sometimes along with lymph nodes under the arm; *modified radical mastectomy*, the most common form of mastectomy, in which the breast, many of the lymph nodes under the arm, the lining over the chest muscles, and sometimes part of the chest wall are removed; and *radical mastectomy* (also called the *Halstead radical mastectomy*), in which the breast,

biopsy (open biopsy)
Usually referred to as an open biopsy, a minor surgical procedure during which tissue of a tumor is removed and examined for presence of cancer.

needle biopsy
Insertion of a needle into a lump in a breast to see whether fluid (which indicates a cyst rather than a tumor) can be removed.

carcinoma
A type of cancer emanating from epithelial cells.

metastasis
Spread of cancer from a primary site to other parts of the body.

lumpectomy
Removal of a lesion, benign or malignant.

mastectomy
Removal of the breast and/or other tissue. *Simple:* Removal of only the breast (sometimes with removal of lymph nodes under the arm). *Modified radical:* Removal of the breast, lymph nodes, lining of the chest muscle, and sometimes part of the chest wall. *Radical:* Removal of the breast, lymph nodes, and chest muscle.

chemotherapy
Use of chemicals (medication) to treat disease; may be oral, intravenous, intramuscular, or topical.

radiation therapy
A form of treatment for cancer that uses carefully directed radiation to destroy cancer cells.

hormone therapy
Form of treatment for cancer that uses hormones to combat cancer cell growth.

TABLE 4.3 **Breast Cancer Screening Controversy**

In November of 2009, the U.S. Preventive Services Task Force issued new guidelines regarding breast cancer screening. These guidelines generated a good deal of discussion with some experts and organizations agreeing and others disagreeing with the task force. The recommendations of the task force and several other organizations are summarized below.

Procedure	Organization(s)	Recommendation
Breast self-exams	USPSTF	Not recommended
	American Cancer Society	Optional
	American Medical Association	Recommended
	National Comprehensive Cancer Network	Recommended
	Canadian Task Force on Preventive Services	Not recommended
	American College of Obstetrics and Gynecology	Optional
	World Health Organization	Not recommended
Clinical breast exams	USPSTF	Not recommended
	American Cancer Society	Recommended
	American Medical Association	Recommended
	National Comprehensive Cancer Network	Recommended
	Canadian Task Force on Preventive Services	Not recommended
	American College of Obstetrics and Gynecology	Optional
	World Health Organization	Not recommended
Mammograms	USPSTF	Only for ages 50–74
	American Cancer Society	For age 40+
	American Medical Association	For age 40+
	National Comprehensive Cancer Network	For age 40+
	American College of Physicians	Optional for age 40+
	Canadian Task Force on Preventive Services	For age 40+
	American College of Obstetrics and Gynecology	For age 40+
	World Health Organization	Only ages 50–69

Given the variance in these recommendations, it is suggested that women discuss the best screening procedures for their individual circumstances with their physicians considering such factors as their family history, health status, and age.

Source: Data from U.S. Preventive Services Task Force. Screening for breast cancer: U.S. Preventive Services Task Force recommendation statement. *Annals of Internal Medicine, 151* (2009), 716–726.

chest muscles, and all lymph nodes under the arm are removed. Radical mastectomy used to be the most frequently performed operation for breast cancer but now is used only when the tumor has spread to the chest muscles.

For patients with no lymph node involvement, hormone therapy may be prescribed as a preventive measure against recurrence of cancer. The most commonly used hormones are tamoxifen and special "designer estrogens," which may be administered for 5 years. There presently remains a question regarding the increased risk of development of cancer of the uterus for women on hormonal therapy. For early-stage breast cancer, long-term survival rates after lumpectomy plus radiation therapy are similar to survival rates after modified radical mastectomy, and, therefore, this less invasive procedure is being used more often—except for those women who choose not to experience the side effects of radiation and thus choose mastectomy.

We live in a society in which breast size and shape are mistakenly seen as contributing greatly to a

Multicultural DIMENSIONS

Breast Cancer More Deadly in African Americans

Although breast cancer develops more often in white women, African American women are more likely to die of it (American Cancer Society, 2010a). Researchers and epidemiologists have been perplexed as to why. It was originally assumed that this difference was due to the disproportionately high number of African American women who live in poverty, resulting in lack of access to health care. That, in turn, would lead to later diagnosis and, consequently, less effective treatment. However, having studied this dilemma for several years, scientists have concluded that, although poverty status plays a role (it is estimated that poverty accounts for approximately 50% of the cause), biology is significantly involved. Tumors in African American women are just more virulent.

Evidence for this conclusion can be found in a study that compared African American and white women who belonged to health maintenance organizations (HMOs) in which health care was readily available (access to mammograms and other medical care). Still, the African American women HMO members had larger and more advanced tumors when diagnosed. The suspicion was that these tumors grew faster, and that is why at the time of diagnosis they were larger and more advanced.

Research also indicates that African American women do not wait any longer to seek medical diagnosis when identifying a breast abnormality than do white women. Consequently, that is not a significant variable in the difference in tumor size or death rates between African American and white women.

A review of research of breast cancer in African American women published in the *New York Times* (Kolata, 1994) summarized what is known about this situation. Cited are several studies in which tumors in African American women were found to be more actively dividing than those in white women, and more lacked hormone receptors and had tissue features indicative of unfavorable diagnosis.

Although it is wise for all women to obtain regular medical examinations, given what we know about tumors in African American women, it is particularly prudent for them to do so.

woman's sexuality. Thus a woman who loses a breast through amputation can be devastated. Many women who have had mastectomies, whether or not they are sexually active, suffer feelings of loss, fear of rejection, and, of course, fear of the cancer's recurrence. Community support systems such as the Reach to Recovery Project of the American Cancer Society (ACS) and the Breast Referral Service, founded by Rose Kushner, who herself recovered from a mastectomy, give invaluable support to women in adjusting to the treatment of their cancers. The involvement of lovers or husbands and children is of great importance, because all of them, not just the woman, must adjust to her changed appearance and emotional sensitivity. Breast reconstruction after a mastectomy is also available. It offers a woman a more normal appearance and often eases her acceptance of the change in her body. This option should be discussed with the surgeon before breast surgery, if possible.

Reconstructive breast surgery can create a breast-like structure by using saline (salt) water encased in a silicone pouch that is implanted under a woman's skin and chest muscle.

Cystic Mastitis Also called *chronic cystic mastitis, fibrocystic condition,* and *mammary dysplasia* (cell change), **cystic mastitis** is the most common breast condition. It is usually found in women 40 to 60 years of age (California Pacific Medical Center, 2008). Because cystic mastitis is uncommon in postmenopausal women, it is believed to be related to estrogen activity.

> **cystic mastitis**
> Known also as fibrocystic disease, a condition characterized by fluid-filled lesions (cysts) that are tender and believed to be related to estrogen activity.

In cystic mastitis small and large cysts form in the breast tissues. The cysts are generally filled with fluid and may have to be drained frequently. Sometimes the cysts must be removed. Studies have concluded that "fibrocystic breasts" occur frequently in women and are not associated with significant increases in risk for breast cancer (Mayo Clinic Staff, 2010). One research report indicated a possible link between cystic mastitis and coffee, tea, cola, and chocolate consumption. On the basis of this study, some practitioners recommend that women decrease or eliminate the consumption of these products. But because this treatment approach has not been tested by using randomized double-blind studies, medical researchers and practitioners have questioned its validity.

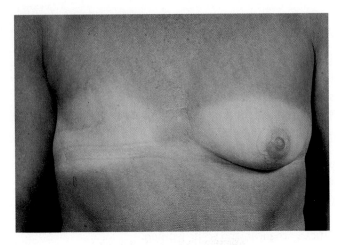

After mastectomy.

After reconstructive surgery after mastectomy.

Fibroadenoma   **Fibroadenoma** is a benign (noncancerous) tumor that may develop in white women in their early 30s and in black women somewhat earlier (there are no data on other groups). The tumor is usually firm, round, and somewhat movable. Generally the treatment is surgical removal.

Nipple Discharge   A discharge from the nipples of women who are not nursing can be due to cystic mastitis, to a small benign tumor (called a *papilloma*) in a duct leading to the nipple, or to an uncommon condition *(ectasia)* in which the ducts of the breast enlarge and distend, allowing fluid to accumulate and escape. Occasionally the use of hormones—such as oral contraceptives and postmenopausal estrogen supplements—can cause nipple discharge, which should cease when the drugs are discontinued. Any discharge from the nipples should be checked by a physician.

fibroadenoma
A benign (noncancerous) tumor that is firm, round, and somewhat movable.

breast abscess
Infection of the breast characterized by redness, swelling, and a painful or tender mass.

invasive cervical cancer
Cancer that has invaded a wide area of cervical tissue.

Breast Abscess   Generally **breast abscesses** (infections) are seen in nursing women, but they occur in nonnursing women as well, and in either case should be treated by a physician. Redness, swelling, or a tender, painful mass is symptomatic of breast infection. If the infection is not stopped, an abscess can develop. These are usually treated by incision and drainage, antibiotics, or both.

The Cervix

Rates of **invasive cervical cancer**, which involves deep-tissue layers of the cervix and sometimes spreads to other organs, have decreased steadily over the past several decades. This decline is attributed to the increase in Pap smear screening, which leads to early detection and subsequent early treatment. Still, an estimated 12,200 cases of invasive cervical cancer were diagnosed in 2010 with 4,210 deaths (American Cancer Society, 2010a), in spite of a steady decline in death rate from cervical cancer since 1982. Cervical cancer death rates declined for African Americans more rapidly than for whites. However, in 2010 the mortality rate for African American women (4.6 per 100,000) was twice as high as it was for white women (2.2 per 100,000). The 5-year relative survival rate for the earliest stage of invasive cervical cancer is 92%. The overall (all stages combined) 5-year survival rate for cervical cancer is about 71% (American Cancer Society, 2010a).

Although the exact cause of cervical cancer is unknown, several factors can put you at risk. Among these are having your first intercourse at an early age, having multiple sex partners, having many pregnancies, having a mother who took diethylstilbestrol (DES) while pregnant with you, and having a sexually transmitted infection caused by the human papillomavirus (HPV).

The American Cancer Society (2010b) recommends a **Pap smear** be performed annually with a pelvic exam in women who are, or have been, sexually active or who have reached the age of 18 years. After three consecutive annual exams have normal findings, the Pap test

Pap smear
A test of the tissue of the cervix for cervical cancer (named after its founder, Dr. Papanicolaou).

may be performed less frequently at the discretion of the woman and her physician. Pap smear screening is a simple procedure that involves swabbing a small sample of cells from the cervix, transferring these cells to a slide, and examining them under a microscope.

Regular gynecological screening is advised for all women, particularly because early cell changes in the cervical tissue do not present symptoms a woman can recognize herself—although invasive cervical cancer sometimes does cause a bloody discharge between periods and/or bloody spotting after intercourse. Unfortunately, data indicate that not enough women are getting regular Pap tests. In 2008, only 75% of women had a Pap smear within the past 3 years (National Center for Health Statistics, 2009).

Other procedures have been developed to screen for cervical cancer. One of these is called *PapSure* (Redfran, 2002). This procedure involves a visual inspection of the cervix using a scope and a blue chemical light, and is performed in conjunction with a traditional Pap smear. Another cervical cancer detection test is the experimental *LUMA Cervical Imaging System* (McMillan, 2004). In this procedure, the cancerous tissue absorbs light differently than healthy tissue, showing possible problematic areas. Certainly, even more advanced screening techniques will be developed in the coming years.

Treatment for invasive cervical cancer generally consists of surgery and radiation, or both. Ninety percent of patients survive 1 year after diagnosis, and 73% survive 5 years. When detected at an early stage, invasive cervical cancer is one of the most successfully treated cancers, with a 5-year survival rate of 92% for cancers that have not spread. Unfortunately, only 57% of invasive cervical cancer in white women and only 49% in African American women are diagnosed at this stage. Again, this points to the value of getting a Pap test regularly (American Cancer Society, 2008).

At the time of this writing, it was estimated that 43,470 cases of cancer of the uterus, most often of the endometrium, would be diagnosed in 2010. Incidence rates of uterine cancer have varied since the mid-1980s. In 2006, the incidence rate for white women was 24.3 per 100,000, and 17.5 per 100,000 for African American women (National Center for Health Statistics, 2010). Although incidence rates are higher among white women than African American women, the relationship is reversed for mortality rates: African American women have mortality rates that are nearly twice as high as rates among white women.

Estrogen is the major risk factor for uterine cancer. Women who choose estrogen replacement therapy to combat the effects of menopause, who are administered tamoxifen to prevent breast cancer or its recurrence, who experience an early menarche, who have a late menopause, who never have children, or who do not ovulate have been shown to be at increased risk. Conversely, pregnancy and the use of oral contraceptives appear to provide protection against uterine cancer.

The Pap test is rarely effective in detecting uterine cancer early. It is with this realization that the American Cancer Society recommends that women older than 40 years have an annual pelvic exam and that women at high risk have an endometrial biopsy at menopause and periodically thereafter. Early warning signs include uterine bleeding or spotting; pain is a later symptom. Treatment, which depends on the stage of the cancer, consists of surgical removal of the uterus and/or ovaries, radiation therapy, hormonal therapy, and chemotherapy. The 5-year survival rate is 96% if the cancer is discovered at an early stage, when it is contained regionally. Survival rates for whites exceed that for African Americans.

The Ovaries

Ovarian cysts and tumors can occur when a female is any age. A cyst is an abnormal cavity that is filled with fluid. The most common ones are called **functional cysts**; these occur on the follicle or corpus luteum and are usually caused by the failure of the follicle to rupture and discharge the egg. Generally they are small and not particularly significant. They usually disappear spontaneously within a month or two.

Dermoid cysts are common in young women. They contain hard, fatty material, and sometimes remnants of teeth. These are believed to be embryonic in nature and are considered benign. Most ovarian cysts and tumors are usually benign, but if they cause symptoms such as pain, tenderness, and internal bleeding, they can require surgery. Because there is always the possibility of future problems, such as malignancy, a woman should remain under medical supervision once cysts or tumors have been diagnosed.

In the **Stein–Leventhal syndrome** the ovaries become enlarged and have cysts on them. Infertility and secondary amenorrhea also result. This condition affects one in ten women of childbearing age and is the most common cause of female infertility. Although its causes are not specifically known, genes are thought to be one factor because women experiencing this condition tend to have a mother or sister with it as well. Researchers also think insulin could be a cause given that Stein–Leventhal syndrome affects the ovaries and ovulation (The National Women's Health Information Center, 2010). Symptoms include infrequent menstrual periods,

functional cyst
An ovarian cyst that occurs on the follicle or corpus luteum, usually caused by the failure of the follicle to rupture and release an egg.

dermoid cyst
A type of benign ovarian cyst commonly found in young women.

Stein–Leventhal syndrome
Reproductive malfunction in women; a syndrome of endocrine origin that involves ovarian cysts, amenorrhea, and infertility.

no menstrual periods, and/or irregular bleeding; infertility; increased hair growth on the face, chest, stomach, back, thumbs, or toes; and pelvic pain. Treatment may include birth control pills; medications such as Clomid and Serophene to stimulate ovulation; surgery ("ovarian drilling") that involves puncturing the ovary and administers an electrical current to destroy a small portion of the ovary; and lifestyle changes (eating a healthy diet, exercise, and weight loss) to improve the body's use of insulin. Most patients respond to therapy, and frequently fertility is restored to normal.

Ovarian cancer killed an estimated 13,850 American women in 2010. In fact, ovarian cancer causes more deaths than any other cancer of the female reproductive system. An estimated 21,880 new cases of ovarian cancer were diagnosed in 2010. One of the reasons ovarian cancer is so deadly is that its symptoms are "silent": They may go unnoticed until late in development. Rarely does abdominal swelling occur and even more rarely abnormal vaginal bleeding. Stomach gas, discomfort, and distention that cannot be explained by other causes may indicate a need to have a thorough medical examination with ovarian cancer in mind.

> **ovarian cancer**
> Cancer of the ovaries; it causes more cancer deaths than any other cancer of the female reproductive system.

Risk factors include never having children, being older (ovarian cancer occurs more frequently in women in their 80s), and having had certain other cancers such as colon and endometrial cancers. As with all cancers, early detection is important. Pelvic exams are most valuable, because Pap tests rarely are effective in uncovering ovarian cancer. In 2000 a new technique using sonography was developed that has the potential of diagnosing ovarian cancer earlier than is presently possible. This new method, *transvaginal ultrasonography*, was able to diagnose stage 1 ovarian cancer in 59% of women, whereas other methods could detect only 30% of these stage 1 cancers (Sato et al., 2000). Treatment can include surgical removal of one or both of the ovaries and/or the fallopian tubes (called a *salpingo-oophorectomy*) and the uterus (*hysterectomy*). If disease is detected early and the tumor is small, only the involved ovary is removed. This consideration is especially important to young women who want to have children. Radiation therapy and chemotherapy are also used in the treatment of ovarian cancer. The 5-year survival rate varies by the stage when diagnosed. If cancer is diagnosed and treated early, the survival rate goes up to 94%. Unfortunately, only 15% of cases are detected in their localized stage. Five-year survival rates vary from 28% to 94%, depending on the stage of the cancer.

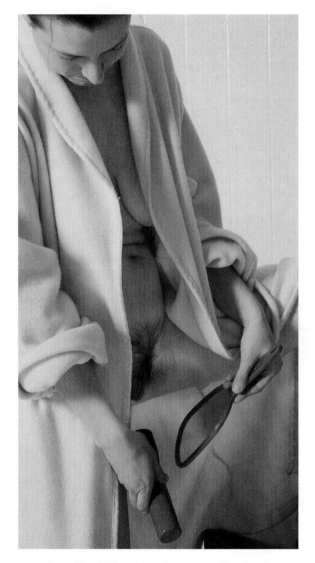

Sexual health begins with routine self-exams.

The Vagina

Normal vaginal secretions are odorless, and the acidity of the vagina helps it to cleanse itself. Nevertheless, some women choose to cleanse the vagina by **douching**—that is, by rinsing with water or a vinegar and water solution. A vaginal douche, the value of which has been questioned, is not recommended and can be harmful if not done correctly.

> **douche**
> Cleansing of the vagina by inserting a nozzle that secretes a recommended cleansing substance, a controversial procedure.

Damage can occur in two main ways: (1) Improper insertion of the douching material may actually damage the tissue, resulting in an increased chance of infection; (2) the chemical balance of the vagina can be altered, affecting contraceptive function. For instance, if a woman is using a spermicidal cream or other form of spermicide as a means of contraception, douching may destroy its effectiveness.

Smegma, a cheeselike substance secreted by the glans penis of males, may have effects on women's health. A female engaging in coitus with a male who has not washed away smegma could be subjecting herself to vaginal infections. There is also some concern that smegma may contribute to cancer of the cervix. It seems prudent, therefore, for sexually active women to make sure that their male sexual partners engage in the routine hygiene care necessary to remove smegma. Although it may be embarrassing, this may be a small price to pay for the prevention of vaginal infection and cervical cancer. Signs of sexually transmitted infections should also be given attention. Make sure to check your vulva routinely. See a healthcare provider if you have unusual discharges, abdominal pain, or open sores on your genitalia.

Toxic Shock Syndrome (TSS)

In the late 1970s several young women died of a previously little-known disease called **toxic shock syndrome (TSS)**. The toxins that cause this syndrome are produced by the *Staphylococcus aureus* bacteria, which may grow in the vagina and are absorbed by the body. These toxins enter the bloodstream and cause high fever (above 102°F), nausea, vomiting, diarrhea, a rapid drop in blood pressure, and sometimes aching muscles and peeling skin on the palms and feet. The exact mechanism of transmission is unknown. The syndrome appears to be linked to the use of tampons—particularly those made of superabsorbent material. It is thought that the presence of the tampon in the vagina for a prolonged period (6 hours or more) may provide an environment conducive to proliferation of the toxin-producing bacteria. When some tampons are inserted into the vagina, small irritations of the vaginal mucosa may occur and promote entry of the bacteria.

> **toxic shock syndrome (TSS)**
> A syndrome caused by *Staphylococcus aureus* bacteria in which symptoms include high fever, nausea, vomiting, diarrhea, and a drop in blood pressure; a potentially fatal syndrome that has been linked with the use of superabsorbent tampons.

It is recommended that superabsorbent tampons not be used because they pack the vagina tightly, prevent air circulation, and allow bacteria to proliferate. It has also been suggested that women using other types of tampons leave them in place for no longer than 2 hours and not use them at all during the night while sleeping.

Toxic shock syndrome has been seen in both genders among postsurgical patients, burn victims, and patients with boils and abscesses. Nonmenstrual cases constitute about half of all reported cases (Nemours Foundation, 2007).

Care from Medical Specialists

All health-related specialists agree that you should report any unusual signs or symptoms related to the reproductive system to a specialist in women's reproductive health—a **gynecologist** or a gynecological nurse practitioner. Furthermore, the American College of Obstetrics and Gynecology recommends that women have a routine gynecological exam every year, even when no signs or symptoms appear. Routine checkups, usually conducted on a special table with the woman's knees up and her feet in stirrups, consist of the following procedures:

> **gynecologist**
> A physician specializing in women's reproductive health.

1. An inspection of the external genitals for any irritations, discolorations, unusual discharges, or other abnormalities.

2. An internal check for cystoceles (bulges of the bladder into the vagina) and rectoceles (bulges of the rectum into the vagina). The examiner also looks for pus in the Skene's glands and for the strength of the pelvic and abdominal muscles. He or she also tests urine control by asking the patient to cough while checking to see whether urine flows involuntarily.

3. An inspection of the vagina and cervix by means of a **speculum**, a plastic or metal instrument that is inserted into the vagina to hold the walls apart during the examination (Figure 4.12). (At this point and throughout the remainder of the examination, if you are interested in seeing your genitals and watching the exam, ask the examiner to set up a mirror for you and to point out the various organs. If the examiner is not sympathetic to this request, you might consider looking for another practitioner.) The examiner will look for anything unusual, such as lesions (sores) or inflammation affecting the vagina or cervix. Next the practitioner will scrape a tiny amount of tissue from the cervix by using a small wooden instrument called a *spatula*. This tissue will be used for the Pap smear. *If requested by the patient*, the smear can also be tested for signs of gonorrhea.

> **speculum**
> A metal (or plastic) instrument that is inserted into the vagina to hold the walls apart, allowing for medical examination.

FIGURE **4.12** Medical examination with speculum and spatula in place.

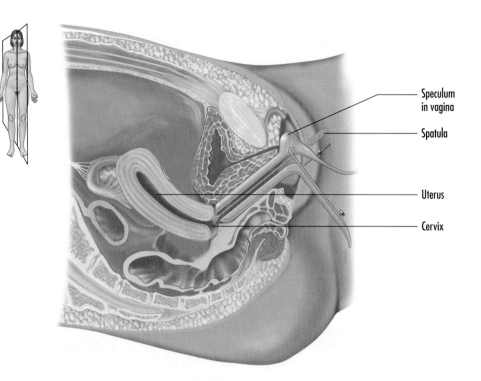

Speculum in vagina

Spatula

Uterus

Cervix

4. A bimanual examination (Figure 4.13). By sliding the index and middle fingers of one hand into the vagina and pressing down on

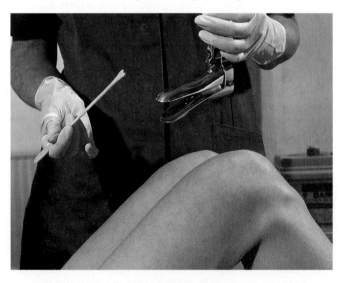

Speculum and spatula.

the abdominal wall from the outside, the examiner feels for the uterus, fallopian tubes, and ovaries to determine their position, their size, and the presence of pain or inflammation. The examiner may also examine the internal genitals by inserting one finger into the rectum and another into the vagina.

5. An examination of the breasts for lumps or thickenings.

Two additional points should be noted about the routine gynecological exam. First, although the checkup may be uncomfortable, it should not be painful. Second, before beginning the physical examination, the practitioner should take a gynecological history. Noted on the history should be information regarding the regularity, flow, and any changes in the menstrual cycle; any pregnancies, miscarriages, or abortions; all birth-control methods used; the incidence of breast cancer in close female relatives; and whether the woman's mother took the drug DES during her pregnancy with the patient—that is, whether the patient is a "DES daughter." DES is a drug that was given in the 1940s and 1950s to women with a history of miscarriage. It is no longer used for miscarriages, because it has been found that vaginal cancer is more prevalent in DES daughters than in other women (Centers for Disease Control and Prevention, 2011a), and that women who took DES have breast cancer in greater numbers than non-DES women. If the patient's mother did take DES, a periodic **colposcopy**, a check for changes in the vagina and cervix, should be conducted. The examiner uses an instrument called a *colposcope* to

colposcopy
An examination of the vagina and cervix using an instrument—a colposcope—to detect abnormal tissue growth.

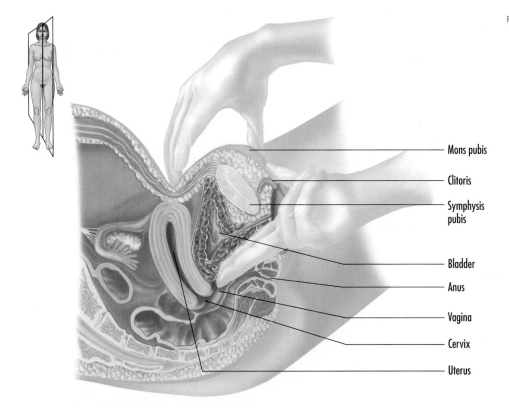

FIGURE **4.13** Bimanual examination.

Mons pubis

Clitoris

Symphysis pubis

Bladder

Anus

Vagina

Cervix

Uterus

view the vagina for abnormal tissue growth. The examiner might also perform a biopsy.

The most consistent research finding for DES sons is that they have an increased risk for noncancerous epididymal cysts, which are growths on the testicles (Centers for Disease Control and Prevention, 2011b).

Care from Organizations and Available Publications

For women, the ACS, the National Organization for Women, the March of Dimes, the National Women's Health Network, women's health centers and clinics, as well as local organizations of women who have had breasts removed due to cancer are but a few of the groups devoted to improving women's reproductive health. These groups function in various ways: Some publish written material, others lobby for legislation and funds, and still others provide social support for women with reproductive health problems. In addition, clinics conduct medical examinations, test and care for STIs, and offer premarital blood tests and other services for women.

Exploring the Dimensions of Human Sexuality

Our feelings, attitudes, and beliefs regarding sexuality are influenced by our internal and external environments. Go to go.jblearning.com/dimensions5e to learn more about the biological, psychological, and sociological factors that affect your sexuality.

The physiological development of a female starts when a sperm with an X chromosome fertilizes an egg. But socioeconomic status of the mother influences whether prenatal care is received, good nutrition will be available, and medical help will be sought. If the mother smokes, drinks, or abuses drugs during pregnancy, the fetus will be affected.

A woman's physiology is further altered during puberty and menopause. The increased fat content at puberty negatively affects many women's body image, which in turn negatively affects self-concept.

Unable to control the changes taking place within her body, the pubertal girl sometimes resorts to controlling the one thing she can control: food intake. Dieting is common, but excessive food control, or self-induced vomiting after meals, can result in a serious eating disorder.

Biological Factors

When a sperm with an X chromosome meets an egg (all of which have X chromosomes), a female will develop. Biological factors continue to influence development throughout life.

- Genetic coding affects physical appearance, including height; coloration of skin, hair, and eyes; breast size; and many aspects of health.
- Female physical appearance changes at puberty, when the lean-body-mass-to-fat ratio changes from about 5:1 to about 3:1, signaling the body to commence menarche.
- Hormonal changes affect mood.
- At menopause, lower estrogen levels increase a female's risk for heart attack.

Sociocultural Factors

Sociocultural factors interact with biological factors to influence health.

- Socioeconomic status influences prenatal care and nutrition.
- Ethnic heritage influences health. African American women tend to get a more virulent form of breast cancer, resulting in a higher death rate. Jewish women are genetically at risk for scoliosis (curvature of the spine).
- Culture influences women's health. Fear of Western medicine prevents some immigrants from seeking treatment at early stages of a problem.
- Media and ads that present ultrathin women as ideals can influence the eating patterns and health of women.

Psychological Factors

Psychological factors interact with other factors and can influence health.

- Women tend to have nearly twice the rate of depression of men.
- Teen women with low self-concept have a higher probability of having an unwanted pregnancy and birth.
- Expressiveness of emotions helps women stay mentally and physically healthy.
- Learned attitudes and behaviors about gender roles can prevent a woman from fulfilling her potential.
- Body-image problems in women can lead to long-term disorders, such as bulimia and anorexia nervosa.

Summary

- The external female genitals (the vulva) consist of the mons pubis, labia majora, labia minora, clitoris, vestibule, and urethral opening.

- The clitoris is protected by the clitoral hood and is very sensitive because it contains many nerve endings.

- The internal female genitals consist of the vagina, uterus, fallopian tubes, and ovaries.

- In the vagina, the outer one-third contains the most nerve endings. As a result, the length of the penis is generally irrelevant to sexual satisfaction. Furthermore, the vagina contracts around an object inserted in it, making the width of the penis also generally irrelevant to sexual satisfaction.

- The uterus consists of three layers: the perimetrium, which is elastic, thereby enabling the uterus to stretch during pregnancy; the myometrium, which is made up of smooth muscle, thereby helping to push the baby through the cervix; and the endometrium, which is loaded with blood vessels, thereby providing the nourishment needed to sustain a developing fetus.

- Hormones control menstruation. Follicle-stimulating hormone (FSH) stimulates the ovary to ripen an ovum, luteinizing hormone (LH) signals the Graafian follicle to release the ripened ovum, estrogens signal the pituitary gland to release LH, and progesterone released by the corpus luteum prepares the uterus for implantation of the fertilized ovum.

- Menstrual problems include dysmenorrhea (painful menstruation), which can be either primary or secondary; amenorrhea (a lack of menstruation); and premenstrual syndrome (menstruation associated with bloating cramping, fatigue, depression, headache, and other symptoms).

- The breast is the leading site of cancer in women, and breast cancer is the second leading cause of cancer deaths among women. Breast care consists of breast self-exams (although some groups recommend not doing breast self-exams), annual clinical breast exams, and mammograms as recommended. In addition, women should have annual gynecological exams and Pap smears as recommended.

Discussion Questions

1. List and describe the parts of the female reproductive system, including external and internal genitalia.

2. Compare the roles of breasts as child nurturer and sexual organ.

3. Describe how hormones react to sexual stimuli and make a person aroused.

4. Which physiological changes occur in a woman's body during the menstrual cycle? What are the resulting psychological effects?

5. For which diseases of the reproductive system is a woman at risk? How can she prevent these diseases?

6. Describe the self-care and preventive medicine that a woman should practice to ensure her sexual health.

Application Questions

Reread the anecdote that opens the chapter and answer the following questions.

1. How could you use your understanding of the parts of the human body to improve your sexuality? Is such knowledge as important as the ability to communicate or to understand the diverse needs of a partner? Put another way, would an expert on sexuality be a better lover?

2. Describe how you feel when you look at anatomical drawings of genitalia. Do you feel sexually excited? Embarrassed? Bored? Explain why you feel that way.

Critical Thinking Questions

1. Some women argue that only another woman can really understand the feelings and sensations that a woman feels, that male gynecologists are likely to discount some female concerns, and that it is easier to talk with another woman than a man about their sexual health. Others may argue that medical competency and compassion are not limited by gender. Should a gynecologist be a woman? Explain your answer.

2. If you look at the women on TV, in movies, and in magazines, the pervasive image is clear: lean and busty. Yet the psychologist G. Terence Wilson, an eating disorder specialist, points out that a woman cannot be lean and have large breasts—it is not biologically possible. As a woman loses fat, her breasts reduce in size.

Should a woman who finds herself lean and flat get breast implants or regain weight so her breasts will be larger? Explain your answer.

Critical Thinking Case

As discussed in the chapter, some researchers believe that onset of menarche occurs on the basis of body composition—namely, when a woman reaches a certain percentage of body fat. It also appears that amenorrhea (cessation of menstruation) occurs in women athletes with low body fat and in women with anorexia nervosa.

Consider the negative connotations associated with body fat in our society, especially as portrayed in the mass media. What reaction might prepubescent girls have to learning that they will gain body fat and then reach menarche? How could middle and high school students be taught in a positive manner about the body composition changes associated with the onset of menarche? Would such knowledge lead young girls to diet to prevent menarche?

One final question: A very athletic person in your dormitory tells you that she has heard about the relationship between body fat and amenorrhea. She tells you that she does strenuous aerobic exercise as a means of what she calls "natural birth control." What would you tell her?

Exploring Personal Dimensions

For Women Only

Taking charge of self-care and prevention greatly increases your chance of achieving sexual health and wellness. If you are a female, for the following statements, circle YES or NO. Then fill in the dates to help you keep track of your self-care activities.

I do vaginal self-examinations on a   YES   NO
regular basis.
    My last vaginal exam was on _____.
    My next vaginal exam is due on _____.

I have regular gynecological   YES   NO
examinations.
    My last gynecological exam was on _____.
    My next gynecological exam is due on _____.

I have regular Pap smears.   YES   NO
    My last Pap smear was on _____.
    My next Pap smear is due on _____.

I have regular mammograms   YES   NO
(if applicable).
    My last mammogram was on _____.
    My next mammogram is due on _____.

I keep track of my menstrual cycle.   YES   NO
    My last period began on _____.
    My next period is due on _____.

I practice safer sexual activities.   YES   NO

I understand that vaginal intercourse   YES   NO
during menstruation increases the
risk of transmitting HIV.

I have a family medical tree listing   YES   NO
diseases.

I discussed my family's medical   YES   NO
history with my doctor.

Suggested Readings

Alexander, L. L., LaRosa, J. H., Bader, H., & Garfield, S. *New dimensions in women's health.* Sudbury, MA: Jones & Bartlett Learning, 2009.

Carlson, K. J., Eisenstat, S. A., & Ziporyn, T. D. *The new Harvard guide to women's health.* Cambridge. MA: Harvard University Press, 2004.

Goldberg, N. *Dr. Nieca Goldberg's complete guide to women's health.* New York: Ballantine Books, 2009.

Heffner, L. J., & Schust, D. J. *The reproductive system at a glance,* 3rd ed. Hoboken, NJ: Wiley-Blackwell, 2010.

Morris, D. *The naked woman: A study of the female body.* New York: St. Martin's Press, 2007.

Schuiling, K. D., & Likis, F. E. *Women's gynecologic health.* Sudbury, MA: Jones & Bartlett Learning, 2011.

Staff of Boston Women's Health Book Collective. *Our bodies, ourselves: A new edition for a new era.* New York: Simon & Schuster, 2005.

World Health Organization. *Mental health aspects of women's reproductive health: A global review of the literature.* Geneva, Switzerland: World Health Organization, 2008.

Web Resources

For links to the websites below, visit go.jblearning. com/dimensions5e and click on Resource Links.

Inner Body: Your Guide to Human Anatomy Online: Female Reproductive System
www.innerbody.com/image/repfov.html

An overview of the female reproductive system with diagrams and detailed information about each structure, including the mammary glands, cervix, fallopian tubes, labia minor, ovary ligaments, ovaries, uterus, vagina, and vulva.

SexualHealth.com
www.sexualhealth.com/channel/view/women-sexual-health/

Presents information on women's sexual health topics such as desire, pleasure, orgasm, medications and supplements, gynecological concerns, pain during intercourse, menopause, menstruation and breast health, infertility, pregnancy and childbirth, masturbation, body image, and contraception.

National Woman's Health Network
http://nwhn.org/

The National Women's Health Network seeks to improve the health of women by developing and promoting a critical analysis of health issues in order to affect policy and support consumer decision making. The Network aspires to a healthcare system that is guided by social justice and reflects the needs of diverse women. On the website, women's health information and resources, as well as health alerts, are provided.

National Women's Health Information Center
www.4women.gov

A website maintained by the U.S. government that provides resources and information about women's health issues. Includes health topics, health organizations, statistics, publications, and other links.

Society for Women's Health Research
www.womenshealthresearch.org

The Society for Women's Health Research is a nonprofit organization whose mission is to improve the health of women through research, education, and advocacy. The society encourages the study of sex differences between women and men that affect the prevention, diagnosis, and treatment of disease. The information provided on this site is designed to support, not replace, the relationship that exists between a woman and her doctor.

References

Adams, D. B., Gold, A. R., & Burt, A. D. Rise in female-initiated sexual activity at ovulation and suppression by oral contraceptives. *New England Journal of Medicine, 299* (1978), 1145–1150.

Addiego, F., Belzer, E., Perry, J., & Whipple, B. Female ejaculation: A case study. *Journal of Sex Research, 17* (1981), 13–21.

Alzate, H., & Hoch, Z. The G spot and female ejaculation: A current appraisal. *Journal of Sex and Marital Therapy, 12* (1986), 211–220.

Alzate, H., & Londono, M. Vaginal erotic sensitivity. *Journal of Sex and Marital Therapy, 10* (1984), 49–56.

American Cancer Society. *Breast cancer screening: The American Cancer Society and Living Well, October module,* 2007a.

American Cancer Society. *Cancer facts & figures 2010.* Atlanta, GA: Author, 2010a.

American Cancer Society. *Cervical cancer: Prevention and early detection.* 2010b. Available: http://www.cancer.org/acs/groups/cid/documents/webcontent/003167-pdf.

American Cancer Society. *Detailed guide: Cervical cancer—what are the key statistics?,* 2008. Available: http://www.cancer.org/docroot/CRI/content/CRI_2_4_1X_What_are_the_key_statistics_for_cervical_cancer_8.asp.

American College of Obstetricians and Gynecologists. *Dysmenorrhea.* San Francisco: Medem, 2009. Available: http://www.medem.com/medlib/article/ZZZH7MGV77C.

American Psychiatric Association. *Diagnostic and statistical manual of mental disorders, fourth edition, text revision.* Washington, DC: American Psychiatric Association, 2000.

AskMen. *Have great sex while she's menstruating,* 2011. Available: http://www.askmen.com/dating/love_tip_60/61_love_tip.html.

Ballagh, S. A., & Heyl, A. Communicating with women about menstrual cycle symptoms. *Journal of Reproductive Medicine, 53* (2008), 837–846.

Barnard, N. D., Scialli, A. R., Hurlock, D., & Bertron, P. Diet and sex-hormone binding globulin, dysmenorrhea, and premenstrual symptoms. *Obstetrics and Gynecology, 95* (2000), 245–250.

Barrack, M. T., Van Loan, M. D., Rauh, M. J., & Nichols, J. F. Physiologic and behavioral indicators of energy deficiency in female adolescent runners with elevated bone turnover. *American Journal of Clinical Nutrition, 92* (2010), 652–659.

Baxter, N. Preventive health care, 2001 update: Should women be routinely taught breast self-examination to screen for breast cancer? *Canadian Medical Association Journal, 164, no.13* (2001), 1837–1846.

Belzer, E. G. Orgasmic expulsions of women: A review and heuristic inquiry. *Journal of Sex Research, 17* (1981), 1–12.

Belzer, E. G., Whipple, B., & Moger, W. On female ejaculation. *Journal of Sex Research, 20* (1984), 403–406.

Boston Women's Health Collective. *Our bodies, ourselves: For the new century.* New York: Simon & Schuster, 1998.

Brooks, J., Ruble, D., & Clark, A. College women's attitudes and expectations concerning menstrual-related changes. *Psychosomatic Medicine, 39* (1977), 289–298.

Bullivant, S. B., Sellergren, S. A., Stern, K., Spencer, N. A., Jacob, S., Mennella, J. A., & McClintock, M. K. Women's sexual experience during the menstrual cycle: Identification of the sexual phase by noninvasive measurement of luteinizing hormone. *Journal of Sex Research, 41* (2004), 82–93.

Burri, A. V., Cherkas, L., & Spector, T. D. Genetic and environmental influences on self-reported G-spots in women: A twin study. *Journal of Sexual Medicine, 7* (2010), 1842–1852.

California Pacific Medical Center. *Breast cysts.* San Francisco, CA: Author, 2008. Available: http://www.cpmc.org/services/women/breast/breast_cyst.html.

Centers for Disease Control and Prevention. *About DES: Known health effects for DES daughters,* 2011a. Available: http://www.cdc.gov/DES/consumers/about/effects_daughters.html.

Centers for Disease Control and Prevention. *About DES: Known health effects for DES sons,* 2011b. Available: http://www.cdc.gov/DES/consumers/about/effects_sons.html.

Centers for Disease Control and Prevention. *Behavioral risk factor surveillance system survey data*. Atlanta, GA: U.S. Department of Health and Human Services and CDC, 2008. Available: http://apps.nccd.cdc.gov/brfss/list.asp?cat+WH&yr=2008&qkey=4421&state=All.

Clayton, A. H. Symptoms related to the menstrual cycle: Diagnosis, prevalence, and treatment. *Journal of Psychiatric Practice, 14* (2008), 13–21.

Dalton, K. *Once a month*. Ramona, CA: Hunter House, 1979.

Daw, J. Is PMDD real? *Monitor on Psychology*, 33 (2002). Available: http://www.apa.org/monitor/oct02/pmdd.html.

Endometriosis Association. What is endometriosis? *Endo-Online* (2005). Available: http://www.endo-online.org/endo.html.

Foldes, P., & Buisson, O. The clitoral complex: A dynamic sonographic study. *Journal of Sexual Medicine, 6* (2009), 1223–1231.

Friedman, R., Hurt, S., Arnoff, M., & Clarkin, J. Behavior and the menstrual cycle. *Signs, 5* (1980), 719–738.

Goldberg, D. C., Whipple, B., Fishkin, R., Waxman, H., Fink, P., & Weisberg, M. The Grafenberg spot and female ejaculation: A review of initial hypotheses. *Journal of Sex and Marital Therapy, 9* (1983), 27–37.

Grafenberg, E. The role of urethra in female orgasm. *International Journal of Sexology, 3* (1950), 145–148.

Greenberg, J. S. *Comprehensive stress management*, 12th ed. New York: McGraw-Hill Higher Education, 2011.

Greenwood, S. Women's health: Menstrual cramps. *Medical Self-Care* (November/December 1986), 20–21.

Heath, D. An investigation into the origins of a copious vaginal discharge during intercourse—enough to wet the bed—that is not urine. *Journal of Sex Research, 20* (1984), 194–215.

Holmes, M., et al. Association of dietary intake of fat and fatty acids with risk of breast cancer. *Journal of the American Medical Association, 281* (1999), 914–920.

Hortobagyi, G. N., McLelland, R., & Reed, F. M. Your key role in breast cancer screening. *Patient Care, 24* (1990), 82–113.

Jannini, E. A., Whipple, B., Kingsberg, S. A., Buisson, O., Foldès, P., & Vardi, Y. Who's afraid of the G-spot? *Journal of Sexual Medicine, 7* (2010), 25–34.

Kaplan, H. S. *The evaluation of sexual disorders*. New York: Brunner/Mazel, 1983.

Kegel, A. Sexual functions of the pubococcyngeus muscle. *Western Journal of Surgery, Obstetrics, and Gynecology, 60* (1952), 521–524.

Kolata, G. Deadliness of breast cancer in blacks defies easy answer. *The New York Times* (August 3, 1994), C10.

Korda, J. B., Goldstein, S. W., & Sommer, F. The history of female ejaculation. *Journal of Sexual Medicine, 7 (2010):*1965–1975.

Koutedakis, Y., & Jamurtas A. The dancer as a performing athlete: Physiological considerations. *Sports Medicine, 34* (2004), 651–661.

Mallon, R. *Demonstration of vestigial prostate tissue in the human female*. (October 1984). Paper presented at the Annual Regional Conference of the American Association of Sex Educators, Counselors, and Therapists, Las Vegas, NV.

Masters, W. H., Johnson, V. E., & Kolodny, R. C. *Human sexuality*, 2nd ed. Boston: Little, Brown, 1985.

Matteo, S., & Rissman, E. Increased sexual activity during the midcycle portion of the human menstrual cycle. *Hormones and Behavior, 18* (1984), 249–255.

Mayo Clinic. *Ask a women's health specialist: Premenstrual dysphoric disorder (PMDD): A severe form of PMS*. Rochester, MN: Author, 2008. Available: http://www.mayoclinic.com/health/pmdd/AN01372.

Mayo Clinic. *Fibrocystic breasts*, 2010. Available: http://www.mayoclinic.com/health/fibrocysticbreasts/DS01070/DSECTION=complications.

Mayo Clinic. *Women's health: Amenorrhea*. Rochester, MN: Author, 2007a. Available: http://www.mayoclinic.com/health/amenorrhea/DS00581/DSECTION=causes.

Mayo Clinic. *Women's health: Premenstrual syndrome (PMS)*. Rochester, MN: Author, 2007b. Available: http://www.mayoclinic.com/health/premenstrual-syndrome/DS00134.

Mayo Health Clinic. *Dietary suggestions for premenstrual syndrome*, 1998.

McMillan, M. Cervical scanner. *Washington Post* (September 14, 2004), HE2.

menstruation.com.au. *Libido and your cycle*, 2008. Available: http://www.menstruation.com.au/periodpages/libido.html.

National Cancer Institute. *Breast cancer screening modalities: Mammography*. Washington, DC: Author, 2008a. Available: http://www.cancer.gov/cancertopics/pdq/screening/breast/HealthProfessional/page5.

National Center for Health Statistics. *Health, United States, 2009*. Hyattsville, MD: Author, 2010.

National Women's Health Center. *Premenstrual syndrome*, 2010. Available: http://www.womenshealth.gov/faq/premenstrual-syndrome.cfm.

Nemours Foundation. *Toxic shock syndrome*. Jacksonville, FL: Author, 2007. Available: http://kidshealth.org/teen/sexual_health/girls/tss.html.

Patterson, J. Killer cramps. *Shape* (August 1990), 20–22.

Perry, J. D., & Whipple, B. Pelvic muscle strength of female ejaculators: Evidence in support of a new theory of orgasm, *Journal of Sex Research, 17* (1981), 22–39.

Phalen, K. F. PMS: Pretty miserable symptoms. *Washington Post Health* (August 1, 2000), 19.

Redfran, S. Pap plus: Some ob-gyns are adding a visual screen to aid cancer detection. *Washington Post* (April 4, 2002), F1.

Research Forecasts, Inc. *The Tampax report: A summary of survey results on a study of attitudes toward menstruation*. New York: Tampax, 1981.

Reuters. Study again clears silicone, *Washington Post* (June 22, 1999), A2.

Ruble, D., & Brooks-Gunn, J. Menstrual myths. *Medical Aspects of Human Sexuality*, 13 (June 1979), 110–127.

Sato, S., et al. Transvaginal ultrasonography screening detects early-stage ovarian cancer. *Cancer 2000, 89* (2000), 582–587.

Sevely, J., & Bennett, J. Concerning female ejaculation and the female prostate. *Journal of Sex Research*, 14 (1978), 1–20.

Skene, A. Two important glands of the urethra. *American Journal of Obstetrics*, 265 (1980), 265–270.

Slob, A. K., Ernste, M., & Van der Werff ten Bosch, J. J. Menstrual cycle phase and sexual arousability in women. *Archives of Sexual Behavior, 20* (1991), 567–577.

Smith, H. S. *How common are menstrual cramps?* 2012. Available at http://www.sharecare.com/question/common-menstrual-cramps.

Sommerfield, J. Lifting the curse: Should monthly periods be optional? *MSNBC Online*.

Tanfer, K., & Aral, S. Sexual intercourse during menstruation and self-reported sexually transmitted disease history among women. *Sexually Transmitted Diseases, 23* (1996), 395–401.

Torstveit, M. K., & Sundgot-Borgen, J. Low bone mineral density is two to three times more prevalent in non-athletic pre-menopausal women than in elite athletes: A comprehensive controlled study. *British Journal of Sports Medicine, 39* (2005), 282–287.

U.S. Preventive Services Task Force. Screening for breast cancer: U.S. Preventive Services Task Force recommendation statement. *Annals of Internal Medicine, 151* (2009), 716–726.

UNICEF. *Female genital mutilation/cutting*, 2011a. Available: http://www.unicef.org/protection/index_genitalmutilation.html.

UNICEF. *The state of the world's children, 2011*. New York: United Nations, 2011b.

Van Goozen, S. H. M., Wiegart, V. M., & Helmond, F. A. Psychoendocrinological assessment of the menstrual cycle: The relationship between hormones, sexuality, and mood. *Archives of Sexual Behavior, 26* (1997), 359–382.

Wimpissinger, F., Stifter, K., Grin, W., & Stackl, W. The female prostate revisited: Perineal ultrasound and biochemical studies of female ejaculate. *Journal of Sexual Medicine, 4* (2007), 1388–1393.

World Health Organization. *Fact sheet: Female genital mutilation*. Geneva, Switzerland: Author, 2008. Available: http://www.who.int/mediacentre/factsheets/fs241/en/print.html.

Zaviacic, M., Zaviacicova, A., Holoman, I. K., & Molcan, J. Female urethral expulsions evoked by local digital stimulation of the G-spot: Differences in the response patterns. *Journal of Sex Research,24* (1988), 311.

CHAPTER 5

Male Sexual Anatomy and Physiology

FEATURES

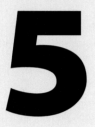

Global Dimensions
Male Genital Mutilation and Circumcision Practices

Ethical Dimensions
What Are a Dead Man's Rights?

Ethical Dimensions
Should Physicians Have to Provide Care Regardless of Their Personal Values or Moral Convictions?

Multicultural Dimensions
PSA Cancer Screening

Gender Dimensions
Testicular Self-Examination

CHAPTER OBJECTIVES

1 Name and describe the parts of the male reproductive system to include the external and internal genitalia, including the pathway of the sperm.

2 Discuss the role of hormones in males as they enter puberty.

3 Cite various diseases that can affect the male reproductive system and the self-care procedures, as well as medical treatments, associated with these diseases.

go.jblearning.com/dimensions5e

Global Dimensions: Male Genital Mutilation and
  Circumcision Practices
Prostate Cancer
Care from Organizations and Available Publications

INTRODUCTION

*A*n economics professor recently told me that a father had come in to talk about his son's mediocre academic performance. The father asked for a second chance for his son, explaining that "too often he thinks with his other head." Of course, this is not the first time I had heard this suggestion that men "think with their penises."

The notion goes back to the fifth century. In the Greek comedy Lysistrata, *the women of the city decide to withhold sex from their men until all wars are ended. The men quickly put their civic pride aside in favor of their women—thinking with their "other heads," no doubt!*

However, today's man may think more about his penis than with it. And the great obsession seems to be size. In the mid-1900s a national sex survey found that men thought the average length of a penis was 14 inches; women thought it was 12 inches. However, the average length is really about 6 inches!

Magazines like Penthouse Forum *do not help, either. Chock-full of large appendages—10 inches here, 8 inches there, a "foot long" here, as "thick as his arm" there—the stories are meant to present fantasy, not reality.*

The writer Susan Minot provides an interesting perspective in her short story "Lust."

> Tim's was shaped like a banana, with a graceful curve to it. They're all different. Willie's like a bunch of walnuts when nothing was happening, another's as thin as a thin hot dog. But it's like faces; you're never really surprised.

As you will read in this chapter, for all the worry that men may feel, it is quite natural for men's penises to vary considerably, just as their faces do.

■ The Male Reproductive System

As females do, males have both external and internal genital organs. Figure 5.1 depicts a side view of the male external and internal genitalia, and Figure 5.2 shows a view from the rear. We begin our study of the male reproductive system with the external genitals.

The External Genitals

The male external genitals are the penis and the scrotum.

The Penis

The **penis** is a male sexual organ consisting of the root, the shaft, and the glans. As we have mentioned, penis size concerns many students, who often ask about the "average-size penis." As a *general* guideline, the average penis is about 2–5 inches long when relaxed (flaccid) and about 4–7 inches long when erect. When sexually aroused, the penis becomes stiff and enlarged (erect) because its tissues fill with blood. The penis shaft is attached to the body by its root. The head of the penis is called the **glans penis**. The glans contains the

> **penis**
> Structure of the male external genitalia consisting of the root, shaft, and glans; also contains the urethra, through which urine is excreted.

urethral opening, or **meatus**, where both seminal fluid (which contains sperm) and urine are passed. Marking the end of the glans is a raised ridge called the **coronal ridge**, or **corona**. The coronal ridge helps to form a seal with the walls of the vagina during sexual intercourse. Below the corona the body, or shaft, of the penis begins. Although the entire penis is sensitive and sexually excitable, the glans and corona are particularly sensitive; in fact, they are the most sensitive parts of the male anatomy.

Historically penis size has been a matter of fascination. The **_Kamasutra_**, an ancient Indian book on erotica, classified men according to penis size in three categories: hare-men (erect penises of approximately 4.5 inches [11 centimeters]), bull-men (erect penises of approximately 6.75 inches [17 centimeters]), and horse-men (erect penises of approximately 9 inches [23-centimeters]). Other sources correlated penis size with personality traits or with the size of some other part of the body. Penises that are short when **flaccid** gain more size during **erection** than those that are

> **glans penis**
> The head of the penis.
>
> **meatus**
> The opening of the urethra in the head of the penis, where both seminal fluid and urine are passed.
>
> **coronal ridge (corona)**
> The raised ridge where the glans penis ends and the penile shaft begins.
>
> *Kamasutra*
> Ancient sex manual from India.

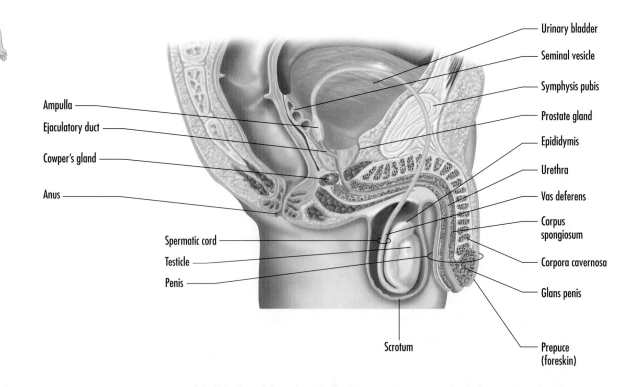

Ampulla
Ejaculatory duct
Cowper's gland
Anus
Spermatic cord
Testicle
Penis
Scrotum

Urinary bladder
Seminal vesicle
Symphysis pubis
Prostate gland
Epididymis
Urethra
Vas deferens
Corpus spongiosum
Corpora cavernosa
Glans penis
Prepuce (foreskin)

FIGURE **5.1** Side view of the male reproductive organs.

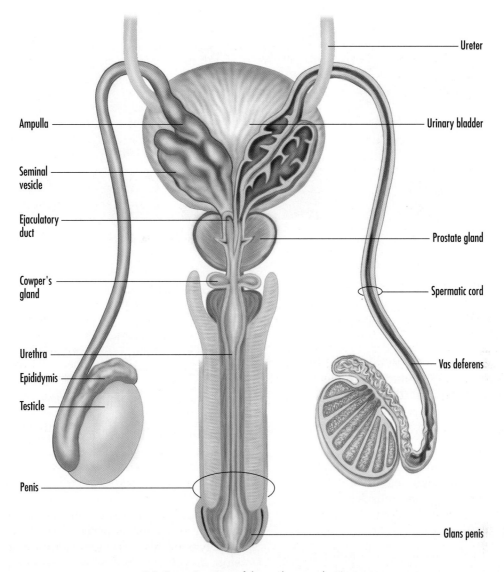

FIGURE **5.2** Posterior view of the male reproductive organs.

Ampulla

Seminal vesicle

Ejaculatory duct

Cowper's gland

Urethra

Epididymis

Testicle

Penis

Ureter

Urinary bladder

Prostate gland

Spermatic cord

Vas deferens

Glans penis

flaccid
The relaxed, unerect state of the penis.

erection
The extension of the penis and its engorgement with blood when the male is sexually stimulated.

longer when flaccid. Thus, although flaccid penises may differ significantly in length, erect penises are of similar lengths (Delvin & Webber, 2008). One way this has been described is that some men are "showers" and others are "growers" (Haffner & Schwartz, 1998).

Two contradictory views regarding penile size flourish in our time: "The larger the penis, the more satisfied the sexual partner" and "Sexual partners don't care about the size of a man's penis." It is not clear which is nearer the truth. Because the vagina adapts to the penis regardless of its size, some people have argued that size is unrelated to the sexual satisfaction of the female. However, part of our response to another's body is visual, and it seems reasonable

to assume that if people have preferences for breasts of certain sizes and shapes, so might they react differently to penises of different shapes and sizes. None of these preferences has anything to do with function unless it causes anxiety. The vagina contracts around the penis, regardless of its width or circumference. Furthermore, the inner two-thirds of the vagina has very little sensitivity. Both of these facts lead most authorities to conclude that penile width or length is unrelated to sexual satisfaction. Some people do, however, report preference for penises of a certain width or length. Whether these preferences are physiological or psychological is unknown at this time.

Just as women can strengthen the pelvic musculature with Kegel exercises, so can men strengthen the muscles surrounding the penis. Because these muscles are usually contracted only during ejaculation, they tend to be weak. By strengthening the muscles surrounding the penis, men may experience

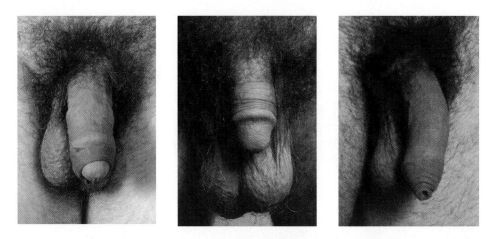

Many variations exist in the size and shape of the male genitals.

more satisfying orgasms and maintain better control of ejaculation. To do male Kegel exercises (National Kidney and Urologic Diseases Information Clearinghouse, 2007):

1. Identify the right muscles by imagining that you are trying to stop yourself from passing gas or urinating. Squeeze the muscles you would use. If you sense a "pulling" feeling, those are the right muscles for pelvic exercises.

2. Do not squeeze other muscles at the same time or hold your breath. Also, be careful not to tighten your stomach, leg, or buttock muscles. Squeezing the wrong muscles can put pressure on your bladder control muscles. Squeeze just the pelvic muscles.

3. Pull in the pelvic muscles and hold for a count of 3. Then relax for a count of 3. Repeat, but do not overdo it. Work up to 3 sets of 10 repeats.

4. Start doing your pelvic muscle exercises lying down. This position is the easiest for doing Kegel exercises because the muscles then do not need to work against gravity. When your muscles get stronger, do the exercises sitting or standing. Working against gravity is like adding more weight.

5. Be patient. Do not give up. It takes just 5 minutes, 3 times a day. Your ejaculatory control may not improve immediately, but most people notice an improvement in approximately 1 month.

Circumcision

The glans penis is covered by a **foreskin** (sometimes called the **prepuce**). For hygienic, cultural, or religious reasons, the foreskin is sometimes surgically removed. Removal of the foreskin—called **circumcision**—is more usual in the United States than in European countries. Circumcision takes place in the hospital approximately 2 days after birth or, if performed according to Jewish custom, 8 days after birth. In addition to Judaism, the Muslim faith requires circumcision. Figure 5.3 shows how circumcision is performed.

Hygiene also provides a rationale for circumcision. Several preputial glands—glands that secrete hormones only after puberty—are located in the foreskin and under the corona (Tyson's glands). These glands secrete an oily substance that, if not removed from under the foreskin, can combine with dead skin cells to form a cheesy substance called **smegma**. If this smegma is not regularly removed from under the foreskin, it becomes granular and irritates the glans penis, causing discomfort and possibly infection. Removing the smegma requires washing the glans penis. This becomes more difficult if the foreskin is not removed, because it has to be retracted manually to expose the glans.

Since 1971, the American Academy of Pediatrics (AAP) has released several statements noting that there is no medical reason for circumcision. As a result, circumcision rates in the United States dropped from a high of 95% of newborn males in the mid-1960s to an estimated 58% in 1987 (Rovner, 1990). However, in 1990, the Academy (Brower, 1989) reversed its position, citing advantages based on the work of Dr. Thomas Wiswell and colleagues (1985).

foreskin (prepuce)
The covering of the glans penis, which is removed during circumcision.

circumcision
The surgical removal of the foreskin covering the glans penis.

smegma
A cheeselike substance secreted by the glans penis that must be removed from below the foreskin of uncircumcised males to prevent irritation and/or infection.

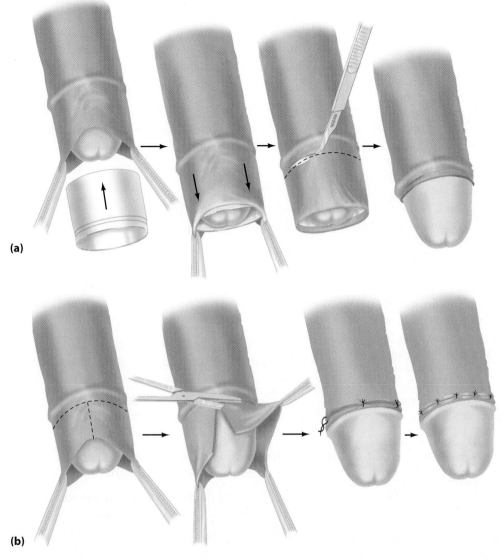

FIGURE **5.3** Methods of performing circumcision. (a) In this method, a piece of plastic is placed over the glans, and the foreskin is stretched over the plastic and trimmed off. (b) In this method, the foreskin is carefully cut "freehand" and then stitched.

(a)

(b)

Wiswell found that uncircumcised infants were 10 times more likely to have urinary tract infections than circumcised babies. Wiswell also reported that of 50,000 cases of cancer of the penis over a 50-year period, only 10 occurred in circumcised men.

However, not everyone agrees with the AAP's 1990 position. For example, Smith and colleagues (1987) found no difference in rates of urinary infections, and other researchers have reached similar conclusions over the years (Samuels & Samuels, 1983; Wallerstein, 1980). More recently, however, AAP has advised that the benefits of circumcision are not significant enough to recommend it as a routine procedure (American Academy of Pediatrics, 1999). This policy was reaffirmed by the AAP in 2005 and is the current policy of the AAP (American Academy of Pediatrics, 2011).

But another argument attempts to justify circumcision: The foreskin interferes with sexual stimulation because it serves as a barrier to the glans penis. There are no data to support this argument and, in fact, logic would indicate otherwise. The foreskin retracts when the penis becomes erect, and the glans penis is, therefore, able to be stimulated just as it is for the circumcised male. Furthermore, some people have argued the opposite: That is, if the glans is not usually protected by a foreskin, it may become insensitive because of its repeated contact with clothing. Therefore, the circumcised penis may, in fact, be *less* sensitive than the uncircumcised penis. Neither viewpoint is conclusive.

Still other reasons have been offered to justify circumcision. For example, uncircumcised males may be at greater risk of penile cancer, and their female sexual partners may be at greater risk of vaginal infections, cervical cancer, genital warts, and other sexually transmitted infections. However, for every study that supports these concerns, there appear to be studies that refute them.

There are more reasons for not being circumcised. First is concern about the trauma the infant experiences. Because infants cannot be administered general anesthesia or pain-relieving narcotic agents, circumcision is often performed without the benefit of anesthesia. To respond to this concern, some physicians inject a local anesthetic directly into the penis in an attempt to diminish or eliminate the pain associated with circumcision. Another issue is the risk of infection, hemorrhage, emotional trauma, and other effects associated with any surgical procedure.

Yet, there is agreement among medical experts that when the foreskin is so tight that an erection hurts or pain is experienced during sexual intercourse, removal of the foreskin is recommended. This condition is known as **phimosis**.

phimosis
Condition resulting when penile erection causes pain because the foreskin is too tight.

To summarize, here are reasons parents might consider circumcising their son:

- They are Jewish or Muslim. Infant circumcision is part of these religious traditions.

- If the father is circumcised, parents might want their son's penis to be like his father's penis.

- Parents do not want to have to teach their sons to clean their foreskins.

- Circumcised men have a lower incidence of urinary tract infections.

- Some uncircumcised men have problems as they grow up, for example, pain during intercourse, requiring circumcision during adulthood. This is much more painful and dangerous than newborn circumcision.

- The rate of cancer of the penis, though extremely rare, is higher in uncircumcised men.

- Uncircumcised men may be more susceptible to sexually transmitted infections.

Here are reasons parents might not want to circumcise their son:

- Circumcision is not part of their cultural tradition.

- Circumcision is painful for infants.

- If the father is not circumcised, parents might want their son's penis to be like his father's penis.

- As with any surgery, circumcision poses some risks. In rare cases (less than two times in 1,000) infection or even damage to the penis occurs.

- They think circumcision is not natural. Boys are born with penises with foreskins; their intact penises should be left alone.

- Circumcision is done without the infant's permission. This should be an adult choice.

- The child is ill at birth. Circumcision should never be done on a sick or medically unstable infant.

The Scrotum
The other external structure of the male reproductive system is the **scrotum**, which is located below the

Global DIMENSIONS

Male Genital Mutilation and Circumcision Practices

Around the world and throughout history there have been many societies that have practiced male genital mutilation. For example, castration, the removal of the testes, was common in ancient Rome; eunuchs, castrated men, dressed as women and became priests. Islamic societies are forbidden by the Koran to castrate men. Yet they used men castrated by the Christians as keepers of the harem, because they posed no threat of engaging in sexual activities. In addition, boys were castrated in the Middle Ages in Europe to maintain their soprano singing voices after puberty.

In some societies in the Pacific, men are circumcised, but the foreskin is not totally removed; instead, it is slit lengthwise and folded back. This is called *supercision*. Sometimes the foreskin is stretched tightly over a piece of bamboo, and then the incision is made. Circumcision is often associated with entry into manhood in these cultures and is usually celebrated with a ceremony of some sort.

scrotum (scrotal sac)
A sac of skin that contains the testes and spermatic cords.

testes
Male gonads contained within the scrotal sacs that produce sperm cells and the male sex hormone testosterone. Singular form: testicle.

spermatic cord
The cord from which the testicle is suspended that contains the vas deferens (defined later), blood vessels, nerves, and muscle fibers.

penis. The scrotum is a sac of skin containing the **testes** and the **spermatic cords**. It comprises two layers: the outer layer, which is covered with hair and sweat glands, and the inner layer (called the *tunica dartos*), which contains muscle and connective tissue. This organ regulates the temperature in the testes by drawing them up toward the body when the body is cold and letting them hang lower, away from the body, when it is hot. As a consequence the temperature of the testes is always approximately 5.6°F (3.1°C) cooler than the internal body temperature. This temperature-control function is necessary for the production of viable sperm. The scrotum also contracts when the inner thigh is stimulated or when it is chilled. This effect, is due to the contraction of the cremasteric muscles located in the spermatic cord, which is known as the *cremasteric reflex*.

The Internal Genitals

The male internal genitals contain numerous organs housed within the penis, the scrotum, and the pelvis (refer again to Figure 5.1).

The Urethra
The **urethra** is a tube through the penis that begins at the bladder and ends at the meatus. Its function is to provide a route for both semen and urine to exit the body. **Urine** is a waste product of the body that is stored in the bladder until it is expelled through the urethra. **Semen**, which is discussed later in this section, contains **spermatozoa**, or **sperm**, as well as other substances.

urethra
The tube through which the bladder empties urine outside the body and through which the male ejaculate exits.

urine
The body-waste product stored in the bladder and eliminated through the urethra.

semen
The male ejaculate, which contains sperm and other secretions.

spermatozoa (sperm)
The mature male sperm cell.

The Corpora Cavernosa and the Corpus Spongiosum
In addition to the urethra, the penis contains three spongy bodies: two **corpora cavernosa** and the **corpus spongiosum**, which are structures filled with networks of blood vessels and nerves. It is these columns of tissue, which

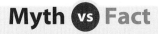

Myth vs Fact

Myth: Whereas females can strengthen their pelvic muscles, thereby exercising better control of their sexual response, there is not much males can do.
Fact: Males can strengthen their pelvic muscles also. They can perform Kegel exercises to strengthen the muscles surrounding the penis, thereby achieving more satisfying orgasms and maintaining better control of ejaculation.

Myth: There is no medical reason for males to be circumcised.
Fact: Recommendations regarding circumcision have changed over the years. More recently, it has been suggested that uncircumcised males may be at greater risk of penile cancer and that their female partners may be at greater risk of reproductive health problems. However, circumcision poses the risk of infection, hemorrhage, emotional trauma, and other conditions. Whether to be circumcised is a decision that needs a great deal of consideration.

Myth: Breast cancer affects women; men do not have to worry about contracting it.
Fact: Men can also contract breast cancer. In 2010 approximately 1,970 new cases of breast cancer were diagnosed, and 390 men died of it.

Myth: The ejaculate is made up predominantly of sperm.
Fact: The ejaculate, semen, consists mostly of seminal vesicle and prostate gland secretions. The volume of sperm is approximately the size of a pinhead.

Myth: A male with a small flaccid penis has much to worry about.
Fact: First, small flaccid penises tend to expand more during erection than do large flaccid penises. Second, the nerve endings in the vagina are in the outer third, making the length of the penis somewhat superfluous, at least as far as sexual satisfaction is concerned.

fill with blood during sexual arousal, that make the penis grow hard and erect. During ejaculation the muscle surrounding the corpus spongiosum (the bulbocavernosus muscle) contracts and forces semen outward through the urethra.

The Testes
As mentioned, the testes (Figure 5.4) are suspended in the scrotal sac by spermatic cords, the **vas deferens** (through which sperm leave the testes), blood vessels, nerves, and muscle fibers. The testes produce sperm (about 50,000 every minute) and **testosterone**, a male sex hormone generally responsible for male secondary sexual characteristics

corpora cavernosa
A spongy body in the penis that contains a network of blood vessels and nerves.

corpus spongiosum
A spongy body in the penis that contains a network of blood vessels and nerves.

vas deferens
The duct, through which sperm stored in the epididymis (discussed later) is passed, that is cut or blocked during vasectomy.

testosterone
The male sex hormone produced in the testes that is responsible for the development of male secondary sex characteristics.

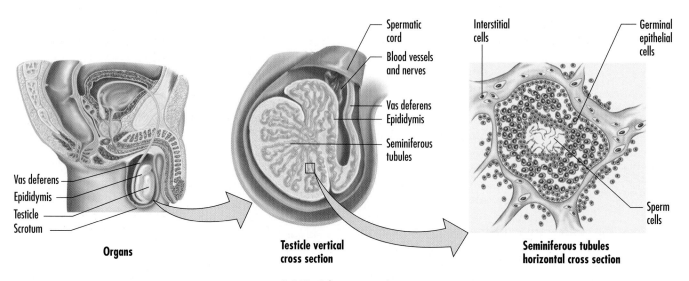

FIGURE 5.4 Testicle cross section.

seminiferous tubules
The structures located within the testes that actually produce the sperm.

spermatogenesis
The manufacturing of sperm in the seminiferous tubules.

interstitial cells
The cells (sometimes called Leydig's cells) between the seminiferous tubules, where testosterone is produced.

vasa efferentia
The duct through which sperm produced in the seminiferous tubules travel to the epididymis.

epididymis
The location where sperm are stored in the testes and where nutrients are provided to help the sperm develop.

(for example, deep voice, facial hair, and body hair). Within each testicle are approximately 1,000 **seminiferous tubules**, which are responsible for producing sperm, in a process called **spermatogenesis**. The cells between the seminiferous tubules, called **interstitial cells**, produce testosterone.

Once sperm are produced in the seminiferous tubules, they travel through the **vasa efferentia** to the epididymis, where they are stored and nourished for up to 6 weeks.

The Pathway of the Sperm

A mature sperm is about 0.0024 inch (0.0060 centimeter) long, with a head, neck, midpiece, and tail. The normal sperm contains 23 chromosomes. Each sperm contains a sex chromosome that determines the sex of the offspring. Sperm can be stored for up to 6 weeks in the epididymis before proceeding up the vas deferens to the **ampulla** (an enlarged portion of the vas deferens). Here in the ampulla the sperm receive more nutrients from the **seminal vesicles**, two sacs, each about 2 inches (5 centimeters) long, that secrete a substance believed to activate the sperm's **motility** (ability to move spontaneously).

ampulla
The enlarged portion of the vas deferens where sperm are provided nutrients from the seminal vesicles; also, the part of the fallopian tube of women containing the cilia.

seminal vesicles
Two sacs of the male internal genitalia that secrete nutrients to nourish sperm.

motility
The ability to move spontaneously, which is required for fertilization.

? Did You Know . . .

1. Testosterone causes bones to thicken and for this reason is sometimes administered to elderly people who have osteoporosis.

2. Excessive concentrations of sex hormones are metabolized primarily in the liver, with the products excreted in the bile and urine. Consequently, people with liver disorders experience the effects of excessive sex hormones (for example, the development of excessive body hair, development of breasts, or aggressiveness).

3. Sex hormones stimulate growth, thereby explaining the rapid growth that occurs during puberty. However, they also stimulate ossification (hardening) of the epiphyseal disks (a band of cartilage at the end of the bone), which causes bones to stop growing. Because estrogens produce greater effects on the disks than androgens, females stop growing earlier than males.

With sufficient sexual stimulation, the ejaculatory process begins. Fluid from the **prostate gland** mixes with the sperm and with the secretions of the seminal vesicles, further aiding sperm motility and prolonging sperm life. The prostate fluid is an alkaline medium that offsets the acidity in the vagina that would otherwise kill the sperm. The **Cowper's glands**, two pea-sized glands adjacent to the urethra, empty into the urethra another alkaline fluid, which serves to neutralize the acidity caused by the urethra's transport of urine. The Cowper's glands secretions are the tiny droplets that sometimes appear on the tip of the penis before ejaculation. This secretion may contain some sperm left over from a previous ejaculation; therefore, it can cause pregnancy to occur even if the penis is withdrawn before ejaculation.

Ejaculation itself is the expulsion through the penis of semen, the mixture in which the sperm are carried. Ejaculation results from muscular contractions of the glands and ducts of the reproductive system. The expelling of semen is usually accompanied by **orgasm**, the climax of a growing complex of pleasurable sensations. Both the ampulla and seminal vesicles contract, as does the bulbocavernosus muscle surrounding the corpus spongiosum in the penis. The ejaculated semen contains sperm (the volume is about the size of a pinhead) and about a teaspoonful of secretions from the seminal vesicles, the prostate gland, and the Cowper's glands. Approximately 300 million sperm are expelled in a single ejaculation. According to some authorities, semen contain at least 20 to 35 million sperm per cubic centimeter in a male who is fertile—that is, able to fertilize an ovum.

During ejaculation a valve at the bladder's entrance closes to prevent urine from entering the urethra.

Table 5.1 reviews the functions of the male reproductive system.

■ Hormones

At some time during puberty, boys become capable of reproduction. This capability is accompanied by the ability to ejaculate, although initially the male's ejaculate does not contain mature sperm. The cause of male reproductive capacity is the increased secretion of androgens, followed by the development of secondary sex characteristics. Accompanying male reproductive capacity, and also a result of increased androgen production, is a heightened interest in sex. This can be considered double jeopardy, because an increase in sexual appetite in a person newly capable of fertilizing an ovum can create problems—such as unplanned pregnancy or frustrated **libido**. The majority of both males and

prostate gland
A structure of the male internal genitalia that secretes a fluid into the semen before ejaculation to aid sperm motility and prolong sperm life.

Cowper's glands
Two pea-sized glands adjacent to the urethra that secrete a lubricating fluid before ejaculation.

ejaculation
The ejection of semen from the penis during orgasm.

orgasm
The peak release of sexual tension, accompanied by sensory pleasure and involuntary rhythmic muscular contractions; ejaculation in the male.

libido
Sexual desire, or drive.

TABLE 5.1 Functions of the Organs of the Male Reproductive System

Organ	Function
Testes	
Seminiferous tubules	Produce spermatozoa
Interstitial cells	Produce and secrete male sex hormones
Epididymis	Stores and allows maturation of spermatozoa; conveys spermatozoa to vas deferens
Vas deferens	Conveys spermatozoa to ejaculatory ducts
Ejaculatory ducts	Receive spermatozoa and additives to produce seminal fluid
Seminal vesicles	Secrete alkaline fluid containing nutrients and prostaglandins
Prostate gland	Secretes alkaline fluid that helps neutralize acidic seminal fluid and enhances motility of spermatozoa
Cowper's gland	Secretes fluid that lubricates urethra and end of penis
Scrotum	Encloses and protects testes
Penis	Conveys urine and seminal fluid outside the body; acts as the organ of copulation

What Are a Dead Man's Rights?

The Center for Bioethics at the University of Pennsylvania documented 25 cases in which sperm were taken from dead men and preserved by deep-freezing. Furthermore, a survey of 273 fertility centers in the United States identified 82 requests for taking sperm from dead men, of which 25 had been honored. It is possible to remove sperm up to 24 hours after death, and the person most often making the request is the widow. However, there also are records of social workers and even an intensive care nurse who made such a request.

Who has a right, if anyone at all does, to have such a request honored? Only the spouse, or a parent as well?

Should men have the right to decide whether they will have children and with whom, even after they are dead?

Should sperm taken from dead men be used by women unrelated to them, whose husbands do not produce viable sperm? Who else should have access to this sperm?

Should the sperm be sold and the proceeds go to the man's family? What should be done with the frozen sperm if the dead man's family decides not to use them?

These are tough decisions that should be guided by ethical principles.

females seem to adjust to this new condition and pass through this phase of life unscarred. Unfortunately some do not, as evidenced by the high rate of pregnancy in unmarried teenage girls.

During puberty, increased testosterone level leads to growth of the penis, prostate, seminal vesicles, and epididymis. The reason males cannot ejaculate before puberty is that the prostate and seminal vesicles are not functional until they are "turned on" by the increased level of testosterone. Late-developing boys (15 to 16 years old) have been found to experience less sexual activity during adolescence than do early developers (Kinsey, Pomeroy, & Martin, 1948; Masters, Johnson, & Kolodny, 1982, 169). This difference has been attributed to the effect of testosterone on increasing the sexual appetite in males. No long-lasting effect on sexual behavior has been reported, however.

Hormone Therapy

Hormone therapy is sometimes administered to men. For instance, testosterone supplements are sometimes administered to treat erectile dysfunction in

older men (although testosterone levels are not low in all men who have trouble maintaining erection). Sometimes this treatment for erectile dysfunction is effective; other times it is not. The reason for this inconsistency is unclear; however, it is safe to say that the complex nature of sexuality makes it only partially responsive to hormone treatment. Testosterone supplements may not have much effect when personality, past experiences, the sexual partner, effectiveness in communication, setting, and so on, continue to have negative effects.

Self-Care and Prevention

Male reproductive care is as specialized as female reproductive care. Men should learn proper hygiene and methods of monitoring their reproductive health. When problems arise, males should consult their own medical specialists (internists or urologists). As with females, there are many organizations and publications that focus exclusively on issues of male reproductive health.

? Did You Know . . .

Androstenedione is the supplement that Mark McGwire made famous during his 70-home-run season. Touted as an artificial steroid, it was said to raise testosterone levels. But researchers at the University of Iowa found that it did not raise testosterone levels or increase strength. A side effect was lower levels of "good" cholesterol (high-density lipoproteins), raising the risk of heart disease. Preliminary results of a further study by the Harvard researcher Hoel Finkelstein for Major League Baseball showed that androstenedione raised estrogen levels in men—and could result in breast enlargement!

Source: Data from Body-building aid questioned, CBSNews (June 3, 1999). Available: www.cbsnews.com/2100-204_162-493000.html.

¿? Ethical DIMENSIONS

Should Physicians Have to Provide Care Regardless of Their Personal Values or Moral Convictions?

One month before George W. Bush's presidency was to end, he finalized a regulation allowing health professionals to refuse to provide any medical service they objected to on moral grounds (Meckler, 2008). This "right of conscience" regulation was interpreted to mean that abortion, family planning, providing prescriptions for emergency contraception (the "morning after pill"), giving certain information or advice, or any other service the medical provider deemed immoral—even referrals for such services—could be withheld from the patient.

Those favoring such a regulation argue that no one—not even a health professional—should be required to behave in a manner that the person considers immoral. Furthermore, if the patient is denied a medical service, there will always be other medical staff willing to provide the desired service. Lastly, medical providers should not face the threat of being fired or losing a promotion because they refuse to do something they believe to be against their religious or moral beliefs.

Those opposed to the "right of conscience" regulation believe that because medical providers are licensed by the state, they are obligated to serve the medical needs of *all* citizens of that state. They also argue that the rule sacrifices the patient's health to the religious belief of the providers (Savage, 2008). Furthermore, not providing a medical service requested by a patient, and not referring the patient to another healthcare provider from whom those services could be obtained, is doing harm to the patient and, therefore, is itself immoral and unethical.

Would you support a "right of conscience" regulation or do you agree with President Obama who rescinded it? What reasoning would you use when making this decision?

Breast Cancer in Men

Cancer of the breast occurs in men as well as women, although it is considered rare. An estimated 1,970 new cases of male breast cancer were diagnosed in 2010, and 390 men died of it that same year (American Cancer Society, 2010). Breast cancer is seen in men as early as their 30s. Although this cancer is rare, men are wise to examine their breasts for lumps. The procedure is the same for men and women.

It appears that several factors are related to the development of breast cancer in men. Among these are obesity, a lack of regular physical activity, and tobacco use (Brinton et al., 2008). Also, African American males have a higher incidence of breast cancer than do white males (Nahleh et al., 2007). In addition, as with women, breast cancer is more prevalent in men who carry the BRCA1 and BRCA2 genetic mutations (Tai et al., 2007). Another cause of concern is that male breast cancer is associated with a higher incidence of prostate cancer, suggesting careful screening for prostate cancer should be performed in men with breast cancer (Lee & Jones, 2008). In one large-scale study (Nahleh et al., 2007), male breast cancer patients survived an average of 7 years as compared to 9.8 years for female breast cancer patients. However, males in this study were diagnosed with breast cancer at a more advanced stage and with more lymph node involvement compared to the female patients. Furthermore, the male patients were diagnosed at a mean age of 67 years, whereas the female patients were diagnosed at a mean age of 57 years.

Treatment for male breast cancer is similar to that of female breast cancer with one major difference: The psychological and emotional consequences of breast removal are not as significant for males as for females. Consequently, men seldom need counseling or a cosmetic means of disguising breast-tissue removal.

The Prostate

An important self-care procedure involves the prostate gland. The symptoms of **prostatitis** (inflammation of the prostate) are pain in the lower back, pain in defecation, pain during a rectal exam, and pus in the urine. Prostatitis usually affects younger men and can be cured with antibiotic drugs. If you experience these symptoms, consult a physician.

prostatitis
Infection of the prostate gland.

An estimated 217,730 new cases of prostate cancer were diagnosed in the United States in 2010, and an estimated 32,050 men died of it that same year. Prostate cancer is the second leading cause of cancer deaths in men in the United States (lung cancer is the first). Between 1989 and 1992, prostate cancer

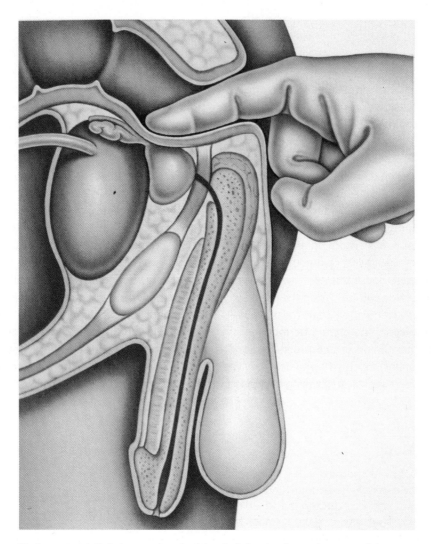

During a rectal digital exam, the physician feels for the size and texture of the prostate gland in an attempt to discover any abnormalities that need follow-up evaluation.

rates increased dramatically, probably because of the use of a blood test developed to identify an antigen produced when prostate cancer is present. The blood test measures the presence of prostate-specific antigen (PSA). Since 1993, prostate cancer incidence rates have declined. It should be pointed out that prostate cancer incidence rates are one and one half times as high for African American men as they are for white men. The reason for this difference is not known, but some experts have conjectured that diets high in fat and/or the presence of a gene that may make the prostate more susceptible to the effects of testosterone may be the cause.

There are several factors that place a man at risk of development of prostate cancer. One of these is age. As a man gets older he becomes more susceptible to prostate cancer, although the cancer may have been present at a younger age but not fully developed. More than 70% of prostate cancers are

diagnosed in men who are older than 65 years of age. Heredity is suspected of playing a role in perhaps 5% to 10% of cases.

Signs and symptoms include weak or interrupted urine flow; the need to urinate frequently, especially at night; blood in the urine; pain or burning when urinating; and persistent pain in the lower back, pelvis, or upper thighs. However, some of these symptoms may be caused by an enlargement of the prostate, which is common as men age, without the presence of a tumor. This condition is called *benign prostatic hyperplasia (BPH)* and can be treated with medications. The only way to distinguish BPH from prostate cancer is by a medical examination that includes a **digital rectal examination (DRE)**, PSA blood

digital rectal examination (DRE)
A rectal examination whereby a physician inserts a finger into the rectum of a male patient to check for any abnormalities of the prostate.

Multicultural DIMENSIONS

PSA Cancer Screening

There is disagreement among healthcare specialists about the advisability of men obtaining PSA screening for prostate cancer. The U.S. Preventive Services Task Force does not recommend PSA screening for men. By comparison, the American Cancer Society recommends annual screening for men 50 years of age and older. To further complicate matters, the American Medical Association and several other respected medical organizations suggest that clinicians discuss the potential benefits and known harms of PSA screening with their patients, and consider their patients' preferences rather than routinely ordering PSA screenings.

One ethical principle guiding this kind of decision making is *paternalism*. Medical care providers who are advocates of paternalism argue that they are experts in health and, therefore, know more than their patients. It follows, then, that they can make a more informed and appropriate medical decision than can their patients. As a result, they are reluctant to discuss the pros and cons of screening *with* their patients and more comfortable making these decisions *for* their patients. This feeling of paternalism becomes even more pronounced when patients are minorities, or poorly educated. Given that some studies have found African American males are less knowledgeable about prostate cancer screening than white males (Chan et al., 2003; Barber et al., 1998), in spite of their higher incidence and mortality rates, the paternalism argument takes on added validity for some healthcare providers.

It seems to your authors that all men deserve to be informed about medical procedures available to them. After all, it is the patient—not the healthcare provider—who has to live with the outcomes of these procedures. If there is potential harm associated with PSA screening, we believe the patient should know that before consenting to the procedure.

test, and biopsy of the prostate. On June 12, 1997, the American Cancer Society published updated guidelines for prostate cancer screening (American Cancer Society, 1997). The guidelines state, "Both prostate specific antigen (PSA) and digital rectal examination (DRE) should be offered annually, beginning at age 50 years, to men who have a life expectancy of at least 10 years. Men at high risk (African American men and men with a family history of one or more first-degree relatives diagnosed with prostate cancer at an early age) should begin treatment at age 45." The reason a 10-year life expectancy is cited is that prostate cancer is usually a slow-growing cancer; thus it is thought prudent for men to refrain from having treatment if they are not expected to live long enough to benefit from that treatment. These men would likely die of some other condition before the prostate cancer killed them. An abnormal PSA test result is one with a value above 4 ng/mL (some suggest above 2 ng/mL), which would then lead to follow-up evaluation and subsequent procedures. These may include a biopsy of tissue extracted from the prostate gland.

In 2008, the U.S. Preventive Services Task Force, which evaluates medical screenings and makes recommendations regarding those screenings, published new guidelines for the use of the PSA test. It stated that men age 75 years of age and older should not be screened for PSA because the length of time one would die of prostate cancer is greater than 10 years, and a 75-year-old man's average life expectancy is only 10 years. Therefore, older men should not be subjected to the test, as it could lead to other medical procedures. For men younger than 75 years, the Task Force stated, "Current evidence is insufficient to assess the balance of benefits and harms of screening." In 2011, the Task Force went further and stated that all men, regardless of age, should not be routinely tested for PSA because the exam does not save lives and subjects men to unnecessary harm. The harms referred to relate to unnecessary medical procedures, such as biopsies and surgery; anxiety; and medical complications. The reasoning behind these recommendations pertains to the lack of evidence of the validity of PSA screening when a cutoff score of 4.0 ng/mL is used, as was standard practice. To respond to the lack of sensitivity of the screening at a score of 4.0 ng/mL, lowering the score to 2.5 ng/mL has been increasingly used. However, lowering the score leads to more false positives and, therefore, subjects men to more unnecessary biopsies and other medical procedures. Furthermore, two recent large-scale, long-term studies have concluded that PSA screening does not affect the prostate cancer death rate (Andriole et al., 2009; Schroder et al., 2009). The researchers found that the rate of death from prostate cancer was very low and did not differ significantly between the group of men who were screened and the group of men who were not.

Recognizing the controversy and lack of clear guidance, most major medical organizations recommend that clinicians discuss the potential benefits and known harms of PSA screening with their patients, and consider their patients' preferences rather than routinely ordering PSA screening. Among these organizations are the American Academy of Family Physicians, American College of Physicians, American College of Preventive Medicine, and American Medical Association. In contrast, the American Urological Association recommends digital rectal examinations and PSA screening to men annually beginning at age 50 years.

If cancer is suspected, treatment consists of surgery, radiation, and/or hormonal therapy and chemotherapy if the cancer is in a late stage. However, because there is significant potential for serious side effects of these treatments (such as erectile dysfunction and/or incontinence), if the cancer is classified as low-grade and/or at an early stage, careful observation over a period without immediate treatment (called "watchful waiting") may be advised.

Eighty-five percent of all prostate cancers are diagnosed while still localized, and these patients have a 100% 5-year survival rate. During the past 20 years, the 5-year survival rate for all prostate cancers increased from 67% to 97%. Seventy-nine percent of men with prostate cancer survive 10 years, and 57% survive 15 years.

The Testes

testicular cancer
Cancer of the testicles; the most common form of cancer in men aged 29 to 35 years.

Testicular cancer is the most common form of cancer in men during late adolescence and early adulthood. Most cases occur in men aged 15 to 40 years. It is estimated that about 8,480 new cases of testicular cancer were diagnosed in 2010 and that 350 men died of testicular cancer that year (American Cancer Society, 2010). The testicular cancer risk is four times greater for white men than it is for African American men. The rate has doubled among white Americans in the past 40 years and has remained the same for African Americans.

Among the risk factors for testicular cancer are undescended testes (cryptorchidism). Approximately 14% of cases of testicular cancer occur in men with a history of cryptorchidism. Other risk factors include a family history of testicular cancer, certain occupations (miners, oil and gas workers, leather workers, food and beverage processing workers, janitors, and utility workers), cancer of the other testicle, and infection with HIV. Testicular cancer is not related to injury or to vasectomy.

Treatment consists of surgery, radiation therapy, and/or chemotherapy. Surgery involves removal of the testicle. A cut is made in the groin, and the spermatic cord and the testicle are withdrawn from the scrotum through the opening. This procedure is called a *radical inguinal orchiectomy*. Depending on the stage of the cancer, some lymph nodes may also be removed. With only one testicle removed, the patient remains fertile. However, if two testicles need to be removed, the patient will no longer be able to produce sperm. Another side effect of the surgery is the possibility of damage to the nerves that control ejaculation. Damage to these nerves may also cause infertility. Men who still wish to have biological children can store sperm in a sperm bank for use after the surgery.

Treatment is highly effective if the cancer is diagnosed early. Ninety-five percent of stage 1 cancers can be cured, 90% to 95% of stage 2 cancers can be cured, and approximately 70% of stage 3 cancers can be cured. The lower the stage number, the earlier the cancer was diagnosed.

Gender
DIMENSIONS

Testicular Self-Examination

In the recent past, males were advised to perform testicular self-examinations in the hope of identifying testicular cancer at its earliest stage. However, after examining the pros and cons of such self-exams, the United States Preventive Services Task Force (2010) recommended that such tests not be performed. As with breast self-exams, the Task Force concluded that the potential harms outweighed the potential benefits of testicular self-exams. Still, any abnormalities found in the testicles should be immediately reported to a physician.

Any lumps, masses, or thickened areas may be symptoms of abnormality, not always cancerous; however, medical diagnosis and consultation are imperative. As with other forms of cancer, early diagnosis increases your chance of survival.

The Penis

Penile discharges of pus, painful urination, itching, or sores or warts on the genitals may indicate the presence of a sexually transmitted infection. Also, as suggested earlier in this chapter, men should make sure that smegma is washed away daily to prevent irritation or infection in themselves and their partners. For circumcised males, keeping the penis smegma-free is easy, involving rolling only a little of the remaining foreskin out of the way during normal showering. Uncircumcised men have to be more careful, pulling back the foreskin and washing the glans and the inside of the foreskin.

Bicycle Riding and Sexual Health

The area between the penis and the anus is called the perineum; it is where the perineal nerve is located. Researchers have found that the perineal nerve is compressed during bicycle riding of three hours per week or longer and that blood flow to the area can be impaired as a result (Huang, Munarriz, & Goldstein, 2005). That can lead to numbness in the penis and perineum and is associated with the onset of erectile dysfunction (Marceau et al., 2001). Erectile dysfunction is the inability to achieve penile erection.

The possibility that this problem might occur does not mean, however, that men should not ride bicycles for protracted periods of time. A minor adjustment in the bicycle saddle can prevent this condition. The bicycle saddle should be changed from the traditional one with a protruding nose to no-nose saddle (Lowe, Schrader, & Breitenstein, 2004). In a study of bicycle police officers, who spend a considerable amount of time riding their bicycles, a no-nose saddle was found to reduce perineum pressure and decrease symptoms (Schrader, Breitenstein, & Lowe, 2008).

Care from Organizations and Available Publications

Several organizations aid men in caring for their reproductive health: The American Cancer Society publishes brochures and pamphlets; local health departments operate clinics providing medical examinations, testing, and care for STIs, premarital blood tests, and counseling about birth control and sexual problems. Other organizations, such as the National Cancer Institute, keep track of the incidence and frequency of diseases related to reproductive health. And still other organizations, such as the Health Research Group, a nonprofit group devoted to studies to improve health care, conduct research to prevent and treat various conditions affecting the male reproductive system.

Exploring the Dimensions of Human Sexuality

Our feelings, attitudes, and beliefs regarding sexuality are influenced by our internal and external environments. Go to go.jblearning.com/dimensions5e to learn more about the biological, psychological, and sociological factors that affect your sexuality.

Biological Factors

When a sperm with a Y chromosome meets an egg, a male offspring will develop. Biological factors continue to influence development throughout life.

- Genetic coding affects physical appearance, including height; coloration of skin, hair, and eyes; muscularity; and many aspects of health.
- Physiological changes result at puberty from the hormone testosterone, which in turn affects muscle development and body size. Testosterone also increases aggression and leads to increased rates of heart attacks.
- Toward middle age, testosterone levels begin to drop, resulting in decreased muscle mass, increased fat, and a reduced sex drive.

Case Study

The physiological development of a male starts when a sperm with a Y chromosome fertilizes an egg. More male than female pregnancies occur, but because male fetuses are weaker, a greater number of miscarriages result. Also, more male infants die than do female infants.

Socioeconomic status of the mother determines whether prenatal care is received, appropriate prenatal and postnatal nutrition is available, and medical help is sought. If the mother smokes, drinks, or abuses drugs during pregnancy, the fetus can be adversely affected.

A man's physiology is altered during puberty. The increased testosterone levels result in greater muscularity and a slimmer body. But testosterone also causes increased aggression.

Male gender roles are often hard for many men to uphold and can result in unhealthy behaviors. Repression of emotions also results in increased stress.

Sociocultural Factors

Sociocultural factors interact with biological factors to influence health.

- Religion may affect the decision as to whether to circumcise the penis.
- The cultural bias allowing men to be sexually permissive can compromise a man's sexual health and wellness.
- Ethnic heritage influences health; for example, African American males tend to have higher levels of stress and heart disease than white males.
- Media and ads portray the ideal man with extreme muscularity, achievable only with tremendous work and, in many cases, illegal steroids.
- Family, neighbors, and friends often reinforce gender stereotypes.
- Behavior proscribed by society as illegal can influence health; for instance, a man can compromise his health by using anabolic steroids.

Psychological Factors

Biological and sociocultural factors combine to influence psychological factors.

- Body image and self-concept are enhanced for many men through exercise and competitive sports.
- In men who suppress their emotions, increased levels of stress can result.
- Learned attitudes and behaviors about gender roles can lead to unhealthy lifestyles for men.

Summary

- The male external genitals consist of the penis and the scrotum. The penis contains the urethra, through which urine and the ejaculate is omitted; the scrotum houses the testes.

- Surgical removal of the foreskin (prepuce) is called circumcision. Over the years there have been differing views on the necessity for circumcision. In some cultures and religions, circumcision is recommended and, therefore, frequently performed.

- The male internal genitals contain numerous structures. The urethra is the tube through which the ejaculate is ejected. The corpora cavernosa and corpus spongiosum fill with blood during sexual arousal, resulting in erection of the penis. Sperm are produced in the seminiferous tubules in the testes, stored in the epididymus, and travel out of the testes through the vasa efferentia.

- The ejaculate consists of secretions from the prostate gland, the seminal vesicles, and sperm. It travels through the vas deferens to the urethra, where it is eventually ejected through the meatus of the penis.

- During puberty, boys become capable of reproduction. This is a result of increased secretion of androgens, followed by the development of secondary sex characteristics. Males are not capable of reproduction before puberty because the prostate and seminal vesicles are not functional until they are activated by the increased production of testosterone that occurs during puberty.

- Males are susceptible to a variety of reproductive system illnesses and conditions. Among these are breast cancer, inflammation of the prostate (prostatitis), enlargement of the prostate (benign prostatic hyperplasia), and prostate cancer.

- Males should regularly care for their reproductive systems. These measures include screenings as appropriate, medical examinations by healthcare providers, and behaviors to prevent illnesses and diseases (for example, eating a nutritional diet, maintaining the recommended weight, exercising regularly, and adjusting the bicycle seat if one is a bicycle rider).

Discussion Questions

1. Name and describe the parts of the male reproductive system, including external and internal genitalia.

2. Explain how the increase and decrease of testosterone level affect the male reproductive system, including physiological and psychological effects.

3. Describe the self-care and preventive practices that a man should use to ensure his sexual health.

Application Questions

Reread the story that opens the chapter and answer the following questions.

1. The phrase "Most men think with their penis" clearly derives from the belief that hormones (physiology) control the man, and not vice versa. Do you believe this is correct? Or do sociocultural and psychological factors help balance a man's thinking?

2. The notion of penis size has generally been shown in research to be of little importance to women. Why does size continue to be a matter of jokes and of apprehension among men?

3. Can the male concern with penis size be compared to a woman's concern about her breast size? (After all, more than 100,000 women have breast enhancements each year.) If men could get relatively safe penis-enlargement surgery, do you believe that many would?

Critical Thinking Questions

1. In many schools throughout the country, sexuality education classes mention the concept of menstruation in a mixed-gender group. But the real discussion of menstruation occurs only in the follow-up "girls only" groupings. Consider whether boys should be taught about menstruation. Without factual knowledge, how can boys comprehend the physical and emotional issues surrounding menstruation? How can they be prepared for safer sexual practices during menstruation if they have not learned about it? Finally, how would you explain menstruation to a group of fifth-grade boys?

Critical Thinking Case

Dad has not been feeling like himself lately. He is unusually tense and easy to upset. It may be due to his lack of sleep. He goes to bed at the same time he always has, but he wakes up often in the middle of the night to urinate. When you ask him about it, he says that he really does not excrete a great deal of urine, just enough to relieve the feeling of having to urinate. As you try to help Dad, answer the following questions.

1. What are some possible causes of Dad's waking up often in the middle of the night to urinate?

2. What would you suggest Dad do about his dilemma? How could you help facilitate his taking this action?

3. What other reproductive system health issues would you expect Dad to encounter as he gets older? What can he do to prevent or postpone the occurrence of these conditions? What can he do to respond to them as they arise?

Exploring Personal Dimensions

For Men Only

Taking charge of self-care and prevention greatly increases your chances of achieving sexual health and wellness. For the following statements, circle YES or NO. Then fill in the dates to help you keep track of your self-care activities.

I have regular physician's examinations. YES NO
My last physician's exam was on _____.
My next physician's exam is due on _____.
My physician perfoms a digital YES NO
    rectal exam.

I practice safer sexual activities. YES NO

I have a family medical tree listing YES NO
diseases.

I discussed my family's medical history YES NO
with my doctor.

Suggested Readings

Bostwick, D. G., Crawford, E. D., Roach III, M., & Higano, C. (eds.). *American Cancer Society's complete guide to prostate cancer*. Atlanta, GA: American Cancer Society, 2004.

Bubley, G. J., & Conkling, W. *What your doctor may not tell you about prostate cancer: The breakthrough information and treatments that can help save your life*. New York: Warner Books, 2005.

Danoff, D. S. *Penis power: The ultimate guide to male sexual health*. Bloomington, IN: Author House, 2011.

Fisch, H., & Braun, S. *The male biological clock: The startling news about aging, sexuality, and fertility in men*. New York: Free Press, 2004.

McCarthy, B. W., & Metz, M. E. *Men's sexual health: Fitness for satisfying sex*. New York: Routledge, 2007.

Peate, I. *Men's sexual health*. Chichester, UK: Whurr Publishers, 2003.

Scardino, P. T., & Kelman, J. *Dr. Peter Scardino's prostate book: The complete guide to overcoming prostate cancer, prostatitis, and BPH*. North Stratford, NH: Avery Publishing Group, 2005.

Taguchi, Y., & Weisbord, M. (ed.). *Private parts: An owner's guide to the male anatomy*. Toronto, Canada: McClelland & Stewart/Tundra Books, 2003.

Vergel, N. *Testosterone: A man's guide*. Newburg, PA: Milestones Publishing, 2010.

Web Resources

For links to the websites below, visit *go.jblearning.com/dimensions5e* and click on Resource Links.

Male Reproductive System
www.training.seer.cancer.gov/anatomy/reproductive/male

Diagram of the male reproductive system with links providing more information. Links include testes, duct system, accessory glands, penis, and male sexual response and hormonal control.

National Cancer Institute
www.cancer.gov

A federal government website providing information about cancer, including prostate and testicular cancers. Includes links to cancer topics, clinical trials, cancer statistics, research and funding, and current news pertaining to cancer.

American Cancer Society
www.cancer.org

A resource for all matters pertaining to cancer, including prostate and testicular cancers. Includes links to types of cancers, making informed treatment decisions, statistics, resources, and recent news.

The Male Health Center
www.malehealthcenter.com

An Internet education site providing information about male health. Included is information about sexual dysfunction, male sexual health problems, sexually transmitted infections, sexual hormones, and sexual aging issues.

Men's Health Network
www.menshealthnetwork.org

Men's Health Network (MHN) is a nonprofit educational organization comprised of physicians, researchers, public health workers, individuals, and other health professionals. MHN is committed to improving the health and wellness of men through education campaigns, partnerships with retailers and other private entities, workplace health programs, data collection, and work with healthcare providers to provide better programs and funding for men's health needs.

References

American Academy of Pediatrics. Circumcision policy statement. *Pediatrics, 103* (1999), 686–693.

American Academy of Pediatrics. *Where we stand: Circumcision,* 2011. Available: http://www.healthychildren.org/English/ages-stages/prenatal/decisions-to-make/pages/Where-We-Stand-Circumcision.aspx.

American Cancer Society. *American Cancer Society updates prostate cancer screening guidelines,* June 12, 1997.

American Cancer Society. *Cancer facts & figures 2010,* 2010.

Andriole, G. L., et al. Mortality results from a randomized prostate-cancer screening trial. *New England Journal of Medicine, 360* (2009), 1310–1319.

Barber, K. R., et al. Differences between African American and Caucasian men participating in a community-based prostate cancer screening program. *Journal of Community Health, 23* (1998), 441–451.

Brinton, L. A., Richesson, D. A., Gierach, G. L., Lacey, J. V., Park, Y., Hollenbeck, A. R., & Schatzkin, A. Prospective evaluation of risk factors for male breast cancer. *Journal of the National Cancer Institute, 100* (2008), 1477–1481.

Brower, V. Circumcision's back. *American Health* (September 1989), 126.

Chan, E. C. Y., Vernon, S. W., O'Donnell, F. T., Ahn, C., Greisinger, A., & Aga, D. W. Informed consent for cancer screening with prostate-specific antigen: How well are men getting the message? *American Journal of Public Health, 93* (2003), 779–785.

Delvin, D., & Webber, C. Facts about penis size. *Net Doctor,* 2008. Available: http://www.netdoctor.co.uk/sex_relationships/facts/penissize.htm.

Haffner, D. W., & Schwartz, P. *What I've learned about sex.* New York: Perigee Books, 1998.

Huang, V., Munarriz, R., & Goldstein, I. Bicycle riding and erectile dysfunction: An increase in interest (and concern). *Journal of Sexual Medicine, 2* (2005), 594–595.

Kinsey, A. C., Pomeroy, W. B., & Martin, C. E. *Sexual behavior in the human male.* Philadelphia: Saunders, 1948.

Lee, U. J., & Jones, J. S. Incidence of prostate cancer in male breast cancer patients: A risk factor for prostate cancer screening. *Prostate Cancer and Prostatic Diseases* (May 27, 2008).

Lowe, B. D., Schrader, S. M., & Breitenstein, M. J. Effect of bicycle saddle designs on the pressure to the perineum of the bicyclist. *Medicine and Science in Sports and Exercise, 36* (2004), 1055–1062.

Marceau, L., Kleinman, K., Goldstein, I., & McKinlay, J. Does bicycling contribute to the risk of erectile dysfunction? Results from the Massachusetts Male Aging Study (MMAS). *International Journal of Impotence Research, 13* (2001), 298–302.

Masters, W. H., Johnson, V. E., & Kolodny, R. C. *Human sexuality.* Boston: Little, Brown, 1982.

Meckler, L. Bush-era abortion rules face possible reversal. *The Wall Street Journal* (December 17, 2008), A5.

Nahleh, Z. A., Srikantiah, R., Safa, M., Jazieh, A. R., Muhleman, A., & Komrokji, R. Male breast cancer in the Veterans Affairs population: A comparative analysis. *Cancer, 109* (2007), 1471–1477.

National Kidney and Urological Diseases Information Clearinghouse. *Urinary incontinence in men.* Bethesda, MD: Author, 2007. Available: http://kidney.niddk.nih.gov/kudiseases/pubs/uimen/#kegel.

Rovner, S. A reversal on circumcision. *Washington Post Health* (May 15, 1990).

Samuels, M., & Samuels, N. All about circumcision. *Medical Self-Care* (Spring 1983), 20–23.

Savage, D. "Conscience" rule for doctors may spark abortion controversy. *Los Angeles Times* (December 2, 2008).

Schrader, S. M., Breitenstein, M. J., & Lowe, B. D. Cutting off the nose to save the penis. *Journal of Sexual Medicine, 5* (2008), 1932–1940.

Schroder, F. H., et al. Screening and prostate-cancer mortality in a randomized European study. *New England Journal of Medicine, 360* (2009), 1320–1328.

Smith, G. L., Greenup, R., & Takafuji, E. T. Circumcision as a risk factor for urethritis in racial groups. *American Journal of Public Health, 77* (1987), 452–454.

Tai, Y. C., Domchek, S., Parmigiani, G., & Chen, S. Breast cancer risk among male BRCA1 and BRCA2 mutation carriers. *Journal of the National Cancer Institute, 99* (2007), 1811–1814.

U.S. Preventive Services Task Force. Screening for prostate cancer: U.S. Preventive Services Task Force recommendation statement. *Annals of Internal Medicine, 149* (2008), 185–191.

U.S. Preventive Task Force. *Screening for testicular cancer,* 2010. Available: http://www.uspreventiveservicestaskforce.org/uspstf10/testicular/testicuprs.htm.

Wallerstein, E. *Circumcision.* New York: Springer, 1980.

Wiswell, T. E., Smith, F. R., & Bass, J. W. Decreased incidence of urinary tract infections in circumcised male infants. *Pediatrics, 75* (1985), 901–903.

CHAPTER 6

Sexual Response and Arousal

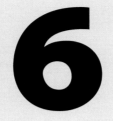

CHAPTER OBJECTIVES

1 Describe the role of the brain in sexual response, including the hormones involved and the role they play.

2 Describe the four phases of the Masters and Johnson sexual response cycle, as well as other theoretical models of sexual response.

3 Describe the physiology of orgasm in both males and females, differentiating between the different types of orgasm.

go.jblearning.com/dimensions5e

The Brain and Sexual Response
Aphrodisiacs
The Masters and Johnson Sexual Response Cycle

INTRODUCTION

*B*rian was sitting in his social studies class paying more attention to the attractive Tanya than to the teacher's lecture. Since
he had entered high school he found himself more and more
interested in girls, whose presence distracted him from his school work
at times that were inappropriate. It was during one of these times that
his social studies teacher asked Brian to identify a particular geographical region on the map in the front of the room. This was a problem for
two reasons, both related to Tanya. First, Brian had no idea where that
geographical region was, and, second, Brian's infatuation with Tanya and
the accompanying fantasies resulted in Brian's having an erection. Now,
erections are not something that high school students, or anyone else for
that matter, choose to display before peers, so understandably Brian was
embarrassed. What was he to do?

This has happened to many high school males, who somehow manage to use textbooks to shield their erections or find some excuse to delay
walking to the front of the room until "it is safer." Some high school
girls and older females also experience sexual excitement that results in
an erection, in this case, of the clitoris. Yet, they are not as vulnerable as
males to being exposed because clitoral erection is not evident through
women's clothes. Women also experience vaginal lubrication when sexually excited, but this too is not readily identifiable when one is dressed.

If this reaction has happened to you, perhaps you wondered whether
you are "normal"—you are. Perhaps you discussed this concern with your
close friends. Most of us probably did not discuss it with our parents.
That would have been too embarrassing. Maybe you read about these
reactions in a magazine or saw them depicted in a movie. Unfortunately,

too many young people rely on these sources for information about sex—and magazines and movies often relay misconceptions and misinformation. But how were you to know that? Where else could you go? Whom else could you speak with?

This chapter provides the information you may have wondered about since that time when your body first responded sexually. Included is a description of the typical human sexual response and the means of eliciting that response. Our goal is to help you establish and maintain a satisfying and effective sexual relationship when you decide you are ready for one. We begin with the study of the usual human sexual response.

■ Sexual Arousal and Response

When unaroused, the penis is flaccid; the skin of the scrotal sac is wrinkled, thin, and loose; and the testes hang down from the body. In females, the labia are thin and enclose the vestibule, the clitoris extends from under the clitoral hood, the inner part of the vagina remains elongated, and the nipples of the breast are not erect.

After sexual excitement diminishes, these structures return to their prearoused state. This takes some time, which varies from person to person.

Sexual pleasure and satisfaction are both psychologically and physiologically based. Without the subjective feeling of pleasure, physiological arousal will not occur. For example, if you dislike the body odor of your partner, it will be difficult for you to develop an erection if you are a male or lubrication of the vagina if you are a female. As we shall soon see, pleasurable sexual stimulation will lead to an identifiable sexual response cycle. Knowing what this response cycle is can help you view your sexuality as a normal part of your functioning, for it suggests that sexual responses can be understood, predicted, and studied in the same way that other physiological processes can. Furthermore, learning to discern and distinguish your own bodily responses can enable you to pay attention, tell your partner about your responses, and thus increase your enjoyment.

How the Mind and Body Control Sexual Response

When a person becomes sexually aroused, several different parts of the body work together to create the psychological feeling of arousal and the accompanying physiological reactions. When Brian fantasized about Tanya, his brain, glands, nervous system,

circulatory system, and reproductive system were only some of the bodily parts involved. Before we discuss the particular response to sexual stimulation, let us look more closely at what happens between the body and mind on such occasions.

The Brain: The Master of the Body

As with most vital functions, the brain is a key player during sexual arousal (Greenberg, 2011). It is the brain that interprets the stimulation—be it visual, olfactory, or other—and begins the process of "activating" other body parts.

The brain includes two major components: the **cerebral cortex** (the upper part) and the subcortex (the lower part). Figure 6.1 shows the structures of the brain and their locations. The subcortex includes the cerebellum (coordinates body movements), the medulla oblongata (regulates heartbeat, respiration, and other such basic physiological processes), the pons (regulates the sleep cycle), and the diencephalon. The diencephalon has many purposes, including the regulation of the emotions. It is made up of the thalamus and hypothalamus. The thalamus relays sensory impulses from other parts of the nervous system to the cerebral cortex. The hypothalamus, a key structure in sexual arousal, is the primary activator of the autonomic nervous system, which controls basic body processes such as hormone balance, temperature, and the constriction and dilation of blood vessels.

The **limbic system**, called the "seat of emotions," consists of the thalamus and hypothalamus

cerebral cortex
The part of the brain called the *gray matter* that controls higher-order functioning such as language and judgment.

limbic system
The part of the brain referred to as the "seat of emotions," which produces emotions in response to physical and psychological signals.

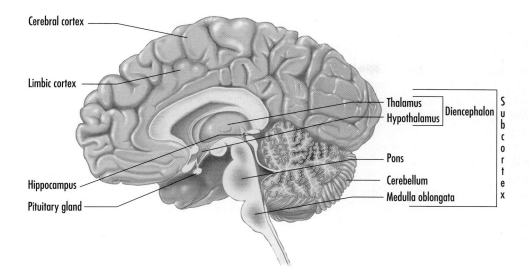

FIGURE **6.1** Many areas of the brain are involved in interpreting and determining each person's reaction to sexual stimulation.

(the diencephalon) and other structures important in sexual arousal. The limbic system is connected to the diencephalon and is primarily concerned with emotions and their behavioral expression. The limbic system is thought to produce such emotions as fear, anxiety, and joy in response to physical and psychological signals.

The cerebral cortex (called the *gray matter*) controls higher-order abstract functioning, such as language and judgment. The cerebral cortex can also control more primitive areas of the brain. When the diencephalon recognizes fear, for instance, the cerebral cortex can use judgment to recognize the stimulus as nonthreatening and override the fear.

Last is the **reticular activating system (RAS)**. In the past, cortical and subcortical functions were considered dichotomized; that is, human behavior was thought to be a function of one area of the brain or the other. Now, brain researchers believe that neurological connections between the cortex and subcortex feed information back and forth. This network of nerves, the RAS, can be considered the connection between mind and body. The reticular system is a kind of two-way street, carrying messages perceived by the higher-awareness centers to the organs and muscles and also relaying stimuli received at the muscular and organic levels up to the cerebral cortex. In this manner, a sexually stimulating touch can generate physiological responses.

reticular activating system (RAS)
A network of nerves that connect the cortex and the subcortex—the connection between mind and body.

The Brain and Sexual Response

When you encounter a sexual stimulus of whatever kind, this message is passed to the brain via nerves. Once it reaches the brain, the message passes through the reticular activating system either from or to the limbic system and the thalamus. The limbic system is where emotion evolves, and the thalamus serves as the switchboard, determining what to do with the incoming messages. Next, the hypothalamus is activated and, in turn, activates the autonomic nervous system and the endocrine system through messages sent via nerves or substances released into the bloodstream.

All of this is generalized, of course. No two people are exactly the same, so no two people should be expected to react in exactly the same manner to sexual stimulation. First, what one person finds sexually arousing, another might not. As a result, one person might experience erection or vaginal lubrication when seeing pictures of people engaged in sexual activities, whereas another person might be "turned off" by this material. Second, because of illness or injury, some typical responses may be precluded for some people. For example, a male with a spinal cord injury might not be able to achieve an erection in spite of what might usually be sexually arousing for others. Furthermore, some people have little control over apparently involuntary responses; however, other people are able to exercise some control. For example, although ejaculation is considered an involuntary response to sexual stimulation, we know that people can learn to control (that is, delay) ejaculation should they choose to. So, in general, there is a great deal of variation in sexual response, even though there are certain typical means of reacting to sexual stimulation.

The Autonomic Nervous System

The autonomic nervous system consists of the sympathetic nervous system and the parasympathetic nervous system. These "subnervous systems" connect to various parts of the body through nerves. Consequently, as sexually arousing stimuli are experienced, messages are sent via the nerves to body parts, instructing them to react. The heart rate increases, muscles tense, perspiration occurs, and the mind starts racing. In addition, certain arteries are instructed to open (dilate) and allow more blood to flow through. That is why, for instance, the penis and the clitoris become erect. Arteries in these structures dilate, allowing blood to flow to the area; the nerves instruct veins to constrict, thereby holding the blood in that one place. The result is erection. The increase of blood to the genital area, called *engorgement,* also creates pressure on the walls of the vagina, resulting in vaginal lubrication. Furthermore, muscles contract as a result of messages sent through the nerves that make up the autonomic nervous system. For men, for example, contractions of the Cowper's gland, the seminal vesicles, and the prostate gland result in fluids being secreted into semen; contractions of the abdominal muscles and the muscles surrounding the reproductive organs are experienced by women.

The Role of Hormones in Sexual Arousal

The endocrine system is responsible for the secretion of hormones that travel to various body parts, instructing them how to behave. For example, when you are "stressed out," hormones are deposited into the bloodstream by the pituitary, adrenal, thyroid, and other glands and transported around the body, resulting in an increase in heart rate, muscle tension, blood pressure, and perspiration.

Sexual arousal works similarly. When you encounter a sexually arousing stimulus, your endocrine system is activated; hormones are secreted and changes occur in your body. That is what happens when someone fantasizes about a sexual experience. The fantasy translates into a sexual response that depends on the release of hormones that target certain body parts and bodily functions.

Sexual hormones are produced in the testes and ovaries. Testosterone, an androgen produced predominantly in the interstitial cells of the testes in men and in the ovaries in women (although a small amount is also produced in the adrenal glands), affects sexual interest, or *libido*. The more testosterone, the greater the interest in sex. Conversely, the less testosterone, the less interest in sex. Islamic societies once used castrated men to watch the women in the harem because their lowered interest in sex made them no threat to the women.

Recognizing the influence of testosterone on sexual interest, and in an attempt to enhance sexual satisfaction, some people turn to chemical aids. One of these "aids" is the substance used by the baseball player Mark McGwire during his record-breaking home run season. Popularly referred to as "andro," androstenedione was marketed as a dietary supplement; thus it was not regulated by the U.S. Food and Drug Administration (FDA). Athletes employed androstenedione to help them recover from weight-training workouts. Chemically, androstenedione is a steroid hormone and a near cousin of testosterone. The association with testosterone was enough to convince some people to use it to enhance sexual satisfaction. The problem with doing so is twofold: (1) The amount of testosterone may not be sufficient for the desirable effects, and (2) its use may result in harmful side effects, especially over the long term. Among other potential side effects, steroid use can lead to liver cancer, mood swings, hair growth, masculinization in women, and atrophied testes in men. In spite of these problems, androstenedione's possible effects on sexual arousal seem to override good judgment for some people hell-bent on making their sex lives ever richer.

The Role of Culture in Sexual Arousal

Whereas sexual arousal involves a physiological reaction to sexual stimulation, that reaction depends on the interpretation of the stimulant. For example, penis and clitoral erections are physiological responses to something interpreted as sexually stimulating. And yet, what someone finds sexually stimulating in one culture may have just the opposite reaction in another culture. For example, one culture might value a "full-bodied" woman, whereas another might value thinness. Furthermore, perceptions of what is sexually stimulating may differ within the same culture over time. In the United States, for instance, the actress Marilyn Monroe was a sexual icon in the 1950s. Today, she would probably be viewed differently because we now place a higher value on thinness than we did back then.

Subcultures also may have different perceptions of what is sexually stimulating. One of your authors' graduate students conducted a study of what African Americans and Caucasians considered to be the ideal body type. Research subjects were given silhouettes to evaluate. Whites reported that a thinner silhouette was more attractive, whereas African Americans stated a more full-figured body type was more desirable.

In some Muslim societies, women are required to be covered from head to toe. In contrast, in many Western societies, scantily clad women evoke a sexual response. In some subcultures, pornographic material is sexually stimulating while in others it is considered disgusting.

Thus, although sexual stimulation is a physiological process, it has a cultural and societal component to it that starts the physiological reaction in the first place.

The Masters and Johnson Sexual Response Cycle

The research of Masters and Johnson (1966) revealed a great deal about human sexuality. One of their major contributions was their description of the four phases of the human sexual response.

Excitement Phase

During the first phase of the Masters and Johnson **sexual response cycle**, the *excitement phase*, sexual stimuli result in a number of specific changes in the bodies of men and women. Heart rate, blood pressure, and muscle tension all increase. Blood engorges the abdominal area, resulting in an increase in penile and clitoral erection, as well as an increase in size of the labia minora, vagina, and nipples. The testes move closer to the body, and the scrotal skin thickens and tightens during the excitement phase. In women, vaginal lubrication occurs, and the labia majora spread and separate so as to make the vestibule more accessible. Some of these structures also deepen in color as a result of the increased blood to the area. The engorgement of blood is also responsible for the darkening of the skin on the chest and breasts called the *sex flush*. Although the sex flush occurs in both genders, it is more common in women and occurs in all ethnic groups, although it may be more evident in whites than in people of color.

Transudation is the process resulting in vaginal lubrication. When a female is sexually aroused, blood flows into the area surrounding the walls of the vagina in a process called *vasocongestion*. The pressure of the increased blood causes a seepage of moisture from the spaces between cells. This moisture crosses the vaginal lining, first appearing as droplets. Eventually the fluid builds up in sufficient quantity to moisten the entire inner walls of the vagina. The amount of moisture may even be enough, depending on the woman's position, to leak out of the vagina and lubricate the labia and introitus.

The excitement phase may be short or last for several hours. The longer it lasts, the more variability occurs. For example, changes in the penis and the vagina vacillate over time during an extended excitement phase, so that the penis may occasionally become less erect, and vaginal lubrication may diminish periodically as well. The exciting aspect of excitement (pun intended) is the great variability among people. Some respond quickly; others need more time. Some favor moving to the next phase quickly; others desire more time. Some focus on their own reactions and feelings and satisfaction; others are more concerned with the partner's satisfaction. Furthermore, any one person may experience the excitement phase differently from one sexual encounter to another.

Plateau Phase

The second phase of Masters and Johnson's sexual response cycle is called the *plateau phase*. During the plateau phase, excitement becomes enhanced. Heart rate quickens, blood pressure rises, muscle tension increases, and breathing is faster. In men, Cowper's gland secretions may result from muscular contractions. The penis becomes fully erect, and the testes move closer to the body cavity. In women, the clitoris retracts under the clitoral hood; the inner two-thirds of the vagina fully extends, forming a "tenting" effect and creating a receptacle for semen; and the outer third of the vagina engorges with blood, forming the orgasmic platform. Although the plateau phase usually lasts but a few minutes, there are reports of more intense orgasms by people who have purposefully extended the plateau phase. And yet, orgasm is not the necessary follow-up to plateau. Although for men the loss of erection is unlikely once plateau is reached, in women as we shall soon see, reaching the plateau phase may be sufficient for sexual satisfaction.

Orgasm Phase

The *orgasm phase* for males consists of two stages: the *emission stage* and the *expulsion stage*. During the emission stage, muscular contractions of the vas deferens, the seminal vesicles, and the prostate gland create a buildup of semen in the urethral bulb located at the base of the penis. At the same time, the external urethral sphincter contracts, holding in the semen. Concurrently, the internal urethral sphincter contracts, thereby preventing semen from entering the bladder (a condition known as *retrograde ejaculation*) and urine from entering the urethral bulb where the

sexual response cycle
The sequence of physiological and psychological reactions as a result of sexual arousal.

transudation
The process of vaginal lubrication resulting from engorgement of blood that creates pressure that forces moisture to seep from the spaces between the cells.

semen has accumulated. The accumulation of semen in the urethral bulb creates a sensation of imminent and inevitable ejaculation, which usually lasts only a few seconds. Soon the second stage, expulsion, occurs.

During the expulsion stage, the **internal urethral sphincter** remains contracted, so urine and semen do not mix. However, the **external urethral sphincter** relaxes, and muscles surrounding the urethral bulb and the urethra contract, with the result that the accumulated semen is expelled from the urethral opening. Although there is some variation from one person to another, males generally experience intense sensations during the first couple of contractions and less sensation during later contractions. The degree of sensation appears also to be related to the amount of semen expelled.

internal urethral sphincter
The valve that prevents urine from entering the urethra and sperm from entering the bladder during ejaculation.

external urethral sphincter
The valve that closes during the emission stage, resulting in a buildup of semen, and that opens during the ejaculation stage, allowing semen to be expelled.

orgasmic platform
The narrowing of the outer third of the vagina during orgasm caused by contractions of the muscles in that area.

In women, the orgasm phase also consists of muscular contractions and intense sensations. The pelvic muscles that surround the vagina, in particular those that make up the **orgasmic platform**, contract 3 to 15 times, each contraction lasting less than 1 second. Other weaker and slower contractions follow. In addition, uterine contractions occur, beginning from the top of the uterus and proceeding downward.

In both males and females, other changes occur during orgasm. For example, heart rate increases dramatically, blood pressure rises, and breathing becomes rapid and shallow. Muscles throughout the body contract, and perspiration is evident. And an intense, pleasant psychological feeling associated with the release of sexual tension afforded by orgasm occurs.

Resolution Phase

During the *resolution phase*, there is a return to the unaroused state. In males, there is a decrease in the size of the penis as the erection is lost. This occurs in two stages: The first lasts about 1 minute as the blood exits the corpora cavernosa; the second takes several minutes as the blood leaves the corpus spongiosum. This is a result of the opening of the veins in the penis, which allows blood to be removed from the area. The testes become smaller and move down from the body cavity, and the scrotal skin becomes thinner and looser.

In women, muscles relax, and the uterus, vagina, and labia return to their unaroused positions and color.

As a result of the uterus's returning to its unaroused position, the cervix lowers into the seminal pool. If sperm is present in the seminal pool, the cervix is likely to have contact with them, and fertilization is possible. If one is trying to become pregnant, then the woman should lie on her back after intercourse to encourage this contact. Of course, the best way to prevent pregnancy if engaging in sexual intercourse is to use some method of contraception.

In addition to the preceding changes, during the resolution phase the clitoris returns from under the clitoral hood and the sex flush dissipates. In both males and females, heart rate, blood pressure, and breathing rate return to normal, and muscle tension decreases. Males then experience a **refractory (recovery) period** during which they are incapable of another orgasm. This period may be only several minutes for young males but is usually longer in older males. Females, however, are capable of having **multiple orgasms** before needing to recover.

refractory (recovery) period
The time needed by males for recovery between orgasms.

multiple orgasms
Orgasms that occur without the need for a refractory, or recovery, period.

sex flush
A darkening of the skin of the neck, face, forehead, or chest during sexual stimulation.

myotonia
Muscle tension occurring during sexual arousal.

hyperventilation
Deep and rapid breathing that occurs during sexual excitation.

tachycardia
An increase in heart rate that occurs during sexual activity.

vasocongestion
Increased blood flow to an area of the body; which occurs in the pelvic area during sexual arousal.

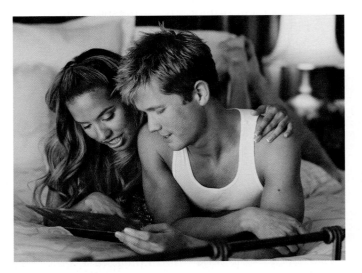

Females and males have many sexual responses in common, as well as many that differ. One of the differences is that males need a refractory period in which to recover before being capable of another orgasm, whereas females do not.

Gender DIMENSIONS

Male–Female Differences in Sexual Response

There are many similarities and many differences in how males and females respond to sexual arousal. Masters and Johnson found the following similarities in the response cycle of men and women:

1. *Nipples.* Both males' and females' nipples become erect and wider in diameter when sexually stimulated.

2. *Sex Flush.* Males and females both experience a darkening of the skin of the neck, face, forehead, or chest during sexual stimulation, known as the **sex flush**. This darkening of the skin is a result of the accumulation of blood in these areas.

3. *Muscle Tension.* Commencing during the plateau phase and involving the legs, arms, abdomen, neck, and face, muscle tension (**myotonia**) appears in both sexes. During orgasm, muscles of the abdomen, chest, and face are also tensed. After orgasm, during the resolution phase, there is a release of all muscular tension in both sexes.

4. *Breathing.* During sexual excitation, both sexes experience deep and rapid breathing, called **hyperventilation**.

5. *Heart Rate.* Heart rate increases from a normal resting rate of about 72 up to 180 or more beats per minute during orgasm are not unusual in either sex. Such an increase is termed **tachycardia**.

6. *Blood Pressure.* Blood pressure rises in both males and females during sexual excitation.

7. *Perspiration.* Approximately one-third of both males and females perspire after orgasm.

8. *Blood Flow.* Increased blood flow to the pelvic area results in clitoral and penile erection and vaginal lubrication. This increased blood flow is termed **vasocongestion**.

9. *Orgasm.* During orgasm there is a rapid contraction of muscles in both sexes, with a relaxing of the muscles after orgasm.

The following listing describes the differences in the sexual responses of males and females:

1. *Nipples.* Whereas females are most likely to experience nipple erection during the excitement phase, males usually experience it during the plateau phase. Further, female nipple erection appears to disappear soon after orgasm (although this is an illusion caused by the swelling of the areolae), whereas male nipple erection is often obvious long after.

2. *Sex Flush.* Whereas males experience sex flush only in the plateau phase, in females sex flush can occur either late in the excitement phase or in the plateau phase. And though it may occur on the neck, forehead, and chest of both males and females, the sex flush occurs over the lower abdomen, thighs, lower back, and buttocks of females only.

3. *Muscle Tension.* In females, muscular tension causes an increase in the length and width of the vagina and expansion of the diameter of the cervix. In males, it causes elevation of the testes; that is, they are moved closer to the body by the contraction of muscles supporting them.

4. *Breathing.* Hyperventilation has different effects on males and females. After orgasm, males must wait for hyperventilation to diminish before being able to have another orgasm or even to achieve another erection; this period while breathing slows is referred to as a *refractory period*. Females, however, may have another orgasm before hyperventilation subsides—that is, without a refractory period and without entering a resolution phase. Consequently some females are capable of many orgasms in a short period.

5. *Blood Pressure.* Blood pressure increases somewhat more in males than in females. In males systolic blood pressure has been found to increase 40 to 100 mm Hg and diastolic blood pressure 20 to 50 mm Hg during sexual stimulation. In females the increase ranges from 30 to 80 mm Hg systolic and 20 to 40 mm Hg diastolic.

6. *Perspiration.* In men, sweating is usually limited to the soles of the feet and palms of the hands. Women are more likely to perspire over the back, thighs, chest, and sometimes the trunk, head, and neck.

7. *Orgasm.* Women are more likely than men to be multi-orgasmic. Further, orgasm for the woman usually lasts longer than for men. There is disagreement about female ejaculation; it is sufficient to say here that, at the very least, female ejaculation does not occur as often during orgasm as does male ejaculation.

Each of us, male and female, progresses sequentially through the preceding four phases if we experience orgasm. Clearly, many body processes are involved during sexual activity, and each phase of the response affects the body somewhat differently. Even if we do not reach the orgasmic phase, we may pass through the earlier phases. For example, you may be engaged in sexual stimulation and quickly reach the excitement phase. The plateau stage may occur next, but—just your luck—the telephone rings and your excitement dissapates when you find out a loved one needs your help.

In studying the sexual response cycle in males and females, Masters and Johnson found both startling differences and amazing similarities. Knowing how females and males compare and contrast sexually is important to reinforcing the notion that we all have much in common while still preserving our differences.

If any of these responses is new to you, do not be surprised. You probably do not know everything about your digestive functions or nervous system, for instance, so why would you know everything about your sexual responses without studying them? The next time you are sexually aroused (either physically or by thoughts or fantasies), stop for a moment and attempt to identify the responses just discussed—or reflect now on some past sexual experience. Remember, no two of us are exactly alike. Consequently you may not experience all the sexual responses as we have described them. This is to be expected. Generally,

though, you will find that your sexual responses are similar to the ones described.

Figure 6.2 depicts the typical male sexual response according to Masters and Johnson. Males start with the excitement phase, move to the plateau phase, proceed to have an orgasm, and then either move through the resolution phase, in which they return to the pre-aroused state, or to a refractory period (a part of the resolution phase), during which they recover from the orgasm and prepare themselves for another orgasm. Masters and Johnson found this pattern to be standard, although men report variations on this model.

Females were described by Masters and Johnson as being more varied in their sexual responses. Figure 6.2 also shows this variability. Pattern (a) is similar to the male pattern with a progression from excitement to plateau to orgasm and then resolution, except that it depicts a female's ability to have multiple orgasms without a refractory period. Pattern (b) shows the woman's progressing from excitement to an enhancement of this excitement during the plateau phase and then moving directly to resolution (bypassing orgasm). This pattern implies that women may be sexually satisfied without experiencing an orgasm. Pattern (c) depicts another possible female sexual response cycle in which there is no definitive plateau phase but a rapid escalation to orgasm and a very quick resolution.

Figures 6.3 and 6.4 summarize changes that occur in males and females during the four phases of the Masters and Johnson sexual response cycle.

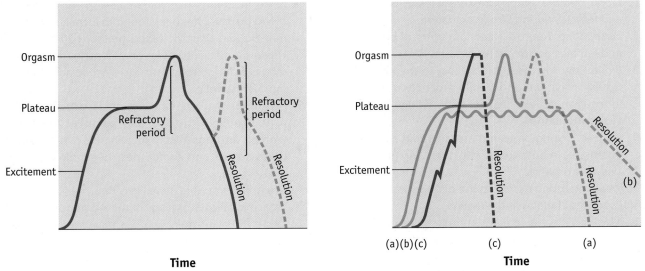

FIGURE 6.2 According to Masters and Johnson, the male sexual response cycle (a) is much more predictable than is the female response cycle (b), and females can have a similar response to males—that is, moving through the four phases and experiencing orgasm—or can maintain the plateau phase without orgasm. Females can also be multiorgasmic without experiencing a refractory period.
Source: Data from Masters, W. H., & Johnson, V. E. *Human sexual response.* Boston: Little Brown, 1966.

(a) Unaroused State

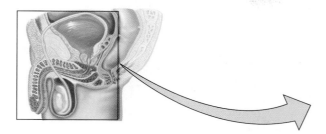

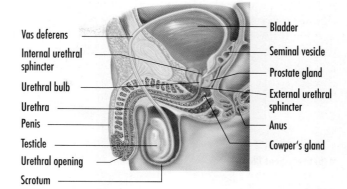

Vas deferens
Internal urethral sphincter
Urethral bulb
Urethra
Penis
Testicle
Urethral opening
Scrotum

Bladder
Seminal vesicle
Prostate gland
External urethral sphincter
Anus
Cowper's gland

(b) Excitement Phase

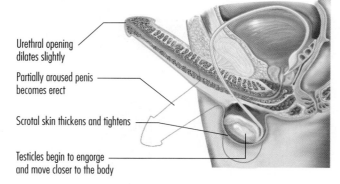

Urethral opening dilates slightly

Partially aroused penis becomes erect

Scrotal skin thickens and tightens

Testicles begin to engorge and move closer to the body

(c) Plateau Phase

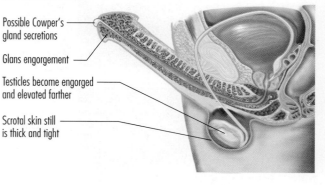

Possible Cowper's gland secretions

Glans engorgement

Testicles become engorged and elevated farther

Scrotal skin still is thick and tight

(d) Orgasm Phase: Emission Stage

Contractions of ampulla of vas deferens

Internal urethral sphincter contracts

Urethral bulb expands

External urethral sphincter contracts

Contractions of prostate gland

Contractions of seminal vesicle

(e) Orgasm Phase: Expulsion Stage

Semen expelled

Internal urethral sphincter stays contracted

Contractions of urethra

External urethral sphincter relaxes and opens

Contractions of muscles around base of penis

Contractions of rectal sphincter

(f) Resolution

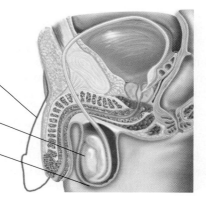

Rapid partial decrease in size of penis; then slow return to unaroused state and size

Testicles become smaller and move down from the body

Scrotal skin thins and becomes more loose

FIGURE **6.3** Male sexual response cycle, in detail.

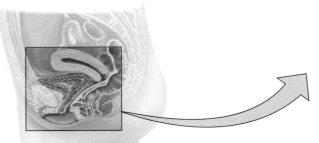

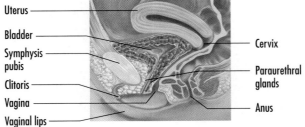

(a) Unaroused State

- Uterus
- Bladder
- Symphysis pubis
- Clitoris
- Vagina
- Vaginal lips
- Cervix
- Paraurethral glands
- Anus

■ (b) Excitement Phase

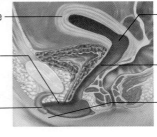

- Uterus increases in size and elevates
- Labia minora become engorged and darken and swell
- Clitoris increases in size
- Inner two-thirds of vagina tents and lengthens
- Vagina walls begin to lubricate
- Labia majora separate to make vestibule accessible

■ (c) Plateau State

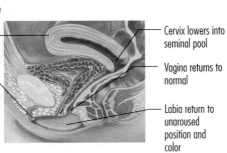

- Inner two-thirds of vagina is fully distended to form the seminal pool
- Clitoris retracts under hood
- Labia become darker
- Outer third of vagina engorges and forms the orgasmic platform

■ (d) Orgasm Phase

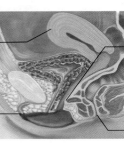

- Uterine contractions occur beginning from the top
- Clitoris is still retracted under hood
- Contractions occur in orgasmic platform
- Anal sphincter muscle contracts

■ (e) Resolution State

- Uterus returns to its normal position
- Clitoris returns from under the clitoral hood to normal position
- Cervix lowers into seminal pool
- Vagina returns to normal
- Labia return to unaroused position and color

■ (f) Breast Changes

- *Unaroused State*
- *Excitement State* Breast size increases; nipples become erect
- *Plateau and Orgasm Phase* Breast size increases more; areolae increase in size (making nipples appear less erect); skin color may become flushed from vasocongestion (called the sex flush)

FIGURE **6.4** Female sexual response cycle, in detail.

Other Theoretical Models of Sexual Response

Other models descriptive of the human sexual response have been proposed. These models are the product of years of experience in sexual counseling and therapy.

Kaplan's Triphasic Model

Originally, the noted sex therapist Helen Singer Kaplan (1974) proposed a biphasic model of the human sexual response. That model conceptualized sexual response as having two identifiable phases. The first phase involved vasocongestion of the genitals, and the second phase consisted of the reflexive muscular contractions of orgasm. Kaplan argued that the two phases were each controlled by a different part of the nervous system: vasocongestion, by the parasympathetic nervous system, and orgasm, by the sympathetic nervous system (both are components of the autonomic nervous system). Furthermore, she explained, different structures are involved in each of these phases: the blood vessels for vasocongestion and the muscles for orgasm. Kaplan gave other justifications for the biphasic model, but space limits our discussion to the justification that derived from Kaplan's observations in her professional practice. Kaplan noted that the interference with vasocongestion resulted in erection problems in the male, whereas different sexual dysfunctions (premature ejaculation and retarded ejaculation) were the result of orgasm impairment. In some females, normal vasocongestion and sexual excitement were experienced in spite of the presence of orgasm problems. Because problems with vasocongestion were quite different from and mutually exclusive with problems with orgasm, Kaplan believed the biphasic model to be valid.

Over the years Kaplan's biphasic model evolved into a triphasic one. Kaplan (1979) now conceptualizes human sexual response as consisting of a **desire phase**, an **excitement phase**, and a **resolution phase**. During her practice as a sex therapist Kaplan had found that sexual dysfunctions fall into one of these three categories and that these categories are separate and distinct (that is, it is possible to function well in one or two phases while having problems in another). The unique component of Kaplan's triphasic model is the desire phase—a psychological prephysical sexual response stage. Masters and Johnson's model ignores this part of the sexual response.

Sexual desire is not always present during sexual activity, however. Sometimes a person may engage in sexual activity to satisfy his or her partner rather than because he or she feels desire. A speaker in one of our sexuality classes described how when his wife complains of some ache or pain (or the proverbial headache) when he is interested in sex, he asks where she feels bothered. When he finds the spot, he gently massages that area, soon turning the massage into a sensual experience. Shortly, he relates, the desire phase is reached.

Zilbergeld and Ellison's Model
Another model of human sexual response consists of five components. The therapists Bernie Zilbergeld and Carol Ellison (1980) were concerned that Masters and Johnson's model ignored the cognitive and subjective aspects of the sexual response, while focusing

desire phase
The first stage of the sexual response cycle, as described in Helen Singer Kaplan's model, which consists of psychologically becoming interested in sex before any physical changes occur.

excitement phase
The second stage of Kaplan's model of sexual response, which consists of physiological arousal and changes and, possibly, orgasm.

resolution phase
A stage of the sexual response cycle consisting of a return to the prearoused state.

exclusively on the physiological aspects. They argued that the subjective elements of sexual desire and sexual arousal were omitted from the Masters and Johnson model. *Sexual desire* is defined in this five-component model as the frequency with which a person wants to engage in sexual activity; *sexual arousal* is defined as how excited one becomes during sexual activity. The five components of this model are as follows.

1. Interest, or desire
2. Arousal
3. Physiological readiness (for example, erection or vaginal lubrication)
4. Orgasm
5. Satisfaction (one's evaluation of how one feels)

As with Kaplan's model, Zilbergeld and Ellison's model allows for sexual dysfunctions that pertain to desire although other responses may be normal. Consequently, this component can be isolated from the other components for treatment by a sex therapist. One might describe the triphasic and five-component models as being more inclusive of the psychological aspects of the sexual response, whereas the Masters and Johnson model is more concerned with the physiological aspects.

Walen and Roth's Model
The contribution of Walen and Roth (1987) relates to the inclusion of perception as the beginning of the sexual response. They argue that without perceiving a potential stimulus as sexually exciting, no sexual response is elicited. Further, they state that a stimulus that is sexually arousing in one situation may not be in another situation. For example, having one's genitals fondled in private may be arousing, but having one's genitals fondled in public may only be embarrassing.

Further, Walen and Roth's model of sexual response includes people evaluating the situation and their response to it to determine if everything is going according to plan. They might evaluate the amount of vaginal lubrication, the presence of penile erection, or heavy breathing. Expecting these to occur and finding that they have occurred validates that the encounter is progressing as expected. The partners can then relax and enjoy the situation, thereby becoming more sexually aroused. However, determining things aren't going as planned can interfere with the sexual response as we try to decide what the problem is and how to solve it. The result might be an inability to have an orgasm, or even to just enjoy the sexual encounter. Recognizing that evaluating one's performance or the situation too critically can interfere with sexual arousal, Walen and Roth advise not placing too high an expectation on performance, not spending too much time observing what is occurring, and relaxing and being fully involved in a manner that will enhance sexual arousal and the enjoyment of the sexual encounter.

Thayton's Model

Wiliam Thayton (2002) is a Baptist minister, and the model of sexual arousal he developed, understandably, has a spiritual and theological perspective. Thayton acknowledges that sex is pleasurable. He proposes that God intended for humans to respond to sex with pleasure and to enjoy the blessing of sexual arousal. Thayton offers evidence of this view by stating that Jesus never preached that sexual pleasure was sinful or to be avoided, in spite of advocating self-denial in other areas of life. Therefore, Thayton concludes that spirituality, sexuality, and love are bound together in God's creation of people who are sexual by nature. As a result, when one is sexual, one is also spiritual. However, love is an important component in this mix for Thayton. Love is the glue that binds sexuality, spirituality, and pleasure. After all, he argues, love allows us to be one with the universe and what is more spiritual than that?

Lastly, Thayton considers sex researchers as sexual guides, just as clergy and theologians are spiritual and religious guides. They all study their area of expertise to understand it better, and then communicate their findings and recommendations to the public at large.

Basson's Model

Basson (2000) is a sex therapist and, as such, her model of sexual response stems from her experience in treating sexual disorders. Basson has no argument with the models offered by Masters and Johnson or Kaplan. However, like Walen and Roth, she believes that how one perceives and interprets a situation is an important component of sexual response. Basson states that feeling positive toward one's partner is necessary for sexual arousal to occur. If one hates one's partner or doesn't trust one's partner, sexual arousal will not occur.

Basson also believes there is a difference in sexual response between males and females. In females, she argues, emotions and intimacy are important precursors of sexual response. Whereas sexual response begins with desire or arousal in males, Basson believes it begins with intimacy in females. In other words, women desire being close to their partners, whereas men desire a physical release of sexual tension. Once women feel intimate toward their partners, desire and arousal are then possible. In fact, Basson believes that intimacy leads to arousal, which

in turn leads to desire. Desire creates greater intimacy, which then results in even more arousal and desire. All along the way, though, there are interpretations and evaluations of what is occurring, similar to the recognition of perceptions in the Walen and Roth model. These interpretations and evaluations affect intimacy, arousal, and desire.

Orgasm is a possible result of this cycle, but not a necessary one for women to feel sexually satisfied, which is the key for Basson. Some people may experience orgasm but not feel the sexual encounter was satisfying. Others may not experience orgasm but feel the encounter was extremely satisfying. Basson believes that should be the goal of the encounter—being satisfied, not orgasm.

Erotic Stimulus Pathway

An important contribution to our knowledge of sexual response is that of the Erotic Stimulus Pathway (ESP) theory of David M. Reed (Haffner & Stayton, 1998). The ESP theory enhances our understanding and ability to treat sexual dysfunctions. Reed divides the sexual response cycle into four phases that correspond to those of Kaplan and Masters and Johnson. For many people, these phases are learned developmentally. Figure 6.5 compares the Masters and Johnson model with the Reed model.

In the *seduction phase* a person learns how to get aroused sexually and how to attract someone else sexually. Seduction translates into memories and rituals. For example, adolescents may spend much time on personal appearance, choice of clothes, and mannerisms, all of which can enhance positive self-esteem if the adolescents like the way they feel. If the adolescents feel good about the way they look and feel, then attracting another person will be much easier. As the adolescents get older, these positive feelings are translated into sexual desire and arousal. These seductive techniques are stored in memory and can be activated later on in life.

In the *sensations phase*, the different senses can enhance sexual excitement and ideally prolong the plateau phase. The early experiences of touch (holding hands, putting arms around a loved one) become very important. The sense of vision (staring at a loved one, holding an image of him or her when absent) is a way of maintaining interest and arousal. Hearing the loved one in intimate conversation or over the telephone becomes very important. Hearing the sounds of a partner responding to sexual stimulation can be titillating. The smell of the loved one, either a particular scent he or she wears or the sexual smell, produces additional excitement. Finally, the taste of a food or drink or the taste of the loved one becomes important to memory and fantasy. All these senses

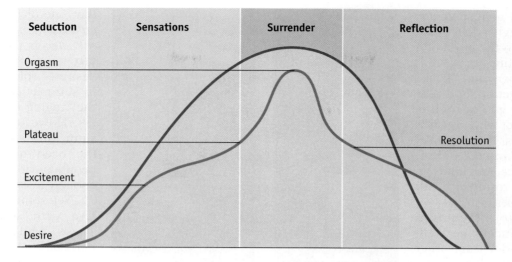

| Seduction | Sensations | Surrender | Reflection |

FIGURE **6.5** Sexual response curve. *Source:* Data from Masters, W. H., & Johnson, V. E. *Human sexual response.* Boston: Little Brown, 1966; Kaplan, H. S. *Disorders of sexual desire.* New York: Simon & Schuster, 1979.

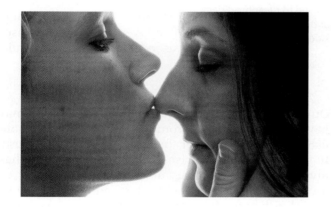

Many senses can evoke a sexual response. The soft touch, kiss, sight, or smell of a partner can be quite sexually stimulating.

extend the excitement into a plateau phase, which makes one want to continue the pleasurable moment over a longer period. These seduction and sensation experiences are the psychological input to the physiology of sexual response. They are the precursors to sexual climax and orgasm.

In the *surrender phase,* orgasm is a "psychophysiological surprise." The psychodynamic issues surrounding orgasm are power and control. Persons with orgasmic dysfunction may be in a power struggle with themselves or with their partners or with the messages received about sex. Overcontrol or undercontrol can affect orgasmic potential and the ability to allow all of the passion to be expressed.

In the *reflection phase,* meaning is given to the experience. Whether the sexual experience is interpreted as positive or negative may determine the

desire for subsequent sexual activity—at least with that sexual partner, under those circumstances, or with those behaviors. Recognize, though, that not every sexual experience can be, or should be, a "10." As the authors have heard it expressed, "Sometimes sex is a four-course gourmet meal, and sometimes it's like having cereal for dinner. Most of the time it's like having hamburgers or chicken. When it's cereal, you have to remember that there are better times ahead."

Aphrodisiacs: Seeking the Ultimate in Sexual Pleasure

An *aphrodisiac,* named after the Greek goddess Aphrodite, the goddess of love, is any substance that arouses sexual desire and/or enhances sexual response. For centuries people have searched for a safe and effective aphrodisiac without much luck. This search has led to "Spanish fly" (*canthardin*), which results in irritation of the urinary tract. Now, is that sexually arousing? It has led to substances to make one "horny," such as ground-up rhinoceros horns or elephant tusks, which just do not work. Oysters, clams, and even the testicles of bulls ("prairie oysters") have been tried without the desired effect.

Even toxic substances have been ingested in the hope of enhancing sexual desire and response; *amyl nitrate* is one of these substances. Amyl nitrate is designed for use by heart patients to reduce chest pain. Its container is "popped" open when chest pain occurs; thus the containers are often called "poppers." Amyl nitrate became popular among some gay men as an aphrodisiac because it facilitated anal intercourse by relaxing the anal sphincter muscle. Although it does dilate blood vessels in the brain and genitals, resulting in warmth in the abdomen and pelvis, facilitating erection, and possibly prolonging orgasm, it is also associated with disturbing side effects. For example, amyl nitrate can cause dizziness, headaches, and fainting, and can even result in death in extreme cases.

Bupropion (acquired under the brand name Wellbutrin) and L-dopa are other substances that have been ingested for their aphrodisiac effects. Bupropion is an antidepressant drug, and L-dopa is a drug used for treating patients with Parkinson's disease. Both of these drugs act on the brain receptors that produce dopamine and so can increase libido. However, unsupervised use of a drug that affects the brain is dangerous; it must be monitored by a physician and prescribed for a specific medical purpose.

Alcohol and *marijuana* have also been ascribed aphrodisiaclike qualities. However, if they work at all, they diminish judgment and make people feel less stress about sex. That may be good, or that may be bad. A decrease in inhibitions may result in high-risk sexual behaviors (such as vaginal or anal intercourse without a condom) that may transmit a sexually transmitted infection (STI) or cause an unwanted pregnancy. Furthermore, alcohol is a central nervous system depressant that can interfere with sexual arousal rather than enhance it. Marijuana can distort perceptions and make one think that the sexual experience continued longer than it really did. Both of these substances can lead to problems in the short run and over prolonged use; in addition, marijuana is illegal.

One substance that appears to have potential as an aphrodisiac is *yohimbine hydrochloride*, from the sap of a West African tree, the yohimbine tree. Yohimbine has been reported to aid some men with erectile dysfunction to achieve and maintain an erection for a long-enough period to engage in sexual intercourse (Senbel & Mostafa, 2008). However, it does not work for all men with erectile dysfunction, and whether it enhances the sexual response of other men is unknown.

Even drugs that inhibit sexual desire have been the focus of researchers for many years. These drugs are called *anaphrodisiacs*. For years, rumor has had it

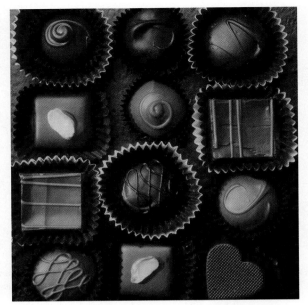

For centuries, people have searched for substances that arouse sexual desire and/or enhance sexual response. Many substances have been proposed to be aphrodisiacs, even chocolate. However, most of these substances either do not work or have disturbing side effects. Still, the search continues.

that one of these substances, *potassium nitrate*, known as *saltpeter*, is used by the military to diminish the sexual desire of soldiers and is used in summer camps to control the "raging urges" of teenagers. However, all that potassium nitrate does is increase the need to urinate; some people obviously think that is enough to interfere with sex.

Yet some drugs do interfere with sexual response. These tend to be central nervous system depressants such as opiates (for example, heroin), tranquilizers, antihypertensive medications, antipsychotic and antidepressant drugs (such as Prozac), and, surprisingly to many people, nicotine, which constricts blood vessels and decreases vasocongestion in the genitals.

Orgasm

Our nonsexual lives tend to be goal oriented. We may have goals to graduate from college, to become established in a good career, or to live in a large house. It should be no surprise that goal orientation has invaded our sexual lives as well. For too many of us, orgasm becomes the goal of almost all of our sexual behavior. We forget about the pleasure that can be derived from sexual activity that does not lead to orgasm, and we forget that the communication and the quality of our relationships can be enhanced through sexual activity that does not result in orgasm. The question "Did you come?" tends to be as much a part of the sexual experience as removing one's clothes.

Orgasmic Sensation

The feelings that accompany orgasm are quite different from the physiological responses and may even contradict what we know is occurring physiologically. For example, women may experience a physiologically intense orgasm (a dozen or so measurable muscular contractions) but report the orgasm to be of mild intensity, or they may experience a mild orgasm physiologically (four muscular contractions) but report the sensation of an intense orgasm. The reason for this discrepancy lies in the understanding that sexual experience is interpreted by the mind as well as the body. When the relationship is a healthy

Global DIMENSIONS

Aphrodisiacs and Tigers: A Strange Mix

Some of the most expensive aphrodisiacs in the world are made from parts of male tigers. The most prized and valuable aphrodisiacs are made from the tiger's penis—often made into a soup! Less expensive "love potions" are made from everything else down to the tiger's crushed bone. Such aphrodisiacs are extremely popular, predominantly in Asian countries.

The net result is that the last several thousand of the world's tigers are endangered—and all for naught. As with many other aphrodisiacs, no physiological sexual response results from ingesting tiger parts.

To help debunk the myth of the tiger as aphrodisiac, the Wildlife Conservation Society hired a Singapore ad agency to create the ad shown here. The TV ad (intended for an Asian audience) shows mating tigers. The voice-over reads, "The last 5,000 tigers in the world are being killed. All because some men believe that eating tiger penis will give them legendary sexual prowess. Perhaps they too can make love for a full 15 seconds."

What psychological effects might such an "aphrodisiac" have in a country where there is a long-standing cultural belief that it works? Might the ability to pay a great deal of money for such an aphrodisiac have a psychological boosting effect? Will the ad help to "destroy the myth," as it claims? Explain your answer.

Image source: Courtesy of Wildlife Conservation Society.

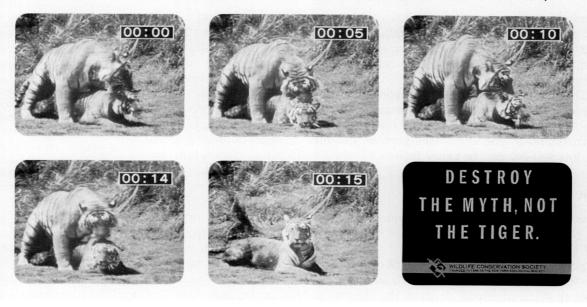

one, sexual partners may experience a great deal of pleasure from a mild orgasm because the experience was shared and made them feel closer. Other factors such as mood, expectations, and the setting can also affect one's subjective judgment regarding the intensity of the orgasm.

Generally, sensations from orgasms are experienced similarly by males and females, but there are exceptions (Silverberg, 2008). In women, there is a highly pleasurable feeling that usually begins at the clitoris but quickly spreads to the whole pelvic area. The genitals often feel warm and tingly, and then a sensation of throbbing in the lower pelvis may be noticed. In men, the experience is also highly pleasurable. They usually experience warmth, pressure, and sometimes a throbbing during the moment when they have reached the "point of no return" (that is, ejaculatory inevitability), at which point men cannot prevent ejaculation. In many men, ejaculation itself is experienced as a sensation of pumping.

The similarity of male and female orgasms was vividly demonstrated by two studies involving college students (Proctor, Wagner, & Butler, 1974; Wiest, 1977). In these studies, students wrote descriptions of their orgasms, and these descriptions were analyzed by a group of experts. The experts could not distinguish between the male and female descriptions, and the researchers concluded that males and females experience similar sensations as a result of orgasm. Although males and females do not generally differ

Researchers (Rubenstein, 1991) asked 5,000 readers of *American Health* magazine, admittedly a biased sample, what they might do to feel more sexually attractive and to respond better sexually. Just over half the women (58%) and almost half the men (49%) surveyed said they would be willing to exercise 1 hour a day to be better lovers, but relatively few of either the women (9%) or the men (12%) would take an aphrodisiac. To enhance their sexual response, 61% of the women and 55% of the men listened to music while engaged in sexual intercourse at some time during the month before the survey, and 19% of the women and 23% of the men watched an X-rated videotape during coitus. What was surprising is that 38% of the women and 34% of the men watched television during intercourse.

In a more recent online survey of almost 1,500 people (757 women and 694 men), only 21% of the women and 15% of the men reported just enjoying the moment. Others were wondering if they were pleasing their partners and what they could do next (15% of the women and 31% of the men). Interestingly, 6% of the women and 7% of the men were imagining they were with another person.

Sources: Data from Rubenstein, The American health sex survey. *American Health* (December 1991), 56–57; Queendom. Polls: General sexual behavior. What do you generally think about during sex? Available: http://www.queendom.com/polls/poll.htm, 2009.

in the sensations they report accompanying orgasm, orgasms *do* differ. That is, an individual may experience an orgasm today that is either more or less intense than one yesterday, and one person may experience orgasms generally more intensely than another person. These differences are not a function of gender; rather, a less pleasurable experience may be a result of guilt, shame, embarrassment, an uncomfortable setting, frustrations with the sexual partner, hostility, distrust, low self-esteem, or other factors.

Controversies About Orgasm

Several controversies surround the topic of orgasm.

Types of Orgasm

First, experts disagree about the types of orgasms that exist. In the early 1900s, Freud theorized there were two different types of female orgasm: the clitoral and the vaginal. He viewed the clitoral orgasm as an immature sexual response that women outgrew. Because he considered the clitoris to be a stunted penis, Freud believed the clitoral orgasm was an expression of masculine sexuality rather than feminine sexuality. If at adolescence the woman had not transferred her erotic focus from the clitoris to the vagina, Freud believed that psychotherapy was in order. When Freud's theory was operationalized, surgical removal of the clitoris (**clitoridectomy**) was actually performed on girls who were too clitorally focused, as determined by their masturbating by stimulating the clitoris.

Masters and Johnson's (1966) research identified but one type of orgasm. Regardless of the point of stimulation—clitoris or vagina—and regardless of the method of stimulation—penile insertion or vibra-

tor—Masters and Johnson reported the same physiological occurrences during orgasm. However, Masters and Johnson did report a difference in the sensations of orgasm that depended on whether they were a result of coital or noncoital activities. They found orgasms from coitus to be less intense than orgasms from noncoital means. This finding was validated by Hite (1976), who found the clitorally stimulated orgasm to be more intense than the orgasm from coitus. Hite also found the coital orgasm to be more diffused throughout the body than was the locally intense clitoral orgasm.

To complicate matters further, other researchers (Singer & Singer, 1972) have reported three distinct types of orgasms: vulval, uterine, and blended. Singer and Singer included emotional satisfaction as a consideration in their research. **Vulval orgasm** is the same as the orgasm described by Masters and Johnson and includes contractions of the orgasmic platform; however, the vulval orgasm is not sexually satiating, and therefore another orgasm can be experienced immediately. A **uterine orgasm** can occur only in the presence of vaginal penetration and involves a woman's holding her breath just before orgasm and then exhaling when the climax occurs. In contrast to the vulval orgasm, the uterine orgasm is sexually

clitoridectomy
Surgical removal of the clitoris.

vulval orgasm
An orgasm in a female that includes the contractions of the orgasmic platform, which is not sexually satisfying and, as a result, allows another orgasm to occur almost immediately.

uterine orgasm
An orgasm in a female that can occur only in the presence of penile penetration and that involves a woman's holding her breath just before orgasm and then exhaling when the climax occurs.

Communication
DIMENSIONS

Discussing Sexual Desires

Communicating sexual desires is embarrassing for many people. After all, sex is not something we are taught to talk about openly. The irony for many of us is that we are taught at a very young age that sex is so "dirty" that we should save it for someone we love. Does not make much sense, does it? Of course, sex is not dirty, although it may make sense to refrain from certain sexual activities altogether and to engage in others only when you are ready. When the time is right, if we could share what we find sexually arousing with a partner, we would be that much more satisfied. To help you along in this process, we have prepared the following guidelines. We recognize, though, that not all of you have chosen to engage in sexual activities with a partner. Still, these guidelines will be useful if and when you decide the time is right for you to do so.

- Speak about what you like sexually at times in which you are not engaged in sexual activity. This allows for a conversation that can be more rational than one carried on while emotions are running high.
- Be specific. State what you like and how you like it, what you dislike and why you dislike it.
- Ask your partner to do the same. Let your partner know that you want to please him or her as well as yourself. If your partner realizes you are concerned about his or her pleasure, he or she will be more likely to be concerned about your pleasure.
- During sex, let your partner know how you feel about what he or she is doing. Reinforce the behaviors you like by letting him or her know they are pleasing.
- Do not hesitate to refrain from any sexual activity you find unpleasant, uncomfortable, or distasteful. When doing so, explain your reasons to your partner.

Remember, you can have a more satisfying sexual relationship, when you are ready to do so, by being able to communicate freely about sex and what you find pleasurable and what you find displeasing.

---

satiating and is therefore usually followed by a refractory period. The **blended orgasm** is a combination of these two; that is, there are contractions of the outer third of the vagina as well as breath holding. These researchers make it clear that no one form of orgasm is better than another, just different.

> **blended orgasm**
> An orgasm in a female in which there are contractions of the muscles in the outer third of the vagina as well as breath holding; a combination of the vulval and uterine orgasms.

How many forms of orgasm are there? As with other areas of human sexuality, there is disagreement. The important point is that orgasm can be conceptualized as merely a physiological reaction to sexual stimulation or as a complex of interactions between partners (the setting, the mood, and a host of other variables). To consider an orgasm as solely a bodily reaction is to ignore the interactive nature of the human mind and the human body and the impossibility of separating them. Without a mind to realize that sexual stimulation is, in fact, stimulating, there is no orgasm.

Recognizing Orgasms

At the beginning of the sexuality classes we teach, we ask students to write questions they would like answered before the semester ends. A common question asks how a man can recognize when his female partner is faking an orgasm. The women in the class are astute enough to know that when their male partners ejaculate, they experience orgasm. What they do not usually know is that sometimes orgasm can occur without an ejaculate—for example, in men with disease of the prostate or in prepubescent boys. Men, however, want to know how to recognize that their partners are sexually satisfied.

This question has several implications that deserve some attention. First, it expresses a concern for the woman's sexual satisfaction. On the surface, that appears to be healthy; however, it is our experience that when asked by men, this question is more related to a man's ego than to a woman's satisfaction. That is, if the male can "give" the woman an orgasm, he must be a good lover. Another interpretation of this question could be that men are afraid their female sexual partners might fake orgasms. A woman may fake an orgasm to meet her partner's expectation, to feed her partner's ego, to end the sexual encounter, to present herself as "normal," or to meet the "goal."

Beyond the fact that faking an orgasm is dishonest and deceitful, it may lead your partner to think that something unsatisfying to you was great and should be repeated the next time. However, if what

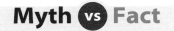

Myth vs Fact

Myth: It is easy to tell when a male has an orgasm because the ejaculate gives it away.
Fact: Although it is usually true that a male will ejaculate during orgasm, this is not always the case. Males may have an orgasm without ejaculating.

Myth: During the plateau phase of the Masters and Johnson sexual response cycle, conditions remain pretty much the same.
Fact: Although Masters and Johnson chose to call the second phase of the sexual response cycle the *plateau phase,* changes do occur. What occurred during the excitement phase is intensified during the plateau phase.

Myth: Whereas women can be multiorgasmic, men cannot.
Fact: Although it occurs relatively infrequently, some men do report needing very little time before being able to have another orgasm.

Myth: Males and females differ tremendously in their responses to sexual excitation.
Fact: There certainly are many differences between males and females in their responses to sexual excitement. Still, there are many similarities as well.

Myth: The clitoris can be stimulated easily during sexual intercourse.
Fact: Relatively early in the sexual response of women, the clitoris retracts under the clitoral hood. Therefore, it is not easily accessible to touch and/or stimulation unless the clitoral hood is purposefully pulled back.

a partner does is pleasurable but does not result in a climax, that might be enough. If so, why not tell your partner? Sexual activity can be enjoyed for itself without being directed toward the goal of orgasm.

Men are also prone to faking orgasms if they are unable to achieve one. When a man has been drinking alcoholic beverages, for example, and cannot reach the orgasmic phase, he might feel threatened by how this may be interpreted by his partner. Will his partner think he is less than a real man? Will his partner think he is sexually dysfunctional? Will his partner think he does not find him or her sexually attractive? Some men believe it is easier to fake an orgasm than to allay these fears.

Whether a man or woman fakes orgasm regularly, the person would be well advised to discuss the situation candidly with his or her partner. Such a discussion can often result in a closer relationship and the understanding that setting up sexual performance goals is self-defeating. Some women do not reach orgasm, some have an orgasm once during intercourse, and some are multiorgasmic. Some men do not reach orgasm, some have an orgasm once during intercourse, and some are multiorgasmic (although some recovery time between orgasms is necessary). For people of either gender who do not reach orgasm, pleasure from coitus can still be attained. Rather than asking,

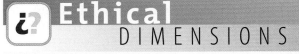

Ethical DIMENSIONS

Should Sexual Enhancements Be Used to Increase Sexual Arousal?

How far should people be allowed, or encouraged, to go in their search for sexual satisfaction and sexual arousal? Some people argue that anything that does not negatively affect another person is appropriate to enhance sexual arousal. They believe the use of X-rated movies, sexually explicit written material, and erotic clothing is within the bounds of acceptability. They also suggest that engaging in sexual relations with a number of different people can provide the experience necessary to reach one's sexual potential. Further, any physical barriers to sexual arousal should be eliminated at any cost. So if a man has blockage of the penile arteries, he should undergo bypass surgery to provide the penis with the blood it needs to become erect. And if there is damage to the penis as a result of an accident, options should include Viagra, artificial penises, surgery to implant rods in the penis to provide an erection, or penis transplantation (from someone who has recently died—similar to heart, kidney, and other organ transplantation).

Others believe that enhancing sexual arousal is appropriate, but only within certain limits. They argue that sexually explicit material is pornographic and/or obscene. Its use is unacceptable for any reason, and it should be outlawed. Furthermore, altering the body "merely" for sexual purposes goes against nature, is therefore "unnatural," and should not be tolerated. Sexual arousal should be enhanced through improving the relationship between the couple, and that can be accomplished only in a marriage, and one in which the spouses remain sexually faithful to each other. Only then, advocates of this view argue, can the couple engage in "lovemaking" as opposed to "sex-making," because sex without love can never achieve the level of arousal that sex with love can.

What do you think? What is appropriate and what is inappropriate when trying to enhance sexual arousal?

Global DIMENSIONS

Age of First Intercourse

A study by the London International Group (1998) found that men and women worldwide are starting to engage in sexual intercourse at ever earlier ages. The study queried 10,000 sexually active adults from 14 developing and developed countries. The average age at first intercourse was 17.4 years (down slightly from the previous year's 17.6 years). However, there was a great deal of variability from country to country. For example, the average age at first intercourse in the United States was 15.8 years, whereas it was 19.0 years in Hong Kong. In a subsequent study, average age at first intercourse was 16.8 years in Kenya, 19.0 years in Bolivia, 18.8 years in Brazil, 18.6 years in Guatemala, and 22.8 years in the Philippines (Population Reference Bureau, 2000). Differences also occurred in the frequency of intercourse. Whereas the average adult reported engaging in coitus 112 times a year, French and Americans reported more frequent intercourse (151 and 148 times per year, respectively) than did men and women from Hong Kong and Thailand (77 and 69 times per year, respectively). In addition, 40% of Americans wanted coitus more often, whereas only 7% of Mexicans expressed that desire.

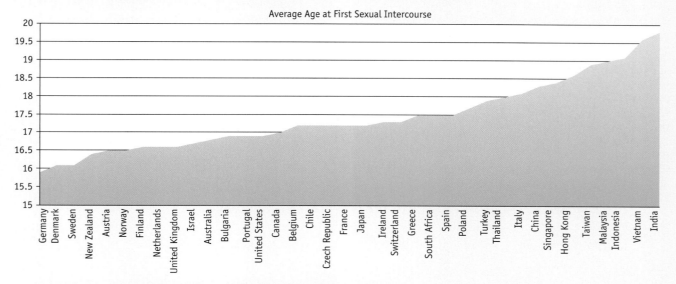

Average Age at First Sexual Intercourse

Source: Adapted from Durex Global Sex Survey. Cambridge, UK: SSL International, 2005.

? Did You Know . . .

An ancient Indian philosophy rebelled against the tenets of organized religion that restricted sexual practices. *Tantra* taught that sexuality was a doorway to the divine and that earthly pleasures were sacred acts. Becoming more popular in Western culture, *tantric sex* seeks to teach means of pleasuring one's lover and connecting with him or her fully, rather than simply to achieve an orgasm. It is seen as a dance with no beginning or end, and the goal is to be in the present moment. One of the outcomes of tantric sex, however, is to extend orgasm and to enjoy multiple orgasms. Among the tantric sex techniques are these (Painter, 2009):

- Welcoming love (making time for each other), creating an inviting atmosphere (for example, candles and flowers), and dressing provocatively

- Using ritual for intimacy (for example, bathing together)
- Experimenting with erotic touch
- Maintaining a deep level of intimacy (for example, gazing into each other's eyes)
- Keeping it slow
- Varying positions
- Pumping the pubococcygeal (PC) muscles
- Stimulating the clitoris and labia during sex
- Stimulating the G spot, called the sacred spot in tantra

"Did you come?" we should ask, "What did I do that you liked?" "How can I pleasure you more?" "How can we feel more intimate?" "How can we improve our relationship?"

Did You Know...

Did you know that women who experience vaginal orgasms can be identified by how they walk? When women were videotaped walking on the street, trained sexologists were 85% accurate in judging whether they were vaginally orgasmic or anorgasmic (Nicholas et al., 2008). They were not, however, able to identify women who were clitorally orgasmic. The observational keys were greater pelvic and vertebral rotation and stride length. In addition, vaginally orgasmic women's gaits were fluid, energetic, sensual, free, and absent of locked muscles.

Simultaneous Orgasm

Another question students often ask is how they and their partners can achieve an orgasm together. Unfortunately, some couples have as an ideal a choreographed orgasmic release, timed so that it occurs at the same time for both partners. Not only is this difficult to achieve, but concentrating on this goal detracts from the enjoyment of the coital experience. As long as each person is satisfied, the exact timing of the orgasm is of no particular importance. Although simultaneous orgasm is an undeniably exciting event, it is only one of a wide range of satisfying sexual patterns.

Exploring the Dimensions of Human Sexuality

Our feelings, attitudes, and beliefs regarding sexuality are influenced by our internal and external environments. Go to go.jblearning.com/dimensions5e to learn more about the biological factors that affect your sexuality.

Case Study

Although the human sexual response cycle is a physiological pattern, many factors influence the ways individuals actually experience the stages. Physical differences, including age, illness, injuries, and disabilities, may alter the response. Illicit drugs, alcohol, and aphrodisiacs also may alter the physical sensation we experience. Some drugs, such as Viagra, may enhance the response cycle.

The stimuli that we react to differ with culture and ethnic group, media exposure, even hygiene. Education and religious beliefs may also have an effect; a person who feels guilty about sexuality may have a more repressed reaction.

Finally, our self-image and our feelings about our partner greatly influence sexual response and arousal. Many people believe that happy times—experiencing a loving relationship, being successful professionally, and so on—make for better sex.

Biological Factors

- Sexual arousal and response are physiological reactions to sexual stimuli.
- Masters and Johnson showed that some aspects of the human sexual response cycle are similar in men and women; however, differences exist.
- The body releases hormones when a person is sexually stimulated.
- Physical disabilities, injuries, or illness may alter the ability to respond to sexual stimuli.
- Male testosterone levels decline with age, affecting sexual response.
- Drugs, alcohol, and some aphrodisiacs may alter sexual response.

Sociocultural Factors

- Biological factors are influenced by sociocultural and psychological factors. For example, some people are turned on by pornography; others are turned off.
- Religious beliefs influence our feelings about sexuality in general.
- Culture and ethnic heritage influence what we find sensual or attractive.
- Media and ads influence the types of sexual stimulation to which we react.
- Family, neighbors, and friends provide information about and influence our sexuality.
- Ethical decisions must be made regarding how far you and your partner are willing to go to achieve sexual arousal.

Psychological Factors

- Our feelings toward our partner influence the sexual response derived.
- Our level of experience influences our response to sexual stimuli.
- Learned attitudes and behaviors include discovering the stimuli to which we respond.
- Body image influences our self-concept. The better we feel about ourselves, the sexier an image we portray to others.

Summary

- When a sexual stimulus is encountered, a message is sent via nerves to the brain. Upon reaching the brain, the message passes through the reticular activating system either from or to the limbic system and the thalamus.

- During sexual arousal, the autonomic nervous system is responsible for sending signals through nerves that result in blood vessels in the penis and clitoris dilating. The effect of the dilation is that these structures become engorged with blood and, consequently, become erect.

- Sexual hormones are produced in the testes and ovaries and affect many different sexually related functions. For example, testosterone affects sexual interest, also known as libido.

- Masters and Johnson described the human sexual response cycle as consisting of four phases: excitement, plateau, orgasm, and resolution. Kaplan described the human sexual response cycle as being triphasic: desire, excitement, and resolution.

- The female sexual response cycle is more varied than the male sexual response cycle. Females sometimes experience a sexual response cycle similar to males except they are more capable of having multiple orgasms without having to pass through a refractory period. In addition, females can move from the excitement phase to the plateau phase and, without having an orgasm, return to resolution; they can also experience rapid escalation from excitement to orgasm without passing through a plateau phase.

- Orgasm is the release of sexual tension resulting in muscular contractions and, at least in males, ejaculation. In most males, orgasm is followed by a refractory (recovery) period in which orgasm is not possible. In many females, orgasm can occur without a refractory period.

- Orgasm in females is preceded by the uterus increasing in size and elevating, the inner two-thirds of the vagina lengthening and expanding, lubrication of the vaginal walls, engorgement of blood in the outer third of the vagina, and retraction of the clitoris under the clitoral hood.

- In males, orgasm is a two-stage process: emission and expulsion. Emission involves contractions of the vas deferens, seminal vesicles, prostate, and external and internal urethral sphincters. Expulsion consists of relaxation of the external urethral sphincter, contractions of the urethra and muscles at the base of the penis and the anus, and the expulsion of the ejaculate from the penis.

Discussion Questions

1. Describe the reaction of the mind and the body when one is aroused by a sensual stimulation. How might artificial hormones or aphrodisiacs alter the response cycle? How would alcohol or other mood-altering drugs affect the cycle?

2. Compare and contrast the Masters and Johnson human response cycle with the models proposed by Kaplan, Zilbergeld and Ellison, and Reed. Why does the Masters and Johnson model continue to attract the most attention?

3. Explain how understanding types of orgasms and recognizing orgasms could lead to a better sexual relationship.

Application Questions

Reread the story that opens the chapter and answer the following questions.

1. Assuming that Brian and Tanya start dating, which visible signs of sexual arousal (aside from erection) might Tanya detect in Brian? Which signs might Brian detect in Tanya?

2. Do you think Brian's feelings about Tanya might differ if he met her after gym class and she reeked of sweat? Explain.

Critical Thinking Questions

1. Laurie Cabot, a well-known practicing witch, often suggests that love potions or spells do work. She writes that a "spell is a thought, a projection, or a prayer." Thus Cabot implies that the psychological effort that you put into a spell can produce a physiological response. Given this idea, would a love potion work? Put another way, would the extra attention you lavish on someone make that person more attracted to you?

2. The drugs Viagra and Cialis positively affect sexual response, especially in older men. However, increased sexual response is accompanied by higher blood pressure and a faster heartbeat—which has resulted in heart attacks and some deaths. Explain why 30 million U.S. males have been willing to take this risk, albeit a small one. Also consider why their partners would want them to risk their health for sexual pleasure.

3. Sexy soap operas are some of the most-viewed TV shows in the world, with more than 1 billion viewers per week. Apply what you learned in the chapter to explain why.

Critical Thinking Case

It has been argued that too much emphasis is placed on orgasm and not enough on the total sexual experience, including talking and nongenital touch. Because sexual intercourse is a way of expressing love for another, the argument proceeds, the emphasis during the experience should be on the total relationship, the love expressed, whole-body sensations, and the feeling of closeness. Concentrating exclusively or primarily on the orgasm is self-defeating and narrows one's experience of sexuality.

In contrast, some people believe that sexual intercourse (or mutual masturbation or oral–genital sex) certainly includes all of the above but, in addition, has a culmination—orgasm. This culmination is so satisfying and, given effective sexual therapy, so available that it should be sought. Although sexual intercourse and other modes of sexual expression can be satisfying without orgasm, an orgasmic conclusion certainly adds to the experience and satisfaction.

What do you think? Why?

Exploring Personal Dimensions

Sexual Stimuli
Once the senses encounter sexual stimuli, the brain takes over, deciding how to respond. You become sexually aroused, although you may decide, for many reasons, not to act on that sexual arousal. Which of the following sexual stimuli do you find arousing? If you have a partner, which does your partner find arousing? More importantly, with which stimuli do you share sexual arousal?

What other sexual stimuli can you think of?

	YOU		YOUR PARTNER	
SIGHT				
Sexually explicit movies	Y	N	Y	N
Sexually explicit magazines	Y	N	Y	N
Romantic movies	Y	N	Y	N
Books	Y	N	Y	N
Lingerie	Y	N	Y	N
Skin	Y	N	Y	N
TOUCH				
Satin sheets	Y	N	Y	N
Leather	Y	N	Y	N
Massage	Y	N	Y	N
Scratching	Y	N	Y	N
SMELL				
Perfume (or cologne)	Y	N	Y	N
Flowers	Y	N	Y	N
Scented candles	Y	N	Y	N
TASTE				
Kissing	Y	N	Y	N
Oral sexual activities	Y	N	Y	N
Whipped cream	Y	N	Y	N
SOUND				
Whispering	Y	N	Y	N
Moaning (or groaning)	Y	N	Y	N
Music	Y	N	Y	N
Silence	Y	N	Y	N

Suggested Readings

Bakos, S. C. *The orgasm bible: The latest research and techniques for reaching more powerful climaxes more often.* Beverly, MA: Quiver, 2008.

Barbach, L. *For yourself: The fulfillment of female sexuality.* New York: New American Library, 2000.

Barbach, L. *For each other: Sharing sexual intimacy.* New York: New American Library, 2001.

Bodansky, V. *To bed or not to bed: What men want, what women want, how great sex happens.* Alameda, CA: Hunter House, 2005.

Carrellas, B., & Sprinkle, A. *Urban tantra: Sacred sex for the twenty-first century.* Berkeley, CA: Celestial Arts, 2007.

Chance, R. S. To love and to be loved: Sexuality and people with disabilities. *Journal of Psychology and Theology, 30* (2002), 195–209.

Chia, M., Chia, M., Abrams, D., & Abrams, R. C. *The multi-orgasmic couple: Sexual secrets every couple should know.* New York: HarperCollins, 2002.

Corwin, G. *Sexual intimacy for women: A guide for same-sex couples.* Berkeley, CA: Seal Press, 2010.

Hathaway, C. *Erotic massage: Sensual touch for deep pleasure and extended arousal.* Chanhassen, MN: Quiver, 2007.

Herbenick, D. *Because it feels good: A woman's guide to sexual pleasure and satisfaction.* Emmaus, PA: Rodale Books, 2009.

Keesling, B. *Sexual pleasure: Reaching new heights of sexual arousal and intimacy,* 2nd ed. Alameda, CA: Hunter House, 2004.

Lacroix, N. *Tantric sex and lovemaking.* London, UK: Lorenz Books, 2008.

McCarthy, B. W., & McCarthy, E. *Discovering your couple sexual style: Sharing desire, pleasure, and satisfaction.* New York: Routledge, 2009.

Stanway, A., & Geary, J. *The art of sensual loving.* Emeryville, CA: Avalon Publishing Group, 2003.

Taylor, S. *101 sex positions: Steamy new positions from mild to wild.* Berkeley, CA: Amorata Press, 2008.

Winston, S. *Women's anatomy of arousal: Secret maps to buried pleasure.* Kingston, NY: Mango Garden Press, 2010.

Web Resources

For links to the websites below, visit *go.jblearning .com/dimensions5e* and click on Resource Links.

SexTutor.com
www.sextutor.com

Sex Tutor offers accurate, clearly written, helpful sex advice on such topics as anal sex, cunnilingus, fellatio, female ejaculation, female masturbation, male masturbation, kissing, sex positions, prolonging sex, adult toys, and others.

iVillage.co.uk: The Website for Women
http://iVillage.co.uk/relationships/sex

Provides articles discussing various sex-related topics for women. Among these topics are sexual dilemmas, hot sex, talk about sex, sex and health, oral sex, orgasms, bedroom basics, and others.

Better Sex Network
www.bettersexnetwork.com

Includes articles with advice to enhance sexual pleasure, as well as data related to sexuality. Recent articles include "Sex Surveys: What's Normal"; "Letting Your Pleasures Be Known"; "Sex on the

Beach: "The Joys of Vacation Sex"; and "Titillate with Touch."

Sexual Arousal Guide
www.sexualarousalguide.com

Includes advice on topics such as sexual arousal, sexual arousal exercises, sexual arousal tips for men and women, sexual arousal roadblocks, frequently asked questions about sexual arousal and sexual dysfunction, the male sexual arousal cycle, the female sexual arousal cycle, sexual arousal and performance tips, and how to improve sexual health.

The Science of Sexual Arousal
www.apa.org/monitor/apr03/arousal.aspx

A site of the American Psychological Association that describes what research has found regarding the cognitive, physiological, and subjective aspects of sexual arousal.

References

Basson, R. The female sexual response: A different model. *Journal of Marital Therapy*, 26 (2000), 51–65.

Greenberg, J. S. *Comprehensive stress management*, 12th ed. New York: McGraw-Hill Higher Education, 2011.

Haffner, D. W., & Stayton, W. R. Sexuality and reproductive health, in *Contraceptive technology*, 7th revised ed., Hatcher, R. A., et al. New York: Ardent Media, 1998.

Hite, S. *The Hite report.* New York: Macmillan, 1976.

Kaplan, H. S. *The new sex therapy: Active treatment of sexual dysfunction.* New York: Brunner/Mazel, 1974.

Kaplan, H. S. *Disorders of sexual desire.* New York: Simon & Schuster, 1979.

Masters, W. H., & Johnson, V. E. *Human sexual response.* Boston: Little, Brown, 1966.

Nicholas, A., Brody, S., de Sutter, P., & de Carufel, F. A woman's history of vaginal orgasm is discernible from her walk. *Journal of Sexual Medicine*, 5 (2008), 2119–2124.

Painter, A. *Tantric sex techniques to reinvigorate lovemaking.* Discovery Health. Sexual Health Center: Tantric Sex, 2009. Available: http://health.discovery.com/centers/sex/tantric/ tantricsex.html.

Population Reference Bureau. *The world's youth 2000.* Washington, DC: Author, 2000.

Proctor, F., Wagner, N., & Butler, J. The differentiation of male and female orgasm: An experimental study, in *Perspectives on human sexuality*, Wagner, N., ed. New York: Behavioral Publications, 1974.

Senbel, A. M., & Mostafa, T. Yohimbine enhances the effect of sildenafil on erectile process in rats. *International Journal of Impotence Research*, 20 (2008), 409–417.

Silverberg, C. Are male and female orgasms different? *About. com: Sexuality*, 2008. Available: http://sexuality.about.com/ od/sexualhealthqanda/f/sex_question41.htm.

Singer, J., & Singer, I. Types of female orgasms. *Journal of Sex Research 8* (1972), 255–267.

Thayton, W. R. A theology of sexual pleasure. *SIECUS Report, 30* (2002), 393–400.

Walen, S. R., & Roth, D. A cognitive approach to sex therapy, in *Theories of human sexuality*, Geer, J. H., & O'Donohue, W. T., eds. New York: Plenum, 1987.

Wiest, W. Semantic differential profiles of orgasm and other experiences among men and women. *Sex Roles, 3* (1977), 399–403.

Zilbergard, B., & Ellison, C. R. Desire discrepancies and arousal problems in sex therapy, in *Principles and practices of sex therapy*, Lieblum, S. R., & Pervin, L. A., eds. New York: Guilford, 1980.

CHAPTER

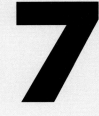

7

Contraception

FEATURES

Ethical Dimensions
Abstinence-Only Versus Comprehensive Sexuality Education

Communication Dimensions
Condom Use and Consistency: Talking About Condom Use

Multicultural Dimensions
Ethnic and Age Differences in Access to Emergency Contraception

Gender Dimensions
Gender Equality in Contraception Use

Gender Dimensions
Margaret H. Sanger: A Woman of Influence

Global Dimensions
Emergency Contraception: How Is NorLevo in France Different from Plan B in the United States?

Global Dimensions
Unmet Need for Contraception in Developing Countries

CHAPTER OBJECTIVES

1 Discuss the reasons to use contraceptives, ways to choose a contraceptive, and the difference between perfect use and typical use.

2 Evaluate the nonprescription methods of contraception, including the effectiveness, the reversibility, and the advantages and disadvantages of each. Explain why some have higher rates of user effectiveness than others.

3 Evaluate the prescription methods of contraception, including the effectiveness, the reversibility, and the advantages and disadvantages of each. Explain why some have higher rates of user effectiveness than others.

4 Discuss the viability of future contraceptive methods. Consider the impact of gender issues, pharmaceutical industry costs for litigation, federal regulation compliance, and FDA approval.

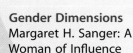

go.jblearning.com/dimensions5e

Ethical Dimensions: Abstinence-Only Versus Comprehensive Sexuality Education
Emergency Contraception
The Future of Contraceptives

INTRODUCTION

*T*hroughout life, people's use of and need for contraceptives change. The case history of Susan presents a typical contraceptive user. During her first sexual encounter at age 18 years, Susan's high school boyfriend used withdrawal.

During her freshman year at college, she began a steady sexual relationship with Jack. Because she was in a monogamous relationship and believed she did not have to worry about sexually transmitted infection (STI) transmission, Susan began to use oral contraceptives (the pill). After she had difficulty remembering to take her pill every day, Susan switched to injectable medroxyprogesterone acetate (Depo-Provera). Every 3 months she would receive her birth control shot at a clinic.

After she and Jack broke up, she was abstinent for a year—the most foolproof method of contraception available. Susan graduated from college and was fitted with a diaphragm; she also used condoms with her two partners.

By age 25 years she married Stephen and had etonogestrel (Implanon) inserted into her upper arm. Implanon releases a steady stream of contraceptive into the reproductive system and is effective for up to 3 years. When she was starting to think about having a child, at her doctor's suggestion, she switched to a non-hormone-based contraceptive (foam and condoms) for 3 months before trying to conceive a child.

After the birth of her first child, she was fitted with an intrauterine device (IUD). Two years later it was removed when she planned to conceive a second child. After the birth of their second child, Stephen had a vasectomy. After several follow-up tests to assure that no sperm were left in his ejaculate, Susan and Stephen enjoyed monogamous, unprotected sex.

Five years later, Susan and Stephen divorced. As one of her first acts as a newly divorced woman, Susan had a laparoscopy—a method of female sterilization. Although she could not become pregnant, she also began to practice safer sex and insisted that her partners wear latex condoms.

In other words, it is possible for a woman to use nearly every contraceptive method available during her more than 30 years of fertility. The method may change, depending on where she is in the life cycle.

This chapter reviews the currently available methods of contraception, their effectiveness, and their advantages and disadvantages.

■ Contraception

Contraception is the prevention of conception. You may already have thought hard about the consequences of such decisions as whether to become pregnant, have an abortion, or adopt a child. If you have considered or do consider such matters, you will understand how significant contraception can be to your life. Many babies are born each year to mothers who are too young or too emotionally immature to raise them well, or to mothers who are too old to carry a fetus to term without a high probability of a birth defect. Many pregnant teenagers and their sexual partners never finish their schooling because of the need to support and care for their child. Some couples who marry in response to pregnancy are soon divorced. Married couples who have already raised children may find yet another pregnancy a threat to their economic and psychological health. Managing this financial burden, as well as dealing with the time and energy necessary to care for an infant, can be as harmful to them— though perhaps in different ways—as to teenagers. But clearly the economic burden a child entails can present problems for people in various age groups and income levels.

Contraceptive and condom use should be routine for sexually active young people and adults unless they are seeking pregnancy *and* they are in a mutually monogamous relationship. Yet, too many people use contraception inconsistently or ineffectively. The result is that the United States has a higher rate of unintended pregnancies than all other developed countries. Currently, it is estimated that every year 1 in 20 American women has an unintended pregnancy

contraception
Means of preventing pregnancy.

(Finer & Henshaw, 2006). Researchers know that many factors increase one's motivation to use contraception. These factors include the following:

- Ability to communicate with a partner
- Cost and accessibility of a method
- Frequency of sexual intercourse
- Motivation to avoid pregnancy
- STI concerns and risks
- Contraceptive's side effects
- One's attitudes and openness about sexuality (Frost, Darroch, & Remez, 2008; Hatcher et al., 2007)

Ask yourself these questions as you read this chapter: Am I ready to have sexual intercourse? Am I committed to avoiding pregnancy myself or preventing a partner's pregnancy at this time? Am I committed to avoiding passing on a sexually transmitted infection? Am I committed to using a contraceptive method every time I have intercourse? Is my partner? If the answer to any of these questions is no, ask yourself another question: What will I do when a pregnancy occurs? Remember, almost 9 in 10 heterosexual couples who do not use a contraceptive method become pregnant within a year.

Contraceptive Effectiveness

We begin our discussion of contraception methods with a warning: The effectiveness of each method is difficult to determine precisely, so you should consider the rates cited for each method as being *approximations only*. Also note that for each method we provide both the percentage of women experiencing an unintended pregnancy during the first year of contraceptive method use when the method is used perfectly (consistently and correctly) and the percentage when it is used typically (Trussell, 2011).

In the latter setting, mistakes are often made—for example, a condom may be put on incorrectly. Consequently, **typical use** is always less effective than **perfect use**. A good contraceptive method is one that limits the gap between the way it is prescribed to be used and the way it is actually used. As can be seen in Table 7.1, there is usually a vast difference between these two measures of contraceptive effectiveness.

Use is measured by the number of women in 100 who will become pregnant during the first year of use of the particular method. Table 7.1 shows the effectiveness of varied methods of contraception.

> **typical use**
> The ability of a method of contraception to prevent pregnancy as actually used at home by people not being monitored.
>
> **perfect use**
> The ability of a method of contraception to prevent pregnancy as measured by consistent and correct use.

Contraception Versus Safer Sex

Couples today need to discuss how they will prevent both pregnancy and transmission of STIs. Many of the most effective methods of preventing pregnancies—oral contraceptives, hormonal implants, sterilization—provide *no* protection against STIs. The IUD, which is highly effective at preventing pregnancies, is not recommended for women who have either gonorrhea or chlamydia (WHO, 2008). The male condom provides the best protection available against STIs but has a lower rate of effectiveness against pregnancy. There are two ways to achieve maximal effectiveness against both STIs and pregnancies relative to sexual intercourse: abstain from all types of intercourse or use a condom and a hormonal contraceptive together. Because STIs pose a threat to the future fertility and health of college students, and because emergency contraception (EC) and abortion are available, many experts recommend that if only one method is used, it should be a condom.

■ Nonprescription Methods

Abstinence

People define **abstinence** in different ways: For some it means no sexual contact of any kind; for others it means no **penetrative behaviors**, including penile–vaginal sex, oral sex, or anal sex. Many adolescents, young adults, and adults choose to abstain. People choose abstinence for a variety of reasons:

> **abstinence**
> Avoidance of any type of sexual intercourse.
>
> **penetrative behaviors**
> Any behavior whereby penetration occurs—for example, penile–vaginal sex, oral sex, or anal sex.

- Their religion teaches that penetrative behaviors are appropriate only in marriage.

- They are not in a loving, committed relationship.

- They do not have a partner.

- They want to avoid the risk of pregnancy or STI.

- The relationship they are in is not ready for the intimacy of penetrative behaviors.

- They are not ready to experience penile–vaginal, oral, or anal sex.

- They are ill or their partner is ill.

- They or a partner have been exposed to an STI.

- They feel that a sexual relationship would complicate their life.

Choosing abstinence does not necessarily mean forgoing sexual pleasure. There are many ways to give and receive sexual pleasure without the risks of sexual intercourse. These include deep kissing, massages, fondling, dancing, masturbating alone, masturbating together, and showering together.

However, for these activities not to end in oral, penile–vaginal, or anal sex, couples must communicate their desire not to engage in such behaviors and must agree to stick to sexual limits.

Effectiveness

Abstinence is the only 100% effective method of fertility control and STI prevention—if the couple or individual is truly committed to refraining from oral, penile–vaginal, and anal sex. Actual user effectiveness rates are unknown. A popular saying is that vows of abstinence fail much more frequently than condoms do; people say that they are practicing abstinence but have penile–vaginal sex in spite of their intention. Communication and commitment are essential. Because abstinence has never had the scientific scrutiny given other methods to determine user or typical use effectiveness, there are no data to make a fair comparison between abstinence effectiveness and other methods. Proponents of abstinence may cite typical use of various contraceptive methods to demonstrate their risk of failure and yet claim the perfect use effectiveness rate of abstinence as 100%.

TABLE 7.1 **Contraceptive Effectiveness: Rates of Unintended Pregnancies per 100 Women**

Method	Consistent and Correct (Perfect) Use	As Commonly Used (Typical Use) (U.S.; Trussell, 2011; Zieman et al., 2010)	As Commonly Used (Typical Use) (Developing Countries; Cleland & Ali, 2004)
Implants (Implanon)	0.05	0.05	—
Male sterilization (vasectomy)	0.1	0.15	—
Levonorgestrel IUD (Mirena IUS)	0.2	0.2	—
Female sterilization	0.5	0.5	—
Copper-bearing IUD (ParaGard copper T)	0.6	0.8	2
Injectables			
Progestin only	0.3	6	2
Combined pill and progestin-only pill	0.3	9	7
Combined patch (Evra Patch)	0.3	9	—
Combined vaginal ring (NuvaRing)	0.3	9	—
Condom[1]			
Male	2	18	
Female (Reality)	5		—
Fertility awareness-based methods			
Ovulation method[2]	3	—	—
Two-day method[2]	4	—	—
Standard days method[2]	5	—	—
Diaphragm with spermicide	6	12	
Sponge			
Nulliparous women[3]	9	12	—
Parous women[4]	20	24	—
Withdrawal	4	22	
Spermicides[5]	18	28	
Cervical caps			
Nulliparous women[3]	9	16	—
Parous women[4]	26	32	—
No method[6]	85	85	85

Key

0–0.9	1–9	10–25	26–32
Very effective	Effective	Moderately effective	Less effective

LAM (lactational amenorrhea method) is a highly effective, *temporary* method of contraception. However, to maintain effective protection against pregnancy, another method of contraception must be used as soon as menstruation resumes, the frequency or duration of breastfeeding is reduced, bottle feeding is introduced, or the baby reaches 6 months of age. Prospective studies have shown pregnancy rates of 0.5% to 1.5% for 6-month perfect use with LAM (Kennedy & Trussell, 2008).

1. Without spermicides.
2. The ovulation and 2-day methods are based on evaluation of cervical mucus. The standard days method avoids intercourse on cycle days 8 through 19.
3. Pregnancy rate for women who have never given birth.
4. Pregnancy rate for women who have given birth.
5. Foams, creams, gels, vaginal suppositories, and vaginal film.
6. These percentages are based on data from populations where contraception is not used and from women who cease using contraception in an effort to become pregnant. Among such populations, approximately 89% become pregnant within 1 year. This estimate was lowered slightly (to 85%) to represent the percentage who would become pregnant within 1 year among women now relying on reversible methods of contraception if they abandoned contraception altogether.

Sources: Data from Trussell, J. Contraceptive failure in the United States. *Contraception, 83* (2011), 397–404; Cleland, J. & Ali, M. M. Reproductive consequences of contraceptive failure in 19 developing countries. *Obstetrics and Gynecology, 104, 2* (2004), 314–320; Zieman, M., Hatcher, R. A., Cwiak, C., Darney, P. D., Creinin, M. D., & Stosur, H. R. *A pocket guide to managing contraception, 2010–2012 edition.* Tiger, GA: Bridging the Gap Foundation, 2010. Available: http://www.managingcontraception.com/downloader.php?file=MC-2010.pdf.

Such a comparison is inappropriate from a public health perspective unless perfect use effectiveness rates are used for the other methods (for example, male condom, 98%; withdrawal, 96%) (Dailard, 2003).

Reversibility
Abstinence does not affect fertility.

Advantages and Disadvantages
Abstinence is an excellent method of fertility control and STI prevention. It is free, you always have it with you, and there are no side effects. It is 100%

effective but only if you use it every time and only if your partner is equally committed to its use. Just as with any method, one should occasionally reconsider whether it is still the method of choice. Research demonstrates how difficult it is to practice abstinence consistently over time. One study showed that 60% of college students who pledged virginity had broken their vow to remain abstinent until marriage. Such a high risk of failure would be concern enough, but another study showed that teens who promised to abstain from sex until marriage were more likely to have unprotected sex when they broke their pledge

¿? Ethical DIMENSIONS

Abstinence-Only Versus Comprehensive Sexuality Education

For more than three decades, "abstinence-only-until-marriage" was the government-sanctioned approach to reducing U.S. rates of teen pregnancy and STIs. More than $1.5 billion in federal and mandated state matching grants supported sexuality education (some say "values education" is a more appropriate label) that restricts or ignores the effectiveness of contraceptives and safer-sex behaviors (SIECUS, 2011).

A study published in the January 2009 issue of *Pediatrics* (Rosenbaum, 2009) found that teens signing virginity pledges are just as likely to engage in sexual behavior as those who do not sign such pledges. Moreover, they are less likely to use contraception, are less likely to get tested for STIs, and may have STIs for longer periods of time when they do break their pledges. Two other major studies, Mathematica findings (Trenholm et al., 2007) and *Emerging Answers 2007* (Kirby, 2007), demonstrated that the evaluated abstinence education programs have no statistically significant beneficial impact on the sexual behavior of young people.

Only one abstinence-only program—targeted at middle school students—has been shown to delay sexual initiation. However, this program does not meet the federal (A-H) abstinence-only criteria in that it focuses on delaying sexual activity "until a later time in life when the adolescent is more prepared to handle the consequences" and not specifically marriage. In addition, facilitators of this program were instructed to correct misinformation about condoms and were not allowed to criticize the benefits of condoms, which differs from most other abstinence-only programs (SIECUS, 2010b).

Given these findings, it is not surprising that many leading health professional groups have raised serious ethical concerns about U.S. support for abstinence-only sexuality

education programs. Policy apprehension is based on questionable science, medical inaccuracies, withholding health- and life-saving information, and being antithetical to informed consent and free choice (SIECUS, 2008). Concern at the state level is evidenced by the trend to no longer accept and match funding that supports abstinence-only education programs (SIECUS, 2010c). In addition, as part of the Patient Protection and Affordable Care Act of 2010, the Personal Responsibility Education Program (PREP) was created. The PREP is the first of its kind—a dedicated streaming fund for comprehensive, medically accurate sexual health education. The program provides $75 million a year for the 2010–2014 period. Unlike the abstinence-only funding, this program requires no matching funds from the states. In addition to the PREP funding, in March 2011 a bill was introduced in the both the U.S. Senate (S 578) and House of Representatives (HR 1085) to repeal the abstinence-only funding stream from the Social Security Act (SIECUS, 2011). Unfortunately, neither bill advanced beyond its introduction during the session.

This change in direction matches what Americans say they want for their children. A 2005–2006 nationally representative survey of U.S. adults, published in the *Archives of Pediatrics and Adolescent Medicine* (Bleakley, Hennessy, & Fishbein, 2006), demonstrated strong support for comprehensive sexuality education (favored by 82% of those polled); 68% favored instruction on how to use a condom; only 36% supported abstinence-only education.

The goal underlying this fundamental change is to make sure that young people have the information and skills they will need to make healthy choices about sexual behavior. If adolescents are sexually active, or will be shortly, they need information to protect themselves. Where there is a need to know, medically incomplete is medically inaccurate (Boonstra, 2009).

Continued

Ethical DIMENSIONS

Abstinence-Only Versus Comprehensive Sexuality Education—cont'd

Abstinence Versus Sex Education

Abstinence-Only Education, as Defined by 1996 Federal Law

According to Title V of the Social Security Act, an eligible abstinence education program is a program that

(A) has as its exclusive purpose, teaching the social, physiological, and health gains to be realized by abstaining from sexual activity;

(B) teaches abstinence from sexual activity outside marriage as the expected standard for all school-age children;

(C) teaches that abstinence from sexual activity is the only certain way to avoid out-of-wedlock pregnancy, sexually transmitted diseases, and other associated health problems;

(D) teaches that a mutually faithful monogamous relationship in the context of marriage is the expected standard of human sexual activity;

(E) teaches that sexual activity outside of the context of marriage is likely to have harmful psychological and physical effects;

(F) teaches that bearing children out of wedlock is likely to have harmful consequences for the child, the child's parents, and society;

(G) teaches young people how to reject sexual advances and how alcohol and drug use increases vulnerability to sexual advances; and

(H) teaches the importance of attaining self-sufficiency before engaging in sexual activity.

Sexual Education, as Defined by the Personal Responsibility Program

According to the Personal Responsibility Program, a sex education program is a program that

(1) covers both abstinence and contraception to prevent pregnancy and STIs;

(2) addresses at least three of the following adulthood preparation topics: healthy relationships, adolescent development, financial literacy, educational and career success, and healthy life skills;

(3) replicates evidence-based effective programs or substantially includes elements of effective programs;

(4) includes medically accurate information and is complete;

(5) provides age-appropriate information and activities;

(6) includes activities to educate sexually active youth on both abstinence and contraception;

(7) is implemented in a cultural context that is appropriate for the participants.

Sources: Data from Boonstra, H. D. Advocates call for a new approach after the era of "abstinance-only" sex education. *Guttmacher Policy Review, 12, no 1.* (Winter 2009). Available: http://www.guttmacher.org/pubs/gpr/12/1/gpr120106.pdf; SIECUS. End funding for the failed Title V Abstinence-Only-Until-Marriage program. Support comprehensive sex education. 2011. Available: http://www.siecus.org.index.cfm?fuseaction=Page.ViewPage&PageID=1271.

---

than those who never made such a promise. Perhaps strategies to promote abstinence are actually increasing the risks for people when they eventually become sexually active (Dailard, 2003). For that reason, it is particularly important for anyone using abstinence as a contraceptive method to choose a different method *before* they stop using abstinence.

withdrawal
Removing the penis from the vagina before ejaculation.

coitus interruptus
The Latin term for *withdrawal*, which means "interrupted intercourse."

Withdrawal

Withdrawal is probably the oldest contraceptive method on record. In the Bible, Onan practices withdrawal, or **coitus interruptus**, so as not to impregnate his brother's widow. To practice withdrawal, the couple has penile–vaginal sex until the man feels that he is about to ejaculate. He withdraws his penis and ejaculates away from the woman's vulva.

Effectiveness
Many people assume that withdrawal is an ineffective method of contraception. However, many contraceptive experts believe that withdrawal is an underrated method. It is about as effective as most barrier methods. When practiced correctly, the rate of efficacy for withdrawal is 4 pregnancies per 100 per year.

When practiced incorrectly, the rate of efficacy lowers to 22 pregnancies per 100 per year (Trussell, 2011).

Many people have been taught that preejaculate fluid might contain sperm. However, preejaculate fluid is a neutralizing solution produced by the Cowper's glands. The results of studies examining sperm levels in the preejaculate vary. Some have shown no sperm (Zuckerman, Weiss, & Orvieto, 2003; Zukerman & Orvieto, 2007) whereas others have detected enough motile sperm to potentially impregnate a partner (Killick et al., 2011).

To quote the authors of *Contraceptive Technology* (Hatcher et al., 2007), "Withdrawal is definitely better than using no contraceptive at all." However, it is no guarantee, and if the man does not withdraw in time and the woman is at a fertile point in her cycle, emergency contraception should be considered (covered later in this chapter).

Advantages and Disadvantages

Withdrawal is free, always available, and relatively easy to use. It has no medical side effects, and it encourages male involvement.

The major disadvantage to withdrawal is that some men, particularly young men, do not recognize impending ejaculation and thus ejaculate inside their partner, putting her at risk of pregnancy. Thus it has a relatively high failure rate among typical users and does not adequately protect against STIs. However, it may reduce the risk of fluid-borne infection. Some couples report that withdrawal reduces the sexual pleasure of the woman and intensity of orgasm of the man. It requires the man to think about what is happening during intercourse.

Male Condom

Condoms are one of the oldest contraceptive methods (Hatcher et al., 2007). Today most condoms are made of **latex**, a synthetic form of rubber. About 5% of condoms are made from the intestines of lambs; these are known as *skin* or *lambskin condoms*. Skin condoms, because they are more porous than latex condoms,

condom
A sheath that covers the penis.

latex
A synthetic rubber.

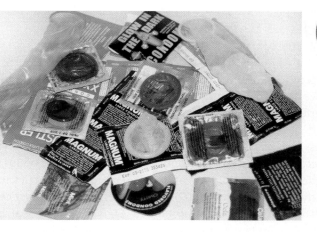

A wide variety of condoms are available in various colors, sizes, and even flavors. Latex, polyurethane, and polyisopropene have been shown to prevent transmission of STIs, including HIV. Animal skin or natural skin condoms only reduce the risk of pregnancy; they provide no protection from STIs.

polyurethane
A type of plastic.

do not provide protection against many STIs and are not recommended for that purpose.

In 1997, the U.S. Food and Drug Administration (FDA) approved the first condom made of **polyurethane**, a type of plastic. Initial studies show that polyurethane condoms are as effective as latex condoms for both contraception and STI prevention but more comfortable to use (Kalichman & Cherry, 1999). Condoms are now available in polyisoprene, a synthetic rubber that allows those allergic to latex to use them without concern. The condoms are said to stretch more and be more comfortable than polyurethane condoms (GoAskAlice, 2009).

There are more than 100 brands of condoms available in the United States today. The U.S. Centers for Disease Control and Prevention provides the following directions for the consistent and correct use of condoms. Individuals who use condoms to prevent unwanted pregnancies and STIs must understand the meaning of *consistent* and *correct* condom use.

CONSISTENT USE

- Use a condom every time, from start to finish, for penile–vaginal sex, oral sex on a male, and anal sex. A new condom must be used for each sex act.

CORRECT USE

- Store condoms in a cool place out of direct sunlight (not in wallets or glove compartments). Latex will become brittle as a result of changes in temperature, rough handling, and age. Do not use damaged, discolored, brittle, or sticky condoms.

- Check the date on the condom. If it is an expiration date, do not use the condom beyond that date. If it is a date of production, the condom may be used for several years beyond that date (2 years for spermicidal condoms, 5 years for nonspermicidal latex condoms) (Zieman et al., 2010).

Communication
DIMENSIONS

Condom Use and Consistency: Talking About Condom Use

Except for withdrawal, condoms have the greatest gap between perfect use (98% effectiveness) and typical use (82% effectiveness) of all the contraceptive methods (see Table 7.1). Because this method is popular and its use is increasing (the rate of condom use at first sex increased from 22% in the 1970s to 67% in 2002), factors associated with its use and consistency are important to know (Guttmacher, 2008). Among teens, high rates of both STIs and unintended pregnancy could be reduced with condom use. A study examining condom use patterns among sexually experienced male adolescents, age 15–19, found multiple domains of influence. Those who had formal sex education, had positive attitudes about condoms, were younger, had a partner close in age, and were committed to a relationship had greater odds of correct and consistent condom use. Recommendations include providing programs with targeted services that address condom use attitudes and that help teens negotiate condom use decision making with sexual partners (Sonenstein, 2008). The following scenario could be helpful with decision making.

You are on your third date in a nice restaurant with a new friend. You are attracted to each other; on the last date, you spent a pretty hot half hour kissing and touching each other. You are pretty sure that you are ready to have sex and are hoping that your new friend feels the same way. But how do you know? And, how do you bring up condom use or other safer sex techniques?

The waiter just delivered dessert. Dinner is coming to an end. Your date says, "Hmmm, do you want to come back to my place?" You say, "I think there are a few things we need to talk about first."

Here's how a successful discussion about condoms with a new partner might go.

Chris: I really like you. I've been fantasizing a lot since our last date about us having sex.

Pat: Me, too. But, it's important to me that we use condoms and practice safe sex.

Chris: Of course. I always use condoms. And because I was hoping you were interested, too, I bought some today.

Pat: I bought some today, too! How about we skip dessert?

But of course, it is not always that easy (although it should be). Chris might have said, "I hate condoms." Here are some ways that Pat might answer.

1. "Not with me you won't. I've learned how to make condom use really fun. I hope you want me to show you."

2. "I'm really sorry to hear that. I would never have sex with someone unless we use a condom."

3. "Tell me which condoms you've used. Maybe we can try a different brand or type."

4. "Well, it looks as if we have an important decision to make. We can agree not to have any kind of sex and just mess around. Or, we can just be friends. But, I won't have sex with you without a condom."

Condom use with a new partner is essential until you have both been tested for STIs and have decided to be monogamous. Remember, "A man who doesn't want to use a condom with you probably didn't use one with his last partner either" (Haffner & Schwartz, 1998).

- Carefully open the condom package—teeth or fingernails can tear the condom.

- Use a new condom for every act of oral, penile–vaginal, and anal sex. If engaging in oral sex first, use a new condom for penile–vaginal sex. If using penetrative sex toys, use a new condom between partners.

- Put on the condom after the penis is erect and before it touches any part of a partner's body. A man who is uncircumcised must pull back the foreskin before putting on the condom.

- Put on the condom by pinching the reservoir tip and unrolling it all the way down the shaft of the penis from head to base (see Figure 7.1). If the condom does not have a reservoir tip, pinch it to leave a half-inch space at the head of the penis in which semen can collect after ejaculation.

- Withdraw the penis immediately if the condom breaks, and put on a new condom before resuming. When a condom breaks, speak to a healthcare provider or pharmacist about emergency contraception.

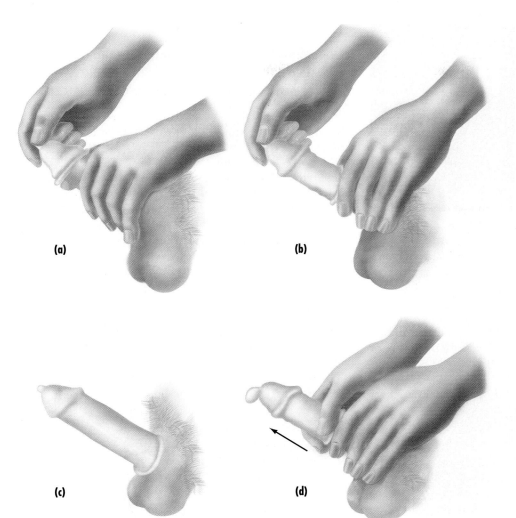

(a)

(b)

(c)

(d)

FIGURE **7.1** If you have never used a condom, you should practice before the first time you use one during oral, penile–vaginal, or anal sex. To put a condom on: (a) Put on the condom by pinching the reservoir tip and unrolling it all the way down the shaft of the penis. (b) Be sure that there are no air bubbles, which could cause the condom to break. (c) The condom should have extra rubber at the top and should be unrolled to the very base of the penis. (d) After ejaculation, hold the rim of the condom so that it does not accidentally slip off or leak and withdraw the penis.

- Use only water-based or silicone-based lubrication with latex or polyisoprene condoms. Use oil-based lubricants such as cooking/vegetable oil, baby oil, hand lotion, or petroleum jelly only with polyurethane condoms. Spermicidal condoms are no longer recommended, although spermicides do not damage latex.

- Immediately after ejaculation, while the penis is still erect grasp the rim of the condom between the fingers, and slowly withdraw the penis (with the condom still on) so that no semen is spilled.

- Check for breakage; dispose of condom (Zieman et al., 2010).

Effectiveness
Condoms are very effective: Only 2% of couples using a condom correctly and for every act of intercourse become pregnant in the first year of use. It is 82% effective in typical users. The major reason condoms fail is that people forget to use them for each act of intercourse (Trussell, 2011). Breakage, slippage, or leakage can also reduce effectiveness. Condom fit may be a factor. Do not use lubricant inside a condom or use one that is too large; it may slip off. If the condom is too small, breakage or reduced sensation may be a problem. Condoms are also highly effective at preventing the spread of HIV, gonorrhea, chlamydia, and trichomoniasis (Zieman et al., 2010).

Advantages and Disadvantages
Advantages of condoms include the following: They are relatively inexpensive, they are easy to obtain, they do not require a visit to the doctor, they may help a man control ejaculation, they provide protection from STIs (with consistent use, risk of HIV transmission is reduced tenfold), and they have none of the unhealthy side effects associated with some of the other methods of contraception. Finally, condom use takes some of the burden of birth control off women. As the women's movement works toward female–male equality, more and more women seek to share the practice of birth control with their partners.

Posters have been part of media campaigns to raise awareness and overcome societal taboos about condom use. The American Indian Health Care Association developed this one. The effort to increase condom use acceptance is central to AIDS prevention programs.

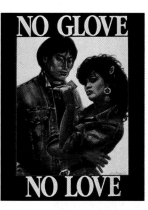

The major disadvantage is that many men complain that condoms reduce sensitivity and spontaneity. Trying different brands can improve sensation, and putting the condom on as foreplay can make it more fun. Another potential problem is a latex allergy or reaction to spermicide. Discontinue spermicide use first. If that does not help, try polyurethane or polyisoprene condoms.

Female Condom

One vaginal barrier is the **female condom** (Figure 7.2). The female condom appeared on the market in the United States in 1993. Originally the female condom was a loose-fitting sheath made of polyurethane with rings on both ends.

> **female condom**
> A polyurethane or synthetic rubber sheath with flexible inner and outer rings worn inside the vagina.

One ring covers the cervix; the other ring remains outside the vagina and partially covers the vulva. A new version of the female condom, the FC2, was approved by the U.S. Food and Drug Administration (FDA) in March 2009. Although it looks similar to its predecessor, it is made from synthetic rubber, making it cheaper to produce. The FC2 is also less noisy during use. In addition to cost, complaints about squeaky noises were among the factors that slowed acceptance of the original version. For now, the price is about 60 cents compared to less than 4 cents for mass-distributed male condoms, a difference that is an issue in the developing world (Crary, 2009).

The female condom is like the male condom in that it can be used only for one act of intercourse. It

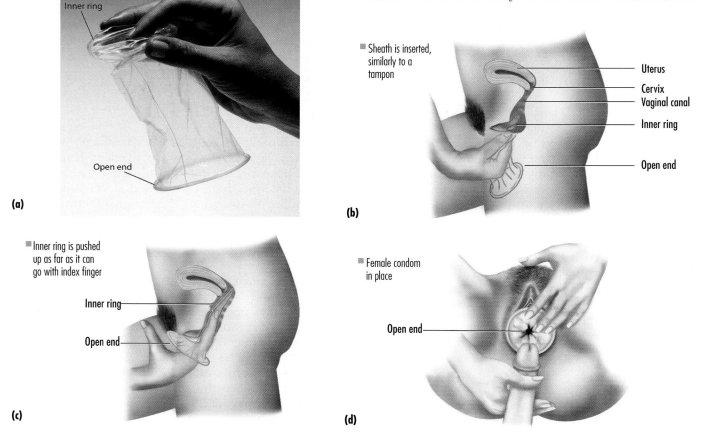

FIGURE **7.2** Inserting a female condom. (a) Photo of a female condom. (b) The inner ring is squeezed for insertion and the sheath inserted into the vagina similarly to a tampon. (c) With the index finger, push the inside of the inner ring as far as it will go. Make sure the sheath is not twisted during insertion. The outer ring should remain outside the vagina. (d) Hold the outer ring in place while inserting the penis, making sure the penis is inserted into the condom and not next to it. Be careful when removing the condom to ensure semen does not spill out.

Multicultural DIMENSIONS

Ethnic and Age Differences in Access to Emergency Contraception

Background Information

Emergency contraception (EC) includes any method used after intercourse to prevent pregnancy. None of the current methods is an abortifacient and none disturbs an implanted pregnancy. Currently, three methods are in widespread use worldwide:

- Hormonal contraceptive pills: high-dose progestin pills (Plan B) and combined oral contraceptive pills (Yuzpe method)
- Progesterone receptor modulator (ella)
- Copper IUD insertion (Paragard)

Only the hormonal methods and the progesterone receptor modulator are utilized to any significant degree in the United States. Unfortunately, many women are not aware of EC. One survey of postpartum U.S. women reported that only 25% knew about EC at the beginning of their pregnancy. This knowledge can affect use; 10% of women ages 15–44 reported use of EC at least once between 2006 and 2008, an increase from 4% in 2002 (Kaiser Family Foundation, 2010).

Research Findings

- Studies have found women getting EC in advance are not more likely to have unprotected sex.
- Women in EC studies often underutilize EC. Inconvenience and fear of the side effects were reasons for nonuse cited in one study.
- A recent review found increased access to EC enhanced use but did not decrease pregnancy rates.
- EC is an appropriate backup option for adolescents. Having EC available does *not* make teens less likely to use regular contraception or more likely to have unprotected sex.

Accessibility

Plan B can be provided from behind the counter (i.e., directly from the pharmacist without a prescription) for people ages 17 and older. At the time of this writing, the states with EC available directly from pharmacies for people of any age are Alaska, California, Hawaii, Maine, Massachusetts, New Hampshire, New Mexico, Vermont, and Washington (Guttmacher Institute, 2012).

Equal Access?

In California, EC is available without a prescription to females younger than 18 through pharmacy access. Timely access to this method of contraception is critical to reduce the rate of unintended pregnancy among adolescents. One study was designed to explore barriers adolescents might face and differences in access to EC by age, ethnicity, and region.

In 2005–2006, researchers posing as English- and Spanish-speaking females—who said they either were 15 and had had unprotected intercourse last night or were 18 and had had unprotected sex 4 days ago—called 115 pharmacies in California. Each pharmacy received one call using each scenario; a call was considered successful if the caller was told she could come in to obtain the method. Statistical measures were used to assess differences between subgroups. In-depth interviews with 22 providers and pharmacists were also conducted, and emergent themes were identified.

Thirty-six percent of all calls were successful. Spanish speakers were less successful than English speakers (24% versus 48%), and callers to rural pharmacies were less successful than callers to urban ones (27% versus 44%). Although rural pharmacies were more likely to offer Spanish-language services, Spanish-speaking callers to these pharmacies were the least successful of all callers (17%). Spanish speakers were also less successful than English speakers when calling urban pharmacies (30% versus 57%).

Interviews suggested that little cooperation existed between pharmacists and clinicians and that dispensing the EC method at clinics was a favorable option for adolescents. Adolescents face significant barriers to obtaining emergency contraception, but the expansion of Spanish-language services at pharmacies and greater collaboration between providers and pharmacists could improve access (Sampson et al., 2009).

---

is unlike the male condom because it can be inserted up to 8 hours before intercourse, although it may not be comfortable for everyday wear. Female and male condoms should *not* be used together because they can stick together and dislodge each other.

Effectiveness

The effectiveness rates for the female condom are based on the original version. No studies have been conducted on FC2. For perfect use, it is 95% effective in preventing pregnancies. In typical use, studies have found it to be 79% effective. Although it is not as effective as the male condom, the female condom is a valuable option to empower women who want to prevent STIs and unintended pregnancy (SexReally, 2009).

Advantages and Disadvantages

This method is available without prescription, is controlled by the woman, can be inserted in advance of intercourse, and is a safe alternative for people with latex allergy or sensitivity. Its disadvantages include somewhat difficult insertion requiring practice for new users and noise during intercourse that may be distracting. The noise can be reduced with additional lubricant, however.

Contraceptive Sponges

The Today contraceptive sponge is made of polyurethane foam (latex-free) and is prefilled with nonoxynol 9 spermicide (discussed in the next section) that is continuously released into the vagina during use. The sponge acts both as a mechanical barrier to sperm migration into the cervical canal and as a chemical agent by applying spermicide directly to the cervix. It is not reusable. The sponge is sold over the counter, without the need for a prescription (three sponges for around $17). When used as a primary method, this barrier method should be coupled with counseling to have EC pills on hand at home.

This contraceptive method was originally introduced in 1983. The manufacturer stopped distributing the product over a dispute not related to its quality or efficacy. In spring 2009, the new, exclusive distributor of the Today Vaginal Contraceptive Sponge for the United States, Canada, and European Union announced that the sponge has been relaunched in the United States (Mayer Laboratories, 2009).

Effectiveness

When the sponge was introduced originally, its perfect-use failure rate in the first year of use was 9% to 11%; the typical-use failure rate in the first year was not much different, at 13% to 16% (Edelman, 1987). Table 7.1 reports that the sponge is twice as effective for women who have never given birth (nulliparous women: perfect use 9% and typical use 12%) as for those who have given birth (parous women: 20% perfect use and 24% typical use).

Advantages and Disadvantages

The contraceptive sponge method is controlled by the woman, is active immediately after placement, can be inserted several hours before sexual intercourse to permit spontaneity, can remain in place for multiple acts of intercourse up to 24 hours, and

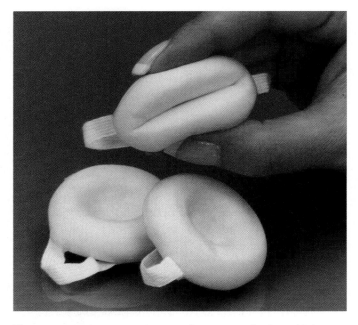

The contraceptive sponge is a one-time use method combining a barrier that prevents sperm from entering the cervix with a chemical spermicide.

is entirely reversible. Studies vary on the sponge's potential in reducing cervical infections, including gonorrhea, chlamydia, and pelvic inflammatory disease. It offers no protection from HIV. Because the evidence is unclear, the sponge should not be used for STI prevention.

Some disadvantages are that the sponge requires placement prior to genital contact, which may reduce spontaneity of sex; some women do not like placing their fingers or an object into their vagina; the sponge does not provide protection against HIV and some STIs; failure rates are higher than with hormonal contraception; odor may develop if the sponge is left in place too long; and severe obesity or arthritis may make insertion or removal of the sponge difficult. No cases of toxic shock syndrome have been reported, but theoretically the risk may be increased if this method is left in too long or used during menses. An increase in uterine tract infections is another possible complication (Zieman et al., 2010).

Spermicides

A **spermicide** kills and/or immobilizes sperm on contact and acts as a cervical barrier, thereby preventing their movement toward an egg (Figure 7.3). Spermicides are available as vaginal creams, films, foams, gels, suppositories, sponges,

spermicide
Chemical detergent compound that immobilizes or kills sperm on contact; as a barrier, prevents sperm from entering the uterus through the cervical os.

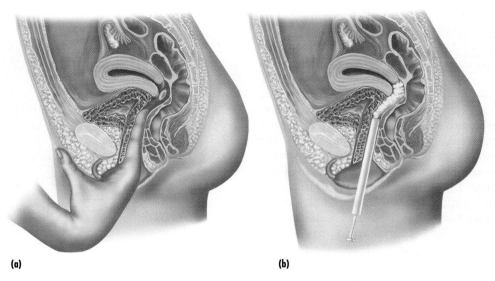

(a)   (b)

FIGURE **7.3** (a) Read the instructions for use of suppositories carefully and follow them. Be sure to wait the proper time for the suppository to dissolve. (b) Insert the plastic applicator into the vagina as far as possible to make sure that the foam covers the cervical opening, and press the plunger.

and tablets. Foams and creams are placed against the cervix by means of a plastic applicator. Spermicidal films (small squares coated with spermicides) and suppositories are inserted manually, high into the vagina. Most spermicides must be inserted within 1 hour of intercourse, and some are not effective for the first 10 to 15 minutes after insertion. Users should read the packet insert instructions carefully.

Effectiveness

The perfect use effectiveness rate of spermicides is 82%, meaning that only 18% of women using spermicides perfectly would become pregnant in 1 year. However, the typical user effectiveness rate is only 72%. Just as for condoms, their ineffectiveness is probably due to inconsistent use of the spermicide with every act of penile–vaginal sex or incorrect use (for example, putting it in too soon or too late). By using condoms and spermicide together, effectiveness rates almost equal those of oral contraceptives. Unfortunately, few couples use both methods simultaneously.

Reversibility

Spermicide use has no effect on future fertility.

Advantages and Disadvantages

There are many advantages to spermicide use. They are easy to use, are available at drug stores and supermarkets without a prescription, and do not require partner involvement.

The major disadvantages of spermicides are the relatively high failure rates for both perfect use and typical use as well as the recent reversal in recommendations involving **nonoxynol 9**. It is the major spermicidal ingredient sold over the counter in the United States. Although several other spermicides (menfegol, benzalkonium chloride, sodium ducosate, and chlorhexidine) are used in products available in Canada and in Europe, these compounds are not available in the United States.

> **nonoxynol 9 (N-9)**
> The major spermicidal ingredient in U.S.-made products.

Women are advised to avoid products with nonoxynol 9 because several studies showed vaginal irritation due to this spermicide, actually increasing the possibility of acquiring HIV and other STIs from an infected partner. Although a potentially effective method, use during anal sex or repeated penile–vaginal sex in one day should be avoided.

Fertility Awareness Methods

Natural family planning (NFP) is also known as **fertility-awareness methods**, or the *rhythm method*. There are several fertility-awareness methods: the *calendar method, ovulation method*, and *symptothermal method*. Each of these methods is based on the identification of the days in the woman's menstrual cycle when she is most likely to be fertile and the avoidance of

> **natural family planning (NFP)**
> Calculation of a woman's fertile times and abstention from penile–vaginal sex on fertile days.
>
> **fertility-awareness methods**
> Methods used to determine fertile days.

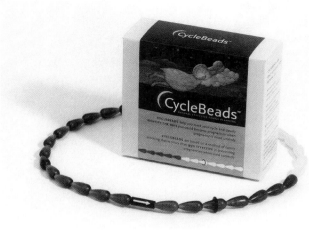

CycleBeads are used as part of the calendar method. Using a string of 33 colored beads, women keep track of their cycle. When used correctly, the efficacy rate is 5 pregnancies per 100 per year.

fertility-awareness-combined methods
Calculation of a woman's fertile times and use of a barrier or withdrawal on fertile days.

penile–vaginal sex during those days (natural family planning) or use of a barrier method or withdrawal during those days (**fertility-awareness-combined methods**).

Fertility-awareness methods are based on the knowledge that there are only about 6 days in a cycle during which a woman can become pregnant. The ovum lives less than 1 day; sperm can live up to 6 days inside the woman's genital tract (Zieman et al., 2010).

People interested in using these methods need to see a trained educator for help in learning to observe, chart, and recognize the woman's fertility signs and patterns. It is estimated that it requires 4 to 6 hours to learn fertility-awareness methods so that they can be used effectively (Jennings & Arevalo, 2008). For that reason, detailed instructions are not included in this text.

People using the **calendar method**, first developed in the 1930s, keep track of the woman's menstrual cycles for several months and then, with the help of a trained person, determine which days she is most likely to ovulate. It is the least effective of the fertility-awareness methods; even with perfect use, there is a 5% chance of becoming pregnant.

calendar method
Charting of the length of a woman's periods for several months to determine the days she is most likely to be fertile.

ovulation methods
Observation of signs of ovulation to calculate fertile days.

basal body temperature
A woman's body temperature immediately upon waking.

basal body thermometer
A special thermometer used to measure changes in basal body temperature.

cervical secretions
Normal fluids from the cervix that change consistency during the month.

Ovulation methods are much more effective. Women can chart their **basal body temperature** or their cervical secretions or both. Basal body temperature is a person's temperature upon awakening. Temperatures usually drop immediately before ovulation and then rise sharply during and after ovulation (Figure 7.4). Thus a woman takes her temperature by using a specially calibrated **basal body thermometer** before she gets up each morning. The temperature is then charted on a monthly graph, and after 3 days of elevated temperature, it is considered safe to have intercourse without the risk of pregnancy.

Cervical secretions can also be monitored and charted. After menstruation, cervical secretions are scant. As estrogen levels increase, cervical mucus becomes thick and cloudy. When estrogen peaks at midcycle, the secretions become clearer, stretchy,

and slippery. In fact, at ovulation, the mucus can be stretched 2 to 3 inches between the thumb and forefinger. After ovulation, the secretions become thick again, and some women may notice a cervical mucus plug. At this point, it is considered safe to have intercourse without worrying about pregnancy.

The **symptothermal method** involves checking both basal body temperatures and cervical secretions and charting them to identify fertile periods (begins as soon as cervical secretions are noticed) and nonfertile times (beginning the fourth day after the last day of wet, clear, slippery mucus—post ovulation). When this method is used perfectly, less then 1% of women become pregnant, making it as effective as the most effective prescription forms of contraception (Trussell, 2011).

symptothermal method
A combination of natural family-planning methods, in which both temperature and signs of ovulation are observed and charted.

Costs involve training and supplies (such as special digital basal body thermometer, cycle beads, and charts) (Jennings & Arevalo, 2008).

Effectiveness
Natural family-planning methods can be highly effective methods of contraception. If they are used perfectly, only 1% to 9% of women using these methods in a year have an unintended pregnancy. The symptothermal method is the most effective natural family-planning method; using a calendar alone is only 87% effective in typical use; however, many of the studies have design flaws, so a true effectiveness is difficult to determine (Jennings & Arevalo, 2008). Fertility-awareness methods can also be used effectively to help couples become pregnant.

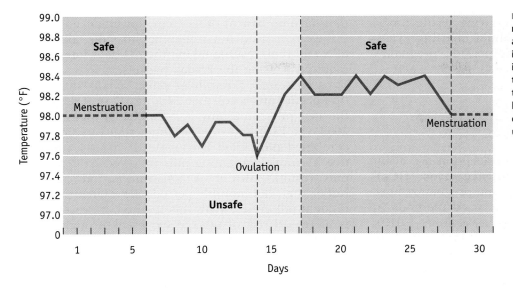

FIGURE **7.4** The basal body temperature method of contraception involves charting a woman's body temperature each morning to determine when unprotected sexual intercourse is safe. Once the basal body temperature has risen for three consecutive days, she can assume that ovulation has taken place and that the rest of the days in that menstrual cycle are safe for unprotected intercourse.

Gender DIMENSIONS

Gender Equality in Contraception Use

During most of human history, contraception was a male responsibility. The only methods available were the condom and withdrawal. Oral contraceptives became available in 1961, and many women were elated. They could now control contraceptive use and thus their risk of becoming pregnant. The pill was effective, was easy to use, and did not require partner participation. Many men who came of age during the 1960s and 1970s never thought much about contraception.

In the 1990s, the HIV/AIDS epidemic and the epidemic of STIs once again shifted the responsibility. Men who are not in monogamous committed relationships now have to use condoms on a regular basis. But many women are unwilling to rely on condoms for pregnancy prevention because they are only 85% effective in preventing pregnancies in typical users. Some men are unwilling to use condoms once they find out that their partner is using the pill. And many men do not like to use condoms, claiming that they reduce sensitivity and sensation.

Heterosexual couples today need to negotiate how they will prevent an unwanted pregnancy *and* how they will protect themselves against STIs. Couples need to discuss who has primary responsibility for contraception. They need to address such questions as, Who will buy the condoms? Who will pay for contraception? Should the man accompany the woman to the clinic visit? And, perhaps most important, what will they do if an unplanned pregnancy occurs?

There are ways that couples can share the responsibility for contraceptive and condom use. Men can remind their partners to take their pills or check their IUD strings. They can learn to insert the diaphragm or female condom as part of foreplay. Women can learn to place the condom on the man's penis as part of foreplay. Contraceptive use and safer sex practices can truly be a shared responsibility.

Reversibility

Natural family-planning methods stop preventing pregnancies as soon as they are discontinued.

Advantages and Disadvantages

Fertility-awareness methods have many advantages. They are an excellent way for men and women to learn about their own fertility. They require both partners' involvement, they are free, and they may alert women to the need for some kind of medical attention. Their primary disadvantage is that they provide no protection against STIs, cervical mucus techniques may be complicated by vaginal infections, and the couple must be vigorously committed to abstaining from intercourse during fertile times. If the couple is not rigorous about charting cycles or has intercourse during fertile periods, pregnancy is likely to occur.

■ Prescription Methods

Oral Contraceptives

Although many methods of contraception are available to U.S. women, **oral contraceptives (OCs)**, which are pills taken daily to prevent pregnancy, have been one of the most commonly used methods in the United States since 1982 (Mosher & Jones, 2010). Oral contraceptives can be categorized as monophasic formulations, in which all the active pills contain the same amount of hormone, and multiphasic formulations, in which the active pills throughout the cycle contain varying amounts of progestin and/or estrogen. The monophasic formulation accounts for the majority of the oral contraceptives available (Nelson, 2008).

oral contraceptive (OC)
A daily pill taken to prevent pregnancy.

combined pill (COC)
Oral contraceptive containing estrogen and progestin.

The **combined pill (COC)**, used since the 1960s, contains both estrogens and progestin (synthetic progesterone). To use the combined pill, a woman ingests the first pill in the packet and takes a pill each succeeding day. Most packets contain 28 pills, but some contain only 21. Most 28-pill packets contain 7 pills that have no benefit other than convenience: That is, the woman need not remember to stop taking her pills and then resume taking them 7 days later—as is required if using the 21-day packets. A few formulations have only 5 reminder pills. Usually menstruation occurs on the 23rd or 24th day (2 or 3 days after the last pill containing a hormone is ingested). In 2003, the FDA approved a long-acting version of the combined pill called Seasonale. It has 84 consecutive hormone-containing pills followed by 7 placebo pills, resulting in only 4 menstrual periods per year rather than the monthly periods associated with traditional pill cycles. With this method, however, there is increased risk of unexpected breakthrough bleeding, especially in the first months of use (Zieman et al., 2010; WHO, 2008), though newer formulations minimize that issue (Nelson, 2010).

The combination pill's estrogen signals the brain's hypothalamus to prevent the pituitary gland from producing FSH and LH; the progesterone also inhibits LH production. Ovulation is suppressed. This suppression mimics the changes that occur in pregnancy.

The progestin-only pill was introduced in 1972. In spite of its lack of estrogen (high dosages of which were found to be related to physical complications), the **minipill (POP)** never achieved a great deal of popularity, and the percentage of women using it remains relatively low to this day. To use this type, a woman takes a pill on the first day of menstruation and every

minipill (POP)
A progestin-only pill.

CONTRACEPTIVE TIMELINE

Ancient Practices—Coitus interruptus (the withdrawal method) was first mentioned in the Biblical Book of Genesis (Genesis 38:8).

1564—The earliest published description of the "condom" was by the Italian anatomist Gabriel Fallopius in 1564. The term "condom" was likely derived from the Latin word *condus*, meaning "receptacle" (Birth control, 2009).

1873—State and federal legislation, collectively referred to as the Comstock Laws, prohibited the importation or mailing of obscene matter. Obscene matter included contraceptive products as well as information about those products.

1350 b.c.—As one of the earliest forms of the condom, Egyptian men may have placed linen sheaths on the penis before intercourse. It is difficult to determine the accuracy of this claim; this time period covers prehistorical events, and evidence suggests that Egyptians worshipped the god of fertility (Youssef, 1993).

1840 through 1870s—Paralleling Charles Goodyear's vulcanization of rubber in the first half of the 19th century, the rubber condom became a popular choice of contraception. Other rubber-made contraceptive products, such as the earliest intrauterine devices, douching syringes, and diaphragms, were referred to as "womb veils" (Birth control, 2009; *Timeline*, 2002).

1879—Margaret H. Sanger was born Maggie Louise Higgins (*Timeline*, 2002).

1881—Surgical occlusion of the fallopian tubes (e.g., the first female sterilization) was performed by an Ohio surgeon (Birth control, 2009).

Gender DIMENSIONS

Margaret H. Sanger: A Woman of Influence

In 1931, the futurist H. G. Wells said Margaret H. Sanger (1879–1966) started the most influential movement of all time (Lehfeldt, 1967). In 1998, she was recognized among the 100 most important people of the 20th century by *Time* magazine. Today, early in the 21st century, her life concerns—health disparities due to poverty, the burdens of unintended pregnancy, and women's access to safe methods of birth control—are still problems, but are now recognized public health priorities. In her lifetime, Margaret Sanger was a catalyst for contraceptive research, an emancipator of women, and a practicing nurse among the marginalized and poor who eventually became known as the woman who established the American birth-control movement.

Margaret H. Sanger was born in 1879, the sixth child of a working-class, Irish Catholic family in New York. As a young nurse tending to the poor on the Lower East Side, Sanger witnessed the severe illness and even death that women suffered when attempting self-induced abortions (Hymowitz & Weissman, 1978). Seeing such tragedy combined with "revolting conditions," where extreme poverty and child labor added to the misery, moved Sanger to find the "secret" of preventing unwanted pregnancies (Lehfeldt, 1967).

The barriers she faced were huge. At first, Sanger began in earnest by writing her radical journal *The Woman Rebel* as well as the *Family Limitation* pamphlet. Even though she did not give instructions regarding specific methods for contraception, the Comstock Laws' definition of "obscene, lewd, lascivious" matter was cited to have her arrested and eventually jailed (Jensen, 1981). Sanger temporarily fled to Europe, where she was introduced to the various contraceptive technologies currently available, as well as several European benefactors and professionals who championed her cause, including British sexologist Havelock Ellis. Based on these experiences, Sanger believed that the diaphragm, along with spermicidal jellies, were the secrets to having a simple, cheap, harmless contraceptive that could be used throughout the world (Lehfeldt, 1967).

In the latter part of Sanger's career, she concentrated on the development of new contraceptive technologies—specifically oral contraceptives. Through the Planned Parenthood Foundation, she arranged for the first grant supporting investigation of progestinal compounds for the purpose of contraception. She obtained additional funding for the scientists who would later be recognized as the inventors of the oral contraceptive (Lehfeldt, 1967). Although she received neither the Nobel Peace Prize nor the Presidential Freedom Award for which she was nominated, she was successful in searching for safe, effective forms of birth control, offering the leading voice in the development of oral contraceptives, as well as providing the foundations for Planned Parenthood.

20th Century—*Hormones*, from the Greek *hormaô*, meaning "stir up" or "incite," were isolated (e.g., estrogen). This development opened the door for the hormonally based methods of contraception in the latter half of the 20th century (Birth control, 2009).

1916—Sanger opened the first birth control clinic in the United States. Ten days after the opening, the clinic was raided, all birth control devices were confiscated, and Sanger was arrested and jailed (Hock, 2007).

1950s and 1960s—Strong arguments were made for the acceptance and use of oral contraceptives. Factors included advancements in hormonal/synthetic research, growth in pro-contraceptive sociopolitical movements, and federal government policy decisions supporting an individual's right to personal privacy.

1914—Pioneer Margaret Sanger published the first major statement on birth control and contraception in her pamphlet *Family Limitations* (Jensen, 1981). She coined the term "birth control" and challenged women to use the term from the pages of her radical journal *The Woman Rebel* (*Timeline*, 2002).

1923—Sanger opened the first legal birth control clinic in the United States (*Timeline*, 2002).

1936—In the *United States v. One Package of Japanese Pessaries*, the court ruled that contraceptives could be sent through the mail if they were to be intelligently employed by conscientious physicians for (1) the purpose of saving life or (2) promoting the well-being of their patients (Birth control, 2009). This decision marked a reversal of one of the last surviving Comstock Laws (Hock, 2007)

1951—The Roman Catholic Church sanctioned the use of the rhythm method, but remained opposed to any other form of birth control, including "the pill." Pope Paul VI issued the encyclical *Humanae Vitae* ("Of Human Life") in 1968 as the authoritative guide for birth regulation among many Catholics (Catholic Church, 1968).

Continued

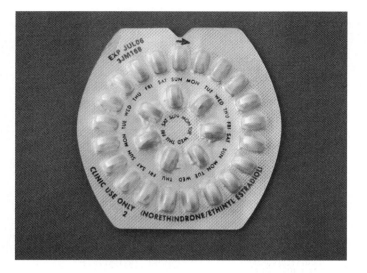

Although oral contraceptives are effective in preventing pregnancy, they offer no protection against STIs or HIV. For protection against pregnancy and STIs, try combining the use of oral contraceptives and latex condoms.

day thereafter. Because progestin is included in every pill, the hormone is ingested daily. With minipills, ovulation is suppressed in about 50% of the cycles (Zieman et al., 2010). However, even if fertilization occurs, the progestin inhibits implantation. Moreover, the progestin causes the cervical mucus to inhibit to some degree the sperm's movement and ability to penetrate the ovum. Minipills are appropriate for women who cannot use estrogen.

The chemical composition of oral contraceptives has changed over the years in response to research on their effects and side effects. In early birth control pills, the typical amount of estrogen was 0.15 milligrams (mg) and 10 mg of progestin. In 1968, fewer than 1% of retail prescriptions for oral contraceptives contained less than 0.05 mg of estrogen. In 1988 approximately 82% of retail prescriptions contained less than 0.05 mg of estrogen. In the 1970s it was found that use of the higher-dosage pills (more than 0.05 mg) was related to cardiovascular complications. Today those higher-dosage pills are still available and used by women with specific medical problems such as uterine bleeding and endometriosis. However, most oral contraceptives using estrogen now contain between 0.02 and 0.035 mg and 1.0 mg to 1.2 mg of progestin.

Regardless of which pill is used, a backup method of contraception should be employed for the first 7 days of pill use and as a precaution if a pill is forgotten for 2 or more days in a row. If a pill is forgotten one day, that pill should be taken immediately and the next pill taken as regularly scheduled. Some medications interfere with the effectiveness of oral contraceptives. Check with your healthcare provider before taking any medication. Previously, some antibiotics were thought to affect pill function, but further research has shown that pregnancy risk is not affected (Nelson, 2008).

It is a good idea for a woman using oral contraceptives to have regular medical exams. Most

CONTRACEPTIVE TIMELINE—cont'd

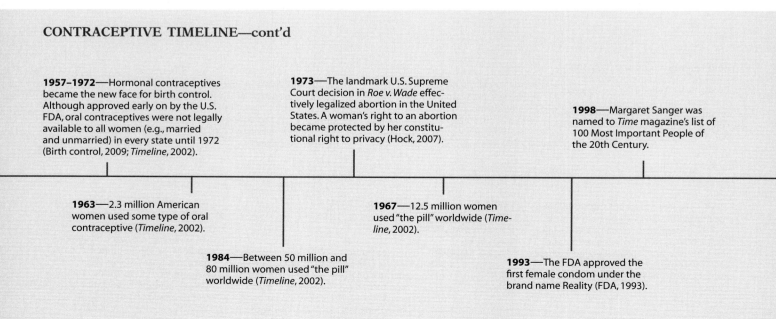

1957–1972—Hormonal contraceptives became the new face for birth control. Although approved early on by the U.S. FDA, oral contraceptives were not legally available to all women (e.g., married and unmarried) in every state until 1972 (Birth control, 2009; *Timeline*, 2002).

1973—The landmark U.S. Supreme Court decision in *Roe v. Wade* effectively legalized abortion in the United States. A woman's right to an abortion became protected by her constitutional right to privacy (Hock, 2007).

1998—Margaret Sanger was named to *Time* magazine's list of 100 Most Important People of the 20th Century.

1963—2.3 million American women used some type of oral contraceptive (*Timeline*, 2002).

1967—12.5 million women used "the pill" worldwide (*Timeline*, 2002).

1984—Between 50 million and 80 million women used "the pill" worldwide (*Timeline*, 2002).

1993—The FDA approved the first female condom under the brand name Reality (FDA, 1993).

physicians require a visit 3 or 6 months after a woman starts OCs, followed by an annual exam thereafter. There is no medical reason for a woman to "take a break" from pill use (WHO, 2008).

Effectiveness

Oral contraceptives provide one of the most effective means of preventing pregnancy. Only 3 in 1,000 women using oral contraceptives becomes pregnant in 1 year of perfect use. Among typical users—for example, some who forget to take their pills as directed—as many as 9% become pregnant in the first year (Trussell, 2011).

It cannot be overemphasized that oral contraceptives provide *no* protection from STIs. Unless you are in a 100% monogamous relationship with a partner who has been tested for STIs and HIV, a condom must be used for each act of intercourse.

Reversibility

Some women who have been on the pill may require slightly more time to become pregnant than women using nonhormonal methods; however, the return to fertility for oral contraceptive use is in a similar range as other hormonal methods (Barnhart & Schreiber, 2009).

Advantages and Disadvantages

Birth control pills have been reported as being 92% effective as actually used and 99.7% effective if used correctly all the time (Trussell, 2011). Besides being

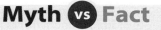

Myth vs Fact

Myth: Birth control pills cause cancer.
Fact: Birth control pills are very safe. Although there may be a slightly increased short-term risk of being diagnosed with breast cancer, it is believed that this is due to (1) detection bias (more breast exams and more mammography) or (2) promotion of already-present cancer cells. In the long term, women who have taken birth control pills have a 25% reduction in risk for benign breast disease. Furthermore, the pill is protective against other cancers such as ovarian and endometrial cancer as well as death from colon cancer. Thus, women using the pill are less likely to contract cancer than women who have never been on the pill.

Myth: You need to take a break from the pill.
Fact: Women can stay on oral contraceptives as long as medical side effects do not develop. There is no need to take a break.

Myth: All condoms protect against STIs.

Fact: Only latex and polyurethane condoms protect against STIs. Animal skin condoms provide no protection against STIs.

Myth: Condoms protect against all STIs.
Fact: Condoms are highly effective at preventing the spread of such diseases as HIV infection, syphilis, and gonorrhea. They do not provide protection against genital warts, crabs, or lice, which can be transmitted through contact with the pubic hair or other parts of the genitals that are not covered by the condom.

Myth: Withdrawal is not a method of birth control.
Fact: Withdrawal is about as effective as barrier methods. It is much better than using nothing.

Myth: Once a person has had penile–vaginal sex, he or she can no longer practice abstinence.
Fact: Abstinence is always a choice. Many teens, college students, and adults choose abstinence even though they have already had oral, penile–vaginal, or anal sex.

1999—The FDA approved the emergency contraceptive Plan B by prescription only. Although emergency contraceptives had been available since the 1970s, Plan B found a new generation of consumers.

2002–2004—New forms of hormonal contraceptives (extended-use pills, implants, patch, vaginal ring) were introduced. Many of these methods either reduce or eliminate a woman's menstrual cycle.

2009–2010—ella, a single-dose EC pill, is approved by the FDA. ella can protect against pregnancy for up to 5 days after unprotected penile–vaginal sex. Plan B is available on an over-the-counter basis to women 17 and older and to women younger than age 17 by prescription only.

1999—Wal-Mart refused to sell the "morning-after pill" with the brand name Preven (Canedy, 1999). Under mounting pressure, Wal-Mart began to sell the emergency contraceptive Plan B in 2006 (Barbaro, 2006).

2008—Four federally funded longitudinal studies showed abstinence-only sex education is associated with (1) no significant impact on teen sexual activity, (2) no differences in rates of unprotected sex, and (3) some impacts on knowledge of STIs and perceived effectiveness of condoms and birth control pills (Trenholm et al., 2007).

effective, the pill does not necessitate interrupting sexual activity. An added benefit for some women is that it helps to regulate the menstrual cycle. Birth control pills are available in the United States only by prescription from a physician, because they have other effects as well. For example, the combination pill may enlarge the breasts, may reduce acne, often eliminates mittelschmerz (a sensation of abdominal pain that sometimes occurs during ovulation), and reduces menstrual cramps. For estrogen-related problems with the combination pill, the progestin-only pill is recommended, because it contains no estrogen, and its low progestin dosage is thought to reduce adverse effects that progestin might otherwise cause.

Combined pills are very safe. In addition to protecting a woman against pregnancy, they lower a woman's risk of ovarian cancer, endometrial cancer, breast masses, and ovarian cysts. They also lessen menstrual blood loss, cramps, and acne. Their primary disadvantage for sexually active college students is that they provide *no* protection against STIs, including HIV.

Symptoms usually develop within 3 to 6 months of starting the pill, but they can develop later. Abdominal pain, chest pain, shortness of breath, headaches, eye problems such as blurred vision, and severe leg pain are examples of such symptoms. If any of these is encountered, call the doctor. Other possible side effects exist. For example, the combination pill has been associated with a greater risk of circulatory system diseases, including heart attacks and strokes. If a woman is obese, diabetic, or hypertensive, the risk of circulatory system diseases is greatly increased. These women should use a different method (Nelson, 2008). Smoking is also a factor, especially for heavy smokers and smokers older than 35 years. In addition, women with liver function problems, hypertension, circulatory problems, heart disease, breast cancer, asthma, varicose veins, or migraine headaches should avoid using combined oral contraceptives (Nelson, 2008).

There has been considerable debate over the years about whether oral contraceptive use can lead to breast cancer. After more than 50 studies and 50 years, most experts believe that pills have little, if any, effect on the risk of developing breast cancer. The Women's Care Study of 4,575 women with breast cancer and 4,682 controls found no increased risk for breast cancer among women currently using pills and a decreased risk of breast cancer for those women who had previously used pills. Use of pills by women with a family history of breast cancer was not associated with an increased risk of breast cancer, nor was initiation of pill use at a young age. Breast cancers diagnosed in women currently on pills or women who have taken pills in the past are more likely to be localized (less likely to be metastatic). By the age of 55, the risk of having had breast cancer diagnosed is the same for women who have used pills and those who have not. While there are still unanswered questions about pills and breast cancer, today, five decades after their arrival on the contraceptive scene, the overall conclusion is that pills do not cause breast cancer (Nelson, 2008).

Emergency Contraception

Condoms sometimes slip or break; women forget more than two contraceptive pills in a row; the man ejaculates too close to the vulva even though he withdraws; a couple vowing abstinence has intercourse anyway. For all these cases, **emergency contraception** is available.

> **emergency contraception**
> The use of oral contraception or insertion of an IUD after unprotected sex has occurred at midcycle.

In addition, emergency contraception is available in cases of rape or incest.

Oral contraceptive pills have been used for emergency contraception (EC) since the 1960s. Various amounts of ordinary combined (estrogen and progestin) birth control pills can be prescribed and cut the chance of pregnancy by 79% (Trussell & Raymond, 2011).

Many different formulations of combined oral contraceptives have been approved for use as emergency contraception. Because these pills contain estrogen, nausea may be a side effect. An over-the-counter or prescription antinausea medication should be taken before the first dose, especially if nausea has been a problem in the past. Check with your healthcare provider about the types of OCs that can be used, dosing instructions, and antinausea options.

Two types of dedicated products (intended specifically for emergency contraception) are marketed in the United States: Plan B One Step (with original Plan B being phased out) and ella.

Plan B and Plan B One Step (generic version Next Choice) are progestin-only pills. The original Plan B formulation consisted of taking two pills (containing levonorgestrel) within 72 hours after having unprotected penile–vaginal sex; this would reduce the risk of pregnancy by 89%. The labeling for Plan B One Step, a single-dose pill, is to take the pill within 72 hours after unprotected penile–vaginal sex; however, recent research shows that it can be effective for up to 120 hours after penile–vaginal sex (Office of Population Research & Association of Reproductive Health Professionals, 2011a).

A single-dose pill, ella contains 30 milligrams of ulipristal acetate, a progesterone receptor modulator. It is available by prescription only and is approved

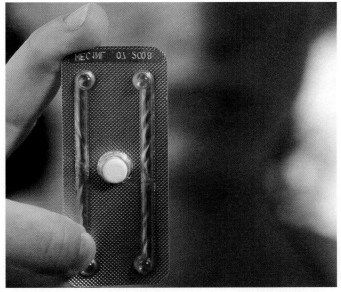

Two types of emergency contraception are available in the United States. Plan B One Step is a progestin-only one-pill dose available directly from pharmacies for individuals older than 17 years. Some states allow over-the-counter distribution for individuals without a prescription through state-approved protocols or collaborative practice agreements with a physician. The second type, ella, is also a one-pill formulation. It is a progesterone receptor moderator and is available with a prescription.

by the FDA for use up to 120 hours after unprotected penile–vaginal sex.

Regardless of the type of EC used, the sooner the pills are taken, the greater the chance that pregnancy will be avoided. If a woman is already pregnant or becomes pregnant following the use of EC, there are no documented negative impacts on fetal development.

Another method is insertion of an intrauterine device (Copper T/ParaGard IUD) that reduces the pregnancy risk by 99% and can be left in place to provide continuous contraception for up to 10 years. While all women are not equally good candidates for IUD use, especially those at risk for STIs (Trussell & Raymond, 2011), results from a recent review concluded that IUDs as emergency contraception should be presented as an option to more women (Cleland, Zhu, Goldstuck, Cheng, & Trussell, 2012).

How emergency contraception prevents pregnancy depends on the day of the menstrual cycle on which the pills are taken. Several mechanisms are possible—inhibition of ovulation, prevention of fertilization, or interference with implantation. It is important to differentiate that emergency contraception is not an **abortifacient**, meaning that it does not disrupt an implanted fertilized ovum (Zieman et al., 2010).

abortifacient
A medical method that causes an embryo or fetus to die.

Knowledge and access are critical barriers that keep emergency contraception from being widely used. Yet, research has clearly demonstrated that access does not increase sexual behavior nor does it diminish use of other methods of contraception (Zieman et al., 2010).

Some university clinics offer emergency contraception as part of their reproductive health services. If they do not, a good resource to learn more about EC and how to access it in the United States and other countries is http://ec.princeton.edu and its companion hotline 888-NOT-2-LATE.

Effectiveness

In order to be most effective, emergency contraception should be used before ovulation. Taking the pills as soon as possible after an unprotected act of penile–vaginal sex will also increase the effectiveness. Studies indicate that using combined OC pills for EC can reduce pregnancy risk by 74%, with progestin-only emergency contraceptive pills (Plan B One Step and Next Choice) being more effective (89%) within 72 hours after unprotected penile–vaginal sex. In addition, recent studies have indicated that the medication can be moderately effective if taken between 72 and 120 hours. The newer ella is the most effective pill option, especially on days 4 and 5 after the unprotected coitus. However, because it is available through prescription only and has a higher cost, access to the medication may not be as easy as other options. The most effective method is the insertion of a copper IUD, which prevents pregnancy 99.9% of the time (Trussell & Raymond, 2011).

Advantages and Disadvantages

The advantage to emergency contraception is that it is the only method available if unprotected intercourse has occurred when fertility is likely. Emergency contraception should not be used as a regular method of contraception. It is significantly less effective than other methods, and its long-term use has not been studied. It also provides no protection against STIs. Because EC has no impact on existing pregnancies, there is no need to test for pregnancy before taking the first dose. However, if menses do not occur within 21 days, a pregnancy test should be done. Another method of contraception should be used following EC (Zieman et al., 2010).

The Combined Contraceptive Patch

In December 2000, Johnson and Johnson applied for approval to market the first contraceptive patch. In March 2003, the patch became available to women seeking a method of contraception that released a steady delivery of hormones over time.

Similar to the use of the nicotine patch, users wear it on the lower abdomen, buttocks, or upper arm. The patch is about the size of a matchbook and delivers a combination of estrogen and progestin through the skin. Each patch is used for 7 days, but contains sufficient hormone for 9 days; then it is removed and discarded. Patches are worn for 3 weeks, followed by a patch-free week to allow menstruation to occur.

Effectiveness

The patch is approximately as effective as birth control pills. It is 99.7% effective when used perfectly; for typical use it has a 91% user effectiveness rate. Some clinicians recommend using another method if the patient weighs over 198 pounds. The patch prevents pregnancy by preventing ovulation, thickening the cervical mucus, and suppressing endometrial growth (Nanda, 2008).

The FDA suggests that women who use or are considering the contraceptive patch work with their health care providers to balance the potential risk related to increased estrogen exposure against the risk of pregnancy (FDA News, 2005). This view would concur with that of researchers who compared the user-effectiveness and cost-effectiveness of the contraceptive patch and the combined oral contraceptive pill. They found both methods to be highly effective in preventing pregnancy with perfect use. Therefore, differences were due to user-effectiveness. The difference was greatest in the youngest age group (15–19 years) for whom the annual probability of pregnancy was 13.1% with combined oral contraceptives and 7.5% for the contraceptive patch. As the age group increased, the probabilities of pregnancy decreased for both methods and the differences between methods also decreased. For example, in the 30–34 age group, the rates were 4.8% and 4.1% for the pill and the patch, respectively. In summary, the researchers view the contraceptive patch as a regimen that holds promise for improving correct use and thus reducing the risk and cost of pregnancy because it requires only 3 weekly applications per month compared with 21 days of active pill taking (Sonnenberg et al., 2005).

Advantages and Disadvantages

This method is comparable to combined pills in menstrual advantages. It adheres well to the skin. The Ortho Evra patch is light colored, which may not be comfortable for women with darker skin tones. Although weight is a restricting factor, age is not. Compliance among teens is good. Disadvantages include breakthrough bleeding and spotting in early use, lack of STI protection, and visibility on the skin. The primary side effects of the patch are headache, nausea, and skin reactions at the application site (Nada, 2008).

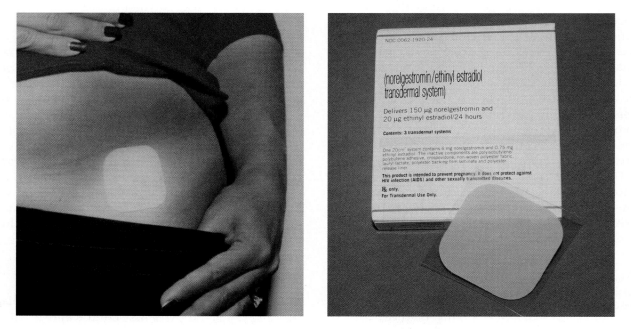

Ortho Evra is the first birth control patch approved by the FDA. Although the patch contains hormones similar to those in combined birth control pills, the patch needs to be changed only once a week, minimizing the margin of error and subsequent decreased effectiveness that is often the case with oral contraceptives.

Injectables

Combined injectables—that is, injectable contraceptives that contain both a progestin and an estrogen—are gaining new attention among family planning clients and providers. Combined formulations are generally injected once a month compared with once every 2 or 3 months for progestin-only injectables such as norethindrone enanthate (NET-EN) and depot-medroxyprogesterone acetate (DMPA/Depo-Provera). Compared with progestin-only injectables, combined injectables disturb vaginal bleeding patterns less and allow earlier return to ovulation after women discontinue use. Although combined injectable contraception has been available worldwide for years, none are currently available in the United States. (The FDA approved Lunelle in 2000, but it is no longer available.) Worldwide, the combined injectable contraceptives are supported by the WHO and other organizations (WHO & Johns Hopkins University, 2011).

Depo-Provera (DMPA)
An injectable progestin-only contraceptive.

Depo-Provera is another form of a progestin-only contraception method. It is a shot that is given every 12 weeks. Depo-Provera suppresses ovulation by inhibiting production of FSH and LH.

Effectiveness

Depo-Provera is even more effective than the pill. In 1 year, only 0.2% of women using Depo-Provera become pregnant. And because it is an injection, there is no chance that a typical user can use it incorrectly, unless she does not return in 3 months for her next shot. Many couples prefer Depo-Provera because its use does not affect the spontaneity of sexual activity.

Reversibility

Fertility may resume immediately after 13 weeks has passed since the last injection. However, studies show that women generally do not conceive for an average of 10 months after the date of the last shot (Zieman et al., 2010). In contrast, women who stop using combined injectables can become pregnant as soon as 6 weeks after their last injection (WHO & Johns Hopkins University, 2011).

Advantages and Disadvantages

Depo-Provera is easy for a woman to use, simply requiring that she return to the clinic every 3 months. It is not used during coitus, and it is one of the most effective methods of preventing pregnancies.

Depo-Provera has few practical disadvantages. Women do need to have injections every 3 months, which may be difficult for some to schedule. Some women report minor weight gain, and many report changes in their periods. Some women have no periods on Depo-Provera; some have frequent bleeding. Spotting between periods is common in the first months of use. Temporary and reversible bone density loss is also associated with Depo-Provera. After discontinuing the medication, bone density returns to normal levels. A major disadvantage to Depo-Provera is that it provides no protection against STIs.

Implants

Implants are small plastic rods or capsules that are inserted into the nondominant upper arm of a woman by her healthcare provider. This contraceptive method helps to greatly reduce the risk of pregnancy by releasing the hormone progestin. Subsequently, the implant works by (1) thickening the cervical mucus, which blocks the sperm from meeting the egg, and (2) disrupting the menstrual cycle and preventing ovulation (WHO & Johns Hopkins University, 2011). Depending on the brand of implant, implants last anywhere from 3 to 7 years. They may be replaced immediately following the end of life of the previous implant. Implants are available under the brand names Implanon, Norplant, Jadelle (Norplant II), and Sino-Implant (II). Currently, Implanon is the only implant available in the United States. It is considered effective for at least 3 years.

Effectiveness

The efficacy rate for implants is less than 1 pregnancy per 100 users per year (5 per 10,000 women). However, some evidence suggests that the effectiveness of some implants decreases for women who weigh more than 150–176 pounds. As with all implants, the risk of pregnancy increases slightly after the first year of use and continues during its lifespan (WHO & Johns Hopkins University, 2011).

Reversibility

Implants are considered a reversible form of birth control, as the woman returns to normal fertility once the implant is removed.

Advantages and Disadvantages

Implants are safe for nearly all women, including women who cannot take estrogen. Irregular bleeding (e.g., between 6 and 12 months) is the primary side effect, but is not harmful. Once the implant is in place, very little maintenance by the user is required. The disadvantages include unpredictable or irregular menstrual bleeding, hormonal side effects (of which headache is most common), and lack of STI protection (WHO & Johns Hopkins University, 2011).

Intrauterine Devices and Systems

Intrauterine devices (IUDs) and **intrauterine systems (IUSs)** are reversible methods of contraception. They are synthetic devices that are inserted by a medical provider into the uterus to prevent pregnancy (Figure 7.5). Currently only one IUD and one IUS are available in the United States. The ParaGard Copper-T 380A is also labeled for use as an emergency contraceptive and can remain in place for 10 years. During that time, women experience regular menstrual cycles that may even involve heavier flow or more cramping than prior to insertion of the IUD. Mirena is a levonorgestrel-releasing intrauterine system (LNG-IUS) introduced in 2000 that is labeled for 5 years of effectiveness. This method reduces or may eliminate menstrual flow over time, although some initial irregular spotting or breakthrough bleeding may occur after insertion of the device (Ramchandran & Salem, 2008).

The intrauterine copper contraceptive works primarily as a spermicide, immobilizing sperm so they rarely reach the fallopian tube, to prevent fertilization. Evidence suggests that IUDs do not work after fertilization. The hormone levonorgestrel in the IUS operates somewhat differently. It causes cervical mucus to thicken so sperm cannot enter the upper reproductive tract to reach an ovum. Changes in uterotubal fluid also restrict sperm movement. Finally, the endometrium is altered to prevent implantation. In the first years of use, this method is also shown to inhibit ovulation in some users (Zieman et al., 2010).

IUDs are a highly effective method of birth control and are a good alternative to hormone-based methods. Although worldwide IUD use has increased steadily, use in the United States rapidly declined as IUD-related product liability litigation peaked in the 1980s. This concern was compounded by the perceived risk of pelvic inflammatory disease. Recent studies confirm the safety and efficacy of IUDs for the great majority of women (Doyle et al., 2008). Misperceptions about potential infertility also help explain the low U.S. rates of IUD use in general and particularly among women who have never had children. Nevertheless, well-designed studies have found that former IUD users are no more likely than other women to be infertile (WHO & Johns Hopkins University, 2011). Additionally, 72% to 96% of women conceived within 1 year of having their IUD removed; this rate is comparable to levels among women who never used contraception (85%) (Ramchandran & Salem, 2008).

Effectiveness

The IUD/IUS is one of the most effective contraceptive methods. Because compliance is not an issue, actual-use efficacy and perfect-use efficacy are nearly the same. For the ParaGard IUD with copper, the pregnancy rate has been less than 1 pregnancy per 100 women each year. The Mirena IUS, which contains the progestin levonorgestrel, has contraceptive efficacy comparable to female sterilization (0.01%).

> **intrauterine device (IUD)**
> Synthetic device that is inserted into the uterus to prevent the sperm from fertilizing the ovum.
>
> **intrauterine system (IUS)**
> Synthetic device placed in the uterus that releases a continuous amount of hormone (levonorgestrel) to prevent ovulation, fertilization, or implantation.

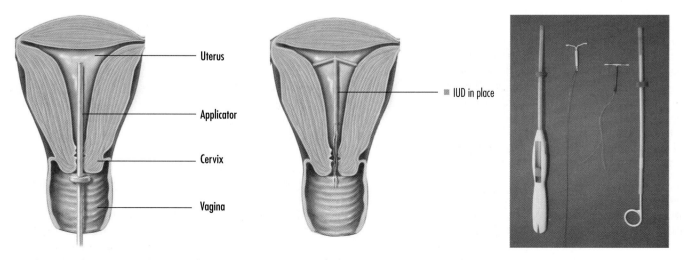

Uterus

Applicator

Cervix

Vagina

IUD in place

FIGURE **7.5** The IUD is inserted past the cervix into the uterus. Before insertion, the length of the uterus is measured with an instrument called a *sound*. Upon insertion, the arms of the IUD gradually unfold. Once the inserter is removed, the threads attached to the IUD are clipped to extend into the vagina through the cervical opening.

In addition to preventing pregnancy in general, the progestin-releasing system (Mirena or LGN-IUS) reduces the chances of ectopic pregnancy, which is the leading cause of pregnancy-related death (Doyle et al., 2008). Women are advised to check the strings to assure the IUD/IUS is still in place; not doing so accounts for the minor difference in effectiveness rates.

Reversibility

Once the IUD/IUS is removed, fertility resumes immediately. Compared to possible detrimental effects of various hormonal contraceptives (oral contraceptives, implants, injectables) on subsequent fertility, the use of LNG-IUS does not affect conception rate; all users in one study conceived within 1 month of discontinuation of the IUS (Backman et al., 2004).

Advantages and Disadvantages

The IUD/IUS is an excellent method for most women. In addition to being highly effective, it is easy to use and has no systemic side effects.

A major advantage of the IUD/IUS is that once inserted it remains in place, so planning before intercourse is unnecessary. (When it is in place, a string attached to the IUD/IUS emerges through the cervix. The woman feels for the string to make sure the IUD/IUS is present, because it is possible for it to pass out of the uterus with the menstrual flow or at other times. The device can also be removed by a physician by means of this string.) Other advantages of the IUD include probable protection against endometrial cancer and possible protection against cervical cancer, its availability for women who cannot use hormonal

methods, and use as an EC. Both the IUD and the IUS offer a rapid return to fertility, convenience as a single insertion that provides 5–10 years of protection depending on the type, cost-effectiveness in terms of the greatest net benefit of any contraceptive if used for more than 2 years, and high level of user satisfaction.

In terms of disadvantages, the copper Para-Gard IUD may cause increased monthly blood loss (menorrhagia) and possibly anemia due to lowered hemoglobin levels in some users. Conversely, the progestin-delivering Mirena (LNG-IUS) actually increases hemoglobin levels over the years of usage by reducing or eliminating menstrual flow (amenorrhea). This method requires an office procedure for both insertion and removal; both can be uncomfortable. Some protocols recommend a chlamydia/gonorrhea check before insertion, as these STIs could lead to the development of pelvic inflammatory disease (PID) as a consequence of the insertion process. This contraceptive method offers no protection from HIV or other STIs. Expulsion of the device, either obviously with cramping or bleeding, or silently without the user's awareness, places the woman at risk for pregnancy (Zieman et al., 2010). The likelihood of expulsion declines over time, but women who have expelled one IUD have about a one in three chance of expelling another (Doyle et al., 2008).

Women who receive extensive counseling on the possibilities of amenorrhea and bleeding problems, occurrence of PID, hormonal adverse effects, and expulsion of the device and risk of pregnancy are significantly more likely to be very satisfied with this method. Modest weight gain could be viewed as a hormonal effect, except that women not using contraception experience virtually the same weight gain (Inki, 2007).

Diaphragm

When in place, the **diaphragm** prevents the sperm from traveling through the uterus and up the fallopian tubes to fertilize an egg, and it holds spermicide against the cervix (Figure 7.6). The diaphragm is a shallow rubber, or synthetic rubber, cap surrounding a flexible metal ring that covers the cervix.

> **diaphragm**
> Shallow rubber cap that covers the cervix and prevents sperm from entering the uterus.

Diaphragms are available in several sizes and styles. Because the diaphragm's purpose is to prevent sperm from going beyond the vagina, its size and shape are very important. If the diaphragm does not fit exactly right, a chance exists that sperm can

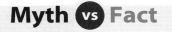

Myth (vs) Fact

Myth: Providing birth control to young people encourages them to have sexual relationships.
Fact: There are no studies that indicate that young people who have access to family-planning methods are more likely to have sexual intercourse. They are more likely to use contraception.

Myth: You can borrow a friend's diaphragm in a pinch.
Fact: Diaphragms are fitted to an individual woman. You cannot borrow another woman's diaphragm.

Myth: If you roll on the condom the wrong way, reverse it and put it on the right way.
Fact: Microscopic tears can occur when you roll on a condom. Throw it out and start with a new one.

Myth: There is nothing you can do but hope and pray if you forget to use your method.
Fact: If you forget to use a method, there is emergency contraception available. It must be used within 120 hours (5 days) of the act of unprotected penile–vaginal sex. Visit a pharmacy or call your healthcare provider.

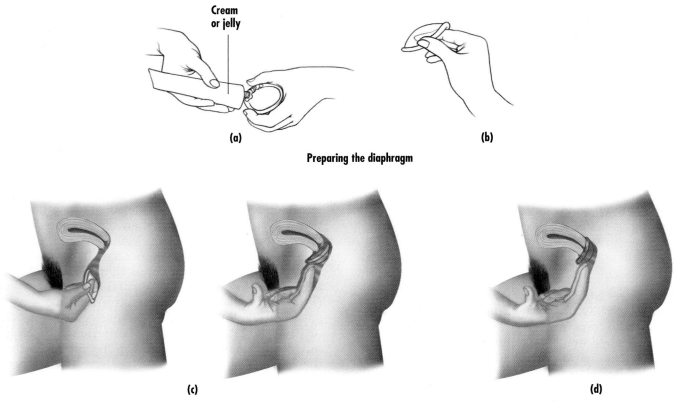

FIGURE **7.6** Procedure for inserting a diaphragm: (a) Before inserting the diaphragm, coat the rim and cup with a spermicidal cream or jelly. (b) Squeeze the rim of the diaphragm together between your thumb and index finger. (c) Insert the diaphragm into the vagina with the rim facing up and push it toward the small of your back. As you let go of the diaphragm, it will spring open. Continue to guide it to your cervix with the tips of your fingers. (d) Be sure to check that the diaphragm completely covers the cervix.

bypass this barrier. Clearly, using someone else's diaphragm is a poor idea. Diaphragms are fitted by a clinician and refitted after women give birth or gain or lose a significant amount of weight. Fit should also be checked during the yearly gynecological exam, and the diaphragm should be replaced every 2 years or with any signs of wear or damage.

The diaphragm must remain in place for at least 6 hours after intercourse, and spermicide must be added for *each* act of intercourse. This combination of requirements, besides increasing effectiveness, allows the male and female to share the responsibility for contraception. (Diaphragms should be removed at least once every 24 hours to reduce the risk of toxic shock syndrome.)

Effectiveness

When inserted properly and used with spermicide, the diaphragm is theoretically 94% effective and 88% effective as actually used. The contraceptive effectiveness of diaphrams without a spermicide containing nonoxynol-9 (N-9) has been insufficiently studied. However, this combination should be assumed to

A diaphragm is a barrier method of contraception that can be used repeatedly with spermicidal cream or jelly. It requires a physician to fit the diaphragm initially.

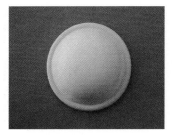

decrease effectiveness. Women infected with or at high risk for HIV, however, should *not* use spermicides containing N-9. Conversely, routine use of N-9 by women not at high risk of HIV does not pose any known increased risk (WHO & Johns Hopkins University, 2011; Zieman et al., 2010).

Reversibility

The diaphragm does not affect fertility (except when it is in place).

Advantages and Disadvantages

The major advantages of the diaphragm are that it is highly effective if used correctly and consistently, is easy to learn to use, and has no systemic side effects unless latex allergy is involved. Some couples make diaphragm insertion part of foreplay. The man can insert it into the woman's vagina before penile–vaginal sex.

One disadvantage of the diaphragm is that it must be inserted before penile–vaginal sex and inserted properly, requiring the woman or couple to plan ahead. Some women are not comfortable touching their genitals and therefore find diaphragm use uncomfortable. Diaphragms provide only limited protection against certain STIs, so condoms must also be used to prevent STI transmission. In addition, some users may experience an increased risk of urinary tract infections. Oil-based lubricants should not be used with diaphragms as they erode the rubber. Odor may develop if the diaphragm is left in place for more than 24 hours. Severe arthritis or obesity may make insertion or removal difficult. A reaction to latex or superficial cervical erosion may cause vaginal spotting or discomfort in some women (Zieman et al., 2010).

Cervical Cap

The **cervical cap** is a silicone rubber, latex-free, dome-shaped device that covers the cervix and holds spermicidal cream or jelly. It is similar to, but smaller than, the diaphragm; is meant to stay in place longer; and is slightly less effective than the diaphragm (Figure 7.7). In 1988, the FDA approved the sale of cervical caps in the United States, although they have been used in Europe for decades. Currently, the FemCap is available through Planned Parenthood, in the United States.

> **cervical cap**
> Shallow silicone rubber device, smaller than a diaphragm, that covers the cervix to prevent sperm from entering the uterus.

The cervical cap can be left in place for 48 hours. However, it must be removed during menstruation to allow the menstrual flow to leave the body.

Although the cap is available in three different sizes, not all women can use it because of the variation in shapes and sizes of cervixes.

Effectiveness
Overall, the cervical cap and the diaphragm have similar rates of effectiveness. Theoretical effectiveness of the cervical cap ranges from 91% to 74%. The cap is much more effective in women who have never been pregnant (nulliparous women). User effectiveness for the cap is 84% for nulliparous women compared to only 68% in women who have been pregnant. In nonmonogamous couples, condoms should also be used to prevent STI transmission. The same precautions and uncertainties regarding the use of N-9 apply to cervical caps (Zieman et al., 2010).

Reversibility
The cap does not affect fertility (except when it is in place).

Advantages and Disadvantages
The cap is easy to use and has no systemic side effects unless spermicide sensitivity is present. Many women like the fact that it can be kept in place for up to 48 hours and that spermicide use for additional acts of intercourse is optional.

There are also disadvantages associated with use of the cap. The cervical cap may occasionally irritate the cervix, may cause an unpleasant odor or vaginal dryness, and has the potential for becoming dislodged during coitus. It can also cause toxic shock syndrome if it is not removed regularly.

Combined Vaginal Ring

The NuvaRing provides protection from pregnancy by emiting ethinyl estradiol (the estrogen component) and etonogestrel (the progestin component) daily for 21 days. In contrast, low-dose estrogen contraceptive pills contain slightly more estrogen, and other contraceptive pills contain almost twice as much estrogen. Additionally, with oral contraceptives, there is a daily spike in hormone levels when the pill is swallowed, followed by a gradual drop throughout the day. In contrast, the ring provides a steady rate of hormone release. Whereas the diaphragm and cervical cap must be positioned correctly to provide maximal protection, NuvaRing cannot be inserted incorrectly. Also, it comes with a timer to use as a reminder of when it needs to be replaced. Even if it is not removed immediately, protection remains for 35 days.

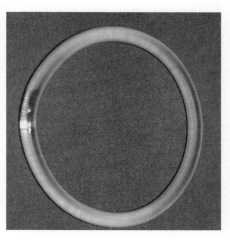

NuvaRing is a flexible, transparent, odorless ring that is about as big as a silver dollar and is inserted into the vagina, where it continuously releases low doses of estrogen and progestin that prevent pregnancy. Heralded for its convenience, NuvaRing leaves even less room for error than the contraceptive patch.

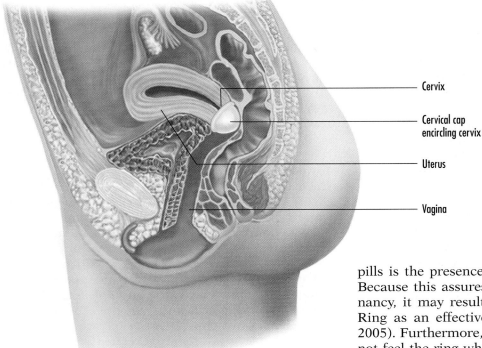

Cervix

Cervical cap
encircling cervix

Uterus

Vagina

FIGURE 7.7 It is important that your cervical cap is always inserted correctly. You should practice inserting before using the cap during penile–vaginal sex.

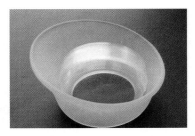

The FemCap is available in three sizes based on pregnancy and birthing history.

NuvaRing costs approximately the same as a cycle of pills in pharmacies and requires a prescription to be purchased.

Effectiveness

NuvaRing is an effective hormonal contraceptive with many advantages. It has a theoretical or perfect-use effectiveness rate of 99.7%. Because once it is in place there is nothing else to do (contrasted, for example, with oral contraceptives, which require remembering to take a pill), effectiveness is greatly enhanced. User effectiveness is not yet established but is expected to be approximately 91% (Trussell, 2011).

Reversibility

Fertility is not affected after NuvaRing is removed.

Advantages and Disadvantages

NuvaRing contains the lowest serum levels of estrogen and progestin in any combined hormonal method, thereby decreasing the risks associated with synthetic estrogens. In addition, the ring does not require any daily action, as does taking a pill each day. All that is required is replacement of the ring after 21 days or 1 month. With this method, privacy is maintained; there is no visible patch or pill package. Another advantage compared to combined oral contraceptive

pills is the presence of regular withdrawal bleeding. Because this assures women of the absence of pregnancy, it may result in greater acceptance of Nuva-Ring as an effective contraceptive method (Sarkar, 2005). Furthermore, the vast majority of women cannot feel the ring when it is in place and report being satisfied with this method of contraception.

As with all methods of contraception, there are also disadvantages associated with NuvaRing. The risk of synthetic estrogen is not eliminated; it is merely reduced. Therefore, as advised by the manufacturer, smokers and those susceptible to blood clots should not use the ring. Other side effects, such as nausea and headache, are similar to the combined pills. Vaginal discomfort and vaginitis may also occur. Partners may feel the ring during penetration, although most reported they did not perceive that to be a problem. If necessary, it can be removed for up to 3 hours without losing its effectiveness. Another disadvantage of the ring for women who are uncomfortable touching their genitalia is the need for the user to insert it manually through the vagina. These women may prefer another contraceptive method that does not entail touching the genitalia. In addition, NuvaRing does not offer any protection against STIs (Zieman et al., 2010).

■ Permanent Methods

Sterilization

Sterilization is a form of contraception that renders a person biologically incapable of reproducing. Men and women both may choose to be sterilized—made infertile—because they have all the children they

> **sterilization**
> A procedure that makes a person biologically incapable of reproducing.

want or because they do not want to have children. Women in ill health, perhaps those with serious heart conditions, may choose to prevent life-threatening pregnancies and births. Couples may choose not to have children if their genetic makeup, when passed to their offspring, would be likely to result in birth defects (for example, sickle-cell anemia or Tay-Sachs disease).

Individual methods of sterilization for men and women are described shortly. Contraceptive choices vary markedly with age. By age 35, more women rely on sterilization than on the pill. Of all women aged 40–44 who practice contraception, 50% have been sterilized and another 18% have a partner who has had a vasectomy. If both male (9.2%) and female (27%) sterilization percentages are combined, then sterilization (36.2%) exceeds oral contraceptives (30%) as the leading contraceptive method of choice (Guttmacher, 2008).

Effectiveness

Male and female sterilization is highly effective. In the first year after sterilization, only 1 woman out of every 1,000 sterilized becomes pregnant, and only 1 in every 2,000 sterilized men causes a pregnancy.

Reversibility

Both men and women should consider sterilization procedures as permanent and irreversible. Thoughtful consideration should be given before undergoing any sterilization procedure. Even with counseling, some individuals may experience regret due to a change in life circumstances or other reason. Microsurgical techniques can be used to reverse male and female sterilization procedures with varying levels of success. For men, a **vasovasectomy** can result in a return of sperm to ejaculate in 75–100% of men, but the pregnancy rate ranges from 35–89%. Reversibility rates decrease as time since the procedure increases, especially after 10 years. Other factors affecting reversal are the skill of the microsurgeon, the presence of antisperm antibodies (man), the partner's fertility, and the type of vasectomy performed (Pollack, Thomas, & Barone, 2008). More recently, microsurgery is being used to reverse laparoscopy; original studies showed wide ranges of success, but more recent studies report a pregnancy rate of around 70%, with one study having an ongoing pregnancy rate of 59% and another having a birth rate of 62%. In all cases, the female's age played a critical role in the ability to become pregnant (Caillet et al., 2010; Gordts et al., 2009; Schepens et al., 2011).

> **vasovasectomy**
> Reversal of a vasectomy, so that sperm can be ejaculated.

Advantages and Disadvantages

Sterilization is only for people who are certain that they do not want more children and who are fertile. Both female and male sterilizations have the same advantages. They are permanent, highly effective (99.9%), are cost-effective, lack side effects, do not interfere with intercourse, and are very safe. Their primary disadvantage is they provide no protection against STIs.

Male Sterilization

In men, sterilization entails interruption of the vas deferens in a procedure called a **vasectomy** (Figure 7.8). Vasectomy became popular as a method of contraception in the late 1960s and early 1970s. The interest in vasectomy was a result of several factors, including concern about the health hazards of the oral contraceptive and extensive promotion by several national organizations (Association for Voluntary Sterilization, Planned Parenthood Federation of America, and Zero Population Growth). In addition, the medical community announced its support for vasectomy as a contraceptive method that was safe and effective.

> **vasectomy**
> Cutting or cauterizing of the vas deferens to prevent sperm from being ejaculated; a means of sterilization.

Despite acceptance among the medical community, vasectomy continues to be an underused method. Only about 500,000 vasectomies are performed annually in the United States (Eisenberg et al., 2009). Low-income and minority men are less likely to receive a vasectomy. By recognizing these underserved groups, providers may be able to reduce the large difference in utilization, which could help close the gap between male and female sterilization rates (Eisenberg et al., 2009).

Vasectomy is a simple, minor surgical procedure that takes about 30 minutes. A small opening is made in the scrotum, and the vas deferens is severed. This severing blocks sperm from entering the ejaculate, because it has no route out of the testes. Clips and plugs can also be used to interfere with the vas deferens passageway; the most widely used technique involves cutting the vas and sealing off its ends (by suturing or cauterization). Vasectomies are done under local anesthesia and require minimal care afterward. Vasectomized men are instructed to avoid hard work or strenuous exercise for several days, to wear a scrotal support for a week, and to apply ice and take mild painkillers for postoperative discomfort. As soon as the man feels ready, he may resume sexual intercourse.

FIGURE **7.8** Vasectomy.

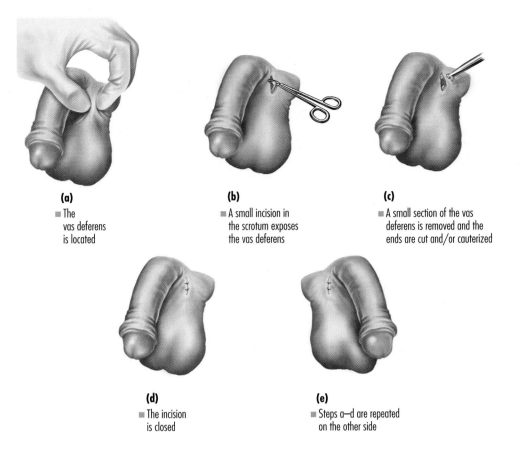

(a)
- The vas deferens is located

(b)
- A small incision in the scrotum exposes the vas deferens

(c)
- A small section of the vas deferens is removed and the ends are cut and/or cauterized

(d)
- The incision is closed

(e)
- Steps a–d are repeated on the other side

Unlike female sterilization, a vasectomy does not provide immediate infertility. Sperm may still be stored in the urethra or elsewhere in the reproductive tract and may not be expelled for 10 weeks or more. The amount of time required to expel this sperm depends partly on the frequency of ejaculation. For this reason, men are asked to return to the physician twice after the vasectomy with a semen specimen to be tested for the presence of motile sperm. Until the absence of sperm is verified, a condom, diaphragm, or other method of contraception is required to prevent conception. Usually two consecutive negative sperm analysis results are required before a backup method of contraception is no longer necessary.

Female Sterilization

Female sterilization takes several forms; the goal is to prevent the egg from moving down the fallopian tube to be fertilized by a sperm. Currently, most female sterilization procedures involve tubal ligation, in which the woman's fallopian tubes are surgically cut or blocked by applying clips, rings, or heat. The two most common surgical approaches are the minilaparotomy and laparoscopy. These approaches require skilled medical professionals and sterile conditions. Local or general anesthesia is also required. The newer approaches not involving surgery can increase access to sterilization (Pollack et al., 2008).

A recent approach to transcervical sterilization called Essure is a nonsurgical method using a spring-like device (microcoil) inserted through the uterus into each fallopian tube. This causes gradual tubal blockage over a 3-month period by encouraging local scar tissue growth with polyesther (PET) fibers. At 5 years, effectiveness is 99.74%. However, Essure is unlikely to be introduced in developing countries soon because of the high cost and complexity of the insertion instruments (WHO & Johns Hopkins University, 2011; Zieman et al., 2010).

Minilaparotomy

A **minilaparotomy**, sometimes called a *minilap*, requires a small incision just above the pubic hairline. An instrument is then inserted into the cervix to move the uterus and pull each fallopian tube into

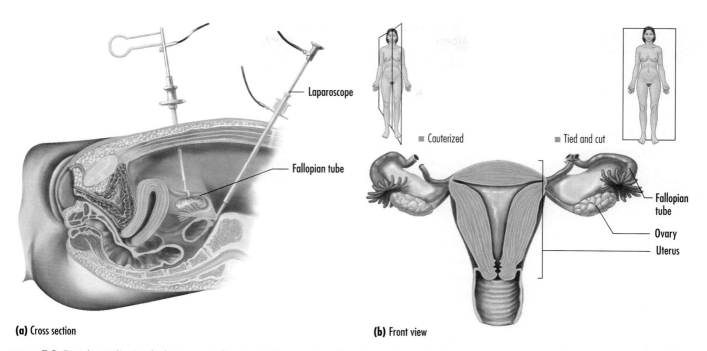

(a) Cross section

Laparoscope

Fallopian tube

Cauterized

Tied and cut

Fallopian tube

Ovary

Uterus

(b) Front view

FIGURE **7.9** Female sterilization by laparoscopic ligation. (a) Cross section: The tubes are located using a laparoscope and cut, tied, or cauterized through a second incision. (b) Front view: The tubes after ligation.

the incision. Part of the tube is taken out of the incision, where it is blocked by **ligation**, clips, or rings, and then replaced in the abdomen. This procedure takes about 20 minutes, and the woman can usually leave the medical setting in 2 or 3 hours. Because the incision is very small (about 3 cm), few complications develop.

Laparoscopy

A **laparoscopy** involves inserting into the abdomen a narrow stainless steel tube with fiber-optic cylinders that transmit light (Figure 7.9). This tube is called a *laparoscope*. Two types of laparoscopes can be used. With one, the physician can insert forceps and other instruments through the tube itself; therefore, only one incision is necessary. With the other type of laparoscope, two incisions are required because the tube does not permit other instruments to be inserted through it. Ligation by electrocoagulation (high-frequency electrical current) or application of clips or rings can take

> **minilaparotomy**
> Female sterilization procedure that involves a small incision in the abdomen through which the fallopian tubes are pulled so they can be blocked.
>
> **ligation**
> The tying of the fallopian tubes to prevent the sperm–egg union.
>
> **laparoscopy**
> Female sterilization procedure that involves inserting a narrow viewing instrument—a laparoscope—through an incision in the abdomen and then performing ligation or applying clips or rings to block the fallopian tubes.

place during this procedure to prevent the passage of the egg.

Transcervical Methods

Other sterilization techniques that do not involve surgery have recently been developed. These techniques permanently prevent pregnancy by blocking the fallopian tubes through the vagina and the uterus. In addition to Essure, another nonsurgical method is the Adiana procedure, which involves implanting a porous plastic matrix into a superficial lesion in each fallopian tube to block the tube. Both Adiana and Essure require skilled use of an expensive hysteroscope for insertion and follow-up X ray or ultrasound imaging 3 months after insertion (Hologic, 2010; Zieman et al., 2010).

Reversibility

As with male sterilization, female sterilization should generally be considered irreversible. As previously discussed, surgical techniques can be successful in opening up the fallopian tubes, highly skilled surgeons and modern microsurgical equipment are required and are very costly. Therefore, women seeking sterilization must expect it to be permanent because reversal is costly and failure rates are high. In vitro fertilization may be possible but many cannot afford this procedure and it is not always successful (Zieman et al., 2010).

Global DIMENSIONS

Emergency Contraception: How Is NorLevo in France Different from Plan B in the United States?

NorLevo is the same postcoital pill as Plan B. Each is a progestin-only emergency contraceptive. Introduction of NorLevo in France in 1999 led quickly to a change in the country's constitution; by 2002 NorLevo could be distributed free in middle and high schools. Minors can also obtain NorLevo free of charge in pharmacies without parental consent. Adult women can be reimbursed up to 65% of the cost of NorLevo by insurance. No adverse effects of NorLevo have been reported. The interest in emergency contraception has created "more open discussion among pharmacists, nurses in schools, and across all society about what to do to prevent pregnancy and sexually transmitted disease" (Boonstra, 2002).

Contrast the above picture with the Plan B story in the United States. Approved at the end of the 1990s, it took almost 20 years to have Plan B available without a prescription for those 17 and older. State laws have needed to be enacted to require pharmacies and pharmacists to distribute EC medication. Less than half the states require information about EC to be presented to sexual assault survivors in emergency rooms, and even fewer are required to dispense it if requested by a patient (Guttmacher Institute, 2012). No high schools or middle schools give it to students. As an over-the-counter medication, Plan B can cost anywhere from $35 to $60 (Office of Population Research & Association of Reproductive Health Professionals, 2011a). The hoops women must jump through to obtain Plan B increase the time from unprotected sex until Plan B is taken or lead to it not being used at all. In contrast to France, where discussion of emergency contraception has fostered increased discussion (and presumably use) of other contraceptives, controversy over emergency contraceptive pills has fueled debate over how pills, minipills, and Depo-Provera injections work, jeopardizing the availability of these traditional contraceptives in some places.

The result? Pregnancy rates in U.S. teens are almost three times higher than teens in France (71.5 versus 25.7 per 1,000 teens), and teen birth rates are four times higher (39.1 versus 7.1 per 1,000 teens) (Advocates for Youth, 2011).

What is wrong with this picture? What seems to underscore the differences in how the United States and France approach teen sexuality—specifically, how they approach sexual activity in teenagers—is the word "responsibility."

Parents, teachers, and community leaders in France and throughout Europe seem to be able to express the sentiment: "A teenager who is having intercourse must be responsible about this potentially dangerous activity."

Why is it that we can say to a 20-year-old who is drinking illegally: "If you drink, don't drive." Or a parent can say to his or her child: "If you drink, call me and I'll come get you."

So NorLevo and Plan B are exactly the same drug, but France and the United States are as different as night and day in the access women have to this drug.

Source: Data from Hatcher, R. A., Zieman, M., et al. *A pocket guide to managing contraception.* Tiger, GA: Bridging the Gap Foundation, (2004), 74.

The Future of Contraceptives

Research to find better methods of contraception continues. The perfect method of contraception, which will probably never exist, would:

1. Be 100% effective
2. Be very inexpensive (or even free)
3. Have no side effects
4. Be reversible
5. Involve no remembering to do something
6. Be convenient (not messy)
7. Prevent STIs
8. Be religiously and morally acceptable
9. Not interrupt sexual behaviors

During the 2000s, several new methods were approved for use in the United States. These included two different nonlatex male condoms, an improved female condom, Implanon, the patch, the vaginal ring, long-lasting emergency contraceptive pills, extended oral contraceptives, and new methods of female sterilization. However, some new methods and some of the old standbys were removed from the market. It seems the driving influence behind business decisions to withdraw a product are based on costs—profit and loss—rather than a product's safety and efficacy. It would be ideal if there was a way for useful methods to still be made available after a manufacturer decides they are no longer a profit maker.

The contraceptive methods now being researched include the following:

1. *Male contraceptive methods:* Most male contraceptive development is focused on blocking hormones. Interfering with the development or transport of sperm has been investigated, but no efforts have been successful, and many of the substances used have been toxic (Nieschlag, 2010). Adjusting testosterone levels is complicated because of the side effects of testosterone on males (Gabelnick, Schwartz, & Darroch, 2008). Some researchers are examining synthetic steroids that resemble testosterone but that protect the prostate; the largest successful study used one such product, testosterone undecanoate, as a monthly injection. Though successful, the frequency of the injections was considered burdensome. Some believe that male contraceptive use is not supported by the pharmaceutical companies; without their support, new methods will not developed quickly (Nieschlag, 2010).

2. *New types and new uses of vaginal rings:* Some research organizations are examining how vaginal rings could be used as emergency contraception (Population Council, 2011a). Vaginal rings could act as dual-protections systems, protecting against sexually transmitted HIV in addition to pregnancy (Friend, 2010).

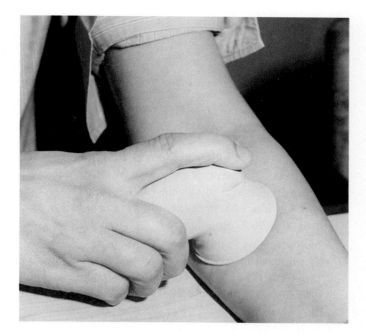

Spray-on contraception is a new way to supply a preset dose of hormones.

3. *Transdermal spray:* Researchers in the United States and Australia have developed a spray-on contraceptive that contains a progestin called Nesterone. The spray-on approach is a new technique for transferring a preset dose of fast-drying hormones onto the skin where it is almost instantly absorbed. It slowly diffuses into the bloodstream over a 24-hour period. Advantages include lower or equivalent cost compared to other hormone-based methods, as well as being easy, convenient, and discreet to use. If estradiol (a form of estrogen) is added to the hormone formulation, this would be the first non-oral contraceptive delivering natural estradiol, which would reduce the risk of blood clots by four times compared to oral delivery (Population Council, 2011b).

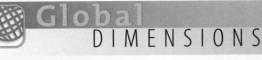

DIMENSIONS

Unmet Need for Contraception in Developing Countries

What is unmet need?

If a woman is not using any method of contraception, either modern or traditional, she has unmet need if she is married and in a consensual union, or never married and sexually active; able to become pregnant; and does not want a child in the next 2 years or wants to stop childbearing.

How extensive is unmet need?

- In 53 developing countries surveyed, 15% of married women aged 15–49 had unmet need for contraception, and 7% of never-married women in 36 countries had unmet need.

- Approximately 71 million married women are at risk of an unplanned pregnancy in 53 countries, as are 4.2 million never-married women in 36 countries. Without access to contraceptive services and supplies, millions of these women will become pregnant unintentionally each year.

- Unmet need in sub-Saharan Africa declined less than 10% between 1990–1995 and 2000–2005. By contrast, unmet need declined by a third or more in the other three regions surveyed.

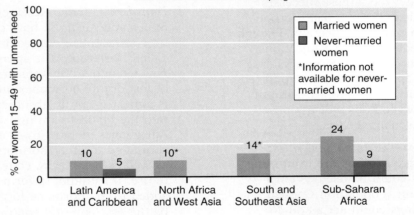

Unmet need for contraception is higher in sub-Saharan Africa than elsewhere in the developing world.

![Global] DIMENSIONS

Unmet Need for Contraception in Developing Countries—cont'd

- In most developing countries, women who are rural, uneducated, poor, and married are more likely to be at risk for unplanned pregnancies than are urban, educated, or nonpoor married women. In sub-Saharan Africa, however, there is no single pattern of unmet need.
- In many countries, women who have had more than three children tend to have higher levels of unmet need as compared to women who have never had a child or who have had one to three children.
- Variations in unmet need reflect patterns of social and economic development. Women who are urban and nonpoor are the first to want smaller families and have unmet need. Eventually, this desire extends to rural and poor women as well, increasing their unmet need.

Why do women not use or discontinue using contraceptives?

- The most prevalent reason is that women do not believe they are at risk of becoming pregnant.
- Lack of access and concerns about methods account for a third of the nonuse.
- Among never-married women, infrequent sexual activity and belief they should be married before seeking contraception accounts for nonuse and discontinuation.

Who are the women with unmet need?

Recommendations for meeting unmet need:

- Focus on places where the gap between fertility desires and contraceptive practice is greatest—many countries in sub-Saharan Africa.
- Enhance effectiveness by including counseling and education to clarify issues of health and side effects.
- Ensure as many options are available as possible; help women match their method with their needs.
- Improve both contraceptive technologies and access to them.
- Promote societal receptivity to contraceptive use to help women overcome cultural and social barriers to achieving their desired family size.

Source: Data from *Facts about unmet need for contraception in developing countries: Guttmacher Institute in brief,* May 2007; data from Sedgh, G., Hussain, R., Bankole, A., & Singh, S. Women with an unmet need for contraception in developing countries and their reasons for not using a method. *Occasional Report, 37.* New York: Guttmacher Institute, 2007.

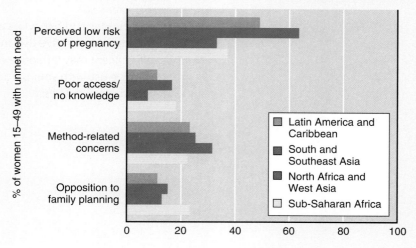

Many are not using a method because they think they will not get pregnant or they are concerned about health or side effects.

Exploring the Dimensions of Human Sexuality

Our feelings, attitudes, and beliefs regarding sexuality are influenced by our internal and external environments. Go to go.jblearning.com/dimensions5e to learn more about the biological, psychological, and sociological factors that affect your sexuality.

Case Study

When choosing a method of contraception, you must consider the effectiveness, side effects, convenience, cost, and protection from STIs and HIV. However, your partner's willingness to use the same method also comes into play, because contraceptives are ineffective if not used properly over time.

Many factors influence your contraceptive use. Legally, the federal government regulates which contraceptives you can buy in the United States. Socioeconomic status also is a factor, because most contraceptives are neither free nor covered by all types of health insurance. Also, people of higher socioeconomic status have greater access to prescription contraceptive methods and are more likely to receive more education about contraceptive methods.

Religion also plays a role in contraceptive choice, because some religions only officially sanction natural family-planning methods. Communication skills also are involved as you negotiate your contraceptive use with a partner.

Biological Factors

- Gender may affect contraceptive decision making. Males have only the option of condoms or vasectomy available; women have to deal with the fact that only they can become pregnant.
- STIs and HIV can be prevented only through strict use of latex, polyurethane or polyisoprene condoms, abstinence, or 100% monogamy.
- Natural family planning relies on using physiological cycles and changes to monitor ovulation.
- Hormones such as estrogen and progesterone prevent the pituitary gland from producing FSH, without which the ova do not develop in the ovaries.

Sociocultural Factors

- Socioeconomic status affects contraceptive availability and use.
- Laws and government regulations limit contraceptive approval and availability.
- Religion affects contraceptive decisions, limiting some couples to natural family planning.
- Media and ad information can affect both contraceptive choice and brand choice.

Psychological Factors

- Experience may determine the contraceptive you choose.
- Emotions often get in the way of practicing contraceptives and safer sex.
- Learned attitudes and behaviors affect your willingness to negotiate contraceptive use and practice safer sex.
- Your self-concept may influence whether you negotiate contraceptive use with your partner or simply accept what your partner desires.

Summary

- Contraception is used to avoid unplanned pregnancy. User motivation accounts for much of the variability in the effectiveness of different methods.

- Perfect use of a contraceptive method reflects the number of pregnancies likely to occur among 100 women in a year's time if the method is always used consistently and correctly. Often typical use effectiveness is less because of human error.

- Except for abstaining from oral, penile–vaginal, and anal sex, condom use (male or female) is the only readily available and widely used contraceptive method that protects against sexually transmitted infections (STIs).

- Of the nonprescription methods, both abstinence and withdrawal are free, always available, and theoretically easy to use with no side effects. However, in practice, both methods have low effectiveness because intentions and practice don't always match.

- More than 100 brands of male condoms are available. All materials protect against pregnancy if used consistently and correctly; latex, polyurethane, and polyisoprene protect against many STIs, but lambskin condoms do not. Female condoms, made of synthetic rubber, are more costly.

- The vaginal contraceptive sponge and spermicides in the form of gels, foams, films, and inserts all use Nonoxynol-9; the FDA has mandated a warning label that this spermicide does not protect against HIV or other STIs and may actually increase risk among susceptable women.

- Fertility awareness methods depend on tracking a woman's fertile time using the calendar, basal body temperature, cervical secretions, cycle beads, or combinations; effectiveness can be high but requires careful record keeping.

- Prescription methods are for females; they include combination oral contraceptive pills containing both estrogen and progestin to suppress ovulation and mimic pregnancy, progestin-only pills, and other mechanisms to deliver hormones such as the patch, injections, implants, and vaginal rings.

- Emergency contraceptive pills may be used effectively (up to 120 hours or 5 days) after intercourse to prevent pregnancy. None of the current methods is an abortifacient, and none disturbs an implanted pregnancy. Plan B is available in the United States over the counter to those 17 and over and in some states to anyone; a generic version is also available. ella is available with prescription.

- Intrauterine devices are highly effective and reversible. The ParaGard IUD can be used for EC and then can remain in place for up to 10 years; the Mirena IUS delivers a hormone that reduces or eliminates menstrual flow and is effective for up to 5 years.

- Diaphragms and cervical caps are barrier methods that are clinically fitted to cover a woman's cervix and used in combination with a spermicide to prevent sperm from entering the uterus.

- Sterilization for males and females is a permanent method of contraception that is almost 100% effective and widely used among adults over age 35 who are fertile but certain they do not want more children.

Discussion Questions

1. List six key considerations in choosing a contraceptive method, and rank their relative importance. Which method did you use to rank their importance?

2. Describe the nonprescription methods of contraception. Discuss the relationship issues that affect the choice of these methods.

3. Describe the methods of contraception requiring prescriptions. Which types of information should be disclosed to a doctor when making a selection?

4. Discuss the varied methods of female and male sterilization. Should the possibility of reversibility be part of the decision process?

Application Questions

Reread the chapter-opening story and answer the following questions.

1. Discuss how Susan altered her contraception use in light of her changing lifestyle. Which other contraceptive methods could she have used at each point? Which suggestions would you have for her?

2. If Susan had a family history of diabetes, high blood pressure, or breast cancer, how would her choices of contraceptive be altered?

3. Consider Stephen's decision to have a vasectomy. Although it may have seemed the perfect method for him at the time—married, monogamous, finished with childbearing—it also leaves him without the ability to father more children, should he remarry. In light of this, should men routinely postpone sterilization until a later age—just in case? Or should they have sperm frozen for the future?

Critical Thinking Questions

1. Assume that you began a relationship with a partner who wanted to use natural family planning because of religious convictions. What advantages and disadvantages would that hold for you from a contraceptive and safer sex standpoint? Answer this question from both male and female viewpoints.

2. The prescription methods of birth control are all female based. What role, if any, should the male partner have in the decision to use these methods?

Critical Thinking Case

Ben and Allie, both age 25 years, had been dating for 6 months and using latex condoms as their contraception method. Because their relationship was monogamous and increasingly dedicated, they had talked about switching to a different method but had never taken the time to discuss the options and how they would fit their lifestyle.

Then one evening, a condom broke. Allie pulled out the calendar on which she mapped her period, but the news was bad: It was right around the time of ovulation. Although committed to one another, they were not prepared to face the possibility of parenthood.

First consider what Allie and Ben should do immediately. Then outline some options for the couple's future, so that they do not face this situation again.

Exploring Personal Dimensions

Choosing a Contraceptive

There is no such thing as a 100% safe, 100% convenient, 100% easy-to-use contraceptive. Every contraceptive has advantages and disadvantages. People need to weigh these advantages and disadvantages for themselves.

Some questions that people need to ask themselves are as follows:

1. *Effectiveness.* What are the relative effectiveness rates for each method considered? How important is it to

prevent pregnancy now? Is using abortion as a backup acceptable to you and your partner, or is an unplanned pregnancy acceptable at this time?

2. *Side effects.* Are you a good candidate for this method? Will you experience adverse side effects? Do you have a medical condition that should prevent you from using this method?

3. *Convenience.* Is this method easy for you to get? Is it easy to use? Will you use it every time?

4. *Cost.* Can you afford it? Does your campus health center provide it? Does your insurance cover it?

5. *STI protection.* Are you in a monogamous relationship? Are you sure? Do you have more than one partner? Do you know your partner's HIV status? Are you willing and committed to using a condom in addition to this method?

6. *Partner.* What does your partner think about this method? Will he or she want to use it every time? Do you want contraception to be a shared responsibility, or is it yours alone?

Suggested Readings

Boston Women's Health Book Collective & Norsigian, J. *Our bodies, ourselves: Informing and inspiring women across generations*. New York: Touchstone/Simon & Schuster, 2011.

Chesler, E. *Woman of valor: Margaret Sanger and the birth control movement in America*. New York: Simon & Schuster, 2007.

Guttmacher Institute. *Perspectives on sexual and reproductive health*, 2012. Available at: http://www.guttmacher.org/archive/PSRH.jsp.

Web Resources

For links to the websites below, visit http://go.jblearning.com/dimensions5e and click on Resource Links.

The Emergency Contraception Website: NOT-2-LATE.com
http://ec.princeton.edu/questions/dose.html

This website is operated by the Office of Population Research at Princeton University and by the Association of Reproductive Health Professionals. Funding is provided by the William and Flora Hewlett Foundation. This website provides accurate information about emergency contraception derived from the medical literature. This website has no connection whatsoever with any companies that manufacture or sell emergency contraceptives.

Guttmacher Institute: Resources: Contraception
www.guttmacher.org/sections/contraception.php

The Guttmacher Institute helps advance sexual and reproductive health worldwide through research, policy analysis, and public education. Its website takes a comprehensive look at contraception in the United States and abroad. As such, it provides access to media kits, fact sheets, state policies, policy articles, research articles, reports, statistics, slide shows, and audio clips.

Planned Parenthood: Health Topics: Birth Control

www.plannedparenthood.org/health-topics/birth-control-4211.htm

Planned Parenthood provides a broad, up-to-date list of safe and effective methods of birth control for both women and men. Covering methods from sterilization to withdrawal and from intrauterine devices to emergency contraception, its website describes how the contraceptive works, what the advantages and disadvantages of using the method are, and what research says about its effectiveness, safety, and reversibility.

Association of Reproductive Health Professionals: Method Match

www.arhp.org/methodmatch/

This simple and interactive tool allows individuals to identify their preferences about contraception and selects possible methods to consider. The site also has the capability of comparing various methods to help visitors decide what method is best for them.

References

Advocates for Youth. *Adolescent sexual health in Europe and the U.S.*, 2011. Available: http://www.advocatesforyouth.org/storage/advfy/documents/adolescent_sexual_health_in_europe_and_the_united_states.pdf.

Backman, T., Raumaro, I., Huhtala, S., & Koskenvuo. Pregnancy during the use of levonorgestrel intrauterine system. *American Journal of Obstetrics and Gynecology, 190* (2004), 50–54.

Barbaro, M. In reversal, Wal-Mart will sell contraceptive. *The New York Times* (2006). Available: http://www.nytimes.com/2006/03/04/business/04walmart.html?_r=2&scp=1&sq=walmart%202006%20plan%20b&st=cse.

Barnhart, K. T., & Schreiber, C. A. Return to fertility following discontinuation of oral contraceptives. *Fertility and Sterility, 91* (2009), 659–663.

Birth control. *Encyclopaedia Britannica*, 2009. Available: http://www.britannica.com/EBchecked/topic/66704/birth-control.

Bleakley, A., Hennessy, M., & Fishbein, M. Public opinion on sex education in US schools. *Archives of Pediatrics and Adolescent Medicine, 160* (November 2006), 1151–1156.

Boonstra, H. Emergency contraception: Steps being taken to improve access. *The Guttmacher Report on Public Policy, 5,* 5 (2002). 10–13. Available: http://www.guttmacher.org/pubs/tgr/05/5/gr050510.pdf.

Boonstra, H. D. Advocates call for a new approach after the era of "abstinence-only" sex education. *Guttmacher Policy Review, 12, 1* (Winter 2009). Available: http://www.guttmacher.org/pubs/gpr/12/1/gpr120106.pdf.

Caillet, M., Vandromme, J., Rozenberg, S., Paesmans, M., Germaya, O., & Degueldre, M. Robotically assisted laproscopic microsurgical tubal reanastomosis: A retrospective study. *Fertility and Sterility, 94* (2010), 1844–1847.

Canedy, D. Wal-Mart decides against selling a contraceptive. *The New York Times* (1999) Available: http://www.nytimes.com/1999/05/14/business/wal-mart-decides-against-selling-a-contraceptive.html.

Catholic Church. *Encyclical of Pope Paul VI, humanae vitae, on the regulation of birth, and Pope Paul VI's credo of the people of God.* Glen Rock, NJ: Paulist Press, 1968.

Cleland, K., Zhu, H., Goldstuck, N., Cheng, L., & Trussell, J. The efficacy of intrauterine devices for emergency contraception: a systematic review of 35 years of experience. *Human Reproduction, 27, 7,* (2012), 1994–2000. doi: 10.1093/humrep/des140.

Crary, D. Health advocates tout new model of female condom. *Associated Press* (April 16, 2009).

Dailard, C. Understanding "abstinence": Implications for individuals, programs and policies. *The Guttmacher Report, 6, no. 5* (December 2003).

Doyle, J., Stern, L., Hagan, M., Hao, J., & Gricar, J. Advances in contraception: IUDs from a managed care perspective. *Journal of Women's Health, 17, 6* (July 2008), 987–992.

Eisenberg, M. L., Henderson, J. T., Amory, J. K., Smith, J. F., & Walsh, T. J. Racial differences in vasectomy utilization in the United States: Data from the national survey of family growth. *Urology, 74* (2009), 1020–1024.

FDA news. FDA updates labeling for Ortho Evra contraceptive patch, U.S. Food and Drug Administration, P05-90 (November 10, 2005). Available: http://www.fda.gov/bbs/topics/news/2005/NEW01262.html.

Finer, L. B. & Henshaw, S. K. Disparities in rates of unintended pregnancy in the United States, 1994 and 2001. *Perspectives on Sexual and Reproductive Health, 38* (2006): 90–96. doi: 10.1363/3809006.

Food and Drug Administration. Female condom, 1993. Available: http://www.fda.gov/ForConsumers/ByAudience/ForPatientAdvocates/HIVandAIDSActivities/ucm126373.htm.

Friend, D. Pharmaceutical development of microbicide drug products. *Pharmaceutical Development and Technology, 15* (2010), 562–581.

Frost, J. J., Darroch, J. E., & Remez, L. Improving contraceptive use in the United States. *Guttmacher—In Brief, 1* (2008).

Gabelnick, H. L., Schwartz, J., & Darroch, J. E. Contraceptive research and development. In R. A. Hatcher et al., *Contraceptive technology*, 19th revised edition. New York: Ardent Media, 2008.

GoAskAlice. *Five kinds of condoms: A guide for consumers*, 2009. Available: http://www.goaskalice.columbia.edu/1835.html.

Gordts, S., Campo, R., Puttemans, P., & Gordts, S. Clinical factors determining pregnancy outcome after microsurgical tubal reanastomosis. *Fertility and Sterility, 92* (2009), 1198–1202.

Guttmacher Institute. *Emergency contraception*, 2012. Available: http://www.guttmacher.org/statecenter/spibs/spib_ED.pdf.

Guttmacher Institute. *Facts on contraceptive use.* January 2008a. Available: http://www.guttmacher.org/pubs/fb_contr_use.html.

Haffner, D. W., & Schwartz, P. *What I've learned about sex.* New York: Perigee Books, 1998.

Hatcher, R. A., Trussell, J., Nelson, A. L., Stewart, F. H., & Kowal, D. *Contraceptive technology*, 19th revised ed. New York: Ardent Media, 2007.

Hock, R. R. *Human sexuality*, 2nd ed. New York: Prentice Hall, 2007.

Hologic. How does Adiana permanent contraception work? 2010. Available: http://www.adiana.com/info/what_is_adiana/adiana-permanent-contraception-works.html.

Hymowitz, C., & Weissman, M. *A history of women in America: From the founding mothers to feminists—how women shaped the life and culture of America.* New York: Bantam Books, 1978.

Inki, P. Long-term use of the levonorgestrel-releasing intrauterine system. *Contraception, 75, suppl 6* (2007), s161–166.

Jennings, V. H., & Arevalo, M. Fertility awareness-based methods. In R. A. Hatcher et al., *Contraceptive technology*, 19th revised edition. New York: Ardent Media, 2008.

Jensen, J. M. The evolution of Margaret Sanger's *Family Limitation* pamphlet, 1914–1921. *Journal of Women in Culture and Society, 6, 3* (Spring 1981), 548–567.

Kaiser Family Foundation. *Emergency contraception*, 2010. Available: http://www.kff.org/womenshealth/upload/3344-04.pdf.

Kalichman, S. C., & Cherry, C. Male polyurethane condoms do not enhance brief HIV-STD risk reduction interventions for heterosexually active men: Results from a randomized test of concept. *International Journal of STD & AIDS, 10, 8* (1999), 548–553.

Kennedy, K. I., & Trussel, J. Postpartum contraception & lactation. In R. A. Hatcher et al., *Contraceptive technology*, 19th revised edition. New York: Ardent Media, 2008.

Killick, S. R., Leary, C., Trussell, J., & Guthrie, K. A. Sperm content of pre-ejaculatory fluid. *Human Fertility, 14* (2011), 48–52.

Kirby, D. *Emerging answers 2007: Research findings on programs to reduce teen pregnancy and sexually transmitted diseases.* Washington, DC: National Campaign to Prevent Teen and Unplanned Pregnancy, 2007.

Lehfeldt, H. Margaret Sanger and the modern contraceptive techniques. *Journal of Sex Research, 3, 4* (November 1967), 253–255.

Mayer Laboratories. Mayer labs acquires Today sponge distribution rights, April 6, 2009. Available: http://www.mayerlabs.com/images/pdf/today-media-kit.pdf.

Mosher, W. D., Jones, J. Use of contraception in the United States: 1982–2008. National Center for Health Statistics. *Vital Health Statistics, 23, no. 29* (2010).

Nanda, K. Contraceptive patch and vaginal contraceptive ring. In R. A. Hatcher et al., *Contraceptive technology*, 19th revised edition. New York: Ardent Media, 2008.

Nelson, A. L. Combined oral contraceptives. In R. A. Hatcher et al., *Contraceptive technology*, 19th revised edition. New York: Ardent Media, 2008.

Nelson, A. New low-dose, extended-cycle pills with levonorgestrel and ethinyl estradiol: an evolutionary step in birth control. *International Journal of Women's Health, 2* (2010), 99–106.

Nieschlag, E. The struggle for male hormonal contraception. *Best Practice and Research Clinical Endocrinology & Metabolism, 25* (2011), 369–375.

Office of Population Research and Association of Reproductive Health Professionals. *Plan B One Step*, 2012a. Available: http://ed.princeton.edu/pills/plan-BOneStep.html.

Office of Population Research and Association of Reproductive Health Professionals. *When would I use ella instead of Plan B One-Step or Next Choice?* 2011b. Available: http://ed.princeton.edu/questions/ella-vs-levo.html.

Pollack, A. E., Thomas, L. J., & Barone, M. A. Female and male sterilization. In R. A. Hatcher et al., *Contraceptive technology*, 19th revised edition. New York: Ardent Media, 2008.

Population Council. *Emergency contraceptive potential of products under development*, 2011a. Available: http://popcouncil.org/projects/19-ECPotential.asp.

Population Council. *Transdermal delivery systems for women: Spray-on contraceptive*, 2011b. Available: http://popcouncil.org/projects/249_TransdermalWomenSpray.asp.

Ramchandran, D., & Salem, R. M. New findings on contraceptives. *Population Reports, Series M (20)* (June 2008). Baltimore, MD: INFO Project, Johns Hopkins Bloomberg School of Public Health.

Rosenbaum, J. E. Patient teenagers? A comparison of the sexual behavior of virginity pledgers and matched nonpledgers. *Pediatrics, 123, 1* (January 2009), e110–e120.

Sampson, O., Navarro, S. K., Khan, A., Hearst, N., Raine, T. R., Gold, M., Miller, S., & Thiel de Bocanegra, H. Barriers to adolescents' getting emergency contraception through pharmacy access in California: Differences by language and region. *Perspectives on Sexual and Reproductive Health, 41, 2* (June 2009), 110–118.

Sarkar, N. N. The combined contraceptive vaginal device (NuvaRing(R)): A comprehensive review. *European Journal of Contraception & Reproductive Health Care, 10, no. 2* (June 2005), 73–78.

Schepens, J., Mol, B., Wiegernick, M., Houterman, S., & Koks, C. Pregnancy outcomes and prognostic factors from tubal sterilization reversal by sutureless laproscopical re-anastomosis: A retrospective cohort study. *Human Reproduction, 26* (2011), 354–359.

Sex. Really. *The female condom: Could it be for you?* 2009. [transcript]. Available: http://sexreally.com/the-show/female-condom-could-it-be-for-you.

SIECUS Policy and Advocacy. Statement of Sexuality Information and Education Council of the United States (SIECUS) on the public health and ethical concerns regarding abstinence-only-until-marriage programs and the need for comprehensive sexuality education, 2008a. Available: http://www.siecus.org/index.cfm?fuseaction=feature.showFeature&FeatureID=1156&varuniqueuserid=75184022109.

SIECUS. *End funding for the failed Title V Abstinence-Only-Until-Marriage program: Support comprehensive sex education*, 2011. Available: http://www.siecus.org/index.cfm?fuseaction=Page.ViewPage&PageID=1271.

SIECUS. *In brief: Personal responsibility program*, 2010a. Available: http://www.siecus.org/index.cfm?fuseaction=Page.ViewPage&PageID=1191.

SIECUS. *New abstinence program shows some results, shortcomings*, 2010b. Available: http://www.siecus.org/index.cfm?fuseaction=Feature.showFeature&featureID=1856.

SIECUS. *State-by-state decisions: The personal responsibility program and Title V Abstinence-Only program*, 2010c. Available: http://www.siecus.org/index.cfm?fuseaction=Page.ViewPage&PageID=1272.

Sonenstein, F. L. Can we afford to be complacent about teens' use of condoms. *Journal of Adolescent Health, 43* (October 2008), 313–314.

Sonnenberg, F. A., Burkman, R. T., et al. Cost-effectiveness and contraceptive effectiveness of the transdermal contraceptive patch. *American Journal of Obstetrics and Gynecology, 192* (2005), 1–9.

Timeline—the pill. The American Experience by PBS, 2002. Available: http://www.pbs.org/wgbh/amex/pill/timeline/index.html.

Total Access Group. *Polyisoprene condoms*. Available: http://www.totalaccessgroup.com/Polyisoprene-condoms_c_186.html.

Trenholm, C., Devaney, B., Fortson, K., Quay, L., Wheeler, J., & Clark, M. *Impacts of four Title V, Section 510 abstinence education programs, final report*. Princeton, NJ: Mathematica Policy Research, 2007. Available: http://aspe.hhs.gov/hsp/abstinence07/report.pdf.

Trenholm, C., Devaney, B., Fortson, K., Quay, L., Wheeler, J., & Clark, M. *Impacts of four Title V, Section 510 abstinence education programs, final report*. Princeton, NJ: Mathematica Policy Research, 2007. Available: http://aspe.hhs.gov/hsp/abstinence07/report.pdf.

Trussel, J. Contraceptive failure in the United States. *Contraception, 83* (2011), 397–404.

Trussell, J., & Raymond, E. G. *Emergency contraception: A last chance to prevent unintended pregnancy*, 2011. Available: http://ec.princeton.edu/questions/ee_review.pdf.

World Health Organization (WHO) Department of Reproductive Health and Research & Johns Hopkins Bloomberg School of Public Health/Center for Communication Programs (CCP), INFO Project. *Family planning: A global handbook for providers (2011 update)*. Baltimore & Geneva: CCP & WHO, 2011.

World Health Organization. *Fact sheet: Female genital mutilation*. Geneva, Switzerland: Author, 2008. Available: http://www.who.int/mediacentre/factsheets/fs241/en/print.html.

Youssef, H. The history of the condom. *Journal of the Royal Society of Medicine, 86* (April 1993), 266–228.

Zieman, Z., Hatcher, R. A., Cwiak, C., Darney, P. D., Creinin, M. D., & Stosur, H. R. A pocket guide to managing contraception, 2010–2012 edition. Tiger, GA: Bridging the Gap Foundation, 2010.

Zukerman, Z. & Orvieto, R. Letter to the Editor. *Journal of Andrology, 28*(5) (2007), 635. doi: 10.2164/jandrol.107.003434.

Zuckerman, Z., Weiss, D. B., & Orvieto, R. Does preejaculatory penile secretions originating from the Cowper's gland contain sperm? *Journal of Assisted Reproduction and Genetics, 20* (2003), 157–159.

CHAPTER

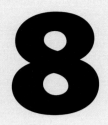

8

Conception, Pregnancy, and Birth

FEATURES

Global Dimensions
The Couvade Syndrome

Communication Dimensions
Communicating About Pregnancy

Gender Dimensions
Fathers and Childbirth

Multicultural Dimensions
Differences in Infant Mortality

Ethical Dimensions
Surrogate Mothers

CHAPTER OBJECTIVES

1 Explain what happens during the process of conception and implantation.

2 Explain what happens developmentally to the mother and embryo and fetus during the three trimesters of a pregnancy.

3 Describe the concept of prenatal care, and discuss the options for birth attendants and place of birthing.

4 Explain the many behaviors that can affect pregnancy outcomes, including use of drugs, diseases, and Rh incompatibility.

5 Identify maternal health problems that may be experienced during pregnancy.

6 Describe the physical and emotional reactions common during the three stages of giving birth.

7 Cite the causes of infertility, and describe various methods of treating it.

go.jblearning.com/dimensions5e

Birthing Alternatives
Nutrition and Weight Gain
Breastfeeding

Mary was in her late 30s when she and her husband, Rich, decided to have another child. For a while, they did not expect to be successful. Month after month of unprotected penile-vaginal sex resulted in no pregnancy. They began to think they might have waited too long.

Finally, all their efforts paid off. Mary's period was late, and an at-home pregnancy kit confirmed their hopes. Mary immediately set up a doctor's appointment to confirm the pregnancy. When she received the positive results, she set up a series of prenatal care appointments with her obstetrician.

At the first appointment, Mary checked out well. The doctor wanted her to have a sonogram—just as in her previous pregnancies. But, because Mary was now older than 35 years, the doctor also encouraged her to consider having an amniocentesis to check the fetus for potential congenital abnormalities.

Mary had the sonogram and was told everything was fine. She had amniocentesis during the 16th week of pregnancy. The doctor called and scheduled an appointment to discuss the results, and Mary and Rich knew that prospects were not good.

The doctor explained that the test detected abnormal results, which could indicate a number of conditions—including mental retardation of the child. The doctor explained the problems of raising a mentally challenged child to the stunned couple and suggested they discuss whether to continue the pregnancy.

Mary and Rich pondered what to do. They believed this would be their last chance to have a child. And Mary, although very much in favor of a woman's right to choose to have an abortion, did not want to do so.

Although Mary and Rich knew in their hearts from the start that they wanted the baby, they were both still nervous as the due date *neared. Mary went into labor. Because of the questions raised by the amniocentesis, the baby was to be delivered in an operating room; extra support staff stood by just in case.*

The attending obstetrician delivered the baby and announced, "The first one is a bouncing baby boy." Now Rich and Mary were really stunned—what do you mean, "the first one"? Within a few minutes, the fraternal twin was delivered. Both children were born without any birth defect.

At the first follow-up appointment with her doctor, Mary wanted to know why she was not told she was pregnant with twins. The doctor said that during the sonogram, the one child must have been hidden behind the other. Because there was no indication of twins, the amniocentesis abnormalities were not attributed to a twin pregnancy.

In spite of Rich and Mary's experience, most conceptions and birth deliveries proceed as planned. Still, others result in unique circumstances, as did Rich and Mary's. In this chapter we discuss the usual and the unusual aspects of conception, pregnancy, and birth.

Creating a New Life

After the man ejaculates, the sperm move through the cervical mucus into the uterus, reaching the fallopian tube within about 5 minutes. Propelling movements of the uterus and fallopian tubes help the sperm to move. Also, prostaglandin, a hormone found in semen, may intensify uterine contractions—not felt by the woman—and shorten the sperm's travel time. Sperm stay alive in the female reproductive tract for 72 to 120 hours. During the first 24 hours after ejaculation, they are at a peak level of health and fertility. The egg's peak fertile period lasts 8 to

12 hours, though an egg can be fertilized for up to 24 hours after ovulation.

Most frequently the millions of sperm in the ejaculate meet an egg in one of the fallopian tubes. For egg and sperm to unite, at least one sperm must penetrate the transparent outer layer of the egg. The sperm secretes an enzyme, hyaluronidase, that dissolves this outer layer, allowing the sperm to enter and fertilize the egg. The union of the egg and the sperm is called **conception**, and the product of that union is called a **conceptus**. At this point the sex of the potential offspring has already been determined by the absence or presence of a Y chromosome in the sperm. It is also possible, though not certain, that the number of offspring has been determined (more than one conceptus may have been conceived).

Implantation

Once the egg is fertilized, the conceptus is known as a **zygote**. The one cell of the zygote begins to divide even as it travels down the fallopian tube on its way to implant itself in the uterus. One cell divides into two cells, the two become four, and so cell division continues. By a week after

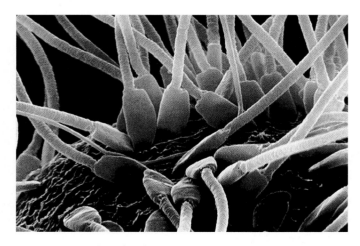

Although many sperm cells may reach the egg cell, usually only one will fertilize it.

conception
The union of the sperm and ovum; also called *fertilization*.

conceptus
The fertilized ovum; the product of conception.

zygote
A fertilized egg.

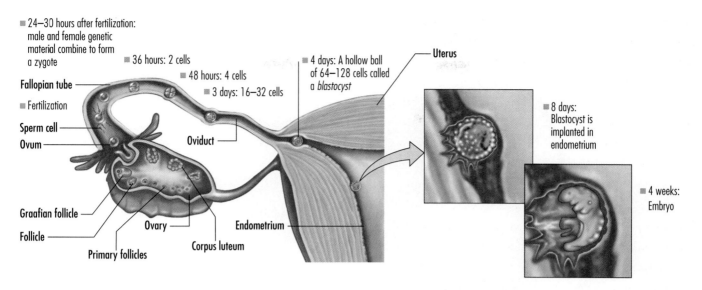

FIGURE **8.1** Following the ovum from ovulation through fertilization and implantation. After being ruptured from the ovary, the ovum is fertilized within the fallopian tube. It then travels to the uterus, where, as a blastocyst, it is implanted on the endometrium (lining) of the uterus.

conception, the zygote is a hollow ball of 100 cells. At this point it is termed a *blastocyst*. Now two layers of cells begin to form. The inner layer of cells will become the **embryo**; the embryo is the zygote from the time of implantation through the first 8 weeks of development. The outer layer of cells, called *trophoblasts*, secretes enzymes that erode the uterine lining so that the blastocyst can attach itself to the endometrium 7 or 8 days after fertilization (Figure 8.1). After implantation these trophoblasts and other cells proliferate and eventually form the placenta, the umbilical cord, and the amniotic sac, a membrane filled with **amniotic fluid**, which surrounds the developing fetus and embryo by the end of the eighth week and absorbs shocks (Shier, Butler, & Lewis, 2003).

Immediately after implantation, the embryo begins receiving nourishment from the endometrial tissue of the mother. Progesterone acts on this tissue to produce the necessary nutrients—glycogen, proteins, lipids, and some minerals. The embryo is nourished from this source for 8 to 10 weeks until the placenta has developed sufficiently to take over.

The **placenta** is a disc-shaped organ that attaches to the uterine wall and is connected to the fetus by the **umbilical cord**. Together the placenta and the umbilical cord (which is attached to the baby at the navel and to the mother at the placenta) form the lifeline between the mother and the fetus. Nutrients, oxygen, and chemicals pass through the walls of the placenta to the fetus. Waste from the fetus is returned to the mother's blood. The placenta, which by the end of the pregnancy will reach a diameter of 8 inches (about 20 centimeters), contains two sets of blood vessels (Figure 8.2). Fetal circulation occurs within the fetus and the inner part of the placenta, while the mother's circulation flows in the walls of the uterus and the uterine side of the placenta. The fetus's blood flows through two umbilical arteries to the placenta and back from the placenta to the fetus by one vein. One important function of the placenta is to keep the blood systems of the mother and child separated from each other. It does this even though the placenta has *permeability*—that is, it allows some substances to pass between mother and fetus. Throughout the pregnancy, besides allowing nourishment and waste to pass between mother and child, the placenta helps to keep bacteria away from the fetus and allows antibodies (disease fighters) to cross to the fetus. These antibodies make the baby immune to diseases to which the mother is immune for about 6 months after birth.

As the embryo develops, the placenta secretes the hormone **human chorionic gonadotropin (HCG)**. This hormone is detectable

embryo
The developing fetus during the 2 months after conception.

amniotic fluid
The fluid inside the amniotic sac in which the fetus floats; it acts as a shock absorber, maintains the fetus at a constant temperature, and serves as a nutrient.

placenta
An organ of interchange between mother and fetus; oxygen, nutrients, and waste are exchanged through its cells.

umbilical cord
The lifeline between mother and fetus, which contains two arteries and one vein. Food, oxygen, and chemicals are transported to the child through the arteries, and waste is returned to the mother through the vein.

human chorionic gonadotropin (HCG)
The hormone that appears in the blood and urine, providing evidence that a pregnancy has occurred.

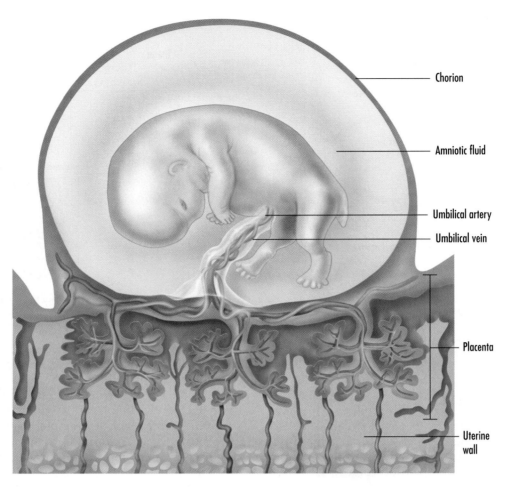

Chorion

Amniotic fluid

Umbilical artery

Umbilical vein

Placenta

Uterine wall

FIGURE 8.2 The embryo and placenta as they appear during the seventh week of development.

through blood tests 8 days after fertilization, just as the blastocyst is implanting, and its presence confirms pregnancy. HCG reaches its maximal level 7 weeks after fertilization and its lowest level about 9 weeks later (16 weeks after fertilization). The function of HCG is to keep the corpus luteum of the ovum alive so that it can continue to secrete estrogen and progesterone. Estrogen and progesterone maintain the uterine endometrium, which nourishes the early pregnancy. By about the 11th week of pregnancy, the placenta itself secretes enough progesterone and estrogen to maintain the pregnancy, and the corpus luteum dies.

Pregnancy

In the preceding section we focused on the developing zygote almost as if it were a being apart. But the development of a new person involves physiological changes in two human beings: the forming fetus and the mother. Let us back up now to account for the change in a woman after an egg is fertilized within her body.

After conception a woman is in a state of pregnancy, which lasts for the time the fetus takes to develop. This period can vary, but the time span from the last menstrual period to the birth of the baby is usually 9 calendar months (10 lunar months, 40 weeks, or 280 days). Most women deliver their babies within 2 weeks of the predicted date, sometimes called the **expected date of confinement (EDC)**. About 4% deliver on the exact date. The EDC is calculated by a formula called *Nägele's rule:* Establish the first day of the last normal menstrual period, add 7 days, and subtract 3 months from this date. The date is the EDC. Nägele's rule is based on a 28-day cycle, however, and, as we have noted, not all women have this cycle. Therefore, a medical practitioner will calculate each patient's EDC to the best of his or her ability, adapting the rule as necessary. At the point at which the fetus has the optimal chance for survival outside the uterus, the pregnancy has reached term, or completion.

> **expected date of confinement (EDC)**
> Due date for normal pregnancy that is usually estimated by Nägele's rule.

Ectopic Pregnancy

An **ectopic pregnancy** is characterized by implantation of the blastocyst in a site other than the uterus. Most often these occur in the fallopian tubes, although ectopic pregnancies can develop in other body parts. Blockage in the fallopian tubes prevents the fertilized egg from traveling down the fallopian tube; this blockage is often caused by past ectopic pregnancy, past infection in the fallopian tubes (such as **pelvic inflammatory disease**), and surgery of the fallopian tubes (such as tubal sterilization) (National Center for Biotechnology Information, 2010).

> **ectopic pregnancy**
> The development of the zygote in a location other than the uterus.
>
> **pelvic inflammatory disease (PID)**
> Infection of the reproductive organs, particularly the uterus, fallopian tubes, and pelvic cavity.

The rate of ectopic pregnancy ranges from 1 in 40 to 1 in 100 pregnancies. Although death due to an ectopic pregnancy in the United States has dropped in the last 30 years to less than 0.1% (National Center for Biotechnology Information, 2010), it is still the leading cause of maternal death in the first trimester of pregnancy (Centers for Disease Control, 2009).

Other factors, such as being over 35 years of age, having many sexual partners, having surgery to reverse a tubal sterilization, smoking, becoming pregnant while using an IUD, and in vitro fertilization, may increase the risk of an ectopic pregnancy (National Center for Biotechnology Information, 2010).

It is essential that an ectopic pregnancy be diagnosed quickly. If a woman experiences symptoms of an ectopic pregnancy, such as abnormal vaginal bleeding, amenorrhea, breast tenderness, low back pain, mild cramping on one side of the pelvis, nausea, or pain in the lower abdomen or pelvic area, she should seek medical treatment. Ultrasound can confirm the presence of an ectopic pregnancy by 6 weeks' gestation, allowing for treatment that is the least destructive and costly. If the area of the abnormal pregnancy ruptures and bleeds, symptoms may get worse and include feeling faint or actually fainting (about 1 in 10 women faint), intense pressure in the rectum, pain that is felt in the shoulder area, and severe, sharp, and sudden pain in the lower abdomen (National Center for Biotechnology Information, 2010).

Confirming Pregnancy

The signs of pregnancy known long before our current methods of testing were available are divided into three categories: presumptive, probable, and positive. Because many of the signs and symptoms of pregnancy may also be attributed to other conditions,

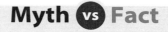

Myth: The peak period for sperm and egg to be fertilized is 1 week after they are released.
Fact: The peak period for sperm is about 24 hours after ejaculated, and the peak period for the egg is approximately 12 hours after release.

Myth: The egg is fertilized by the sperm in the uterus.
Fact: The egg–sperm union occurs in the fallopian tube.

Myth: Obstetricians are very accurate at predicting the date of delivery.
Fact: Only approximately 4% of women actually deliver on the expected date of confinement; most women do deliver within 2 weeks of their predicted due date.

Myth: To protect the fetus, pregnant women should refrain from exercising during their pregnancy.
Fact: Pregnant women can exercise without causing harm to the fetus. However, they should follow the exercise guidelines of the American College of Obstetrics and Gynecology.

Myth: As long as drugs are available over the counter, a pregnant woman can feel safe taking them.
Fact: All drugs have the potential to cause harm to fetuses. Therefore, pregnant women should refrain from taking all medications without the advice of their doctors.

medical practitioners proceed with caution to avoid a wrong conclusion. Emotional, endocrine, or systemic conditions can cause symptoms identical to the early signs of pregnancy.

Presumptive Signs
Presumptive signs and symptoms are those that may indicate pregnancy but that may occur when a woman is not pregnant. The presumptive signs and symptoms include missed menstrual periods, nausea and vomiting, a tingling feeling in the breast (*mastodynia*), increased urinary frequency, some weight gain, fatigue, a rise in the basal body temperature, some skin changes, slight abdominal enlargement, and some vaginal discoloration and discharge. It is important to note that not all pregnant women experience all these symptoms.

Probable Signs
Probable signs and symptoms include the presumptive symptoms plus enlargement of the abdomen and the uterus, some painless uterine contractions, *ballottement* (at 16 to 20 weeks, bimanual examination gives the physician an impression that a floating object is in the uterus), and *uterine souffle* (a rushing sound, which the physician hears through a stethoscope placed on the woman's abdomen). Uterine souffle in pregnant women is caused by blood filling placental blood vessels and spaces.

Positive Signs
What are conventionally called the positive signs of pregnancy are not present until the 17th week after

Global
DIMENSIONS

The Couvade Syndrome

Around the globe, men whose partners are pregnant are experiencing pregnancy symptoms. Called *couvade syndrome*, cases have been reported across cultures, continents, and centuries (Polinski, 2009). Symptoms include indigestion, increased or decrease appetite, weight gain, diarrhea or constipation, headache, nausea, and bloating. Symptoms typically occur during the late stages of the first trimester, with an increase during the late stage of the third trimester. Symptoms generally resolve with childbirth (Budur, Mathews, & Mathews, 2005).

Prevalence estimates range from less than 20% to 80% of expectant fathers (Wynne-Edwards, 2006); however, the exact cause of modern couvade is unknown. One challenge in determining the cause is that researchers—and their studies—often define couvade differently (Wynne-Edwards, 2006). In spite of this challenge, possible social and biological causes have been identified: lifestyle changes that the couple experiences together during pregnancy; social attachment, as fathers who have strong empathy for their partner are more likely to demonstrate symptoms; and hormonal (prolactin) changes in the father. Men with higher levels of prolactin, the hormone that causes lactation in women, report more couvade symptoms. In men, the prolactin causes a decrease in testosterone and sperm production; prolactin levels peak just before delivery. Similarly, levels of cortisol (a hormone related to stress), estradiol (a form of estrogen), and progesterone also change in the father, though not as much as do those in the mother (Storey et al., 2000; Berg & Wynne-Edwards, 2001). The conclusion was that men experience hormonal changes similar to changes experienced by their pregnant partners, though it is unknown if these hormonal changes are cause-and-effect or simply a correlation (Wynn-Edwards, 2006).

Even if men don't experience pregnancy symptoms, support for a pregnant partner is always welcome!

---

conception. There are three of these signs, any one of which can confirm a pregnancy: fetal heartbeat, which can be monitored at 17 to 18 weeks; active fetal movement, at about the fifth month or between the 20th and 24th weeks; and palpation of the abdomen, by which the practitioner can detect the fetus. X ray would reveal a fetal skeleton, but this procedure is rarely used, because it can harm the developing fetus.

Women today do not need to wait months to confirm a pregnancy, and for the health of both the woman and the developing fetus it is best not to do so. Echography or ultrasonography (which measures sound waves as they pass through tissues of various densities, each returning its own echo) can be done as early as 4 weeks, and laboratory tests on urine and blood samples can now be done as early as 8 days after conception.

Pregnancy Tests

Pregnancy is confirmed by the presence of the hormone human chorionic gonadotropin (HCG), which is found in the blood and urine if a pregnancy exists. Currently the most frequently used laboratory test has the intimidating name of *beta subunit HCG radioimmunoassay*. This test measures the HCG in a blood sample and can confirm pregnancy, as mentioned earlier, about 8 days after conception occurs.

Two other laboratory pregnancy tests currently in use are the slide test and the test tube test. The slide test is a urine test that can be performed 2½ weeks after a missed menstrual period. Results are obtainable in about 1 or 2 minutes. The test tube test is performed, at the earliest, 2½ weeks after a missed menstrual period. In both the slide and tube tests, urine is mixed with a chemical reagent. The slide test is less sensitive and the blood test more sensitive to the presence of HCG.

Home pregnancy testing is also available. Commercial test kits that measure the presence of HCG in urine can be used as early as the day menstruation should have started. When used according to directions, they are considered to be quite accurate. The problem is that accurate use of a test by an inexperienced person can sometimes be difficult. Nervousness, possible misreading of directions, and improper handling of the kit's components can lead to inaccurate results. Often people feel the tests should be repeated. This can increase the cost considerably and still does not guarantee accurate findings. If one has a choice, a professional laboratory procedure is preferred. Professional testing is done by private, health-department, clinic, and hospital laboratories. Choose a pregnancy testing facility carefully. Some "Crisis Pregnancy Centers" offer free pregnancy testing but do not provide balanced information abut pregnancy options.

Due Date and Delivery Date

As mentioned earlier, to determine the approximate due date, obstetricians use what is called Nägele's rule. They identify the first day of the last period, count back 3 months, and then add 7 days. For example, if the first day of the last missed period was January 1, 2013, the approximate due date would be October 8, 2013. If the pregnancy exceeds 40 weeks and more urgently after 41 weeks, concern for the health of the fetus may necessitate inducing labor. Pregnancies of that length are associated with a higher risk of infant mortality and injury to the mother and baby (Bruckner, Cheng, & Caughey, 2008; Kaimal et al., 2011; Oros et al., 2012). In addition, induction may be recommended if there is a maternal illness such as high blood pressure, diabetes, or uterine infection.

Labor can be induced in several ways. One method involves the intravenous administration of pitocin, an artificial version of the hormone oxytocin. Generally, the amount is increased every 15 to 30 minutes until a good contraction pattern is achieved. Induction can also occur by the administration of prostaglandin gels or suppositories. These are used when the cervix is not favorable, meaning that it is dilated less than 3 centimeters, is hard, posterior, not effaced, or barely effaced, or any combination of these characteristics (Weiss, 2009). Another method of inducing labor is to artificially rupture the membrane ("breaking the bag of waters"). Lastly, some midwives or other holistic providers practice *natural induction*, which may include use of herbs, castor oil, or other agents to stimulate or advance a stalled labor.

■ Fetal Development

Prenatal development is commonly regarded as having two stages: the **embryonic stage** (from the Greek *embryo*, "to swell"), which lasts 2 months, and the **fetal stage** (from the Latin *fetus*, "the young one"), which lasts from the beginning of the third month to birth (Figure 8.3). The 9-month pregnancy, however, is commonly viewed as consisting of three 3-month developmental periods called **trimesters**.

embryonic stage
The stage of prenatal development that includes the first 8 weeks of pregnancy.

fetal stage
Period from the ninth week of pregnancy to birth.

trimester
A 3-month period of the 9-month pregnancy, which is typically divided into three trimesters.

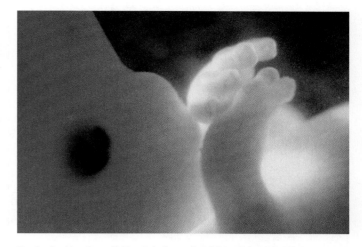
By the beginning of the eighth week of development, the embryonic body has recognizable human features.

The First Trimester

During the first trimester, weeks 1 through 12, most of the embryo's physiological systems and body parts begin to form. At the end of the first month, the embryo is about 0.25 inch (0.6 centimeter) long. By this time, three cell layers have formed: the *ectoderm* (outer layer), from which the skin, sense organs, and the nervous system will grow; the *mesoderm* (middle layer), from which the muscular, circulatory, and excretory systems will form; and the *endoderm* (inner layer), from which the digestive system, glandular systems, and lungs will develop.

At the end of the second month, the embryo is about 1¼ inches (3 centimeters) long and weighs 1/30 ounce (0.9 gram). The head represents almost half the embryo's total bulk. Facial features such as eyes, ears, nose, lips, and tongue are visible, and the forehead is prominent because of the brain size (Figure 8.4).

When the third month begins, as mentioned, the developing child is called a **fetus**. At the third month the fetus, afloat in the amniotic fluid, is 3 inches (7.6 centimeters) long and 1 ounce (2.8 grams) in weight. It can move, but its motions are not yet felt by the mother. The fingers and toes have nails, and the genitals can be seen as male or female. By the end of the first trimester, the fetus is a miniature human. During the next two trimesters, organs mature and general growth occurs.

fetus
The developing child from the ninth week after conception until birth.

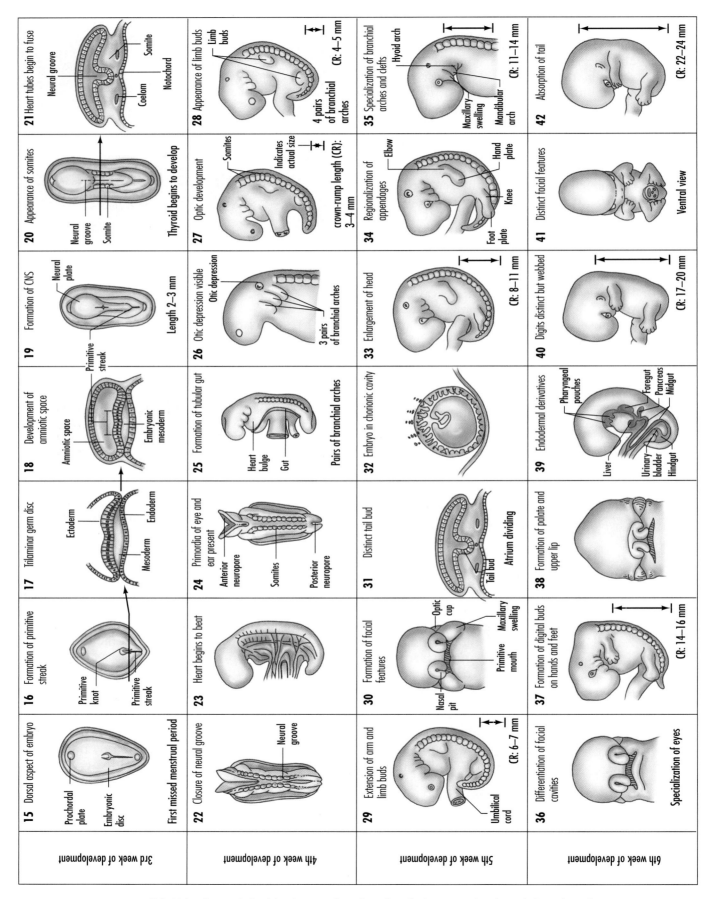

FIGURE 8.3 Major changes in fetal development from the 3rd week after conception through the 10th week.

49 Well-established placenta

Placenta
Amniotic cavity

56 Delineation of appendicular muscles

63 Development of the cerebellum

70 Accelerated growth in body length

CR = 45–50 mm

48 Formation of undifferentiated external genitalia

Genital tubercle
Urogenital membrane
Anal membrane ♂ or ♀

55 Formation of dental buds for teeth

All principal body organs are formed

62 Development of accessory reproductive organs within male

69 Developing ear bones

47 Distinction of toes

Toes

CR = 26–27 mm

54 Distinction between anus and genitalia

Genital tubercle
Urethral groove
Anus ♂ or ♀
Testes and ovaries distinguishable

61 Differentiation of male genitalia

Phallus
Urogenital fold
Labioscrotal fold
Perineum

68 Further differentiation of male genitals

Glans penis
Urethral groove
Scrotum
Fusion of urethral groove

46 Ossification centers begin to form

Appearance of nipples

53 Well-developed facial features

60 Differentiation of female genitalia

Phallus
Urogenital fold
Labioscrotal fold
Perineum

67 Further differentiation of female genitalia

Clitoris
Labium minus
Urogenital groove
Labium majus

45 Distinction of fingers

CR = 23–25 mm

52 Anal membrane perforated

59 Distinct nails on digits

66 Enlargement of cerebrum

44 Formation of eyelids

51 Marked development of brain

58 Position of fetus within uterus

65 Differentiation of inner and outer layers of the eye

43 Formation of extraembryonic membranes

Placenta
Yolk sac
Decidua capsularis
Uterus
Lumen of uterus

50 Trunk elongating and straightening

CR = 28–30 mm

57 Beginning of fetal stage

CR = 34–40 mm

64 Refined facial profile

7th week development

8th week development

9th week development

10th week development

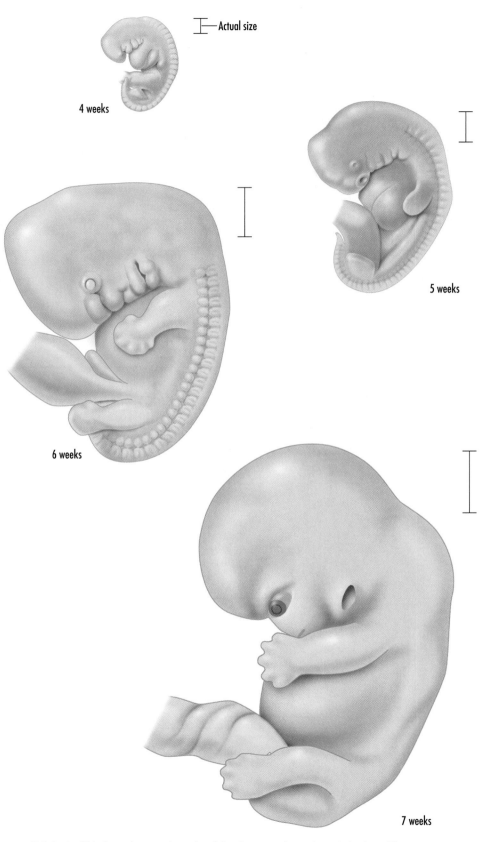

4 weeks

Actual size

5 weeks

6 weeks

7 weeks

FIGURE 8.4 In the fifth through seventh weeks of development, the embryonic body and face start to develop a humanlike appearance.

The Second Trimester

During the fourth month, the first month of the second trimester, the greatest amount of fetal growth occurs. The fetus is now 6 inches (15 centimeters) long, the lower body is growing increasingly larger, and the head is now one-third the length of the body. The fetus moves and can suck, and its motion, called **quickening**, is felt by the mother. During the fifth month, the halfway point of the pregnancy, the fetus weighs about 1 pound (454 grams) and is about 12 inches (30 centimeters) long. It sleeps and wakes and has a preferred body position. During the sixth month the fetus grows about 2 inches (5 centimeters) and gains another pound. By this point the fetus's eyes are formed, it is sensitive to light, and it can hear uterine sounds. The skin is wrinkled and covered with fine hair. Though development is well under way, a baby born at this stage probably would not survive.

> **quickening**
> Movements of the fetus felt by the mother; usually occurs about the fourth month of pregnancy.

By the end of this trimester, refinement of body features has occurred, movement is stronger, and further growth has been achieved.

The Third Trimester

During the period of the third trimester, the fetus positions itself more or less for birth. The most common fetal position, or *presentation*, is head down (Figure 8.5).

As a fat layer is laid underneath the skin, the fetus takes on a more babylike form. By the end of the seventh month, it is generally agreed, the baby can live outside the uterus, although babies have survived when born much earlier and cared for in neonatal intensive care units. By the end of the eighth month, the fetus weighs about 5 pounds and 4 ounces (2,384 grams) and is about 20 inches (51 centimeters) long. During the eighth and ninth months, skin redness lessens and wrinkles begin to disappear as the fetus begins to gain about 1½ pound (227 grams) a week. The nails reach the end of the fingers and toes and

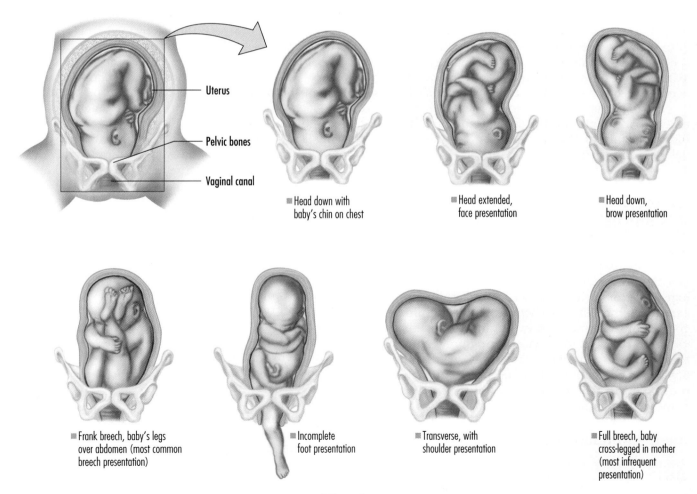

FIGURE **8.5** Fetal positions.

Communication
DIMENSIONS

Communicating About Pregnancy

Although it is not routinely discussed, most women do not have an easy time with pregnancy: Morning sickness, continual tiredness, and new physical sensations may bring about momentary feelings of "Did I do the right thing?" This is balanced against society's view of happy pregnant women, who work until the last days of pregnancy and always smile.

From our experience, pregnant women who talk to other women who have been pregnant gain a great sense of relief. They find that their experience is not unique. Few women go through a "perfect" pregnancy. Ironically, women who have been pregnant usually wait for the pregnant woman to discuss an issue before opening up about their experience.

But pregnant women who talk to those who have not had children (a group that includes men) are often chided for their complaining. One pregnant woman recently said that after she had morning sickness at work—every day for weeks on end—most colleagues would smile and remind her of how "lucky" she was. Any complaining during lunch or breaks was met with reproachful glares—how dare she have a negative thought about the fetus inside her! She soon learned to keep her feelings to herself.

Explain why people have such a hard time talking about pregnancy. Is it because it is the result of sexual activity? Or because of the special roles that young children play in our society?

---

the fetus's actions become limited because of its tight fit in the uterus. As birth becomes imminent, in the 38th to 40th weeks, the head is 60% of its full size, the fine body hair has about disappeared, and the skin becomes smoother and is now covered with a waxy protective substance called the *vernix caseosa.*

During this last trimester, the fetus will have reached a weight and size that prepare it to live independently of the mother. The baby is ready for delivery and birth.

Bearing a Healthy Infant: Prenatal Choices

Staying as healthy as possible is the pregnant woman's chief responsibility to her developing child. Pregnancy is a time of great change. Both physical and psychological factors affect the health and well-being of an expectant mother and her developing child. Many choices must be made by expectant parents, including whom to seek out for advice during pregnancy, where the birth will take place, and what health-enhancing lifestyle modifications they can make throughout the pregnancy. In the sections that follow, we discuss the many decisions facing today's expectant parents.

Birth Attendant Options

Even though pregnancy is a normal physiological event, there is still no question that a woman's general health affects not only her own experience of pregnancy but also the health of her developing child.

The best advice for a healthy pregnancy is supervision by a health practitioner trained to give prenatal (prebirth) care. Thus, the selection of a health professional who will advise during the pregnancy and serve as the birth attendant during labor and delivery is an important decision that should be made by the expectant parents early in the pregnancy.

In the United States all physicians are trained in medical school in the procedures involved in pregnancy and birth. Generally, however, the family-practice specialist (a newer term for general practitioner) and the **obstetrician** are the primary providers of pregnancy care. The obstetrician has had specialized advanced training in this area. Many women physicians specialize in obstetrics, and a considerable number of pregnant women purposely seek women obstetricians. Some women feel that a female physician is more empathetic and understanding of the variety of body changes that occur during pregnancy and delivery. There is the possibility that the female physician has experienced parturition (the process of giving birth), and many pregnant women find this reassuring and relaxing. **Midwifery** has also been used in the

obstetrician
A physician who specializes in the care of pregnant women and the process of childbirth. Because these physicians are also gynecologists, they are often referred to as obstetrician– gynecologists or OB–GYNs.

midwifery
The practice by nonphysicians of assisting in the process of pregnancy and childbirth. Lay midwives are not trained healthcare professionals; nurse midwives are registered nurses who have received advanced training and often certification in the techniques of the birthing process.

United States. Historically, American midwives were laypeople who helped with birth deliveries. Today nurse–midwives are registered nurses (RNs) or certified nurse–midwives (CNMs) who receive advanced training in childbirth processes. Many states require nurse–midwives to pass a national certification exam given by the American College of Nurse–Midwives to be licensed.

Whereas midwife-attended births steadily increased from less than 1% in 1975 to 8% in 2004, the rate has remained constant since then in this country (Martin et al., 2009). In 2009, 8.1% of all births in the United State were attended by midwives—93% of whom were CNMs. Because midwives are not typically involved in surgery (like cesarean sections), the percentage of midwife-attended births increases to 12.1% when considering vaginal births only. As a result, in 2009, more than 1 in 8 vaginal births was attended by a midwife (Declercq, 2012). Most midwife-attended births occur in hospitals (91.7%) (Martin et al., 2010).

Nurse–midwifery is often chosen by families who consider birthing to be a natural process that does not require highly technological interventions. Nurse–midwives routinely practice in freestanding birth centers and in hospitals. Some nurse–midwives work with an obstetrician present at the delivery; some work alone but have an affiliation with an obstetrician who is on call for problem deliveries. Some nurse–midwives assist in home deliveries with a physician present or on call.

Increasingly couples are planning their deliveries, making decisions that suit them, and choosing birth attendants and facilities to match their needs.

Birthing Alternatives

To receive the kind of care they want before, during, and after delivery, future parents should investigate the birthing alternatives available in their area as soon as possible. Often the choice of a birth attendant is tied to the setting in which that birth attendant chooses to or is allowed to practice. Currently in the United States there are three major settings where labor and delivery typically occur: hospitals, the home, and freestanding birth centers. Each setting has advantages and disadvantages that should be considered by prospective parents.

Hospital Birth

Not many years ago most babies were born in hospital delivery rooms with the mother heavily drugged and the father barred from participating. Nowadays expectant parents often have a wide range of choices regarding the kind of delivery they will experience in the hospital setting.

Perhaps the most marked change is the increased participation of fathers in the birth of their children. Even in traditional births, fathers are now allowed to be present in the delivery rooms of many hospitals, and in less conventional setups fathers often

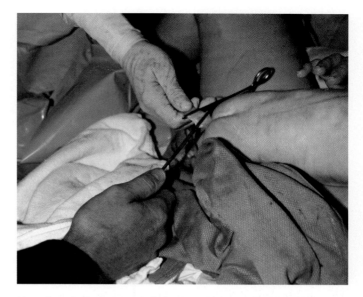

Many hospitals encourage fathers to participate in the birth of their children. Some even allow the father to hold the newborn as it emerges from the birth canal, or to help cut the umbilical cord.

participate—perhaps by helping to hold the newborn as it emerges from the birth canal or by cutting the umbilical cord (under guidance, of course). This trend reflects a new appreciation for the role of fathers in child rearing. Although long considered "women's work," childbearing and raising are increasingly being recognized as joint undertakings, involving father and mother equally. The benefit of this new trend is that fathers share openly not only in the work and responsibility of parenting but also in the joys and satisfactions. Many believe that this form of "male liberation" results in sounder father–child relationships and that strong father–infant bonds begin, as do mother–child bonds, at the moment of birth.

Most traditional hospital maternity facilities consist of separate rooms for labor, delivery, and recovery. Physicians, usually obstetricians, serve as the primary birth attendant, with assistance from nurses. Emergency equipment and trained personnel are quickly accessible should the need arise. **Analgesics** and **anesthetics** are options typically available only in this setting. High-risk pregnancies especially benefit from technological advances found in the hospital setting.

Although traditional labor and delivery rooms are still the standard in many hospitals, some hospitals provide the option of a more homelike birth setting for their clients. Typically this takes the form of a **birthing room**, which is attached to a labor and delivery suite and is often run by nurses and nurse midwives.

analgesics
Substances that decrease pain locally, such as topical creams.

anesthetics
Substances that elicit unconsciousness and thereby relieve pain.

birthing room
A homelike birth setting now available in some hospitals.

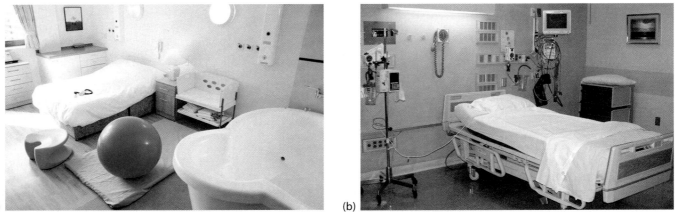

(a)   (b)

Many hospitals now offer a birthing room alternative (a) in addition to the traditional hospital delivery room (b).

The birthing room is decorated in a homelike style, often including soft lighting, wallpaper, a rocking chair, and a private bath. Mothers labor, deliver, and recover in one room with a support person, such as a spouse or other family member, present. Regulations regarding the use of a birthing room vary from one hospital to the next, and not uncommonly birthing rooms are used only for low-risk pregnancies. Couples interested in using a hospital birthing room need to find out whether this option is available at local hospitals and whether they are likely candidates for its use.

Home Birth
Home birth with a nurse–midwife is another birth alternative. Home birth is an option for only healthy women with low-risk pregnancies, and nurse–midwives are trained to screen out women who might be at risk of complications during labor and delivery. For low-risk women, several studies have found home birth to be as safe as hospital delivery (de Jonge et al., 2009; Janssen et al., 2009; Johnson & Daviss, 2005). A recent meta–analysis did find a risk for home births (Wax et al., 2010), but it has been criticized for methodological issues (Davey & Flood, 2011; Gyte, Dodwell, & Macfarlane, 2011; Johnson & Daviss, 2011; Kirby & Frost, 2011; Zohar & De Vries, 2011).

Home birth candidates are watched closely during pregnancy for signs of possible risk. In addition, individuals need to consider what nearby services are available should complications arise during delivery. While home births are common in Europe (for example in the Netherlands about 30% of women give birth at home) (Royal College of Obstetricians and Gynaecologists, 2009), the practice is controversial in the United States, and the American College of Obstetricians and Gynecologists does not support home births (ACOG, 2011a).

If a couple chooses the home birth option, the midwife or physician—though relatively few physicians support home birth—goes to the couple's

home and delivers the baby in a previously selected room. Children and other family members may be present. In 2009, only 0.72% of women in the United States had their babies at home. While the rate is less than 1%, it has increased almost 30% since 2004. White women choose home births more than women of other ethnicities with about 1 in 90 births to white, non-Hispanic women occurring in the home (MacDorman, Mathews, & Declercq, 2012).

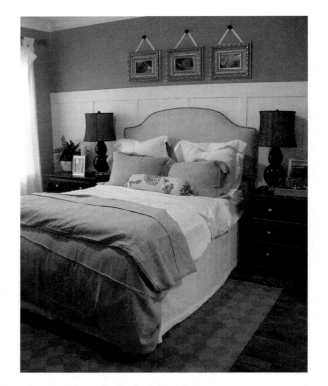

Many hospitals have built plush birthing centers to attract patients to this highly profitable area. Consumers have many options to choose from and should shop around and ask people they know for referrals before making a final selection.

Freestanding Birth Centers

The birth center is a birthing alternative available to prospective parents that represents a compromise between the traditional hospital delivery and the option of home birth. Birth centers are facilities that offer a homelike birth experience outside a hospital setting. Most birth centers are licensed by the state and are often run by nurse–midwives. Typically, birth centers limit their clientele to low-risk pregnancies. Women are monitored throughout the pregnancy by a nurse–midwife and may be referred to a hospital for delivery if complications arise during the prenatal period. Some emergency equipment is available in birth centers, and most birth centers are located in close proximity to a hospital for ready access if medical care is needed. It has been estimated that approximately 13% of women who begin delivery at a birth center are transferred to a hospital setting to complete the delivery (Reinberg, 2005).

Prenatal and postnatal care are provided by the birth center's staff, and this continuity of care is a major benefit offered by birth centers. Freestanding birth centers are family oriented, encouraging family participation throughout the prenatal period. Couples are active participants in designing their personal birth plan, and family members are allowed to stay near the mother during labor and delivery.

Additionally, the infant remains with the mother after delivery. Although birth centers have increased in popularity and availability, they are not available in every city or even every state. Couples who wish to use a birth center must investigate the availability of this birth alternative in their community.

Nowadays it is acknowledged that childbirth is an emotional experience as well as a physical one—and not just for the mother and child but for the father as well. The many birthing options available reflect this perspective and make responsible decision making by expectant parents increasingly important. If a birthing center option is chosen, a center that is accredited by the Commission for the Accreditation of Birth Centers (CABC) should be selected. In addition, some states regulate birth centers; therefore, only those facilities sanctioned by the state should be considered.

Prenatal Care

Traditionally, **prenatal care** consists of monitoring fetal development, screening for high-risk pregnancy, and educating those involved about pregnancy and childbirth. For most normal pregnancies 10 to 12 prenatal care visits, beginning at about the 6th week of pregnancy, are optimal. For a high-risk pregnancy more frequent visits may be necessary. Studies show that the risk of very low birth weight increases when women do not receive comprehensive prenatal care.

prenatal care
Care given to an expectant mother before the birth of her child that typically consists of monitoring fetal development, screening for high-risk pregnancy, and providing education for pregnancy and childbirth.

The prenatal evaluation begins, as most medical visits do, with the taking of a personal health history, relevant social and emotional factors, employment of the parents, conditions of their work environment, and the stability of their relationship itself. The practitioner is usually interested in knowing what sort of support system the woman and her new child will have, for many factors—both medical and nonmedical—can affect the well-being of a pregnant woman and her child. Additionally, a series of laboratory tests is usually completed at the first prenatal examination. These laboratory tests normally include examination for hemoglobin levels, glucose or protein in the urine, evidence of a current syphilis infection, antibodies for rubella (German measles), and blood type and Rh determination (discussed shortly). An examination of the cervix is also done at this time.

A family history is taken as well. Is the woman on her own—and thus possibly facing much stress and financial anxiety—or does she live with a partner? Is the father involved in the pregnancy? Is the baby wanted or unwanted? Was the pregnancy planned or unexpected? All these factors can place stress on the mother, and thus they have a bearing on her prenatal care. The medical practitioner overseeing her care will—or should—take an interest in these matters from the start. On the basis of this medical and social history, the practitioner will also determine how much information the expectant parents lack, what sort of guidance they need to adapt to the pregnancy, and, of course, what sort of delivery they favor. When pregnancy is concerned, the practitioner–client relationship is unique. If the couple, and particularly the mother, feel misgivings about their first choice, seeking another practitioner early in the pregnancy is highly advisable.

Nutrition and Weight Gain

Maternal nutrition directly affects fetal growth and development. The developing fetus depends on the mother for nutrition and can deplete her supply of necessary nutrients. For example, the mother usually needs iron supplements to prevent anemia. Iron is a major component of hemoglobin, which carries oxygen to the cells of both mother and baby. Protein influences tissue building in both the mother and baby and contributes to maintaining a healthy placenta and uterus. Vitamins ensure better resistance to infection, influence energy level, and aid in the absorption of calcium. Calcium is needed by the mother to prevent muscle irritability and by the baby to allow bone growth. Trace minerals, such as zinc and cobalt, build enzymes that influence chemical actions. The food intake of the mother fuels the development of the baby and directly influences the baby's weight gain.

Among the most important nutrients to obtain during pregnancy is folate (a B vitamin), which helps prevent serious abnormalities of the brain and spinal cord. Lack of folate also may increase the risk of preterm delivery, low birth weight, and poor fetal growth. Folate obtained through vitamin supplements is called folic acid. At mentioned, other necessary nutrients include calcium for strong bones and teeth, protein for growth and repair of body tissue, and iron.

Even if they eat healthfully, women may miss out on key nutrients. A daily prenatal vitamin, ideally starting 3 months before conception, can compensate for any missed nutritional needs. In addition, healthcare providers may recommend special supplements for women who follow a strict vegetarian diet or who have chronic health conditions.

In the past it was the fashion in prenatal care to place pregnant women on strict regimens to prevent them from gaining more than about 20 pounds. Obese patients were even put on weight-reduction programs. New attitudes suggest that dieting during pregnancy can be harmful in that breakdown of fat produces toxic substances (called *ketones*) that can impair the mental and physical development of the fetus. Current recommendations for a healthy weight gain during pregnancy vary with the prepregnancy weight of the mother (National Academy of Sciences, 2009). Those mothers who were considered by their physician to be at a normal weight before conception should gain between 25 and 35 pounds. Those women who were underweight should gain slightly more (28 to 40 pounds); those who were overweight before pregnancy should gain less weight (15 to 25 pounds). Women identified as obese before pregnancy

should gain 11 to 20 pounds during the pregnancy. This weight gain includes a variety of components for both the mother and the fetus (see Figure 8.6). As has been noted in this discussion, extra nutrients are needed in pregnancy, and a wide variety of foods is needed to provide them.

Exercise During Pregnancy

Previously, the safety of aerobic exercise during pregnancy was questioned. However, studies to date indicate that exercise is safe for both the pregnant woman and the fetus. Exercise during pregnancy has been found to have both psychological and physiological benefits (ACOG, 2011b; DeMaio & Magann, 2009; Lewis et al., 2008). For example, the physical discomforts of pregnancy, such as backaches, bloating, constipation, and swelling, are reduced with exercise. Risk for gestational diabetes and treatment of the condition can also be helped with regular exercise. Energy and mood are both elevated. In addition to benefits during pregnancy, because individuals who exercise regularly are more fit, they can often handle the physical efforts of labor and have an easier labor (ACOG, 2011b).

To ensure the safety of both the mother and the developing infant, pregnant women should follow the exercise guidelines of the American College of Obstetrics and Gynecology (ACOG, 2011). ACOG recommends that pregnant women engage in 30 minutes or more of moderate exercise on most, if not all, days of the week. The exceptions to this recommendation include proscriptions against scuba diving (due to the risk of fetal decompression sickness); contact activities that carry a risk of abdominal injury (for example, hockey, basketball, and soccer); and activities

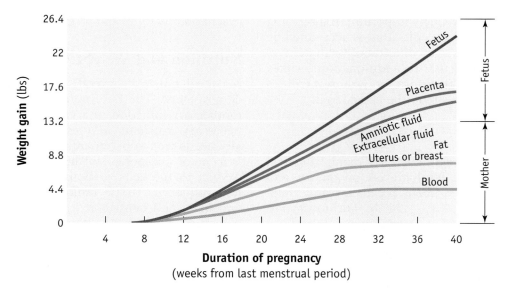

FIGURE **8.6** Pattern and components of maternal weight gain during pregnancy.

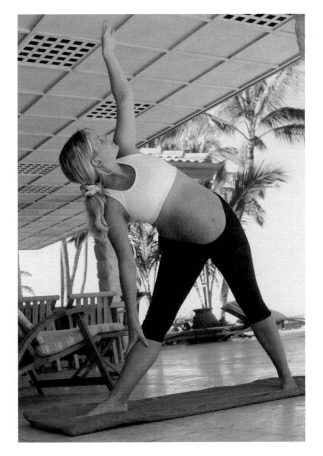

There is no reason that pregnant women should not maintain an exercise regimen. In fact, the American College of Obstetrics and Gynecology recommends pregnant women engage in 30 minutes or more of moderate exercise on most days.

that have a risk of falling (for example, gymnastics, skiing, and horseback riding).

Before exercising during pregnancy, a woman should consult her physician or nurse–midwife. There are certain conditions, such as cardiac disease, a history of three or more spontaneous abortions (miscarriages), or abnormal bleeding, that are contraindications to exercise during pregnancy. This consultation is especially important for women with high-risk pregnancies. If a woman has been sedentary before her pregnancy, she should not attempt to take up a strenuous aerobic exercise program. Walking and swimming are appropriate activities for pregnant women who are beginning to exercise. Runners can continue to run, though their program may need to be modified (ACOG, 2011b). Consult with your clinician before starting other types of exercise programs.

Regular intake of fluids during exercise and consumption of adequate calories daily (usually an additional 200 to 300 calories) are essential for maintaining a safe exercise program. Pregnant women should not start or stop exercising suddenly; like anyone exercising, gradual warm-up and cool-down periods

of 5 to 10 minutes are recommended. Proper clothing, especially a support bra and good athletic shoes, should be worn during exercise sessions. The pulse should be checked every 10 to 15 minutes during exercising and should not exceed 140 beats per minute.

If a woman experiences fatigue, shortness of breath, dizziness, nausea, uterine contractions, pain, vaginal bleeding, or decreased fetal movement during exercise, she should stop exercising immediately and call her physician or nurse–midwife. Pregnant women who follow these guidelines improve their chances of experiencing a satisfying pregnancy and delivering a healthy baby.

■ Threats to Having a Healthy Infant

Mothers- and fathers-to-be often worry about whether their baby will be born healthy. In our technological society we are exposed to a larger number of risks to healthy pregnancy than ever before. Exposure to chemicals and radiation at the work site and in the home, lifestyle factors such as cigarette smoking and other drug use and abuse, and exposure to infectious agents are just some of the factors currently posing a risk to bearing healthy children. Although the great majority of infants are born healthy, both public health professionals and parents-to-be have legitimate concerns about infant morbidity and mortality.

In 2010, the National Center for Health Statistics reported an infant death rate of 6.1 deaths per 1,000 births in the United States (Centers for Disease Control & Prevention, 2011d). This represents a significant decrease from the 1988 rate of 10.1 deaths per 1,000 births. Still, compared with other developed countries, the United States ranks 41st in neonatal deaths or deaths of infants less than 28 days old (Oestergaard et al., 2011). Additionally, the U.S. infant death rate is more than twice as high for African Americans as for whites.

Birth defects are the leading cause of infant mortality in the United States. Approximately 120,000 children are born every year with a birth defect (March of Dimes, 2011), and while many of these babies will die during the first year, the majority must cope with a range of defects throughout their lives. A pregnant women can take steps to reduce the chance of a birth defect; however, about 70% of the causes of birth defects are unknown (March of Dimes, 2011). **Teratology** is the branch of research that searches for causes of birth defects. Some known causes include chromosomal defects, mutant genes, and environmental causes, such as exposure to harmful chemicals and

teratology
The study of causative factors of birth defects.

drugs. Education can decrease risk of birth defects by environmental factors.

Birth defects are one of the important causes of infant death in the United States; the second leading cause of infant deaths is low birth weight (Mathews & MacDorman, 2011). Low birth weight, which is considered to be a birth weight of less than 5 pounds, 8 ounces, and very low birth weight (less than 3 pounds, 4 ounces) substantially increase an infant's chances of dying during the first year of life. This is especially true for African Americans, for whom low birth weight is the leading cause of infant death in the United States.

There are two types of low birth weight. The first involves infants who are born prematurely (before 37 weeks of gestation) and are thus underweight. A second type of low birth weight is known as *fetal growth restriction*. These infants are born full term, but they are underweight. Some of these babies are healthy, whereas others have low birth weight because something slowed or halted their growth in utero. Risk factors associated with low birth weight include smoking, alcohol and other substance use, chronic health problems in the mother, infections in the mother or fetus, low pregnancy weight gain, and socioeconomic factors such as low income, low educational levels, maternal age younger than 18 or older than 35, or being black (March of Dimes, 2008b).

Research into the causes and prevention of birth defects and low birth weight is greatly needed. Yet there is much we already know about preventing these conditions. Reducing these risk factors is the focus of our attention here.

Drugs and Other Substances

Any drug taken by a pregnant woman can potentially pass through the placenta to the fetus. If the drug (whether medically prescribed or self-prescribed) affects the mother in some way, it will also affect the developing baby. A danger of taking drugs during pregnancy is that an adult dose can be an overdose for a fetus. The liver of the fetus cannot metabolize drugs as can the adult liver, and the unchanged drug can affect the fetus differently from the mother. Furthermore, drugs can alter the metabolism of the mother, influence hormones in the bloodstream, and affect placenta functioning.

Over-the-Counter Drugs

Many Americans are polydrug users. *Over-the-counter drugs (OTCs),* sold legally without a prescription, are widely used for self-medication purposes. The use of many OTCs causes special concerns for pregnant women. Because of the extensive number of OTCs available, it is beyond the scope of this chapter to provide a complete review. The safest course of action

for pregnant women is to avoid self-medication and OTC drugs until their use is approved by the clinician providing prenatal care.

Cigarette Smoking

Smoking during pregnancy has been identified as the most preventable cause of illness and death among infants (Centers for Disease Control and Prevention, 2007); unquestionably it is harmful to the unborn baby. One study showed 13.8% of U.S. women in 2005 still smoked during pregnancy, which was a decrease from 15.2% in 2000 (Tong, 2009). In general, smoking during pregnancy is associated with ectopic pregnancy, higher rates of spontaneous abortion, lower birth weight, structural changes in and decreased functioning of the placenta, stillbirth (March of Dimes, 2010), and some congenital heart defects (Clinton et al., 2011). After birth, babies whose mothers smoked during pregnancy are more susceptible to childhood illness, especially development of respiratory problems such as asthma (Midodzi et al., 2010) and are more likely to die of SIDS (Sudden Infant Death Syndrome) (Centers for Disease Control and Prevention, 2007). Some studies have indicated a link between smoking and the development of attention deficit hyperactivity disorder in children (Knopik, 2009; Pinkhardt et al., 2009).

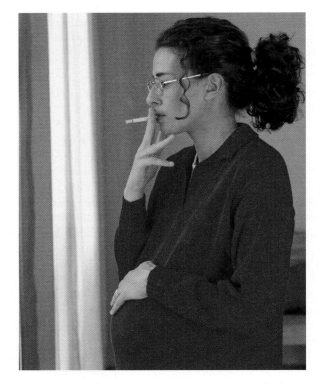

Cigarette smoke is one of the most toxic substances for fetuses and newborns. Smoking before birth exposes the fetus to a range of health risks, including low birth weight and birth defects. Smoking after birth exposes the infant to breathing problems and other health risks.

Marijuana

Tetrahydrocannabinol (THC), the primary psychoactive agent in marijuana and other cannabinoids, can pass through the placental barrier and affect the ability of the placenta to function.

Prenatal exposure to marijuana has been associated with decreased development in utero. For women who use marijuana six or more times a week, there appears to be an increased risk of slow fetal growth and premature birth. After birth, some babies born to mothers who used marijuana during pregnancy display altered responses to visual stimuli, trembling, and a high-pitched cry, which could indicate problems with neurological development. Other studies have linked marijuana use in pregnancy to lower intelligence in children (Goldschmidt et al., 2008) and use of marijuana as an adolescent (Day, Goldschmidt, & Thomas, 2006). Some researchers question the specific impact of marijuana, because it is difficult to isolate the effect of marijuana from environmental factors (Schempf & Strobino, 2008) unless only animal studies are considered. Animal studies have shown that marijuana is a teratogen (an agent capable of causing birth defects); pregnant women should refrain from using marijuana to ensure as healthy a pregnancy as possible.

Alcohol

Many women realize that consuming large quantities of alcohol during pregnancy is a risk to the developing fetus. **Fetal alcohol syndrome (FAS)**, more recently referred to as **fetal alcohol spectrum disorders (FASD)**, are a range of problems and abnormalities that can appear as a result of heavy alcohol consumption during pregnancy. An estimated 40,000 babies are born in the United States each year with FASD. Infants suffering from FASD may have unusual facial features, such as small eye slits; deep epicanthic folds (a fold of skin from the eyelid to the inner corner of the eye, giving it a slanted effect); upturned nose and a thin flattened upper lip; and a flattened or decreased groove in the upper lip. They may also have heart defects, dysfunctions of the central nervous system, or growth deficiency. Most often, some level of mental challenges exist, ranging from learning problems and below average intelligence to mental retardation. Impaired memory development (Pei et al., 2008) has also been recently identified in children with FASD. The typical low math skills in FASD

fetal alcohol syndrome (FAS)
Impaired psychological and physical characteristics common in infants born to alcoholic women.

fetal alcohol spectrum disorders (FASD)
The full spectrum of birth defects that are caused by prenatal alcohol exposure.

children have been linked to brain structure differences (Lebel et al., 2010).

There is some debate about the safety of low or moderate amounts of alcohol consumption during pregnancy, with some media reports and pregnancy books stating that small amounts of alcohol are safe. Almost all U.S. health organizations (for example, the U.S. Surgeon General, the American College of Obstetrics and Gynecologists, and the March of Dimes) recommend no alcohol be consumed if someone is trying to become pregnant, might be pregnant unintentionally, or is pregnant. Alcohol does cross the placental barrier and can affect fetal cells and tissues. At least one review study showed effects on socioemotional and cognitive development in children with low to moderate alcohol consumption (Swedish National Institute of Public Health, 2009).

Cocaine

In the early months of a pregnancy, cocaine use has been associated with miscarriages. In later months, cocaine use can trigger preterm labor (labor that occurs before a completed pregnancy of 37 weeks). Placenta problems, like placenta abruption when the placenta disconnects from the uterine wall, can also occur and cause life-threatening complications (March of Dimes, 2008a).

After birth, some babies who were regularly exposed to cocaine during pregnancy may have mild behavioral disturbances. Some are jittery and irritable, and they may startle and cry at a soft touch or sound; it may be difficult to comfort these children. Others may avoid surrounding stimuli by sleeping heavily for long periods during the day. Usually, these behaviors are temporary and resolve during the first few months after birth (March of Dimes, 2008a).

Like marijuana use, the effects of cocaine use by a pregnant woman may be difficult to separate from other environmental factors, such as poverty, malnutrition, and other substance use. At the same time, of all illicit substances, cocaine is most consistently associated with poor birth outcomes, especially those related to fetal growth (Gouin et al., 2011), such as low birth weight, intrauterine growth restriction, and reduced head circumference.

Later in life, some of the effects of prenatal cocaine exposure include impaired gross motor development at 4 months (Bigsby et al., 2011); impaired motor development at age 2 and a slower rate of growth through age 10 (Richardson et al., 2008); less ability to self-regulate one's behavior (Ackerman, Riggins, & Black, 2010); impaired language development and processing (Beeghly et al., 2006); attention deficits in preschool and elementary school (Ackerman, Riggins, & Black, 2010); and an increased likelihood of being in a special education program (Levine et al., 2008).

Heroin and Other Narcotics

Today several types of narcotic drugs are used on a prescription basis, including morphine, codeine, paregoric, hydramorphone hydrochloride, laudanum, meperidine, methadone, and others. Pregnant women should not take these drugs without the consent and approval of their healthcare provider. Another type of narcotic—heroin, an illegal street drug—will be the focus of this section.

Use of and addiction to heroin and other opiates in a pregnant woman result in a narcotized fetus who must go through withdrawal. The mother's withdrawal from heroin while pregnant can lead to fetal death. Rapid withdrawal of the mother during the first trimester may result in miscarriage and result in life-threatening fetal distress if done during the third trimester. Pregnant women using heroin should consult with their healthcare provider about potential treatment plans during pregnancy.

In addition to the specific risk of drug addiction, heroin use during pregnancy is also associated with poor fetal growth (about half of all babies of heroin users have low birth weight), premature birth, and stillbirth. There is some association with heroin use and birth defects, but it is not clear if the drug is the causative factor or if the poor health behaviors of the mother and the substances that heroin is often mixed with contribute to this connection. Some research does suggest that prenatal exposure to heroin is related to increased risk of learning and behavioral problems in childhood (March of Dimes, 2008a).

Steroids

Steroids are prescribed drugs such as sex hormones and other specific chemicals (cortisol and prednisone) used to treat kidney inflammations, joint inflammation, and tissue damage caused by rheumatic fever and other serious diseases. They can cross the placenta and cause fetal distress.

Diethylstilbestrol (DES)

DES is a synthetic nonsteroid estrogen first prescribed in the 1950s to prevent miscarriage. In 1971 it was discovered that DES caused a specific vaginal cancer in some female offspring of women who took the hormone during their pregnancy before the 18th week of gestation. Additionally, approximately 35% of exposed women exhibit benign vaginal epithelial cell changes. There is also a risk of problems with fertility and pregnancy. Male offspring are possibly vulnerable to infertility and prostatic problems.

Diseases

Certain diseases can be passed from mother to fetus, but their significance varies with the stage of pregnancy. No matter how severe or how innocuous a disease might be in the pregnant woman, the effect on the fetus depends on the stage of fetal development at the time. Common diseases that can be transmitted to the fetus with harmful consequences follow.

German Measles (Rubella)

The disease rubella is most harmful to the fetus in the first trimester (the effect is almost nil after the third or fourth month). If a pregnant woman contracts rubella early in her pregnancy, there is an 80% chance her baby will be born with a birth defect (Centers for Disease Control and Prevention, 2011e). Common effects on the infant include hearing loss or deafness, eye defects, mental retardation, and liver and spleen damage. Death sometimes occurs shortly before or after birth. To prevent rubella and its effects, it is recommended that women who have not had rubella be vaccinated well before they decide to conceive. Additionally, vaccines should be given to children at 12 to 15 months of age, because children are the major sources of rubella infection of pregnant women.

Diabetes

Diabetes is an insulin deficiency that affects sugar metabolism and can influence fetal weight and complicate delivery. Infants of diabetic women may have a high birth weight (10 pounds or more) and a higher than average mortality rate.

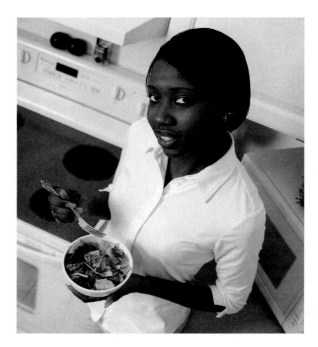

Staying as healthy as possible is the pregnant woman's chief responsibility to her developing child. Many choices must be made by expectant parents, including which health-enhancing lifestyle modifications, such as following a healthy diet, they can make throughout the pregnancy.

Human Immunodeficiency Virus

A fetus can become infected when the human immunodeficiency virus (HIV) crosses the placenta of an infected woman or during the birth process, when the infant might have contact with the mother's infected blood during delivery. It is currently estimated that without treatment 15–30% of infants born to HIV-positive women will also be HIV-positive and may contract AIDS. An additional 5–20% will become infected with HIV through breastfeeding (AVERT, n.d.). Acquired immune deficiency syndrome (AIDS) is a viral disease characterized by depression of the immune system and the presence of certain opportunistic infections and malignancies. However, with systematic HIV testing of pregnant women, antiretroviral (ARV) medications given to the female during pregnancy and labor and to the infant in the first weeks plus a complete avoidance of breastfeeding, the risk of mother-to-child transmission has been reduced to 2% in high-income countries. In developing countries, a variety of other protocols may be used based on availability of medications, availability of resources, and cultural ideas (Johri & Ako-Arrey, 2011).

Syphilis

The STI syphilis is a common cause of stillbirth and can infect a fetus when the spirochetes cross the placenta. The infected fetus may show signs of syphilis at birth or may appear normal until adolescence, when signs of late syphilis appear. The fetus is unaffected if the mother receives penicillin before the fourth month.

Gonorrhea

This STI affects the eyes as the baby passes through the vagina and can, by transmission through the placenta, eventually cause a form of arthritis.

Genital Herpes

Genital herpes is an STI caused by the herpes simplex virus (HSV). If lesions are present on the genitals of the mother at the time of delivery, the virus can be absorbed by the baby, causing encephalitis, inflammation of the brain, and possible death. A woman with a history of genital herpes will be followed closely from 32 weeks of gestation until delivery. If herpes lesions are present on her genitals, delivery will be by cesarean section.

Chlamydia

The STI chlamydia is caused by the intracellular parasite *Chlamydia trachomatis*. Infants born to mothers with chlamydia infections have a chance of acquiring either inclusion conjunctivitis (an eye infection) or chlamydial pneumonia during delivery. All pregnant women should be screened for chlamydia at their first prenatal visit. The infection is easily treated with antibiotics.

Genital Warts

Genital warts, another STI, are caused by the human papillomavirus (HPV). Infected mothers may transmit HPV to the fetus in utero or during the birth process. Infected mothers may transmit HPV to the fetus during the birth process, but this is rare. If transfer does occur, it is most commonly associated with respiratory papillomatosis, which causes hoarseness and respiratory distress in the infant. If a pregnant woman has genital warts that are large, they may interfere with the birth process, requiring a cesarean delivery; however, this is uncommon.

Rh Incompatibility

The **Rh factor** is a substance in the blood of about 85% of the population. If the Rh factor is present, the person's blood type is Rh positive (Rh+); if it is not present, the blood type is Rh negative (Rh–).

> **Rh factor**
> The presence of Rh agglutinogens (antigens) in the blood, which indicates that a person is Rh positive, whereas its absence designates the person as Rh negative.

A problem in pregnancy exists when an Rh– mother is pregnant with an Rh+ child, a child who has inherited the positive factor from the Rh+ father. The mother's body develops anti-Rh agglutinins, antibodies to the presence of the Rh+, similar to the antibodies that fight disease. These anti-Rh antibodies enter the fetus and cause its red blood cells to clump together—that is, agglutinate. During the first such pregnancy, the mother's body does not develop many agglutinins. However, in subsequent pregnancies her body develops the anti-Rh agglutinins rapidly, and the babies of these pregnancies may be born anemic and jaundiced, with red blood cells and hemoglobin below normal. This condition can be prevented if the woman is given an injection of Rh immunoglobulin (RhIg), which prevents the sensitization of the Rh factor. RhIg is used during pregnancy and after delivery, which includes any miscarriage, ectopic pregnancy, or induced abortion. If the preventative treatment is not given to the mother, the newborn infant will receive a blood transfusion (Medline Plus, 2011).

Testing for Disorders

Many different tests can be performed during a pregnancy. Some of these tests are virtually risk-free and as simple as a blood test. Others are more invasive and carry more risk to the pregnancy.

An early blood test used at 7 week's gestation (called cell-free fetal DNA testing) can screen for sex-related disorders without invasive testing. The cell-free fetal DNA testing looks for the Y chromosome; the results can help parents who may be worrying about male-only genetic disorders such as hemophilia or a specific type of muscular dystrophy (Devaney et al., 2011). Currently these tests are not regulated in the United States, and many practitioners do not prescribe them because labs are not federally certified to use them. They are available over the counter and through drug stores, with total costs (materials, lab fees, shipping, etc.) ranging from $250 to $330. Although the purpose is to assist with prenatal care, some are concerned that individuals may use the test to screen only for sex, with the intent of aborting nonmale fetuses (Benn & Chapman, 2010). Some corporations do not sell the tests in China or India, where males are valued over females and there is concern that female fetuses are regularly aborted (Belluck, 2011).

Another almost risk-free procedure is the ultrasound, or **sonogram**; during this procedure, high-frequency sound waves are directed at the pregnant woman's uterus. The echo from the waves is transformed into a visual representation of the uterus and fetus, including the internal structures of the fetus. This technique can provide indication of the sex of the fetus, the number of fetuses, and some abnormalities. If the ultrasound shows a possible abnormality, a fetal MRI might be used to provide a more detailed and clear image (Obenauer & Maestre, 2008). A fetal MRI uses the same techniques

> **sonogram**
> A diagnostic picture revealing the fetal outline. In ultrasonography, sound waves are bounced off the fetus. With a scanner, the image is then projected onto a computer screen, revealing whether certain defects are present.

as brain imaging and can better detect some internal abnormalities, such as those found in the central nervous system, gastrointestinal tract, genital area, and chest (Baysinger, 2010; Weston, 2010).

Amniocentesis is the drawing of fluid from the amniotic sac for the purpose of diagnosing fetal abnormalities (Figure 8.7). The procedure cannot be safely performed until the 16th week of pregnancy. A sonogram picture is taken to show the outline of the fetus so that the needle used will not touch the baby. Under sterile conditions and using a local anesthetic, a physician inserts a long needle through the abdominal and uterine walls into the amniotic sac and withdraws up to 20 milliliters (2/3 ounce) of fluid. The fluid, which contains cells sloughed off by the fetus, is analyzed for a variety of fetal abnormalities. The test analysis takes 10 days or longer. Chromosomal disorders, genetically induced metabolic disorders, sex-linked diseases, and genetics-linked inherited conditions can be determined by this procedure. Maternal age older than 35 years carries a higher risk of chromosomal disorders (such as Down syndrome), and amniocentesis is often recommended for these pregnant women. The sex and exact age of the fetus can also be determined by means of this procedure, although amniocentesis is rarely performed for these reasons alone because it always entails some risk to the fetus. Even though the procedure is performed under sterile conditions, there is always the risk of introducing infection into the uterine environment, inducing miscarriage, or damaging the fetus.

> **amniocentesis**
> Withdrawal by syringe of amniotic fluid to determine the presence of fetal abnormalities.

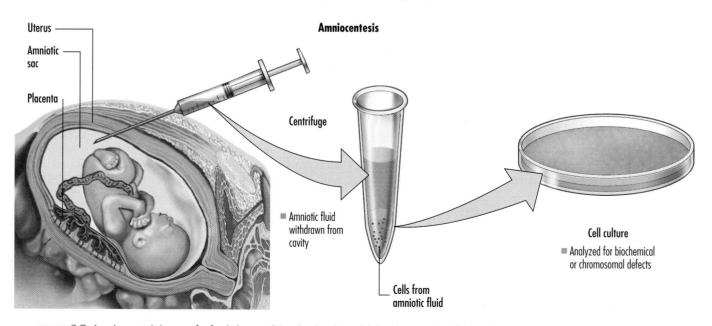

Uterus

Amniotic sac

Placenta

Amniocentesis

Centrifuge

Amniotic fluid withdrawn from cavity

Cells from amniotic fluid

Cell culture

Analyzed for biochemical or chromosomal defects

FIGURE **8.7** Amniocentesis is a test for fetal abnormalities that involves withdrawing amniotic fluid and inspecting the cells contained within it.

Another technique for prenatal detection of genetic defects, **chorionic villi sampling (CVS)**, is performed ideally at 8 to 10 weeks into the pregnancy. The chorion is the outermost protective covering of the growing embryo. The villi are thread-like, vascular (containing blood) protrusions growing on the outer surface of the chorion. In the procedure a plastic catheter is passed through the vagina into the uterus to these villi. Ultrasound is used to guide the insertion of this catheter. About 30 milligrams (0.001 ounce) of tissue is suctioned and then studied. If an abortion would be considered, CVS has the advantage of providing information several weeks earlier in a pregnancy than an amniocentesis. A first-trimester abortion is less risky to the mother than is one done in the second trimester. However, certain defects, such as neural tube defects, cannot be detected by this technique. If such a problem is suspected, amniocentesis must be performed. CVS does carry a slightly higher risk of miscarriage than amniocentesis (1.0% and 0.3% (Mayo Clinic 2010a, 2010b), respectively).

Another prenatal screening test is available for detection of fetal abnormalities early in pregnancy. Maternal serum alpha-fetoprotein (MSAFP) testing is a blood test, performed at 16 to 18 weeks of pregnancy, to detect neural tube defects such as spina bifida (an open spine) and anencephaly (lack of higher brain structures). Abnormal levels of MSAFP could indicate several other conditions, such as twin pregnancy, ventral wall (heart) defects, Down's syndrome, and fetal demise. This test, however, is a screening test that detects *potential* problems; it is *not* a diagnostic test that can confirm these conditions with certainty. Abnormal levels of MSAFP are an indication that a diagnostic test such as amniocentesis should be performed. MSAFP could be an important screening test for pregnant women aged 35 years and older. If such a pregnant woman, who would normally be placed in a high-risk category, had the MSAFP test and it indicated a low risk for fetal abnormalities, it could spare her from having amniocentesis and its inherent risk of miscarriage.

chorionic villi sampling (CVS)
A technique for prenatal detection of genetic defects that involves removal of some of the villi growing on the outer surface of the chorion and examining their chromosomes.

Maternal Health Problems During Pregnancy

Over 20% of all pregnant women and their babies are "at risk." When a practitioner deems a pregnancy to be a high-risk one, the label indicates that the mother and/or child could suffer some adverse effects during pregnancy, labor, or delivery. The mother's health, economic status, and access to medical care, as well as the genetic history of both parents, influence the risk status of the pregnancy. The mother's age, too, has a major effect: Those younger than 18 years and older than 35 years are at greatest risk. The most common causes of maternal deaths in pregnancy and childbirth in the United States are due to hemorrhage, infection, preeclampsia, eclampsia, and convulsions.

Hypertension

Blood pressure that is above normal while the heart is contracted or relaxed, or both, is the condition called *hypertension*. Women who have a history of hypertension or who become hypertensive in pregnancy need attentive medical supervision, but their condition by no means precludes a successful pregnancy.

Hypertensive conditions induced by a pregnancy have been traditionally called the **toxemias of pregnancy**. Despite the term, however, these conditions are not caused by toxins—poisons—circulating in the blood, as some people believe. Toxemias are also called *preeclampsia* and *eclampsia*. **Preeclampsia** is pregnancy-induced hypertension accompanied by swelling of the face, neck, and upper extremities. These body parts swell when tissues retain too much fluid. Proteinuria, an abnormal amount of protein in the urine, is another symptom of preeclampsia. The term **eclampsia** refers to the preeclampsia events, plus convulsions or coma, which can be fatal. At present the causes of preeclampsia and eclampsia are unknown.

It is important to state that edema—swelling of the tissues—does not always indicate an abnormal condition in pregnancy. In fact, it is quite common among pregnant women. There is more than one type and cause of edema in pregnancy.

toxemias of pregnancy
Hypertensive conditions, subdivided into preeclampsia and eclampsia.

preeclampsia
Pregnancy-induced hypertension; symptoms include swelling of the face, neck, and upper extremities; and excess levels of protein in the urine.

eclampsia
Pregnancy-induced hypertension accompanied by swelling of the face, neck, and upper extremities, plus convulsions or coma, which may be fatal.

morning sickness
The condition of nausea and vomiting that is common in early pregnancy; thought to be caused by hormonal changes.

Nausea and Vomiting

Although the exact cause is unknown, the nausea and vomiting common to early pregnancy are thought to be caused by hormonal changes. **Morning sickness** is the usual term applied to these conditions, because the nausea often occurs early in the day and dissipates relatively quickly. Small meals, avoidance of strongly flavored foods, and eating of toast and jelly before moving around in the morning are suggested. As the body adjusts to the pregnancy, the nausea and vomiting disappear.

Severe, continuous vomiting in pregnancy (*hyperemesis gravidarum*) can be serious. Dehydration, loss of electrolytes, and dietary insufficiency can result and threaten the pregnancy. Bed rest and sedation are frequently necessary, and, in extreme cases, hospitalization and intravenous feeding are required. The treatment usually includes a search for the physiological or psychological causes, because most practitioners favor limiting the use of medication in pregnancy.

Hemorrhoids

Hemorrhoids are varicose veins of the anal area. They are caused by the same pressures that create varicose veins in the legs. The increased flow of blood to the pelvic area during pregnancy results in added pressure of blood flow, which stresses the inelastic veins. In an effort to accommodate the increased blood flow, the veins are stressed, resulting in swelling, pain, and bleeding. The usual treatment employs sitz baths (a bath in which only the hip area is immersed) and topical creams. A pregnant woman who has hemorrhoids should tell her practitioner and allow him or her to prescribe treatment.

Other Conditions

A number of conditions frequently associated with pregnancy, although not serious, are often irritating. **Chloasma**, or the "mask of pregnancy," is a usually yellow to brown patch of skin pigmentation that appears on the faces of white women. The mask is thought to be caused by hormonal action that increases the number of pigment cells. Estrogen and progesterone can also produce these skin changes, as can ultraviolet light. When the pregnancy ends, the chloasma disappears.

chloasma
A yellow to brown patch of skin pigmentation that may appear on the faces of pregnant white women; sometimes referred to as the "mask of pregnancy."

Stretch marks, also more common in white women than in others, are visible white streaks in the skin of the abdomen and breasts, which enlarge during pregnancy. They are thought to be caused by a weakening of fibers in the tissue under the skin. It is believed that some people have a predisposition to this condition. In most instances stretch marks do not disappear, although they may fade or lighten in time.

Hair loss sometimes occurs because of an increase in hormone production. It is temporary when it does occur, and as long as no significant health problems exist, normal growth recurs within 6 months after delivery.

Reddish branchlike vascular "spiders" in the neck, chest, face, and arms are due to high estrogen levels and vascular weakness. Small capillaries under the skin surface break, and uneven streaks become visible on the surface. These streaks also fade, but in some women they do not disappear completely.

During the last few months of a pregnancy, weak and slow contractions of the uterus occur. Known as **Braxton-Hicks contractions**, these contractions become more frequent as the pregnancy proceeds. Some researchers consider this a means through which the uterus practices for labor.

■ Childbirth

Parturition, derived from a Latin term meaning "to produce," is the process of giving birth. It begins with **labor**—contractions of the uterus, a gradual opening of the cervix, and purposeful bearing down by the woman—and ends in **delivery**—the expulsion of a child and the placenta. Sometimes women experience what is called *false labor*. False labor, common in late pregnancy, is characterized by brief uterine **contractions**, sometimes accompanied by mild back and abdominal pain and involving no changes in the cervix. **True labor** is characterized by (1) regularly spaced contractions of the uterus that gradually gain in intensity, (2) thinning and **dilation** (gradual opening) of the cervix, and (3) descent of the presenting part of the fetus into the vagina (Figure 8.8). The presenting part of the fetus is that part of its body that can be felt through the cervix during a vaginal examination. Usually the cervix begins to soften and dilate a few days to a few weeks before the actual delivery time.

Braxton-Hicks contractions
Weak and slow uterine contractions that occur during the last few months of pregnancy.

parturition
The process of giving birth.

labor
The process of expelling a child by uterine contractions, dilation of the cervix, and bearing-down pressure.

delivery
The stage of childbirth characterized by the expulsion of the infant and the placenta.

contraction
The shortening or tension of uterine muscles during labor.

true labor
Characterized by regularly spaced contractions of the uterus, thinning and dilation of the cervix, and a descending of the presenting part of the fetus into the vagina.

dilation
In childbirth, the gradual opening of the cervix during labor.

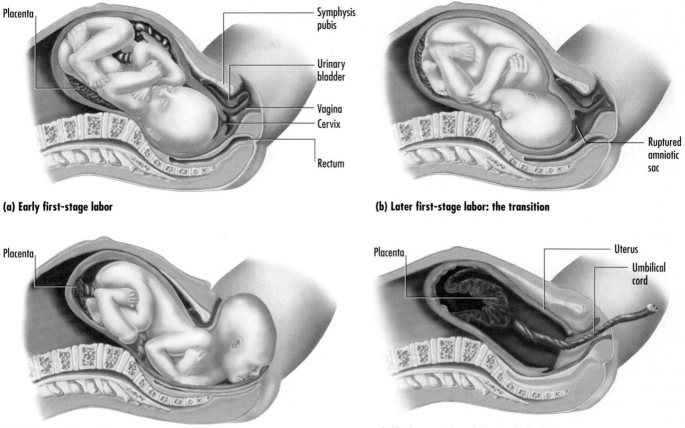

Placenta

Symphysis
pubis

Urinary
bladder

Vagina

Cervix

Rectum

(a) Early first-stage labor

Ruptured
amniotic
sac

(b) Later first-stage labor: the transition

Placenta

(c) Early second-stage labor

Placenta

Uterus

Umbilical
cord

(d) Third-stage labor: delivery of afterbirth

FIGURE **8.8** Childbirth: The stages of labor. (a) First stage: The cervix is dilating. (b) Late first stage (transition stage): The cervix is fully dilated, and the amniotic sac has ruptured, releasing amniotic fluid. (c) Second stage: The birth of the infant. (d) Third stage: Delivery of the placenta (afterbirth).

Labor

Labor takes place in three distinct stages—at least from an obstetrician's point of view. Stage I is the period from the onset of labor to the point at which the cervix is fully dilated; that is, when the cervix is opened to 4 inches (10 centimeters) across. The average length of the first stage in a first pregnancy is 8 to 12 hours, but it often lasts up to 20 hours. Stage II is the period from full cervical dilation through the birth of the child. This stage can last from a few minutes to 2 hours in a normal delivery, though the longer time is most common. Stage III is the period from the infant's birth to delivery of the placenta, or **afterbirth** (usually taking up to half an hour).

Labor usually begins with the first of the contractions that will mark the whole of the first stage. Often the contractions are irregular at first and of unequal length. But in true labor, they eventually occur in a settled pattern: for example, contractions of 30 to 40 seconds occurring every 2 to 3 minutes. Along with the onset of contractions, a **bloody show** occurs—the disintegration of the mucus plug at the cervix. Usually the **amniotic sac** (the "bag of waters") ruptures spontaneously near the beginning of labor, experienced as either a rush or trickle of fluid through the vagina. Sometimes, however, contractions increase, but the amniotic sac remains unruptured; in such cases the attending physician or midwife breaks the sac. In some situations in which labor is overdue or dilation is progressing poorly, the drug oxytocin (Pitocin) is used to start labor or to increase the frequency of the contractions.

The medical attendants monitor the heartbeat of the fetus regularly by placing a stethoscope on the mother's abdomen, and they perform vaginal examinations periodically. If giving birth in a hospital, an **electronic fetal monitor** is also used to assess fetal heart

afterbirth
The delivery of the placenta.

bloody show
The expelling of the mucus plug (often streaked with blood) that has closed off the cervix during pregnancy.

amniotic sac
A fluid-filled membrane that surrounds the developing infant in the uterus.

electronic fetal monitoring
A technique used during labor whereby a physician places an electrode on the woman's abdomen to monitor the fetal heart rate for signs of fetal distress.

Gender DIMENSIONS

Fathers and Childbirth

One of us vividly remembers driving his wife to the hospital when she went into labor and being met by a very accommodating nurse. She took us immediately into the labor room, an area in which women could scream and shout and kick. The comfort I was able to offer my wife was not immediately acknowledged—she had other things on her mind—but was nonetheless helpful and appreciated in retrospect. Yet, when it came time for her to deliver our son, my wife was wheeled into the delivery room and I was escorted to the waiting room. That was how it was done in those days.

Since then, more and more fathers are accompanying the mothers of their babies into the delivery room and observing the birth. Some even view the birth through a camera lens as they try to capture the moment for posterity. In this way they feel involved in all phases of childbirth and, some research indicates, develop a greater sense of closeness—bonding—with their children as well as with their spouses.

Although this trend may be welcomed by most men, it places a burden on others. Akin to the pressure on women to work outside the home or to have a "natural childbirth delivery," the one-model-fits-all approach ignores those men who prefer not to be in the delivery room. Some men may feel squeamish about medical procedures and fear fainting during the delivery, and others may feel uncomfortable observing their partners in pain. Which types of accommodations could a hospital or birthing center provide for fathers who do not feel comfortable attending a delivery?

---

rate. The nurse attaches an electrode to the woman's abdomen, and electrocardiographic impulses are transmitted to paper, giving a tracing (a reading) of the fetal heartbeat. Fetal heart rate can be influenced by such conditions as uterine contractions, problems with the placenta, and problems with the umbilical cord.

If anesthesia is used to reduce or eliminate the pain of contractions, it is administered late in the first stage or in the second stage. We discuss some of the choices women have regarding anesthesia later in the chapter.

Delivery

The physician or midwife may try to control the delivery to prevent a too sudden or too forceful ejection of the baby. The goal is to prevent injury to the central nervous system of the baby or injury to the mother's perineum, the area between the vulva and the anus.

Sometimes there is a need to enlarge the vaginal opening to permit the baby to pass through and to prevent the mother's tissue from tearing. In this event an incision is made into the perineum, a procedure called an **episiotomy**. Although in the past episiotomy was performed routinely in all hospital births, recently many physicians and midwives have been challenging the need for routine episiotomies, making the incision only when absolutely necessary (ACOG, 2006).

The usual delivery is divided into three phases: delivery of the head, of the shoulders, and of the body and legs. **Crowning** is the presentation of the baby's head at the vaginal opening. In a **breech delivery**, the baby presents the hip, body, shoulder, and head, in that order. Though rare, a breech delivery can be hazardous to the mother or baby, or both, for several reasons. The membranes can rupture prematurely, predisposing the mother to infection; because the buttocks of the baby do not conform to the contours of the lower uterus, labor can be prolonged; manipulation of the baby is more involved than in a head presentation; and lacerations may occur in the cervix, vagina, and perineum, possibly causing infection or hemorrhage. A breech delivery can be hazardous to the baby in that the umbilical cord may separate or be compressed between the baby and the inner wall of the uterus, depriving the baby of oxygen; intracranial hemorrhage can occur because of stress on the head as it is delivered last; and injuries to the head, neck, and upper arms can occur during manipulations of delivery. Each breech delivery is managed according to its need.

Under certain conditions in which resistance inhibits the normal delivery mechanism, a forceps delivery may be necessary. Such conditions include the mother's exhaustion, cardiac or pulmonary problems, or illness; fetal distress; or certain obstetrical conditions (such as

episiotomy
Incision between the vulva and anus to enlarge the vaginal opening at the time of birth.

crowning
The presentation of the baby's head at the vaginal opening.

breech delivery
A delivery in which the infant is born with another body part first, rather than head first. This form of delivery can be hazardous for both mother and infant.

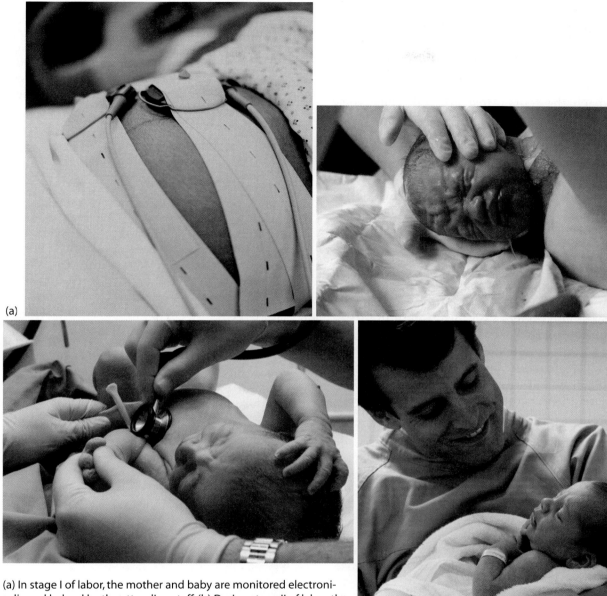

(a) In stage I of labor, the mother and baby are monitored electronically and helped by the attending staff. (b) During stage II of labor, the child is born, with the head appearing first. (c) The baby, 1 minute old, with umbilical cord. (d) After delivery and checking over of the baby, the parents begin to bond with their newborn child.

certain positions of the baby's head). The forceps is a tool designed to deliver the baby's head and is used to gain traction and to rotate the baby. A forceps must be used carefully, however, because it exerts force and can cause fetal damage.

After delivery of the baby, the umbilical cord is clamped and cut.

Delivery of Placenta

The third stage, delivery of the placenta and the membranes, usually occurs about 5 minutes after the baby is born. When the placenta emerges—again through contractions of the uterus—the doctor or midwife examines it carefully to be sure it is completely smooth. If the placenta is not smooth, it is likely that some placental tissue has remained in the uterus. Any tissue left behind may cause uterine bleeding or infection. If contractions stop before the placenta is expelled, manual techniques or injection are used to facilitate its delivery. If an episiotomy has been performed, it is repaired after the placenta is delivered.

Drugs Used in Childbirth

Expectant parents must grapple with the question of whether drugs will be used during delivery. Decisions about drugs in childbirth require some homework, because many kinds of drugs are available, all having different effects. Anesthetics inhibit perception, not just of pain but of touch and all other sensations, in the mother. General anesthetics not only affect the mother but also cross the placental barrier and reach the fetus. Most are central nervous system depressants and can act as such on the fetus. Some general anesthetics are used in pain-reducing concentrations, in which case they are less powerful depressants. These are usually inhaled. Among them are continuous nitrous oxide and enflurane.

Whereas general anesthetics put the individual to sleep, local anesthetics and local and regional analgesics (reducers of pain perception) inhibit feelings and sensations in specific parts of the body. They can be used to reduce pain without placing the fetus in jeopardy. Hypnosis is an example of what is called an **obstetrical analgesia**, a nondrug pain reliever.

A local anesthetic injected around the nerves in a given spinal area reduces sensory feeling in a specific area of the body. A local anesthetic is generally administered during the later part of the first stage of labor and during all of the second stage. Single or multiple injections are administered via a catheter into the spinal area. Drugs commonly used for local pain relief include tetracaine, lidocaine, and bupivacaine. Different areas of the pelvic region are anesthetized by different procedures. **Saddle blocks**, or **epidural blocks**, anesthetize the area of the buttocks, perineum, and inner thigh (the area that literally sits on a saddle). In a **paracervical block**, injections are given at positions around the cervix.

Drugs have been used successfully and safely during labor for many years. Therefore, their use is not cause for alarm. Still, as with all drugs, there are potential, though minimal, risks. Spinal anesthesia, for example, can cause headache, nausea and vomiting, and a drop in blood pressure. A reduction in blood pressure can reduce the oxygen supply to the baby and can change the fetal heartbeat.

Because pregnancy is a 9-month experience, expectant parents have plenty of time to discuss alternatives. Talks with the physician or midwife, with friends who have used different methods, and, most important, with each other, will yield a well-thought-out decision.

> **obstetrical analgesia**
> A nondrug pain reliever used in delivery (e.g., hypnosis).
>
> **saddle (epidural) block**
> An anesthetic used during childbirth that blocks pain sensations in the buttocks, perineum, and inner thigh.
>
> **paracervical block**
> An anesthetic used during childbirth that blocks pain sensations in the pelvic area, in which injections are given at positions around the cervix.

Natural Childbirth

Drug-free childbirth gained support in the latter part of the 20th century, particularly as the adverse effects of some drugs on the newborn were discovered. This mode of giving birth is **natural childbirth**—or *prepared childbirth*, as it is sometimes called, because it involves education and practice. Electing to have a natural delivery often means that both parents are more involved in the pregnancy than they would be in a more traditional approach.

> **natural childbirth**
> Drug-free childbirth; sometimes called *prepared childbirth*.

Within the natural childbirth movement, a number of specific options exist. The movement began early in the 1930s with Dr. Grantly Dick-Read, an English physician. He developed a method of childbirth with no anesthetics or analgesics and published his approach in *Childbirth Without Fear*. At the heart of his method were techniques for relaxing tension to reduce the pain of labor. In 1950 a Russian named Velvoski published a work on his theory of psychoprophylaxis, which was taken up in France by Fernand Lamaze. Psychoprophylaxis is based on the premise that with the aid of a supportive coach (usually a partner, but any concerned, interested adult friend can play this role), a woman who has

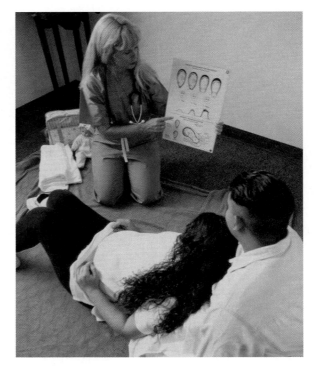

Natural, or prepared, childbirth involves both of the prospective parents being educated in techniques—exercise and breathing techniques among them—to decrease the likelihood that anesthetics will be required during childbirth.

(?) Did You Know . . .

Some women choose to give birth immersed in a pool of water as a way to relax, alleviate pain, and minimize the need for medications during childbirth (Maude & Foureur, 2007). The baby receives oxygen via blood passing through the placenta, so the fact that birth occurs under water is not a cause of concern. A healthy baby, one not in distress, will only take a breath as soon as it feels cold air on its nose and mouth. Therefore, it is imperative that the woman's hips and pelvis be fully submerged to ensure that no cold air is on the baby as it arrives. The child is immediately brought out of the water by an attendant, usually seconds after birth. To ensure safety, water births should be attended by a nurse–midwife or other healthcare provider who is trained in water births. Some water births occur at home, whereas others occur in a birthing center or hospital setting.

As with any delivery procedure, a number of aspects need to be considered. The temperature of the water needs to be close to 98 degrees so that it is close to human body temperature. Water that is too hot or too cold can cause stress to the baby (Oregon Health and Science University, 2011).

Many professionals recommend that women are dilated by 4 or 5 centimeters before entering the water, because this practice seems to speed labor. Entering the water too early may actually extend and slow labor (Oregon Health and Science University, 2011). Some individuals are concerned about infection (because of fecal matter released from the mother into the water during labor), but at least one study showed that infection risk to the infant is no greater than a conventional vaginal delivery (Thöni, Mussner, & Ploner, 2010).

Although more research is needed, studies have shown water births to provide some potential benefits. For example, women having water births had significantly shorter labor duration (Qiu & Liu, 2008; Zanetti-Dällenbach et al., 2007); were less likely to need an episiotomy (Jin et al., 2009; Thöni, Mussner, & Ploner, 2010; Zanetti-Dällenbach et al., 2007); and experienced less pain and/or were less likely to request pain relievers (Jin et al., 2009; Thöni, Mussner, & Ploner, 2010; Zanetti-Dällenbach et al., 2007). Overall, when the procedure is used for low-risk pregnancies and attended by a trained health professional, risk to mother and fetus have not been demonstrated.

---

positive attitudes can reduce the stress and tension of parturition and relax the pelvic muscles. The objective is to reduce the pain of labor to the point where painkilling drugs become unnecessary. Exercise and breathing techniques are integral to what has come to be called the **Lamaze method**. The woman and her coach attend classes together once a week for approximately 6 to 8 weeks before the expected delivery date. Both adults participate in the birth process, with the coach guiding the mother in performing the exercises appropriate to the stage of labor.

> **Lamaze method**
> An approach to childbirth in which exercise and breath control are central to reducing anxiety and discomfort.

With this approach the woman receives both emotional support and coaching, particularly during the delivery itself. As was noted earlier, an effort to include the father has many advantages, particularly regarding his relationship to the newborn. Because some men may feel frightened or uncomfortable at the prospect of being present at a birth, a couple must discuss the option thoroughly. Does the man eagerly look forward to participating? Is the woman willing to undergo a natural birth without her partner

present and perhaps with another coach? As do most other aspects of reproductive behavior, the natural childbirth option requires free and open communication between partners.

Although natural childbirth can be extremely satisfying, it is important to realize that natural methods are not suited to every pregnancy. The mother's health, as well as her pain threshold, will influence the decision. It is particularly important for expectant parents to realize that even when they have made the decision to have a drug-free delivery, the woman may decide during labor that she needs something for pain. In such a case the mother may be given a mild tranquilizer. Women ought not to feel guilty about asking for drugs in labor. Natural childbirth is not a contest!

Cesarean Section

Cesarean section (C-section) is the delivery of the fetus and placenta through an incision in the walls of the abdomen and uterus. The procedure is performed when a

> **cesarean section (C-section)**
> Surgical intervention to deliver the fetus, placenta, and membranes through an incision in the walls of the abdomen and uterus.

delivery through the vagina would be of risk to mother or to baby. Possible reasons for a C-section include fetal distress, failure of labor to progress, or problems with the umbilical cord or placenta. Sometimes reasons for a C-section may be identified in advance, such as a breech presentation, a multiple pregnancy (especially for three or more fetuses), a baby that is 9 or 10 pounds, maternal infections, other maternal health conditions (such as high blood pressure), or a previous C-section. C-sections are also performed if the mother has an STI that can be transmitted to the baby during a vaginal delivery, if the baby is too large to pass easily through the vaginal canal and opening, and if a vaginal delivery will cause potential harm to the mother because of certain illnesses (such as diabetes). In 2008, C-sections accounted for 32.3% of all deliveries in the United States (Martin et al., 2010). This is an all-time high and nearly a 2% increase from 2007. There is much debate about the high rates of C-sections in the United States and other parts of the world. The World Health Organization (WHO) states that there is no reason for any country to have rates higher than 10–15%. A recent WHO study of 137 countries showed only 14 countries in that range, with 69 countries above that range, accounting for 6.2 million medically unnecessary procedures (Gibbons et al., 2010).

A 2011 editorial in *Obstetrics & Gynecology* outlined several strategies to decrease the cesarean rate. Some suggestions include increasing the number of VBAC (vaginal birth after cesarean delivery) procedures, compensating clinicians equally for vaginal deliveries and cesearean section deliveries (but more for VBAC procedures), increasing education and training with regard to breech vaginal deliveries, changing litigation practices so that clinicians do not resort to the cesareans as protection from possible lawsuits, increasing the use of midwives in the birthing process, and educating patients about the risks of the surgical procedure (Queenan, 2011).

There are disadvantages to having a C-section. It is expensive; the mother needs a recuperative period that may interfere with her caring for her baby; there is scarring of the uterus; and there is the possibility, though slight, of hemorrhage or infection. It must be pointed out, however, that many babies and mothers would die without surgical intervention. The same WHO study previously mentioned also showed that worldwide 3.18 million cesarean section procedures were needed but did not happen, causing severe complications and death for those involved (Gibbons et al., 2010). Cesarean intervention is an alternative delivery method to be considered in certain complicated situations.

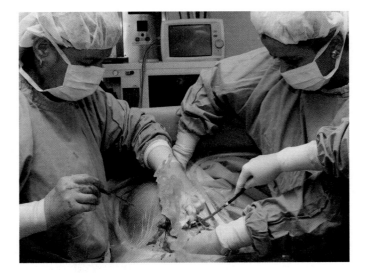

The number of cesarean sections has increased among Americans in recent years. Some argue that this is the result of fear of lawsuits on the part of obstetricians, whereas others believe it is less traumatic for the mother than the strains of natural childbirth and is best for the newborn. Whether C-sections are performed too often is still being debated by the experts.

Premature Birth

When a child is born before the normal gestation period is completed but still has a chance of surviving, its birth is regarded as **premature**. In 2008, 12.3% of all babies born in the United States were premature (Martin et al., 2010). A premature infant is usually between 28 and 36 weeks gestation, although some are as young as 24 weeks. Gestational age is associated with low birth weight, and 43.5% of these infants weigh less than 5.8 ounces (2,500 grams), with about 11.6% weighing less than 3.3 pounds (1,500 grams). This weight average drops dramatically when looking at births at less than 28 weeks. Over 90% have a very low birth weight, and 96% have a low birth weight (Martin et al., 2010).

> **premature**
> Type of birth in which an infant is born before the complete term of gestation but late enough in the pregnancy that it has a chance to survive.

Prematurity is caused by many factors. One common cause is a maternal age younger than 17 years or older than 35 years. Other causes include maternal malnutrition, cigarette smoking and alcohol consumption, inadequate prenatal care, and a history of a previous premature delivery.

The premature baby is born before some of its body systems can perform adequately. The respiratory system in particular is immature in these babies. They may forget to breathe and may have difficulty in moving the air through the respiratory tract. Sometimes their lung surfaces are unable to work with the necessary amounts of oxygen needed for survival because of immaturity of the lungs. These infants are usually placed in incubators, which are special cribs with controls to monitor temperature and oxygen levels. Because oxygen is necessary to sustain life, on the one hand, and because an excess of oxygen can cause eye damage (retrolental fibroplasia [RLF]), on the other hand, oxygen levels must be carefully controlled. A device has been developed that, when put on the baby's skin, can measure blood oxygen levels continuously.

Premature infants often have difficulty swallowing and digesting food, so they may require special intravenous feedings. Small amounts of breast milk are fed to the baby as he or she begins to mature, both for nutrition and for the antibodies provided by the milk. Chemical tests that can detect some metabolic problems are used in the monitoring techniques.

Neonatal intensive care is the name given to the medical specialty of premature infant care. It

is costly because it requires the talents of trained specialists and special equipment. Given this care, however, most premature babies develop normally and catch up to their peers somewhere between the end of the first year and the third year. The investment to child, family, and ultimately society certainly justifies the time and costs involved.

neonatal intensive care
A medical specialty that focuses on the care of premature infants.

Psychological and Physical Adjustment After Childbirth

Psychological reactions after childbirth can occur. One of these reactions is depression, called *postpartum depression*. It is not unusual for women to have the "blues" after childbirth, in which they experience mood swings; feel sad, anxious, or overwhelmed; or have crying spells, loss of appetite, or trouble sleeping. These symptoms usually go away after a few weeks. When they persist or include thoughts of hurting the baby or oneself, or having no interest in the baby, postpartum depression may exist. About 13% of women experience postpartum depression (U.S. Department of Health and Human Services, 2009).

Hormonal changes may trigger symptoms of postpartum depression. During pregnancy, levels of the hormones estrogen and progesterone increase greatly. In the first 24 hours after childbirth, these hormones' levels quickly return to normal. Researchers think this major change in hormone levels may

lead to depression, similar to the way smaller hormone changes can affect women's moods before their periods. Levels of thyroid hormones (thyroxin) may also drop after giving birth. Low levels of thyroxin can cause symptoms of depression (U.S. Department of Health and Human Services, 2009).

Certain factors may increase a woman's risk of developing postpartum depression. These include a personal history of depression or another mental illness, a family history of depression or another mental illness, lack of support from family and friends, anxiety or negative feelings about raising the child, problems with a previous pregnancy or birth, marriage or money problems, stressful life events, young age, and substance abuse. Women who are depressed during pregnancy have a greater risk of depression after giving birth.

The two common types of treatment for depression are counseling and medication. Counseling involves talking to a therapist, psychologist, or social worker to learn to change how depression makes one think, feel, and act. Medication includes a variety of antidepressant medicines that appear to be safe for breastfeeding women (Logsdon, Wisner, & Hanusa, 2009). Some research has indicated that regular exercise may also help in treating postpartum depression (Daley, Macarthur, & Winter, 2007). The interaction between partners may play a role in postpartum depression; one study indicated that when fathers are highly supportive the mother is less likely to develop postpartum depression (Smith & Howard, 2008).

Physical changes also occur after childbirth (U.S. Department of Health and Human Services, 2010). For example, women will have a discharge of blood, called *lochia*. This shedding of the uterine lining will begin as bright red but will become lighter and eventually stop before the 6-week postpartum checkup.

Pain in the perineum (the area between the vaginal opening and the rectum) may also occur because of stretching, tearing, or if an episiotomy was performed. Although uncomfortable, this should heal quickly, even if an episiotomy was performed. Uterine contractions, sometimes called *afterpains*, may also occur. This is a normal part of involution, the process by which the uterus returns to its prepregnancy state. After birth, the uterus weighs 2 or 3 pounds; by 5 or 6 weeks after birth, it only weighs 2 to 4 ounces.

Changes in the breast will also occur. Breast milk comes in 3 to 6 days after delivery. Even if a woman is not breastfeeding, milk can leak from nipples and the breasts might feel full, tender, or uncomfortable. Breastfeeding regularly is the best strategy to address engorgement; cold compresses and a supportive bra can also help.

In addition to these and other changes, one of the most critical physical issues is sleep—or lack thereof

(Gunderson et al., 2008). Fatigue can contribute to a woman's poor self-concept and confidence in her abilities as a mother (Runquist, 2007).

▨ Breastfeeding

To ready the breasts for producing milk (**lactation**), glandular tissue and ducts proliferate during pregnancy as a result of the placenta's secretion of estrogen, progesterone, and **lactogen**. These developments account for the increase in breast size in pregnancy. Large amounts of estrogen and progesterone secreted by the placenta prevent milk production before birth, but after the placenta is delivered, both estrogen and progesterone levels drop significantly, and the level of the pituitary hormone prolactin rises. Prolactin secretion activates the breast cells to produce milk. A second pituitary hormone, **oxytocin**, acts as a stimulant for the breasts to eject milk.

Twenty-eight to 48 hours after delivery, the lactation process begins. For the first 3 or 4 days, a thin, yellowish liquid called **colostrum** is secreted by the breasts. Colostrum is a high-protein substance containing many antibodies. Actual milk production begins between the fourth and seventh days, and by the seventh day mature milk production begins. The infant's sucking stimulates nerve cells in the nipples; the mother's brain receives the message and stimulates the pituitary to secrete oxytocin, which in turn stimulates ejection of milk from the breasts. When the milk is forced out, the mother feels a tingling sensation known as a **letdown** about 30 to 60 seconds after suckling begins. This feeling is produced by a neurogenic reflex that is necessary for adequate milk supply to reach the infant. Continued milk supply is dependent on sucking. The infant's demand regulates the breasts' supply. When the baby sucks longer, the breasts produce more milk to meet the increased demand. When the baby sucks less, milk production decreases.

Breastfeeding benefits the baby by providing a diet of balanced, uncontaminated nutrients and antibodies against disease. It has also been shown to have a variety of protective benefits,

lactation
Production of breast milk.

lactogen
A hormone that stimulates the production of milk, the principal one being prolactin.

oxytocin
A pituitary hormone that stimulates the breasts to eject milk so that breastfeeding may occur after childbirth.

colostrum
The yellow fluid secreted by the breasts just before and after childbirth until milk production begins.

letdown
The tingling sensation in the breasts when milk is forced out about 30 to 60 seconds after the infant begins to suckle.

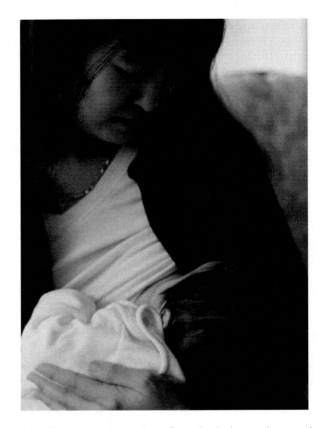

Breastfeeding conveys many benefits to both the newborn and the breastfeeding mother. Breastfeeding provides newborns with uncontaminated nutrients and antibodies against infection. It also helps the mother's uterus return to its nonpregnant shape and postpones the return of menstruation.

including reduced risk of ear infections, gastroenteritis, and severe lower respiratory infections and lower rates of sudden infant death syndrome, childhood obesity, type 2 diabetes, and leukemia (U.S. Department of Health and Human Services, 2011). The breastfeeding mother benefits, too. Nursing helps the uterus to return to its nonpregnant shape and postpones the return of menstruation (although it is not a sufficient contraceptive by itself). In addition, women who breastfeed have lower rates of breast cancer (Akbari et al., 2010), ovarian cancer (Stuebe & Schwartz, 2010), and a small reduction in the risk of type 2 diabetes (Stuebe & Schwartz, 2010). Other studies have indicated that women with a lifetime history of breastfeeding of at least 12 months have a decreased risk of developing hypertension, diabetes, high serum cholesterol, or cardiovascular disease (Gunderson et al., 2010; Schwarz et al., 2009). But probably most important, breastfeeding encourages the close attachment, or **bonding**, of infant and mother. Perhaps not incidentally, breast milk is less expensive than formula milk. Because of these

bonding
A sense of close emotional attachment.

multiple benefits, the American Academy of Pediatrics and the U.S. federal government recommend breast-feeding over formula feeding.

Currently, a woman's right to breastfeed in public is protected by law, and the Patient Protection and Affordable Care Act provides protection for pumping and storing breast milk at work for up to the first year after birth. In addition, support through organizations such as the La Leche League can also help women with the practical, how-to aspects of breastfeeding. Many times a woman will use a breast pump to extract milk that is stored for use by fathers and other caregivers during bottle feeding.

While breastfeeding is recommended for the first year, with exclusive breastfeeding recommended for 6 months of life, most women do not follow the recommendation. Almost 75% of women start breastfeeding, but only 44% are still breastfeeding at 6 months, with only 14.8% of those using breast milk exclusively, the others supplementing with formula (Centers for Disease Control and Prevention, 2011c).

Women may not breastfeed initially or continue to breastfeed for a variety of reasons. For example, some women may not produce sufficient milk to breastfeed; this may be true for women who have multiples. Others may experience pain or discomfort during breastfeeding. For those women, bonding can be experienced by holding an infant close during bottle feeding.

■ Sexual Activity During Pregnancy and After Delivery

Some, perhaps many, pregnant couples are afraid to have intercourse for fear of hurting the fetus. The frequency and kinds of sexual activity that are safe during and after pregnancy are determined both by personal preference and by health. A woman with no medical problems can continue to have the kind of sexual and sensual life she had before pregnancy (Figure 8.9). Even for healthy women, though, changes in body size and sense of comfort might dictate alterations in sexual habits. In advanced pregnancy some couples tend to replace intercourse with manual stimulation.

When certain physical conditions are present, however, coitus might add risk to the pregnancy. For example, when spotting, bleeding, pain, or past history of spontaneous abortion is present, a medical practitioner should decide whether intercourse is permissible. In healthy women, orgasmic contractions are not harmful to the fetus and will not initiate labor.

Sexual feelings can change during pregnancy. A woman's desire may be influenced by her personal involvement with the baby late in pregnancy, her individual personality, her attitudes about sexuality, her feelings about her physical appearance, and so on. Here again, the necessity for free-flowing sexual communication, both trustful and honest, cannot be stressed enough.

Penile–vaginal sex or other vaginal penetration after delivery depends on many factors: whether there were complications during and after delivery, whether a C-section was performed, and of course, whether the woman is comfortable, particularly after a difficult delivery. Most obstetricians prefer that couples delay vaginal penetration until after the first postdelivery examination, which usually takes place 4 to 6 weeks after delivery. This is to be sure that the vulva has healed if there was a tear or an episiotomy and to allow time to discuss the choice of a method of birth control.

Couples should be sure to resume contraception before penile–vaginal sex after childbirth. Despite the

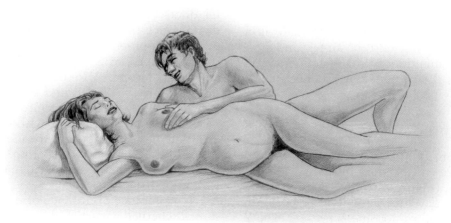

FIGURE **8.9** Pregnancy need not mean the end of sexual intercourse.

Multicultural
DIMENSIONS

Differences in Infant Mortality

Infant mortality comprises deaths occurring within the first year of life. The good news is that the infant mortality rate continues to decline. Whereas in 1983 it was 10.9 per 1,000 live births, in 2010 the infant mortality rate was 6.1 per 1,000 live births (Centers for Disease Control & Prevention, 2011d).

The bad news was that the infant mortality rate for African Americans is still much higher than that for other subgroups in the population. In 2007, the white infant mortality rate was 5.63 per 1,000 live births, but the African American infant mortality rate was 13.1 per 1,000 live births. The reasons for the high rate among African Americans are many and varied; poverty is foremost. Poverty rates are proportionately higher among African Americans than among whites. Consequently, African Americans cannot as readily afford health care, proper nutrition, and other services and behaviors that are conducive to birth of healthy babies. For example, whereas 86% of white mothers began prenatal care during the first trimester, only 76% of African American mothers did. And, though only 3.0% of white mothers began prenatal care either during the third trimester or not at all, 5.7% of African American mothers began prenatal care late or not at all (National Center for Health Statistics, 2008). In addition, data show that the rate of preterm births is higher for black, non-Hispanic women, and this difference accounts for 78% of the increased infant mortality (MacDorman & Mathews, 2011). If women were able to access prenatal care earlier, than a decrease in black, non-Hispanic infant mortality might occur.

To respond to this infant mortality rate gap between African American and white Americans, communities have instituted educational campaigns encouraging early prenatal care, particularly targeted at African American populations. Some of these programs rely on public service advertisements in newspapers, on signs on buses, or as messages over radio or television. Other programs employ women who live in the targeted communities to identify pregnant women, meet with them, and encourage them to see a healthcare provider. Still other programs employ a combination of these and other methods in conjunction with free or low-cost health care to help pregnant moms be healthier and deliver healthier children.

---

fact that breastfeeding delays the return of menstruation, that alone is not a dependable form of birth control.

Hormonal Influences on Prenatal Development: Becoming Male or Female

The process of becoming a male or a female is a complicated one, involving chromosomes and hormones. As we have mentioned, a key influence on sex determination is the presence or absence of a Y chromosome.

Typical Sexual Differentiation

Sexual differentiation, or the process of gonad and duct development, does not start until the seventh week of development (Figure 8.10). In the uterus, the fertilized egg always develops as if it were going to be female unless the Y chromosome is present. The Y chromosome contains the SRY gene. This gene gives instructions for the development of the testes; specifi-cally, it tells the indifferent gonads (neither male nor female) to develop testis-determining factor (TDF). The TDF causes the indifferent gonads to develop into testes. Because there is no SRY gene in females, no TDF is produced, and therefore ovaries develop (Hospital for Sick Children, 2011).

A similar process occurs for the development of the urogenital ducts. Before the seventh week of fetal development, embryos have two sets of urogenital ducts. These are called Müllerian and Wolffian ducts. Once the gonads have formed, they influence duct development. In a male fetus, the testes make two hormones, MIS (Müllerian inhibiting substance) and testosterone. MIS makes the Müllerian ducts disappear by week 10, and testosterone causes the Wolffian ducts to develop into spermatic ducts by week 12. In a female fetus, without testosterone, the Wolffian ducts disappear around week 10, and by week 20 the Müllerian ducts have developed into the uterus, fallopian tubes, and vagina (Hospital for Sick Children, 2011).

The presence or absence of male hormones determines whether a particular piece of tissue becomes a penis or a clitoris, a prostate gland or a Skene's gland, a Cowper's gland or a Bartholin's gland, or

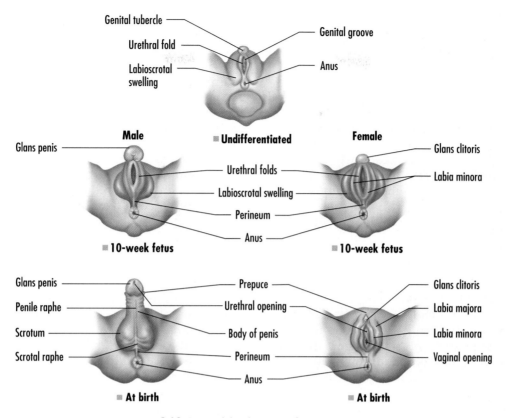

FIGURE **8.10** Prenatal development of external genitalia.

a scrotum or a labia majora. Structures that develop from the same tissue in this way are called **homologous** structures (see Table 8.1).

homologous
Organs that differ but that developed from the same tissue—for example, the glans penis and clitoris.

The differentiation of the male and female brain is called *brain dimorphism*. Brain differentiation may extend into the first few days or weeks after birth. Interestingly, it appears that brain differentiation allows for the coexistence of both masculine and feminine nuclei and pathways in some, if not all, parts of the brain. Some researchers, in fact, postulate that differentiation between males and females in many areas of the brain is not that great (Joel, 2011). While many continue to be believe that males and females differ greatly, this research shows how men and women may be more alike than previously thought.

Variance of Sexual Differentiation

The description of sexual differentiation assumes that everything goes according to plan, and it usually does. However, once in a while, development does not follow the typical path. In fact, it is possible for

TABLE 8.1	Homologous Structures	
Female	**Male**
Clitoral glans	Penile glans
Clitoral shaft	Penile shaft
Clitoral hood	Penile foreskin
Labia majora	Scrotum
Labia minora	Bottom of penile shaft
Ovaries	Testes
Bartholin's gland	Cowper's gland
Skene's gland	Prostate gland

the genetic sex, or *genotype* (the chromosomes); the gonadal sex, or *phenotype* (testes or ovaries); and the internal sexual structures (uterus, fallopian tubes, prostate gland, and vas deferens) to differ. For example, a person could be born with two X chromosomes, have a penis, an empty scrotum (without testes), two ovaries, a uterus, and a fallopian tube. Another individual may have male chromosomes (XY), male gonads (testes), and female external genitalia, as in complete androgen insensitivity syndrome.

Androgen insensitivity syndrome (AIS) is a condition in which individuals with XY chromosomes do not respond to androgens, or male hormones, in a typical way. People with complete AIS (CAIS) do not respond to androgens at all. They have testes and typical female external genitals. People with partial AIS (PAIS) do respond to androgens, but only partially and to varying degrees. They have testes and can have a range of different body types. Their genitals may not look exactly like typical female or typical male genitals.

These conditions are examples of **disorders of sexual development (DSD)**, anomalies of the sex chromosomes, the gonads, the reproductive ducts, and the genitalia. This term was initiated at an international consensus conference

> **disorders of sexual development**
> Anomalies of the sex chromosomes, the gonads, the reproductive ducts, and the genitalia.

(Hughes et al., 2006). Previously the term *intersex* was used to describe individuals who had chromosomal or anatomical differences that made them not clearly male or female. (And before that, the term *hermaphrodite* was also used.) Today, many organizations use DSD because of the lack of precision with the term *intersex* (Accord Alliance, 2008). However, others—especially many international groups—still use intersex because of dislike for the "disorder" component of DSD (Diamond, 2009) and a variety of other concerns with the term (for example, that it is not inclusive for adults living with these conditions; it does not translate clearly to other languages).

Within DSD there is much variation. Some individuals have typical male or female chromosome structure but exhibit physical differences. Examples of these include: *46, XY, micropenis*, in which an individual has male chromosome makeup but an extremely small penis; *clitoromegaly*, in which an individual has an enlarged clitoris; and *MRKH syndrome* where ovaries are present but the uterus is absent, misshapen, or small (Accord Alliance, 2008).

Other examples of DSD can be traced to the chromosomes. For example, in a condition called *Turner's Syndrome*, which is caused by the presence of only one X chromosome (instead of two), the female may be infertile, have short stature, and may be at risk for some cardiac or renal anomalies. In another condition, *Klinefelter's syndrome*, caused by an XXY genetic makeup, boys appear normal until puberty but then do not develop the normal secondary sex characteristics and may develop breasts at that time. Individuals with Klinefelter's may also have low levels of sperm.

Accord Alliance (formerly known as the Intersex Society of North American) is one organization helping educate families and clinicians about treatment options and psychological needs of children with DSD. In the past, genital surgery was often performed for cosmetic reasons, resulting in physical and emotional damage. Today, more informed decisions about gender assignment are made with the hope of lessening the emotional toll. Likewise, nonmedically needed surgeries may be delayed until the individual with DSD can consent. Hormonal therapy may also be part of the treatment; counseling for the child with DSD and the family is recommended.

Still another problem associated with sexual differentiation is called an *inguinal hernia*. The testes descend into the scrotum through a structure called the *inguinal canal*. This normally occurs by the seventh month of fetal development. If the inguinal canal does not close properly after the testes descend or if it opens up afterward, it is possible for the intestine to move down the canal and enter the scrotum. An inguinal hernia can be corrected surgically.

If the testes do not descend down the inguinal canal, as occurs in about 2% of male newborns, the condition is called *cryptorchidism* (more commonly called *undescended testes*). Usually the testes will descend during early childhood or by puberty. If they do not, however, either surgery or hormonal therapy is necessary for two reasons: (1) Testes in the abdomen are at too high a temperature to produce viable sperm, and if they are left undescended, infertility is likely to result; and (2) there is a greater risk of testicular cancer if testes are left undescended.

■ Infertility

Infertility, or the inability to reproduce, can cause great emotional anguish for people who want children. This unhappiness, accompanied by tension, frustration, and even resentment, can damage the health

> **infertility**
> The inability to reproduce.

and the relationships of infertile couples. The situation may be further complicated by an inability or unwillingness to adopt a child. It is important to add, however, that while adoption may relieve the stress of wanting to raise children, it may not eliminate the stress related to infertility.

More than 5 million people of childbearing age experience infertility. Primary infertility is defined as inability to conceive despite having unprotected intercourse for at least 1 year or 6 months if older than age 35. Secondary infertility is defined as inability to conceive despite having unprotected intercourse for at least 1 year and having previously conceived (Nelson & Marshall, 2008). It is estimated that 10% to 15% of couples experience primary infertility.

Women and men can both contribute to infertility. Infertility related to sperm and other male problems

¿? Ethical DIMENSIONS

Surrogate Mothers Some couples who attempt to conceive children cannot. In some cases, the cause is a lack of viable sperm. In other cases, the problem is a blockage of the fallopian tubes, which prevents the sperm–ovum union. In still other cases, the woman does not produce an ovum to be fertilized or, because of some medical condition, cannot carry a fetus in her uterus until delivery. In the latter circumstance, the woman's ovum can be fertilized by her partner's sperm outside the womb and implanted in the uterus of another woman, a *surrogate womb* or gestational carrier. However, when a woman does not produce ova for fertilization, sometimes another woman's egg is fertilized by her partner and develops in that other woman's uterus. Upon delivery, the baby becomes the child of the father and his partner rather than of the father and the woman whose eggs and uterus were used for

9 months or so. The woman whose eggs and uterus were used is the biological mother, referred to as a *surrogate mother.*

When surrogate motherhood occurs without complications, it provides for everyone's needs. However, every once in a while, circumstances requiring creative solutions develop. For example, what do you think should happen if the surrogate mother does not want to give up the child after delivery? (Maybe she develops an attachment to the baby, or her situation has changed and she now wants a child of her own.) What should happen if the father and his partner do not want to accept the baby? (Maybe the baby has a birth defect, the couple has separated or divorced, or they just changed their minds about wanting children.) Each of these situations has actually occurred. What is your opinion?

is indicated in 30–40% of cases, ovarian dysfunction is attributed in 10–15%, and tubal and pelvic issues indicated in 30–40%. Unexplained infertility accounts for 10% of infertility (Nelson & Marshall, 2008). In addition, women older than 35 may also encounter diminished ovarian reserve, meaning that their remaining eggs are few and/or of poor quality.

Causes of Infertility

In women, the most common cause of infertility is related to problems with ovulation, and therefore no eggs to fertilize (Department of Health and Human Services, 2009). Other, less common conditions can include blocked fallopian tubes due to pelvic inflammatory disease (PID), endometriosis, or surgery for an ectopic pregnancy; physical anomalies with the uterus, and uterine fibroids (non-cancerous build-up of tissue and muscle on the walls of the uterus). PID can be caused by untreated chlamydia or gonorrhea infections. Sexually active college students can reduce their risk of future infertility by using condoms, practicing safer sex behaviors, and getting regularly tested for STIs.

STIs are not the only diseases that affect fertility. Health problems in women cause hormonal changes, such as polycystic ovarian syndrome, and an increased risk of infertility. In men, mumps, kidney disease, or hormone problems can be related to infertility issues. People with sickle-cell disease have higher infertility rates. In both males and females, radiation and

chemotherapy treatment related to cancer can affect fertility. Several drugs may inhibit sperm production or sperm function, including antimalarial drugs, antihypertensives, and calcium-channel blockers.

One of the largest factors affecting infertility is age. Women are most fertile in their mid-20s and after age 30, fertility potential gradually declines. Men older than age 40 may be less fertile than younger men. Substance use is another component of infertility; if either partner smokes, the chance of pregnancy decreases, and it also reduces the benefit of any fertility treatment. Miscarriages are also more frequent in women who smoke. For women, moderate to heavy levels of alcohol use make it more difficult to become pregnant. For women, weight—either being overweight or underweight—may affect fertility. Some studies have found excessive exercising—more than 7 hours a week—to be associated with ovulation problems (Mayo Clinic, 2011). Environmental exposure to chemicals such as pesticides, herbicides, and some insecticides can also affect male and female reproductive functioning (Woodruff, Carlson, Schwartz, & Giudice, 2008). Although infertility can cause stress, there is no conclusive evidence that stress can cause infertility (American Society for Reproductive Medicine, 2011b).

Finally, in some couples, a lack of knowledge about anatomy, physiology, and reproduction leads to infertility. These couples may not know when conception is most likely to occur, they may not have penile–vaginal sex frequently enough to conceive, and they may not know how to time intercourse.

The ovum is alive for less than 1 day; sperm can live as long as 5 days inside the woman. Couples must have penile–vaginal before ovulation to maximize the possibility of pregnancy.

Testing and Treatment for Infertility

As couples focus on education, careers, and other aspects of life, delayed parenthood is more common, and with that, the increased risk of infertility. While media reports often focus on specific reproductive technologies in isolation, the path to addressing infertility can be quite long for many couples.

Some individuals prefer to try "natural" ways to enhance their fertility. Unfortunately, research has shown that there is very little related to the act of sex that changes the likelihood of conceiving. Specific timing of sex, positioning during sex, or having the female rest on her back after sex have no significant impact on fertility (American Society for Reproductive Medicine, 2008). Penile–vaginal sex every 1 to 2 days yields the highest pregnancy rates, but having sex only 2 or 3 times per week is nearly the same. For those who have penile–vaginal sex less frequently, devices that help identify when ovulation occurs may be helpful. In reality, age, lifestyle factors, and frequency of sex are the most important ways to influence fertility (American Society for Reproductive Medicine, 2008).

If a couple has been trying to conceive for more than 12 months without success (or more than 6 months if the woman is 35 years or older), they should consult with a clinician about testing. In many cases, infertility can be successfully treated. In fact, most infertility cases—85–90%—are treated with conventional medicine, such as medication and surgical repair of the reproductive organs (American Society for Reproductive Medicine, 2011a). In all cases, the first step is to determine why a couple is unable to conceive. At present, several basic infertility screening procedures may be used in this examination phase:

1. *Semen analysis.* The man is asked to masturbate and collect the ejaculate in a container. The ejaculate is then examined to determine the number of sperm present, the sperm's motility, and the amount of fructose (nourishment for the sperm) in the semen.

2. *Basal body temperature (BBT) recordings.* The woman is required to record her body temperature (with an oral or BBT thermometer) daily. The decrease in estrogen production as ovulation nears causes the basal temperature to drop about 0.3 degree. When ovulation occurs, basal temperature rises about 0.6

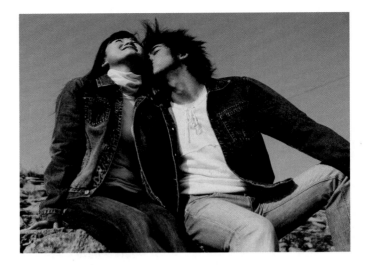

In spite of their love for one another, their understanding of the menstrual cycle and ovulation, and their ability to effectively engage in sexual intercourse, some couples are not able to conceive. There are several reasons for this, and several screening tests to determine the reason for any particular couple. Once the reason is uncovered, treatment can begin to increase the likelihood of conception.

degree as a result of the corpus luteum's production of the hormone progesterone. Thus a physician can determine whether ovulation is occurring normally by monitoring the basal temperature.

3. *Endometrial biopsy.* A biopsy (microscopic examination of excised tissue) of the endometrium is performed. This procedure helps identify uterine abnormalities.

4. *Tubal patency tests.* Dye is projected through the fallopian tubes and observed by X ray to detect any blockage; this test is also called a *hysterosalpingogram.*

5. *Postcoital examination.* Two to 4 hours after the couple has had penile–vaginal sex, the cervical mucus is examined microscopically. The physician checks for several conditions of the cervical mucus that can be fatal to sperm (for example, too much viscosity or too little salt). The sperm are counted and their ability to travel determined, because the more motile the sperm, the greater the likelihood of conception.

6. *Hormone monitoring.* Several ovulation prediction kits are currently sold over the counter. These kits measure the level of luteinizing hormone (LH), the hormone causing ovulation midway through the menstrual cycle. Urine tests can also be used to

measure the amount of progesterone during various phases of the cycle. Other hormones (such as prolactin, thyroid hormones, and follicle-stimulating hormone [FSH]) can be monitored as well.

7. *Cervical mucus evaluation.* The cervical mucus can be evaluated for its elasticity, its nature just before ovulation (it should be thin, watery, salty, and stretchy), and the presence of cells, debris, and proper pH level (degree of acidity or alkalinity).

8. *Ultrasonography.* High-frequency sound waves are transmitted and reflected by internal organs and structures. From the resulting pattern, detailed outlines of the reproductive system can be obtained.

9. *Hysteroscopy.* The uterus is expanded with carbon dioxide gas or liquid and is observed through a hysteroscope—a long, narrow, illuminated instrument that is inserted through the cervix into the uterus. Abnormalities such as polyps, fibroids, and adhesions can be identified in this manner.

10. *Laparoscopy.* In this minor surgery, a small incision is made in the lower abdomen and a laparoscope (small tool with a light) is inserted. The ovaries, fallopian tubes, and uterus can be checked for disease and physical problems, such as scarring or endometriosis.

Depending on the couple's medical history, personal factors, and other available medical information, a couple may be asked to undergo some but usually not all of these screening procedures. Generally, male semen analysis is almost always done to determine any male factors. Once the cause or causes are determined, treatment can be prescribed. Cessation of ovulation can be restarted through hormone therapy or by increasing body fat through nutritional therapy. Blocked fallopian tubes can be cleared through microsurgical techniques. In some cases, more complicated and advanced procedures are required. Depending on the patient's age, reason for infertility, and other medical factors, a doctor may recommend **intrauterine insemination (IUI)** and/or artificial reproductive technologies (ART), such as in vitro fertilization (IVF).

> **intrauterine insemination**
> Introduction of semen into the uterus by noncoital means.

In IUI, specially prepared sperm are injected into a women's uterus. Sometimes in this procedure the woman uses medication to stimulate ovulation, though this can increase the number of eggs released. IUI is often used to treat mild male factor infertility, cervical mucus problems in females, and couples with unexplained infertility. For men who produce no sperm (a condition called *azoospermia*) or who have a sperm count too low to ensure fertilization (*oligospermia*) or for females without male partners, a donor could also be used for the sperm.

If the woman does use medications to increase the number of follicles maturing and the potential number of eggs, it is not possible to control the number of eggs that will be fertilized. Therefore, IUI increases the chance for a pregnancy of multiple fetuses. As the number of fetuses increases, concern about health issues for the mother and the fetuses also increases. Babies born as part of a multiple pregnancy are more likely to be born premature and with low or very low birth weights. In some cases, a woman may opt for selective abortion, in which one or more fetuses are aborted to give the remaining fetuses a better chance to develop.

The group of procedures in which the clinician handles both the sperm and the egg are called **assisted reproductive technologies (ART)**. In these methods, eggs are removed from a woman's body, fertilized with sperm, and allowed to develop into embryos in a laboratory. The embryos are then put back in the woman's body (U.S. Department of Health and Human Services, 2009). Common methods of ART include:

> **assisted reproductive technologies (ART)**
> Procedures in which the clinician handles both the sperm and the egg.

- In vitro fertilization (IVF) is often used when a woman's fallopian tubes are blocked or when a man produces too few sperm. The woman takes medication that causes the ovaries to produce multiple eggs. Once mature, the eggs are removed from the woman and put in a dish in the lab along with sperm for fertilization. After 3 to 5 days, if healthy embryos have been produced, they are implanted in the woman's uterus. Recommendations for the number of embryos to transfer have been established (American Society for Reproductive Medicine & Society for Assisted Reproductive Technology, 2009). These guidelines are based on the woman's age, the maturity of the embryo, and other medical factors, but in most cases implanting fewer than four embryos is recommended. There is increasing emphasis to limit transfers to one embryo because of the increased risk of a multiple pregnancy. IVF is the most successful ART and is also the most common.

- Zygote intrafallopian transfer (ZIFT) or tubal embryo transfer is similar to IVF. Fertilization occurs in the laboratory; however, a very young embryo is transferred to the fallopian tube instead of the uterus.

- Gamete intrafallopian transfer (GIFT) involves transferring eggs and sperm into the woman's fallopian tube. In this case, fertilization occurs in the woman's body. Because of lower success rates, few clinics provide GIFT as a procedure.

- Intracytoplasmic sperm injection (ICSI) is often used when there are serious problems with the sperm or if there are genetic disorders that an individual does not want to pass on to a child. ICSI may also be used for older couples or for those with failed IVF attempts. In ICSI, a single sperm is injected into a mature egg. Then the embryo is transferred to the uterus or fallopian tube.

In 2006, 44% of ART transfer procedures resulted in a pregnancy, and 36% in a delivery of one or more live-born infants; this equates to approximately 1% of U.S. infants (Sunderman et al., 2009). However, the success rate declines with the age of the eggs. For women using their own eggs, the success rate is 41% in women younger than 35 years, 32% in women aged 35–37 years, 22% in women aged 38–40 years, 12% in women aged 41–42 years, and 5% in women aged 43–44 years (Centers for Disease Control and Prevention, 2011b). The age of the eggs is so critical that if everything else was equivalent a 38-year-old woman using her own eggs would likely have less success with IVF than a 42-year-old woman using the eggs from a 25-year-old egg donor.

While many women are able to successfully conceive with ART, it is not without risk. Studies show that preterm deliveries and low/very low birth weight are increased with ART, largely because of the increased risk of a multiple pregnancy. A multiple pregnancy can also cause additional strain on the mother, such as increased risk for complications during pregnancy and delivery. In addition, adverse prenatal and postbirth outcomes are more common among singleton ART infants than among naturally conceived singletons (Centers for Disease Control and Prevention, 2011a).

With any of the ART procedures, individuals could use donor eggs (eggs from another woman), donor sperm, or previously frozen donor embryos. Individuals may choose these paths because of health conditions, such as not being able to produce sperm or eggs themselves, or when one has a genetic condition that can be passed to the child. Donor embryos were either created by couples who were already undergoing infertility treatment or were created from donor sperm and donor eggs. The donor embryos would be transferred into the uterus. Procedures are in place to screen sperm and egg donors for communicable infections; egg donors also receive a genetic screening both via a detailed family history and specific blood tests that are determined by ethnic/racial background (Resolve, 2011).

Others may consider surrogacy. In this situation, a woman agrees to become pregnant using sperm from a male and her own egg. After birth, the surrogate will give up the baby for adoption by the parents. Some same-sex male couples may also choose this option. While similar, using a gestational carrier may be an option for a woman with ovaries but no uterus, a uterus that cannot support a pregnancy, or who should not become pregnant because of a serious health problem. In this situation, a woman's own egg is fertilized by the man's sperm and the embryo is placed inside the carrier's uterus. The carrier will give the baby to the parents at birth.

All of these scenarios can include legal and potentially ethical issues. In many clinics, more eggs are harvested and fertilized than the number needed for a single cycle. These embryos are then frozen so they can be used for future IVF procedures. However, in some cases couples have divorced before the transfer of the embryos, and so couples have fought over these embryos as part of a divorce settlement. In a few widely publicized cases, embryos have been implanted after the man has died. Is the child in that case born to a married couple or to a single mother? And should insurance companies and Medicaid pay for IUI and ART? In most cases, they do not. A basic IVF procedure (without special circumstances such as genetic testing, donors, etc.) costs $12,000 to 15,000 per cycle. Should ART only be available to the wealthy?

In some of these cases, clinics are taking steps to minimize legal issues, such as having couples decide if embryo use requires the consent of both partners and what happens to the eggs and the decision making if one partner dies. Regarding costs associated with ART, some states require ART be covered by insurance. A number of health organizations are interested in working on an action plan to address infertility and access to treatments in the United States (CDC Infertility Working Group, 2010).

In reality, it is has only been a little over 30 years (1981) since the first baby was conceived by IVF in the United States. We are just beginning to understand the potential of these technologies and the complications they bring.

Exploring the Dimensions of Human Sexuality

Our feelings, attitudes, and beliefs regarding sexuality are influenced by our internal and external environments. Go to go.jblearning.com/dimensions5e to learn more about the biological factors that affect your sexuality.

Case Study

Pregnancy is a time of wonder and joy. For first-time parents, the world is forever changed after their infant is born. But even the degree of responsibility and emotional attachment to the child are influenced by many dimensions.

Biological age of the mother plays a factor. Teen pregnancies tend to have more medical complications for both mother and child. Risk of Down syndrome increases with age, from 1 in 940 births at age 30 years, to 1 in 85 births at age 40 years, to 1 in 35 births at age 45 years (Morris et al., 2003).

Socioeconomic status plays a role in the health care of children. Parents on the low end of the socioeconomic scale may lack resources for parental and infant care, as well as the education and resources for raising healthy children.

Social pressure about child rearing is exerted by grandparents as well.

When disposable diapers were introduced, Pampers advertised them as "easier." But grandparent pressure—"What was wrong with the diapers we used on you?"—caused many parents to return to cloth diapers. Pampers had to change its marketing strategy from being easier to being better for the baby.

Working parents tend to rely on a far-flung network of day care providers, friends, family, and peer parents for emotional and practical advice. Without such support, the emotional impact of raising a child can be overwhelming.

Biological Factors

- Hormones create gender differentiation during the second month of prenatal development.
- Physiological cycles and changes in the fetus take place at an extremely fast pace.
- Physical appearance of the mother changes (for example, clearer skin) as hormonal changes take place.
- Parents' genetic characteristics determine many attributes of their children, such as height and hair color.

Sociocultural Factors

- Socioeconomic status influences infant and maternal health, because poor people have less access to prenatal care than well-off people do.
- Laws restrict access to abortions during the third trimester.
- Religion, culture, and ethnic heritage influence many beliefs about pregnancy, childbirth, and parenting.
- Media and ads may influence the choice of where to have a child or whether to use the services of a midwife or a physician.
- Family, neighbors, and friends who have children can provide invaluable advice and assistance to new parents.

Psychological Factors

- A pregnant woman's emotions can swing wildly because of hormonal shifts. The postpartum period can be associated with the "baby blues" or more severe depression.
- Experience counts in pregnancy; subsequent infants go through labor faster and breastfeed more readily.
- Self-concept usually increases as a result of the responsibility of caring for another person.
- Learned attitudes and behaviors are often exhibited by pregnant couples.
- A woman's body image can suffer if she views herself as "getting fat" rather than as "carrying a child."

Summary

- Conception occurs in the fallopian tube. Sperm stay alive in the female reproductive tract for 72 to 120 hours. The ovum's peak fertile period is 8 to 12 hours, although an egg can be fertilized for as long as 24 hours after ovulation.

- The conceptus is known as a zygote until 8 weeks of development, when it is known as an embryo. At the beginning of the third month of development, the conceptus is known as a fetus. The embryo develops in the amniotic sac cushioned with amniotic fluid.

- Sometimes an ectopic pregnancy occurs in which the blastocyst becomes implanted in a site other than the uterus. Ectopic pregnancies are the main cause of maternal morbidity and mortality in the first trimester.

- Childbirth can occur under the supervision of a physician or a nurse–midwife. It can take place in a hospital, in a free-standing birthing center, or at home.

- Among the threats to a normal birth delivery are the use of over-the-counter drugs and alcohol, cigarettes, marijuana, cocaine, heroin and other narcotics, and birth control pills. Disease such as diabetes, HIV infection, and other STIs are additional threats. The pregnant woman may also experience hypertension, nausea and vomiting, hemorrhoids, and other conditions.

- Labor occurs in three stages. Stage I is the period from the onset of labor to the point at which the cervix is fully dilated. Stage II is the period from full cervical dilation through the birth of the child. Stage III is the period from the infant's birth to the delivery of the placenta, or afterbirth.

- Infertility, or the inability to reproduce, can be caused by occlusion of the fallopian tubes, blocked sperm ducts, low sperm production, or poor semen quality. Infertility can be treated by assisted reproductive technologies such as intrauterine insemination, in vitro fertilization, or gamete intrafallopian transfer.

Discussion Questions

1. Explain the process by which life begins, citing as much detail as possible.

2. What are the characteristics of fetal development that differentiate the three trimesters?

3. What can a pregnant woman do to increase the chance of having a healthy pregnancy and child?

4. Describe how various drugs and diseases can threaten infant health.

5. Which maternal problems may occur during pregnancy? What can be done to alleviate some of these problems?

6. Differentiate the three phases of labor and methods of reducing the pain of labor.

7. Describe the benefits of breastfeeding an infant.

8. Is sex safe during pregnancy? Explain the situations in which it is or is not.

9. Compare and contrast the prenatal undifferentiated and sex-differentiated external genitalia, including the hormones that create the sexes.

10. Explain the most common causes of infertility and the methods to treat such problems.

Application Questions

Reread the chapter-opening story and answer the following questions.

1. The Rich and Mary story underscores how the many dimensions of human sexuality play into our decision making. Although Mary believed in the social and ethical right of women to have abortions, her personal convictions and the psychological desire for another child led her to continue her pregnancy. What would you have done in Rich and Mary's situation? Which of the dimensions of human sexuality mentioned here would influence you?

2. The Rich and Mary story also underscores the fact that medical personnel often work with less than perfect information—they did not know she was carrying twins! If you had been in their situation, where could you find more information on analyzing amniocentesis test results? Would you pursue such avenues?

Critical Thinking Questions

1. A premature baby born at 24 weeks gestation (5½ months), weighing about a pound, can be saved—at a cost of more than $300,000. But that is just the start. Many "preemie" children continue to have problems in school, requiring special-education programs. Choose a side and debate for or against saving children born more premature than 35 weeks. (*Note:* This question was submitted by a parent of two premature babies to provoke discussion.)

2. Hospitals have found that birthing centers are enormously profitable ventures. In major cities, hospitals compete for patients by having birthing rooms designed to look like homes with extra amenities and "freebies" (such as a champagne breakfast the morning after). Yet to maintain profits, patients are sent home as soon as state laws allow—usually 24 to 48 hours after birth. Do patients benefit from such an arrangement—or is it simply a business deal for the hospitals?

Critical Thinking Case

For many years, there had been concern that too many cesarean birth deliveries were being performed in the United States. In 2008, the U.S. cesarean rate of nearly 32.3% of all births was higher than that of other industrialized nations. Interestingly, the data indicated that the increase in the cesarean rate did not contribute to the decline in infant mortality rate. Making matters worse, maternal morbidity and mortality rates are higher in cesarean deliveries than in routine vaginal deliveries. One of the *Healthy People 2010* national health objectives was to decrease the rate of cesarean deliveries in women giving birth the first time to 15% of live births and to 63% of women giving birth who had a prior cesarean. The continued increase in C-section rates eliminated the possibility of reaching that goal.

The Healthy People 2020 objectives aim for a decrease of 10% in the cesarean section rates by 2020, with a new goal of 23.9% for first-time births and 81.9% for women with a prior cesarean section (U.S. Department of Health and Human Services, 2012).

It had previously been thought unwise and unhealthy for women who had a previous cesarean delivery to attempt a vaginal birth. The concern was for tearing of the tissue and possible infection for the baby. The standard practice was "Once a cesarean, always a cesarean." However, it was found that, barring complications, many women who had a cesarean delivery could deliver vaginally the next time without endangering their or their baby's health.

Are the high rates of C-sections the result of the current medicolegal climate in the United States, which causes physicians to perform C-sections more often than in the past to protect themselves against a lawsuit?

Is the fact that C-sections earn the obstetrician more money a factor in the decision to perform them?

Given the increased risk to the mother of a cesarean delivery, and the evidence that it has little effect on infant mortality rate, is the relatively high rate of cesarean deliveries ethical?

Exploring Personal Dimensions

How Much Do You Know About Pregnancy and Birth?

For each of the statements that follow, indicate whether you think the statement is true or false. The correct answers and explanations appear after the questions.

True _____ False _____   1. Pregnant women should stop exercising as soon as they discover they are pregnant.

True _____ False _____   2. Once a woman has had a C-section, she should have C-sections for subsequent deliveries to prevent tearing of the abdominal tissue.

True _____ False _____   3. The use of midwives has decreased in recent years.

True _____ False _____   4. Breastfeeding is covered by the Patient Protection and Affordable Care Act, which guarantees that working women may breastfeed.

True _____ False _____   5. Teen birth rates have steadily increased and are of significant concern.

True _____ False _____   6. In terms of a newborn baby's health, the length of time before its mother becomes pregnant again does not matter.

Answers and Explanations

Each of the statements above is false.

1. Pregnant women are encouraged to continue exercising if they exercised before becoming pregnant. Some studies have suggested that exercise during pregnancy helps make the labor and delivery easier and shorter, promotes earlier recovery after delivery, and reduces the chance of C-sections. However, women who have not maintained an exercise regimen before

becoming pregnant should not begin after becoming pregnant. Rather, they should exercise by adopting a mild walking or swimming program or by consulting an expert on exercise and pregnancy for other activities that will be beneficial for them and their fetuses.

2. There is no reason why, as a matter of routine, women who have had one C-section need to have C-sections for subsequent pregnancies. C-sections need be performed only if the woman has an STI that can be transmitted during childbirth, if the baby is too large to pass through the vaginal opening, or if the stress of the delivery has the potential to cause harm to the mother.

3. Contrary to popular belief, the proportion of women who use a nurse–midwife rather than an obstetrician to deliver their babies has remained constant. Eight percent of births are attended by a midwife.

4. Many women have been fired or discriminated against for breastfeeding at work. The Patient Protection and Affordability Care Act, coupled with increased support for breastfeeding, provides clear guidelines for employees about their rights regarding breastfeeding at work. The Act also provides clear guidelines for employers about the actions and policies they are required to follow.

5. The birth rate for teenagers increased in 2006 for the first time after 14 straight years of decline. The rate in 2006 was 41.9 births per 1,000 females aged 15–19 years, up from 40.5 births in 2005. The teen birth rate had dropped 34% from 1991 (61.8 births per 1,000) to 2005 (Martin et al., 2010). The rate increased again in 2007, but did decline in 2008 to 41.5 birth per 1,000 (Martin et al., 2010). Teen birth rates are still too high and are, rightfully, of national concern.

6. Research has shown that a short interpregnancy interval is a risk factor for infant mortality; low birth weight; being small for one's gestational age; and, less consistently, preterm birth (Conde-Agudelo, Rosas-Bermudez, & Kafury-Goeta, 2006; de Weger et al., 2011; Thompson & Clark, 2011). Two explanations have been offered to explain this finding. The *maternal depletion hypothesis* suggests that at least 1 year between the birth of one child

and subsequent conception is essential to restore maternal nutritional resources necessary for a successful pregnancy. The postpartum stress hypothesis states that caring for an infant can be so stressful that the physical or emotional strain can interfere with the growth of the fetus. In any case, an 18-month interpregnancy interval is recommended (Conde-Agudelo, Rosas-Bermúdez, & Kafury-Goeta, 2006).

Suggested Readings

Almeling, R. *Sex cells: The medical market for eggs and sperm.* Berkeley and Los Angeles, CA: University of California Press, 2011.

American College of Obstetricians and Gynecologists. *Your pregnancy and child birth,* 5th ed. Atlanta, GA: American College of Obstetricians and Gynecologists, 2010.

Boston Women's Health Book Collective & Norsigian, J. *Our bodies, ourselves: Informing and inspiring women across generations.* New York: Touchstone/Simon & Schuster, 2011.

Goldberg, L. *Pea in a pod: Your complete guide to pregnancy, childbirth, & beyond,* 2nd ed. Garden City Park, NY: Square One Publishing, 2011.

Simkin, P. *The birth partner: A complete guide to childbirth for dads, doulas, and all other labor companions,* 3rd ed. Boston, MA: Harvard Common Press, 2008.

Tsigdinos, PM. *Silent sorority: A barren woman gets busy, angry, lost, and found,* 2nd ed. Charleston, SC: BookSurge Publishing, 2010.

Web Resources

For links to the websites below, visit *go.jblearning.com/dimensions5e* and click on Resource Links.

Accord Alliance
www.accordalliance.org

As the focus of the organization narrowed to helping clinicians and families address issues of disorders of sexual development, the Intersex Society of North America transitioned into Accord Alliance. The website contains guidelines for clinicians and documents for families that are living with a child with DSD. The ISNA website (www.isna.org) is still available as a historic document for those who may be interested.

RESOLVE: The National Infertility Association
www.resolve.org

Established in 1974, this nonprofit organization is a national network mandated to promote reproductive health and to ensure equal access to all family building options for men and women experiencing infertility or other reproductive disorders. The website includes current information and support for people who are experiencing infertility. RESOLVE also works to increase awareness of infertility issues through public education, such as National Infertility Awareness Week, and advocacy.

Maternal and Child Health Bureau
www.mchb.hrsa.gov

A bureau of the Health Resources and Services Administration of the U.S. Department of Health and Human Services, this site provides links to information pertaining to issues of the health of mothers and their children. Included are links to programs, funding opportunities, data, and resources and publications.

National Campaign to Prevent Teen and Unplanned Pregnancy
www.teenpregnancy.org

Presents information on programs that have been successful in preventing teen pregnancy and other links to assist in this endeavor. Provides information to acquire materials to support a National Day to Prevent Teen Pregnancy.

Association of Reproductive Health Professionals
www.arhp.org

Provides information and resources pertaining to many aspects of reproduction. Among the topics about which information is provided are abortion, contraception, emergency contraception, menopause, politics and reproductive health news, international reproductive health news and issues, and patient education materials.

National Center for Fathering
www.fathers.com

Seeks to inspire and equip men to be the involved fathers, grandfathers, and father figures their children need. The center provides practical, research-based training and resources, and reaches more than 1 million dads annually through seminars, small-group training, the WATCH D.O.G.S. (Dads of Great Students) program, a daily radio program, and weekly email.

References

Accord Alliance. *Clinical guidelines for the management of disorders of sex development in childhood*, 2008. Available: http://www.accordalliance.org/dsd-guidelines.html.

Ackerman, J. P., Riggins, T., & Black, M. M. A review of the effects of prenatal cocaine exposure among school-aged children. *Pediatrics, 125* (2010), 554–565.

American Congress of Obstetrics and Gynecology. *ACOG recommends restricted use of episiotomies*, 2006. Available: http://www.acog.org/from_home/publications/press_releases/nr03-31-06-2.cfm.

American Congress of Obstetrics and Gynecology. Committee opinion #476: Planned home births. *Obstetrics & Gynecology, 117, no. 2* (2011a), 424–428.

American Congress of Obstetrics and Gynecology. *Frequently asked questions: Exercise during pregnancy*, 2011b. Available: http://www.acog.org/publications/faq/faq119.pdf.

American Congress of Obstetrics and Gynecology. *Frequently asked questions: Ectopic pregnancy*, 2011c. Available: http://www.acog.org/publications/faq/faq155.pdf.

American Society for Reproductive Medicine. *Frequently asked questions about infertility*, 2011a. Available: http://reproductivefacts.org/awards/index.aspx?id=3012.

American Society for Reproductive Medicine. *Stress*, 2011b. Available: http://www.asrm.org/topics.detail.aspx?id=1738.

American Society of Reproductive Medicine & Society for Reproductive Technology. Guidelines on the number of embryos transferred. *Fertility and Sterility, 95* (2009), 1518–1519.

AVERT. *Preventing mother-to-child transmission of HIV (PMTCT)*. n.d. Available: http://www.avert.org/motherchild.htm.

Baysinger, M., Martin, B., Rose-Jacobs, R., Cahral, H., Heeren, T., Augustyn, M., et al. Prenatal cocaine exposure and children's language functioning at 6 and 9.5 years: Moderating effects of child age, birth weight, and gender. *Journal of Pediatric Psychology, 31* (2006), 98–115.

Belluck, P. Test can tell fetal sex at 7 weeks, study says. *New York Times* (August 9, 2011). Available: http://www.nytimes.com/2011/08/10/health/10birth.html?_r=0

Benn, P. A., & Chapman, A. R. Ethical challenges in providing noninvasive prenatal diagnosis. *Current Opinion in Obstetrics and Gynecology, 22* (2010), 128–134.

Berg, S. J., & Wynne-Edwards, K. Changes in testosterone, cortisol, and estradiol levels in men becoming fathers. *Mayo Clinic Proceedings, 76, no. 6* (2001), 582–592.

Bigsby, R., LaGasse, L. L., Lester, B., Shankaran, S., Bada, H., Bauer, C., & Liu, J. Prenatal cocaine exposure and motor performance at 4 months. *American Journal of Occupational Therapy, 65, no. 5* (2001), e60–e68.

Bruckner, T. A., Cheng, Y. W., & Caughey, A. B. Increased neonatal mortality among normal-weight births beyond 41 weeks of gestation in California. *American Journal of Obstetrics and Gynecology, 199,* (2008), 421.e1–421.e7. doi: 10.1016/j.ajog.2008.05.015.

CDC Infertility Working Group. *Outline for a national action plan for the prevention, detection, and management of infertility,* 2010. Available: http://www.cdc.gov/art/PDF/National ActionPlan.pdf.

Centers for Diseases Control and Prevention. *Assisted reproductive technology,* 2011a. Available: http://www.cdc.gov/ART/.

Centers for Diseases Control and Prevention. *Assisted reproductive technology (ART) report, 2009 national summary,* 2011b. Available: http://apps.nccd.cdc.gov/art/Apps/NationalSummaryReport.aspx.

Centers for Diseases Control and Prevention. *Breastfeeding among U.S. children born 2000–2008, CDC National Immunization Survey,* 2011c. Available: http://www/cdc/gov/breastfeeding/data/NIS_data/index.htm.

Centers for Diseases Control and Prevention. *Female sterilization: Risk of ectopic pregnancy after tubal sterilization fact sheet,* 2009. Available: http://www.cdc.gov/reproductivehealth/unintendedpregnancy/ectopicpreg_factsheet.htm.

Centers for Diseases Control and Prevention. *Preventing smoking and exposure to secondhand smoke before, during, and after pregnancy,* 2007. Available: http://www.cdc.gov/nccdphp/publications/factsheets/Prevention/pdf/smoking .pdf.

Centers for Diseases Control and Prevention. *Provisional monthly and 12-month ending number of live births, deaths, and infant deaths and rates: United States, January 2009–December 2010,* 2011d. Available: http://www.cdc.gov/nchas/data/dvs/provisional_table01_2010Dec.pdf.

Centers for Diseases Control and Prevention. *Rubella disease in-short (German measles),* 2011e. Available: http://www.cdc.gov/vaccines/vpd-vac/rubella/in-short-adult.htm.

Clinton, J., Alverson, C. J., Strickland, M. J., Gilboa, S. M., & Correa, A. Maternal smoking and congenital heart defects in the Baltimore-Washington infant study. *Pediatrics, 127, no. 3* (2011), e647–e653.

Daley, A. J., Macarther, C., & Winter, H. The role of exercise in the treatment of postpartum depression: a review of the literature. *Journal of Midwifery and Women's Health, 52* (2007), 56–62.

Davey, M., & Flood, M. M. Perinatal mortality and planned home birth. *American Journal of Obstetrics and Gynecology, 204, no. 4* (2011), e18.

Day, N. L., Goldschmidt, L., & Thomas, C. A. Prenatal marijuana exposure contributes to the prediction of marijuana use at age 14. *Addiction, 101* (2006), 1313–1322.

de Jonge, A., van der Goes, B., Ravelli, A., Amelink-Verburg, M., Mol, B., Nijhuis, J., Gravenhorst, J., & Buitendijk, S. Perinatal mortality and morbidity in a nationwide cohort of 529,688 low-risk planned home and hospital births. *BJOG, 116, no. 9* (2009), 1177–1184.

de Weger, F. J., Hukkelhoven, C., Serroyen, J., te Velde, E. R., & Smits, L. J. Advanced maternal age, short interpregnancy interval, and perinatal outcome. *American Journal of Obstetrics and Gynecology, 204, no. 5* (2011), 421.e1–421.e9.

Declercq, E. Trends in midwife-attended births in the United States, 1989–2009. *Journal of Midwifery & Women's Health, 57,* (2012), 321–326. doi:10.1111/j.1542-2011.2012.00198.x

DeMaio, M., & Magnann, E. F. Exercise and pregnancy. *Journal of the American Academy of Orthopaedic Surgeons, 17, no. 8* (2009), 504–514.

Devaney, S. A., Polamaki, G. G., Scott, J. A., & Bianchi, D. W. Noninvasive fetal sex determination using cell-free DNA systematic review and meta-analysis. *Journal of the American Medical Association, 306, no. 6* (2011), 627–636.

Diamond, M. Human intersexuality: Difference or disorder? *Archives of Sexual Behavior, 38, no. 2* (2009), 172–173.

Gibbons, L., Belizan, J. M., Lauer, J. A., Betran, A. P., Merialdi, M., & Althabe, F. The global numbers and costs of additionally needed and unnecessary caesarean sections performed per year: Overuse as a barrier to universal coverage. *World Health Report, Background Paper, 30* (2010). Available: http://www.who/int/healthsystems/topics/financing/healthreport/30C-sectioncosts.pdf.

Goldschmidt, K., Richardson, G. A., Willford, J., & Day, N. L. Prenatal marijuana exposure and intelligence test performance at age 6. *Journal of the American Academy of Child and Adolescent Psychiatry, 47, no. 3* (2008), 254–263.

Gouin, K., Murphy, K., Shah, P. S., et al. Effects of cocaine use during pregnancy on low birthweight and preterm birth: Systematic review and meta-analyses. *American Journal of Obstetrics and Gynecology, 204, no. 4* (2011), e1–e12.

Gunderson, E. P., Jacobs, D. R., Chiang, V., Lewis, C. E., Feng, J., Quesenberry, C. P., & Sidney, S. Duration of lactation and incidence of the metabolic syndrome on women of reproductive age according to gestational diabetes mellitus status: A 20-year prospective study in CARDIA (Coronary Artery Risk Development in Young Adults). *Diabetes, 59, no. 2* (2010), 495–504.

Gunderson, E. P., Rifas-Shiman, S. L., Oken, E., Rich-Edwards, J. W., et al. Association of fewer hours of sleep at 6 month postpartum with substantial weight retention at 1 year postpartum. *American Journal of Epidemiology, 167* (2008), 178–187.

Gyte, G., Dodwell, M. J., & Macfarlane, A. J. Home birth meta-analysis: Does it meet AJOG's reporting requirements? *American Journal of Obstetrics and & Gynecology, 204, no. 4* (2011), e15.

Hospital for Sick Children. *Sexual differentiation,* 2011. Available: http://www.aboutkidshealth.ca/En/HowTheBodyWorks/SexDevelopmentAnOverview/SexualDifferentiation.

Hughes, I. A., Houk, C. P., Ahmed, S. F., Lee, P. A., & International Consensus Conference on Intersex organized by the Lawson Wilkins Pediatric Endocrine Society and the European Society for Paediatric Endocrinology. Consensus statement on management of intersex disorders. *Archives of Disease in Childhood, 91, no. 7* (2006), 554–563.

Janssen, P. A., Saxell, L., Page, L. A., Klein, M. C., Liston, R. M., & Lee, S. K., Outcomes of planned home birth with registered midwife versus planned hospital birth with midwife or physician. *Canadian Medical Association Journal, 181, no. 6–7* (2009), 377–383.

Jin, W., He, X., Liu, P., et al. Maternal and neonatal outcomes in water birth. *Journal of Practical Obstetrics and Gynecology, 11* (2009) [abstract retrieved from http://en.cnki.com.cn/Article_en/CJFDTOTAL-SFCZ200911016.htm].

Joel, D. Male or female? Brains are intersex. *Frontiers in Integrative Neuroscience, 5, no. 57* (2011), 1–5.

Johnson, K. C., & Daviss, B. International data demonstrate home birth safety. *American Journal of Obstetrics and Gynecology, 204, no. 4* (2011), e16–e17.

Johnson, K. C., & Daviss, B., Outcomes of home births with certified professional midwives: Large prospective study in North America. *BMJ, 330* (2005), 1416.

Johri, M., & Ako-Arrey, D. The cost-effectiveness of preventing mother-to-child transmission of HIV in low- and middle-income countries: Systematic review. *Cost-Effectiveness and Resource Allocation, 9, no. 3* (2011).

Kaimal, A. J., Little, S. E., Odibo, A. O., Stamilio, D. M., Grobman, W. A., Long, E. F., Owens, D. K., & Caughey, A. B. Cost-effectiveness of elective induction of labor at 41 weeks in nulliparous women. *American Journal of Obstetrics and Gynecology, 204,* (2011), 137.e1–9. doi:10.1016/j.ajog.2010.08.012

Kirby, R. S., & Frost, J. Maternal and newborn outcomes in planned home birth vs. planned hospital births: a meta-analysis. *American Journal of Obstetrics and Gynecology, 204, no. 4* (2011), e16.

Knopik, V. S. Maternal smoking during pregnancy and child outcomes: Real or spurious effect? *Developmental Neuropsychology, 34* (2009), 1–36.

Lebel, C., Rasmussen, C., Wyper, K., Andrew, G. & Beaulieu, C. Brain microstructure is related to math ability in children with fetal alcohol spectrum disorder. *Alcoholism, Clinical and Experimental Research, 34* (2010), 354–363.

Levine, TP, Liu, J., Das, A., Leter, B., Lagasse, L., Shakarna, S. et al. Effects of prenatal cocaine exposure on special education in school aged children. *Pediatrics, 122* (2008), e83–e91.

Lewis, B., Avery, M., Jennings, E., Sherwood, N., Martinson, B. & Crain, A. L. The effect of exercise during pregnancy on maternal outcomes: Practical implications for practice. *American Journal of Lifestyle Medicine, 2, no. 5* (2008), 441–445.

Logsdon, M. C., Wisner, K., & Hanusa, B. H. Does maternal functioning improve with antidepressant treatment in women with postpartum depression? *Journal of Women's Health, 18* (2009), 58–90.

MacDorman, M. F., & Mathews, T. J. Understanding racial and ethnic disparities in U.S. infant mortality rates. NCHS data brief, no 74. Hyattsville, MD: National Center for Health Statistics, 2011.

MacDorman, M. F., Mathews, T. J., & Declercq, E. Home births in the United States, 1990–2009. NCHS data brief, no. 84. Hyattsville, MD: National Center for Health Statistics. Available: http://www.cdc.gov/nchs/data/databriefs/db84.htm.

March of Dimes. *Birth defect research,* 2011. Available: http://www.marchofdimes.com/research/birthdefectresearch.html.

March of Dimes. *Illicit drug use during pregnancy,* 2008a. Available: http://www.marchofdimes.com/pregnancy/alcohol_illicitdrug.html.

March of Dimes. *Low birth weight,* 2008b. Available: http://marchofdimes.com/professionals/medicalresources_lowbirthweight.html

March of Dimes. *Smoking during pregnancy,* 2010. Available: http://www.marchofdimes.com/pregnancy/alcohol_smoking.html.

Martin, J. A., Hamilton, B. E., Sutton, P. D., Ventura, S. J., Menacker, F., Kirmeyer, S., & Mathews, T. J. Births: Final data for 2006. *National Vital Statistics Reports, 57, no. 7* (January 7, 2009), 102.

Martin, J.A., Hamilton, B.E., Sutton, P.D., Ventura, S.J., Mathews, T.J., Osterman, M. Births: final data for 2008. *National Vital Statistics Reports, 59, no. 1* (2010). Available: http://www.cdc.gov/nchs/data/nvsr/nvsr59_01.pdf.

Mathews, T. J., & MacDorman, M. F. Infant mortality statistics from the 2007 period linked birth/infant death data set. *National Vital Statistics Reports, 59, no. 6* (2011). Available: http://www.cdc.gov/nchs/data/nvsr59/nvsr59_06.pdf.

Maude, R. M., & Foureur, M. J. It's beyond water: Stories of women's experience of using water for labour and birth. *Women and Birth, 20, no. 1* (2007), 17–24.

Mayo Clinic. *Amniocentesis: Risks,* 2010a. Available: http://www.mayoclinic.com/health/amniocentesis/MY00155/DSECTION=risks.

Mayo Clinic. *Chorionic villus sampling: Risks*, 2010b. Available: http://www.mayoclinic.com/health/chorionic-villus-sampling/MY00154/DSECTION=risks.

Mayo Clinic. *Infertility: risk factors,* 2011. Available: http://www.mayoclinic.com/health/infertility/DS00310/DSECTION=risk-factors.

Medline Plus. *Rh incompatibility,* 2011. Available: http://www.nlm.nih.gov/medlineplus/ency/article/001600.htm.

Midodzi, W.K., Rowe, B. H., Majaesic, S. M., Saunders, L. D., & Senthilselvan, A. Early life factors associated with incidence of physician-diagnosed asthma in preschool children: results from the Canadian Early Family Childhood Development cohort study. *Journal of Asthma, 47, no. 1* (2010), 7–13.

Morris, J. K., Wald, N. J., Mutton, D. E., & Alberman, E. Comparison of models of material age-specific risk for Down syndrome live births. *Prenatal Diagnosis, 23, no. 3* (2003), 252–258.

National Academy of Sciences. Weight gain during pregnancy: Reexamining the guidelines, 2009. Available: https://download.nap.edu/catalog/php?record_id=12584.

National Center for Biotechnology Information. *Ectopic pregnancy,* 2010. Available: http://www.ncbi.nlm.hih.gov/pubmedhealth/PMH0001897/.

National Center for Health Statistics. *Health, United States, 2008.* Hyattsville, MD: Author, 2008.

Nelson, A. L., & Marshall, J. R. Impaired fertility. In R. A. Hatcher, et al. *Contraceptive technology,* 19th revised edition. New York: Ardent Media, 2008.

Obebauer, S., & Maestre, L. Fetal MRI of lung hypoplasia: Imaging findings. *Clinical Imaging, 32* (2008), 48–50.

Oestergaard, M. Z., Inouel, M., Yoshida, S., Mahanani, W. R., Gorel, F. M., Cousens, S., Lawn, J. E., & Mathers, C. D. Neonatal mortality levels for 193 countries in 2009 with trends since 1990: A systematic analysis of progress, projections, and priorities. *PLoS Med, 8,* no. 8 (2011).

Oregon Health and Science University. *Waterbirth,* 2011. Available: http://www.ohsu.edu/xd/health/services/women/services/midwifery/out-services/waterbirth.cfm.

Oros, D., Bejarano, M. P., Cardiel, M. R., Oros-Espinosa, D., Gonzalez de Agüero, R., & Fabre, E. Low-risk pregnancy at 41 weeks: When should we induce labor? *Journal of Maternal-Fetal and Neonatal Medicine, 25, 6,* (2012), 728–731. doi:10.3109/14767058.2011.599079

Pei, J. R., Rinaldi, C. M., Rasmissen, C., Massey, V., & Massey, D. Memory patterns of acquisition and retention of verbal and nonverbal information in children with fetal alcohol spectrum disorders. *Canadian Journal of Clinical Pharmacology, 15,* no. *1* (2008), e44–56.

Pinkhardt, E. H., Kassubek, J., Brummer, D., Koelch, M., Ludolph, A. C., Feget, J. M., & Ludolph, A. G. Intensified testing for attention-deficit hyperactivity disorder (ADHD) in girls should reduce depression and smoking in adult females and the prevalence of ADHD in the long term, *Medical Hypothesis, 72,* no. *4* (2009), 409–412.

Qiu, J., & Liu, X. A clinical study on 280 cases of water birth. *Chinese Journal of Woman and Child Health Research, 5,* 2008. [Abstract retrieved from http://en.cnki.com.cn/Article_en/CJFDTOTAL-SANE2008805021.htm].

Queenan, J. T. How to stop the relentless rise in cesarean deliveries. *Obstetrics and Gynecology, 118* (2011), 199–200.

Reinberg, S. Childbirth at home as safe as hospital delivery: Study review finds no increased problems for low-risk women. *HealthDay News* (June 16, 2005).

Resolve. *Using donor sperm,* 2011. Available: http://www.resolve.org/family-building-options/donor-options/using-donorsperm.html.

Richardson, G. A., Goldschmidt, L., & Willford, J. The effects of prenatal cocaine use on infant development. *Neurotoxicology and Teratology, 30* (2008), 96–108.

Royal College of Obstetricians and Gycnaecologists. *BJOG release: New figures on the safety of home births,* 2009. Available: http://www.rcog.org.uk/news/bjog-releasenew-figures-safety-home-births.

Runquist, J. Persevering through postpartum fatigue. *Journal of Obstetric, Gynecologic, and Neonatal Nursing, 36* (2007), 28–37.

Schempf, A. H., & Strobino, D. M. Illicit drug use and adverse birth outcomes: Is it drugs or context? *Journal of Urban Health, 85,* no. *6* (2008), 858–873.

Shier, D., Butler, J., & Lewis R. *Hole's essentials of human anatomy and physiology.* New York: McGraw-Hill, 2003.

Smith, L. E., & Howard, K. S. Continuity of paternal social support and depressive symptoms among new mothers. *Journal of Family Psychology, 22* (2008), 763–773.

Storey, A. E., Walsh, C. J., Quintone, R. L., & Wynne-Edwards, K. E. Hormonal correlates of paternal responsiveness in new and expectant fathers. *Evolution and Human Behavior, 21, no. 2* (2000), 79–95.

Sunderam, S., Chang, J., Flowers, L., Kulkarni, A., Sentelle, G., Jen, G., & Macaluso, M. Assisted reproductive technology surveillance—United States, 2006. *Morbidity and Mortality Weekly Report, 58, no. SS05* (2009), 1–25.

Swedish National Institute of Public Health. *Low-dose alcohol exposure during pregnancy—does it harm?* 2009. Available: http://www.fhi.se/PageFiles/7261/R2009-14-low-dose-alcohol-exposure-pregnancy.pdf.

Thompson, D. R., & Clark, C. L. *Short birth intervals: Associated maternal factors and subsequent risk of adverse birth outcomes,* 2011. Florida Department of Health, Division of Family Services. Available: http://doh.state.fl.us/family/mch/docs/birthintervalpaper09-29-11-final.pdf.

Thoni, A., Mussner, K., & Ploner, F. Water birthing: Retrospective review of 2625 water births. Contamination of birth pool water and risk of microbial cross-infection. *Minerva Ginicologica, 62, no. 3* (2010), 203–211.

Tong, V. T., Jones, J. R., Dietz, P. M., D'Angelo, D., & Bombard, J. M. Trends in smoking before, during, and after pregnancy—Pregnancy Risk Monitoring System (PRAMS), United States, 31 sites, 2000–2005. *Morbidity and Mortality Weekly Report, 58, no. SS04* (2009), 1–29.

U.S. Department of Health and Human Services. Depression during and after pregnancy. *Womenshealth.gov,* 2009. Available: http://www.womenshealth.gov/FAQ/depression-pregnancy.cfm#d.

U.S. Department of Health and Human Services. *Infertility fact sheet,* 2009. Available: http://www.womenshealth.gov/publications/our-publications/fact-sheet/infertility.cfm#d.

U.S. Department of Health and Human Services. Office of Disease Prevention and Health Promotion. Healthy People 2020: Maternal, Infant, and Child Health Objectives. Washington, DC. Available: http://www.healthypeople.gov/2020/topicsobjects2020/pdfs/MaternalChildHealth.pdf.

U.S. Department of Health and Human Services. *Pregnancy: Recovering from birth,* 2010. Available: http://www.womenshealth.gov/pregnancy/childbirth-beyond/recovering-from-birth.cfm.

U.S. Department of Health and Human Services. *The Surgeon General's call to action to support breastfeeding.* Washington, DC: Author, 2011.

Wax, J. R., Lucas, F. L., Lamont, N., Pinette, M. G., Cartin, A., & Blackstone, J. Maternal and newborn outcomes in planned home birth vs. planned hospital births: A meta-analysis. *American Journal of Obstetrics and Gynecology, 203, no. 3* (2010), e1-e8.

Weiss, R. E. Couvade syndrome: Sympathetic pregnancy. *About.com,* 2009. Available: http://pregnancy.about.com/cs/forfathersonly/a/couvade.htm.

Weston, M. J. Magnetic resonance imaging in fetal medicine: A pivotal review of the current and developing indications. *Postgraduate Medicine Journal, 86* (2010), 42–51.

Woodruff, T. J., Carlson, A., Schwartz, J. M., Guidice, L. C. Proceedings of the Summit on Environmental Challenges to Reproductive Health and Fertility: Executive summary. *Fertility and Sterility, 89* (2008), 281–300.

Wynne-Edwards, K. Ask the brains: Why do some expectant fathers experience pregnancy symptoms such as vomiting and nausea? *Scientific American Mind, 17, no. 3* (2006).

Zanetti-Dallenbach, R., Lapaire, O., Maertens, A., Holzgreve, W., & Hösli, I. Water birth, more than a trendy alternative, a prospective, observational study. *Obstetrical & Gynecological Survey, 62, no. 4* (2007), 222–223.

Zohar, N., & De Vries, R. Study validity questioned. *American Journal of Obstetrics and Gynecology, 24, no. 4* (2011), e14.

I»N»T»E»R chapter FOCUS

Unexpected Pregnancy Outcomes

FEATURES

Ethical Dimensions
Should Intact Dilation and Evacuation (D&E) Be Banned?

Communication Dimensions
Debating the Abortion Issue

Global Dimensions
A Worldwide Preference for Boys

Gender Dimensions
Baby "Richard"

Multicultural Dimensions
International Adoptions

CHAPTER OBJECTIVES

1 Discuss abortion issues, including abortion procedures, legal history, and current attitudes toward abortion.

2 Describe the various types of adoptions and the laws surrounding them, including closed and open adoptions, public and private agency adoptions, independent adoptions, and facilitated adoptions.

go.jblearning.com/dimensions5e

Global Dimensions: A Worldwide Preference for Boys
Emotions and Abortion
Multicultural Dimensions: International Adoptions
Foster Care and Adoption

INTRODUCTION

*T*oo many pregnancies are unplanned and unwanted. The dilemma this causes for some men and women is eloquently described by the author Anna Quindlen (1988, 209–212).

It was always the look on their faces that told me first. I was the freshman dormitory counselor and they were freshmen at a women's college where everyone was smart. One of them would come into my room, a golden girl, a valedictorian, an 800 verbal score on the SATs, and her eyes would be empty, seeing only a busted future, the devastation of her life as she knew it. She had failed biology, messed up the math; she was pregnant. That was when I became prochoice.

Quindlen then describes the birth of her own son.

It was the look in his eyes that I will always remember, too. They were as black as the bottom of a well, and in them for a few minutes I thought I saw myself the way I had always wished to be—clear, simple, elemental, at peace. My child looked at me and I looked back at him in the delivery room, and I realized that out of a sea of infinite possibilities it had come down to this: a specific person, born on the hottest day of the year, conceived on a Christmas Eve, made by his father and me miraculously from scratch.

Once I believed that there was a little blob of formless protoplasm in there and a gynecologist went in there with a surgical instrument, and that was that. Then I got pregnant myself—eagerly, intentionally, by the right man, at the right time—and I began to doubt. My abdomen still flat, my stomach roiling with morning sickness, I felt not that I had protoplasm inside, but, instead, a complete human being in miniature to whom I could talk, sing, make promises. Neither of these views was accurate; instead, I think, the reality is something in the middle. And that is where I find myself now, in the middle—hating the idea of abortions, hating the idea of having them outlawed.

For I know it is the right thing in some times and places. I remember sitting in a shabby clinic far uptown with one of those freshmen, only three months after the Supreme Court had made what we were doing possible, and watching with wonder as the lovely first love she had had with a nice boy unraveled over the space of an hour as they waited for her to be called, degenerating into sniping and silences. I remember a year or two later seeing them pass on campus and not even acknowledge each other because their conjoining had caused them so much pain, and I shuddered to think of them married, with a small psyche in their unready and unwilling hands....

I don't feel all one way about abortion anymore, and I don't think it serves a just cause to pretend that many of us do. For years I believed that a woman's right to choose was absolute, but now I wonder. Do I, with a stable home and marriage and sufficient stamina and money, have the freedom to choose abortion because a pregnancy is inconvenient just now? Legally I do have the right; legally I wanted always to have that right. It is the morality of exercising it under those circumstances that makes me wonder....

I have taped on my VCR a public television program in which somehow, inexplicably, a film is shown of a fetus in utero scratching its face, seemingly putting up a tiny hand to shield itself from the camera's eye. It would make a potent weapon in the arsenal of the antiabortionists. I grow sentimental about it as it floats in the salt water, part fish, part human being. It is almost living, but not quite. It has almost turned my heart around, but not quite my head.

Many people are surprised to learn that nearly half of all pregnancies in the United States are unintended. Yet, that is the case. When an unintended pregnancy occurs, decisions are required. Should the pregnancy be terminated? If so, which method of abortion should be used? What are the legal, moral, and health implications of this decision? Should the fetus be brought to term and a baby born? If so, should the child be raised by the biological parents? Should it be placed for adoption? If placed for adoption, should adoption be arranged through an agency or through a relative? What are the legal and moral implications of this decision? This chapter explores the alternatives presented to people who experience an unintended pregnancy.

■ Abortion

For unplanned pregnancies, the first decision to be made is whether to continue the pregnancy. Sometimes the woman or the couple decide to allow the pregnancy to continue, but something goes wrong and the fetus stops developing. Such natural cessations of the pregnancy are called **spontaneous abortions**, or miscarriages. Abortions requiring intervention to end the pregnancy are technically called **induced abortions**.

Abortion is safest in the earliest weeks of pregnancy. If a woman thinks she is pregnant and does not want to continue the pregnancy, she should perform a home pregnancy test or go to a clinic as soon as she misses a period.

Abortion Procedures

Vacuum Aspiration

Almost all abortions in the United States are performed during the first trimester of pregnancy, using a surgical procedure called **vacuum aspiration**. It is a surgical procedure that uses suction equipment to evacuate the contents of the uterus. It can also be used in the first weeks of the second trimester. Almost 90% of abortions are performed in the first 12 weeks of pregnancy, with about 1.5% occurring after 21 weeks (Guttmacher Institute, 2011).

spontaneous abortion (miscarriage)
The natural termination of a pregnancy.

induced abortion
Purposeful termination of a pregnancy.

vacuum aspiration
Surgical procedure that uses a suction tube to evacuate the contents of the uterus, which can be used through the first weeks of the second trimester.

Manual vacuum aspiration (MVA) is a variation of vacuum aspiration that can be used from the detection of pregnancy to up to 12 weeks since the last menstrual period (LMP). In contrast to traditional vacuum aspiration procedures, it uses nonelectric suction instruments. The procedure takes 5 to 15 minutes, and the woman usually leaves the clinic within 2 hours.

manual vacuum aspiration (MVA)
A variation of vacuum aspiration that uses nonelectric suction instruments and can be used from detection of pregnancy through 12 weeks.

medical abortion
A procedure that uses drugs to induce abortion.

mifepristone
A drug that blocks the hormone progesterone, which is needed to maintain a pregnancy.

methotrexate
A drug that blocks the hormone progesterone, which is needed to maintain a pregnancy.

misoprostol
A prostaglandin that causes uterine contractions.

Medical Abortions

Medical abortions are procedures that use drugs to induce abortion, including **mifepristone** or **methotrexate** in combination with **misoprostol**. Mifepristone was discovered by a French pharmaceutical company in 1978 and was known as RU 486. (*RU* refers to Roussel Uclaf, the French pharmaceutical company.)

In the fall of 2000, mifepristone was approved by the U.S. Food and Drug Administration (FDA). Mifepristone blocks the hormone progestrone, which is needed to maintain a pregnancy. In the FDA-approved protocol, a woman who is no more than 49 days LMP takes mifepristone at a clinic visit. She returns to the clinic 2 days later and takes misoprostol, a prostaglandin that causes uterine contractions. Early studies showed that using this protocol successfully terminated the pregnancy approximately 92% of the time. More recent studies have shown that a lower dose of mifepristone—200 milligrams orally—followed by 800 micrograms of misoprostol taken vaginally at home can be equally effective through 63 days LMP, has fewer side effects, and allows women more privacy. Another evidence-based method uses 200 milligrams of mifepristone orally followed by 800 micrograms buccally (between the gum and the cheek)(Paul & Stewart, 2008). Some have also advocated for a misoprostol regimen alone because of its lower cost and easier access, but a recent study showed much lower rates of abortion completion (76.2%) than when using both mifepristone and misoprostol (96.5%)(Ngoc et al., 2011).

Methotrexate blocks folic acid and prevents cell division. A woman who is no more than 49 days past her last missed period receives an injection of methotrexate at a clinic and then 3 to 7 days later inserts 800 micrograms of misoprostol vaginally. After 24 hours without bleeding or if an abortion has not occurred in 1 week, she may repeat the dose of misoprostol. Most women (92–96%) successfully abort within 4 weeks of initiating the procedure, but in 15–25% of the cases it can take up to 4 weeks. (Paul & Stewart, 2008).

Currently, in the United States, methotrexate medical abortions are available only on an "off-label" basis. When drugs are approved by the U.S. FDA, their safety and efficacy are judged to warrant their use for specific conditions. Often, however, physicians discover other uses for those drugs and prescribe them for these other purposes. This practice, termed *off-label use*, is perfectly legal. Methotrexate is currently approved by the FDA for use by physicians for psoriasis and for rheumatoid arthritis (Paul & Stewart, 2008). Although approved for these conditions, it is used off-label by physicians for medical abortions.

While most abortions in the United States are performed surgically, the percentage of medical abortions is increasing. (Jones & Kooistra, 2011). Many women prefer the privacy of being at home. A recent study examining the experience of medical abortion showed that most (81%) of the women stated that bleeding was either "as expected" or "not as bad as expected," and 58% of the women stated that the pain was "as expected" or "not as bad as expected." The majority (84%) of the women said that they would recommend this method to a friend (Cameron et al., 2010), and a Dutch study reported that 80% of women would choose medical abortion again (over surgical procedure) (Loeber, 2010). Another study indicated that the pain associated with medical abortion was correlated with the pain during menstruation (Suhonena et al., 2011), and the authors recommended that clinicians and women seeking an abortion consider this factor when choosing between a medical or surgical procedure.

Dilation and Evacuation

During the second trimester of pregnancy, **dilation and evacuation (D&E)** is the abortion procedure used. It involves dilating the cervix, scraping the walls of the uterus, and removing the endometrial lining with suction. The D&E procedure does require surgical expertise, but it is safer than injecting a saline or prostaglandin into the uterus to induce premature labor (Paul & Stewart, 2008).

> **dilation and evacuation (D&E)** Surgical procedure that involves dilating the cervix, scraping the walls of the uterus, and removing the endometrial lining with suction.

As previously mentioned, almost 90% of all abortions are performed during the first trimester and only about 1.5% are performed at 21 weeks or more (Guttmacher Institute, 2011). Third trimester abortions are very rare, but occasionally a clinician might perform an intact D&E, which has been dubbed by opponents of legal abortion as a "partial birth abortion." This procedure is required when the fetus is too large for other abortion procedures to be performed safely and effectively (see the box on page 278).

The Law and the Debate

Because abortion is an issue debated by citizens, ruled on by the judiciary, and legislated by elected representatives—not to mention it being a major decision for people who become directly involved in unplanned pregnancies—it is a topic that needs the fullest possible study and consideration.

For more than four decades, abortion has been vehemently debated in the political sector. Although in vitro fertilization, contraception, and sterilization all have their controversial aspects, none of them generates the political, religious, and emotional heat that abortion does. Some people believe induced abortion to be murder of a baby, whereas others see it as a medical intervention into a biological process. Some people feel that the question of when life begins is central to this debate: Is it at conception, at some point when the fetus could (with help) exist outside the uterus, or at birth? But a person's view of when life begins is only one factor in shaping his or her attitudes on whether induced abortion is morally acceptable. Another central issue is whether the individual woman has the right to make a decision so basic to her own life or whether the government has that right and power. Other attitudes also enter into the debate—for instance, attitudes regarding world population, religious issues, women's "place," political power, poverty, public and private child care, and the degree of responsibility people should assume for their sexual behavior.

At this writing political groups generally typed pro-life are actively supporting candidates who are

Ethical DIMENSIONS

Should Intact Dilation and Evacuation (D&E) Be Banned?

Intact dilation and evacuation is performed late in the second trimester when, in the judgment of the physician, it is deemed the best means of abortion—that is, the most effective and safest. Some reasons for this type of abortion are concern for the health of the pregnant woman, late determination of birth defects in the fetus, or the woman's delay in seeking abortion as a result of fear of letting others know that she is pregnant. Objections have been raised to this method of abortion because it is performed at or near viability of the fetus. Those opposed to abortion at any time in any form are understandably opposed to D&E. However, even some Americans supportive of a woman's right to abortion during the first trimester and through the second trimester until the fetus could live outside the womb are disturbed by abortions occurring so late in the pregnancy. In their desire to secure support for their position, opponents have dubbed D&E "partial birth abortion," attempting to have D&E viewed as the interference with the birth of a live baby, rather than the termination of a pregnancy.

Those opposed to placing restrictions on the type of abortion allowed argue that the most qualified person to make this decision is the physician. Therefore, they believe a ban on any type of abortion procedure would limit physicians' options at a time when performing it would be most effective and safest. Opponents to restrictions also believe that once restrictions are allowed, Right to Life supporters will use them as a wedge to introduce more restrictions, eventually eroding a woman's right to abortion.

In 1997, Congress passed a law banning D&Es. However, President Bill Clinton vetoed that law, and Congress could not muster the votes required to override the veto. The following year, Congress again passed a similar law, but it was again vetoed by President Clinton. However, this time the House overrode the veto. Once the bill arrived back in the Senate, the veto was sustained, thereby preventing the legislation from becoming law.

In June 2000, the U.S. Supreme Court ruled in *Stenberg v. Carhart* that bans on intact D&E abortion were unconstitutional. However, in 2007, the Supreme Court, in *Gonzales v. Carhart*, upheld the federal Partial-Birth Abortion Ban Act of 2003, which prohibits this type of abortion without any exemptions (that is, regardless of concerns for the woman's health). As a result, dilation and evacuation abortions are banned by the federal government. Confusion still exists, because the federal law does not provide a precise description of what is banned. Consequently, states have proposed their own laws. As of 2012, 31 states had enacted bans on "partial birth" abortions (13 of which were blocked by a court and are not in effect); all of them include some sort of exemption if the woman's health is jeopardized by the pregnancy (Guttmacher Institute, 2012a).

Do you believe D&E should be banned as an abortion procedure? Why do you believe as you do?

---

totally opposed to abortion. Their goal is to pass legislation making abortion illegal or even to pass a constitutional amendment prohibiting abortion in the United States. Groups labeled pro-choice, however, believe that women should have the right to decide for themselves what they will do with their bodies. Consequently they oppose legislative restrictions on the availability of abortion to women who choose that option, and they wish to uphold the Supreme Court decision of 1973, which established the current legal status of abortion in the United States. The Court ruled (in *Roe v. Wade*) that abortion should be available to women during the first trimester (the first 3 months) of pregnancy. The decision is made by the pregnant woman and her physician. With regard to abortion during the second trimester, the Court ruled that the states can develop the regulations they deem necessary to maintain the pregnant woman's health. In the third trimester the states can limit or prohibit abortions if the mother's health is not in jeopardy.

In 1983 the Supreme Court reaffirmed its 1973 decision and stated that the government could not interfere with abortion unless such interference was clearly justified by "accepted medical practice." In effect this ruling prohibited governmental interference even into the second trimester and invalidated state laws that required abortions during the second trimester to be performed in a hospital.

However, in 1989 a Court made more conservative by new presidential appointments revisited this issue. The justices decided in *Webster v. Reproductive Health Services* that a Minnesota law requiring physicians to test fetuses to determine whether they could survive outside the womb before performing abortions was constitutional. That opened up the possibility that other regulations of abortion would be reviewed positively by the Court. Subsequently, two other cases were taken before the Supreme Court and decided in 1990. In *Hodgson v. Minnesota*, the Court rejected a law requiring a physician to notify both parents of a minor before an abortion could be performed. The rationale for this ruling was that some minors either do not live with both parents or have abusive or otherwise uncaring parents. The Court made it clear that if this law included a judicial bypass (in which a judge could approve the abortion if the parents were not the ones most appropriately notified), this law would be considered constitutional. In fact, in *Ohio v. Akron Center for Reproductive Health*, the Court held that a similar law that required notification of one parent and that did include a judicial bypass was constitutional.

In 1992, the Supreme Court reaffirmed the constitutionality of states attaching regulations to abortions, although it also reaffirmed the right of a woman to have an abortion if she chooses. In *Planned*

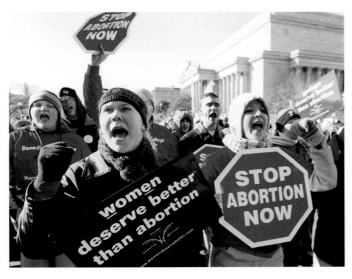

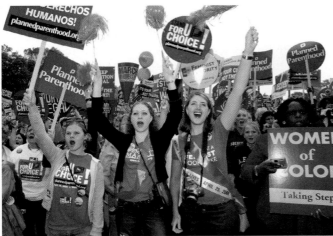

Both sides of the abortion issue attempt to show their strength in numbers with annual marches on Washington coinciding with the anniversary of *Roe v. Wade*. The marches do not happen on the same day, to minimize conflict as well as to accommodate the huge influx of people to Washington.

Parenthood of Southeastern Pennsylvania v. Casey, the Court ruled that Pennsylvania could require a woman seeking an abortion to receive counseling; to wait 24 hours before an abortion could be performed; and, if a minor under 18 years old, to obtain a parent's informed consent or a judge's approval. The Court also ruled that a physician had to keep detailed records of abortions and reasons for performing late-term abortions. However, the Court refused to overturn *Roe v. Wade*, as many opposed to abortion had hoped a conservative Court would do.

In June 2000, the Supreme Court returned its most significant abortion ruling since the *Casey* case (NARAL, 2011). In *Stenberg v. Carhart*, the Court ruled that bans on intact D&E (referred to as partial birth abortions) were unconstitutional since they did not take into account the health of the pregnant woman. Still, in 2003, the federal government passed the Partial-Birth Abortion Ban Act, which prohibited D&E abortions. In 2007, the Supreme Court upheld the constitutionality of that law.

While not directly affecting *Roe v. Wade*, in 1980 the Supreme Court made a decision that profoundly affected the availability of legal abortions. It ruled that the federal government could refuse to fund abortions for the poor, even though it funded other health care (Hyde Amendment). The consequence of this action has been to prohibit poor women from obtaining safe abortions—the same abortions that middle- and upper-class women can receive by paying for them—with Medicaid funds. People who oppose abortion acknowledge that an inequity exists between poor and affluent women regarding the availability of abortion, but they view this circumstance as leaving the fetuses of more wealthy women unprotected by law. Some states have taken on the financial costs of abortion for poor women who are denied federal assistance by the Hyde Amendment.

Current Laws on Abortion Services

People who oppose legalized abortion have unsuccessfully tried to outlaw abortion services completely. However, they have been successful at limiting the availability of abortion under many circumstances.

The federal government has restricted access to abortion by denying abortion coverage to military personnel and their families, women receiving care from Indian Health Services, and people on disability insurance. In fact, military health insurance does not cover abortion in cases of rape or incest, and personnel stationed overseas are not permitted to use personal funds to pay for abortions at overseas military facilities; this means that servicewomen must use local services (but potentially incur safety issues and language barriers) or take vacation leave to fly back to the United States to get an abortion.

Communication
DIMENSIONS

Debating the Abortion Issue

Because of the intense emotions associated with abortion, as well as the moral and ethical implications, pro-choicers and pro-lifers tend to talk past one another. Often, this is because they are using different ethical principles as a basis for their beliefs. Many pro-life individuals use nonmaleficence (do no harm) as a guide that abortion should not be allowed at all. Pro-choice proponents often cite autonomy and liberty as the principle that factors most prominently and therefore allows women to make their own decisions. These different principles can be in conflict however. About half (47%) of U.S. adults favored permitting abortion under "some [but not all] circumstances," and 50% believed abortion should be legal under certain, but not all, circumstances. (Gallup Inc., 2011; Harris Interactive, 2011).

The vocal minority—on both sides—attracts media attention and often takes the extreme positions. For example, extreme pro- lifers emphasize late-term abortions, whereas these abortions constitute only approximately 1% of all abortions. However, extreme pro-choicers oppose any restrictions on abortion through all three trimesters of pregnancy.

The result is a figurative—and too often a literal—shouting match rather than a conversation, and this form of communication can unfortunately lead to extreme actions. The National Abortion Federation reports that between 1977 and 2011, there were 6,461 attacks on abortion providers (National Abortion Federation, 2012).

Is this an effective way of communicating? Is this the way to resolve an ethical dilemma? How might groups such as clergy, citizens, or politicians work together to employ communication techniques that require listening as well as speaking?

In addition, many states have also passed laws limiting abortion services. These include limiting funding for abortion, parental consent laws, waiting periods, and bans on certain procedures (see Tables IF1.1 and IF1.2 for state laws regarding parental consent and waiting period laws). Interestingly, one study has shown that in areas of the United States with more restrictive abortion policies and less access to abortion, the rates of searching for abortion information on the Internet are higher compared to areas with fewer restrictions and greater access (Reis & Brownstein, 2010). The Guttmacher Institute (www.guttmacher.org) is a good resource for updated information about state policies

Who Has Abortions?

In 2008 (the latest data available at the time of this writing), an estimated 1.21 million abortions were performed in the United States, down from 1.31 million in 2000 (Jones & Kooistra, 2011). From 1995 through 2005, more than 45 million legal abortions occurred in this country. The decline in abortion procedures in the United States has slowed, with rates changing little since 2005 (Jones & Kooistra, 2011). At current rates, each year approximately 2% of women ages 15–44 have an abortion, and surprising to most people, half of them have had at least one previous abortion (Jones, Finer, & Singh, 2010). By these same rates, it is estimated that nearly 1 in 10 U.S. women will have an abortion by age 20, one-quarter by age 30, and nearly one-third by age 45 (Jones & Kooistra, 2011).

The Alan Guttmacher Institute monitors abortion laws and the characteristics of those having abortions. It reports that about half (49%) of all pregnancies of American women are unwanted and that 40% of these are terminated by abortion. What surprises some people is that of these women 61% have had a previous birth (Jones et al., 2010).

Fifty-one percent of abortions are performed for women younger than 25 years. One-third of abortions are performed for women aged 20 to 24 years, and teenagers have 17% of all abortions.

Of the women who have abortions, 30% are black, 36% are white, 25% are Hispanic, and 9% are other races. Income is another characteristic that varies greatly among women seeking abortion; 42% of women obtaining abortions in 2008 reported income levels that would classify them as poor, which is a significant increase from the 27% in 2000. In addition to this general increase, poor women have five times the abortion rate compared to women who are considered "better off" with incomes at 200% or more of the poverty level (Jones et al., 2010). One factor in the difference of abortion rate is the difference in unintended pregnancy rates among women of different incomes. The overall rate of unintended pregnancy in the United States has remained around 50%; however, the unintended pregnancy rate for poor women is more than five times the rate for women in the

TABLE IF1.1 Parental Involvement in Minors' Abortions

State	Parental Involvement			Judicial Bypass				Exceptions	
	Consent Only	Notification and Consent	Notification Only	Available	Specific Criteria	"Clear and Convincing" Evidence	Other Adult Relatives	Medical Emergency	Abuse, Assault, Incest or Neglect
Alabama	X			X				X	
Alaska			X	X				X	X
Arizona	X*			X	X	X		X	X
Arkansas	X*			X				X	X
California	▶								
Colorado			X	X		X		X	X
Delaware			X†,‡	X†,‡			X‡	X‡	
Florida			X	X	X	X		X	
Georgia			X	X				X	
Idaho	X			X		X		X	X
Illinois			§	§			§	§	§
Indiana	X			X				X	
Iowa			X	X			X	X	X
Kansas	Both parents*			X	X	X		X	
Kentucky	X			X	X			X	
Louisiana	X*			X		X		X	
Maryland			X†						X†
Massachusetts	X			X				X	
Michigan	X			X				X	
Minnesota			Both parents	X				X	X
Mississippi	Both parents			X		X		X	
Missouri	X			X					
Montana			▶						
Nebraska	X*			X		X			X
Nevada			▶						
New Hampshire			X	X				X	
New Jersey			▶						
New Mexico	▶								

Continued

TABLE IF1.1   Parental Involvement in Minors' Abortions—cont'd

State	Parental Involvement			Judicial Bypass				Exceptions	
	Consent Only	Notification and Consent	Notification Only	Available	Specific Criteria	"Clear and Convincing" Evidence	Other Adult Relatives	Medical Emergency	Abuse, Assault, Incest or Neglect
North Carolina	X			X			X	X	
North Dakota	Both parents			X		X		X	X
Ohio	X			X	X			X	
Oklahoma		X		X		X		X	X
Pennsylvania	X			X				X	
Rhode Island	X			X					
South Carolina	X†			X‡			X†	X†	X†
South Dakota			X	X		X		X	
Tennessee	X			X				X	X
Texas		X*		X				X	
Utah		X		XΩ				X	X§
Virginia		X*		X			X	X	X
West Virginia			X†	X*				X	
Wisconsin	X†			X*			X	X	X
Wyoming	X			X		X		X	
Total	21	5	11	36	5	13	6	33	15

Note: Except where indicated, policies require the involvement of one parent.

▶ Enforcement permanently enjoined by court order; policy not in effect.

§ Enforcement temporarily enjoined by court order; policy not in effect.

* Requires parental consent documentation to be notarized.

† Allows specified health professionals to waive parental involvement in limited circumstances.

‡ While most states' laws apply to all minors, Delaware's law applies to women younger than 16 and South Carolina's law applies to those younger than 17.

Ω The provision only applies to parental consent requirements.

ξ The provision only applies to the parental notice requirements.

Source: Reproduced from Guttmacher Institute, Parental Involvement in Minors' Abortions, State Policies in Brief, New York: Guttmacher, 2012, http://www.guttmacher.org/statecenter/spibs/spib_PIMA.pdf, accessed August 2, 2012.

TABLE IF1.2 Abortion Counseling and Waiting Periods

State	Length of Waiting Period (in hours)	In-Person Counseling Necessitates Two Trips to Clinic	Writing Materials Given or Offered	Woman Informed that Abortion Cannot Be Coerced	Description of Procedure		Fetal Development		Ability of a Fetus to Feel Pain	Accessing Ultrasound Services
					Specific	All Common	Gestational Age of Fetus	Throughout Pregnancy		
States with Detailed Abortion-Specific Information Consent Requirements (28 states)										
Alabama	24		Given	V,W	V	W	V	W		
Alaska			Offered		V	W	V	W	W*	
Arkansas	Prior day		Offered	V,W	V	W	V	W	V,† W	
Georgia	24		Offered		V	W	V	W	V,W	V
Idaho	24		Given		V	W		W		
Indiana	18	X	Given		V	W	V	W	V‡	V
Kansas	24		Given	W	V	W	V	W		W
Kentucky	24		Offered		V	W	V	W		
Louisiana	24	X	Given	W	V	W	V	W	V,W	
Massachusetts	▶									
Michigan	24		Given		V,W	V,W	V,W	W		W*
Minnesota	24		Offered		V	W	V	W	V,‡ W	
Mississippi	24	X	Offered		V	W	V	W		
Missouri	24	X	Given	W	V	W	V	W	W†	W
Montana	▶									
Nebraska	24		Offered		V	W	V	W		V,W
North Carolina	24		Offered	V^Φ	V	W	V	W		W
North Dakota	24		Offered		V	W	V	W		
Ohio	24	X	Given		V	W	V	W		
Oklahoma	24		Offered		V	W	V	W	V,‡ W	V,W
Pennsylvania	24		Offered	W	V	W	V	W		
South Carolina	24		Offered		V	W	V	W		W
South Dakota	24^Ω	§	Given	V	V	W*	V	W	W*	
Texas	24	X^ξ	Offered		V	W*	V	W	W*	
Utah	72	X^Ↄ	Given	W	V	W	V	W	V	V
Virginia	24	X^ξ	Offered		V	W	V	W		‡
West Virginia	24		Offered	W*	V	W	V	W		
Wisconsin	24	X	Offered	W	V	W	V	W		V,W

Continued

TABLE IF1.2 Abortion Counseling and Waiting Periods—cont'd

State	Length of Waiting Period (in hours)	In-Person Counseling Necessitates Two Trips to Clinic	Writing Materials Given or Offered	Woman Informed that Abortion Cannot Be Coerced	Description of Procedure		Fetal Development			
					Specific	All Common	Gestational Age of Fetus	Throughout Pregnancy	Ability of a Fetus to Feel Pain	Accessing Ultrasound Services
States with Customary Informed Consent Provisions (9 states)										
Arizona	24	X	‡	V	V	‡	V	‡		
California					V					
Connecticut					V		V			
Delaware		▶			V		V			
Florida					V		V			
Maine					V		V			
Nevada					V		V			
Rhode Island					V		V			
Tennessee^Ψ		▶					V			
Total	**26**	**10**	**26**	**12**	**34**	**21**	**33**	**25**	**11**	**12**

All states waive mandatory waiting period requirements in a medical emergency or when the woman's life or health is threatened. In Utah, the waiting period requirement is waived if the pregnancy is the result of rape or incest, the fetus has grave defects, or the patient is younger than 15. The counseling requirement is waived in cases of ectopic pregnancy or severe fetal impairment (Alabama) and in cases of a medical emergency (Georgia and Rhode Island).

V = verbal counseling; W = written materials.

▶ Enforcement permanently enjoined by court order; policy not in effect.

* Included in written counseling materials although not specifically mandated by state law.

§ Enforcement temporarily enjoined by court order; policy not in effect.

† Information given only to women who are at 20 weeks' gestation or more; in Missouri the law applies at 22 weeks gestation.

‡ Required by law to be included in the written materials, but the materials have not yet been updated. In Indiana, the provision is not enforced against Planned Parenthood of Indiana due to a court case.

Φ Counseling includes discussion of coerced abortion and counselors must provide resources and private access to a phone for woman who are believed to be coerced into the abortion. These resources are not developed by the state.

Ω A law that would extend the waiting period to 72 hours and mandated in person counseling is blocked during a court case.

Ψ Enforcement of a provision of the Tennessee law requiring that a woman be told that an abortion constitutes major surgery is enjoined.

ξ In person counseling is not required for women who live more than 100 miles from an abortion provider.

Ↄ Counseling must be conducted "face-to-face" at "any location in the state."

Continued

TABLE IF1.2 Abortion Counseling and Waiting Periods—cont'd

State	Counseling On Health Risks of Abortion						Counseling on Health Risks of Pregnancy
	Future Fertility		Breast Cancer		Mental Health		
	Accurately Portrays Risk	Inaccurately Portrays Risk	Correctly Reports No Link	Inaccurately Asserts Possible Link	Correctly Reports Range of Emotional Responses	Describes Negative Emotional Responses	
Alabama					W†		W
Alaska	W†			W†	W		W
Arkansas	W†				W		V,W
Georgia	W†				W		V,W
Idaho	V				W†		V,W†
Indiana	V‡						V
Kansas		W†		W†		W†	V,W
Kentucky							V
Louisiana	W†				W†		V,W
Massachusetts							
Michigan						W	W
Minnesota	V,W†		V,W†		W		V,W
Mississippi	V,W†		V	W†		W†	V,W†
Missouri	V				V		
Montana							
Nebraska	V,W†					W	V,W
North Carolina		W				W	V
North Dakota	V						V
Ohio							V
Oklahoma	W†			W†	W		V,W
Pennsylvania	W†				W		V,W
South Carolina	W†						W
South Dakota	V	W†	V			V,W†	V,W†
Texas	V	W	V	W		W†	V,W
Utah		W				W	V,W
Virginia					W		W
West Virginia	V	W				W	V,W
Wisconsin	V,W		V,W				V,W

Continued

TABLE IF1.2   Abortion Counseling and Waiting Periods—cont'd

State	Counseling On Health Risks of Abortion						Counseling on Health Risks of Pregnancy
	Future Fertility		Breast Cancer		Mental Health		
	Accurately Portrays Risk	Inaccurately Portrays Risk	Correctly Reports No Link	Inaccurately Asserts Possible Link	Correctly Reports Range of Emotional Responses	Describes Negative Emotional Responses	
States with Customary Informed Consent Provisions (9 states)							
Arizona						‡	V
California							
Connecticut							
Delaware							
Florida							V
Maine							V
Nevada					Φ		
Rhode Island							
Tennessee							V
Total	**18**	**5**	**3**	**5**	**12**	**8**	**29**

V = verbal counseling; W = written materials.

† Included in written counseling materials although not specified by state law.

‡ Required by law to be include in the written materials, but the materials have not yet been updated.

Φ Law requires discussion of emotional impact of abortion.

Source: Reproduced from Guttmacher Institute, Counseling and Waiting Periods for Abortion, State Policies in Brief, New York: Guttmacher, 2012, http://www.guttmacher.org/statecenter/spibs/spib_MWPA.pdf, accessed August 2, 2012.

highest income level. Likewise, there is little difference between education levels among women in the highest income bracket, but minorities have the highest unintended pregnancy rates regardless of income level (Finer & Zolna, 2011).

Religion plays a role as well. Women who report no religious affiliation are one and a half times as likely to obtain an abortion as other women. Among specific religions, 37% of women obtaining abortions identify themselves as Protestant, and 28% as Catholic.

Marital status is another variable associated with abortion. Eighty-five percent of abortions are obtained by women who are not married; however, nearly half of women obtaining abortions were living with their male partner (Jones et al., 2010).

There are three primary reasons women give for seeking an abortion (Guttmacher Institute, 2011). Three-quarters say that having a baby would interfere with their work, education, or other responsibilities. Approximately three-fourths say they cannot afford a child. And half say they do not want to be a single parent or are having problems with their husband or partner. In addition, some abortions are performed for health-related reasons.

The Safety of Abortion

Abortion is an extremely safe procedure. Less than 0.3% of abortion patients experience a major complication. Of these, the primary risks are pelvic infection, hemorrhaging, or unintended major surgery. For abortions performed during the first 8 weeks of pregnancy, 1 death occurs per 1 million abortions. The risk rises as the pregnancy progresses to 1 death per 29,000 during weeks 16 to 20, and 1 death per 11,000 after 20 weeks (Guttmacher Institute, 2011). In comparison, the risk of death associated with childbirth is 12 times greater than that associated with abortion (Grimes, 2006). Furthermore, there is no effect on subsequent pregnancies or births in women who have first-trimester abortion procedure.

Although there has been some concern raised about the psychological health of women as a result of experiencing an abortion, there is little evidence that women are negatively affected. A 2009 review of existing studies found that the majority of adult women who terminate a pregnancy do not experience mental health problems and that there is no evidence to support the claim that mental health problems are caused by abortion (Major et al., 2009). A similar study on adolescents showed that abortion does not cause either depression or low self-esteem among young women in the short term or up to 5 years after the abortion (Warren, Harvey, & Henderson, 2010). Likewise, a rigorous research study in Denmark with over 84,000 participants found no evidence of increased risk of mental disorders after a first-trimester abortion (Munk-Olsen et al., 2011). This study has been heralded as the most methodologically sound research study to date. Although these studies show that most do not experience mental health issues, there is great variation among women, and it is important to remember that some women do experience issues after an abortion even if the abortion is not the sole factor (Major et al., 2009).

Attitudes About Abortion: Changing and Unchanging

Since *Roe v. Wade*, attitudes toward abortion have been evolving, and many studies have attempted to identify Americans' attitudes. Many of the studies and polls are limited by study methods and sampling procedures, so it is important to consider survey results as general approximations and not exact percentages. This perspective becomes important, because abortion beliefs are almost equally divided in this country. In the mid-1990s the country had a more pro-choice viewpoint on the issue, but since then more individuals have come to believe in restricting abortion in at least some way.

A 2011 national poll showed an almost equal division between those calling themselves pro-choice (49%) or pro-life (45%) (Gallup Inc., 2011). Interestingly, two national polls conducted within months of each other showed similar results when asked about women's access to abortion or if abortion should be legal. The Harris poll indicated that 36% of adults think women should have access to abortion in "all circumstances," and the Gallup poll indicated that 27% of the respondents wanted abortion legal in all circumstances. Similarly, 17% felt that women should not have access to abortion in any circumstance, and 22% wanted it illegal in all circumstances. The highest percentage for both polls indicated a middle ground philosophy, with 47% of U.S. adults favoring permitting abortion under "some [but not all] circumstances" and 50% continuing to choose the middle position, saying abortion should be legal under certain circumstances (Gallup Inc., 2011; Harris Interactive, 2011).

For both polls, gender was not a factor, but political party affiliation did play a role. Individuals who identified as Republican or Democrat seem to follow party lines, with Republicans more likely to favor laws restricting abortion and limiting access. More Democrats wanted to make access to abortion easier compared to Republicans and were more likely to consider it legal in more circumstances (Gallup Inc., 2011; Harris Interactive, 2011).

Availability of Legal Abortion

It is becoming increasingly difficult for a woman to have an abortion in the United States. While overall the number of abortion providers has declined since 1982, the number of providers remained stable between 2005 (1,787) and 2008, (1,793). At the same time, 87% of all U.S. counties lacked an abortion provider in 2008, with 35% of U.S. women living in those counties (Jones & Kooistra, 2011). These data are not surprising considering that one study found 40% of medical schools do not offer formal education on abortion in the preclinical years, and 25% do not offer it for third-year students doing clinical rotations in obstetrics and gynecology (Espry, 2005). In another study, only 51% of residency programs in obstetrics and gynecology were found to routinely provide abortion training (although residents could opt out if they had religious or moral objections). An additional 39% of programs offered optional abortion training, and 10% did not offer abortion training at all (Eastwood et al., 2006). Access to training about abortion is critical. One study found that regardless of intention

to provide abortion before residency, the availability of abortion training is positively correlated with providing abortions in the future practice of obstetricians and gynecologists (Steinauer et al., 2008).

Further many abortion clinics are picketed on a regular basis. In many cities college students volunteer as escorts at local abortion clinics in order to assure that women can use the clinic without interference. Only 15 states have specific laws protecting abortion clinics (Guttmacher Institute, 2012d). See Table IF1.3 for details.

Violence has also plagued many abortion clinics and abortion providers. Between 1977 and 2011, there were 41 bombings, 175 arsons, 100 attempted bombings and arsons, and 656 bomb threats directed at abortion providers (National Abortion Federation, 2012). Abortion providers have been murdered at the clinics where they work in Florida and Massachusetts. In 2009, Dr. George Tiller was murdered while attending church services because he provided abortions. Table IF1.4 summarizes the incidents of abortion-related violence over the past three decades.

TABLE IF1.3   Protecting Access to Clinics

State	Obstruction	Threat	Damage	Telephone Harassment	Other	Protected "Bubble Zone"
California*	X	X	X			
Colorado						8-ft. zone within 100 ft. of door
Dist. of Columbia	X	X		X	Noise, Trespassing	
Kansas	X					
Maine	X			X	Noise, Odor	
Maryland	X					
Massachusetts						35-ft. zone around entrances and walkways
Michigan		X				
Minnesota	X					
Montana	X					8-ft. zone within 36 ft. of door
Nevada	X					
New York	X	X	X			
North Carolina	X	X			Weapon	
Oregon	X		X			
Washington	X	X		X	Noise, Trespassing	
Wisconsin					Trespassing	
Total	**11 + DC**	**5 + DC**	**3**	**2 + DC**	**4 + DC**	**3**

* Requires the collection and analysis of data by state attorney general's office and training for law enforcement officers by experts on clinic violence.

Source: Reproduced from Guttmacher Institute, Protecting Access to Clinics, State Policies in Brief, New York: Guttmacher, 2012, http://www.guttmacher.org/statecenter/spibs/spib_PAC.pdf, accessed August 2, 2012.

TABLE IF1.4 **Incidents of Violence and Disruption Against Abortion Providers in the United States and Canada**

Violence	1977–1994	1995	1996	1997	1998	1999	2000	2001	2002	2003	2004	2005	2006	2007	2008	2009	2010	2011	Total
Murder[1]	5	0	0	0	2	0	0	0	0	0	0	0	0	0	0	1	0	0	8
Attempted Murder[1]	11	1	1	2	1	0	1	0	0	0	0	0	0	0	0	0	0	0	17
Bombing[1]	29	1	2	6	1	1	0	1	0	0	0	0	0	0	0	0	0	0	41
Arson[1]	124	14	3	8	4	8	2	2	1	3	2	2	0	2	0	0	0	0	175
Attempted Bomb/Arson[1]	64	1	4	2	5	1	3	2	0	0	1	6	4	2	1	1	1	2	100
Invasion	347	4	0	7	5	3	4	2	1	0	0	0	4	7	6	1	0	0	391
Vandalism	585	31	29	105	46	63	56	58	60	48	49	83	72	59	45	40	22	27	1,478
Trespassing	0	0	0	0	0	193	81	144	163	66	67	633	336	122	148	104	45	69	2,171
Butyric Acid Attacks	80	0	1	0	19	0	0	0	0	0	0	0	0	0	0	0	0	0	100
Anthrax Bioterrorism Threats	0	0	0	0	12	35	30	554	23	0	1	0	0	1	3	2	1	1	663
Assault and Battery	95	2	1	9	4	2	7	2	1	7	8	8	11	12	6	9	4	3	191
Death Threats	225	41	13	11	25	13	9	14	3	7	4	10	10	13	2	16	2	2	420
Kidnapping	2	0	0	0	1	0	0	0	0	0	0	0	1	0	0	0	0	0	4
Burglary	34	3	6	6	6	4	5	6	1	9	5	11	30	12	7	12	13	8	178
Stalking[2]	200	61	52	67	13	13	17	10	12	3	15	8	6	19	19	1	7	1	524
Total	1,801	159	112	223	144	336	215	795	265	143	152	761	474	249	237	187	95	113	6,461
Disruption																			
Hate Mail/Harassing Calls	1,833	255	605	2,829	915	1,646	1,011	404	203	432	453	515	548	522	396	1,699	404	365	15,062
Email/Internet Harassment	0	0	0	0	0	0	0	0	24	70	51	77	25	38	44	16	44	17	406
Hoax Device/Susp. Package	0	0	0	0	0	0	0	0	41	13	9	16	17	23	24	17	8	2	170

Continued

TABLE IF1.4   Incidents of Violence and Disruption Against Abortion Providers in the United States and Canada—cont'd

Violence	1977–1994	1995	1996	1997	1998	1999	2000	2001	2002	2003	2004	2005	2006	2007	2008	2009	2010	2011	Total
Bomb Threats	311	41	13	79	31	39	20	31	7	17	13	11	7	6	13	4	12	1	656
Picketing[4]	7,768	1,356	3,932	7,518	8,402	8,727	8,478	9,969	10,241	11,348	11,640	13,415	13,505	11,113	12,503	8,388	6,347	4,780	159,430
Total	9,912	1,652	4,550	10,426	9,348	10,412	9,509	10,404	10,543	11,880	12,166	14,034	14,102	11,702	12,980	10,124	6,815	5,165	175,724
Clinic Blockades																			
Number of Incidents	634	5	7	25	2	3	4	2	4	10	34	4	13	7	8	1	1	5	769
Number of Arrests[3]	33,361	54	65	29	16	5	0	0	0	0	0	0	0	0	1	0	0	0	33,834

All numbers represent incidents reported to or obtained by NAF. Actual incidents are likely much higher. Tabulation of trespassing began in 1999 and tabulation of email harassment and hoax devices began in 2002.

1. Incidents recorded are those classified as such by the appropriate law enforcement agency. Incidents that were ruled inconclusive or accidental are not included.
2. Stalking is defined as the persistent following, threatening, and harassing of an abortion provider, staff member, or patient away from the clinic. Tabulation of stalking incidents began in 1993.
3. The "number of arrests" represents the total number of arrests, not the total number of persons arrested. Many blockaders are arrested multiple times.
4. NAF changed its method for collecting this data in 2011.

Source: Reproduced from National Abortion Federation. Violence and Disruption Statistics, 2011. Available at: http://www.prochoice.org/about_abortion/violence/documents/Stats_Table2011.pdf.

Global DIMENSIONS

A Worldwide Preference for Boys

Around the world, on average, there are 105 boys born for every 100 girls born. Yet in China, there are 118 boys born for every 100 girls. Why is China so different from the rest of the world? Unfortunately, it is not.

Throughout the world, especially in densely populated countries, there are many reasons that boy babies are preferred, most based on long-term gender bias. China has no social security system, leaving elders vulnerable. In a country where couples are encouraged to have only one child, boys are presumed to be more valuable, because they are able to work and support their parents as they age. Either girls are not able to earn enough money to support their parents, or they are married off and assume duties with their new families. This situation is exacerbated as China becomes a more capitalistic country requiring men to travel for business purposes, while women are expected to stay at home. Men's travel earns money and makes them still more valuable in the eyes of many Chinese parents.

So the preference is for boy babies, but what is done to ensure that more boys will be born than girls? The shocking answer is female infanticide. When a Chinese woman delivers a baby, the village midwife sometimes prepares a bucket of water in which, if it is a girl, the baby's head is submerged before she starts to breathe. In India, where boy babies are preferred to girl babies for many of the same reasons as in China, female infanticide takes on a slightly different form. Pregnant Indian women have amniocentesis to determine the gender of their fetus. If the fetus is a girl, they undergo an abortion. Although the Indian authorities attempted to outlaw the use of amniocentesis for this purpose, the populace became outraged and refused to change this practice. A new pregnancy blood test can determine the sex of the fetus as early as 7 weeks. Some are concerned that this new test will increase abortions based on sex.

Looking at the female infanticide practices from the eyes of Western culture, experts have concluded that until gender equality is achieved around the world, female infanticide will be difficult to eradicate. Along with female genital mutilation, female infanticide may be culturally based. Some people believe that Western culture should refrain from interfering with the practices of other cultures. Others believe that in this case interference is warranted. What do you believe?

? Did You Know . . .

On January 22, 2001, President George W. Bush reinstated the Global Gag Rule (also called the Mexico City Policy). This policy restricts foreign nongovernmental agencies that receive funds from the U.S. Agency for International Development from

- Providing legal abortions, except in the case of rape, incest, or endangerment of the woman's life
- Lobbying their governments to legalize abortion or to decriminalize abortion
- Providing advice or information regarding the availability of abortion and referring women to another clinic that offers abortion services

- Conducting educational campaigns regarding abortion

Consequently, healthcare organizations needed to decide whether to give up needed funds for family planning and other reproductive services or to give up their rights of free speech and to provide their patients with complete and accurate medical information.

In 2009, President Barack Obama rescinded the Gag Rule.

Do you think this rule is wise policy? If so, why? If not, why not?

In addition to the lack of providers and clinic violence, age may also affect access to abortion. Thirty-seven states have passed laws requiring that adolescents have parental consent or notification for abortion (Guttmacher Institute, 2012c)(Table IF1.1).

Twenty-seven states have laws requiring a woman to have to make more than one visit to a clinic to have an abortion, insisting on a "waiting period," which can also affect a woman's ability to access services (Guttmacher Institute, 2012e).

Paying for an abortion can also affect access. Public funds may not be available to assist poor or low-income women. The patchwork of state laws concerning public funding for abortion services is complex. As a result of the Hyde Amendment, the use of federal Medicaid funds for abortion is prohibited except in cases in which the woman's life is in danger. The amendment was expanded in 1993 to include situations in which the pregnancy resulted from rape or incest. Each state establishes its own abortion funding policy related to state revenues. In 2012, the Guttmacher Institute reported that 17 states funded abortion in their state medical assistance programs in all or most circumstances (Guttmacher Institute, 2012f), and several states ban insurance coverage for abortion unless women pay an extra premium (Guttmacher Institute, 2012e).

Emotions and Abortion

The emotional reactions to abortion are varied. Some women feel guilty, depressed, angry, and ashamed. Others feel none of these feelings, or feel them just to a limited extent. The same range of emotions may apply to male partners as well.

Religious and moral beliefs; reactions of the medical staff, relatives, and friends; and the strength of the relationship between the partners all affect emotional responses. In addition, the earlier the abortion is performed, the lower the emotional cost. Perhaps the lack of humanlike features of the conceptus is what influences this finding. Realizing this, a film was developed by opponents of abortion and shown widely in the United States. Entitled *The Silent Scream*, this film is a 28-minute depiction of an abortion using ultrasound visualization. The viewers see a 12-week-old fetus being aborted by vacuum curettage and supposedly screaming in pain. The narrator, Dr. Bernard N. Nathanson, makes one feel that abortion is akin to infanticide because, he argues, "The unborn child is just another human being ... all the rest of his human functions are indistinct from any of ours." Many physicians and others have taken issue with Dr. Nathanson. For example, the American College of Obstetricians and Gynecologists responded to *The Silent Scream* with a statement that there is no scientific evidence to support the assertion that a 12-week-old fetus feels pain. Others have argued the following points (Spake, 1985):

1. The cerebral cortex of a 12-week-old fetus is insufficiently developed to feel pain.

2. Fetal movements are the result of reflexive action rather than "frantic activity" away from "the abortionist's instruments."

Myth vs Fact

Myth: Most abortions are performed late in the pregnancy.
Fact: Ninety percent of all abortions are performed during the first trimester. These abortions are usually performed by vacuum aspiration, but an increasing number are medical abortions.

Myth: Abortion is a dangerous procedure.
Fact: The risk of death during childbirth is 12 times greater than it is during abortion procedures. Furthermore, fewer than 0.3% of abortion patients experience a major complication.

Myth: Late-term abortions result in partial birth of the baby.
Fact: Opponents of abortion have labeled late-term abortion "partial birth abortion." This is a political tactic rather than an accurate description of late-term abortions. The correct term for these abortions is intact dilation and evacuation (D&E).

Myth: Adoptions have to be coordinated through an adoption agency.
Fact: Adoptions can be arranged independently, although these adoptions require court approval. In addition, adoptions can be arranged with relatives, although, again, they require court approval.

Myth: The withholding of the names of the birth parents (confidentiality and anonymity) is guaranteed by agencies and courts that arrange adoptions.
Fact: There is a debate taking place in our society regarding the rights of the birth parents versus the rights of the child. Several states have passed or are considering legislation to unseal adoption records.

3. Because the mouth of the fetus cannot actually be identified in the film, and because there is no air inside the fetus's lungs, the "scream" is no scream at all.

4. The fetal model used by Dr. Nathanson as he narrates is much larger than a 12-week-old fetus. In addition, many of the "fetuses" shown in the film are not fetuses but rather stillborn, premature infants.

The Silent Scream is but one example of the extreme emotion associated with the issue of abortion. Abortion facilities have been bombed, and staff and patients have been targets of harassment. Reputable abortion facilities provide counseling before the abortion to help the woman, alone or with her partner, make sure that she does indeed want an abortion performed—it is usually considered the best of several bad choices. In addition, they provide counseling after the abortion to lessen the emotional costs associated with this decision. These functions are difficult to perform well in the face of bomb threats, actual bombings, arson directed at abortion facilities, or picketing and/or harassment of patients seeking services at these facilities. Furthermore, some professionals choose not to subject themselves to this type of treatment and, therefore, refuse to work at

Gender DIMENSIONS

Baby "Richard" In June 1990, Daniella Janikova and Otakar Kirchner, both immigrants from what is now Slovakia, conceived baby "Richard" (his name has been changed to protect his identity). However, before Richard's birth, Otakar returned to his country with a former girlfriend, leaving Daniella in the United States. Before the delivery, Daniella arranged to place Richard for adoption. Daniella was then introduced to the "Warburtons," a pseudonym for a family interested in adopting Daniella's baby. Daniella signed the necessary forms to arrange for the Warburtons to adopt Richard. However, under Illinois law, the father has to agree to an adoption. When Daniella was asked for the name and address of the father, she refused to give it, falsely stating that he had abused her. Richard was born on March 16, 1991.

A few days after Richard's birth, Otakar received a call informing him that Richard had died. One month later, however, he learned that the baby was alive, and soon he returned to Daniella. Otakar then hired an attorney, who started legal proceedings for the return of his child. Subsequently, he and Daniella were married.

The Warburtons, however, contested the return of Richard, and a Cook County Circuit Court judge ruled the adoption valid, declaring Otakar unfit largely

because he had not filed a petition within 30 days of the birth (as required in Illinois) and because the prior testimony of Daniella alleged that he was abusive. However, when this decision was appealed, the Illinois Supreme Court in June 1994—after Richard had been living with the Warburtons for more than 3 years—overturned the adoption, stating that Otakar was led to believe that Richard had died and, therefore, could not have been expected to pursue his parental rights in a timely fashion.

After several appeals to the United States Supreme Court proved unsuccessful, Otakar and Daniella took custody of Richard on April 30, 1995. At the time of the wrenching transfer, Richard appealed to his adoptive mother, "I'll be good. Don't make me leave. I'll be good."

This case, tragic as it was for all parties, was decided on the rights of the father to agree to adoption of his biological offspring. In the mid-1990s, father's rights were often not protected. Because of this case and others, there is a stronger foundation and more awareness about the rights of biological fathers. Each state has different laws regarding the rights of biological fathers, and it is important for all involved in an adoption process to be aware of those rights in order to prevent heartbreaking stories like this one.

abortion facilities. Of course, some refuse to work there because of their own moral objections as well.

Adoption

Another response to an unwanted pregnancy is delivery of the baby, followed by adoption placement. Women who are unwed and choose not to raise a baby or who do not have the financial resources necessary to raise a baby often select adoption as an alternative for providing a good life for their babies.

Types of Adoptions

There are two basic types of adoption. *Closed adoptions* are confidential; there is no contact between the birth parents and the adoptive parents. The identities of the birth parents and adoptive parents are

kept secret. *Open adoptions* allow contact between the birth parents and the adoptive parents. In fact, the birth parents may even select the adoptive parents. Contact can occur regularly or intermittently throughout the child's upbringing.

Although there have been some highly publicized cases of birth parents seeking to reverse them, adoptions are legally binding and irreversible after a limited period. Birth parents sign "relinquishment papers" after the baby is born, and, unless both birth parents have not signed these papers, the courts have refused to reverse adoptions.

Domestic adoptions (adoptions within the United States) can be arranged one of four ways: a public agency, a licensed private agency, an attorney ("independent adoption"), or an adoption facilitator or unlicensed agency (if allowed by state law). Public and licensed private agencies must meet state standards and have more oversight to ensure quality services. Unlicensed agencies and facilitators may

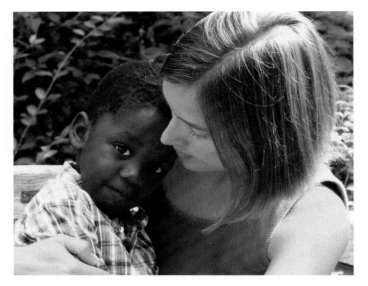

For many reasons individuals or couples may choose to adopt. International adoptions are among many options available.

not be subjected to the same state oversight and, as a consequence, there may be more financial, emotional, and legal risk for adoptive and birth families using unlicensed services (Child Welfare Information Gateway, 2010).

Public agencies mainly handle the adoption of children in a state's foster care system; these children can range from infants to teens. In a licensed agency adoption, the birth parents relinquish their parental rights to the agency, and adoptive parents then work with the agency to adopt. These agencies are licensed by the government and may offer a number of services. They provide counseling, handle legal matters, make hospital arrangements for the birth, select adoptive parents, and refer the mother to agencies if financial assistance is needed. Usually, though not always, adoptions arranged through agencies are open adoptions. Adoption agencies can be located through contacting most religious organizations; several national organizations can also be good resources, such as the National Council for Adoption (www.adoptioncouncil.org) or Independent Adoption Center (www.adoptionhelp.org).

In an independent adoption, attorneys assist prospective parents with the adoption process. Families adopting independently identify the expectant parents (or pregnant woman) without an agency's help. Independent adoptions are usually open adoptions, and attorneys who facilitate independent adoptions must adhere to the standards of the American Bar Association. Some attorneys who specialize in adoption are members of the American Academy of Adoption Attorneys, a professional membership organization with standards of ethical practice. Not all states allow independent adoptions (Child Welfare

Information Gateway, 2010). It is recommended that all prospective parents and birth parents have separate legal representation to ensure that no one is exploited. Often, the adoptive parents agree to pay the medical costs associated with the pregnancy and may even agree to pay for living expenses during that time. At the birth of the baby, the adoptive parents sign a "take into care" form that allows the adoptive parents to take the baby to their home while the state investigates their ability to raise the baby. This investigation usually takes 6 to 8 weeks. At any time while this investigation is occurring, either set of parents can change their minds. At the end of the investigation, the birth parents sign "relinquishment papers."

Adoptive services by facilitators and unlicensed agencies offer the least amount of supervision and oversight. A facilitator is any person who links prospective adoptive parents with expectant birth mothers for a fee. As mentioned previously, these individuals may or may not be regulated in their state, and some states may prohibit their use. Families who work with facilitators often have little recourse if the plan does not work out as they had hoped (Child Welfare Information Gateway, 2010).

Sometimes the birth parents want the child to stay in the family and the baby may be adopted by relatives. Even so, these adoptions require the approval of the courts. As in other adoptions, the relative is investigated by the state to determine ability to provide care for the child. Once the adoption is approved, the birth parents have no more rights pertaining to the child than they would in any other form of adoption.

Contemplating Adoption

Adopting a child is a decision that requires a great deal of consideration. So does the decision to give a child up for adoption. Be familiar with the adoption laws in your state so that you know how much time after birth you have to make or revoke your decision. In addition, anyone considering relinquishing their parental rights should ask these questions:

1. Can you accept your child living with someone else?

2. As a female, will going through pregnancy and delivery change your mind? As a male, will watching your partner go through a pregnancy and childbirth change your mind?

3. Are you willing to get good prenatal care?

4. Does adoption feel like what you should do, not what you want to do?

5. Will you be able to cope with any feelings of loss?

6. Will the child's father approve of adoption?

7. Is anyone pressuring you to choose adoption?

8. Are you confident your child will be treated well?

9. Can you not be jealous of the adoptive parents?

10. Do you respect women who place their children for adoption?

11. How important are other people's opinions of your decision?

Someone contemplating placing a child for adoption may want to discuss these questions with a partner, clergy, professional counselor, or a trusted relative or friend.

Foster Care and Adoption

For parents who are not ready to decide between placing a child for adoption and parenting, many cities and counties provide temporary residences for their children. This arrangement is termed *foster care*. To arrange for this option, the birth parents must sign a legal foster care agreement that allows another family to care for the child. Often, foster care agreements specify the frequency of visits between the child and birth parents that will be allowed, the duration of stay with the foster care family, the amount of money the birth parents will have to provide the foster care parents for caring for their child, and the number and frequency of visits to a professional counselor (usually a social worker). Although foster care arrangements and regulations vary from state to state, if the foster care agreement is violated, the birth parents can lose the child permanently.

Foster care is also provided for children who are taken from their birth parents for abuse, neglect, or other behavior that precludes them from being able to raise their children and places their children at risk. Children placed in foster care permanently are eligible for adoption, and, in fact, that is the goal of state agencies that supervise foster care arrangements.

The U.S. foster care system includes more than 408,000 children, of whom 25% are eligible for adoption (Child Welfare Information Gateway, 2012a). Fortunately, more and more of these children are being adopted. In 2010, 53,364 children in the foster care system were adopted. In 1997, the U.S. Congress passed the Adoption and Safe Families Act, designed to speed up adoption of children in the foster care system. That legislation provided bonuses of $4,000 to states for every child in the child protective system for whom they arranged adoption. For particularly difficult cases—such as older children or those with disabilities—states were provided $6,000 for each adoption. To further the goal of arranging for adoptions of children in foster care, in November 1998 President Clinton announced a plan to create an Internet site that would carry photographs and information about these children (Vobejda, 1998). The hope was that it would facilitate matching children eligible for adoption with parents seeking to adopt. Most states maintain websites to facilitate adoption of children in the foster care system. Still other states provide information to private agencies that maintain such websites.

Multicultural DIMENSIONS

International Adoptions

Many children from other countries are adopted by Americans. These adoptions may be the result of humanitarian concern of people who see children orphaned by war or widespread disease, or difficulty in locating the type of American child they wish to adopt. These international adoptions, though, can be very costly.

Recently, there has also been a lot of controversy about how international adoptions are facilitated. In early 2010, a Tennessee woman placed a 7-year-old boy she had adopted from Russia alone on a one-way flight back to Moscow with a note saying he was violent and had severe psychological problems. The adoptive mother claimed that she was lied to about his mental state; Russian officials said that she had not been lied to and demanded that the U.S. government take action against the woman and considered blocking all future adoptions to the United States.

In 2011, a 6-year-old girl adopted from Guatemala by a U.S. couple was identified as a child kidnapped from her biological mother when she was 2 years old. The U.S. couple had no knowledge of the kidnapping, and the child entered the United States through a valid immigration process, and presumably became a U.S. citizen at that time. A Guatemalan judge issued a court decision that the child be returned to Guatemala and her biological family; this is the first time that the return of an adopted child by a country of origin has been ordered.

Multicultural DIMENSIONS

International Adoptions—cont'd

In May 2012, the U.S. State Department stated that it did not have jurisdiction to help return the girl to Guatemala and that the U.S. state courts were the appropriate venue for hearing the case. At the time of this writing, the child's biological mother in Guatemala was attempting to find representation in the United States to assist in filing a case in the U.S. courts.

More stringent regulations and supervision of international adoption have been in place since the Hague Convention on the Protection of Children and Cooperation in Respect of Inter-Country Adoption went into force in the United States in 2008. However, these only apply to other countries that have also adopted the Hague Convention. Many people adopt from countries that are not part of this agreement; in fact, when considering children adopted internationally in 2011 by U.S. adults, four of the top five countries from which children were adopted were not part of the Hague Convention (Bureau of Consular Affairs 2011a, 2011b).

Another factor of interest is the steady decline of international adoptions. Since a peak in 2004 of 22,991 adoptions, the number of annual international adoptions had decreased almost 60% by 2011 (9,319). The reasons for this are complex and, for many countries, include an increased emphasis on domestic adoptions.

Given that there are American children waiting to be adopted, should the federal government discourage international adoptions? If so, what will happen to children orphaned by war or abused or neglected in other countries? Or should people wanting to adopt children be supported wherever those children come from?

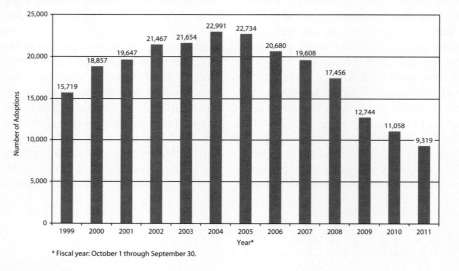

* Fiscal year: October 1 through September 30.

Source: Data from Bureau of Consular Affairs, U.S. Department of State. (2011). Statistics: Adoptions by Year. Available at: http://adoption.state.gov/about_us/statistics.php.

TABLE IF1.A   Top 5 Adopting Countries, 2006–2010

2010	2009	2008	2007	2006
1. China*	1. China*	1. Guatemala**	1. China*	1. China*
2. Ethiopia	2. Ethiopia	2. China*	2. Guatemala**	2. Guatemala**
3. Russia	3. Russia	3. Russia	3. Russia	3. Russia
4. South Korea	4. South Korea	4. Ethiopia	4. Ethiopia	4. South Korea
5. Ukraine	5. Guatemala**	5. South Korea	5. South Korea	5. Ethiopia

* Hague Convention country.

** Hague Convention country, but United States stopped accepting adoptions in 2007.

Source: Reproduced from Bureau of Consular Affairs, U.S. Department of State. (2011). Statistics: Adoptions by Year. Available at: http://adoption.state.gov/about_us/statistics.php.

Finding the Birth Parent

Because they seek to determine their complete history or because they are curious or have some other reason, many adults who were adopted seek to identify their birth parents. There is a good deal of disagreement as to whether and how this process should be facilitated. Some experts believe that contacting the birth parents might make them feel guilty about the adoption. Also, the birth parents might reject the adopted person, who might then have an unhealthy reaction to that rejection.

Before World War II, it was common practice for adoption records to be open. However, after the war, the combination of an increase in out-of-wedlock pregnancies and a conservative mood in the country resulted in adoption going "into the closet." Adoption records became sealed so that secrecy could be maintained. Since then, several states have passed legislation to open these records.

When an adoption is finalized, a new birth certificate for the child is usually issued to the adoptive parents. The original birth certificate is sealed and kept confidential by the state. As of 2009, four states (Alabama, Alaska, Maine, Oregon) and the Virgin Islands allow access to the original, unaltered birth certificate at the request of the adult adoptee, and eight other states may allow access at the request of the adoptee unless the parent had filed a motion denying release of the records (Child Welfare Information Gateway, 2009).

To help facilitate access to records that require consent, many states (about 30 in 2009) offer a mutual consent registry. A mutual consent registry is a means for individuals directly involved in adoptions to indicate their willingness or unwillingness to have their identifying information disclosed. Procedures for mutual consent registries vary significantly from state to state (Child Welfare Information Gateway, 2009). The Child Welfare Information Gateway is a resource with updated information about each state's policies.

Summary

- Abortions can be spontaneous (miscarriages) or induced. Induced abortions can be performed by vacuum aspiration, manual vacuum aspiration, medical abortion, or dilation and evacuation.

- The Supreme Court legalized abortion in the *Roe v. Wade* ruling in 1973. Since then, several restrictions have been placed on abortions by the states and declared constitutional by the Supreme Court. In 2007, the Supreme Court upheld the constitutionality of the 2003 Partial-Birth Abortion Ban Act, which banned intact dilation and evacuation for late-term abortions.

- Forty-nine percent of pregnancies are unwanted in the United States, and approximately 40% of these pregnancies are terminated by abortion.

- Fifty-one percent of abortions are performed in women younger than 25, one-third in women aged 20 to 24 years of age, and 17% in teenagers. Women who report no religious affiliation are one and a half times as likely to obtain an abortion as other women, and 85% of abortions are performed in unmarried women.

- Abortion is a safe procedure, with only 0.3% of abortion patients experiencing a major complication. Abortions are safest when performed during the first 8 weeks of pregnancy.

- Many Americans believe that abortions should be legal under certain circumstances, while less than a quarter believe abortion ought to be legal under all circumstances or believe it ought to be illegal under all circumstances.

- Adoptions can be closed—confidential with no contact between the birth parents and the adoptive parents—or open—allowing contact between birth parents and adoptive parents.

- Adoptions can be public agency adoptions, usually for children in the foster care system; private agency adoptions, in which the parents release the baby to adoption agencies; independent adoptions usually arranged by a lawyer; or facilitated adoptions, which are not allowed in all states and may not be subjected to rigorous oversight.

- Although sealed in the past, adoption records have been opened in several states. Alabama, Alaska, Maine, and Oregon have adopted an unqualified right to review original birth records, and several other states make records available if birth parents have not filed an objection.

Discussion Questions

1. What are the methods of abortion, and in which situations are they used?

2. Create a personal chart showing your own dimensions of human sexuality that relate to the abortion issue. After seeing all the issues involved, have you altered your position on abortion?

3. Explain the types of adoption available and the way each works.

Application Questions

Reread the chapter-opening story and answer the following questions.
1. The author Anna Quindlen appears to take a situational view of abortion: She thought abortion was OK for a bright college student but had second thoughts about an older and financially secure adult (herself). Does situation matter? In which situations is it acceptable to get an abortion? In which situations is it unacceptable?

2. The chapter also mentions the possibility of adoption. Should Quindlen have counseled her freshman with information about adoption? Explain why or why not.

Critical Thinking Questions

1. When the issue of abortion versus adoption is discussed, the father rarely enters into the discussion. Should the father have control over whether a woman can have an abortion or give a child up for adoption?

2. When do you believe that life begins? At conception? At a certain point in fetal development? At about 24 weeks, when the fetus can survive outside the womb (albeit with neonatal intensive care)? At about 35 weeks, when most babies can sustain life without medical intervention? Explain your answer.

3. Because many infertile couples want to adopt a child, why are there not more incentives for women to place children of unexpected pregnancies up for adoption? What could be done to motivate such a practice? Should the federal government be involved in such an effort?

Critical Thinking Case

In the late 1970s, Dr. Milfred Jefferson, an African American surgeon and chairperson of the national Right to Life organization, stated that abortion was genocide. She believed that a federally funded abortion program was aimed at eliminating the poor, African American population of the United States. Dr. Jefferson cited statistics showing that 30% of all abortions funded by Medicaid were performed on African Americans (while African Americans made up about 11% of the population). She said that "abortion is accomplishing what 200 years of slavery and 300 years of lynching didn't."

Opponents argue that the disproportionate number of Medicaid-funded abortions performed on African American women resulted from higher representation of African Americans among the poor in the United States; hence, they would have more need of financial support for abortions. Along these lines, people of lower socioeconomic status have less access to sex education, birth control information, and prescription birth control.

Abortion rates are still disproportionately high for African Americans. In 2008, the abortion rate for whites was 11.5 per 1,000 live births, the abortion rate for Hispanics was 28.7 per 1,000 live births, and the abortion rate for African Americans was 40.2 per 1,000 live births—almost four times the rate for whites (Jones & Kavanaugh, 2011).

Exploring Personal Dimensions

What is your feeling about abortion? Place an A, B, C, D, or E in the blank to the left of each of the following items, using the provided scale:
   A. I *strongly agree* with the statement.
   B. I *tend to agree* with the statement (some reservation).
   C. I am *undecided* (uncertain about my feelings or have no feelings one way or the other).
   D. I *tend to disagree* with the statement (some reservation).
   E. I *strongly disagree* with the statement.

_____ 1. Abortion penalizes the unborn [child] for the mother's mistake.

_____ 2. Abortion places human life at a very low point on a scale of values.

_____ 3. A woman's desire to have an abortion should be considered sufficient reason to do so.

_____ 4. I approve of the legalization of abortion so that a woman can obtain one with proper medical attention.

_____ 5. Abortion ought to be prohibited because it is an unnatural act.

_____ 6. Having an abortion is not something to be ashamed of.

_____ 7. Abortion is a threat to our society.

_____ 8. Abortion is the destruction of one life to serve the convenience of another.

_____ 9. A woman should have no regrets if she eliminates the burden of an unwanted child with an abortion.

_____10. The unborn [child] should be legally protected against abortion because it cannot protect itself.

_____11. Abortion should be an alternative when there is contraceptive failure.

_____12. Abortions should be allowed because the unborn [child] is only a potential human being, not an actual human being.

_____13. Any person who has an abortion is probably selfish and unconcerned about others.

_____14. Abortion should be available as a method of improving community socioeconomic conditions.

_____15. Many more people would favor abortion if they knew more about it.

_____16. A woman should have an illegitimate child rather than an abortion.

_____17. Liberalization of abortion laws should be viewed positively.

_____18. Abortion should be illegal, because the Fourteenth Amendment in the Constitution holds that no state shall "deprive any person of life, liberty, or property without due process of law."

_____19. The unborn [child] should never be aborted no matter how detrimental the possible effects on the family.

_____20. The social evils involved in forcing a pregnant woman to have a child are worse than any evils in destroying the unborn child.

_____21. Decency forbids having an abortion.

_____22. A pregnancy that is not wanted and not planned for should not be considered a pregnancy, but merely a condition for which there is a medical cure, abortion.

_____23. Abortion is the equivalent of murder.

_____24. Easily accessible abortions will probably cause people to become unconcerned and careless with their contraceptive practices.

_____25. Abortion ought to be considered a legitimate health measure.

_____26. The unborn child ought to have the same rights as the potential mother.

_____27. Any outlawing of abortion is oppressive to women.

_____28. Abortion should be accepted as a method of population control.

_____29. Abortion violates the fundamental right to life.

_____30. If a woman feels that a child might ruin her life, she should have an abortion.

To score this instrument, use the following point values for items 3, 4, 6, 9, 11, 12, 14, 15, 17, 20, 22, 25, 27, 28, and 30 only: A = 5, B = 4, C = 3, D = 2, E = 1.

For items 1, 2, 5, 7, 8, 10, 13, 16, 18, 19, 21, 23, 24, 26, and 29, use the following scale: A = 1, B = 2, C = 3, D = 4, E = 5.

Now add your points; the score should fall between 30 and 150. A score of 30 represents an unfavorable attitude, a score of 90 represents a neutral attitude, and a score of 150 represents a favorable attitude toward abortion.

Source: Reproduced from Snegroff, S. _Manual and Guide for the Abortion Attitude Scale and Knowledge Inventory._ Saluda, NC: Family Life Publications, Inc., 1978.

Suggested Readings

Baumgardner, J., & Todras-Whitehill, T. _Abortion & life_. New York: Akashic Books, 2008.

Faundes, A., & Barzelatto, J. _The human drama of abortion: A global search for consensus._ Nashville: Vanderbilt University Press, 2006.

Greenhouse, L., & Siegel, R. _Before Roe v. Wade._ New York: Kaplan Publishing, 2010.

Halfman, D. _Doctors and demonstrators: How political institutions shape abortion law in the United States, Britain, and Canada._ Chicago: University of Chicago Press, 2011.

Pertman, A. _Adoption nation: How the adoption revolution is transforming our families—and America._ Boston: Harvard Common Press, 2011.

Wicklund, S., & Kesselheim, A. _This common secret: My journey as an abortion doctor._ Jackson, TN: Public Affairs, 2008.

Web Resources

For links to the websites below, visit _go.jblearning.com/dimensions5e_ and click on Resource Links.

Alan Guttmacher Institute
www.guttmacher.org

The Alan Guttmacher Institute is a nonprofit organization focused on sexual and reproductive health research, policy analysis, and public education. The website contains links to the Guttmacher Institute publications _Perspectives on Sexual and Reproductive Health, International Family Planning Perspectives, The Guttmacher Report on Public Policy_, and special reports on topics pertaining to sexual and reproductive health and rights. The Institute's mission is to protect the reproductive choices of women and men in the United States and throughout the world. It supports their ability to obtain the information and services needed to achieve their full human rights, safeguard their health, and exercise their individual responsibilities in regard to sexual behavior and relationships, reproduction, and family formation.

National Abortion and Reproductive Rights Action League
www.naral.org

NARAL is committed to protecting the right to choose abortion and electing candidates who will promote policies to prevent unintended pregnancy. The latest laws and political issues pertaining to a woman's right to choose abortion are available on the NARAL website, as well as related issues such as emergency contraception.

Child Welfare Information Gateway
www.childwelfare.gov

Child Welfare Information Gateway connects child welfare and related professionals to comprehensive information and resources to help protect children and strengthen families. They include updated information on a variety of topics, including establishing permanent homes for children, child abuse and neglect, foster care, and adoption.

National Adoption Center
www.adopt.org

Devoted to increasing the number of children adopted, the National Adoption Center works to expand adoption opportunities for children living in foster care throughout the United States and is a resource to families and to agencies who seek the permanency of caring homes for children. Included on the website is information on how to adopt, resources and matching programs for prospective parents and adoption agencies, as well as photolistings of children waiting to be adopted.

References

Bureau of Consular Affairs, U.S. Department of State. *Convention countries*. 2011a. Available: http://adoption.state.gov/hague_convention/countries.php.

Bureau of Consular Affairs, U.S. Department of State. *Understanding the Hague convention*. 2011b. Available: http://adoption.state.gov/hague_convention/overview.php.

Cameron, S. Glasier, A., Dewart, H., Johnstone, A. Women's experiences of the final state of early medical abortion at home: results of a pilot survey. *Journal of Family Planning and Reproductive Health Care, 36* (2010), 213–216.

Child Welfare Information Gateway. *Access to adoption records: Summary of state laws*. Available: http://www.childwelfare.gov/systemwide/laws_policies/statutes/infoaccessapall.pdf.

Child Welfare Information Gateway. *Adoption options*. 2010. Available: http://www.childwelfare.gov/pubs/f_adoptoption.pdf.

Child Welfare Information Gateway. *Foster care statistics 2010*. 2012. Available: http://www.childwelfare.gov/pubs/factsheets/foster.pdf.

Eastwood, K. L., et al. Abortion training in United States obstetrics and gynecology residency programs. *Obstetrics and Gynecology, 108* (2006), 303–308.

Espry, E., et al. Abortion education in medical schools: A national survey. *American Journal of Obstetrics and Gynecology, 192* (2005), 640–643.

Finer, L. B., & Zolna, M. R. Unintended pregnancy in the United States: Incidence and disparities, 2006. *Contraception, 84, no. 5* (2011), 478–485.

Gallup, Inc. *Americans still split along "pro-choice," "pro-life" lines*. 2011. Available: http://www.gallup.com/poll/147734/Americans-Split-Along-Pro-Choice-Pro-Life-Lines.aspx.

Grimes, D. A. Estimation of pregnancy-related mortality risk by pregnancy outcome, United States 1991 to 1999. *American Journal of Obstetrics and Gynecology, 184* (2006), 92–94.

Guttmacher Institute. *Facts on induced abortion in the United States*. 2011. Available: http://www.guttmacher.org/pubs/fb_induced_abortion.html.

Guttmacher Institute. *Bans on "parital-birth" abortion*. 2012a. Available: http://www.guttmacher.org/statecenter/spibs_MWPA.pdf.

Guttmacher Institute. *Counseling and waiting periods for abortion*. 2012b. Available: http://www.guttmacher.org/statecenter/spibs/spib_MWPA.pdf.

Guttmacher Institute. *Parental involvement in minor's abortions*. 2012c. Available: http://www.guttmacher.org/statecenter/spibs/spib_PIMA.pdf.

Guttmacher Institute. *Protecting access to clinics*. 2012d. Available: http://www.guttmacher.org/statecenter/spibs/spib_PAC.pdf.

Guttmacher Institute. *Restricting insurance coverage of abortion*. 2012e. Available: http://www.guttmacher.org/statecenter/spibs_RICA.pdf.

Guttmacher Institute. *State funding of abortion under Medicaid*. 2012f. Available: http://www.guttmacher.org/statecenter/spibs/spib_SFAM.pdf.

Harris Interactive. *American show rising support for abortion rights*. 2011. Available: http://www.harrisinteractive.com/vault/HI-HealthyDay-Abortion-2011-7-25.pdf.

Jones, R. K., & Kavanaugh, M. L. Changes in abortion rates between 2000 and 2008 and lifetime incidence of abortion. *Obstetrics and Gynecology, 117* (2011), 1358–1366.

Jones, R. K., & Kooistra, K. Abortion incidence and access to services in the United States, 2008. *Perspectives on Sexual and Reproductive Health, 43* (2011), 41–50.

Jones, R. K., Finer, L. B., & Singh, S. (2010). Characteristics of U.S. abortion patients, 2008. Available from the Guttmacher Institute: http://www.guttmacher.org/pubs/US-Abortion-Patients.pdf.

Loeber, O. E. Motivation and satisfaction with early medical vs. surgical abortion in the Netherlands. *Reproductive Health Matters, 18* (2010), 145–153.

Major, B., Appelbaum, M., Beckman, L., Dutton, M. A., Russo, N. F., & West, C. Abortion and mental health: Evaluating the evidence. *American Psychologist, 64* (2009), 863–890.

Munk-Olsen, T., Laursen, T. M., Pedersen, C. B., Lidegaard, O., & Motensen, P. B. Induced first-trimester abortion and risk of mental disorder. *New England Journal of Medicine, 364* (2011), 332–339.

NARAL. Roe v. Wade *and the right to choose*. 2011. Available: http://prochoiceamerica.org/media/fact-sheets/government-federal-courts-scotus-roe.pdf.

National Abortion Federation. *Violence and disruption statistics, 2011*. 2011. Available: http://www.prochoice.org/about_abortion/violence/documents/Stats_Table2011.pdf.

Ngoc, N. T., Blum, J., Raghavan, S., Nga, N. T., Dabash, R., Diop, A., Winikoff, B. Comparing two early medical abortion regimens: mifepristone+misoprostol vs. misoprostol alone. *Contraception, 83, no. 5* (2011), 410–417.

Paul, M., & Stewart, F. H. Abortion. In R. A. Hatcher et al. *Contraceptive technology*, 19th revised edition. New York: Ardent Media, 2008.

Quindlen, A. *Thinking out loud*. New York: Random House, 1988.

Reis, B. Y., & Brownstein, J. S. Measuring the impact of health policies using Internet search patterns: The case of abortion. *BMC Public Health, 10* (2010), 514.

Spake, A. The truth about "The Silent Scream." *Ms*. (July 1985), 88, 91–92, 112–114.

Steinauer, J., Landy, U., Filippone, H., et al. Predictors of abortion provision among practicing obstetrician-gynecologists: A national survey. *American Journal of Obstetrics and Gynecology, 198* (2008), 39.

Suhonena, S., Tikkaa, M., Kivinena, S., & Kauppilab, T. Pain during medical abortion: Predicting factors from gynecologic history and medical staff evaluation of severity. *Contraception, 83* (2011), 357–361.

Vobejda, B. Web site to list foster children for adoption. *Washington Post* (November 25, 1998), A5.

Warren, J. T., Harvey, S. M., & Henderson, J. T. Do depression and low self-esteem follow abortion among adolescents? Evidence from a national survey. *Perspectives on Sexual and Reproductive Health, 42* (2010), 230–235.

CHAPTER 9

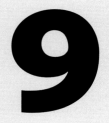

Gender Dimensions

FEATURES

CHAPTER OBJECTIVES

1 Describe the biological, psychological, and sociocultural differences between males and females.

2 Explain the effects of gender identity, gender roles, and gender stereotypes on sexuality.

3 Analyze how the women's movement has affected both females and males.

go.jblearning.com/dimensions5e

Gender and Health
Global Dimensions: The Oppression of Women
Ethical Dimensions: Extreme Gender Roles—The Price of Honor
The Women's Movement

When Mark attended college in the late 1970s, he thought all the talk about gender differences was bunk. Men and women appeared to share equal places in classrooms and in faculty positions. Women appeared to have the same opportunities as men in the outside work world. He and his classmates believed that the wage gap and glass ceiling were things that past generations dealt with. Those were the days.

But Mark still remembers one college guest speaker—a distinguished American composer. During his speech, the aging composer asserted that women were not good composers because their social upbringing left them devoid of technical skills. He told the stunned audience—among whom sat several prominent female composers—that boys take things apart and put things together, while girls play with dolls. Therefore, boys grow up with more technical abilities, which to him included the ability to orchestrate music. It seemed that everyone in attendance wrote off his comments as those of an elderly man from another era.

But as Mark joined the workforce, married, and had children, he began to witness more and more gender differences and biases. As the years passed by, the number of female friends who had experienced sexism in the workplace grew from none to all of them. It became clear that women and men did communicate differently, manage differently, work differently, play differently.

In Mark's marriage, gender roles have been reversed—because of work situations, not a deliberate decision. While his spouse works a managerial "nine-to-five job" (read, 7:00 A.M. to 6:00 P.M.), Mark writes and edits out of his home. He is responsible for raising two young children and for doing most household jobs. Because children cannot be ignored, he often has to put off work until they are in bed.

Mark has become keenly aware of the gender differences among parents. At his son's independent school, where most students' mothers do not have a job, he is one of the few fathers who take the child to school, go to parent–teacher conferences, and volunteer for various events. This creates quite a dilemma in friendships: While playing both the mother and father roles, he really does not fit into either group. Mark also notes that teachers react differently to him: When several mothers voiced a complaint to a teacher, the teacher spoke to them directly; however, the teacher would only communicate with Mark in the presence of a senior administrator.

Suprisingly, gender biases exist even among medical professionals. At his son's first pediatric appointment, the male doctor's first question was a stern "Where is the child's mother?" Some years later, during a hospital emergency room visit, the doctors and nurses clearly listened to every small comment his spouse made—yet brushed off Mark's input as insignificant.

As Mark's experience shows, gender plays a role in many aspects of our lives—at home, at work, and in our social activities. We develop a sexual identity, which is the outgrowth of the interaction of biology—being male or female—and social learning. Society's expectations for the behavior of men and women are conveyed to the individual by a process called socialization, which has a dominant influence on gender roles. As children model adults' behaviors, these gender roles are perpetuated, although traditional gender roles are changing as a broader range of behaviors is accepted by society.

If someone asked you whether you were a woman or a man, your first thought would probably be, What a ridiculous question! You know what gender I am. Still, that question might lead you to ask other questions about gender, such as, How did I learn to act as a man or woman? To what extent is my masculinity or femininity natural, and to what extent is it learned? Are my personal characteristics determined or influenced by my gender? In this chapter we explore some of the forces that influence our conceptions of **masculinity** *and* **femininity**.

■ Gender Differences

When gender differences and similarities are considered, discussions often center on "nature versus nurture." Those who argue from a nature perspective attribute most characteristics to biological differences or similarities. Those who argue more for nurture believe that we become the way we are mostly as a result of social factors and learning. There are persuasive arguments on each side, and some people believe that a combination of nature and nurture makes us the way we are.

People learn attitudes and values and have their personal

masculinity
Those qualities characteristic of and suitable for boys and men according to the rules and expectations of a society.

femininity
Those qualities characteristic of and suitable for girls and women according to the rules and expectations of a society.

experiences in a "gendered world." Gender issues are dealt with differently in different societies. For example, there may be more or less gendered examples in spheres such as occupational roles, child care, clothing styles, and some social and recreational activities.

In this chapter, we discuss some gender differences related to attitude and behavior. Caution is needed when considering such differences, however, because many variations in these attitudes and behaviors exist. Overgeneralization can result in inappropriate stereotypes. At the same time, however, many argue that different genders have their own important characteristics.

Developmental Differences

There is no question that males and females differ biologically in more than their physical structure and biological function. Developmentally, girls are more advanced than boys at birth—that is, their central nervous system is more mature. Boys tend to weigh more when born, but girls have fewer physical defects and a higher survival rate. More male children are conceived, but the miscarriage rate for males is greater than for females, and more males die in the first 12 months of life. The female's two X chromosomes, compared with the XY chromosomes of the male, may be a biological advantage. The X chromosomes are larger than Ys and can supply the female with a greater variety of genetic material. Even if one of the female's X chromosomes is a carrier of genetic defects, the second one can have normal genes that offset any genetic defect.

In infancy and early childhood, growth in boys and girls is similar. The development of language, the growth of body organs and the nervous system, and perceptual and motor development proceed in sequence. The female is more developed prenatally, but the male develops more rapidly postnatally. Until age 8 years the male is heavier and taller than the female, but he reaches puberty more slowly. The onset of puberty occurs approximately 2 years earlier in the female. In the preadolescent period the female, having greater physical maturity, can perform physical and athletic tasks better than the male. With menarche, estrogen influences the increase of **adipose** (fat) tissues and enlargement of the female pelvis. Eventually the estrogen prevents growth in the skeletal long bones, and height stabilizes for girls at about age 17 years.

adipose
Pertaining to fat tissue in the body.

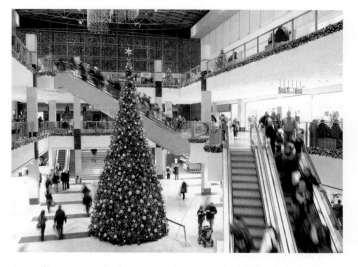

According to one study, men and women also differ in their reaction to holiday shopping. All 36 male subjects showed a dramatic increase in blood pressure when confronted with crowds and lines. But one in four females showed increased blood pressure. What physiological, psychological, and social factors would cause such a result?

When the male reaches puberty, androgen increases his muscle mass and skeletal development, and thus the adolescent boy has more body mass but less fat than the girl. This androgenic effect on male development gives him more strength and more speed. Furthermore, the male's greater lung and heart capacity and greater capacity for oxygen transport to tissues, combined with his predisposition toward being taller and heavier than the female, give him more power.

Many researchers have studied the brains of males and females. Although most researchers agree that men's brains are about 10% bigger than women's, women's brains seem to have more connections between the two brain hemispheres. In some regions, the female brain is more densely packed with neurons. Women tend to use more parts of their brain to accomplish certain tasks. This might help explain why they often recover better from a stroke, because the healthy parts of the brain may more easily compensate for the injured regions. Even though men and women have different brain architectures, we really don't know yet what that might mean (Ripley, 2005).

Gender and Abilities

There are various opinions about similarities and differences in abilities between males and females. Although it is always possible to find someone who disagrees, most experts agree that until about age 11 or 12 males and females have similar verbal abilities. Around age 11 or 12, females have greater abilities in language and verbal tasks, but males perform better on visual–spatial tasks. This difference seems to persist into adulthood (see Figure 9.1). In addition, girls seem to speak sooner than boys. On average, women show more verbal skills than men.

(a) Problem-Solving Tasks Favoring Women

Women tend to perform better than men on tests of perceptual speed, in which subjects must rapidly identify matching items—for example, pairing the house on the far left with its twin:

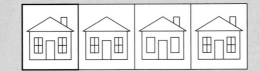

In addition, women remember whether an object, or a series of objects, has been displaced:

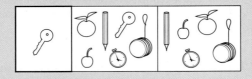

On some tests of ideational fluency, such as those in which subjects must list objects that are the same color, and on tests of verbal fluency, in which participants must list words that begin with the same letter, women also outperform men:

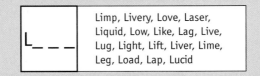

Women do better on precision manual tasks—that is, those involving fine-motor coordination—such as placing the pegs in holes on a board:

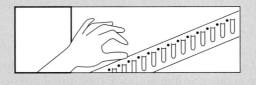

And women do better than men on mathematical calculation tests:

| 77 | $14 \times 3 - 17 + 52$ |
| 43 | $2(15 + 3) + 12 - \frac{15}{3}$ |

(b) Problem-Solving Tasks Favoring Men

Men tend to perform better than women on certain spatial tasks. They do well on tests that involve mentally rotating an object or manipulating it in some fashion, such as imagining turning this three-dimensional object:

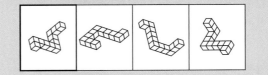

or determining where the holes punched in a folded piece of paper will fall when the paper is unfolded:

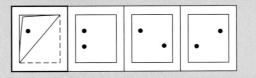

Men also are more accurate than women in target-directed motor skills, such as guiding or intercepting projectiles:

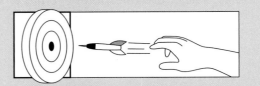

They also do better on disembedding tests, in which they have to find a simple shape, such as the one on the left, once it is hidden within a more complex figure:

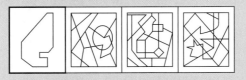

And men tend to do better than women on tests of mathematical reasoning:

| 1,100 | If only 60% of seedlings will survive, how many must be planted to obtain 660 trees? |

FIGURE 9.1 Problem-solving tasks for women and men. Research suggests that some problem-solving tasks may demonstrate gender-related performance differentiation.
Source: Adapted from Kimura, D. Sex differences in the brain. *Scientific American, 267* (1992), 188–195.

Whether boys have better mathematical abilities than girls is still debated. Historically, math was seen as a masculine area of study in which girls were not expected or encouraged to excel. Because many females were raised thinking they should not succeed in math, their performance on math measures tended not to be high. Several decades ago, however, females' perceptions of their ability to do well in math showed signs of change.

Interestingly, math scores on national tests for fourth-graders have been improving for both genders, with no statistically significant differences between boys and girls. However, girls score about 7% lower than boys on the math part of the SAT. It has been suggested that one reason for this might be that more girls than boys from lower-income families take the test (Ripley, 2005).

Looking at a different type of ability, Horgan et al. (2004) found that women more accurately recalled information concerning the appearance of other people, such as physical features, clothing, and postures. Both men and women did better at remembering the appearance of women than remembering how men looked.

Does this mean that biology is destiny when it comes to these abilities? No, because even though each gender seems to have specific abilities, there are also cultural explanations for these differences. These include teachers' assumptions and their treatment of students, parents' attitudes toward their children, the perception of society that math has been for males, each gender's self-perception and ambitions, and social pressures on adolescents—just to name some possibilities.

Gender and Aggression

Some experts believe that boys are more physically and verbally aggressive than girls, beginning at pre-school age. Given that this seems to be true in many cultures, there may be some biological basis for this difference. Males probably remain more aggressive into their college years, but as they mature the trait diminishes. There is some evidence that boys are punished more than girls for aggression.

Intimate-partner violence continues to be a major problem in the United States. Many forms of violence have decreased in recent years, but intimate-partner violence has increased. While traditionally it was thought to be only a male-to-female activity because usually males are bigger and stronger than females, acts of violence against both women and men have increased within intimate relationships.

Tavris (2002) provided an interesting view related to female aggression. She pointed out that many authors have written about hidden and formerly

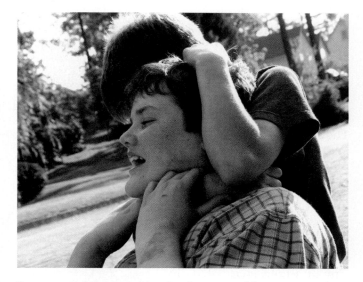

Boys seem to be more aggressive than most girls.

secret female aggressiveness. She said that girls are not sweeter than boys, but just as bad, sexual, and aggressive—maybe even meaner, given the ruthless and sneaky ways they control one another. For example, our culture refuses girls access to open conflict, and it forces their aggression into nonphysical, indirect, and covert forms. Girls use backbiting, exclusion, rumors, name calling, and manipulation to inflict psychological pain on targeted victims. Boys, in short, resort to physical aggression; girls, to "relational" aggression.

Anger and aggression are learned behaviors and are characteristic of humans. Traditionally they have been viewed as more appropriate for males than for females. However, as we move toward humanism and less-defined parameters of what is male and what is female, we must reevaluate our cultural acceptance of these behaviors.

Gender and Health

While there is not unanimous agreement on this point, there seem to be differences in males' and females' health attitudes and behavior. Examples include women being more likely to take action to prevent health problems, men tending to rely on spouses for social support related to their health, and women being more likely to turn to friends and their children for assistance in this area. Women also seem to experience more health problems and make more extensive use of health services.

When it comes to health care, there are also some interesting comparisons between males and females. While women show a preference for a female physician in the fields of general practice and gynecology (probably due to the intimate nature of the clinical intervention), beyond that most people do not have a strong preference for a healthcare provider of a particular gender.

Men are more likely to avoid regular health care than are women (Galdas, Chaeter, & Marshall, 2005). They often say they feel fine and do not need to consult physicians. Because of their needs related to reproductive health, women find it more difficult to avoid the health care system regardless of how well they may feel. Men and women seem to have similar experiences of daily symptoms, but women are more likely to seek medical care for these symptoms. Men also seem to have more trouble adopting the patient role than do women.

Another gender issue related to health is that some health insurance plans provide coverage for prescription drugs, but exclude coverage for prescription contraceptives. This can result in an extra financial burden on women and also make it more likely that some will use less-effective contraceptive methods—making unwanted pregnancy more likely.

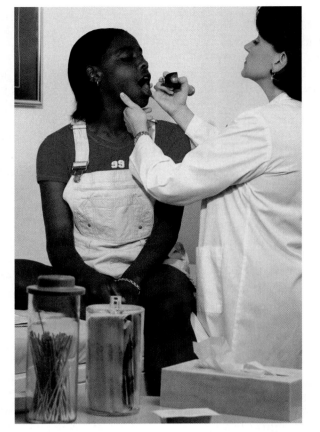

Women seem to prefer a female medical care provider in general practice and in gynecology.

Another issue related to gender and health insurance is the practice of having different rates based on gender. Some have argued that split rates are justified because younger women typically seek healthcare services more often than men. Some women have been paying as much as 20% more than men for the same individual coverage. Federal law prohibits employers that offer health plans from charging different rates based on gender, and in 2009 California became one of 10 states with a similar law (State Politics & Policy, 2009).

On an international level, Guptka (2001) pointed out that power imbalance increases HIV risk. For example, in many societies there is a culture of silence surrounding sexuality that dictates that "good" women are expected to be ignorant about sexual behavior and passive in sexual interactions. This makes it difficult for women to be informed about HIV risk reduction and, even if informed, to be proactive in negotiating safer sexual activity. In addition, the traditional norm of virginity for unmarried females increases young women's risk of infection, because

it restricts their ability to ask for information about sexuality because of fear that they will be thought to be sexually active. In cultures in which virginity is highly valued, some young women practice alternative sexual behaviors, such as anal intercourse, to preserve their virginity. These behaviors may place them at increased risk of HIV. Accessing treatment services for STIs can be highly stigmatizing for women. Finally, using barrier methods as safer options for sexual activity can be a dilemma for women in societies in which motherhood is considered to be a feminine ideal.

Other international examples were given by Billowitz and Kukke (2004). They pointed out that gender roles can have direct implications for health outcomes. For example, in many countries female infants die at a significantly higher rate than boys because they are not as highly valued. Boys are more likely to be immunized, have better nutrition, and receive medical care more promptly. These authors estimated that more than 1 million girls die each year from malnutrition, neglect, and abuse who would not have died had they been male. Sex-selective abortion is also still practiced in some countries where males are more highly valued.

Billowitz and Kukke (2004) also indicated other effects of gender roles. Gender norms may keep males from asking vital questions about sexuality. Men are supposed to demonstrate a bravado that makes it impossible to admit they don't know something about sexuality. In some cultures masturbation is believed to negatively affect a man's "manliness." This leads males to seek casual or commercial sexual activity when they have a desire to ejaculate, resulting in pressure to engage in frequent sexual activity with multiple partners, often without using a condom. Poor females who go to clinics may be intimidated by clinic personnel who show their attitudes about what women should do and not do. Also, in many countries economic inequities leave women few options for their livelihood, which may lead them to engage in transactional sexual activity or formal

Multicultural DIMENSIONS

Examples of Gender Equity Promoting Programs

Nigeria

In Nigeria, girls are traditionally taught to be subservient to their male family members. The Girls' Power Initiative provides girls with information on sexuality, human rights, sexual and reproductive health and rights, leadership, self-esteem, and life skills. The girls are trained to speak out against gender inequities. There is a counterpart program that works with young men to change attitudes toward gender roles and issues.

Kenya

Maendeleo Ya Wanawake Organization, a grassroots women's organization, was the first group in Kenya to advocate for the elimination of female genital cutting (FGC). The Organization goals included raising awareness about the harmful effects of FGC, devising ways to provide a positive image of uncircumcised girls, and developing an alternative rite of passage for girls that would replace initiation by cutting. As a result, the prevalence of FGC dropped among girls ages 14 to 19, and the number of women in favor of discontinuing the practice grew substantially.

Brazil

Project H is a training project based on research into the factors necessary for young men to be "gender equitable." Activities focus on themes of sexuality and sexual/reproductive health, paternity and care, violence prevention, mental health, and HIV/AIDS prevention and care. The project aims to reduce gender-based violence and generally improve health indicators. As a result, young men's attitudes have improved, and fewer young men are agreeing with statements such as "Men need sex more than women" and "I would be outraged if my wife asked me to use a condom." There was also a drop in STI symptoms and an increase in condom use.

India

The Better Life Options Program in India uses an empowerment approach to train low-income girls ages 12 to 20 (married and single) in family life education, literacy and vocational skills, and general and reproductive health. The project stresses leadership and social mobilization through advocacy and community involvement. Goals include building girls' self-esteem and self-confidence, as well as expanding their choices related to marriage, fertility, health, vocation, and civic participation. Girls completing the program were more likely to be literate, have completed secondary education, be employed, have learned a vocational skill, have traveled outside their village or visited the health center alone in the last 6 months, and to make autonomous decisions about going to the market, spending what they earned, and deciding when to marry.

Source: Data from Billowitz, M., & Kukke, S. Doing gender the 'rights' way. *SIECUS Report, 32, no. 3* (Summer 2004), 5–10.

sex work, making them vulnerable to negative health consequences.

Some people think healthcare delivery and research benefit men at the expense of women. They believe that heart disease has been studied more in men and that women have been excluded from major national clinical studies. Others believe that women have benefited from medical research, as shown by improvements in breast cancer research as well as developments in laparoscopic surgery and ultrasound that were initially used on women's bodies (Daniel & Levine, 2001).

Kluger (2003) reported that twice as many women as men suffer from depression and twice as many men suffer from alcoholism. Similarly, women tend to be more prone to anxiety disorders, and men are more likely to have conditions stemming from impulsiveness and violence.

In recent decades it was found that men with a history of heart disease were two to four times more likely than females to die later of sudden cardiac death. However, now women heart attack survivors are becoming almost as likely as men to succumb to sudden cardiac death. This gender gap has narrowed a great deal (Sudden cardiac gender gap closing in on women, 2002).

Some have pointed out a need for more gender-based medicine because of some differences between males and females. (Men, women more different than thought, 2004). For example, major illnesses like heart disease and lung cancer are influenced by gender, and treatment for women may need to be slightly different from the approach used for men. Lung cancer, not breast cancer, is the number one cancer killer among women. The American Heart Association has developed heart disease prevention

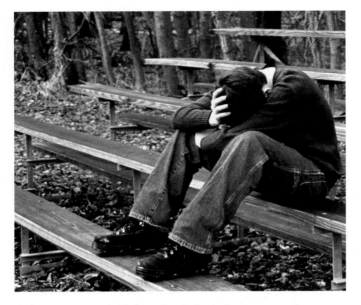

Males report more withdrawal and physical symptoms of depression than females.

guidelines tailored for women. Also, heart attacks in women frequently don't involve chest pain; rather they may exhibit as more vague, flu-like symptoms. Women who do not smoke appear to be more susceptible to lung cancer than nonsmoking men. Women are less likely than men to get oral cancer, and more prone to autoimmune diseases including lupus, rheumatoid arthritis, and multiple sclerosis.

Kulkarni et al. (2011) reported that men are increasing their life expectancy at a higher rate than women. Between 1987 and 2007, life expectancy in the United States increased nationwide from 71.3 years to 75.6 years for men and from 78.4 to 80.8 years for women. Possible reasons given for this include the fact that women are increasing their smoking more than men in general, the obesity epidemic in women is greater, and reducing high blood pressures has been emphasized much more in men than women. Despite this increase, Americans still lag more than 3 years behind the 10 longest-living nations, including Japan, Australia, Singapore, and Sweden. In addition, the researchers pointed out that many women still do not understand that they will be affected by heart disease. They are also more stoic, have a higher pain threshold than men, and often do not say they are in pain.

An interesting gender twist related to nutrition has occurred. Supermarket aisles are filling up with nutrient-rich female-friendly treats (Winters, 2001). There was a nutrition bar called "Luna" decorated with silhouetted dancing girls and packed with ingredients that women are supposed to need. It quickly became the top-selling bar in natural food stores. Then there was a line of breakfast cereals from Zoe foods produced by a woman who wanted to make granola for women who were like her menopausal mother. General Mills produces Harmony cereal for

Communication
DIMENSIONS

Men Are from Mars; Women Are from Venus

John Gray, the author of the bestseller *Men Are from Mars, Women Are from Venus*, explains one reason why men and women may sometimes be frustrated in communicating with each other. He says women expand, and men contract. By this he means that women are likely to expand a topic, whereas men want them to get to the point. For example, he says that generally when a man speaks he has already silently mulled over his thought until he knows the main idea he wants to communicate. Then he speaks. A woman, in contrast (according to Gray), does not necessarily speak to make a point; speaking assists her in discovering her point. When she explores her thoughts and feelings out loud, she figures out where she wants to go.

For example, a man may want to pull away and take a little time to mull over his thoughts so he knows what he wants to say. However, a woman may find greater clarity by expanding and sharing. When she begins sharing, she is not necessarily aware of where it will take her, but she is confident it will take her where she needs to go. For her, this is a process of self-discovery.

There have been mixed feelings about Gray's book. Some feel it is inaccurate and biased, while others feel that while it may have some good points, Gray does not offer enough solutions. For example, Hamson (2004) feels that the book is completely useless as a "fix," but its popularity is invaluable for what it tells us about ourselves as a society. She points out that boys and girls/men and women share more traits than society is willing to admit. She further indicates that while we all have differences as human beings, biases and stereotypes based on gender must be understood to be not only groundless but just as divisive and nonproductive as racial prejudice.

Source: Data from Gray, J. *Men, women and relationships.* New York: Harper Paperbacks, 1996.

women, and Quaker has a Nutrition for Women oatmeal. These foods are alike in that they are supposed to have nutrients that benefit women in particular. Manufacturers are trying to appeal as much to women's emotional needs as to their dietary ones. In reality, the basic laws of nutrition still apply to both men and women.

One final example related to gender and health focuses on college students. A survey of more than 1,400 college students in the Northeast showed that more than 83% reported having had sexual intercourse, with slightly higher rates for females (86%) than males (78%). Females (86%) were more likely than males (79%) to have had sexual intercourse without a condom. Yet, when asked if they would have sexual intercourse with a partner who refused to use a condom, significantly fewer females (8%) than males (24%) reported they would have sexual intercourse without a condom in this situation. Males (53%) were significantly more likely to report frequent condom use than females (44%) (Bontempi et al., 2009).

Gender and Dating

Some experts think there are gender issues related to dating. For example, some have indicated that females assume males will try to deceive them, but males don't seem to feel females will try to deceive them. Two issues related to sexual behavior and dating are frequency of sexual behavior and number of partners. Common sense would indicate that, on average, heterosexual men and women would have about equal numbers of sexual partners. However, males consistently report more partners than females do. Does this discrepancy arise because men are inclined to exaggerate sexual experience, and women to minimize it? Or is it because people have

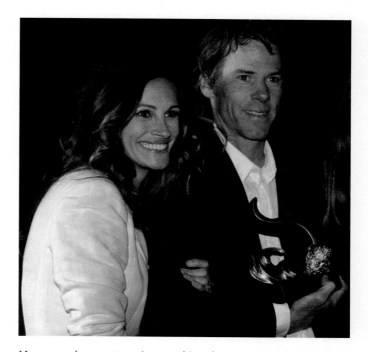

Many people seem to enjoy watching the romantic relationships of celebrities.

faulty memories? Or do women and men view sexual behavior differently?

Some think that the nature of intimacy is also a factor in male–female relationships. Many women tend to derive intimacy from talking and may be disappointed if men do not verbally share their problems, express their emotions, or listen to their feelings. In contrast, men may feel emotional closeness by working or playing side by side.

When the topic of "dating" is discussed with many contemporary college students, talk soon turns to "hanging out" and "hooking up." For some college students, dating is an outdated concept. Instead, they prefer to attend activities in groups or simply

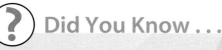 **Did You Know...**

In 2011 the White House issued the first federal report since 1963 on the welfare of women (Women in America, 2011). Among the findings: Although more women than men have college degrees, women still earn only 29% of total household incomes in the United States. Other findings include:

- Women are having children later. The percentage of women in their thirties giving birth for the first time in 1970 was 4%, but in 2007 it was 22%.
- The average age at which women first gave birth in 2007 was 25, compared to 21 in 1970.
- Both men and women are marrying later. Between 1970 and 2010, the average age at first marriage increased from

20.8 to 26.1 years for women and from 23.2 to 28.2 years for men.

- More women than men are enrolled in college. The 2008 college enrollment was 57% women and 43% men.
- Women are less likely than men to be unemployed. In 2010 about 8.5% of women were unemployed, as compared to about 10% of men.
- A pay gap still exists. In 2009 women earned 75% of the salaries earned by men.

"hang out" with one or more people. Interestingly, in a number of sexuality classes one of your authors has asked college students to define "hanging out" and "hooking up." In each of these conversations the conclusion was that college students do not agree on the definition of either of these terms, even though the terms are commonly used.

Other Gender Issues

Various experts have studied what males and females talk about with their friends. It is common to hear that men often discuss work issues, sports, and future goals. For women, the top three topics seem to be children, personal problems and self-doubts, and work issues. People believe that women's speech is more emotional than men's, although that stereotype has decreased in recent years (Popp et al., 2003). People also think women are more likely to show sympathy and communicate their support in problem situations (Basow & Rubenfeld, 2003). However, in a study in which men and women offered supportive communications, few differences appeared between men's and women's styles of communication (Mac-George et al., 2004).

There are also some stereotypical things that seem to bother males and females about the other gender. Women commonly report being disturbed about men making sexual demands (making them feel sexually used or trying to force sexual behavior), making them feel inferior or stupid, and emotional constriction and excess (hiding his emotions, drinking or smoking too much). Men commonly report being disturbed about women's sexual rejection (being unresponsive to sexual advances, being a sexual tease), moodiness, and self-absorption (fussing over appearance or spending too much on clothes).

The division of household labor has long been an interest area for gender researchers because who does the various tasks reveals information about power and equity in relationships. For decades, research has indicated that even when women are employed outside the home, they still do the majority of housework and child care chores. Even though the differences are not as great today as they were in past years, women still perform about twice as much household work and child care as men do. Interestingly, gay couples seem more likely to split tasks, with each partner performing a set of chores. Lesbian couples seem more likely to alternate in sharing

Gender DIMENSIONS

The Social Dimensions of Sexual Behavior

Related to dating, but also to later relationships, Baumeister and Tice (2000) proposed that sexual behavior is a social exchange in which women hold the power card, and that men will do just about anything to get it. They say that the catch is if sexual activity is given too freely, men will take it and run. For women, there is a flip side: If they never have sexual activity, they then lose the value of the power they wield. When vying for attention of men, they have to walk the fine line between being a miser or a vamp.

In simple terms, according to Baumeister and Tice, women have something that men want. Whoever wants sexual activity less has a certain amount of power in a relationship. Reasons for this situation are rooted in culture. Men value women with the least number of sexual encounters, because men tend to see the value of sexual activity decreases for a woman as her sexual encounters increase. This standard does not hold for men, they say, as women gravitate toward physically robust males.

Other points made by the authors follow:
- High self-esteem enables a woman to resist the advances of men.
- Sexual possessiveness may be rooted in nature, and all cultures impose stricter penalties against wifely infidelities.
- Nature instills in people the desire for sexual activity, but culture controls that desire.
- Women prefer sexual activity with stable committed relationships rather than commitment-free sexual activity, but men like both kinds.
- Sexual fluidity affects same-gender relations, where women are more able to move from lesbian to bisexual relationships, whereas men tend to be either heterosexual or homosexual.
1. Which points made by the authors do you agree or disagree with? Why?
2. Are there any points made by the authors that are bothersome to you? If so, why?

tasks, taking turns in performing the same chores (Sayer, 2005).

Fisher (Males, females, and evolution, 2001) has mentioned other gender differences. She says men usually want to cut straight to the point; they do not like getting distracted by side issues. Women have a more contextual view of the world and see issues as part of a larger whole. Also, young males often take many more risks than young females do. Scientists think this may be linked to differing levels of a chemical in the brain. In addition, females are more likely than males to bear grudges, sometimes for a very long time.

Peplau (2003) states that a large body of research documents four important gender differences related to sexuality. First, in many ways, men show greater sexual desire than do women. Second, compared to men, women place greater emphasis on committed relationships as a context for sexuality. Third, aggression is more strongly linked to sexuality for men than for women. Fourth, women's sexuality tends to be more malleable and capable of change over time. Obviously, not all of these differences are absolutes because men and women can vary a great deal. In general, however, these differences affect thoughts, feelings, and behavior. Also, they characterize not only heterosexuals but lesbians and gay men as well.

Gender and the Workplace

Do men and women approach things differently in the workplace? Are women being treated fairly in the workplace? Are salaries and benefits the same for males and females? These, and other interesting issues, have long provided hot topics for research and discussion.

An extensive study showed that women scored higher on orientation to production and getting results, and men scored higher on strategic planning and organizational vision. Women were seen as operating with more energy, intensity, and emotional expression; men were seen as more low-key and quiet through the control of emotional expression. Women were rated higher on people-oriented leadership skills, whereas men were rated higher on business-oriented leadership skills by bosses and peers (Do men and women lead differently?, 2000).

Eagly (2003) analyzed 45 studies of leadership styles and concluded that women in management positions were actually better leaders than men in equivalent positions. Women were more likely than men to be "transformational" leaders, or leaders who try to inspire workers and develop their skills and creativity. They serve as role models, mentor and empower workers, and encourage innovation even when the organization they lead is generally successful. Other kinds of leaders include transactional leaders, who lead by rewarding and punishing, and laissez-faire leaders, who take a hands-off approach. Previous studies indicate that transformational leaders create the most productive and satisfying work environments. Women also scored higher than men on one measure of transactional leadership—rewarding employees for good performance. One reason why women may favor transformational leadership is that such a leader operates more like an excellent teacher than a traditional boss.

Stoker et al. (2011) examined whether the gender of an employee, the gender of the manager, and the management–gender ratio in an organization were related to employees' managerial stereotypes. They found that although the general stereotype of a manager is masculine, and although most employees prefer a man as a manager, female employees, employees with a female manager, and employees working in an organization with a high percentage of female managers have a stronger preference for feminine characteristics of managers and for female managers.

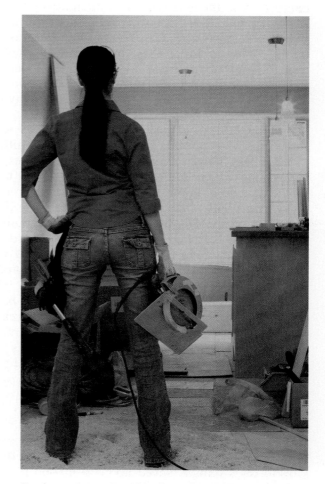

Employment opportunities for males and females have changed in recent years.

Many people have assumed that women would rather work with and be supervised by other women, but some studies (Sachs, 2001) indicate that women can be each other's worst enemies on the job. According to such studies, women often betray and undermine one another; they damage other women's career aspirations; and they often fail to support other women—even actively undermining their authority and credibility. One theory is that for two women to forge a positive relationship, their self-esteem and power must be kept "dead even." When one woman gets more power, it sets off tensions and leads to hostility and sniping. One-third of the women in these studies said they would prefer a male boss.

Relatedly, Meese (2009) reported out that at least 40% of the bullies in the workplace are women. They choose other women as targets more than 70% of the time. Men seem to bully men and women pretty much equally. Reasons given for women's bullying include women believing they need to be aggressive to be promoted, women sabotaging other women because they believe helping female coworkers could jeopardize their own careers, women withholding information such as promotional information from other women to help themselves, and other women supposedly being easier to bully than men because they are less tough than men. Many women have learned they are supposed to be nurturers and supporters, but bullying behavior is antithetical to the way they are supposed to be.

Namie (2010) indicated that 35% of the U.S. workforce report being bullied at work, and an additional 15% witness it. Men make up 62% of the bullies, and 58% of the targets are women. Women bullies target women in 80% of the cases. Bullying is four times more prevalent than illegal harassment, and the majority (68%) of bullying is same-gender bullying. In the study, bullying was defined as "repeated mistreatment: sabotage by others that prevented work from getting done, verbal abuse, threatening conduct, intimidation, and humiliation."

Because more than half the women with babies younger than 1 year are in the workforce, increasing numbers of them want to breastfeed their infants. In response, more companies are meeting this need by setting up a private room and a work schedule so mothers can pump their breast milk (Luscombe, 2001). Some companies provide a private room, a hospital-grade pump, a carrying case for discreet transport of the pumping paraphernalia and expressed milk, plus bottles and access to a refrigerator. One company, Cigna, in which 80% of the workforce is female, saved about $240,000 per year in healthcare expenses for breastfeeding mothers and

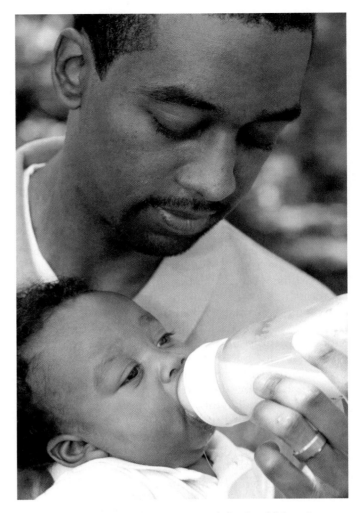
Many men have assumed more responsibility for child rearing.

their children and another $60,000 through reduced absenteeism. This does not include the incalculable goodwill of happy new parents.

The relationship between salaries of men and salaries of women has long been of interest to some people. In 2007, more than 10.4 million men and slightly less than 3.5 million women were paid $100,000 or more. Median earnings were $59,798 for men, compared to $42,340 for women (U.S. Census Bureau, 2007). In 2009, the National Organization for Women indicated that for full-time, year-round workers, women are paid, on average, only 78% of what men are paid, and the gap is significantly wider for women of color. This gap remains despite the passage of the 1963 Equal Pay Act and a variety of legislation prohibiting employment discrimination (On Equal Pay Day NOW calls attention to persistent gender wage gap, 2009). The Bureau of Labor Statistics (2011) reported that women who usually worked full time had median earnings 82.4% of the median for men. It is difficult to interpret the meaning of these data accurately, however, without knowing more about years of experience, academic preparation, levels of responsibility, and other variables that may influence salary levels.

Hilary Lips (2005) argues that there is a gender-based wage gap that exists in virtually every occupational category. She points out that this is at least partly because occupations typically associated with women are less prestigious and pay less than occupations associated with men and masculine skills. After reviewing wage trends over a number of years, she indicates there is no evidence that this wage gap is closing. She feels that employers must be convinced to re-examine assumptions that place higher value on the type of work men do than on the type of work typically done by women.

In 2008, the Center for Women's Business Research reported that women owned 20% of U.S. businesses with revenues exceeding $1 million per year. A total of 10.1 million firms were owned by women, employing 13 million people and generating $1.9 trillion in revenues. Women business owners who exceed the $1 million revenue mark typically are "gutsy," action-oriented women; have a solutions orientation; believe that larger business provides more freedom; are energized by the "business of growing a business"; create their own rules; focus on internal business culture; and are lifelong learners (New study shows women own 20% of businesses with revenues exceeding $1 million, 2008).

An interesting study was reported by McKeen (2005). She surveyed 214 Canadian and 160 Chinese business students regarding their future spouses' employment and family roles relative to their own. Results showed that a large proportion from both countries hoped for equality between the spouses, especially in the distribution of domestic tasks. However, significant discrepancies existed between their ideal hopes and their expectations of what will actually happen. Many men and women of both countries expected that the wives would do more of the domestic work and have less prestigious jobs and lower earnings than their husbands.

Catalyst is a nonprofit organization working globally with businesses and the professions to build inclusive workplaces and expand opportunities for women and business. In 2009, several of its reports provided information on related issues. For example, in 2008 women's representation as corporate officers rose to 16.9%, an increase of 1.8% since 2006 (Jenner & Ferguson, 2009). Because men dominate executive positions, the flow of information from senior leaders tends to perpetuate gender gaps in senior leadership. In addition, gender bias inhibits the establishment of inclusive and effective talent management programs (Warren, 2009). Clearly, men have a critical role to play in inclusion and diversity efforts. Men who are more aware of gender bias are more likely to say that it is important to them to achieve gender equality. Three key barriers that undermine men's support for initiatives to end gender bias are apathy, fear, and ignorance about gender issues. Men must be helped to understand their critical role in gender initiatives (Prime & Moss-Racusin, 2009).

A Catalyst study also found that women's advancement in corporate leadership continues to stagnate, with virtually no growth seen in women's share of top positions. For example, women held 15.2% of board director positions in 2008, compared to 14.6% in 2007. They held 15.7% of corporate officer positions in 2008, compared to 15.4% in 2007 (Catalyst 2008 census of the *Fortune* 500 reveals women gained little ground, 2008). Yet another Catalyst study showed that companies with the most women in senior management had a higher return on equity.

In today's marketplace, the female management style is distinctly different, but it is essential. Women manage more cautiously than men; they focus on the long term. Men thrive on risk, especially when they are surrounded by other men. Women are less competitive, in a good way: They are consensus builders, conciliators, and collaborators (Shipman & Kay, 2009).

Although women have not held a high percentage of leadership positions in industry, in May 2009 a historical event occurred when Ursula Burns became the first African American female to head a *Fortune* 500 company (Xerox). That made her one of about 15 women leading *Fortune* 500 companies. Her ascension marked the first female-to-female transition.

As you can see, some of the facts and observations already mentioned can relate to money and power. Some experts feel that as female economic power grows, it is changing how men and women work, play, shop, share, court, and even love each other (Mundy, 2012). Related information and examples include:

- In dual-earner couples, women now contribute an average of 44% of the family income, up from 39% in 1997.

- In the majority of U.S. metro areas, single, childless women in their 20s make more per dollar than their male peers (from $1.09 in Los Angeles to $1.14 in Atlanta to $1.18 in Dallas).

- In 2012 women earned 57% of the bachelor's, 60% of the master's, and 52% of the doctoral degrees conferred.

- Less than 1 in 5 married-couple families are supported by the husband alone.

- In households where the male brings in more income, buying decisions are made equally, but in households where the female earns more, she typically makes twice as many buying decisions as the male.

- It is predicted that within a generation a majority of working wives will outearn their husbands.

Gender and the Media

Advertising has long contributed to thinking about gender images and roles. Stereotypical examples include females with beautiful bodies often dressed in skimpy clothing being the object of another's gaze much more than their male counterparts. The authoritative male voice is still used in many commercials. It seems that through the years there has been a change in the images of women in commercials—but not the images of men. Today women are shown more often representing managerial and professional occupations. They are shown in more diverse occupations than in the past, whereas images of men have changed little. There is probably only a small increase in images of men parenting and doing housework.

Preidt (2008) has indicated that the way men and women are portrayed in TV commercials can have a major impact on how they behave in their daily lives. Men, in particular, are influenced by commercials that more often depict them in a career setting than doing domestic chores. TV advertisements help to socially construct gender and influence how people think about their own gender as well as other genders. Most commercials featuring women focus on selling home products, such as food, cleaners, personal care items, and furniture. Men are most likely to be engaged in work behavior in commercials, whereas women are least likely to be depicted working outside the home. Only some 2% of commercials show men doing domestic chores, such as cooking, cleaning, or caring for children.

Monk-Turner et al. (2008) looked at how sexual themes are used in magazine ads. Most ads did not use a sexual theme to sell a product. If used, however, this theme was more likely to appear in an ad aimed at a male audience.

Zimmerman and Dahlberg (2008) looked at attitudes of young women toward sexually objectified

advertising and compared their results to findings from earlier studies. Respondents agreed that females were portrayed as sex objects in advertisements, but were less offended by these portrayals than were female respondents in 1991. Respondents also indicated that attitudes toward the advertisement have little influence on whether they intend to purchase the products. This was a significant change from the responses of the 1991 group, who indicated they were influenced by such ads.

Koernig and Granitz (2006) looked at the portrayal of women compared to men in e-commerce magazine ads. They were interested in seeing whether e-commerce ads continue to reflect negative stereotypical gender differences in relation to technology given that such portrayals may propagate harmful stereotypes to men and women. They found that, compared to past studies, ads for e-commerce products and services portray women more equitably.

As the preceding information shows, there have probably been some improvements in the way ads treat gender issues, but a number of gender-based issues remain. For example, Andersen (2009) indicated that ads admonish women to be afraid—afraid of aging, afraid of food, afraid of being alone, or afraid of having a bust that is too small or too big.

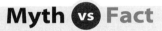

Myth: Females lack achievement motivation compared to males.
Fact: There are no differences here. Females have just as much achievement motivation as males.

Myth: Females have lower self-esteem.
Fact: Self-esteem is influenced by many factors. A person's gender, however, has no effect on self-esteem.

Myth: Females are better at learning roles and simple repetitive tasks.
Fact: The ability to learn roles and simple repetitive tasks is not influenced by gender.

Myth: Males are more analytical.
Fact: There is no difference in analytical skills between males and females.

Myth: All men think about women the same way. (Or all women think about men the same way.)

Fact: It is incorrect to conclude that all people of a certain gender think the same way about anything.

Myth: Females are more social than males.
Fact: The interest in being social, or the ability to be social, does not vary by gender even though it certainly can vary from one individual to another.

Myth: Females are more affected by heredity than males.
Fact: We are all influenced by our heredity, but our gender makes no difference in this situation (except that a few diseases are specific to one gender or the other).

Myth: Males are more affected by environment than females.
Fact: Everyone is influenced by the environment, but we are not affected more or less because of our gender.

They promise that with the right products, a woman can be seductive, change how she looks, and wear the right scent and be more attractive in general for one major purpose—to attract a partner. These are powerful messages that many take seriously. In fact, the impact of these messages is so strong that the American Psychological Association (2007) concluded that "throughout U.S. culture, and particularly in mainstream media, women and girls are depicted in a sexualizing manner. These representations can be seen in virtually every medium."

Taylor and Setters (2011) looked at the impact of media representations of film stars on gender role expectations for women. They found that college students perceived more attractive film leads as better role models than the less attractive leads. Their findings suggested that both men and women expect women to fulfill both feminine and masculine roles, that women generally have higher expectations of women than men, and that watching attractive, aggressive heroines exaggerates these expectations.

Screen star Geena Davis became concerned about the portrayal of females in the media. She observed that male characters largely outnumbered female characters, that female characters hardly ever had powerful roles, and that females were almost always portrayed in skimpy or overly sexualized clothes. She then established the Geena Davis Institute on Gender in the Media. The Institute sponsored the largest study ever done on G-rated movies and on TV shows for kids 11 and younger. Results confirmed her observations. Male characters outnumbered females 3 to 1. In scenes featuring groups, the ratio increased to 5 to 1. In addition, aspirations and occupations of female characters were very limited. The female characters had very narrow stereotypes. Almost the only aspiration for female characters was to find romance. Hypersexualization was common. The female characters in G-rated films wore about the same amount of sexually revealing clothing as the female characters in R-rated movies. Realizing that there was a clear message that girls and women are less important than boys and men to our society, Davis worked with the National Institute of Health to establish a research agenda designed to promote better ways to establish more positive stereotypes and expectations for girls and women in the media (Garnett, 2011).

Myths About Male–Female Differences

Socialization determines a great deal of what many people choose to see as "naturally" masculine or feminine. People look at the ways many women and men and girls and boys *do* behave and conclude that those are the only ways in which females and males *can* behave. Countless myths explain real or apparent differences in male–female feelings, attitudes, aptitudes, and behavior. (See examples of such myths in the box on the previous page.)

■ Gender Identity, Roles, and Stereotypes

Once a baby is delivered and "It's a boy!" or "It's a girl!" rings out, social influences go to work to form the baby's gender identity and mold his or her future role. Each society has a set of rules for how its males and females should behave. Boys and girls learn early to conform to these established behavior standards and take on their accepted roles. Psychologists have tried to explain how children do this in terms of psychoanalytical, social-learning, cognitive-developmental, and gender-schema theories.

According to psychoanalytical theory (explained by Sigmund Freud), appropriate gender typing means that boys grow to identify with their fathers and girls with their mothers. Identification is completed as children resolve the **Oedipus complex** (sometimes called the *Electra complex* in girls). From roughly age 3 to 5 years, children supposedly develop incestuous wishes for the parent of the other gender and see the parent of the same gender as a rival. This is resolved when the child eventually identifies with the same-gender parent and develops behaviors typically associated with that gender. Today the psychoanalytical theory of gender-role development is not widely accepted.

In social-learning theory, the development of gender-typed behavior is explained in terms of processes such as observational learning, identification, and **socialization**. Children learn what is deemed masculine or feminine by observing, experimenting, and being rewarded for certain behaviors.

In cognitive-developmental theory, children form concepts about gender and then make their behavior conform to their gender concepts. This is called **gender typing**. By about age 7 to 8 years, **gender constancy** develops in most children. They realize that gender does not change even if the appearance and actions of

Oedipus complex
A development stage in which the boy wants to possess his mother sexually and sees the father as a rival (similar to the female *Electra complex*).

socialization
The process of guiding people into socially acceptable behavior by providing information, rewards, and punishments.

gender typing
The process whereby children develop behavior that is appropriate to their gender.

gender constancy
The concept that people's gender does not change—even if they change their dress or behavior.

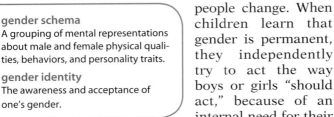

gender schema
A grouping of mental representations about male and female physical qualities, behaviors, and personality traits.

gender identity
The awareness and acceptance of one's gender.

people change. When children learn that gender is permanent, they independently try to act the way boys or girls "should act," because of an internal need for their behaviors to be consistent with what they know.

Gender schema theory indicates that children develop a grouping of mental representations about male and female personality traits, physical qualities, and behaviors. Once they develop a gender schema, they begin to judge themselves according to traits considered relevant to their genders. By doing this, they blend their developing self-concepts with the gender schema of their culture. Many associations can be made between gender and other qualities, such as strength and affection. Traditionally, strength has been viewed as a masculine trait and affection as a feminine trait. Other gender distinctions may be viewed as important—such as men being sexually assertive and women being sexually passive, or men's being in leadership positions and women's being placed in lesser positions.

Gender Identity

Gender involves more than just a biological component; it also includes the biological, social, and cultural norms and something called **gender identity**. Gender identity is one's self-image as a female or a male; it is the attachment one has to one's role. Societal and cultural factors are thought to exert more influence on gender identity than the biological component. At the very least, gender identity should be considered a biopsychosocial process—it is a result of interaction of biological, psychological, and social factors.

Masculinity and femininity are not innate or instinctive. The masculinity or femininity of gender identity needs a healthy human brain in which to take root. However, the developing brain is shaped by the environment in which it grows and from which it takes its mental nourishment (Money, 1988). In this way the biological foundation is shaped by psychological and sociological influences.

Because each society defines its roles for males and females and perpetuates behaviors through gender-role socialization, boys are given reinforcement for behaving in a "masculine" way, and girls receive reinforcement for exhibiting "feminine" behaviors. Should either gender engage in cross-sex conduct, such behavior is labeled gender-role-inappropriate; when each sex behaves as the society

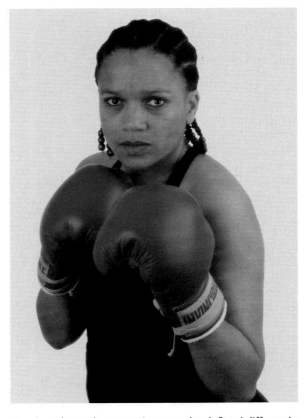

Gender roles and expectations may be defined differently by various people.

deems normal, that behavior is labeled gender-role-appropriate and is rewarded.

Gender roles differ markedly from society to society. Many societies discourage any deviation from the prescribed gender roles; others, such as ours, are now working toward flexibility and individualism in a wide variety of behaviors.

The expectation that people will exhibit certain characteristics and/or behaviors dictated by the customs and traditions of the society is called **stereotyping**. Expecting individuals to behave in particular ways because they are male or female is referred to as **gender-role stereotyping**. There are still many rigid, unyielding traditional attitudes about gender-role behaviors that make it difficult for people to express themselves and for society to implement change. Stereotypical images of people do not take into account individual differences. Until recently the stereotypical woman or wife in our society was passive, quiet, and concerned primarily with home, husband, and

stereotyping
The expectation that individuals will exhibit certain characteristics or behaviors.

gender-role stereotyping
Expectation that individuals will behave in certain ways because they are male or female.

Global
DIMENSIONS

The Oppression of Women

In past years, and even today, there are many international examples of the oppression of women. One example became public in 2001. First, members of a hard-line militant group in Kashmir announced they would throw acid at women who did not wear veils and the traditional *burkah*, a long black cloak that covers a woman from head to toe. Later it was announced that women not wearing the veil would be shot. To prevent trouble, the heads of girls' schools and women's colleges asked their students to dress conservatively and to wear no makeup (Overland, 2001).

Even after American troops invaded Afghanistan, many Afghan women were still mistreated. They continued to be abused, harassed, and threatened all over Afghanistan. For example, a team of 90 women from the Ministry of Religious Affairs harassed women in Kabul's streets for "un-Islamic behavior" such as wearing makeup and, in some instances, followed them home to castigate their parents or spouses (We want to live as humans, 2002).

In 2011 the government of Saudi Arabia moved swiftly to stop a protest movement of women claiming the right to drive. A woman was detained for up to 5 days on charges of disturbing public order and inciting public opinion by twice driving a car. She was arrested after two much-publicized drives to highlight Facebook and Twitter campaigns to encourage women across Saudi Arabia to participate in a collective protest. However, the government blocked the campaigns in the kingdom. The arrest was probably intended to give other women pause before participating in protests in a country where a woman's public reputation, including the ability to marry, can be badly damaged by an arrest. Whether or not women should drive in Saudi Arabia is a highly emotional issue in the kingdom, where women are also not allowed to vote, or even work without their husbands' or fathers' permission (MacFarquhar, 2011).

In 2011 more than 200 experts from five continents ranked countries on their overall perception of danger for women. On the top of the list was Afghanistan, with one of the highest maternal mortality rates in the world, minimal access to basic health care and education, and scarcely any economic rights for women and girls. Eighty-seven percent of Afghan women are illiterate, 1 in 11 dies in childbirth, and as many as 8 in 10 face forced marriages. The Congo was rated second because many threats prevail for women. The levels of sexual violence and rape there are the highest in the world, and a married woman cannot sign any legal documents without her husband's authorization. Pakistan was ranked third, based on religious traditions that are harmful to women. More than 1,000 women a year are victims of so-called honor killings, and many more are victims of acid attacks, child marriage, and abusive punishments, including stoning (Anderson, 2011).

---

children; the stereotypical man was gruff, strong, unfeeling, and concerned mostly with work and money. The danger of such stereotypes is that people take them seriously and act on them, turning a blind eye to the qualities, capabilities, and interests of individuals—frequently denying even their own. People often believe that those who deviate from stereotypes are not as good as those who conform to them. Thus one who accepts as true the stereotypes described might look down on a woman who cared about work or a man who chose to stay home with his children. People become boxed in not only by social pressure to conform closely to the stereotype, but also by rigid customary practice (such as promoting men but not women in business and professions, hiring women but not men to nurse and teach small children, or paying men more than women, regardless of their responsibilities), as well as by law. The assumptions behind such stereotyped behavior are being challenged today, and laws are being changed as well, but popular assumptions and attitudes are slow to change and are still passed on.

Teaching Gender Roles and Stereotypes

Gender roles are taught throughout the life cycle, but parents probably have the greatest effect, especially when children are very young. Very early on, parents reinforce the behaviors deemed acceptable to their child's gender with such remarks as "What a good, sweet girl!" or "What a big, strong boy!" accompanied by smiles and nods of approval. There is no doubt that most, if not all, of the forces of socialization in our culture—parents, teachers, peers, movies, television, and

> **gender role**
> Complex groups of ways males and females are expected to behave in a given culture.

books (targeted at children and adults)—encourage different behaviors in boys and girls. The resulting sets of traits are what we call *masculinity* and *femininity*. Let us look briefly at a few examples of how gender roles and stereotypes are taught.

The Influence of Schools

School personnel pass on social stereotypes in a number of ways. For example, if teachers feel that boys are naturally more aggressive or that girls are naturally more passive, how will this attitude influence the way they treat their students? If gender-role stereotyping exists in teachers' expectations, it can lead to biases in how they treat and evaluate their students.

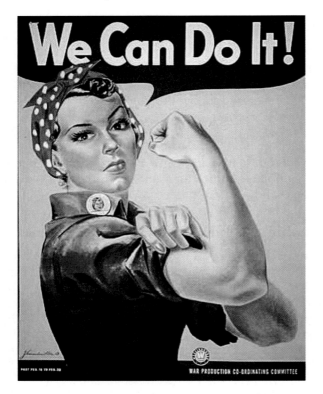

During World War II, Rosie the Riveter was part of the U.S. government's public relations campaign to get women into the workforce. Rosie shows off a strong bicep but still has a perfect manicure.

Berk (2008) mentioned a number of ways teachers and the school environment might contribute to gender stereotyping. For example, younger girls often gather around the teacher, following directions, while boys are attracted to other areas of the classroom where teachers are minimally involved. Consequently, boys and girls engage in different social behaviors. Teachers also use more disapproval and controlling discipline with boys. When girls misbehave, teachers tend to negotiate, coming up with a plan to improve behavior. Teachers seem to expect boys to misbehave more, a belief that seems based partly on boys' actual behavior and partly on gender stereotypes.

If teachers believe in stereotypes, they may expect one gender to excel more than the other in certain subjects, they may encourage one gender more than the other, or they may favor one gender in terms of attention and/or extra help. They may even intentionally or unintentionally promote **sexism**, which is a prejudgment that because of gender a person will possess negative traits. In addition to these prejudgments, sexism can entail discrimination against someone because of gender. For example, not hiring a man for a day care job because it is believed that males cannot nurture children would be sexism. Teachers can help promote the healthy sexual development of children if they provide equal opportunities for girls and boys, do not impose gender stereotypes, and do not use sexist language. Although young children are busy establishing their own identities, and many may exhibit stereotypical behavior, it is the role of the teacher to encourage learning and responsible behavior that does not discriminate.

School materials can also influence gender-role stereotyping. For example, in preschool picture books there has been a trend toward depiction of greater gender equality. At the same time, however, female characters are more likely to be shown as

sexism
The prejudgment that because of gender a person will possess negative traits.

Multicultural
DIMENSIONS

How the Economy Affects Gender Equality

Relations between men and women are influenced by race, class, and sexuality; however, the most pressing issue for men and women of color, especially those who are poor and working class, is the economy. While both the employment rates and real wages of men are down, women are working in greater numbers, and their wages are on the rise.

For working-class African Americans, Hispanics, and Native Americans, the effect of these changes has been harsh. The decline in employment for men has caused an increase in domestic violence, alcohol abuse, and other problems associated with joblessness. However, the increase in women's employment and economic resources is not enough to allow most to support a family, nor has it been accompanied by available, affordable child care.

These changes not only challenge the expectations traditionally associated with gender, but also are reshaping families along distinctive racial and class lines. For example, although families maintained by single women have become a permanent feature in all racial and class categories, this type of family is most prevalent among people of color and the poor.

Among whites, the chief cause of the increase in households headed by women is women's growing economic independence. But the growth in African American households headed by women partly reflects the employment problems of African American men.

In addition, for all immigrant groups, life in the United States leads to increased rates of single parenthood and divorce.

The economic challenges facing poor and working-class African American, Hispanic, and Native American men and women constitute the most pressing issue in relations between the sexes today. This is because racial and ethnic discrimination, combined with economic difficulties, make these groups extremely vulnerable to shifts in the economic and social climate.

Source: Data from Dill, B. T. Economic disparity is key for all minorities, *Chronicle of Higher Education, 45, no. 6* (October 2, 1998), B7–B8.

---

dependent or submissive, and males as independent and creative. Many subtle traditional expectations still exist.

Some people claim bias still exists in achievement tests. Language in the tests has often referred to males and their environments. Women were disproportionately shown to be homemakers, and men to be engaged in directive, leadership, achieving roles. Boys were described in action terms; girls were described in helping or more passive terms. A strong bias against nontraditional behavior in both sexes has been evident in many tests.

Sadker and Zittleman (2005) point out that gender bias lives for both genders. It can be hard to detect because it affects boys and girls in different ways. For example, in school, the boys may be expected to "act out" and rebel at schoolwork, while the girls are expected to be docile. Both of these expectations reflect gender stereotyping, or bias. Other examples of challenges related to gender bias include:

- Boys and girls like and do well in math and science in elementary school, but girls become less positive and do less well in higher grades.

- Boys receive more math- and science-related toys than girls do.

- Girls receive higher report card grades throughout their schooling.

- Boys often regard reading and writing as "feminine" subjects, and report that reading threatens their masculinity.

- Current software products are likely to reinforce gender stereotypes and bias rather than reduce them.

- Teachers call on boys more often than girls, wait longer for boys' answers, and provide more precise feedback to boys.

- Girls are more likely to be quiet in class and praised for neatness.

Even at the college level, educators need to be sensitive to the influence of the classroom environment. It has been thought that female students participate less often and less assertively than male students in college classrooms and that the professors' discriminatory behaviors are partly responsible.

Teachers, books, and tests are powerful forces, but it is important to stress that gender stereotypes are perpetrated by other factors as well. Children take to the classroom notions of gender roles formed through the influence of parents and peers.

Gender DIMENSIONS

Gender Equality on the College Campus

The New England Council of Land-Grant University Women created a document entitled *Vision 2000*, which was a call to high-level university administrators to ensure full and equitable participation by women in New England universities. The gender-equality goals in the document were intended to:

1. Foster faculty and administrative accountability for gender equality in curriculum and pedagogy
2. Implement diversity initiatives
3. Promote family-friendly policies (affordable and available child care, flex time, and parental leave policies)
4. Encourage women's academic and career development
5. Establish and support strong women's centers
6. End sexual harassment of and violence against women
7. Correct inequities in hiring, promotion, tenure, compensation, and working conditions for women employees

Critics of *Vision 2000* claim that it is a plot by women's studies faculty to stifle academic freedom—that they will determine gender-equality standards and impose them on recalcitrant faculty. They worry that feminist "indoctrination" of students will lower academic standards and destroy academic debate. Others believe that it is time to ensure gender equality in higher education. They point out that there are fewer women faculty members overall and they are concentrated in lower ranks, less well-paid career tracks, and part-time and non–tenure track positions.

Are the goals of *Vision 2000* needed at your college or university? How is your institution dealing with each of the seven areas listed? What else might have to be done on your campus?

Sources: Data from *Vision 2000*, New England Council of Land-Grant University Women, February 1997. Available: http://www.umass.edu/wost/articles/vision2k/whole.htm; Ferguson, A. Gender equity on the college campus, *Boston Globe* (Feb. 23, 1997), 27.

The Influence of Parents and Peers

In most cases, as soon as a child is born, interaction between parents and child begins—interaction that differs according to the gender of the child. Traditionally, a girl is thought to be fragile, to need protection, and to have needs that revolve around personal appearance and development. A boy is seen as tough, physically active, and unemotional. Children perceive these expectations, which tend to define their reality. Because the mother is usually the primary caregiver, the female child finds it easier to learn her appropriate gender role than does the male child. The female internalizes feminine behavior and is rewarded for her identification. The male may be in a bind. He may not have a constant role model because his father may not be around as much as his mother. He frequently learns from the mother's telling him that boys "don't do" certain things. Thus boys may learn to be anxious about gender-role identity.

It seems that increasing numbers of parents try to prevent teaching gender-role stereotypes to their children, but this can be hard to achieve. They may act differently toward a child, depending on the child's gender, even if they do not intend to do so. For example, if a boy is asked to participate in sports or

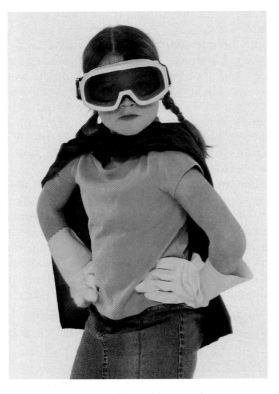

Some parents try to avoid teaching gender stereotypes.

help his father with outside chores while a girl is asked to wash dishes or clean her room, this pattern sends messages about expected gender roles.

What children observe at home in regard to sex roles also sends important messages. For example, even when both parents work outside the home in managerial or professional jobs, the redistribution of roles within the family has not yet clearly or completely occurred. American women—even those employed full time—continue to work more hours than do their husbands on household tasks, and there is little evidence that men's proportionate share of family work has changed much in recent years. Many social scientists feel parents are very influential in regard to establishing gender roles.

The question of whether we can, or want to, raise "gender-neutral" children has been debated. Some argue that it not only is possible, but also can result in more positive self-esteem. They say that children

raised with gender-neutral expectations will have a more open, positive view of the world in general. Others argue that gender and gender-role expectations are tied very closely to familial and cultural expectations. They believe that gender-specific role fulfillment is vital to certain cultures, ensuring the survival of important cultural traditions (Can we raise "gender-neutral" children?, 2003).

Sanchez-Flores (2004) pointed out that young men are exposed to many messages from different sources that inform them about what it means to be a man. Ideals such as "boys don't play with dolls," or "boys don't wear pink" may seem outdated to many adults today, but social groups still successfully transfer messages like this from generation to generation. As a result, boys live in social networks and follow norms that determine both acceptable behaviors and the consequences for not behaving that way. Another message males hear is "boys will be boys." It is most

Ethical DIMENSIONS

Extreme Gender Roles—The Price of Honor

News of an interesting ethical situation related to female sexual behavior was reported in Jordan. Sirhan, a 35-year-old man, was proud to say that he had murdered his younger sister. She had reported to the police that she had been raped. Sirhan said, "She committed a mistake, even if it was against her will. Anyway, it's better to have one person die than to have the whole family die from shame." To Sirhan, it was more ethical to kill his sister than to suffer from the shame that would have sullied his "male honor."

For centuries, Arab men have engaged in "honor killing"—the intrafamily killing of errant females. Honor killing has its roots in the crude Arabic expression "A man's honor lies between the legs of a woman." For Arab women, virginity before marriage and fidelity afterward are considered musts. Men are expected to control their female relatives. If a woman strays, it is widely believed, the dignity of the man can be restored only by killing her. In Jordan the 25 or so cases of honor killing documented every year make up a quarter of all homicides there.

Forbidden sexual activity is not always the issue. Marrying or divorcing against the family's wishes can also provoke murder. The law winks at honor killers.

If a man catches his wife or a close female relative in the act of adultery and kills her, he is exempt from punishment.

Running away is next to impossible for women, because Arab societies are close knit, and few women have the means to live alone. "Rafa," 20 years old, was locked up in prison to protect her after her uncles and brothers vowed to murder her for having a 3-day affair with a coworker. She said, "With the mistake I made, I deserve to die."

Honor killing has started to receive media attention, and a hotline has been created by the Jordanian Women's Union for women in distress. However, honor killings are hard to combat because of the extremely strong feelings related to male and female gender roles in Jordan (Beyer,1999).

The exact origins of honor killings are not known. Among northern Arabian tribes, the practice predates Islam in the seventh century. It is sometimes a problem even in the United States. For example, Faleh al-Maleki was convicted in Arizona of killing his daughter. He ran over her with his car. He was upset with her fondness for tight jeans and makeup and a reluctance to accede to his plans for her. The plans included an arranged marriage to a man in Iraq (Labi, 2011).

? Did You Know . . .

In 2009, Barbara Millicent Roberts turned 50. In case you don't recognize that name, it is the formal name of the doll we all know as "Barbie." In 1959, Barbie debuted as a teenage fashion model—and she still is today. In 1959, 38% of women were in the workforce—today that percentage is 60%. Through the years, Barbie has been an astronaut, gone to medical school, been an Olympic athlete, served in the military, and run for president. She has had more than 108 careers and represented 50 nationalities. Some have called her the first feminist.

Others believe Barbie is not a good role model because of her emphasis on appearance. Barbie is 11.5 inches tall and weighs 7.25 ounces. This apparently translates into a woman who would be 5 feet, 9 inches tall, weighing about 110 pounds. Many have argued that this is an unrealistic and unhealthy build that promotes negative stereotypes in both males and females. Do you think Barbie has been and is a positive or negative role model?

Source: Towner, B. 50 and still a doll, *AARP Bulletin* (March 2009), 35.

often used to dismiss actions that are challenging or seem impossible to change. This gives the impression that gender excuses behavior.

The peer group is also an important influence in learning about sex roles. Even early in life, children choose members of their own sex as playmates most of the time. This segregation by gender continues into the school years and helps contribute to sex-typing in play activities that help prepare children for adult roles.

The influence of peers becomes increasingly important by late childhood and early adolescence. Conformity can be viewed as being very important, and behaving according to traditional gender roles promotes social acceptance by peers. Those who do not behave in ways accepted by the peer group are likely to be pressured and even ridiculed.

There is no question that biology is important. There are biological factors that tilt males and females in different directions related to their interests and behavior, but numerous social factors influence the way the biological tilts can be redirected. In other words, regarding the nature versus nurture debate, biology does matter; however, the way we are treated and what we learn can drastically influence our expression of gender roles.

Gender Identity Difficulty

There are some people who experience **gender dysphoria**. They believe they are trapped in the body of the "wrong sex." They feel they are not really the gender indicated by their genitals. Sometimes the term *gender dysphoria* is used interchangeably with the term **transsexual**. Other times the term

gender dysphoria
Feeling trapped in the body of the "wrong" sex.

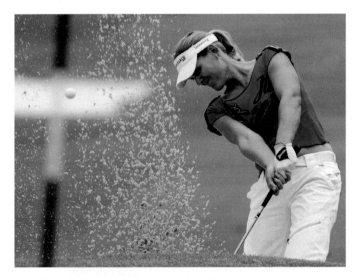

Danish-born Mianne Bagger, a successful amateur golfer, was barred from membership in the Australian Ladies Professional Golf Association because she was born male. Bagger's contention, like that of many transsexuals, was that she was, in fact, born female.

transsexual is used to refer to people who wish to have, or have had, their genitals surgically altered to conform to their gender identity. Therefore, an anatomically male transsexual feels that he is a female but that some quirk of fate provided him with male genitals. He wants to be socially identified as the female he believes himself to be. He does not derive sexual excitement from cross-dressing, as is the case with a transvestite, but views himself as a female.

Sometimes the terminology used related to gender identity difficulty can be tricky. For example, in

transsexual
A person whose gender identity does not match her or his biological sex; also a person who wishes to have, or has had, his or her gender surgically altered to conform to his or her gender identity.

transgender
A general term used when one's identity does not match one's physical/genetic sex. It includes such diverse categories as transsexualism and transvestism.

addition to the terms mentioned previously, in recent years the term **transgender** has become more common. According to the International Foundation for Gender Education (2005), gender is a person's innate sense of themselves as being male or female, which may differ from their biological sex. The terms "sex" and "gender" are often used interchangeably, but they are not the same. People whose sex and gender differ are known as transgender.

Transsexualism, which is a gender orientation, is not to be confused with homosexuality, a sexual orientation. Some transsexuals are homosexual, and some are heterosexual. Unless a transsexual chooses to tell another person, an observer will probably not know whether homosexual or heterosexual behavior is being practiced.

According to the American Psychological Association Task Force on Gender Identity and Gender Variance (2008), the prevalence of gender identity disorder in adults is estimated to be about 1 in 11,900 for male-to-female transsexuals and 1 in 30,400 for female-to-male transsexuals. Male-to-female transsexuality is 1.5 to 3 times more prevalent than female-to-male transsexuality.

Boylan (2003) wrote an interesting book on this subject entitled *She's Not There: A Life in Two Genders*. Even as a child, James Boylan felt that he was supposed to be a woman, but he thought everyone would reject him if he made the transition. So he lived as a man, married, and had children. In spite of his loving family, a successful career, and hobbies he loved, he eventually decided that he couldn't live with being a man. So he made the transition to living as a woman (Jenny Boylan). The book includes a portrait of a loving marriage—the love of James for his wife, Grace, and against all odds, the enduring love of Grace for the woman who became her "sister," Jenny. Jenny's wife, children, mother, and colleagues responded with love and acceptance. Her sister cut off contact. Boylan feels fortunate to have been given a rare gift in life—the gift of being able to see into the worlds of both men and women with clear eyes. Through it all, Boylan was a professor of English at Colby College in Maine.

When an employee switches genders, there can sometimes be difficult issues for employers (Armour, 2005). Issues can relate to how an employee informs coworkers about switching genders, how clients might react, how others will handle a transitioning employee using the restroom, and logistical issues such as changing security badges to reflect a new gender. In many states it is legal to fire employees

because they are transgender. However, many companies have put policies in place to protect against discrimination of transgender employees. Major companies, such as Merrill Lynch, Chevron, BP, and Microsoft are among those with such policies.

In April of 2012 the Equal Employment Opportunity Commission ruled that a refusal to hire or otherwise discriminate on the basis of gender identity is by definition sex discrimination under federal law. This was a groundbreaking decision because it set a national standard of enforcement that offered employers clear guidance on the issue (Rowe & Woodard, 2012).

Wilson (2005) reported on an interesting case at the University of Nebraska where, in 2005, a popular professor named Wally Bacon returned for the fall semester as a female, W. Meredith Bacon. After 29 years in the political science department, and 37 years of marriage, Ms. Bacon decided to become what she thought she was since she was a young child. In an eight-page letter, the professor explained to colleagues the decision to become a woman. Students were told that she would be happy to answer their questions if they desired. Few asked her any questions. The university administration was supportive. This had not been the case in some other situations. In one small college in New Hampshire, one man was fired after he informed the administration that he planned to become a woman. In Indiana, a professor decided to leave after his decision to disclose his sex-change plans to the college's president backfired. He says the president voiced her support, but said that he would lose his job because of the potential loss of contributions from donors who might disapprove. Ms. Bacon's wife, Lynne, remained supportive and the couple stayed together. Lynne mourned the loss of Wally, but also enjoyed counseling her spouse on her new female look.

There have been issues related to transgender athletes. The first famous transgender athlete in the U.S. was a former Yale tennis captain named Richard Raskin who underwent surgery in 1975 and became Renee Richards. She won a landmark legal battle in 1977 that enabled her to play as a female at the U.S. Open. Yet, it is only recently that transgender athletes are gaining sustained recognition from sports' governing bodies. In 2004 the International Olympic Committee ruled that any trans athlete who wants to compete against those not of their birth gender must undergo sex reassignment surgery and two years of hormone therapy to go from male to female. However, in 2011 the National Collegiate Athletic Association (NCAA) took a different approach. It decided against requiring surgery which typically costs five figures and isn't covered by insurance. The NCAA also said that trans females need to undergo only one year of testosterone suppression before they can compete against women, and trans males can receive a medical exemption to take testosterone under a doctor's supervision but can no longer compete on a women's team. Some colleges have created their own transgender inclusion policies (Torre & Epstein, 2012). It will be interesting to see what happens in the future related to policies for transgender athletes.

Wilson (2005) also reported that psychiatrists estimate that 1 in 30,000 men suffer from transgendered feelings. However, groups representing transgendered people say that number of men and boys who experience "intense transsexualism" is closer to 1 in 300 to 500 with about 1 in 2,500 having undergone genital surgery. She further reported that businesses are more likely than colleges to protect employees from discrimination. According to the Human Rights Campaign, an advocacy group for gay, transgendered, and bisexual people, 73 *Fortune* 500 companies do so, compared to 37 universities.

There is no clear understanding of either the causes or the nature of transsexualism. Some theorists believe the causes relate to early parent–child relationships related to gender roles of mothers and fathers and the ways that parents treated a child. Others focus on hormonal imbalances that influenced the brain during prenatal development; however, no one knows for sure.

Gender-Reassignment Surgery

The idea of gender reassignment is controversial, and psychotherapy has not been very useful for most transsexuals. Surgery is part of gender reassignment, but, because it is irreversible, professionals usually require that the transsexual live publicly as a member of the other sex for a year before undergoing surgery. During this time it is easier for the person or the medical personnel to change their minds. Surgery is not something to be taken lightly, and it is usually done only after careful screening of the individual.

A lifetime of hormonal treatment is also necessary. Male-to-female transsexuals take estrogen. It causes fatty deposits to develop in the breasts and hips, inhibits beard growth, and softens the skin. Female-to-male transsexuals take androgens, which promote deepening of the voice, masculine hair distribution, large muscles, and loss of fatty deposits in the breasts and hips. The clitoris may also grow larger.

It is not possible to construct internal genital organs or gonads, so gender-reassignment surgery is mostly cosmetic. Male-to-female surgery is usually more successful because it is easier to construct a vagina than a working penis. The vast majority of transsexuals who undergo surgery are happy with the outcome. Gender-reassignment surgery is done in only a few places in the United States, is very expensive, and is usually not covered by health insurance policies. Indeed, only several thousand such operations have been performed in the United States since 1953. Clearly this is something to be done only with extensive counseling and medical support.

A special case of potential gender-reassignment surgery relates to the question of what should be

Ethical DIMENSIONS

Should Dad Dress as a Woman? Should Dad Participate in His Child's Field Trip While Dressed as a Woman?

In Saint Louis, most of the kids on a fourth-grade field trip did not notice or did not care that a classmate's father was dressed as a woman, in jeans, a sweater, and nice shoes. Most of the teachers were equally untroubled. However, one parent spotted the "cross-dressing" dad and alerted some friends. As a result, one school board member proposed a new policy that would require parent chaperones to wear "gender-appropriate" clothing for school functions.

The father described had dressed as a woman at work for years, kept his hair long, worn slacks and blouses, and used a name that could be either male or female. He had actively participated in his daughters' education and in their schools while in women's attire with no previous problems.

Some people argue that it is ethical to require parents to wear "gender-appropriate" clothing at school functions. Others argue that it is not ethical to do this because it violates the parents' rights to dress as they please—particularly because to qualify for sex-change surgery individuals must first go through a prolonged period of transition when they present themselves in public as the gender they want to become.

What do you think?

Source: Data from Simon, S. After dad dresses as woman, field trip controversy still boils, *The Birmingham News* (January 6, 2003), 4B.

done with intersex infants—those born with ambiguous or mixed genitalia and chromosomal structures. It is estimated that every year in the United States about 65,000 babies are born with ambiguous genitalia. Some people believe that feminizing surgery should be done at birth to ensure that the baby will be able to function later as an adult woman. Others feel that children should remain intact until they are older and decide for themselves what, if anything, to do about their ambiguous genitalia (Should parents surgically alter their intersex infants?, 2003).

Some experts point out that gender depends on more than anatomy or hormones. They feel gender is essentially hard-wired into the brain before birth. A review of 94 intersex children found that over half of the genetic males "transitioned" to become boys despite being raised as girls and undergoing female sex assignment. More doctors seem to be putting off sex-assignment surgery until later, so as to be more certain about the person's gender. The Intersex Society of North America (www.isna.org) is a good place to learn more about personal stories (Surgery may be hasty for unclear gender, 2005).

The Influence of Gender Stereotypes on Sexuality

As you can see, gender-role stereotyping limits self-expression and personal growth and development, and that limiting in turn affects sexuality. When individuals define masculinity and femininity for themselves, they express personal beliefs through gender-role behaviors. The traditional definitions are confining, emphasizing as they do conventional conformity to long-existing gender-role norms. We have referred particularly to males being socialized toward initiating, aggressive, and directive behaviors and females being socialized toward receiving, passive, and compliant behaviors. In descriptions of anatomical function, for example, the vagina has tended to be described as receiver, not for sexual pleasure but for reproduction. The penis is often described in terms of insertion based on need, dominance, and desire. Thus again, men initiate and women are passively receptive.

The pressure to conform to socialization has provoked in both sexes anxieties that we are only now beginning to discuss freely and reevaluate. The emphasis on the macho aspects of male performance tends to obliterate consideration of men as sensitive, gentle, nurturant, and intimate beings who can relate to adult partners on a variety of levels. The emphasis on the passivity of women has long neglected consideration and acknowledgment of them as full sexual beings with the same needs as men for expression and fulfillment.

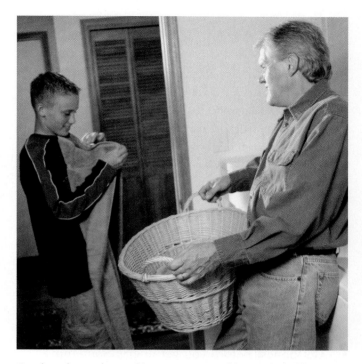

Gender roles are learned in many ways and from many different people.

Each gender needs to be able to express feelings heretofore defined as either masculine or feminine. Both genders need to be directive and sensitive to function effectively. Women need to make decisions in parenting, in controlling their careers, and in their sexual behavior. Men need to accept responsibility for parenting, be comfortable as receivers as well as givers, and accept that sharing intimacy and intimate acts does not mean loss of control.

Many men and women in our society still differ in their expectations for interpersonal relationships. Some women still expect assertive, in-command, successful men; some men still expect supportive, helpful, receiving women. Stereotypes of the dominant male and the submissive female continue to influence the interpersonal dynamics between the genders. Both genders have been socialized into these expectations, and socialization probably accounts for more of these distinctions than does biology.

Men have often learned to equate sexual activity with the fulfillment of their needs for support, tenderness, and the feeling of being loved. Women have often not been taught that receiving sexual pleasure has value. Mixed feelings about what they really feel and what society tells them they are supposed to feel can confuse both sexes.

The popular press suggests that men and women may always have problems because they are so different. Examples often given are in communication (she wants more talk; he wants more action); intimacy (she needs to relax to participate in intimate sexual

? Did You Know . . .

A study of 150 undergraduate students examined how being visually "checked out" (an objectifying gaze) by a member of the other gender affected each student's performance on math problems. The gaze caused decreased math performance for women, but somewhat ironically the same women also wanted more interaction with the person who had objectified them. The men were unfazed when females stared at their chests. The researchers felt that one explanation for the math performance change is stereotype threat. Math performance may decrease because the gaze conveys that women's looks are valued over their other qualities. The objectifying gaze may trigger a vicious cycle in which women underperform but continue to interact with the people who led them to underperform in the first place (Gervais, 2011).

behavior, but he needs to participate to relax); division of household labor and child care (she says she does more; he talks about how much he does); and money and careers (she says he does not value her job as much as his; he notes that he makes more money).

Related to communication, the following are some of the ways to close the gender gap:

• **G**et honest before you get angry: Something deeper than dry cleaning or dishwashing is probably bothering you.

• **E**stablish systems for sharing chores and child care.

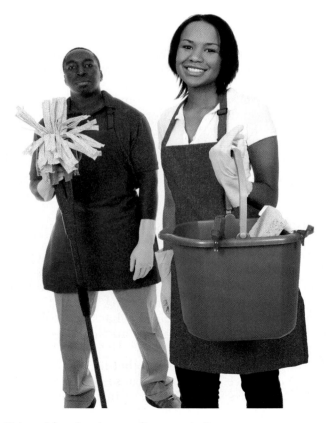

Male and female roles are often very similar.

• **N**egotiate the division of labor and the division of love.

• **D**o not get locked into your role: Try swapping responsibilities on occasion.

• **E**xpress your emotional needs and expectations and really listen to your partner.

• **R**eview the cultural messages of your childhood to help understand the conflicts inherent in your new roles.

• **G**ive each other time to change: Do not monitor or criticize.

• **A**ccept your differences and applaud each other's strengths.

• **P**rotect your intimate time together.

There is increased thinking that similarities between men and women, particularly in the human struggle for intimacy, far outweigh differences. Healthy couples appear to transcend traditional gender roles, and the roles, such as pursuer and distancer, are interchangeable. There is no one definition of an intimate, healthy relationship. Love and respect are essential in a good relationship.

In terms of human sexual expression, both partners need the freedom to be self-disclosing, intimate, and communicative. Restrictive definitions of roles serve only to repress the joy, pleasure, and emotionally fulfilling responses of sexual intimacy. And perhaps equally important is the fact that gender-role stereotyping also restricts personal fulfillment in nonsexual relationships between men and women.

The Possibilities of Androgyny

According to legend, there once were three kinds of humans—the male, the female, and the androgyne. All humans had two sets of arms and legs. The males and females had two faces and two sets of genitalia of the same gender. The androgynes each had one masculine face and one feminine face, one set of female genitalia, and one set of male genitalia. This group of humans had tremendous strength and an arrogant nature, which offended the gods.

Zeus, to punish them, split the androgynes in half and remade them as hemipeople. Thus men and women have lost their other half and seek it in other people.

The word **androgynous** originated from the story of the androgynes. An androgynous person is one who has a combination of masculine and feminine characteristics—one who exhibits some traits of both masculinity and femininity as defined by the society. Thus an androgynous male might be nurturing in addition to providing, and an androgynous female might be assertive as well as soft-spoken. The idea of androgyny can serve as a means of doing away with gender-role stereotyping. Many people believe that they must conform absolutely to society's notions of maleness and femaleness, especially in the ways they acknowledge and express (or repress and deny) their feelings. In conforming, they lose the opportunity to express themselves as individuals. But if, as a society, we were to view people as androgynous, then all of us might consider the expression of a variety of emotions appropriate for everyone. A significant benefit would be that people who expressed their true feelings, unswayed by the demands of gender-role stereotypes, would experience a greater depth of sexual intimacy with their partners than would those concerned solely with how manly or womanly they appear.

androgynous
Exhibiting a combination of masculine and feminine traits as defined by the society.

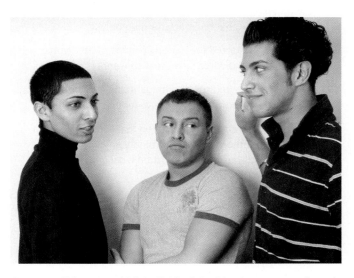

Can you tell for sure which individuals in this picture are male and which are female?

The concept of androgyny has been around a long time. For example, in 1975 Sandra Bem, a noted proponent of androgyny, indicated that stereotypical gender roles were restrictive and unhealthy. She described androgynous people, by contrast, as flexible and healthy. She felt that rigidity in gender-role expectations was reflected in inflexible responses in real-life situations. To test her theory, Bem developed the Bem Sex Role Inventory. She gave a group of men and women a list of personality characteristics—some traditionally masculine (assertiveness, ambition, independence), some traditionally feminine (dependence, sensitivity, gentleness), and some neutral (friendliness, likability)—and asked the subjects to rate the accuracy of each term in describing them. Participants were then placed in situations that tested masculine and feminine behaviors such as nurturance, responsiveness to a troubled person, and conformity. Men who had described themselves as having masculine traits were not comfortable with "feminine" activities, and women who had described themselves as having feminine traits were not comfortable doing "masculine" tasks. But androgynous men and women were able to function in all situations.

It should be noted that not all studies are supportive of the androgyny concept. Yet many experts and numerous studies tend to agree that freedom from stereotypical gender roles allows for greater health and life satisfaction. People continue to do research related to androgyny. However, others criticize the concept and do not place much confidence in it.

The Women's Movement

In recent decades we have seen social upheaval that has changed our society in a variety of ways. Patterns of sexual behavior have been affected, for example, by contraceptive technology, abortion, and sterilization. Divorce has become more acceptable, and changes in leisure pursuits, delays in pregnancy, and the acceptance of intentional childlessness all offer women a greater diversity in lifestyle. But perhaps the single most important effect has been the women's movement. The ability of women to explore their potential has never been as great as at this time. Economic independence, control over reproduction, and choices in relationships and lifestyle have given women freedom from domination by men and the opportunity for self-direction as individuals. Statistics illustrate the increasing inroads into the labor force being made by women as they seek to achieve economic independence and/or to supplement the family's income.

There were at least four groups who converged in the 1960s to help create the modern women's

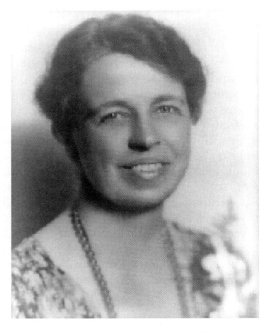

Eleanor Roosevelt helped raise people's awareness about sexism.

movement. First, there were those, such as Eleanor Roosevelt, who used John F. Kennedy's Presidential Commission on the Status of Women to reveal pervasive sexism in American society and law. Second, there were those who were from the civil rights movement, broadening the definition of equality to include women. The third group, working-class women, turned to feminism and the women's movement in their struggle for the Equal Pay Act of 1963. The fourth group was made up of white, middle-class suburban women, who found themselves stifled by gender stereotypes (Kerber, 1999).

The women's movement probably also is responsible for increased attention to victims of sexual assault and other forms of violence. A better understanding of aggressive behavior, improved services for assault victims, and greatly increased education on these topics are all evidence of this increased attention. In addition, the public discussion of sexual harassment throughout recent years must be at least partially attributed to the women's movement. There is also a growing body of literature about many issues related to gender.

? Did You Know . . .

Some people think that the women's movement started in the 1960s. There were actually many significant events prior to that time. Here is a list of selected important events related to the Women's Movement (Imbornoni, n. d.; National Women's History Project, 2005).

1769 American colonies based their laws on English common law. By marriage, husband and wife were considered one person under the law.

1777 All states passed laws taking away women's rights to vote.

1839 The first state (Mississippi) granted women the right to hold property in their own name, with their husbands' permission.

1869 The first woman suffrage law in the United States was passed in the territory of Wyoming.

1908 The first state (Wyoming) granted women the right to vote in all elections.

1916 Margaret Sanger tested New York's anticontraception law by establishing a clinic in Brooklyn. She helped establish a woman's right to control her own body.

1920 The Nineteenth Amendment to the U.S. Constitution, which states that the right to vote shall not be denied based on sex, was ratified.

1938 The Fair Labor Standards Act established a minimum wage without regard to sex.

1963 The Equal Pay Act promised equitable pay for the same work regardless of race, color, religion, national origin, or sex of the worker.

1968 Executive Order 11246 prohibited sex discrimination by government contractors and required affirmative action plans for hiring women.

1969 The Seventh Circuit Court of Appeals ruled that women meeting the physical requirements could work in many jobs that had been for men only.

California adopted the nation's first "no fault" divorce law, allowing divorce by mutual consent.

1972 Title IX prohibited sex discrimination in all aspects of education programs that receive federal support.

1973 The U.S. Supreme Court declared that the Constitution protects women's right to terminate an early pregnancy, thus making abortion legal in the United States (*Roe v. Wade*).

1974 Housing discrimination on the basis of sex and credit discrimination against women were outlawed by Congress.

1978 The Pregnancy Discrimination Act banned employment discrimination against pregnant women.

1984 Sex discrimination in membership policies of organizations such as the Jaycees, Kiwanis, and Rotary was forbidden by the Supreme Court.

1993 The U.S. Supreme Court ruled that the victim did not need to show that she suffered physical or serious psychological injury as a result of sexual harassment.

1994 Congress adopted the Gender Equity in Education Act to train teachers in gender equity, promote math and science learning for girls, counsel pregnant teens, and prevent sexual harassment.

1997 Elaborating on Title IX, the Supreme Court ruled that college athletic programs must actively involve roughly equal numbers of men and women to qualify for federal support.

1998 The Supreme Court ruled that employers are liable for sexual harassment even in instances when a supervisor's threats are not carried out. However, it also said the employer can defend itself by showing it took steps to prevent or promptly correct any sexually harassing behavior and the employee did not take advantage of available opportunities to stop the behavior or complain of the behavior.

1999 The U.S. Supreme Court ruled that a woman can sue for punitive damages for sex discrimination if the antidiscrimination law was violated with malice or indifference to the law, even if that conduct was not especially severe.

2003 The U.S. Supreme Court ruled that states can be sued in federal court for violations of the Family and Medical Leave Act.

2005 The U.S. Supreme Court ruled that Title IX, which prohibits discrimination based on sex, also inherently prohibits disciplining someone for complaining about sex-based discrimination.

2006 The U.S. Supreme Court upheld the ban on the "partial-birth" abortion procedure. It was the first ruling to ban a specific type of abortion procedure.

2009 President Obama signed the Lily Ledbetter Fair Pay Restoration Act, which allows victims of pay discrimination to file a complaint with the government against their employer within 180 days of their last paycheck. Previously, victims (mostly women) were allowed only 180 days from the date of the first unfair paycheck.

Multicultural DIMENSIONS

Has the Women's Movement in France Caught Up?

In 2011, the former International Monetary Fund chief, a Frenchman, was arrested in New York for the alleged sexual assault and attempted rape of a hotel housekeeper. Many key figures in France's intellectual and political elite converged to protect him. They minimized, cast doubt upon, or even ignored the plight of the single mother who had accused him. This angered a consortium of French feminist groups, which in response gathered thousands of signatures on a petition denouncing sexual violence against women, sexist remarks on the French airwaves, and the rise to the surface of sexist and reactionary remarks among leading French figures.

The show of anger by the feminist groups forced the political and media elite to quickly change their tune. Feminist commentary—some written by men—appeared in France's mainstream publications. Women reporters started to share their own stories of harassment and even assault by powerful men. There was talk about how feminist issues could play a prominent role in the election of the next French president. It was pointed out that all of this could mark the end of an era in which talking too forcefully about inequities between men and women was rejected as too old-school, too angry, too American.

Many French people believe that there has not been enough progress in the promotion of equality between men and women. Generous family policies aimed at promoting and allowing women to balance work and family have had the effect of reinforcing old gender stereotypes, as employers were unwilling to hire women of childbearing age on the grounds that they will take too many costly and disruptive maternity leaves. Many younger women and men were raised on the promise of equality, but have grown angry when reality has not met their expectations. For example, political parties are supposed to offer equal numbers of male and female candidates, but that hasn't happened. There have been repeated legislative efforts to promote pay equality, but wage inequality between men and women has persisted or even worsened in recent years. The trend towards workplace flexibility has tended to push women disproportionately into unstable and low-paid part-time positions.

In France, appearances have changed, but real life has not. It remains to be seen whether women's issues will remain front and center, but it seems that the dialogue about gender relations in France has been forever altered.

Source: Data from Warner, J. Cherchez les Femmes: Has the Women's Movement in France Finally Caught Up? *Time, 177, no. 23* (June 6, 2011): 38–39. Available at http://www.time.com/time/world/article/ 0,8599,2074070,00.html.

With the change in the present and potential status of women, new pressures and anxieties about role redefinition and intimate relationships have arisen. Women are more informed about their physiology and their right not only to expect sexual fulfillment and satisfaction but also to initiate or refuse sexual behavior. For many, traditional values concerning virginity, self-sacrifice for children, lifelong commitment to marriage, and the support role of women are giving way to new modes of commitment. These changes can be seen as giving both women and men a chance to explore a number of alternatives.

Some people feel true female empowerment has been shown by women (notably some movie stars) who have chosen as partners men who are less successful than they are. Because many modern women work outside the home and are financially independent, they are empowered enough to make a choice among men based on their personality, as opposed to making a choice only among men who earn as much or more. His career is less important than hers, so when they go out she gets all the attention (Tan, 2001).

The Institute for Women's Policy Research (Overview of the status women in the states, 2001) reported that gains in education and income and an increased presence in politics helped women boost their economic and social status. Yet, even states rated highly in its report must progress for women to gain equality with men. The Institute looked at political participation, employment and earnings, economic autonomy, reproductive rights, and health and well-being in all states. Detailed results can be seen at the Institute's website at www.iwpr.org.

In 2003 an interesting gender-equity issue arose within the sport of golf. In Virginia a 17-year-old girl won the high school boys' golf tournament. However, she won playing from tees set closer to the hole than the tees the boys used. The rules had been changed 4 years earlier to allow girls to compete with this advantage. Earlier, a woman professional golfer won a tournament to qualify to play in a men's professional tournament. She, too, had competed from tees set closer to the hole. It was later ruled that when she played in the men's professional tournament she had to play from the same tees as the men. Whether females should be required to play from the same tees as the men if they are going to compete against men remains a controversial issue. Bowen (2003) has said that once females play against males, they should play by the same rules. If a female is racing against a male in the 100-meter run, for example, she should not be able to start 20 meters ahead just because she is a female. It will be interesting to see how this issue is resolved in the coming years.

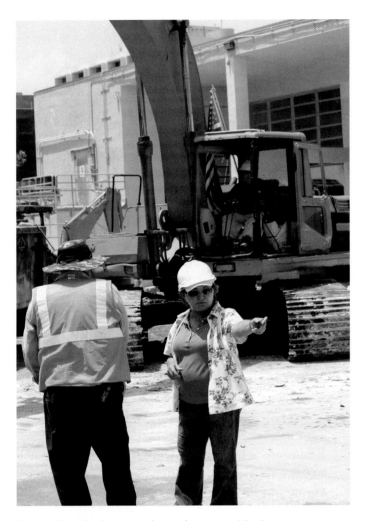

Women have had more and varied opportunities in recent years.

Since the enactment of Title IX in 1972, female high school athletic participation has increased by more than 900% and female college athletic participation has increased by almost 500%. An unprecedented number of girls and women are playing sports and participating in activities that used to be perceived as primarily male (or at least dominated by males), including ice hockey, boxing, wrestling, and football, among others. However, there are still significantly fewer women than men in administrative and coaching positions. Overall, in 2007 only 17.7% of all teams (men's and women's) were coached by a female head coach. Even though many institutions are still not in compliance with Title IX, women continue to gain opportunities to participate and lead in sport. Some of them are thriving even in male-dominated sports and will no doubt continue to push the envelope (Strecker 2010).

Examples of changes since Title IX and some changes that might still needed include:

- In 1972–73, more than 12 times more boys than girls played high school sports. By 2010, while boys' participation was at a record level, they outnumbered girls by a relatively small 29%.

- In 2010 about 8,300 girls played on high school ice hockey teams, up from a total of just 96 in 1974.

- The number of law and medical degrees going to women has jumped from 7% and 9% respectively in 1972 to 47% and 48% in 2010.

- A physical-activity gender gap remains. Almost 40% of young boys exercise 6 or 7 days a week, compared with 26% of young girls.

- Today, women make up about 45% of the athlete population at NCAA schools while accounting for about 55% of the student body.

The topic of women in the military has received increasing attention in recent years. In 1990, the National Board of the National Organization of Women (NOW) adopted a policy about women in the military. It said: "NOW demands equality for women in joining the military and in training, job assignments, and benefits in the military; and NOW actively supports elimination of statutory restrictions on women in the military" (Women in the military, 1990).

Since 1995 a number of significant events have occurred related to women in the military (Chronology of significant legal and policy changes affecting women in the military: 1947–2003, 2005). For example, in 1995, the Marine Corps selected a woman for aviation training for the first time. Between 1996 and 2001, more than 15,000 American servicewomen served in Bosnia. In 1998, women aviators flew combat missions for the first time in Operation Desert Fox. In 1999, the Navy opened Coastal Mine Hunters and Mine Counter Measures ships to women. Also, women aviators participated in combat operations during the air war in Kosovo. In 2000, two women sailors were killed and several wounded in a terrorist attack on the USS *Cole*. In 2001, military women deployed to the Afghan theater as part of Operation Enduring Freedom, the war on terrorism. In 2002, the first woman Marine was killed in Afghanistan. In 2002, the Defense Authorizations Act required the Department of Defense to submit an annual report on the status of women in the services. In 2003, more than 25,400 women were deployed in support of Operation Iraqi Freedom. As of early 2009,

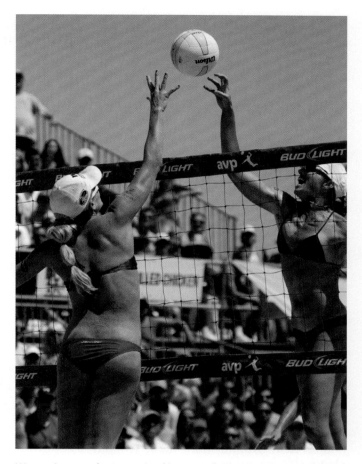

Women's sports have received increased attention in recent years.

there were more than 205,000 women on active duty, accounting for 14.2% of the total active-duty forces. In addition, 80,000 women served in the reserves (24.1% of the total) and 71,000 women were members of the National Guard (15.1% of the total) (Statistics on women in the military, 2009).

As more women began to serve in the military, a practical issue came up. Military gear was made with the male physique in mind. For women, this meant body armor that fit so poorly that it was tough to fire a weapon, combat uniforms with knee pads that hit around mid-shin, and flight suits that made it nearly impossible to urinate while in a plane. New combat uniforms and other equipment for women have been designed (Hefling, 2011).

Women's gains in educational attainment have significantly outpaced those of men since 1970 (Women in America, 2011). Since 1970, the percentage of women with at least a high school education rose from 59% (about the same as men) to about 87% (slightly more than men). In 1970, only about 8% of women and 14% of men were college graduates. Now, it is about 28% for each group. In 2008, for all racial and ethnic subgroups, a higher percentage of bachelor's and master's degrees were earned by

Gender DIMENSIONS

Is There Gender Equality in College Sports?

Since 1972, Title IX of the Education Amendments has forbidden sex discrimination at institutions receiving federal funds. One important, and still controversial, part of this legislation relates to college sports. After nearly 40 years of living with Title IX, there are still many viewpoints about it. Some people believe that men have been penalized for having a higher interest in athletics than women. They point to the fact that in some cases men's sports have been cut to comply with Title IX. Others believe that Title IX has not hurt men's sports, and it has greatly helped women's athletic opportunities. Efforts continue among athletic officials, college administrators, and legislators to see how to deal best with Title IX and its implications.

women than men. Women earned about 57% of all college degrees in 2008, and constituted 57% of total undergraduate enrollment. Women age 25–34 are now more likely than men of that age group to have attained a college degree, reversing the norm from 1968. The percentage of women age 25–34 with 2 or more years of graduate school increased dramatically since the late 1970s to about 11%, while the percentage of men in that age group with 2 or more years of graduate school has remained around 8%. In 1998, more doctoral degrees were conferred to men than to women. A decade later, more doctoral degrees were conferred to women than men. Women account for about 59% of graduate school enrollment.

The Sexuality Education and Information Council of the United States (SIECUS) has issued the following position statement on gender equality and equity:

> SIECUS believes that gender equality and equity are fundamental human rights. Society must recognize how gender-based stereotyping, including prejudice toward transgender, transsexual, and intersex individuals, can result in harmful consequences, such as gender-based violence and sexual, physical, and psychological abuse. Gender-based stereotyping must be eliminated, and the use of gender-inclusive language promoted. The legal system should guarantee the civil rights and protection of all people, regardless of gender, gender identity, or gender expression.

As we have pointed out throughout this chapter, some people have many different feelings about some gender issues. In 2008, the American Psychological Association (APA) adopted a policy statement related to transgender, gender identity, and gender expression nondiscrimination (American Psychological Association, 2008). Here is part of that statement:

> Therefore be it resolved that APA opposes all public and private discrimination on the basis of actual or perceived gender identity and expression and urges the repeal of discriminatory laws and policies;

> Therefore be it further resolved that APA supports the passage of laws and policies protecting the rights, legal benefits, and privileges of people of all gender identities and expressions;

> Therefore be it further resolved that APA supports full access to employment, housing, and education regardless of gender identity and expression.

Exploring the Dimensions of Human Sexuality

Our feelings, attitudes, and beliefs regarding sexuality are influenced by our internal and external environments. Go to go.jblearning.com/dimensions5e to learn more about the biological, factors that affect your sexuality.

Case Study

Your gender plays a major role in how you perceive the world—and how the world perceives you. Gender plays a pervasive role in many areas that define our self-concept, including career opportunities. Men and women communicate in different styles, and they express emotions differently. Physiological differences play out in health—women do live longer, but are sick more often.

Gender roles are influenced by virtually all social and cultural aspects, including religion, ethnic heritage, family traditions, peers, and even the mass media.

In sexuality, a "double standard" still exists, as men are encouraged to be sexually aggressive and women are discouraged from being sexually active.

Biological Factors

- Chromosomes (XX or XY) determine biological gender.
- Primitive gonadal tissues differentiate into prenatal ovaries or testicles.
- At puberty, sex hormones cause emergence of primary and secondary sexual characteristics. Sex hormones continue to act throughout one's lifetime.
- Testosterone plays a role in aggression; estrogen has been linked to heart attack prevention.
- Most medical studies have been completed on men, and findings have been assumed to be the same for women, without taking into account gender differences in hormones and chemical makeup.

Sociocultural Factors

- Gender-role orientation begins at birth. Children are treated differently according to social standards for gender.
- Family, neighbors, friends, and teachers influence our thinking about gender through their actions.
- Ethnic groups pass down gender-specific heritages and gender roles.
- Mass media are often gender-biased, portraying men and women in traditional, stereotypical roles.

Psychological Factors

- Expressiveness and communication style differ between genders, as men withhold feelings and women express them openly.
- Women suffer more from self-esteem issues relating to body image, as they attempt to live up to the biologically impossible "Barbie" standard.
- In a society where men are presented with greater opportunities, motivation and possibility of achievement are more challenging for women.

Summary

- Discussions about gender similarities and differences often focus on "nature versus nurture." Some attribute most of these gender-based characteristics to biological factors; others attribute them to social factors and learning.

- Gender similarities and differences usually fall into certain categories, such as developmental differences, gender and abilities, gender and aggression, gender and health, and gender and dating.

- Many gender issues have emerged related to the workplace in recent years. Issues commonly discussed include different work styles and leadership styles of men and women, rights of males and females in the workplace, and arguments about the existence of a gender-based wage gap.

- There are many feelings about gender and advertising. Some people believe numerous ads promote gender stereotypes just to sell products; others see gender-based ads as nothing very important one way or the other.

- Gender identity, roles, and stereotypes are learned in many ways. Gender roles can differ markedly from society to society.

- Gender roles and stereotypes are taught in a number of ways in society. They are strongly influenced by teachers and the school environment, and by parents and peers.

- Some people experience gender identity difficulty. A transsexual is a person whose gender identity does not match his or her biological sex. Gender-reassignment surgery is usually done only after careful screening of the individual.

- Gender-role stereotyping limits sexuality in many ways. It can limit self-expression, personal growth and development, and healthy feelings about masculinity and femininity.

- The women's movement has had many influences on gender roles as well as social and legal issues.

- Today more women than men receive bachelor's, master's, and doctoral degrees. However, many different feelings about male and female roles still exist.

Discussion Questions

1. Of the many differences between the genders, which do you believe are the most important nonbiological differences? Explain your answer. In your own college or university, are male and female students treated differently? Give specific examples.

2. Compare and contrast the feelings of males and females toward sexuality. Then discuss how the genders can bridge those differences.

3. How can women achieve sexual equality with men without becoming competitive? Does such a change need to begin with women—or with men?

Application Questions

Reread the story that opens the chapter and answer the following questions.

1. Is the writer androgynous? Explain why or why not.

2. Which conflicts has the author experienced from his "reversed" gender role?

3. Is there any merit to the composer's comment that gender play during childhood influences abilities later in life? Which other factors probably influenced the development of women composers?

4. As a student, how do you view the future of gender roles? How will life experiences affect your view of gender roles?

Critical Thinking Questions

1. Consider the expression "Candy is dandy, but liquor is quicker." Explain the gender bias of the expression. Which type of tensions might such thinking create between the genders?

2. Is there a gender bias in the United States toward the male management style? What other reasons might explain the lack of women in high-level executive positions and on boards of directors?

3. Michael Jackson was often cited as an androgynous person. Why did the popular press believe this? Was it true?

Critical Thinking Case

Because of physiological differences, men and women often have slightly different medical symptoms. The same seems true for psychological problems. For example, school-aged boys who act out in class are often considered for the *DSM-IV* diagnosis of attention-deficit/hyperactivity disorder. Boys who receive treatment can learn to do quite well in school. However, girls have been socialized not to act out in class; they tend to have different symptoms and are less often diagnosed. That difference puts those young girls at a disadvantage, leading to poor scholastic achievement and low self-esteem.

In adulthood, depression is diagnosed in women nearly twice as often as in men. Research from the 1990s suggests that when men are faced with negative emotions, they distract themselves through drinking or sports. Women, in contrast, tend to focus attention on the negative mood. If such focus intensifies the negative mood, a woman would be more prone to a diagnosis of depression.

1. Should separate diagnostic manuals for psychiatric disorders be written for men and women? Explain your answer.

2. Should psychiatrists focus their training on one gender? Or should training be generic? Explain your answer.

Exploring Personal Dimensions

Female–Male Differences and Similarities
Females and males respond in similar ways to sexual stimulation. However, in some ways they also respond dissimilarly. To assess your knowledge of these similarities and differences, determine whether each of the following statements describes a response that is similar or dissimilar for females and males. Then place a check mark to indicate your answer. The correct answers appear at the conclusion of the statements.

Similar   Dissimilar

——   ——   1. Erection occurs.

——   ——   2. When a sexual fantasy occurs, hormones are secreted.

——   ——   3. Testosterone is produced by the body.

——   ——   4. During sexual excitement, the nipples become erect.

——   ——   5. Sex flush appears during the excitement phase of the sexual response cycle.

——   ——   6. Males and females can have multiple orgasms without requiring a rest period.

Correct Answers
1. Similar. Both the penis and the clitoris become engorged with blood and become erect.

2. Similar. Hormones in both genders activate various body parts in response to sexual stimulation.

3. Similar. Testosterone is produced in the interstitial cells of the testes in men and in the ovaries of women (although in a small amount).

4. Similar. Although nipple erection is more obvious in women, it occurs in men, too.

5. Dissimilar. In men, sex flush occurs during the plateau phase; in women, it occurs during the excitement phase.

6. Dissimilar. Whereas women have the capacity to be multiorgasmic, males generally need to experience a refractory period before subsequent orgasms.

Suggested Readings

Andersen, M. *Thinking about women*, 8th ed. Boston: Allyn and Bacon, 2009.

Brannon, L. *Gender: Psychological perspectives*, 5th ed. Boston: Pearson, 2008.

Feminist Majority Foundation. Available: www.feminist.org.

Lips, H. *A new psychology of women*, 3rd ed. Long Grove IL: Waveland Press, 2006.

Lips, H. *Sex and gender*, 6th ed. New York: McGraw-Hill, 2007.

Manning, L. *Women in the military: Where they stand*, 5th ed. Washington D.C.: Women's Research & Education Institute, 2005.

Matlin, M. W. *Psychology of women*, 7th ed. Belmont, CA: Waswsorth, 2011.

Mottet, L., & Tanis, J. *Opening the door the inclusion of transgender people: The nine keys to making lesbian gay, bisexual, and transgender organizations fully transgender-inclusive*. New York: National Gay and Lesbian Task Force Policy Institute and the National Center for Transgender Equality, 2008.

Overview of the status of women in the states. Institute for Women's Policy Research (2008). Available at: www.iwpr.org.

Web Resources

For links to the websites below, visit *go.jblearning .com/dimensions5e* and click on Resource Links.

Institute for Women's Policy Research
www.iwpr.org
The Institute for Women's Policy Research conducts rigorous research and disseminates its findings in key program areas: employment, education and economic change; democracy and society; poverty, welfare, and income security; work and family; and health and safety.

Radford University Center for Gender Studies
http://gstudies.asp.radford.edu/

Lists a number of Internet sites and resources relevant to studies and searches where the focus is women, men, and gender expectations. Each listing can be activated for a direct connection to that site. Beneath the tabular summary, a brief overview of each resource is provided along with a direct link to its web address.

Myths, Fallacies, Folderol and Idiotic Rumors About Military Women
http://userpages.aug.com/captbarb/myths.html

Explores reasons often given for why women should not be in military combat. The reasons are treated as myths and refuted.

National Organization for Women
www.now.org

This website contains information about contemporary issues of particular importance to women. The content changes periodically, but issues likely to be discussed include abortion rights, breast implants, tax issues, insurance and child support, emergency contraception, and information about contraceptive options.

WomensMedia.com: Expert Advice for Working Women
http://womensmedia.com

Emphasizes issues that might be of increased interest to women who are employed. Examples include women and investing, gender communication, male–female differences, the "old boy" network, and networking tips.

References

American Psychological Association Task Force on Gender Identity and Gender Variance. *Report of the Task Force on Gender Identity and Gender Variance*. Washington, DC: American Psychological Association, 2008.

American Psychological Association. *Report of the APA Taskforce on the Sexualization of Girls*. Washington, DC: Author, 2007.

American Psychological Association. *Resolution on transgender, gender identity, and gender expression non-discrimination*, August 2008. Available: http://www.apa.org/pi/lgbc/policy/transgender.pdf.

Andersen, M. *Thinking about women: Sociological perspectives on sex and gender*. Boston: Allyn and Bacon, 2009, 54.

Anderson, L. Poll highlights hidden but deadly dangers for women. TrustLaw (June 16, 2011). Available: http://www.trust.org/trustlaw/news/analysis-poll-highlights-hidden-but-deadly-dangers-for-women/.

Armour, S. When an employee switches gender, what's a company to do? *USA Today* (June 10, 2005), 1B–2B.

Basow, S. A., & Rubenfeld, K. "Troubles talk": Effects of gender and gender-typing. *Sex Roles, 48* (2003), 183–187.

Baumeister, R., & Tice, D. *The social dimension of sex*. Boston: Allyn and Bacon, 2000.

Bem, S. L. Androgyny versus the tight little lives of women and chesty men. *Psychology Today* (September 1975), 58–62.

Berk, L. E. *Exploring lifespan development*. Boston: Allyn and Bacon, 2008, 212.

Beyer, L. The price of honor. *Time, 153, no. 2* (January 18, 1999), 55.

Billowitz, M., & Kukke, S. Doing gender the "rights" way. *SIECUS Report, 32, no. 3* (Summer 2004), 5–10.

Bontempi, J. B., Mugno, R., Bulmer, S. M., Danvers, K., & Vancour, M. L. Exploring gender differences in the relationship between HIV/STD testing and condom use among undergraduate college students. *American Journal of Health Education, 40, 2* (March/April 2009), 97–105.

Bowen, F. Is there a case for an uneven playing field? *The Birmingham News* (January 9, 2003), 7E.

Boylan, J. F. *She's not there: A life in two genders.* New York: Broadway Books, 2003.

Bureau of Labor Statistics. *Usual weekly earnings summary.* April, 19, 2011. Available: http://www.bls.gov/news.release/wkyeng.nr0.htm.

Can we raise gender-neutral children? in *Taking sides: Issues in family and personal relationships,* Schroeder, E., ed. Guilford, CT: McGraw-Hill/Dushkin, 2003.

Catalyst 2008 census of the *Fortune* 500 reveals women gained little ground advancing to business leadership positions. Catalyst, 2008. Available: http://www.catalyst.org/press-release/141/catalyst-2008-census-of-the-fortune-500-reveals-women-gained-little-ground-advancing-to-business-leadership-positions.

Chronology of significant legal and policy changes affecting women in the military: 1947–2003. Women's Research & Education Institute (2005). Available: http://www.wrei.org/projects/wiu/wim/wim_chron01.pdf.

Daniel, E. L., & Levine, C. *Taking sides: Clashing views on controversial issues in health and society,* 5th ed. Guilford, CT: McGraw-Hill Dushkin, 2001.

Do men and women lead differently? *Leadership Strategies 3, no. 10* (October 2000): 8.

Eagly, A. H. Transformational, transactional, and laissez-faire leadership styles: A meta-analysis comparing women and men. *Psychological Bulletin, 129, no. 4* (July 2003), 569–591.

Galdas, P. M., Cheater, F., & Marshall, P. Men and health help-seeking behavior: Literature review. *Journal of Advanced Nursing, 49* (2005), 616–622.

Garnett, C. Sharing the sandbox equally: screen star Davis urges gender balance in the media. *NIH Record, 63, no. 11* (2011). Available: http://nihrecord.od.nih.gov/newsletters/2011/05_27_2011/story1.htm.

Gervais, S. J., Vescio, T. K., & Allen, J. What you see is what you get: The objectifying gaze for women and men. *Psychology of Women Quarterly, no. 35* (March 2011), 5–17.

Guptka, G. Gender, sexuality, and HIV/AIDS: The what, the why, and the how. *SIECUS Report, 29, no. 5* (June/July 2001), 6–12.

Hafling, K. They're not guys: New gear to fit female soldiers. ABC News (April 22, 2011). Available: http://abcnews.go.com/US/wireStory?id=13433425.

Hamson, S. The passive/active divide: What the village is teaching our children about gender. *SIECUS Report, 32, no. 3* (Summer 2004), 14–16.

Horgan, T. G., Mast, M. S., & Hall, J. A. Gender differences in memory for the appearance of others. *Personality and Social Psychology Bulletin, 30, no. 2* (2004), 185–196.

Imbornoni, A. A women's rights movement in the U.S. Available: http://www.infoplease.com/spot/womenstimeline3.html.

International Foundation for Gender Education (2005). Available: http://www.ifge.org/.

Jenner, L., & Ferguson, R. 2008 Catalyst census of women corporate officers and top earners of the FP500. Catalyst, March 2009. Available: http://www.catalyst.org/publication/295/2008-catalyst-census-of-women-corporate-officers-and-top-earners-of-the-fp500.

Kerber, L. K. Moving beyond stereotypes of feminism. *Chronicle of Higher Education, 45, no. 33* (April 23, 1999), B6–B8.

Kluger, J. What's sex got to do with it? *Time, 161, no. 3* (January 20, 2003), 35.

Koernig, S. K., & Granitz, N. Progressive yet traditional: The portrayal of women compared to that of men in e-commerce magazine advertisements. *Journal of Advertising, 35, 2* (2006), 81–98.

Kulkarni, S. C., Levin-rector, A., Ezzati, M., & Murray, C. J. L. Falling behind: Life expectancy in U.S. counties from 2000 to 2007 in an international context. *Population Health Metrics, 9, no. 16* (2011). Available: http://www.pophealthmetrics.com/content/pdf/1478-7954-9-16.pdf.

Labi, N. An American honor killing: One victim's story. *Time* (February 25, 2011). Available: http://www.time.com/time/nation/article/0,8599,2055445,00.html.

Lips, H. The gender wage gap: Debunking the rationalizations. Center for Gender Studies (2005). Available: http://www.womensmedia.com/new/Lips-Hilary-gender-wage-gap.shtml.

Luscombe, B. Pumping it up, *Time, 58, no. 11* (September 3, 2001), Y26.

MacFarquhar, N. Saudis arrest women leading right-to-drive campaign. New York Times (May 23, 2011). Available: http://www.nytimes.com/2011/05/24/world/middleeast/24saudi.html.

MacGeorge, E. L., Graves, A. R., Feng, B., & Gillihan, S. J. The myth of gender cultures: Similarities outweigh differences in men's and women's provision of and responses to supportive communication. *Sex Roles, 50* (2004), 143–175.

Males, females, and evolution: An interview with Helen Fisher. *Family Life Matters 43* (Spring 2001), 1, 4–5.

McKeen, C. A. Gender roles: An examination of the hopes and expectations of the next generation of managers in Canada and China. *Sex Roles, 52, nos. 7–8* (April 2005), 533–546.

Meese, M. Backlash: Women bullying women at work. *New York Times* (May 10, 2009). Available: http://www.nytimes.com/2009/05/10/business/10women.html.

Men, women more different than thought. *Intellihealth* (September 27, 2004), Available: http://www.intelihealth.com.

Money, J. *Gay, straight, and in-between*. New York: Oxford University Press, 1988.

Monk-Turner, E., Wren, K., McGill, L., Matthiae, C., Brown, S., & Brooks, D. Who is gazing at whom? A look at how sex is used in magazine advertisements. *Journal of Gender Studies, 17, 3* (September 2008), 201–209.

Mundy, L. Women, Money and Power. *Time, 179, no 12* (March26, 2012), 26–34.

Namie, G. The WBI U.S. workplace bullying survey. Workplace Bullying Institute (2010). Available: http://www.workplace-bullying.org/wbiresearch/2010-wbi-national-survey.

New study shows women own 20% of businesses with revenues exceeding $1 million. Center for Women's Business Research, December 3, 2008. Available: http://www.womensbusinessresearch.org.

On Equal Pay Day NOW calls attention to persistent gender wage gap. National Organization for Women, April 27, 2009. Available: http://www.now.org/press/04-09/04-27.html.

Overland, M. A. In Kashmir, militant group threatens to shoot female Muslim students who do not wear veil. *The Chronicle of Higher Education*, Today's News (September 17, 2001). Available: http://chronicle.com/daily/2001.

Overview of the status of women in the states. Washington, DC: IWPR, 2001. Available: http://www.iwpr.org/.

Peplau, L. A. Human sexuality: How do men and women differ? *Current Directions in Psychological Research, 12, no. 2* (April 2003), 37–40.

Popp, D., Donovan, R. A., Crawford, M., Marsh, K. L., & Peele, M. Gender, race, and speech style stereotypes. *Sex Roles, 48* (2003), 317–325.

Preidt, R. TV commercials color gender choices for careers. *MedicineNet.com*, May 28, 2008. Available: http://www.medicinenet.com.

Prime, J., & Moss-Racusin, C. A. Engaging men in gender initiatives: What change agents need to know. Catalyst, May 2009. Available: http://www.catalyst.org/publication/323/engaging-men-in-gender-initiatives-what-change-agents-need-to-know.

Ripley, A. Who says a woman can't be Einstein? *Time, 165, no. 10* (March 7, 2005), 51–60.

Rowe, S., A. & Woodard, D. L. National Law Review, May 22, 2012. Available: http://www.natlawreview.com/article/eeoc-rules-transgender-employees-are-covered-under-title-vii.

Sachs, A. Work's bad girls. *Time, 158, no. 11* (September 3, 2001), Y7–Y8.

Sadker, D., & Zittleman, K. Gender bias lives, for both sexes. *Education Digest, 70, no. 8* (April 2005), 27–30.

Sanchez-Flores, H. Everything I do, a man does. *SIECUS Report 32, no. 3* (summer 2004), 17–20.

Sayer, L. C. Gender, time and inequality: Trends in women's and men's paid work, unpaid work and free time. *Social Forces, 84* (2005), 285–303.

Shipman, C., & Kay, K. Women will rule business. *Time, 173, 20* (May 25, 2009), 46–47.

Should parents surgically alter their intersex infants? In *Taking sides: Issues in family and personal relationships,* Schroeder, E., ed. Guilford, CT: McGraw-Hill/Dushkin, 2003.

State politics & policy. *Daily Women's Health Policy Report,* National Partnership for Women & Families, May 18, 2009. Available: http://www.nationalpartnership.org/site/News.

Statistics on women in the military. Women in Military Service for America Memorial Foundation, April 7, 2009. Available: http://www.womensmemorial.org/PDFs/StatsonWIM.pdf.

Stoker, J. I., Van der Velde, M., & Lammers, J. Factors relating to managerial stereotypes: The role of gender of the employee and the manager and management gender ratio. *Journal of Business and Psychology* (March 19, 2011). Available: http://www.springerlink.com/content/y3458105hg318322/fulltext.pdf.

Strecker, L. Women in men's sports. *Update Plus* (July/August 2010), 29–31.

Sudden cardiac death gender gap closing in on women. *InteliHealth* (December 20, 2002). Available: www.intelihealth.com.

Surgery may be hasty for unclear gender. *InteliHealth* (2005). Available: http://www.intelihealth.com/.

Tan, C. L. Latest hot accessory for successful women: The lesser boyfriend. *The Birmingham News* (April 22, 2001), 1E, 5E.

Tavris, C. Are girls really as mean as books say they are? *Chronicle of Higher Education, 48, no. 43* (July 5, 2002), B7–B9.

Taylor, L. D., & Setters, T., Watching aggressive, attractive, female protagonists shapes gender roles for women among male and female undergraduate viewers. *Sex Roles, 65, no. 1–2* (2011), 35–46.

The power of play. *Sports Illustrated* (May 7, 2012), 43–66.

Torre, P. S., & Epstein, D. The Transgender Athlete. *Sports Illustrated* (May 28, 2012), 66–73.

U.S. Census Bureau. American community survey: Earnings in the past twelve months, 2007. Available: http://factfinder.census.gov/servlet/STTable?-geo_id=01000US&-qr_name=ACS_2005_EST_G00_S2001&-ds_name=ACS_2005_EST_G00_.

Warren, A. K. Cascading gender biases, compounding effects: An assessment of talent management systems. Catalyst, February 2009. Available: http://www.catalyst.org/publication/292/cascading-gender-biases-compounding-effects-an-assessment-of-talent-management-systems.

We want to live as humans. *Human Rights Watch, 14, no 11* (December 2002), 1–52.

Wilson, R. Second sex. *Chronicle of Higher Education, 52, no. 7* (October 10, 2005), A10–A12.

Winters, R. A food of one's own. *Time, 57, no. 25* (June 25, 2001), 47.

Women in American: Indicators of social and economic well-being. Washington, DC: White House Council on Women and Girls, 2011.

Zimmerman, A., & Dahlberg, J. The sexual objectification of women in advertising: A contemporary cultural perspective. *Journal of Advertising Research, 48, 1* (March 2008), 71–79.

Body Image

FEATURES

Gender Dimensions
Dissatisfaction with Body Parts

Multicultural Dimensions
Weight and Culture

Ethical Dimensions
To Train or Not to Train—That Is the Question

Gender Dimensions
Why Are Eating Disorders Mainly Found in Women?

CHAPTER OBJECTIVES

1 Discuss body image, its role in sexuality, and the way media have created impossible body-image ideals to emulate.

2 Describe how to improve one's self-image.

3 Describe the problems that poor body image cause for females and males, including eating disorders, muscle dysmorphia, steroid use, and cosmetic surgery.

go.jblearning.com/dimensions5e

The Influence of the Media
Genetics: Building on Your Strong Points
Eating Disorders
Sports and Dieting

INTRODUCTION

*I*f you had the privilege of knowing Marc Grabowski for some time, as one of your authors has, you would assume that he must have always been a confident young man. As a graduate of Boston University, with a double major in political science and philosophy, he worked as a trainer at a local gym while applying to law schools. Not only that: The month before he graduated, he placed fifth in the National Physique Committee's New England Body Building Competition as a heavyweight. Marc appears to be a pillar of strength and confidence.

But as with most people, Marc's confidence and bodily self-assurance have been built up over many years. In fact, Marc had very low self-esteem when he started high school. Smaller and lighter than his friends, he was picked on constantly (called "Ostrich Boy" because of his long neck). As his self-image sank, Marc decided to do something about it. He started lifting weights in his basement at age 14 years. By the time he was 16 years old, he had joined a gym. To Marc and his male friends, weight and size mattered. Their perception was that gaining any weight—fat, water weight, anything—was great.

It was not only his friends who pushed the weight issue. Marc would look at magazines like Flex and Muscle & Fitness and believe that he "could get like that": amazing abs or bulging biceps in 30 days! The articles focused on weight lifting but failed to mention nutrition, cardiovascular work, drugs (steroids), and muscle maturity. As Marc has learned, muscles take years to mature and grow dense in fibers so that they can stand out as hard as iron.

Yet those magazines continue to peddle false dreams. As Marc puts it, "They'll intentionally deceive the readers just to sell magazines." Worse than that: As many others do, Marc injured himself, rupturing the capillaries in his chest, by following the training routines in such magazines. And when the cover-boy results do not appear, that is a further blow to one's self-esteem.

Having a better body image has made Marc's social life easier. "Like it or not, the first thing people notice about you is your physical appearance. In social situations, that can be an advantage. But that is balanced against professional situations, where the negative connotations of a large size have to be overcome." Although he readily admits to "hiding behind the weight," Marc also says he enjoys life more. "It's nice to hear someone say, 'You've gotten in great shape.'"

By the time he reached Boston University, Marc set a goal to be in a bodybuilding show by the time he graduated. Although his studies always came first, Marc began the final preparations and dieting in his senior year.

The diet is what does most people in. During the off-season, Marc ate 10,000 calories or more a day. But as the contest drew nearer, he began to diet. By the last month, all Marc ate were 7 to 10 pounds of chicken and six potatoes a day! (And, of course, he drank water.) The diet takes a physical toll by depleting energy. Marc had trouble staying awake while studying for and taking exams.

The strict diet also has psychological effects. He felt "totally miserable" for the final 2 months of dieting. Marc deliberately tried to avoid social situations when he got cranky. He did not date during his final semester of college— and that, he ironically points out, somewhat defeated the original purpose of bodybuilding!

By the show, Marc was down to 206 pounds, with an incredibly low 2.7% body fat. Within 24 hours after the show, he had regained back 18 pounds (mostly water) and he gained an additional 10 pounds over the next 6 days. Marc lost the weight for a specific event but had no problem regaining it. Marc feels comfortable at an off-season weight of about 250 pounds and a body fat percentage of 10%.

As a personal trainer, Marc enjoys seeing the day-to-day growth of his clients—both in muscle and in confidence. The psychological effects of training are clear to Marc: Not only do clients have better body images, but their increased confidence is also seen in their becoming more outgoing. Clearly, a positive body image can improve your self-confidence.

As you will see in this chapter, obtaining your desired body image can be good for you both physically and psychologically. However, as Marc's story should show, it is important to keep your true goals in mind and, as you do so, respect your body and its needs.

Source: Interview with Marc T. Grabowski, June 9, 1999.

There's always a bigger fish in the water! A person in excellent shape for a young adult (bottom) can be dwarfed by a "professional" bodybuilder (top).

Body Image

Body image refers to the mental image we have of our own physical appearance. It is influenced by many factors—among them are weight, our weight distribution, our values about physical appearance, our concepts of a good physical appearance, our ethnic background, and what we see in others around us, what we hear through the media, and what we hear from others. We have previously discussed the importance of self-concept in relation to human sexuality. Self-concept is usually closely related to body image. A better body image contributes to a more confident individual; the better we feel about ourselves, the more likely we are to pursue a potential partner.

> **body image**
> The mental image we have of our own physical appearance.

Body image also affects sexual behavior. People with a positive body image are more likely to be open to sexual expression that exposes the body. Those with a poor body image might be less likely to pursue sexual expressions that cause them to reveal themselves and make them feel uncomfortable. Therefore, body image is an important part of sexual health. People who feel comfortable in their bodies are more likely to make healthy sexual decisions, such as protecting their health by using condoms. Those who feel comfortable about their sex organs are more likely to be comfortable talking openly about sexual behavior and feelings with a partner (Body image, 2009). Also, body satisfaction and, for women, the extent to which they see themselves as possessing characteristics associated with "being a sexual woman" are related to elements of subjective well-being (Donaghue, 2009).

Conversely, concerns about body image can impair sexual function and satisfaction. Sanchez and Kiefer (2007) found that body concerns negatively affect sexual pleasure and promote sexual problems for both men and women. However, Tucker and Irwin (2009) found that college students are very interested in improving their body image.

Many interesting points about body image were presented in the findings of *Psychology Today*'s 1997 body image survey (Garner, 1997). Despite the concerns of feminists and other observers, body image issues seem to be growing in importance. Body image influences much of our behavior and self-esteem. It governs whom we meet and whom we select as life partners, as well as our day-to-day interactions and our comfort level. Despite this importance, there is a growing gulf between actual and preferred shapes. As individuals, we are growing heavier, but our body preferences are growing thinner.

Results of the *Psychology Today* survey indicated that 89% of the women wanted to lose weight, and 22% of the men wanted to gain weight. Some women also reported avoiding pregnancy because of a fear of what a pregnancy would do to their bodies. Sexual experiences affect our body image, and our body image affects our sexual experiences. For example, 40% of men and 36% of women said that unpleasant sexual experiences caused negative feelings about their body. However, 70% of men and 67% of women felt that good sexual experiences contributed to satisfactory feelings about their body. In addition, 23% of women considered sexual abuse very important in negatively shaping their body image. Finally, 93% of women and 89% of men wanted models in magazines to represent the natural range of body shapes.

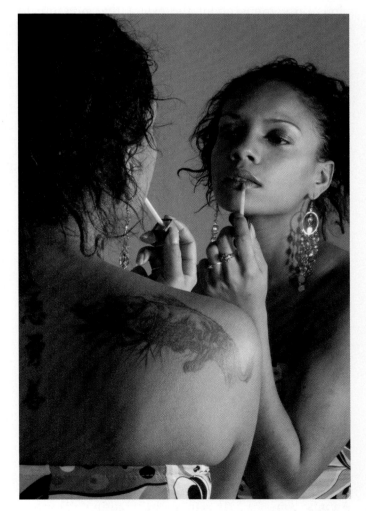

Many women feel pressure to conform to an "ideal" body image.

Women seem to be more likely than men to have poor body image. In a study with more than 3,500 participants who were university employees and bank workers, men were more likely to be overweight than women. However, women were significantly more likely than men to perceive themselves as overweight, even when their weight was within the appropriate range for their height. Overall, female university employees were 3 times as likely as men, and female bank workers 10 times as likely as men, to see themselves inaccurately (Women up to 10 times more likely to have poor body image than men, 2001).

A study of women at Duke University (Lipka, 2004) found that many undergraduate women felt relentless pressure to conform to an ideal. They described a social environment that supported the expectation that a woman would be "smart, accomplished, fit, beautiful, and popular." It was also found that people at other campuses said, "It's the same way at my college." These findings stimulated discussions on campus about the extent that pressure to conform to an ideal influences women's lives.

It is common for women attending college to have body image issues. Research at the Center for Appearance Research (2011) at the University of the West England found that 30% of college women would trade at least 1 year of their life to achieve their ideal body weight and shape. Ten percent would trade 2 to 5 years of their life, and another 2% would trade 6 to 10 years of their life. Seventy-nine percent of the women reported they would like to lose weight, despite the fact that the majority of them (78.4%) were within the underweight or "normal" weight ranges.

Leone et al. (2011) looked at how college students perceive their bodies and to what extent that perception affects their behavior. They found that there was a strong correlation between having lower levels of body image satisfaction and risky behavioral management strategies. For example, those who had lower levels of body image satisfaction were more likely to use more risky behavior management strategies such as excessive dieting, excessive exercise dependence, supplement use, and drug use.

A growing number of researchers say that many men are also suffering from body image problems—and they are often reluctant to seek help (Morgan, 2002). Some say that binge eating has become as prevalent for college men as binge drinking—about 40% of them do it. One group of researchers has named severe body-image problems in men "the Adonis complex." It can include eating disorders and a disorder called *muscle dysmorphia*, in which

men perceive their bodies as perpetually puny. Some researchers argue that almost half of all college men are dissatisfied with their body.

Studies of men's body image have focused mainly on dimensions of adiposity and muscularity. Tiggemann et al. (2008), however, found that men were also dissatisfied with their head hair, body hair, height, and penis size. They were most concerned about their body weight, penis size, and height.

Research indicates that young men's body dissatisfaction increases when they see images of attractive muscular men. Those who are dissatisfied with their bodies are at risk for negative self-evaluations when exposed to idealized images, whereas those who are satisfied with their bodies seem to be protected against negative impacts from seeing such images (Blond, 2008). In addition, lower ratings of overall self-concept and higher levels of depression, anxiety, and interpersonal sensitivity are predictive of body image concerns in men (McFarland & Kaminski, 2009).

Interestingly, research has shown that gay men's body-image concerns are generally similar to those of heterosexual men (Martins, Tiggemann, & Churchett, 2008). Also, an investigation of transsexuals who had gone through sex-change operations (both male-to-female and female-to-male) showed that their body image was much improved as compared to their body image prior to the surgery (Kraemer et al., 2008).

Body image can be a unique problem for physically challenged people, such as those who have any kind of physical difficulty, including changes in body contours due to accident or disease and changes in body functioning that might relate to sexuality. People with disabilities or disease may view themselves as flawed or unattractive.

Depending on the type of physical challenge, various areas of concern need attention, including the feelings of loss of control over one's bodily functions, the inability to care for personal needs, the fear of being less of a person, and the feeling of being unacceptable. Education and counseling about body image are important and ideally should also involve the partners of challenged persons.

For many people, thinking about body image and how they would like to look implies becoming thinner. In recent years, however, there has also been a movement to acknowledge that there is a great range of beauty and attractiveness. For example, Emme became a well-known and sought-after size-16 supermodel. Also, *Mode*, a fashion magazine, was developed for women who wear average and large sizes.

For years the 11-inch-tall blonde, blue-eyed Barbie fashion doll (who celebrated her 50th birthday in 2009) represented the ideal American beauty—even though Barbie's stick-thin figure is impossible to achieve in real life. Now Barbie has some competition: the Emme doll. Based on super-model Emme's size 14–16 figure, it is the world's first plus-size fashion doll. Emme hopes the doll will give girls the "emotional armor" to help them deal with poor body image. The doll is a vehicle for talking about health, fitness, anorexia, and obesity, she says (Mendelsohn, 2002).

There are varying opinions regarding why some people prefer certain body shapes. Research among adults has shown a preference for average weight female figures with waist-to-hip ratios of 0.7, and average weight male figures with waist-to-hip ratios of 0.9 (Connolly, Slaughter, & Mealey, 2004). In one study, more than 500 children from 6 to 17 years of age were asked to select drawings of males and females they thought looked the nicest or most attractive. The youngest children showed preferences for the under-weight figures, changing to consistent preferences for the average weight figures in the teenage years.

Singh (2002) looked at cross-cultural feelings about attractiveness. He asked men and women from the Azores Islands, Guinea-Bissau, Indonesia, and the United States to judge the attractiveness of female figures differing in body weight and waist-to-hip ratio (WHR). There was a strong cross-cultural agreement for attractiveness. Figures with low WHR were judged to be more attractive than figures with high WHR within each weight category. Participants also judged attractive figures as less faithful than less-attractive figures. It was found that, compared to women with high WHRs, low-WHR women reported engaging in more flirting to make dates jealous, suggesting some truth to the attractiveness stereotype.

The AP–iVillage Poll (2009) suggested that there is a big disconnect between body image and true physical condition. Even though many women want to improve their body image, their behavior is often not consistent with that desire. Physical fitness is undervalued and absolute weight and appearance are overvalued. About 60% of Americans are over-weight or obese. Half don't like their weight, but just a third don't like their physical condition, even though being overweight and sedentary are big risk factors for type 2 diabetes, heart disease, and other ailments. The Poll found women putting in a median of 80 minutes of exercise per week, meaning that half do even less. The average adult is sup-posed to get at least 2 ½ hours of exercise a week for good health. In addition, just 8% of women ate the minimum recommended servings of fruits and vegetables—five a day.

As seen already, many factors can influence body image. Even engaging in "fat talk"—the common neg-ative conversations about one's own or others' bod-ies—can result in lower satisfaction with one's body and higher levels of depression. Arroyo and Harwood (2012) found that fat talk predicts changes in depres-sion, body satisfaction, and perceived pressure to be thin. This was true for both males and females. The more often one engaged in fat talk, the lower that person's body satisfaction and the higher the level of depression was likely to be.

Gender DIMENSIONS

Dissatisfaction with Body Parts

It is interesting to compare the feelings of men and women about specific parts of their body. Here are the percentages of 4,000 respondents who reported feeling dissatisfied with parts of their body:

	WOMEN	MEN
1. Overall appearance	56%	43%
2. Weight	66%	52%
3. Height	16%	16%
4. Muscle tone	57%	45%
5. Breasts/chest	34%	38%
6. Abdomen	71%	63%
7. Hips or upper thighs	61%	29%

Some respondents reported that body image and sexual experiences are related. For example, some said that as they feel less attractive, they have less desire for sexual activity.

Source: Data from Garner, D. M. The 1997 Body Image Survey results. *Psychology Today, 30* (1997), 30–44.

The Elusive Perfect Body

What does the perfect body look like? The answer to that question will probably depend on the purpose we have in mind. Taking a look at successful female athletes gives us some excellent examples. The best swimmers tend to be relatively tall and look like a capital *Y* from the front, with wide, flexible shoulders; long arms and hands; a narrow waist; and lightweight legs. Swimmers get by with more body fat than other athletes because it lets them ride higher in the water. Top speed skaters, in contrast, are shorter and look rather average from the waist up. Farther down, however, we see heavily muscled legs with rather short thighs. At the same time, the female gymnast probably has a lean, petite frame; a fine-boned face; small breasts; and long arms. A body that excels in one athletic context can be a hindrance in others.

Of course most of us are not training to be Olympic athletes, but there is a lesson here for all of us. The bodies closest to "perfect" are, to a large extent, born that way. We must take what we have and develop and use it as best we can. We can make the most of the genetic gifts we do have. In the end, the perfect body is the one that will allow you to do things you enjoy and allow you to live your life to the fullest—without compromising your health.

Why Models Look So Perfect

A quick glance at the covers of major fashion and sports magazines—or at the ads therein—seems to bolster the argument that "Some have it, some don't." These models, as well as those in many movies, seem too perfect to be real. Could these people look like that all the time? The answer is, of course, no. But they may look that way only for the millisecond that the camera snaps. However, some of the images in certain magazines may be completely computer generated. They might not even be real people! Some images of models actually consist of body parts from different people.

Getting "the look" begins long before the photo shoot ever takes place. For example, months before a movie begins production, the director (and/or art director) hires a specific personal trainer who will get "the look" that the director wants. Workouts and diet are structured to transform the actor or actress.

Still in preproduction, clothes, makeup, and lighting are chosen to enhance whatever qualities have been chosen. The day of shooting starts with hours of makeup application (sometimes over the entire body), hair styling, and clothes fitting. Ever wonder how clothes can fit so skintight on some people? No problem: The clothes are literally pasted on!

Production is the time when the camera rolls (or snaps). The art director makes clear what is desired from the photographer, who in turn adjusts lighting and the camera lens to make it happen.

Then the fun begins. During postproduction, any alterations at all can be made to the pictures. You have probably heard that blemishes are covered, teeth are routinely whitened, wrinkles in clothes are deleted. But did you know that *Penthouse* routinely augments breast size? *Playboy* thinks nothing of slimming the waist and thighs of models. A knowledgeable source has told one of the authors that when photos of a playmate's rear end were not approved, the postproduction team put a new rear end on her!

To increase the sex appeal of female models, it is not uncommon for art directors to "stretch" legs to give them a longer, thinner look. Just think: You could go from being short and stocky to having the body of Cameron Diaz with a few clicks of a computer mouse!

Eventually, the picture that emerges is one that matches the art director's vision—not one that shows

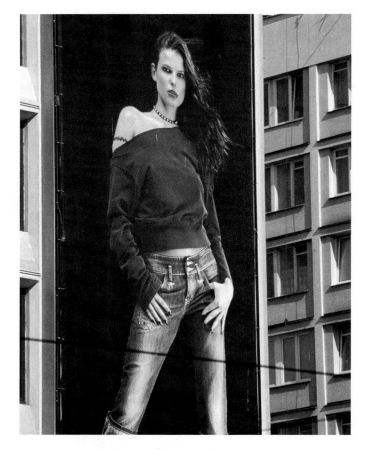

Images we see may be carefully staged and even computer generated.

(?) Did You Know . . .

the person's real body. And that is not always good. To make the point that image retouching can go too far, the retouching artist Kathy Grove redid one of the most famous Depression-era photographs, Dorothea Lange's *Migrant Mother*. Grove's point is simple: Do not believe everything you see.

Some experts believe that the all-too-perfect models who grace magazine covers send powerful—and often negative—signals to figure-conscious adolescent girls. Mind on the Media (2009) provides some interesting related statistics: Roughly $12 billion is spent on advertising and marketing to young people every year, the average young person views more than 3,000 ads per day, the number one wish for girls ages 11–17 is to be thinner, females say the media is the most important source of pressure to be thin, and as early as age 13 approximately 53% of American girls are "unhappy with their bodies." In addition, advertisers admit that they sell more than products: They use images to affect the way we see ourselves.

Concerned about images that children and adolescents see in advertisements, the American Medical Association (AMA) adopted a policy encouraging advertising associations to develop guidelines for advertisements, especially those appearing in teen-oriented publications, that would discourage the altering of photographs in a manner that could promote unrealistic expectations of appropriate body image. In one image, a model's waist was slimmed so severely that her head appeared to be wider than her waist. An AMA spokesperson said, "We must stop exposing impressionable children and teenagers to advertisements portraying models with body types only attainable with the help of photo editing software" (AMA adopts new policies at annual meeting, 2011).

The Influence of the Media

For years, some people have criticized the Barbie doll for presenting children with standards for body size and appearance that are both unrealistic and unattainable for most females. Experts also have become concerned about the impact of the "GI Joe Extreme" action figure, which has a more muscular and defined body than past GI Joe figures. At issue is whether such dolls plant the concept of the ideal body in children's minds—a concept that usually cannot be achieved without using obsessive behaviors to lose weight and gain muscle.

Recently, some clothing manufacturers developed padded bras and bikinis for girls as young as age 7. As a result of pressure from some children's advocates, and concerns that such products sexualize children and encourage them to grow up too fast, in some instances the bras and bikinis have been removed from store shelves. These products also send messages to young girls about their body image.

Relatedly, beauty pageants are another way society defines its ideal of beauty, including weight and shape. Researchers computed the body mass index (BMI) (weight divided by the square of height) of winners of the Miss America Pageant from 1922 to 1999. There was a significant decline in the BMI over that time, placing an increasing number of winners in the range of undernutrition. Pageant winners' height increased less than 2%, but body weight decreased by 12%. (Rubinstein & Caballero, 2000).

Even *Playboy* centerfold models have changed over time (Voracek & Fisher, 2002). A review of *Playboy* centerfold models' body measurements over a 50-year period showed that over time bust size and hip size decreased, while waist size increased. Body mass index and bust-to-hip ratio decreased, while waist-to-hip ratio, waist-to-bust ratio, and androgyny index increased. The study's authors concluded that shapely body characteristics of centerfold models have given way to more androgynous ones.

Interestingly, Bryla (2002) explored the effects of media on female image. She concluded that beyond media exposure, awareness and internalization of sociocultural ideals appear to be significant predictors of body image disturbance. In other words, looking at the effects of media on body image is not a simple matter.

Monro and Huon (2005) studied the effects of media-portrayed idealized images on female college students. They found that these images detrimentally affected the body image of the students.

Ashikali and Dittmar (2011) indicated that psychological research has consistently shown that women feel unhappy with their body after looking at images of thin, idealized models, which are typically represented in the media. However, they also found that materialism in the media is a further factor that makes women more vulnerable to negative body image.

While much of the media influence on body image focuses on women, men experience some similar influences and effects. In addition, we now have "men's shapewear," which are products designed to make men look better. For example, girdles have been specially designed to help men look better. There is also Spanx for Men—undershirts that fit and feel like a wetsuit. The cotton compression undershirt helps men to hide their love handles and beer bellies and gives them the look of having a sculpted chest.

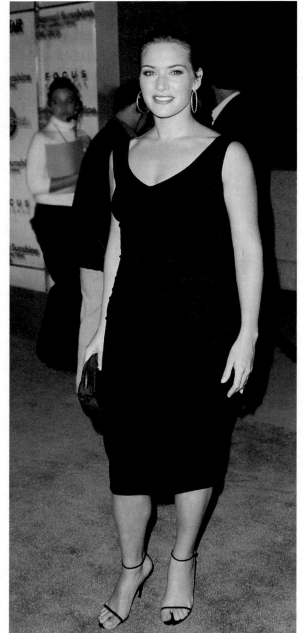

Anything is possible with photo retouching. The February 2001 issue of the U.K. edition of *GQ* magazine features a retouched image of the actress Kate Winslet. Famous for defending the appearance of fuller-figured women, Winslet has received attention not only for her acting, but also for the fluctuations in her weight. Winslet responded to the cover with shock; "I do not look like that," the actress, 37, said at the time. "And, more importantly, I don't desire to look like that." The controversy has highlighted how common it is for magazines to retouch photographs of models and celebrities, male and female. How do you think this practice affects the body image of young people?

There have been some attempts by advertisers to appeal to potential consumers of different sizes. One example in 2005 was the ad campaign for Dove beauty products. In the Dove ads, six women ranging from size 6 to 14 were shown wearing only bras, panties, and big smiles. The Dove marketing director said, "It is our belief that beauty comes in different shapes, sizes, and ages. Our mission is to make more women feel beautiful every day by broadening the definition of beauty" (Babwin, 2005). Dove personnel reported that responses from women of various sizes seemed to indicate that the ads helped them develop a more positive body image.

Long (2005) pointed out that in *Seventeen, Teen People, CosmoGirl!,* and *Teen Vogue,* there are bathing suit sections partially illustrated by girls with less-than- perfect figures and tips on maximizing assets and minimizing defects. More average women and fewer models are being used to reflect changing body types and to help self-conscious teens see that not everyone is perfect. In 2004, *Glamour* broke a barrier of sorts by putting the sizable Queen Latifah on the cover. *CosmoGirl!* shows five skin tones to reflect different ethnic groups. Compared to just a few years ago, there are now many efforts to use models of all shapes and sizes. Presenting a broader range of beauty, even under the guise of selling products, gives people more permission to believe they are attractive.

Even video games may have an influence on body image. Barlett and Harris (2008) conducted two studies to see whether playing video games that emphasized the body would increase negative body image. They found that participants in both studies had significantly lower body esteem after video game play. They concluded that video games have a negative influence on the body image of players.

Diversity and Body Image

In the past in the United States, the idea of beauty involved using the images of Barbie or Ken dolls or the like with the goal of creating some version of a white person. For example, it has been common for the winners of Latin American beauty contests to look "international": tall; not-too-dark hair; light skin; high, girlish bust; and long legs. Hispanic women often have to cope with the way the world would like to change them: if only the earrings were smaller, the makeup not so dramatic, the hair not so wild, the walk not so sexy, the hand gestures not so expressive, the emotions not so on-the-surface, and they were thinner.

Other examples related to diversity and body image are also apparent. For example, African American adolescent females seem to be happier with their bodies and less likely to diet than are European American adolescent females (Wilson et al., 1996). A major problem for some African American women who seek psychological help is their skin color. For Asian American women, eye surgery is sometimes done so they will look more like whites.

However, as the result of pressure from groups interested in emphasizing the diversity of real life, products, methods, and goals relating to beauty have changed. Even plastic surgeons have learned a lot about working with people from diverse backgrounds.

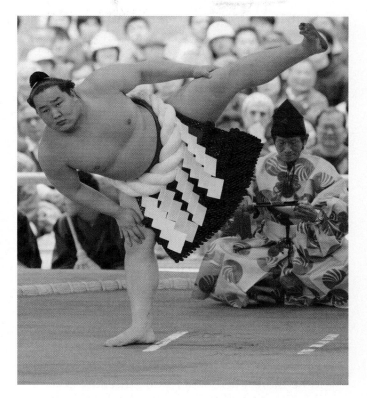

In Eastern cultures, the shape of a powerful body is that of a pyramid—with a strong base as the foundation. In Western culture the shape of a powerful body is that of an upside-down pyramid—broad shoulders and tapered waist.

Multicultural DIMENSIONS

Weight and Culture

The National Health and Nutrition Examination Survey (NHANES), which is conducted periodically by the U.S. Centers for Disease Control and Prevention (CDC), reported in 2011 that, after a quarter-century of increases, obesity prevalence did not measurably increase in recent years. But levels of obesity are still high—at 34% of U.S. adults aged 20 and older. Obesity means weighing at least 20% more than ideal weight. Data also suggest that the weight is not distributed evenly among ethnic and cultural groups:

• There were large race-ethnic disparities in obesity prevalence among women.
• Approximately 53% of non-Hispanic black women and 51% of Mexican American women aged 40–59 were obese, compared with 39% of non-Hispanic white women.

• Among women 60 and older, 61% of non-Hispanic black women were obese, compared with 37% of Mexican American women and 32% of non-Hispanic white women.
• Race/ethnic disparities in obesity were not observed in men.

Other researchers have also looked at cultural differences in body weight and in body image. For example, Grammas and Schwartz (2009) found that more Asian males were dissatisfied with their muscles than were Caucasian, Hispanic, or African American males. Also, Thomas et al. (2008) reported on similarities and differences in black and white women's perceptions about obesity. Black women disagreed with the ideal of being thin and family members' dissatisfaction with their weight. White women were interested in losing weight, but desired support during weight loss from other obese individuals.

Building a Better Self-Image

Given that none of us will be perfect, and given that we all have imperfections in our appearance, we can still look better and improve our body image. It may not always be easy, but small efforts can also make a huge difference.

When we feel good about the way we look, we are happier and likely to feel better about others. Many actions can help you improve your body image. Here are some examples:

1. Do not feel a need to apologize about every blemish you might see in your appearance. Chances are, others do not notice them anyway. None of us is perfect.

2. Be careful about basing your body image on what you see and hear in advertisements. They are carefully produced to send certain messages to sell products. Few people look and act the way the people you see in the ads do.

3. Attractive people are often judged by others to be more warm, interesting, friendly, considerate, and strong than those who are less attractive. In spite of our defects, we can do things to feel more attractive. For example, clothes, styles, and personal hygiene all affect attractiveness. What can you do to feel more attractive?

4. You should be free to be yourself; however, the message you send about your appearance and the ones you receive from others may not always be the same. For example, a person might wear a certain outfit to be comfortable; another person might interpret that as a desire to be sexy. Which messages are you sending in the appearance you present?

5. The way you move your body (body language) can indicate the way you feel about yourself. Watch what others do when they are nervous, happy, or sad. Use this information to control some of your body movements so they send messages you want to send.

Here are some additional tips for a positive body image (Body image, 2009):

- Remember that health and appearance are two different things.

- Accept and value your genes—you probably inherited a lot of traits from your family members, so love those traits as you love your family.

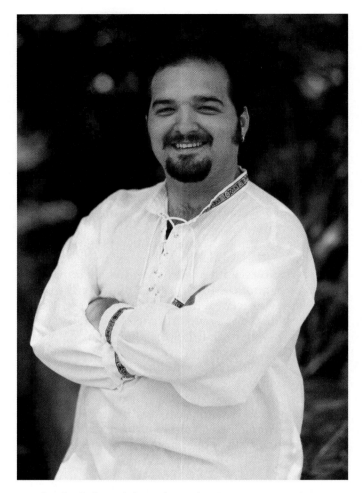

People who feel good about themselves are more attractive to others.

- Keep a list of your positive qualities that have nothing to do with your appearance.

- Surround yourself with people who are supportive and who make you feel good about yourself.

- Treat your body with respect and kindness.

Powerful people use their bodies to convey authority. One high-power pose is sitting at a desk occupying as much space as possible—feet on the desk, fingers interlaced behind the head, and elbows straight out to the sides. Another high-power pose is standing straight and leaning forward on a table or desk while talking with people or listening. These poses are in contrast to low-power poses such as slouching in a chair or standing with arms wrapped around the body. Carney et al. (2010) found that using high-power poses causes hormonal and behavioral changes for both males and females. These changes can help people behave more positively and feel better about their body image. This is another example of the importance of positive body language.

¿? Ethical DIMENSIONS

To Train or Not to Train: That Is the Question

A professionally prepared personal trainer knows how to help people develop the body to look the best it can. The trainer also knows that it is usually not possible to change the body type of a person drastically. So, what should a trainer who runs his or her own business and needs paying clients do when a person asks to look the way someone pictured in a magazine does? If the trainer agrees to help the person resemble the one in the picture, there will be false hopes created; however, you could argue that at least the person will improve his or her appearance and health—and probably body image as well. Or should the trainer tell the client that there is no way he or she can look like the picture and explain how unrealistic expectations can cause a waste of money if he or she tries to obtain objectives that cannot be reached?

Body image is important. People who feel good about themselves are more attractive to others than people who do not. Concentrate on your strengths. Do you have great hair? Eyes? Hands? Play them up. But remember your other strengths, too. Are you funny? Kind? Smart? You are more than just your looks.

There are excellent projects designed to help people improve their body image. One example is WIN Wyoming (www.uwyo.edu/winwyoming/guiding_principles.htm). It is a collaborative effort of educators and health professionals whose mission is to educate people to respect body-size diversity and to enjoy the benefits of active living, pleasurable and healthful eating, and positive self-image. Another example is Full of Ourselves: Advancing Girl Power, Health and Leadership (www.midcoast.com/-megirls/FOO.htm). It is an upbeat educational program designed to help girls improve their mental, physical, and social health and to decrease their vulnerability to the development of body preoccupation, overeating, and disordered eating behaviors. As a result of the program, girls have an improved body image, increased body satisfaction, and better body esteem.

Creating Your Optimal Body

Imagine that you are a personal trainer in a local fitness center. A center member gives you a magazine and says, "I want to look like the person in this picture, and I need you to help me do it!" What should you do?

If you are the one who wants to resemble a person in a magazine picture, it might be wise to remember that you need to optimize your own body. It does us no good to strive to be someone else. There may be qualities of other people—physical as well as others—that we want to obtain, but we cannot be exactly like another person.

Genetics: Building on Your Strong Points

A person who is 5'4" tall may strive to be an Olympic basketball player, but his or her chance of success is not good; the 6'8", 225-pound man will probably not make a good competitive gymnast. Although these examples are extreme, we need to keep them in mind when we consider what is possible and best for each of us.

Many people are not happy with the appearance of their bodies. Al Sabbah et al. (2009) surveyed adolescents in 24 countries and regions in Europe, Canada, and the United States. They found that body weight dissatisfaction was highly prevalent but was more common in girls than boys, among overweight than non-overweight individuals, and among older adolescents than younger adolescents.

Your Body Weight

Most often when we think of body weight, we think about what the scale says when we stand on it. Although this is useful information, if you are serious about reaching your optimal body weight, it would be worthwhile to learn more about some topics beyond the scope of this book: **body mass index (BMI)** and **body composition**. Knowing about these will help you understand your body weight better and have more realistic goals.

> **body mass index (BMI)**
> Weight in kilograms divided by the square of the height in meters.
>
> **body composition**
> The percentage of fat versus lean tissue.

What the scale says is not always the complete truth, and what we see is not always what we are. For example, sometimes overweight people see themselves as heavier than they really are. When they look in a mirror, they see a bigger abdomen, rear end, and thighs than they actually have. This body image may be hard to change, even if body weight decreases.

Other overweight people may see themselves as much slimmer than they really are. They often rationalize away their need to lose weight. However, some people see themselves as they really are. Those with realistic body images tend to have the greatest success with weight control.

Body weight can even continue to influence more established relationships. Meltzer et al. (2011) conducted a 4-year longitudinal study of newlywed couples. They found that husbands were more satisfied initially and wives were more satisfied over time to the extent that wives had lower BMIs than their husbands. They concluded that marriages are more satisfying when wives are thinner than their husbands.

Diet

The diet business is big business in the United States. Despite the interest in diet products and services, few people have long-term weight control success.

To have any hope of long-term success with weight loss, our approach to diets must change. A "diet" must mean permanent changes in eating habits. Do not waste time on dieting if you are not committed to maintaining a healthy weight throughout your life. If you want to change your eating habits, you must pay close attention to the kinds and amounts of foods you eat. There is no substitute for well-balanced diets and a reduction in intake of calories—especially when combined with proper exercise habits.

Exercise

Exercise plays an important role in losing pounds and keeping them off: Researchers have compared the effects of weight loss by diet only and by exercise only. They found that the group who were only exercising lost a higher percentage of fat and had more success keeping off the weight than the group who were only dieting.

Moderate exercise suppresses appetite, rather than increasing it, as many people think. You might want to exercise just before a meal to take advantage of that effect. Another benefit of exercise is that it strengthens muscle tissue. Muscle tissue requires more calories than fat tissue does to maintain itself, so as lean muscle tissue increases, more calories are burned. This is important, because our resting metabolic rate accounts for about 70% of the calories we burn.

The ultimate goal of any weight-loss program should be the loss of body fat, not just body weight. Those who combine diet and exercise lose more fat and are more likely to keep it off. Exercise and sound eating habits result in a steady weight loss that can be maintained on a permanent basis if you maintain your exercise and dietary changes.

Issues Related to Trying to Be Perfect

Although we know it is impossible to be perfect, some people are so concerned about their body image that they run into problems, such as eating disorders, obsessive muscle dysmorphia, and complications of cosmetic surgery.

Eating Disorders

In the quest to be attractive and improve one's body image, some people are willing to pay a high price. It is common to want to look as good as we can, and many people attempt to control body weight by

? Did You Know . . .

How can you tell if someone you love has an eating disorder?

Not all people with eating disorders experience symptoms, and there may be different combinations of symptoms. Someone does not have to have any or all of the following symptoms to have an eating disorder, but it is good to be alert for these symptoms:

1. Weight loss or weight fluctuation
2. Excessive exercise
3. Binging and/or purging
4. Caloric restriction
5. Picky eating
6. Misuse of laxatives or diet pills
7. Caffeine abuse
8. Misuse of ipecac or epsom salts
9. Females may quit menstruating
10. Hair loss
11. Anemia
12. Damaged teeth
13. Fingernails break easily
14. Growth of fine hair on face or body

Source: Data from How to recognize signs of an eating disorder. International Business Times (April 29, 2011). Available at: http://www.ibtimes.com/art/services/print.php?articleid=139835.

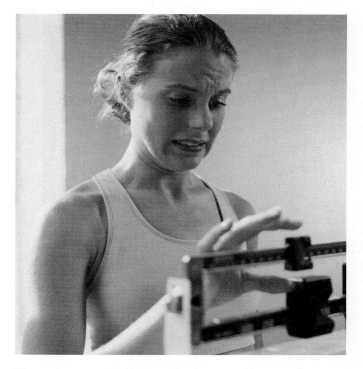

We need to pay attention to our body composition as well as our body weight.

using various diets at some time during their lives. A fear of fat seems to drive some people to extreme forms of eating behaviors. Compulsive overeating (also called *binge eating*) and compulsive dieting are the behaviors known as *eating disorders*. Striegel-Moore et al. (2008) reported that women are more likely to have eating disorders than are men. Women are significantly more likely to participate in fasting, binge eating, and vomiting. Nevertheless, a substantial minority of men have eating disorder symptoms. In addition, many college athletes show disordered eating patterns, with the greatest prevalence occurring in gymnasts and swimmers.

While they probably mean well, sometimes athletic coaches and even parents might contribute to eating disorders. They could do this by encouraging young people to diet or by demeaning their bodies by telling them they are too fat or do not have the "correct" body proportions.

The exact causes of eating disorders are not known for sure, but they seem to be triggered by life's stressors, emotional trauma, tragic events, and the media. Common health problems associated with eating disorders include intestinal problems; decayed teeth; malnutrition; dehydration; stomach ruptures; esophagus tears; serious heart, kidney, and liver damage; and death (Hughes, 2005).

Anorexia nervosa is a condition in which the individual severely limits calorie intake; it is sometimes described as self-induced starvation. The individual fears gaining weight even though he or she may already be underweight. There is also a disturbance in the way personal body weight or shape is viewed by the individual. Anorexia can be fatal. Most people with anorexia are white females younger than 25 years of age who are focused on a goal of extreme thinness and willingly starve themselves and overexercise to reach that goal.

anorexia nervosa
A condition in which the individual severely limits caloric intake.

Over the course of a lifetime, 0.5% to 3.7% of girls and women develop anorexia nervosa. Approximately 0.5% of the female population die each year as a result of their illness, making it one of the top psychiatric illnesses leading to death (Taylor et al., 2006). Although this condition affects females 95% of the time, it may be more common than previously thought among college males. Most males with anorexia are men who depend on their thin physique for employment—such as models. Anorexia results in death in about 10% of all cases in both sexes.

Although the exact cause of anorexia is unknown, it seems to involve a combination of psychological and environmental factors. The female with anorexia might reject food in an attempt to avoid dealing with what she feels are society's demands that she become a superwoman. The severe weight loss can make the female resemble a young girl, in what some researchers feel is a conscious attempt to avoid dealing with issues related to intimacy and sexuality. People with anorexia might feel that their weight is the only factor they can control in a world where expectations of others seem difficult to fulfill. One of the most difficult to understand aspects of anorexia is self-perception. Regardless of how much weight has been lost, the person with anorexia still feels too heavy (Bruess & Greenberg, 2009).

There are more than 500 websites that deal frankly, and sometimes approvingly, with anorexia and other eating disorders. One of these websites, ceruleanbutterfly.com, promotes the idea that an eating disorder is less a disease than a lifestyle choice—"a decision to pursue perfection" (Song, 2005). On the website, people with eating disorders gather for support and companionship, share tips for losing weight and hiding the signs of malnutrition, and provide "thinspiration," like photos of bony fashion models. No one knows for sure how many of the estimated 11 million Americans suffering from anorexia or bulimia visit the websites, but the developer of one of them claims to have had more than 85,000 hits in a period of about 18 months. They are often referred to as "pro-ana forums" (ana being short for anorexia). Most adolescents tend to use the websites without their parents' knowledge, and the sites can be especially

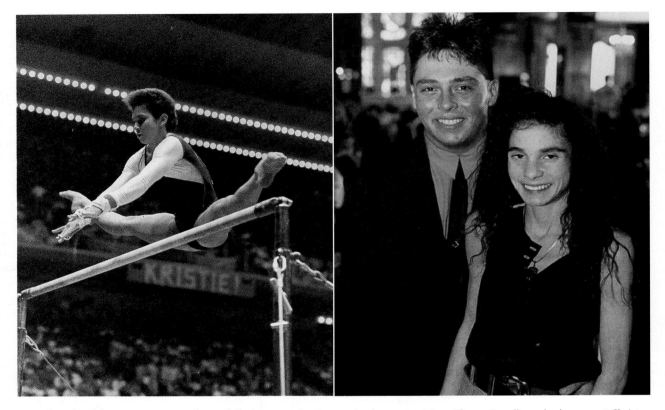

Many female athletes turn to some form of dieting to maintain an edge in competitions. The nationally ranked gymnast Christy Henrich took her dieting too far and struggled with anorexia nervosa for several years before she died of it in 1994. Here she is seen performing in the late 1980s (left) and just before her death in 1994 (right).

seductive. One girl said, "Now I can learn to be an anorexic from the Internet." The pro-ana sites are a world that is comforting to those with an eating disorder, and they provide a sense of belonging.

Bulimia nervosa is a condition in which the person periodically binges and purges, with an obsessive fear of becoming fat. Bulimia (insatiable appetite) has been confused with anorexia nervosa because periodic bingeing is common to both disorders; however, a number of the characteristics are different. People with bulimia are usually older than people with anorexia and may have been anorexic earlier. Whereas people with anorexia are obsessed with being thin, people with bulimia have an obsessive fear of becoming fat.

> **bulimia nervosa**
> A condition in which the individual periodically binges and purges, with an obsessive fear of becoming fat.

Approximately 2% to 3% of the U.S. population has bulimia. Some research indicates the rate is higher for college-age women—around 4%. The illness usually begins in late adolescence or early adult life. Only an estimated 5% to 15% of people with bulimia are male, but the incidence is increasing among males. Bulimia is often perceived to be an affliction of Caucasian girls and young women in middle and upper socioeconomic classes. However, increasing numbers of cases are being seen in men and women of all different ethnic and cultural groups. It is evident that bulimia occurs in all cultures (Schoenstadt, 2007; TieMeyer, 2007).

There is still a lot to be learned about both anorexia and bulimia. Researchers continue to discover new information about both of these eating disorders. For example, Taylor et al. (2006) found that an Internet-based intervention program may prevent some high-risk, college-age women from developing an eating disorder. In addition, Marsh et al. (2009) reported that the brain circuitry involved in regulating impulsive behavior may be less active in women suffering from bulimia. It is not clear if the brain differences are a cause or an effect of the disorder.

During their secretive eating binges, people with bulimia may consume many thousands of calories in only a few hours. Afterward, they try to purge the food through a variety of methods, including vomiting, laxatives, diuretics, and exercise. After bingeing and purging, the person with bulimia may feel discouraged about the behavior.

Binge-eating disorder (BED) is an eating disorder characterized by recurrent binge eating but not by inappropriate weight-control behaviors. Persons with

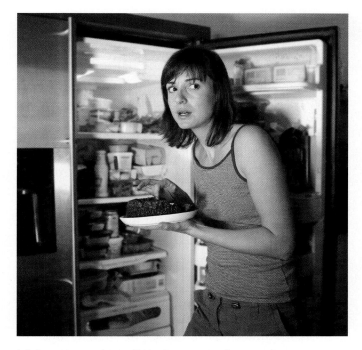

It is important to be realistic about our eating practices.

binge-eating disorder (BED)
Eating disorder characterized by recurrent binge eating but not by inappropriate weight-control behaviors.

BED do not regularly engage in purging, and the majority are obese. They also may be referred to as "compulsive overeaters."

Characteristics of binge eating include eating much more rapidly than normal, eating until feeling uncomfortably full, eating large amounts even though one is not hungry, eating alone because of embarrassment about eating habits, and feeling disgusted or guilty after overeating. There is usually a feeling that one cannot stop eating or control what or how much is being eaten.

Treating Eating Disorders

Many approaches are used in the treatment of anorexia, but the prognosis is not good. Drug therapy is used in about 25% of the cases, and behavior modification in about 45%. A combination of approaches is also used. Most specialists recommend a period of hospitalization to ensure weight gain, and families are often involved in the therapy. The prognosis for people with anorexia is worse than for people with bulimia.

Overcoming bulimia requires establishing a normal eating pattern that eliminates dieting. Although people with bulimia can hide their disorder from others, they are more likely than people with anorexia to seek treatment; however, they might expect immediate results and become frustrated with therapy. Antidepressant drugs are used in the treatment of bulimia, as is psychological therapy. Antidepressant

medication and psychological treatments can also reduce binge eating of BED patients.

Muscle Dysmorphia

Body image and goals related to it may change over time. Thus, as someone makes progress with weights, or in gymnastics or figure skating, the ideal of the perfect body image may become more "perfect." A perpetual chasing of the ideal can cause people to lose perspective about their actual body image. An example of this was given in the opening story of this chapter.

One disorder that afflicts bodybuilders is essentially the opposite of anorexia nervosa. Called **muscle dysmorphia**, also known as bigorexia and reverse anorexia, it involves bodybuilders who, despite their extremely muscular bodies and tip-top shape, consider themselves to be puny. Weight lifting, for some people, can become a dangerous obsession.

muscle dysmorphia
A disorder whereby a bodybuilder in top shape considers himself or herself to be puny.

Dawes et al. (2009) provided an overview of the literature related to muscle dysmorphia (MD). They pointed out that MD is characterized by an overwhelming compulsion with accruing large amounts of lean mass. It occurs mainly in men, but women who are bodybuilders can also have MD. People with MD are preoccupied by irrational thoughts regarding their perceived small musculature despite actually having high levels of muscular development. This preoccupation can lead to increased mood, social, and anxiety disorders. It is not uncommon for people with MD to miss important social, occupational, and/or recreational activities because of a compulsive need to maintain a specific workout and dietary schedule. They might even sever personal relationships and turn down professional opportunities and job promotions to devote more time to their time-consuming training regimes. Supplements and pharmacological interventions (especially steroids) are commonly used to attain greater levels of muscularity. It is hard to determine an exact cause of MD, but research indicates that continuous exposure to idealized male body images portrayed in the media and in male action figures may have a negative impact on male body image satisfaction. Some health risks associated with MD are musculoskeletal injuries from overtraining, increased risk of cardiovascular disease, kidney failure, steroid abuse, drug addiction, eating disorders, infections, disease from the use of dirty and/or shared needles, and even death.

Interestingly, in one study American and European college men were asked to pick a body type that they thought women would find attractive. The

Gender DIMENSIONS

Why Are Eating Disorders Mainly Found in Women?

It seems clear that physical attractiveness is more important for women than men. This is because beauty is often a central aspect of femininity (girls learn early that being pretty draws attention to them), and women's self-worth is often tied to establishing and maintaining close relationships. They can improve their feeling of self-worth based on others' opinions and approval of them.

The ideal standard of physical attractiveness has become thinner over the past few decades. This makes it even harder for women to meet the standard, so they are more likely to resort to extreme ways to control their weight—such as rigid dieting and purging.

Even when men take extreme measures to control their weight, it is usually done to improve their athletic performance (such as with jockeys and wrestlers). Their goal of losing weight is secondary to their goal of performing well. For women, however, dieting to achieve an ideal weight is related to their self-evaluation.

---

average pick had 20 to 30 more pounds of muscle than a normal man. When women were asked the same question, they chose the normal-sized man most of the time (Fahmy, 2004).

A simple test for bigorexia involves questions like: (1) How often do you look at your body in the mirror? (2) Do you think your body needs to be leaner and more muscular? (3) Do you find yourself reading up on new training methods, diets, and supplements? (4) Do you eat special high-protein or low-fat diets or use food supplements to improve muscularity? (5) Do you ever wear baggy clothes to hide the body you feel is too lean—or do you avoid situations where your body might be seen? (6) Do you still train when injured because you fear losing muscle mass? (7) Do you compare yourself to other men and feel envious? (8) Do you ever think others are snickering at your puniness? (9) Would you rather spend time going to the gym than having sex, and has your libido taken a dive? (10) Have you turned down social events, taken time off from work, or skipped family responsibilities so you can work out? Typically, men who have bigorexia will say "yes" to three or more of these questions (Mind over fatter, 2005).

Muscle dysmorphia does not usually involve the serious medical complications of anorexia, but it still can have significant effects. It is certainly normal for people who go to a gym to want to improve their physique and build larger muscles. The turning point from normal goals to muscle dysmorphia occurs when the quest for "massive" size takes over one's life, destroying career, relationships, and, ironically, self-esteem.

Sports and Dieting

Eating disorders may be the gravest health problem facing female athletes, affecting gymnasts, figure skaters, swimmers, distance runners, divers, and even tennis and volleyball players. Given the importance that sport attaches to weight—and, in subjectively judged sports, to appearance—it is not surprising that eating disorders are common among athletes.

But weight—and dieting—also play a major role in endurance sports. As an athlete's weight falls, his or her aerobic power increases. Put another way, it takes less energy to run if you weigh less; thus

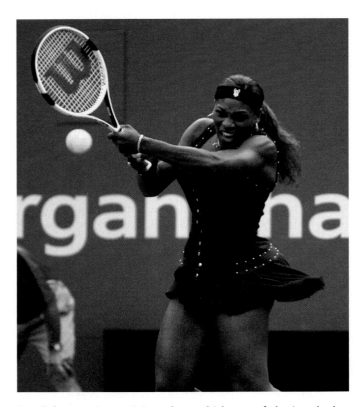

People have various opinions about which type of physique looks attractive.

more energy can be expended on running faster. So runners and swimmers also succumb to the need to diet to win.

Steroid Use

Steroids are synthetic versions of the male hormone testosterone. Steroid abuse is fast becoming a very serious problem among adolescent males, both athletes and nonathletes, who take large doses in an attempt to achieve much greater body mass quickly. In addition to potential to halt growth and bone development, steroid use can cause testicular shrinkage, increased cholesterol levels, infertility, decreased sexual drive, prostate cancer, kidney disorders, liver malfunction, aggression and violence,

> **steroids**
> Synthetic versions of the male hormone testosterone that promote tissue growth.

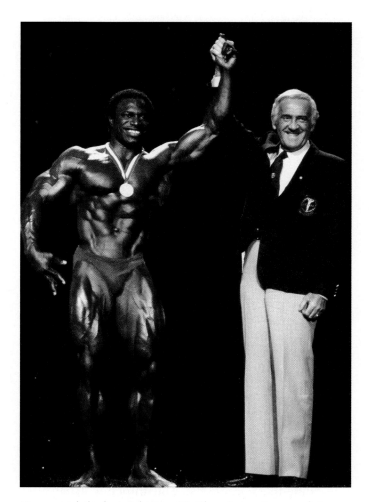

Many people look at eight-time Mr. Olympia Lee Haney only in terms of his muscles. But Haney keeps body image in perspective, placing God, family, and friends above business—and to Haney, bodybuilding was a business.

suicidal tendencies, and extreme moodiness. Steroids can also be psychologically and physically addictive.

Steroid abuse is a problem among teenagers. Johnston et al. (2009) reported that there was a fairly sharp increase in the use of steroids by male teens in the late 1990s, with peak levels reached in 1999 among eighth-grade males, in 2000 among tenth-grade males, and in 2001 and 2002 among twelfth-grade males. Since those peak years, the annual prevalence rate has dropped by more than half among eighth- and tenth-grade males (to 1.2% and 1.4%, respectively), and by one-third among twelfth-grade males (to 2.5% annual prevalence in 2008). Steroid use is not limited to males, however. While the prevalence rates tend to be much lower among females, the trend toward steroid use by females is much the same as for males.

People may go to unhealthy extremes simply to look good. Goodale and coworkers (2001) reported that the most common reason male bodybuilders give for using steroids is to enhance looks.

Women in endurance sports also take steroids. Steroids help a runner in two ways: A thin runner expends less energy in running; by speeding muscle recovery, a long-distance runner is able to recover faster, train more, and thus run faster.

The adverse effects of steroids in women include lowered voice, increased body and facial hair, male-pattern baldness, enlarged clitoris, decreased breast size, and changes in or cessation of menstruation. There are not sufficient studies of female steroid users to fully understand the extent to which a woman's body may be damaged and whether the effects are permanent.

In addition to the many adverse effects of steroids listed, there is a risk of HIV transmission through shared needles. Finally, anabolic steroids are illegal in the United States; their use carries stiff fines and possible imprisonment.

Some feel that a "male body ideal" has caused increasing numbers of males to develop an "Adonis complex"—defined as a condition shared by millions of males who develop eating disorders, abuse steroids, work out compulsively, or otherwise obsess over their physical appearance. The taboo against overt male vanity inhibits men from seeking help for their disorders (Miller & Sharlet, 2000).

Makeovers and Cosmetic Surgery

If we pay attention to our favorite movie and TV stars, we see that they radically change their appearance from time to time. The makeover has become a powerful draw for many stars—they feel it can renew the spirit, save a career, and even mend the heart. Indeed, Hollywood may be in the grip of a redo revolution. Some stars like to re-create themselves,

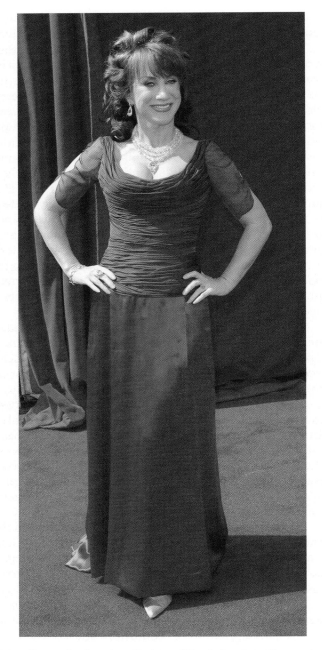

According to the American Society of Plastic Surgeons, liposuction is the most popular cosmetic surgery procedure for men and women, after rhinoplasty. Comedian Kathy Griffin underwent liposuction in an attempt to drop from a size 4 to a size 2. Medical complications during and after the surgery, as she recounts in an article published by *Glamour* magazine, proved to be nearly fatal. Have you ever considered undergoing cosmetic surgery in pursuit of your ideal body? Do you think the benefits outweigh the risks?

increase their confidence by showing that they can wear more than one style, and avoid being linked with a look created by a past role.

According to the American Society of Plastic Surgeons, the number of cosmetic procedures in the United States increased to more than 13.1 million in 2010, a 5% increase from 2009 (American Society of Plastic Surgeons, 2011). Some people feel this increase relates to a surge in reality cosmetic surgery television programming. Viewing reality cosmetic surgery shows is significantly related to more favorable cosmetic surgery attitudes, perceived pressure to have cosmetic surgery, past attainment of a cosmetic procedure, a decreased fear of surgery, and overall body dissatisfaction and disordered eating (Sperry et al., 2009).

In our quest to create the perfect look, we may see the stars radically change theirs and decide we want to do it too. People today often view their body as increasingly malleable. Sometimes, they even want to use ways that look easy, such as liposuction, implants, and plastic surgery.

Liposuction is a technique for removing adipose (fat) tissue with a suction-pump device. A hollow suction tube, which is attached to a special vacuum, is inserted into small incisions in the skin. It is used primarily to remove

> **liposuction**
> A technique for removing adipose tissue with a suction-pump device.

and reduce areas of fat around the abdomen, breast, legs, face, and upper arms. Liposuction can be helpful for the removal of fat in particular areas, but it should not be viewed as a way to lose large amounts of fat or to change one's physique dramatically. Most people lose an average of only 3 pounds as a direct result of the procedure. According to the American Society of Plastic Surgeons (2011), liposuction was the fourth most common cosmetic procedure in 2010, with just over 203,000 such procedures performed. That was a 2% decrease since 2009 and a 43% decrease since 2000. The average physician fee was about $3,000.

Breast implants have been around for quite a few years. Silicone-gel–filled breast implants first went on the market in 1962. They were banned in 1992 by the Food and Drug Administration (FDA). The question of whether they should be used has been greatly debated. In April 2005, an FDA advisory committee voted to recommend allowing them back on the market under certain conditions—making sure women understand potential risk, having women get regular MRI exams, allowing only specially trained plastic surgeons to perform the insertions, and requiring continued research studies related to the implants. Women who wanted a return of the product say silicone-gel implants look and feel more natural than the saline-filled implants. The implants have been exonerated from concerns that they might cause serious or chronic illnesses such as cancer or lupus. Aside from the risk of breakage and pain, however, they can cause infection and development of painful scar tissue. Breast augmentation was the most common cosmetic surgical procedure in 2010, with just over 296,000 performed. This was a 2% increase over 2009 and a 39% increase over 2000. The average physician fee was about $3,400 (American Society of Plastic Surgeons, 2011).

Cosmetic surgery includes the procedures already mentioned, and there are also many other possibilities. Many people elect to have cosmetic surgery when a part of their body makes them self-conscious or uncomfortable. After surgery, many patients say they have a more positive self-image. Statistically, about 9% of the total number of cosmetic operations are done on men. About 89% are done on Caucasians, 9% on Hispanics, 6% on African Americans, and 5% on Asian Americans (American Society for Aesthetic Plastic Surgery, 2009).

> **cosmetic surgery**
> Surgery done for the sole purpose of improving the appearance.
>
> **rhinoplasty**
> Surgery done to change the shape of the nose.

Another common procedure is **rhinoplasty** (surgery done to change the shape of the nose). It usually takes 1 to 2 hours and costs an average of $4,300. It is not covered by insurance unless the nose structure impedes breathing. As with any surgery, there can be undesirable results. The patient may not like the aesthetic result and want a revision, the newly formed nose may make breathing difficult, or fibrous scar tissue may form. In 2010 over 252,000 rhinoplasty procedures were performed. This was a drop of 1% from 2009 and 35% from 2000 (American Society of Plastic Surgeons, 2011).

Some men turn to implants to enhance their pectoral muscles. The average cost for putting in a pair of palm-size silicone discs is just over $3,800. This is a relatively new procedure. In 2010 222 pectoral implants were performed, a 3% drop from 2009. In 2010 more than 1.1 million men elected to have cosmetic procedures, a 2% increase over 2009. Men accounted for 9% of all cosmetic procedures; 91% of all procedures were performed on women (11.5 million—a 5% increase over 2009) (American Society of Plastic Surgeons, 2011).

The top five procedures may be listed differently depending upon the source. The American Society of Plastic Surgeons (2011) lists the top five for women as being breast augmentation (296,000), nose reshaping (189,000), liposuction (179,000), eyelid surgery (177,000), and tummy tuck (112,000). The top five for men were nose reshaping (64,000), eyelid surgery (31,000), liposuction (24,000), breast reduction (18,000), and hair transplantation (13,000).

If you watched the Austin Powers movies, you may have laughed at Austin for having a penis-enlargement pump. Men's magazines and websites are filled with ads for pumps, pills, weights, exercises, and surgeries that are supposed to increase the length and/or the width of the penis. However, no scientific research supports the use of any nonsurgical method to enlarge the penis, and no reputable medical society endorses penis-enlargement surgery performed for purely cosmetic reasons. Many of these techniques can damage the penis and may even cause functional problems. Cosmetic surgeons have developed several enlargement techniques, but none of them are endorsed by medical organizations. Following various procedures, some men have had to undergo additional surgeries to correct deformities caused by the original procedure. Others have had scarring, shorter penises, hair on the base of the penis, low-hanging penis, loss of sensitivity, and bumps and lumps. Other complaints include loss of sexual function, urinary incontinence, and persistent pain. Surgery should only be an option for penises that have been amputated or damaged for some reason (Beware of penis enlargement scams, 2005).

Some women want breast implants; others want to have large, heavy breasts reduced in size. The latter procedure may not necessarily be considered cosmetic surgery, depending on the intention and the situation, because it may be performed to relieve physical ailments such as back and neck pain caused by large, heavy breasts. It involves removal of fat and breast tissue and may leave noticeable scars. The procedure may also affect the ability to breastfeed. It usually takes 2 to 4 hours and costs an average of $5,400. It may be covered by insurance if medical problems are associated with the size of the breasts. In 2010 about 138,000 breast reductions were performed on females, as compared with 48,000 in 1997 (American Society for Aesthetic Plastic Surgery, 2011).

Whereas liposuction only removes fat, the **tummy tuck** is a more extensive surgical procedure that removes excess skin and fat from the lower abdomen and tightens the abdominal muscles. It usually requires a hip-to-hip lower-abdominal incision and takes 1 to 2 hours to complete if fat deposits are below the navel. If a more extensive procedure

> **tummy tuck**
> Extensive surgical procedure that removes excess skin and fat from the abdomen.

is needed, it can take 2 to 5 hours. It costs $5,000 to $9,000, with an average total cost of $6,400, usually not covered by insurance (American Society of Aesthetic Plastic Surgery, 2011).

Other available procedures include face lifts, upper and lower eyelid reduction, and chin implantation. In short, we can have just about any part of our body altered if we are strongly motivated and have the means to pay for it. Because it is legal in most U.S.

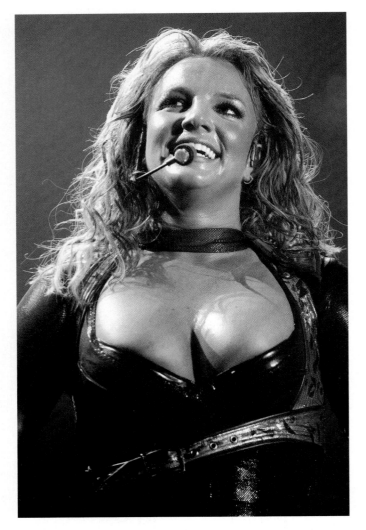

Young girls emulate superstars like Britney Spears, who in 1999 is rumored to have had breast augmentation surgery. In fact, according to the American Society of Plastic and Reconstructive Surgeons, 3,095 girls age 18 and younger had breast implants in 2002, up 19% from 2001 and up 59% from 1999. Breast augmentation surgery is the most common cosmetic surgery procedure for women, with 264,000 operations performed in 2005. Interestingly, most of the surgeries take place in California, Texas, and Florida—why do think that is the case?

states for any physician to advertise himself or herself as a plastic or cosmetic surgeon, candidates for surgery must select a well-trained plastic surgeon for any type of cosmetic surgery.

Several trends indicate that cosmetic surgery will continue to be a growth industry. Younger people are getting more cosmetic procedures, people who have had cosmetic procedures tend to have others, men are becoming more "vain," the number getting surgery has increased rapidly, and the aging of the population is likely to result in more cosmetic surgery (Grant, 2001).

The top five nonsurgical cosmetic procedures in 2009 were Botox injection (2.4 million procedures); injection of hyaluronic acid (a jelly-like substance that softens facial lines and furrows; 1.3 million procedures); laser hair removal (936,000 procedures); microdermabrasion (mechanical scraping of the top layers of the skin to soften sharp edges of surface irregularities; 563,000 procedures), and chemical peel (494,000 procedures). People age 35–50 had the most procedures—4 million (44% of the total). People age 19–34 had 20%, people age 51–64 had 28%, people age 65 and older had 7%, and people age 18 and younger had 1.3% of the procedures (American Society for Aesthetic Plastic Surgery, 2011).

Finally, body piercing and tattoos have been used by some people to enhance their body image. No longer a practice carried out in back rooms, body piercing and tattoos are making their way into socially acceptable studios. Although many people have questioned the motivations behind body piercing, some feel it gives people a strong sense of self and a connection with others by marking relationship events in commitment ceremonies, by enhancing people's feelings about their body, by providing the rush of the piercing experience, and by giving people a way to rebel against mainstream society. The most common places for body piercing are the face or ears; some people pierce their tongues, nipples, abdomen, and genitals. This practice is not risk-free; it sometimes produces infection.

Summary

- Body image refers to the mental image we have of our own physical appearance. It is influenced by many factors, and in turn, influences our attitudes and behaviors.

- The media play a major role in influencing people's body images. Many media images are unattainable in real life.

- People from different cultures may view body image very differently.

- We can do a lot to build a better body image by not apologizing for all our blemishes; not basing our body image on what we see in the media; dressing and acting in ways that make us feel more attractive; and paying attention to our body language.

- Diet and exercise can play major roles related to body image.

- Some people are so concerned about their body image that they develop eating disorders such as anorexia nervosa, bulimia nervosa, and binge-eating disorder.

- Using steroids in an attempt to develop one's body is a very dangerous thing to do. Steroids cause many serious health problems.

- Cosmetic surgery has become much more popular today than it was just 10 to 12 years ago. The most common procedures include liposuction, breast augmentation, eyelid surgery, tummy tuck, and nose reshaping.

Discussion questions

1. Explain how the media have created unrealistic body images for women and men.

2. Which strategies can be used to create a more positive body image?

3. Which problems, both physical and psychological, occur when people try to make themselves more "perfect"?

Application Questions

Reread the story that opens the chapter and answer the following questions:

1. As do many teens, Marc had a poor body image. Teased by his friends ("Ostrich Boy") and haunted by the images in men's magazines, he turned to lifting weights. If you had a chance to talk to a group of 14-year-old boys, what advice would you give them on how to handle body-image issues? What about a group of 14-year-old girls?

2. One of the problems about weight lifting to improve body image is that you can "never be too big." The more muscle you gain, the more you strive for. But as goals are set higher, workouts require more time in the gym, more sleep for recovery, and more time for eating properly. How is it possible to manage the desire for continued physical improvement without becoming obsessive?

3. Consider the changes in Marc's body image as he goes to law school, gets a job, gets married, has children, and so on. How might Marc's body image change across time? If he suddenly found himself divorced and single at age 40 years, should he hit the weights again?

Critical Thinking Questions

1. Because excessive weight has been linked to many health problems, why should we all not strive to be thin? Is it more harmful to diet excessively or to be obese?

2. You are an assistant college coach. An athlete returns from summer vacation, having put on 30 pounds of muscle. He says he spent the summer "lifting his ass off." You think he may have used steroids. Would you report him to the school's athletic director? (If he were found to have taken steroids, he could be expelled from school. However, if he continued to use steroids, he could suffer serious medical problems.)

3. Would your answer to question 2 be different if a female athlete returned in the fall with an additional 15 pounds of muscle? Explain your answer.

4. The noted eating-disorder psychologist G. Terence Wilson has stated that, biologically, women cannot be thin and have large breasts. Yet many women exercise and diet until they have low body fat and then have breast implants to compensate. Role models for the thin-yet-busty type include professional bodybuilders, many of the athletes on daytime TV exercise shows, and many actresses. How do such role models affect women?

Critical Thinking Case

Before attending college, your girlfriend Amanda ran cross-country and track. But with the pressures of college studies, part-time work, and your relationship, she has little time to exercise. She has started to worry more and more about the "freshman 15," the extra weight that many college freshmen gain. She often comments on how good the cover girls on fashion magazines look. That is not all: You have noticed she rarely eats when you go out. When you mention this, she says she is trying to help save money for a vacation. When you find over-the-counter diet pills hidden under her bed, she says, "Everyone takes them." When you tell her that someone heard her throwing up in the bathroom after meals, she flatly denies it. When you tell her she is looking "rather thin," she smiles and says, "Thank you."

You have read the information in this chapter and do not believe that she has an eating disorder. However, you are concerned about Amanda's physical health and psychological well-being. How could you help her to improve her body image?

Exploring Personal Dimensions

Body Image

How do you feel about the appearance of these regions of your body?

	Quite satisfied	Somewhat satisfied	Somewhat dissatisfied	Very dissatisfied
Hair	❏	❏	❏	❏
Arms	❏	❏	❏	❏
Hands	❏	❏	❏	❏
Feet	❏	❏	❏	❏
Waist	❏	❏	❏	❏
Buttocks	❏	❏	❏	❏
Hips	❏	❏	❏	❏
Legs and ankles	❏	❏	❏	❏
Thighs	❏	❏	❏	❏
Chest/ breasts	❏	❏	❏	❏
Posture	❏	❏	❏	❏
General attractiveness	❏	❏	❏	❏

1. Which of your thoughts and actions enhance your body image?

2. Which of your thoughts and actions are detrimental to your body image?

3. Which societal forces (e.g., expectations of friends and parents, advertising, celebrities and professional athletes) influence your body image most strongly?

4. What could you do to become more satisfied with your body image?

Suggested Readings

Anderson, E., Siegel, E. H., Bliss-Moreau, E., & Barrett, L. F. The visual impact of gossip. *Science, 332, no. 6036* (June 2011), 1446–1448.

American Society of Asethetic Plastic Surgery. (2012). Available: http://www.surgery.org/media/statistics.

American Society of Plastic Surgeons. (2012). Available: http://www.plasticsurgery.org.

Cope, M. B., & Allison, D. B. Obesity: person and population. *Obesity Research, 14* (November 2010), 156–159.

Johnson, S. K., Podratz, K. E., Dipboye, R. L., & Gibbons, E. Physical attractiveness biases in ratings of employment suitability: Tracking down the "beauty is beastly" effect. *Journal of Social Psychology, 150, no. 3* (May/June 2010), 301–318.

Lin, L., & Reid, K. The relationship between media exposure and antifat attitudes: The role of dysfunctional appearance beliefs. *Body Image, 6, no. 1* (January 2009), 52–55.

Markey, C. N., & Markey, P. M. A correlation and experimental examination of reality television viewing and interest in cosmetic surgery. *Elsevier 7* (November 2010), 165–171.

Slater, A., & Tiggemann, M. Body image and disordered eating in adolescent girls and boys: a test of objectification theory. *Sex Roles, 63* (2010), 42–49.

Swami, V., Chamorro-Premuzic, T., Bridges, S., & Furnham, A. Acceptance of cosmetic surgery: Personality and individual difference predictors. *Body Image, 6, no. 1* (January 2009), 7–13.

Web Resources

For links to the websites below, visit *go.jblearning* *.com/dimensions/5e* and click on Resource Links.

Club Drug Counselor: Male Body Issues
www.josephlafleur.com/about_Male_Body_Issues.htm

Provides information about male health issues related to body image. Includes some comparisons from different cultures.

Eating Disorder Referral and Information Center
http://edreferral.com

Dedicated to the prevention and treatment of eating disorders. Information and treatment resources are given for all forms of eating disorders.

LiveWell Colorado
www.livewellcolorado.org

Committed to preventing and reducing obesity by promoting healthy eating and active living. LiveWell Colorado inspires and advances policy, environmental, and lifestyle changes that aim to provide access to healthy foods and opportunities for physical activity in the community.

Media Awareness Network
www.media-awareness.ca

Deals with many issues in the media, including stereotypes about females and males. Emphasis is on female stereotypes and their effect on cultural ideas of beauty and social development. The effect of media portrayals of what masculinity means is included.

National Eating Disorder Association
www.nationaleatingdisorders.org

Provides general information about eating disorders and body-image concerns along with possible referrals for treatment, educational materials, and opportunities to help through volunteering.

Women's Issues
www.womensissues.about.com

Contains information on many women's issues including stereotypes, body image, and self-improvement.

References

Al Sabbah, H., Vereecken, C., Elgar, F. J., Nansel, T., Aasvee, K., Abdeen, Z., Ojaia, K., Ahiuwalia, N., & Maes, L. Body weight dissatisfaction and communication with parents among adolescents in 24 countries: International cross-sectional survey. *BMC Public Health, 9, 1* (February 6, 2009), 52.

AMA adopts new policies at annual meeting. *AMA News*, June 21, 2011. Available: http://www.ama-assn.org/amam/pub/mews/news/a11-new-policies-page.

American Society for Aesthetic Plastic Surgery. ASAPS 2010 statistics on cosmetic surgery. Available: http://www.surgery.org/media/statistics.

American Society for Aesthetic Plastic Surgery. Quick facts, 2009. Available: http://www.surgery.org/download/2007QFacts.pdf.

American Society of Plastic Surgeons. Report of the 2010 plastic surgery statistics. 2011. Available: http://www.plasticsurgery.org.

AP–iVillage Poll, May 4, 2009. Available: http://www.msnbc.msn.com/id/30687221/ns/health_diet_and_nutrition/t/poll-women-value-weight-over-physical-health/.

Arroyo, A., & Harwood, J. Exploring the causes and consequences of engaging in fat talk. *Journal of Applied Communication Research, 40, no. 2* (May 2012), 167–187.

Ashikali, E., & Dittmar, H. The effect of priming materialism on women's responses to thin-idea media. *British Journal of Social Psychology*, 2011; DOI: 10.1111/j.2044-8309.2011.02020.x.

Babwin, Don. Dove ads featuring "real women" meant to be an inspiration. *The Birmingham News* (August 3, 2005), 1G, 5G.

Barlett C. P., & Harris, R. J. The impact of body emphasizing video games on body image concerns in men and women. *Sex Roles, 59, 7–8* (October 2008), 586–601.

Beware of penis-enlargement scams. MayoClinic.com (May 24, 2005). Available: http://www.mayoclinic.com/.

Blond, A. Impacts of exposure to images of ideal bodies on male body dissatisfaction: A review. *Body Image, 5, 3* (September 2008), 244–250.

Body image. Planned Parenthood, 2009. Available: http://www.plannedparenthood.org/health-topics/body-image-23374.htm.

Bruess, C. E., & Greenberg, J. S. *Sexuality education: Theory and practice*, 5th ed. New York: Macmillan, 2009.

Bryla, K. Y. Effects of media on female body image: myth or reality? *Health Education Monograph Series, 19, no. 2* (2002), 13–16.

Carney, D. R., Cuddy, A. J. C., & Yap, A. J. Brief nonverbal displays affect neuroendocrine levels and risk tolerance. *Psychological Science, 21, no. 10* (October 2010), 1363–1368.

Centre for Appearance Research. 30% of women would trade at least one year of their life to achieve their ideal body weight and shape. *Science Daily*. March 2011. Available: http://www.sciencedaily.com/releases/2011/04/11040411812.htm.

Connolly, J. M., Slaughter, V., & Mealey, L. The development of preferences for specific body shapes. *Journal of Sex Research, 41, no. 1* (Feb. 2004), 5–15.

Dawes, J., Roozen, M., & Spano, M. Muscle dysmorphia. National Strength and Conditioning Association, June 5, 2009. Available: http://www.nsca-lift.org/HotTopic/download/Muscle_Dysmporphia.pdf.

Donaghue, N. Body satisfaction, sexual self-schemas, and subjective well-being in women. *Body Image, 6, 1* (January 2009), 37–42.

Fahmy, S. Males insecure over muscle mass. *The Spokane Spokesman Review*, (July 27, 2004), C6.

Garner, D. *The 1997 Psychology Today Body Image Survey*. Available: http://www.psychologytoday.com/print/25283.

Goodale, K. R., Watkins, P. L., & Cardinal, B. J. Muscle dysmorphia: A new form of eating disorder? *American Journal of Health Education, 32, no. 5* (September/October 2001), 260–266.

Grammas, D., & Schwartz, J. Internalization of messages from society and perfectionism as predictors of male body image. *Body Image, 6, no. 1* (January 2009), 31–36.

Grant, P. Face Time. *Modern Maturity, 22, no. 2* (March–April 2001), 60–69.

Hughes, Z. Dying to be thin. *Ebony* (July 2005), 72–76.

Johnston, L. D., O'Malley, P. M., Bachman, J. G., & Schulenberg, J. E. *Monitoring the Future national results on adolescent drug use: Overview of key findings, 2008*. Bethesda, MD: National Institute of Drug Abuse, 2009.

Kraemer, B., Delsignore, A., Schnyder, U., & Hepp, U. Body image and transsexualism. *Psychopathology, 41, 2* (December 2008), 96–100.

Leone, J. E., Partridge, J. A., & Maurer-Starks, S. Psychobehavioral attributes of body image in college freshman and seniors: Implications for long-term health. *The Health Educator, 43, no. 1* (Spring 2011), 13–20.

Lipka, S. Feminine critique. *Chronicle of Higher Education, 50, no. 37* (May 21, 2004), A35–36.

Long, C. Female magazines evolve to feature flabby. *Intelihealth.* Harvard Medical School's Consumer Health Information (2005). Available: http://www.intelihealth.com.

Marsh, R., Steinglass, J. E., Gerber, A. J., O'Leary, K. G., Wang, Z., Murphy, D., Walsh, T., & Peterson, B. S. Deficient activity in the neural systems that mediate self-regulatory control in bulimia nervosa. *Archives of General Psychiatry, 66, 1* (2009), 51–63.

Martins, Y., Tiggemann, M., & Churchett, L. The shape of things to come: Gay men's satisfaction with specific body parts. *Psychology of Men and Masculinity, 9, 4* (October 2008), 248–256.

McFarland, M. B., & Kaminski, P. L. Men, muscles, and mood: The relationship between self-concept, dysphoria, and body image disturbances. *Eating Behavior, 10, 1* (January 10, 2009), 68–70.

Meltzer, A. L., McNulty, J. K., Novak, S. A., Butler, E. A., & Karney, B. R. Marriages are more satisfying when wives are thinner than their husbands. *Social Psychology and Personality Science, 2* (July 2011), 416–424.

Mendelsohn, A. You big, beautiful (and realistic) doll. *The Birmingham News* (December 22, 2002), D1.

Miller, D. W., & Sharlet, J. The Adonis complex studies men's obsession with a "male body ideal": Physicist examines "the soul-battering system" that envelops professionals. *Chronicle of Higher Education*, Research & Publishing section, May 26, 2000. Available: http://www.chronicle.com.

Mind on the Media. Inspiring independent thinking and fostering critical analysis of media messages, 2009. Available: http://www.mindonthemedia.org/index.php?type=static&page=shocking.

Mind over fatter: The bulk of bigorexia (2005). Available: http://www.mindoverfatter.co.za/html/bigorexia.htm.

Monro, F., & Huon, G. Media-portrayed idealized images, body shame, and appearance anxiety. *International Journal of Eating Disorders, 38, 1* (July 2005), 85–90.

Morgan, R. The men in the mirror. *Chronicle of Higher Education, 49, no. 5* (September 27, 2002), A53–A54.

People. Scoop. January 27, 2003. Available: http://www.people.com/people/article/0,,20139090,00.html.

Rubinstein, S., & Caballero, B. Is Miss America an undernourished role model? *Journal of the American Medical Association*, Research Letter, *283, no. 12* (March 22/29, 2000), 1569.

Sanchez, D. T., & Kiefer, A. K. Body concerns in and out of the bedroom: Implications for sexual pleasure and problems. *Archives of Sexual Behavior, 36, 6* (December 2007), 808–820.

Schoenstadt, A. Bulimia statistics. *MedTV*, January 29, 2007. Available: http://bulimia.emedtv.com/bulimia/bulimia-statistics.html.

Singh, D. Female mate value at a glance: Relationship of waist-to-hip ratio to health, fecundity, and attractiveness. *Human Ethology & Evolutionary Psychology, 23* (December 2002), 81–91.

Song, S. Starvation on the Web. *Time, 166, no. 3* (July 18, 2005), 57.

Sperry, S., Thompson, J. K., Sarwer, D. B., & Cash, T. F. Cosmetic surgery reality TV viewership: Relations with cosmetic surgery attitudes, body image, and disordered eating. *Annals of Plastic Surgery, 62, 1* (January 2009), 7–11.

Striegel-Moore, R. H., Rosselli, F., Perrin, N., Debar, L., Wilson, G. T., May, A., & Kraemer, H. C. Gender differences in the prevalence of eating disorder symptoms. *International Journal of Eating Disorders* (December 23, 2008).

Taylor, C. B., Bryson, S., Luce, K. H., Cunning, D., Doyle, A. C., Abascal, L. B., Rockwell, R., Dev, P., Winzelberg, A. J., & Wilfley, D. E. Prevention of eating disorders in at-risk college-age women. *Archives of General Psychiatry, 63, 8* (August 2006), 881–888.

TieMeyer, M. Eating disorders: Bulimia statistics. *About.com Eating Disorders*, 2007. Available: http://eatingdisorders.about.com/od/whatisbulimianervosa/p/bulimiastats.htm?p=1.

Tiggemann, M., Martins, Y., & Churchett, L. Beyond muscles: Unexplored parts of men's body image. *Journal of Health Psychology, 13, 8* (November 2008), 1163–1172.

Tucker, P., & Irwin, J. D. University students' satisfaction with, interest in improving, and receptivity to attending programs aimed at health and well-being. *Health Promotion Practice* (February 5, 2009).

Voracek, M., & Fisher, M. L. Shapely centrefolds? Temporal changes in body measures: Trend analysis. *British Medical Journal, 325* (December 21, 2002), 1447–1448.

Wilson, G. T., Nathan, P. E., O'Leary, K. D., & Clark, L. A. *Abnormal psychology: Integrating perspectives*. Needham, MA: Allyn & Bacon, 1996.

Women up to 10 times more likely to have poor body image than men, *InteliHealth: Women's Health* (May 14, 2001). Available: http://www.intelihealth.com.

CHAPTER 10

Sexual Orientation

FEATURES

Multicultural Dimensions
Race and Ethnicity and Same-Gender Sexual Behavior

Gender Dimensions
Gay–Straight Alliances and Gender Activism

Ethical Dimensions
Research on Causes of Homosexuality

Ethical Dimensions
Teaching About Gay History

Global Dimensions
Attitudes About Homosexuality in Other Countries

Communication Dimensions
Communication About Gay and Lesbian Athletes

Communication Dimensions
Coming Out

Multicultural Dimensions
The Chinese Lawyer Who Is Out

Ethical Dimensions
Should Gay Marriages Be Legal?

CHAPTER OBJECTIVES

1 Define sexual orientation, including heterosexuality, homosexuality, situational homosexuality, and bisexuality. Discuss the validity of the Kinsey continuum.

2 Compare and contrast the theories of sexual orientation, including biological, psychological, and sociocultural theories.

3 Discuss homosexual life, including the challenges specific to homosexuality.

4 Discuss social issues that affect homosexuals.

go.jblearning.com/dimensions5e

Theories of Sexual Orientation
Homophobia
Coming Out
The Gay Rights Movement

INTRODUCTION

*B*y all appearances, Brad was an archetypal high school male: a "good" student, a "really nice" guy with a willingness to help out with school projects and panache in fixing cars. He dated several girls. But his relationship with Peggy was extra special. They were best friends, hanging out together and attending high school parties and dances as a couple. They also engaged in a variety of sexual activities.

At first Brad could not quite understand why the idea of sexual intercourse with Peggy did not appeal to him as much as it should. Eventually Brad realized that he was gay. Peggy was hurt at first about the abrupt end of their relationship, but she cared about Brad enough to remain a close friend.

After high school, Brad attended a local college and continued to hang out with his high school friends who had accepted his sexual orientation, rather than venturing out to meet people who might not have been so accepting. Gay bashing was common, and Brad had a legitimate fear for his safety. During this time, he met Brian, whom he has been with ever since.

Brad felt comfortable "coming out" to his friends, but he did not tell his elderly parents for fear of their reaction. This silence caused a bit of a problem, because his parents (and relatives) were forever introducing him to "nice girls" and wondering why nothing ever came of the dates Brad claimed he had. About the time Brad turned 30 years old, over dinner one evening, his father said to him, "You're gay, aren't you?" Although Brad's parents may have initially been hurt or confused, or may have questioned their own parenting, they continued to love and support Brad.

For Brad, as for many gays and lesbians, AIDS took a terrible toll. Many friends became sick and died. Many of Brad's friends learned about *and began practicing safer sexual activities, no longer going to bath-houses or having quick, anonymous encounters. Brad attended rallies to promote governmental funding for AIDS research.*

Brad was lucky: Both he and Brian tested negative for HIV. One thing that HIV did teach Brad, however, was that although he and Brian had been together for many years in a committed relationship, their situation was quite different from that of a legally married couple. When one of Brad's close friends died of AIDS, Brad's friend's parents, who did not want to believe their child was gay, demanded all his assets—which the deceased had intended to leave for his partner. Because the parents had the legal standing in the state in which the death occurred, the grieving partner lost everything. Even while his friend was dying, the parents were allowed to make all medical decisions and legally barred the partner from hospital visits.

In marriages, spouses automatically have each other's power of attorney, which means that if one spouse is incapacitated, the other has control over his or her affairs. A gay couple must go through lawyers to ensure that each partner has power of attorney for the other. Because Brian and Brad had purchased a home together and had made various other investments together, they realized it was imperative for them to complete the proper documentation to protect each other.

Brad's story illustrates many of the dimensions of sexual orientation. Sexual orientation takes time to develop and has an impact on many aspects of a person's life. In this chapter, we look at the ways that the many dimensions of human sexuality interact to determine sexual orientation.

■ Sexual Orientation

People have various feelings about sexual orientation—and even the topic of sexual orientation. The Sexuality Information and Education Council of the United States (SIECUS) position statement on sexual orientation (2012) is as follows:

> *Sexual orientation is an essential human quality. Individuals have the right to accept, acknowledge, and live in accordance with their sexual orientation, be they bisexual, heterosexual, gay, or lesbian. The legal system should guarantee the civil rights and protection of all people, regardless of sexual orientation. Prejudice and discrimination based on sexual orientation is unconscionable.*

A person's **sexual orientation** is one's erotic, romantic, and affectional attraction to the same gender, to the other gender, or to both. **Sexual identity** refers to an inner sense of oneself as a sexual being, including one's identification in terms of gender and sexual orientation. **Sexual preference** is a term once

sexual orientation
One's erotic, romantic, and affectional attraction to the same gender, to the opposite gender, or to both.

sexual identity
Inner sense of oneself as a sexual being, including one's identification in terms of gender and sexual orientation.

sexual preference
Term formerly used to describe sexual orientation that is now outdated, because sexual orientation is no longer commonly considered to be a conscious individual preference or choice, but to be formed by a complicated network of factors.

bisexual
One whose erotic, romantic, and affectional attraction is toward both genders.

heterosexual
One whose primary erotic, romantic, and affectional attraction is toward members of the other gender.

homosexual
One whose primary erotic, romantic, and affectional attraction is toward members of one's own gender.

gay
Male or female homosexual. (*Gay* used alone probably refers to a male, though it is acceptable to refer to a *gay female*.)

lesbian
Female homosexual.

used to describe sexual orientation—**bisexuality** (attracted to both genders), **heterosexuality** (attracted to members of the other gender), and **homosexuality** (attracted to members of the same gender). This term is now outdated because sexual orientation is no longer commonly considered to be one's conscious individual preference or choice; instead, it is thought to be formed by a complicated network of social, cultural, biological, economic, and political factors.

For our purposes, the terms *homosexual* and **gay** are used interchangeably to apply to either males or females. The term **lesbian**, however, applies only to a female homosexual.

The Kinsey Continuum

No clear-cut line separates homosexuality and heterosexuality; in fact, it is more accurate to think of these orientations as being on a continuum.

Figure 10.1 shows a seven-point continuum of sexual orientation originally devised by Kinsey. Most of us probably experience varying degrees of sexual orientation; that is, most of us are attracted to both genders, even though we may act in only one way sexually.

The notion of a continuum of sexual orientation helps explain not only differences among people but also a phenomenon known as **situational homosexuality**—that is, sexual behavior limited to specific circumstances in which members of the same gender are generally deprived of contact with the other gender. Homosexual activity in a single-sex school or in a prison, for example, does not necessarily indicate that the individuals involved are primarily homosexual. They may never participate in homosexual activity in other situations, and their orientation may prefer sexual activity with the other gender. However, because people of the other gender are not available to them, and because they prefer sexual activity with another person to masturbation exclusively, they engage in sexual behavior with people of the same gender. You may have participated in sexual activity with someone of the same gender sometime in your life; however, unless you are sexually attracted to people of the same gender, fall in love with people of the same gender,

situational homosexuality
Homosexual behavior limited to circumstances in which members of the same gender are deprived of contact with the other gender.

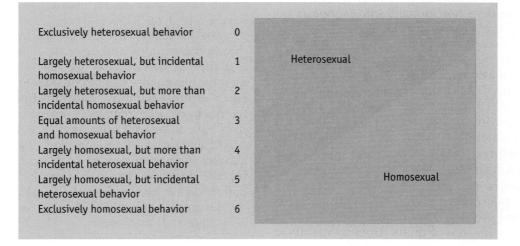

FIGURE **10.1** Kinsey sexual orientation continuum. The Kinsey continuum refers only to homosexual or heterosexual *behavior;* remember that it was developed in the 1950s. If such a continuum were developed today, it would likely refer to erotic, romantic, and affectional attraction, as do our definitions of sexual orientation. It would also probably recognize that a person's behavior and sexual orientation might differ. For example, a person can be heterosexually married, have sexual intercourse with a spouse, and still be a homosexual or a bisexual.

Source: Reproduced from Kinsey, A. *Sexual behavior in the human male.* Philadelphia: W.B. Saunders, 1948. With permission of The Kinsey Institute for Research in Sex, Gender, and Reproduction, Inc.

Multicultural DIMENSIONS

Race and Ethnicity and Same-Gender Sexual Behavior

Laumann and associates (1994) reported some differences in the rates of same-gender sexual behavior for people with different racial and ethnic backgrounds in the United States. For example, the proportion of people reporting same-gender sexual behavior since puberty was as follows:

White = 7.6% of males and 4% of females
African American = 5.8% of males and 3.5% of females
Hispanic = 8.8% of males and 3.8% of females
Asian = no males and 3.3% of females

The same researchers also asked people which sexual behaviors they found "very appealing." The following proportions found sexual activity with a same-gender partner "very appealing":

White = 3.3% of males and 2.7% of females
African American = 2.9% of males and 3.5% of females
Hispanic = 2.9% of males and 4.4% of females
(Sample sizes for other groups were too small to be meaningful.)

Interestingly, in most cases the proportion of people who find same-gender sexual behavior to be "very appealing" is lower than the proportion who have participated in it. We are not certain of the reason(s) for this, but perhaps some of those who participated were experimenting and learned that the behavior did not appeal to them after all.

have sexual behaviors with people of the same gender, and identify yourself as a homosexual, you are not classified as a homosexual.

The distinction we wish to make is between specific behavior and one's sexual orientation. A person's engaging in sexual activity with someone of the same gender does not indicate that person is a homosexual; someone's not engaging in sexual activity with the same gender does not indicate that person is not a homosexual. For example, a heterosexual person might engage in sexual behavior with a person of the same gender for the purpose of experimentation, or because of a situation such as being in prison or in a single-sex school. This does not mean the person is a homosexual. Or, a homosexual might engage in sexual behavior with a person of the other gender to appear more socially acceptable and/or to hide true homosexual feelings. This does not mean that person is a heterosexual. Sexual orientation is not the same as sexual behavior.

Many of us take our sexual orientation for granted; however, about 11% of junior and senior high school students may not be sure of theirs. Uncertainty about sexual orientation declines with age, from about 26% of 12-year-old students to 5% of 17-year-old students. About 20% of gay and bisexual men surveyed on college campuses knew that they were gay or bisexual in junior high school, and 17% said they knew in grade school. Six percent of gay or bisexual women knew that they were gay or bisexual in junior high school; 11% knew in grade school (Gay, lesbian, and bisexual adolescents, 1998).

Bisexuality

If homosexuality is difficult to define accurately given the Kinsey scale, bisexuality is even more so. A bisexual person has erotic, romantic, and affectional attraction to both genders. Looking only at sexual behavior, Kinsey found that 9% of single 30-year-old women and about 16% of single 30-year-old men could be categorized as bisexual (between the numbers 2 and 4 on Kinsey's scale).

The problem with this categorization, though, is that homosexuality and heterosexuality are more than a matter of behavior, as we have discussed. Consequently, bisexuality can be considered to be a relatively equal erotic, romantic, and affectional attraction to members of both genders, even though an individual may have a favorite attraction or behavior.

Bisexuality is enjoying and engaging in sexual activity with members of both genders or recognizing the desire to do so. As with homosexuality, our definition of bisexuality allows that someone who at one time engaged in bisexual behavior may not be a bisexual, and someone who has never participated in bisexual behavior could be a bisexual. For example, someone may fantasize about sexual relations with members of both genders and find himself or herself attracted to people of both genders but may never have engaged in sexual relations with a same-gender partner. This person may nevertheless be bisexual. Bisexuals are referred to in many ways: as "switch hitters," "AC–DC," or "people who swing both ways."

For people who are really homosexual but are unwilling to acknowledge their sexual orientation even to themselves, bisexuality may be a means of coping. Many of these people eventually accept their homosexuality without the need to mask it with bisexual behavior. Others remain bisexual throughout their lives because their sexual attraction is truly to both genders. Still others engage in bisexual behavior for a time but sooner or later revert to heterosexuality.

Bisexuals point to the variety that characterizes their sexual relationships. They are able to fully enjoy the sexual pleasures of both males and females and are open to the most erotic of activities. One of the disadvantages of bisexuality, though, is the suspicion it provokes in both the heterosexual and homosexual communities. In one sense, bisexuals are both like and unlike these groups; however, it is often the "unlikeness" that is the focus. Homosexuals view bisexuals as homosexuals who are afraid to admit to their preference. Some homosexuals reject sexual relations with bisexuals for this reason. It seems that lesbians are even more rejecting of bisexual women than are male homosexuals of bisexual men. Some lesbians want bisexual women to declare openly their lesbianism and insist there is no such thing as a true bisexual.

On some college campuses, new student organizations for bisexuals who feel shunned by gay-student support groups are emerging. Interestingly, supporters of the new groups say many of the previous groups established for gay, lesbian, and bisexual students have exhibited the very kinds of intolerance and discrimination they were designed to fight. The name for this behavior is *biphobia*, or antipathy toward those who identify as bisexual. Supposedly, some gay students belittle bisexuality as a "cop-out" to avoid identification as gay. Others say that bisexuals are confused about their real sexual orientation.

In recent years there has been an increase in the number of research studies related to bisexuality. For example, Saewyc et al. (2009) found that bisexual adolescents had lower levels of most protective factors (family connectiveness, school connectiveness, and religious involvement) than did heterosexual adolescents. They suggested that these factors help explain the higher prevalence of risky behavior among the bisexuals.

The Ontario Consultants on Religious Tolerance (2008) summarized the following points about bisexuality:

- Bisexuality may be a difficult concept to comprehend because we are often taught to look at things as a duality: male and female, light and dark, hot and cold, etc. In this case, at least three classifications (and perhaps more) are needed to represent sexual attractions and activities.

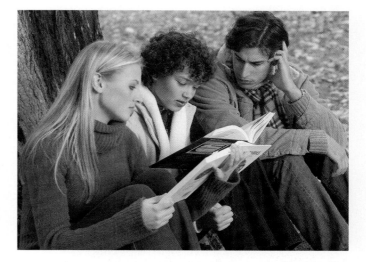

We do not know a person's sexual orientation unless they tell us what it is.

- A bisexual is attracted to both males and females, but not necessarily to the same degree.

- Bisexuality describes how people feel, not necessarily how they act.

- Misinformation about bisexuality is very prevalent.

- Although it has been said that only 2% of the population is bisexual, research indicated that almost 21% of men and 18% of women admitted to same-gender sexual attraction/behavior at some time in their lives.

- Some people believe that bisexuality is just a phase. While this may be true for some people, others regard themselves bisexual throughout their lives.

- It has been said that bisexuals are only satisfied if they have sexual partners of both genders. This is not true because bisexuals do not necessarily act on their feelings of attraction.

- Some openly bisexual individuals may be subjected to prejudice from the homosexual community as well as the heterosexual community. However, this seems to be decreasing.

Pansexuality

Pansexuality includes all kinds of sexual expression and sexual relationships that can exist in humans. It can involve sexual activity in many

pansexual
One whose sexual orientation includes all kinds of sexual expression and sexual relationships that can exist in humans.

forms. A pansexual person can love not only the traditional male and female genders, but also transgendered, transsexual, cross-dressing, androgynous, and gender-fluid people and all other variations of gender identification, including those who feel they do not have a gender. It is often confused with or included within the definition of bisexuality, but it is a more fluid and much broader form of sexual orientation in which the pansexual individual experiences sexual attraction towards members of all genders (not to be confused with sexes; a person's sex is purely physical, gender has to do with a person's psychological orientation).

Asexuality

Asexuality has seldom been discussed, but more attention has been given to it in recent years. For example, the Asexual Visibility and Education Network (AVEN) was founded in 2001 with two distinct goals: creating public acceptance and discussion of asexuality, and facilitating the growth of an asexual community. It has thousands of members and can be reached at www.asexuality.org. According to the AVEN website, asexual people have the same emotional needs as anyone else. Many asexual people experience attraction, but feel no need to act out that attraction sexually. Because they don't see a lack of sexual arousal as a problem to be corrected, asexual people focus their energy on enjoying other types of arousal and pleasure.

> **asexual**
> One who does not experience sexual attraction. Some asexuals may experience attraction but feel no need to act out that attraction sexually.

Barnes (2005) summarized some interesting points about asexuals. He indicated that asexuality isn't celibacy—the refusal to act on attraction. It is the absence of sexual attraction. Asexuals insist that theirs is a valid fourth orientation, like straight, bisexual, and gay orientations. There is nothing wrong, they say; it is simply the way they were born and they are not interested in sexual activity. Many asexuals form deep emotional bonds that they define as "romantic"—resembling those commonly understood as coupledom, except for a lack of sexual behavior. As one asexual said: "In early high school all of my friends started talking about how they were attracted to people, who they had crushes on, and I just didn't understand why sexuality was such a big deal for everyone else."

Statistically speaking, according to Barnes, there may be as many as 4.5 million Americans who are asexual. A study in Britain indicated that more than 1% of the population agreed with the statement, "I have never felt sexually attracted to anyone at all."

Many experts agree that motivation to engage in sexual intimacy is a dimension that runs from zero to extremely high; thus there are probably some people at that zero end. Asexuality seems to exist in the animal world as well.

Homosexuality in the Population

It is hard to know exactly how many homosexuals live in U.S. society; most still choose to keep their sexual orientation hidden. Estimates of how many people identify as lesbian, gay, or bisexual vary widely, and there is not a lot of research on the subject. According to SIECUS (2009), approximately 90.2% of males aged 18–44 identify as heterosexual, 2.3% identify as homosexual, 1.8% identify as bisexual, and 3.9% identify as "something else." Among females aged 18–44, 90.3% identify as heterosexual, 1.3% identify as homosexual, 2.8% identify as bisexual, and 4% identify as "something else." However, some differences arise when people are asked who they are attracted to. For example, 92.2% of males aged 18–44 report being attracted only to females, 3.9% report being attracted mostly to females, 1.7% report being attracted mostly to males, 1.5% report being attracted only to males, 1.0% report being attracted to both males and females, and 0.7% are not sure who they are attracted to. Among females aged 18–44, 85.8% report being attracted only to males, 10.2% report being attracted mostly to males, 1.9% report being attracted to both males and females, 0.8% report being attracted mostly to females, 0.7% report being attracted only to females, and 0.8% are not sure who they are attracted to. Finally, 6% of males aged 15–44 report ever having anal or oral sexual activity with another male, and 4.5% of males aged 15–19 report having done so. Among females, 11.2% of females aged 15–44 report having sexual experience of any kind with another female. Among females aged 15–19, 10.6% report having done so. Note that the question asked of males was of more limited scope, so in this last instance the male and female numbers cannot be directly compared to each other.

In addition to the number of homosexuals who hide their orientation and the difficulty of defining exactly who is included on Kinsey's continuum, another reason for the disparity in the estimated number of homosexuals relates to political implications. For example, those lobbying for greater gay rights need to show that large numbers of people are affected by this issue. If they can demonstrate political clout—that is, a large voting bloc—they can convince politicians to support their causes. That support can translate into legislation that assures gays the rights and privileges they feel have long been denied to them. However, it is in the interest of those opposed

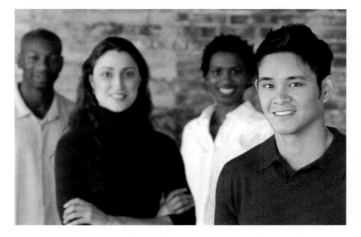

You cannot tell a person's sexual orientation just by his or her appearance.

to gay rights for these estimates to be lower, because such lower numbers would marginalize gay people. That is one reason why some gay rights organizations estimate that 10% of the population is homosexual and others use a much lower figure.

Same-gender couples head nearly 600,000 homes in the United States, according to census data considered the federal government's most thorough count yet of homosexuals (Census shows nearly 600,000 same-sex couple homes, 2001). A gay or lesbian couple heads a household in nearly every county in America. Sixteen percent of the same-gender couple homes are in California, 8% in New York, and 7% in Texas. However, such living arrangements still make up a tiny share of the nation's households—just over 0.005% of the 105.5 million U.S. homes. The results also dispel stereotypes that homosexuality is limited to large urban areas and college towns.

Heterosexuality in the Population

Regardless of the exact numbers of homosexuals and bisexuals in U.S. society, it is safe to assume that the sexual orientation of most people is heterosexual. As was seen in the statistics presented in the previous section, more than 90% of both males and females identify as being heterosexual. Because of this, some heterosexuals may have a difficult time understanding and supporting the need for equal rights and opportunities for people with different sexual orientations. Some heterosexuals may even be guilty of heterosexism, which means they think about human experience only in heterosexual terms and ignore or put down homosexual behaviors. They also may stereotype homosexuals in a negative manner and view them as dangerous to others.

While many people have wondered about the developmental process of those who do not identify

themselves as heterosexuals, only in recent years have some researchers focused more on how heterosexuals develop their sexual orientation identities. For example, Worthington et al. (2002) indicated that heterosexual development encompasses the following six important dimensions to be accomplished over time:

1. Identification and awareness of one's sexual needs, as determined by sexual orientation.
2. Adoption of personal values related to sexual behavior and sexuality in general.
3. Awareness of which sexual activities are preferred.
4. Awareness of the specific characteristics that are preferred in sexual partners.
5. Awareness of preferred modes of sexual expression.
6. Recognition of one's sexual orientation and personal identification with that orientation.

People with a heterosexual orientation seem to go through some rather predictable developmental states as they integrate their sexual orientation into their personalities. Early in life, they realize their heterosexual orientation but have not yet acted on it sexually. This stage is termed *unexplored commitment* to being heterosexual. They may then enter into an *active exploration* phase, where they intentionally try out numerous sexual ideas and fantasies, and often engage in sexual activities with members of the other gender. This helps them clarify which activities and partners they prefer. Some people experience *diffusion*, which may involve sexual exploration, but with less intentionality and goal direction than active exploration. After some exploration along with maturation, heterosexuals enter into the stage of *deepening and commitment*, which is characterized by more intimacy and loving feelings in relationships. People can move through these stages at various times, but the final status of heterosexual identity is *synthesis*, in which the various elements of identity, group membership, and attitudes toward sexual minorities have achieved congruence and meaning in the person, though this may be a difficult status to achieve. All of this helps to explain how heterosexual people gradually integrate their sexual orientation into their sense of self (Hoffman, 2004; Worthington et al., 2002).

■ Theories of Sexual Orientation

Although many studies have been done on the subject, no one knows exactly which factors shape sexual orientation. Some argue that biological factors account for a homosexual, heterosexual, or bisexual orientation. Others claim that psychological factors or learned behavior is responsible. Determining an accurate method for defining and identifying sexual orientation for the purpose of constructing representative samples of homosexuals, bisexuals, and heterosexuals is a goal of researchers. Different definitions and measures have been used to develop samples since the 1860s, when the topic of sexual orientation first attracted widespread research interest. If advances in the understanding of sexual orientations are to be made, it is critical that definitions and measures of sexual orientation be standardized.

Because the vast majority of people are heterosexuals, most theories about sexual orientation relate to homosexuality or bisexuality. It is as though heterosexuality is the "norm" and homosexuality and bisexuality are indications that something went wrong. These theories are described in the following paragraphs.

Biological Theories

Biological theories of the development of homosexuality include genetic factors and hormonal factors.

The Genetic Theory

The genetic theory of the cause of homosexuality states that something in a person's genes causes that person to be sexually attracted to members of the same gender. The most frequently cited evidence for this view is the study by Kallman (1952). Kallman studied twins (both fraternal and identical) who grew up in the same home. Fraternal twins do not share an exact genetic inheritance, whereas identical twins do share the same genetic material (they occupied the same ovum). Consequently, the environments are

the same for both sets of twins, but the difference is in the genetic makeup. Kallman found identical twins had a 95% concordance rate (both twins were homosexual) compared to a 12% concordance rate for fraternal twins. He concluded that homosexuality is a function of genetic predisposition. Whitman and Diamond (1986) reported a concordance rate of 75% for identical twins and a 19% rate for fraternal twins, thereby supporting the genetic theory. However, numerous other studies over the years have not been able to verify Kallman's findings. Furthermore, Kallman's selection of twins for his studies was criticized. He chose twins from prisons, psychiatric settings, and charitable organizations, thereby restricting the ability to generalize his results to twins living in more typical situations.

Bailey and Pillard (1991) also studied twins. They looked at identical twins, fraternal twins, and adopted brothers, among whom one of each pair

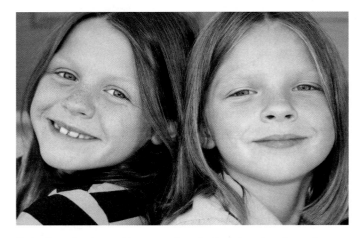

Twins have been used in research to look at theories about the cause of sexual orientation.

Gender DIMENSIONS

Gay–Straight Alliances and Gender Activism

A descriptive case study was conducted within the GSA (Gay–Straight Alliance) Network, a youth-based community organization in the San Francisco Bay Area that provides leadership and networking opportunities for youth in GSA clubs throughout California. Activism focused on sexual identity and rights is a controversial topic. Nevertheless, an increasing number of localities are passing antidiscrimination legislation protecting youth based on sexual identity and expression. Antidiscrimination policies necessitate grounded, comprehensive education and

outreach strategies. The priority is to ensure that all youth remain safe from violence, harassment, and discrimination within schools. Many youth activists' efforts center on educating school communities toward a broader understanding of the diverse ways that all people live their gendered and sexual lives. They are focused on building a community based on difference rather than defining themselves and advocating based on a single group identity.

Source: Data from Schindel, J. Gender 101—Beyond the binary: Gay–straight alliances and gender activism. *Sexual Research & Social Policy,* 5, no. 2 (June 2008), 56–70.

? Did You Know . . .

In *Biological Exuberance* (St. Martin's Press, 1990), the linguist and cognitive scientist Bruce Bagemihl attempts to dispel the myth that humans are the only species who practice homosexuality. In fact, he found that homosexual activity has been documented in more than 20% of the 2,000 species whose sexual activity has been observed. The following are a few examples discussed in his book:

• Male giraffes wrap their necks together until both are sexually aroused.

• Homosexual activities account for 50% of sexual activity among bonobos (chimplike apes).

• A male greylag goose may pair with another male goose for 15 years.

Source: Data from Kluger, J. The gay side of nature, *Time, 153, no. 16* (April 26, 1999), 70.

---

had declared himself to be a homosexual. They found that the more genetically similar each was to his gay brother, the more likely he was to be gay as well. Homosexuality was found in the remaining member of each pair in 52% of the identical twins (who developed from the same ovum), 22% of the fraternal twins (who developed from different ova), and only 11% of the adopted brothers (who shared no common genetic material). The researchers estimated that between 30% and 70% of the determining factors of homosexuality are genetic. However, questions remain: Even if 70% is genetic, what accounts for the other 30%? What role do prenatal hormonal secretions play? What role does environment play once the child is born?

Many researchers feel that the most promising support for a biological reason for sexual orientation comes from genetic studies. There is a great deal of evidence that gay male and lesbian sexual orientations run in families (Bailey et al., 2000; Dawood et al., 2000; Kendler et al., 2000).

Sexuality experts do caution that a specific gene linked to homosexuality has not been identified. Also, because of the complexity of sexual orientation, it is likely that a possible genetic link is only part of the picture.

Demir and Dickson (2005) reported on an interesting genetic study with fruit flies. They showed that a single gene in a fruit fly is sufficient to determine all aspects of the fly's sexual orientation and behavior. This means that instinctive behavior can be specified by genetic programs. However, it is not yet clear if there is a similar master gene for humans.

Burri et al. (2011) indicated that sexual orientation and "gender conformity" in women are both genetic traits. They followed a group of 4,000 British women who were one of a pair of twins. They found a connection between mental traits and how sexual orientation develops, with both factors being connected to genetics.

The Hormonal Theory

The hormonal theory of the cause of homosexuality states that homosexuality is a result of hormonal imbalances that occur before or after birth. Because it is known that prenatal hormonal treatment in animals can lead to different male and female behavior patterns (Dorner, 1968; Hutchinson, 1978; Money & Ehrhardt, 1972), some theorists have concluded that these same conditions might cause homosexuality. Evidence for this view can be found in the work of several researchers. For instance, Dorner and associates (1975) studied the responses of homosexuals and heterosexuals to injections of the hormone estrogen and found these responses to differ. Furthermore, Gladue and colleagues (1983) found that when homosexual men were administered estrogen, their patterns of secretion of luteinizing hormone (LH) changed to be more like those of heterosexual women; in addition, their testosterone levels remained lower for a longer time than did heterosexual men's when both groups were administered estrogen. Studies have also found that a prenatal excess of androgen in females is associated with a greater incidence of lesbianism (Ehrhardt, Evers, & Money, 1968; Money & Schwartz, 1977) and that a prenatal deficiency in androgen production in males is associated with an increased incidence of male homosexuality.

One research project tentatively identified prenatal exposure to the synthetic estrogen diethylstilbestrol (DES) as predisposing female offspring to lesbianism (Ehrhardt et al., 1985). Another researcher alleges the existence of anatomical differences in the size of parts of the brains of homosexual and heterosexual men (LeVay, 1991). Yet another researcher has pointed out that there is little evidence supporting the hormonal theories and that sexual orientation is more likely determined by other personal and cultural factors (Doell, 1995).

Savic et al. (2005) reported that gay men do not respond to the smell of bodily chemicals the same way that straight men do. Previously, they had isolated bodily chemicals from both males and females. When women smelled the male chemicals, their hypothalamuses "lit up," but they had no reactions to the female chemicals. In men, the results were exactly the opposite. Then the researchers included gay men in the study. When gay men were exposed to the smell of male chemicals, their hypothalamuses lit up just like a woman's. The smell of female chemicals did nothing for them. However, this study doesn't show that sexual orientation is biologically hardwired from birth. It could also be that the brains of gay men learn to respond to the smells over time and with experience.

As is the case with the genetic theories, there are problems in research on the hormonal causation of sexual orientation. There is no convincing evidence that sexual orientation is the result of either prenatal or postnatal hormonal imbalances, or that homosexuality causes these imbalances. However, research continues in this area.

Psychological Theories

Psychological theories of the development of sexual orientation consider psychoanalytical factors and the influence of learned behavior. Although these theories were historically believed, they have not been proved valid. Today many experts do not support these theories.

The Psychoanalytical Theory

Psychoanalytical theories of the cause of sexual orientation relate to parental and family characteristics. Sigmund Freud postulated that everyone is born with the potential to be bisexual. Whether someone becomes heterosexual or homosexual is, Freud believed, a result of circumstances that affect the child's psychosexual development. For example, if a young boy is unable to resolve the Oedipal complex (an attraction for his mother) satisfactorily and becomes "fixated" at this phase of psychosexual development, he may become homosexual; or if the boy continues to fear castration ("castration complex"), he may grow up to be homosexual.

Irving Bieber and colleagues (1962) fueled this view of the influence of family background when they compared the family backgrounds of 106 homosexual men and 100 heterosexual men and found differences. Specifically, Bieber found that homosexual men more often had overprotective and dominant mothers and weak, passive, and detached fathers than did heterosexual men. Bieber hypothesized that this family upbringing made men homosexual because they were fearful of interacting with women and unable to identify with their father. The problem with Bieber's study

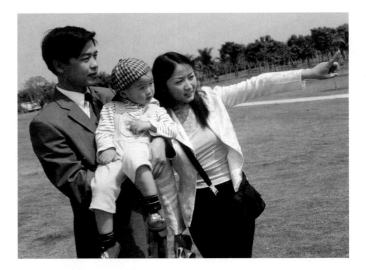

Some experts argue that family relationships influence sexual orientation.

was the manner in which he acquired his sample of homosexual men. Because there is a social stigma associated with homosexuality, thereby making many homosexuals unwilling to admit to their preference, it has often been difficult to find gay men and women to study. Consequently, homosexual samples have in the past too frequently been obtained from either psychiatric settings (patient populations), prisons, or the military. The ability, therefore, to generalize these results to socially functional homosexuals is suspect. Bieber's sample was obtained from patients undergoing psychoanalysis. As Clark and Epstein (1969, p. 575) state:

> One does not go into prisons and mental hospitals or clinics to study normal heterosexuality and then generalize to the population at large; therefore, to do so with homosexuals, as has been done so often in past research dealing with this area, is to study a sample already selectively loaded with psychopathology which may not be truly representative of the whole homosexual population.

On the one hand, evidence supporting Bieber's theory exists in the larger-than-usual population of homosexuals who have such family characteristics. On the other hand, there are many heterosexuals who grew up in similar households but never became homosexual. Clearly this theory remains just that—a theory.

The Learned Behavior Theory

Behaviorists believe that homosexuality is the result of situations experienced usually early in childhood and reinforced throughout one's life. For example, someone may experience an unsuccessful and unsatisfying heterosexual relationship that leads him or her to experiment with homosexuality, with which the person finds satisfaction. The attitude of many

¿? Ethical DIMENSIONS

Research on Causes of Homosexuality

As can be seen from information presented in this chapter, many researchers are interested in what determines sexual orientation or, perhaps for some, what causes homosexuality. They would argue that it is important to know which factors determine sexual orientation because if causes are known, then sexual orientation could be influenced in whatever way might be desired.

Others argue that research into the cause(s) of homosexuality is unethical and should not be undertaken because it assumes more often than not that homosexuality is a form of mental illness or an undesirable deviance from the heterosexual norm, which should be cured (Schuklenk & Ristow, 1996).

Do you think research about the causes of sexual orientation (or homosexuality) is ethical or unethical?

people is that "if they only had an effective lover, they'd never be homosexual." Others believe homosexuals are physically unattractive to the opposite sex, so their only sexual outlet is someone of the same sex. Dew (1985) found that many college students had this view. Others believe that an early childhood homosexual experience "recruits" people to homosexuality.

Studies are not supportive of these viewpoints. Homosexuals do not differ from heterosexuals in terms of their frequency of dating in high school, nor are they seduced into homosexuality as children (Bell, Weinberg, & Hammersmith, 1981), and they often report having had sexual experience with people of the opposite sex (Klach, 1974; Martin & Lyon, 1972). As with the other theories, the learned behavior theory demands further investigation before it can be supported.

Recently some researchers have argued that we have no business trying to determine the cause of homosexuality until we are able to determine what causes any form of sexual orientation. In other words, we are what we are; why we have certain sexual orientations might be scientifically interesting, but it has very little practical significance. Whether or not you accept this type of reasoning, the fact is that we still do not know why some people are homosexual and others heterosexual.

Integrated Theories

The integrated theory of the development of sexuality—homosexuality is just one form—argues that physical, psychological, and learned factors are involved. A good explanation of this view has been offered by the renowned endocrinologist John Money (1987). Money describes societies in which homosexuality is a precursor of heterosexuality. For example, in the large area in the Pacific between Sumatra

through Papua New Guinea and Melanesia, homosexuality is institutionalized. Males between the ages of 9 and 19 years move out of their families' homes into the long-houses in the center of the village. There they engage regularly in homosexual activity until they reach marriage age (19 years). After marriage, homosexual activity stops or is kept to a minimum. Likewise, the Sambian people in the eastern part of New Guinea require a boy just before puberty to give up his mother's milk for the "milk" (semen) of men. That is the only way the boy can grow and mature into a man. In fact, omission of this phase would stigmatize the man as deviant, rather than stigmatizing him as deviant for participating, as it might in American culture.

In the examples cited, homosexuality is a part of society and is learned behavior. Still, there is evidence presented by integrated theorists of the biological aspects of homosexuality. Experiments on certain animals have shown that the brain can develop in contrast to the body's form and structure. In one such study, pregnant lambs were injected with testosterone at a critical point in the pregnancy, and the resulting ewe was homosexual. That is, its brain was masculinized and it acted exactly as a ram acts in its mating and urinating behaviors. However, it possessed ovaries that secreted estrogen.

Integrationists, then, conclude that the prenatal influence on sexuality is important but that it plays out in a social context. Therefore, sexuality (heterosexuality, bisexuality, and homosexuality) is a function of the interaction of all of these factors: biology, hormones, cultural expectations, learned behavior, and psychological variables.

No single scientific theory about what causes sexual orientation has been substantiated. Studies to associate orientation exclusively with genetic, hormonal, or environmental factors have so far been inconclusive.

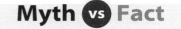

Myth vs Fact

Myth: A homosexual can be easily recognized as being different from heterosexuals.
Fact: Only a small proportion of homosexuals are what can be termed "visible homosexuals." The vast majority look and act just as everyone else does and differ only in their sexual orientation.

Myth: Gay men really want to be women and lesbians really desire to be men.

Fact: Most homosexuals are perfectly happy with their gender; they just prefer relationships with someone of the same gender.

Myth: Homosexual males are effeminate and weak, and homosexual females are masculine and physically strong.
Fact: Sexual orientation has nothing to do with one's body type or style of movement, nor does body type dictate sexual orientation.

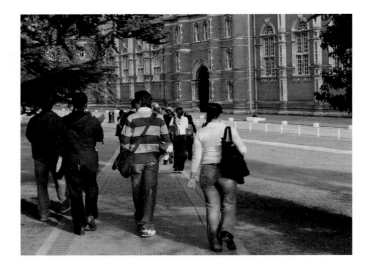

Homosexual students face extra adjustment challenges in schools.

Effect of School Environment

Something not often considered related to sexual orientation is the environment found in educational institutions. For example, how do teachers deal with the topic of sexual orientation or with students with various sexual orientations? How do heterosexual peers treat gays, lesbians, and bisexuals?

Fontaine (1998) pointed out that gay adolescents face the same developmental challenges as their heterosexual counterparts, with the added burden of attempting to incorporate a stigmatized sexual identity with little support from school personnel. Teachers either avoid the topic of homosexuality or, when discussing it, frequently present it in a negative manner.

Ryan and Futterman (2001) pointed out that although the vast majority of lesbian and gay youth become well-adjusted adults who lead satisfying, productive lives, their additional developmental challenges require a range of coping skills and adaptation. Unfortunately, unlike most of their heterosexual peers, they have no built-in support system. They must learn to identify, explore, and ultimately integrate a positive adult identity despite persistent negative stereotypes of lesbian and gay people. They also must learn to protect themselves from ridicule, verbal and physical abuse, and exposure. The social and emotional isolation experienced by gay and lesbian youth is a unique stressor that increases risk for a range of health problems.

Russell (2001) added support to this idea by indicating that gay and lesbian youth have more threats of violence as well as experiences of violence, have substance use and abuse rates well above the national average, and have a higher risk of thinking about and attempting suicide. In addition, Sadowski (2001) indicates that verbal, physical, and sexual harassment of gay and lesbian students is widespread in U.S. schools and that many teachers and administrators do not deal effectively with such incidents.

Staley and coworkers (2001) indicated that the individual consequences of living as an openly gay person can be profound—rejection by family and friends, physical violence and verbal abuse, insensitive health and social services, loss of jobs or housing, and lack of protection under the law. Homosexual boys are more likely than heterosexual boys to report poor body image, binge eating, and suicide attempts.

Frankowski (2004) and the Committee on Adolescence of the American Academy of Pediatrics pointed out that young people are recognizing their sexual orientation earlier than in the past. Nonheterosexual youth are at higher risk of dropping out of school, being kicked out of their homes, and turning to life on the streets for survival. Some of them engage in substance abuse, and they are more likely than their heterosexual peers to start using tobacco, alcohol, and illegal drugs at an earlier age. They are more likely to have had sexual intercourse, to have had more partners, and to have experienced sexual intercourse against their will. This puts them at increased risk of STIs, including HIV infection. They are also more likely to attempt suicide and be victimized. High levels of stress and lack of family support are also common.

Lesbian, gay, and bisexual (LGB) youth have a higher risk of suicidal behavior. They are nearly 1.5 to 3 times more likely to report thinking about suicide than non-LGB youth. They are nearly 1.5 to 7 times more likely to report actually attempting suicide. It is also likely that LGB youth experience higher rates of suicide deaths than their non-LGB peers, though it is difficult to know for sure because most mortality data do not include sexual orientation. Risk and protective factors do help explain suicidal behavior, however, and LGB youth generally have more risk factors and fewer protective factors than heterosexual youth. For example, LGB youth often lack important

Ethical DIMENSIONS

Teaching About Gay History

As of January 2012, California became the first state to mandate that the contributions of gays and lesbians in the state and the country be included in social science instruction and in textbooks. The state already required schools to teach about the contributions of some other minority groups, including African Americans and women. Advocates for the legislation said they believed the shift would help make schools safer for gay and lesbian students. However, one lawmaker indicated that it is a sad day when the government essentially tells people what they should think. He said the law prohibited schools from presenting gays and lesbians "in other than a positive light, and I think that's censorship right there." State textbooks and curriculum will not be updated for several years. In the meantime, teachers will have to use supplemental materials in the curriculum.

Do you think this law is a good idea? Is it needed? Is it ethical to mandate that gay history be taught in schools? Is this any different than mandating other things that must be taught in schools?

Source: Data from Lovett, I. California to require gay history in schools. *The New York Times* (July 14 2011). Available: http:// www.nytimes.com/2011/07/15/us/15gay.html.

protective factors such as family support and safe schools, and more LGB young people appear to experience depression and substance abuse (Suicide Prevention Resource Center, 2008).

Kann et al. (2011) found that sexual minority youth, particularly gay, lesbian, and bisexual students and students who had sexual contact with both genders, are more likely to engage in health-risk behaviors than other students. This was particularly true for behaviors that contribute to violence, behaviors related to suicide, tobacco use, alcohol use, other drug use, sexual behaviors, and weight management.

The Gay, Lesbian and Straight Education Network (GLSEN) (Presgraves, 2010) reports periodically on the national school climate. Key findings about LGBT students include:

- Nearly 9 out of 10 experience verbal or physical harassment in school.

- About 72% heard remarks such as "faggot" or "dyke" frequently at school.

- Nearly two-thirds reported they felt unsafe in school because of their sexual orientation.

- About 30% missed at least 1 day of class in the past month because of safety concerns.

- Grade point averages of students who were more frequently harassed were almost half a grade lower than for those who were less often harassed.

Relatedly, Russell et al. (2011) found that LGBT school victimization is strongly linked to young adult mental health and risk for STIs and HIV. Elevated levels of depression and suicidal ideation among males is also a result of high rates of LGBT victimization.

They concluded that reducing LGBT-related school victimization will likely result in significant long-term health gains and reduce health disparities for LGBT people.

An additional relationship not often heard about is that LGB teens are at a higher risk of becoming pregnant or causing a pregnancy than their heterosexual peers. This is apparently because the discrimination, sexual abuse, and harassment these teens face prompt them to indulge in more sexually risky behavior, such as having sexual intercourse without using condoms, starting to have sexual intercourse before the age of 14, or having multiple sexual partners. Girls who describe themselves as lesbians or bisexuals are 2 to 2.5 times more likely to become pregnant at least once than are heterosexual girls. Males who describe themselves as bisexual or gay are 3 to 4 times more likely than heterosexual males to impregnate a girl. LGB teens may have sexual intercourse with members of the other gender for a variety of reasons. Some engage in this behavior to hide or to deflect the abuse they see inflicted on LGB teens. Others may have been told they are abnormal and wrong, so they may feel that "If I just have sexual intercourse with enough other-gender people, it will cure me" (Saewyc et al., 2008).

More and more universities are signaling to prospective students that they have gay-friendly campuses. For example, in 2003 Stanford University gave every freshman a CD highlighting the campus's gay and lesbian resources, including its community center. San Jose State University regularly features gay and lesbian people in its brochures. Several forces are driving the growing momentum to make gay students feel welcome. Students are coming out earlier and are searching for colleges where they will find social acceptance. As the gay population increases its visibility, students and scholars are demanding the same outreach efforts that ethnic groups and women fought for years ago. Also, school admissions staff are realizing that homosexual students represent an important demographic that should be reached in some way (Vo, 2003).

Lipka (2011) reported that the population of gay applicants is becoming more visible, and colleges are stepping up to recruit them. Students seek campuses where they will fit in, and admissions and other campus officials try to extend a deft welcome. Secondary schools around the country have over 3,000 gay–straight alliances. At least 750,000 high-school students are out of the closet, and 90% of them plan to go to college. The national advocacy group Campus Pride held its first college fair in 2007. In 2011, there were at least six such fairs nationwide, and about 200 institutions took part. As one example of efforts to recruit gay students, the University of Southern California guide indicates that "you should think about our supportive campus climate." The guide highlights LGBT programs and student groups as well as financial aid information.

Archibald (2005) reported that a pro-gay group (Parents, Families and Friends of Lesbians and Gays) presented a workshop at the national PTA convention designed to get teachers and administrators to support gay, lesbian, bisexual, and transgender students in their identity. Presenters pointed out that these students do not feel safe in schools, and they need champions to help them. Goals of the workshop included developing support for diversity and intervening to prevent harassment of sexual-minority students. Attendees at the packed workshop largely supported the presentation, but some said, "I don't know why you need to teach this in schools."

School personnel need to be familiar with legal matters related to sexual orientation. Here are some examples (Student sexuality: How can and should schools respond?, 2004):

- Like all other students, lesbian, gay, bisexual, and transgender (LGBT) students are guaranteed equal protection under the Fourteenth Amendment to the Constitution and free speech and association under the First Amendment.

- The Equal Access Act requires schools to treat student clubs that address LGBT issues the same as other student groups.

- A school cannot refuse to allow a group such as a gay–straight alliance to meet because other students, teachers, administrators, parents, or community members object to the formation of the club.

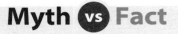

Myth: Homosexuals want to seduce children into a life of homosexuality.
Fact: Although some homosexuals seduce children, most sexual abuse of children is committed by heterosexuals. Both situations are intolerable, but to blame homosexuals alone for the sexual abuse of children is wrong.

Myth: Homosexuals should not be teachers.
Fact: It would be clearly wrong for a teacher of any sexual orientation to seduce students or to encourage them to adopt a particular sexual lifestyle, but there is no reason to expect such behavior to be more or less prevalent among homosexuals.

Myth: Homosexuals are suffering from a mental illness.
Fact: When homosexuals and heterosexuals are matched by age, IQ, and education, mental health experts cannot find differences in adjustment between the two groups.

Myth: Homosexuals are poor security risks.
Fact: There may have been some foundation for this belief in the past because homosexuals were easy targets for blackmail; however, as society grows less homophobic and as many homosexuals identify themselves publicly, the supposed risk should evaporate.

- To be covered by the Equal Access Act, student clubs must be "student initiated." Outside community members may not direct, control, or regularly attend activities of student groups.

There have been attempts at helping homosexual students do better in schools by having a more positive environment for them. For example, in the San Francisco Unified School district there is a LGBTQ (lesbian, gay, bisexual, transgender, or questioning) liaison in place in every school that handles individual student concerns. The program helps to promote students' acceptance of one another. The Milwaukee high school called Alliance (started in 2005) and the Harvey Milk High School in New York City (started in 2003) are both intended specifically for LGBTQ students. Both schools were started to give these youths the chance to attend a public school populated by students like themselves and an environment in which their differences are welcomed. These schools provide much safer environments for the students, but they also reawaken the debate about school segregation (Calefati, 2009).

In 2010 a gay-friendly online high school was established in Maplewood, Minnesota. Supporters indicate that the online nature of the school allows it to reach young people wherever they have Internet access—especially in rural areas, where smaller populations make a physical version of the school impossible. They also say that it removes gay students from potentially hostile school environments and places them in a safe and welcoming educational community. Others feel that the online school is not a good idea because students might become further alienated. Students might stay isolated and feel uncared for. More information about the gay-friendly online school can be found at www.glbtqonlinehighschool.com.

Presgraves (2010) indicated potential positive interventions and support for LGBT students. All of them relate to more positive overall experiences for the students. They include having a gay–straight alliance in school, having supportive staff in school, and having an antibullying policy in the school.

It can be helpful for parents and teachers to talk about sexual orientation with school-age children. Here are some examples of important messages for young people of various ages (Why it's important to talk about sexual orientation, 2004):

Messages for young people age 5–8 include:

- Human beings can love people of the same gender and people of the other gender.

- There are men and women who are homosexual, which means they can be attracted to and fall in love with someone of the same gender.

Messages for young people age 9–12 include:

- Sexual orientation is one part of who we are.

- Gay, lesbian, or bisexual people's relationships can be as fulfilling as heterosexual people's relationships.

Messages for young people age 12–15 include:

- People do not choose their sexual orientation.

- Having discussions about sexual orientation can be difficult for some people.

Messages for young people age 15–18 include:

- The understanding and identification of one's sexual orientation may change over the course of that person's lifetime.

- Civil rights for gay, lesbian, bisexual, and transgender people are being debated in many places across the United States.

Sexual Orientation Issues

As we grow and develop, many challenges confront us regardless of our sexual orientation. Typically homosexuals are happy, well-balanced people just like anyone else. They basically enjoy the same activities as other people, have similar goals in life, and in recent years have been able to enjoy parenthood through adoption or, for some lesbians, through artificial insemination. This is not often the picture that heterosexuals get, however, because it is more commonly problematic behavior that is seen. For example, happy, healthy homosexuals do not seek psychotherapy more often than happy, healthy heterosexuals do; but we often tend to generalize about all homosexuals from those few who do seek help. If we did the same thing with heterosexuals, we would have a very skewed picture of what heterosexuals are really like.

Many homosexuals, however, are more likely to experience certain kinds of challenges than are heterosexuals. Gay, lesbian, and bisexual youth must cope with prejudiced, discriminatory, and violent behavior and messages in their families, schools, and communities. These often result in isolation, fear of stigmatization, and lack of peer or familial support (*Just the facts about sexual orientation and youth*, 2000).

An interesting case of discrimination was reported by Young (2002). A Christian group at Central College in Iowa forced one of its student leaders to give up his position as president of the InterVarsity Christian Fellowship because he would not disavow his homosexuality. The same person was also president of the student government at the college. Leaders of InterVarsity asked him to resign his leadership position because he would not agree to a statement that the only acceptable form of sexual activity is that of a man and a woman who are married. This led to a debate at the college about whether the InterVarsity Christian Fellowship should continue to be recognized on the campus.

One development on some college campuses has been the establishment of fraternities for gay students. The University of South Alabama, Kent State University, and Florida International University (FIU) are among the universities that have them. At FIU the Gamma Lambda Mu men took great pains to spell out the precise limits of their bonding. Their bylaws state that brothers may not date one another. They want to prove to their classmates that gay men can join together in the spirit of service and camaraderie and not for sexual activity. Gay and lesbian groups have gained acceptance on most college campuses, but entry into the Greek system has been much slower (DeQuine, 2003).

An increasing number of gays seek marriage, even though these marriages are not usually legally recognized. Some lawmakers simply ignore the issue, and others have gone out of their way to institute laws prohibiting gay marriages. Sometimes homosexuals decide to have a marriage ceremony even though it may not be legally recognized. This can lead to other interesting issues. We will discuss more about this and other legal issues later in this chapter.

Global
DIMENSIONS

Attitudes About Homosexuality in Other Countries

In 2010 a new Mexico City law went into effect allowing same-gender couples to marry and adopt children (Malkin, 2010). But there was fierce opposition as soon as the law was passed. A leading Catholic Cardinal said that the family was under attack by the equivalence of homosexual unions with marriage between a man and a woman. Others were concerned because this law was contradictory to the law of the country. Some were concerned that the new law would weaken the legal definition of marriage.

The relative freedom of a newly democratic Iraq and improvements in security allowed a gay subculture to flourish. However, in 2009 it was reported (Williams & Maher, 2009) that the bodies of as many as 25 boys and men suspected of being gay turned up over a 2-month period. The killers, the police said, were not just Shiite death squads, but also tribal and family members shamed by their gay relatives. Clerics in Sadr City urged followers to help root out homosexuality in Iraqi society because, as some said, it is against the law and disgusting.

In China, all major religions have codes that have been traditionally interpreted as being against homosexuality. At the same time, none of the major religions condemns homosexuality as a sin. Sodomy was decriminalized in 1997. Homosexuality was removed from the *Chinese Classification and Diagnostic Criteria of Mental Disorders* in 2001. Surveys show that Chinese people are becoming more tolerant toward homosexuality, and gay bashing is rare. However, some people complain that the government is indifferent and does nothing to improve the situation for homosexuals. Many cases show that gays still have to endure prejudice from the justice system and harassment from police. Same-gender marriage is still forbidden in China (Homosexuality in China, 2005).

Homosexuality has never been viewed as a sin in Japanese society and religion, and there is no specific legal prohibition. It is still true that sexual activity is not viewed in terms of morality, but rather in terms of pleasure. Gay male content is common in romantic literature, but lesbian content is much less widespread (Homosexuality in Japan, 2005).

Other examples of attitudes about homosexuality include the following (Breaking the cultural straitjacket, 2005):

- In Nigeria, homosexuality is punishable by flogging or stoning to death. Violence against sexual minorities is promoted. It is almost imperative for homosexuals to live heterosexual lives to avoid having problems.

- In India, homosexuality is prohibited. There is no climate that promotes human rights for sexual minorities. Homosexual behavior is sanctioned.
- In the Dominican Republic, homosexual behavior is considered a mental illness; homosexual activity could lead to psychological treatment including the use of drugs to "cure the disease." Gays and lesbians are a minority stigmatized and discriminated against in every field of life. Only a few people see this as a civil rights issue.

In 2011 the United Nations Human Rights Council passed a resolution supporting equal rights for all, regardless of sexual orientation. The resolution, introduced by South Africa, was the first-ever U.N. resolution on the human rights of lesbian, gay, bisexual, and transgendered persons. Although not everyone was in favor of it, supporters indicated that it sent a clear message that abuses based on sexual orientation and gender must end (Dougherty, 2011).

As would probably be expected, the developed world leads on gay rights. Although laws and rights related to sexual orientation change from time to time, as of 2011 same-gender rights around the globe could be summarized as follows (International Gay and Lesbian Human Rights Commission):

- Same gender marriage is legal in Canada, Spain, the Netherlands, Belgium, Norway, Sweden, and South Africa.
- Homosexual acts are punishable by death in Iran, Saudi Arabia, United Arab Emirates, Yemen, Mauritania, and parts of Nigeria and Sudan.
- Sanctions against homosexuals seem to be easing in China, Singapore, Cuba, and Nepal.
- Sanctions against homosexuals seem to be tightening in Burundi, Nigeria, Russia, and Uganda.

Sources: Data from Homosexuality in China, 2005. Available: www.absoluteastronomy.com/encyclopedia/h/ho/homosexuality_in_china.htm; Homosexuality in Japan, 2005. Available: www.absoluteastronomy.com/encyclopedia/h/ho/homosexuality_in_japan.htm; Breaking the cultural straitjacket, 2005. Commission on Human Rights: Sixty-First Session, March 14–April 22, 2005. Available: www.ngochr.org/view/index.php?basic_entity=DOCUMENT&list_ids=110; Malkin, E. Gay marriage puts Mexico City at center of debate. *The New York Times* (February 7, 2010). Available: www.nytimes.com/2010/02/07/world/americas/07mexico.html; Williams, T., & Maher, T. Iraq's newly open gays face scorn and murder. *The New York Times* (April 8, 2009). Available: www.nytimes.com/2009/04/08/world/middleeast/08gay.html; Dougherty, J. U.N. Council passes gay rights resolution. *CNN World* (June 17, 2011). Available: http://articles.cnn.com/2011-06-17/world/un.lgbt.rights_1_gay-rights-human-rights-gay-pride-event?_s=PM:WORLD; International Gay & Lesbian Rights Commission. Historic decision at the United Nations. Available: www.iglhrc.org/cgi-bin/iowa/home/index.html.

The Social Scene

In the United States the homosexual subculture centers on private clubs, homosexual bars, and homophile organizations. These organizations are designed to help protect homosexuals, promote their rights, promote a positive image of the gay lifestyle, and help the general public better understand homosexuality. Clubs, bars, and organizations give homosexuals opportunities to fraternize with other gays and perhaps develop social and/or intimate relationships.

Although clubs, bars, and organizations are often safe places for homosexuals, there is a fear of police harassment and of possible discovery. In addition, some homosexuals desire to have more open and intimate relationships.

Like people in general who now use the Internet for various social reasons more than in previous years, those interested in same-gender relationships often choose this course. For example, there seems to be an association between online sexual activity seeking and risk for HIV infection among men who have sexual activity with men (MSM). Intention to go online seeking sexual activity has been found to predict more episodes of anal sexual activity. In addition, unprotected anal intercourse is a common activity with online-initiated liaisons. Therefore, MSM who go online to meet sexual partners are important targets for HIV interventions (Horvath et al., 2006).

In a permanent relationship, living together seems to be more important to lesbians than to male homosexuals. Many gays of both sexes believe that steady love relationships are quite meaningful and enjoy the warmth and understanding of such relationships.

Social Issues and Homosexuals

Additional issues related to homosexual life are being considered all the time. For example, the issue of homosexuals becoming parents has been controversial. Some people believe that homosexuals and bisexuals should have the same rights to be parents as others do. Other people believe that the inherent nature of same-gender attraction would prevent homosexuals from "properly raising" children.

Starting in 1994 the U.S. military had a "Don't ask; don't tell" policy. This meant that military officials were not supposed to ask about the sexual orientation of members of the military, but that they were supposed to discharge openly gay troops. This policy was repealed late in 2010. At least 24 other countries now also allow gays and lesbians to serve openly in the military.

In 1993 the American Medical Association (AMA) banned discrimination against gay, lesbian, and bisexual doctors by adding the words *sexual orientation* to the AMA nondiscrimination bylaws. Despite progress such as increasing support services for gay medical

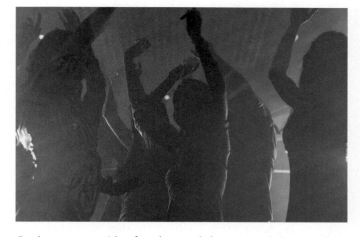

Gay bars cater to either female or male homosexuals, but usually not to both.

students, two-thirds of medical students reported hearing antigay comments from a classroom instructor, 42% said that clinical faculty had made negative remarks about homosexuality, and 7% indicated that their homosexuality had been criticized personally by an instructor. Gay and lesbian patient care needs to be integrated throughout the medical school curriculum (Wallick, 1997).

In 2004 the American Academy of Pediatrics issued a report giving guidance to clinicians in rendering pediatric care (Frankowski, 2004). The Academy reaffirmed the physician's responsibility to provide comprehensive health care and guidance in a safe and supportive environment for all adolescents, including nonheterosexual adolescents and young people struggling with issues of sexual orientation. The report outlined special needs of nonheterosexual youth as well as special considerations for them. It

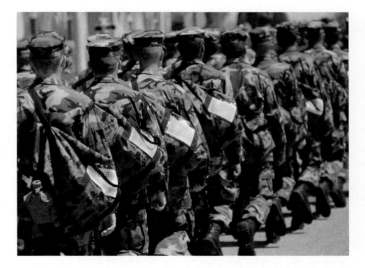

Until 2011, more than 13,000 men and women were discharged from the military because there was a ban on openly gay troops. But this is no longer the case. In fact, in 2012 a woman became the first openly gay general in the U.S. Army.

emphasized the importance of trying to prevent the major physical and mental health problems that may confront nonheterosexual youths in their transition to a healthy adulthood.

Evidence is accumulating that lesbians experience certain elevated health risks when compared to heterosexual women. These include increased risk of breast cancer, untreated STIs, and barriers to health care (Ellingson, 2002). The reasons for these risks are not totally clear. Reasons for increased breast cancer may include childlessness (associated with a 36% increase in the risk of development of breast cancer), higher rates of obesity and alcohol use, and less likelihood to practice breast self-examination and receive clinical breast exams. Although the prevalence of STIs is generally lower among lesbians than among heterosexual women, risk reduction behaviors also seem to be lower. Reasons given for relatively low frequency of early detection behaviors include low perceived need, fears of and experience of homophobic care providers, and lack of insurance.

Trebay (2004) pointed out that lesbians are a powerful presence in fashion, in both predictable and unexpected ways. While old stereotypes about lesbians have not faded, they have slipped into something decidedly "cool." Although lesbians wear a variety of clothing types and styles just like anyone else, one fashion designer referred to a show where "a parade of models appeared in slashed jeans, flat shoes and mannish jackets that were hip and sexy-tough, vulnerable and imposing, just the sort of stuff one might expect a fashionable young lesbian to wear."

Gay and lesbian tourists account for more than 10% of the money Americans spend abroad in a year. However, they have felt very unwelcome close to home in the Caribbean. For example, the Cayman Islands recently turned away gay cruises. Travel agents have had to remind gay tourists to avoid public displays of affection in Barbados (where homosexuality is outlawed) or face fines and harassment. In St. Kitts, gays were thought to be a threat to national security. Partly in response to these incidents, the International Gay and Lesbian Travel Association started a campaign to boycott certain spots, encouraging gay tourists to direct their dollars only to gay-friendly destinations. A more welcoming attitude lately has been shown in St. Thomas (where they advertise gay bed-and-breakfasts and gay weddings) and in Puerto Rico (Padgett, 2005).

In 2005 MTV started a new gay cable TV channel called Logo (MTV launches new gay cable TV channel, 2005). The prospect of a television channel entirely devoted to gay programs for gay people may strike some as unnecessary and others as a sign of immoral times, but media giant Viacom thought there was money in it. A spokesperson for Concerned Women for America, which describes itself as a conservative Evangelical group, said it was "a sad day for America." She said MTV was in a powerful position to influence youth and it was "unconscionable" to present in a positive view a promiscuous lifestyle that causes "illness and diseases." The general manager of Logo cited studies saying there were some 15 million openly gay people in America, an attractive demographic for advertisers, considering that many will have no children, meaning more disposable income.

In July 2005, Oprah Winfrey devoted a show to a lifestyle called living on the "down low." This is an expression to describe men who are married or have girlfriends, but are secretly sleeping with men. The main guest on the show, J. L. King, author of *On the Down Low: A Journey into the Lives of "Straight" Black Men Who Sleep with Men*, said the term applies only to blacks. He also said he doesn't consider himself gay. The behavior is not a social thing. Down low is just about sexual gratification and not a relationship. According to King, down low is on college campuses, too.

In August 2005, black journalists attending a National Association of Black Journalists conference in Atlanta discussed media coverage of the black community and the down low phenomenon (Black journalists criticize media coverage of "down low" phenomenon, 2005). They hotly debated whether media coverage of the phenomenon is a public service to the black community or a "salacious distraction" from other issues affecting the black community. Many said the media coverage unfairly characterized down low as occurring only among black men and often inappropriately linked it with statistics about the increasing number of AIDS cases in the black community. As a result, many black women went on "witch hunts" to determine whether the men in their lives were secretly gay, and people of other races wrongly assumed that this does not apply to them.

Examples of homosexual lifestyles in the media continue to grow. In 2005 a homosexual relationship was portrayed in a place that was probably unexpected—in a western film entitled *Brokeback Mountain*. The main characters, seen as very manly examples, participated in sexual encounters early in the film. Both went on to get married to females and even had children. However, after 4 years they got back together and their relationship flourished.

It has become much more common to see characters in the movies and on TV with various sexual orientations. While many people do not give this a second thought and accept it as part of normal life, others are bothered by the increasing presence of such characters. As stated earlier, the lives of those with different sexual orientations are, for the most part, very similar. The values people have in general,

Communication
DIMENSIONS

Communication About Gay and Lesbian Athletes

Being accepted and being accepting can be issues for college athletes. Traditionally there is an assumption that male athletes are heterosexually virile and desirable. Female athletes can face a very different perception—that they are all lesbians or bisexual. Straight women can go to great lengths to avoid that stereotype, leaving their homosexual teammates out in the cold. After using a series of interviews with lesbian, bisexual, and heterosexual Women's National Basketball Association (WNBA) fans, Dolance (2005) argued that the (perceived) large lesbian attendance at WNBA games enables the construction of a lesbian community by lesbian and bisexual fans in a site very different from traditional locations of lesbian community. Because the WNBA is not an explicitly lesbian space, the process of speculating about which players, coaches, and fans are lesbians is a meaningful part of being a WNBA fan for many lesbian and bisexual fans. Fantasizing a large lesbian presence enables lesbian and bisexual fans to actively and interpretively create lesbian community at the games. The women socialize and connect with other lesbian and bisexual women. WNBA games are defined as a unique space that is different from lesbian bars and other traditional "gay-only" spaces.

The highly visible men's sports of football, basketball, hockey, and baseball remain the most unaccepting of homosexual athletes. Athletes who perform individually, rather than on teams, may have an easier time being accepted (Jacobson, 2002a).

In 2002 the Rice University football coach was quoted as saying that "while he would not necessarily kick a player off the team for being gay, he probably would think hard about doing so." Immediately, the president of Rice University indicated the need for the coach to affirm his commitment to the university's nondiscrimination policy and to apologize for "the damage done by his comments." The coach did so (Jacobson, 2002b).

In 2002, Esera Tuaolo, who had played defensive tackle in the National Football League for 9 years, revealed that he was gay. He said that he retired from pro football in 1999 because of failing knees and shoulders, but also because of the discomfort he experienced hearing players make disparaging remarks about gays. One of his former teammates said, "Had other players known Tuaolo was gay, he would have been eaten alive" (Airing it out, 2002).

Smith (2010) indicated that not one gay male athlete in a major professional team sport in the United States had come out while still playing. He reported that the only gay man in a major professional team sport who was out of the closet was Gareth Thomas, a rugby player in Wales. He's 6'3" and 225 pounds of muscle. He's broken his nose five times, fractured both shoulders, and lost eight teeth. He has also been named to the Welsh national rugby team more times than any other man.

Thomas (2010) reported on the Oneonta College men's lacrosse team. When one of its captains announced in an online essay that he was gay, the team developed a new reputation as a model of tolerance. The gay player was embraced with open arms. Teammates came up to him and gave him handshakes. The team's coach was also very supportive of the player. He said, "If we had a roster of 30 players and 15 of them did not want to play on the team because you are gay, I would tell them to leave the team."

Bishop (2011) pointed out that dozens of gay leagues exist throughout the United States for most sports, from flag football to volleyball, with tens of thousands of participants. For example, the Gay Softball World Series attracts several hundred teams from around the country each year, and it has existed for over 35 years. In the interest of inclusion, some nongay athletes are usually allowed to play. The National Flag Football League sets the limit at 20% of each roster being heterosexual. The National American Gay Amateur Athletic Alliance limits the number of heterosexual players to two per team. But, questions remain. Is it enough to have an honor system where athletes simply indicate their sexual orientation? Should any "proof" of sexual orientation be required? Can bisexuals or those with other sexual orientations play? Rules have been challenged and discussions about appropriate rules and procedures continue.

Communication related to homosexual athletes remains an important social issue.

and the lives that they lead are very much the same, regardless of sexual orientation.

Another social issue is that people with disabilities who identify as LGB represent a population that has received little attention. Awareness of the unique needs and concerns of these individuals is crucial for optimizing their physical and mental well-being. This population is actually a double minority with some

? Did You Know . . .

The National Institutes of Health (NIH) asked the Institute of Medicine (IOM) to assess current knowledge of the health status of LGBT populations. In 2011 the IOM presented its findings in a report entitled *The Health of Lesbian, Gay, Bisexual, and Transgender People: Building a Foundation for Better Understanding*. It is available at www.iom.edu/Reports/2011/The-Health-of-Lesbian-Gay-Bisexual-and-Transgender-People.aspx.

The recommendations of the U.S. Department of Health and Human Services (HHS) based upon the report are available at www.hhs.gov/secretary/about/lgbthealth.html.

A number of actions resulted from the report. Here are a few examples:

- The HHS employment policies already prohibited discrimination based on sexual orientation, but they were updated to explicitly protect against unfair treatment of employees and applicants for employment based on gender identity and genetic information.
- HHS was directed by the president to initiate rulemaking to ensure that hospitals receiving Medicare or Medicaid patients respect the rights of patients to designate visitors, regardless of sexual orientation, gender identity, or any other nonclinical factor.
- HHS was also directed to establish new guidelines allowing patients to designate who they want to make medical decisions on their behalf through advance directives.
- A national technical assistance resource center was funded to support organizations serving the needs of LGBT older adults.
- In cooperation with other federal agencies, the HHS established a national task force on bullying.

experiences similar to those of other minority groups (Fraley, Mona, & Theodore, 2007).

Do you think we need to make changes in society's views, or do you feel conditions are fine the way they are?

Issues Related to Religion/Morality

You are probably aware that many people have religious/moral concerns about sexual orientation. The Ontario Consultants on Religious Tolerance (2005) summarized these concerns as follows:

- Same-gender activity is something that should be criminalized.
- Homosexuality is sinful and immoral, no matter what the relationship.
- Homosexuality is hated by God.
- Homosexuality is indicative of mental illness.
- Homosexuality is a choice that people make.
- Homosexuality is changeable through repentance and being saved, prayer, and/or reparative therapy.
- Homosexuality is abnormal and unnatural for everyone.
- Same-gender marriage is an extreme danger to society.

The Religious Institute on Sexual Morality, Justice, and Healing offered advice to religious foundations on securing the freedom to marry for same-gender couples (An open letter to religious leaders on marriage equality, 2008). Religious leaders within the Institute felt that there are strong civil liberties arguments for ending the exclusion of same-gender couples from the legal institution of marriage. A list of the religious denominations supporting homosexuals is available at http://religiousinstitute.org.

Many religious denominations are debating about how to deal with homosexuality in general, with homosexual religious leaders, and with same-gender marriages, among other issues. For example, in 2005 the Evangelical Lutheran Church in America retained its policy against blessing same-gender unions and ordaining gays, but suggested that sanctions could be avoided for pastors and congregations that chose to do so. Earlier, the United Methodist Church defrocked a minister in Pennsylvania who had admitted to being in a long-term lesbian relationship. She appealed the decision. The Episcopal Church USA also wrestled with how to handle homosexuality. In 2003 the Episcopal Church ordained an openly gay bishop in New Hampshire. Some Episcopal leaders called for a moratorium on ordaining bishops living in gay relationships and to halt public "rites of blessing" for same-gender unions (Banerjee, 2005).

Also in 2005, The United Church of Christ became the first mainline Christian denomination to officially support same-gender marriages (Dewan, 2005). Its ruling body passed a resolution affirming "equal marriage rights for couples regardless of gender." Symbolically, the church passed the resolution on July 4.

In 2011 the Presbyterian Church (U.S.A.) voted to change its constitution and allow openly gay people in same-gender relationships to be ordained as ministers, elders, and deacons (Goodstein, 2011). This was a reversal of only 2 years earlier when a majority of the church's regions voted against ordaining openly gay candidates. This time the vote was 205 to 56. The church's stated clerk, its highest elected official, indicated that they had been having this conversation for 33 years. He said, "Some people are going to celebrate this day because they've worked for it for a long time, and some people will mourn this day because they think it's a totally different understanding of Scripture than they have."

In "Brief Descriptions of the Sex Belief Systems," Ontario Consultants on Religious Tolerance (2009) noted that most people can be divided into one of six groups, depending on their fundamental beliefs about homosexuality. Although these six groups are stereotypical, they illustrate the typical concepts shared by many adults. Of course, some people will fit neatly into a single viewpoint, whereas others will combine the beliefs of more than one point of view. Here are the six groups:

- *Abomination:* This is the most conservative position. Based on Biblical writings, homosexual behavior is to be condemned under all circumstances.

- *Change is expected:* This viewpoint teaches that homosexuality is a product of a sinful world. Gays and lesbians can be cured and converted to heterosexuality through prayer.

- *Celibacy is expected:* This position recognizes that adult sexual orientation is fixed and homosexuals cannot change. For them, God expects a celibate lifestyle, without loving partners with whom to share their lives.

- *Marginally acceptable:* Homosexuality is a psychosexual disability that victims must try to overcome. If they are unable to change and unable to be celibate, then the least horrendous option is a monogamous, long-term, same-gender relationship.

- *Equality:* Equal status and equal rights are the goal. Homosexuals are quite capable of entering into a loving, committed same-gender relationship that is the equal of an other-gender relationship. Morality of acts is judged exactly the same way as in heterosexual relationships.

- *Liberation:* This is the most liberal position. Homosexuality is seen to be equal to heterosexuality.

Homophobia

Although society's attitudes are gradually becoming more accepting, there are still many people who have strong negative feelings about homosexuals. **Homophobia** is an irrational fear of homosexuality in others, a fear of homosexual feelings within oneself, or an unhappiness with one's own homosexuality. Homophobia probably results from ignorance, a belief in the common myths about homosexuality, or even the tendency to judge homosexuals as immoral. People with strong negative feelings often reveal their homophobia by openly insulting homosexuals and even subjecting people suspected of being homosexual to verbal or physical assault. Also, homophobics are often careful to avoid behaving in ways that could be interpreted as homosexual, for example, by shunning certain kinds of clothing or physical activities.

> **homophobia**
> An irrational fear of homosexuality.

Some people have wondered if there is a difference between males and females when it comes to homophobia. Research into this issue has not yielded clear results. However, it is interesting that Davies (2004) reported that on measures of attitudes toward homosexual behavior and homosexual persons, heterosexual men are more negative toward gay men than women are.

Homophobia is an international problem. Every 2 or 3 days a person is killed in Brazil in violence connected with his or her sexual orientation. In Mexico, the reported figure is nearly two fatalies per week. Most of the victims are men who have sexual relations with other men (UNAIDS, 2009). It has been found that gay people in the United Kingdom experience more extreme homophobia as young people than as adults. Two-thirds of young gay, lesbian, and bisexual people experienced direct bullying in British schools, 92% of young people were subject to verbal abuse, and 41% were physically assaulted. In Latin America, a gay man was killed every 2 days because of his sexual orientation (Ruscombe-King, 2009).

It may be that homophobia is more pronounced in individuals with an unacknowledged attraction to the same gender and who grew up with authoritarian parents who forbade such desire. It seems that individuals who identify as straight, but in psychological tests show a strong attraction to the same gender, may be threatened by gays and lesbians because homosexuals remind them of similar tendencies within themselves (Weinstein, et al. 2012).

What can be done to tackle homophobia? Schools have an important role to play. Lesbians and gay students are more likely to feel positive about school if school personnel clearly state that homophobic

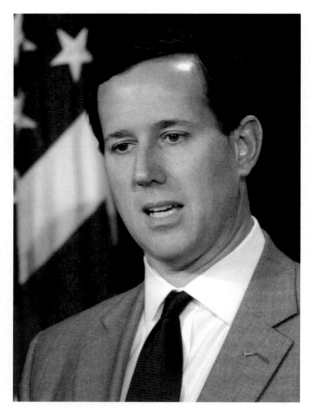

Senator Rick Santorum, also a presidential candidate in 2012, was quoted by the Associated Press as comparing consensual homosexual activity to bigamy, polygamy, adultery, and even incest. He later admitted to having a problem "with homosexual acts" and "acts outside of traditional heterosexual relationship." What message regarding the government's view of homosexuality did this send to the American public?

behavior is against the rules. Also, it is likely that personal attitudes will become more accepting toward gay people if individuals are exposed to educational programs about homosexuality. Community-based organizations can also provide support to gay and lesbian people who might feel isolated and, at the same time, campaign for tolerance toward homosexuality. Other bodies and agencies that could positively influence the way that gay, lesbian, and bisexual people are treated are leaders of political parties, police forces, health services, broadcasters, and employers (Ruscombe-King, 2009).

We talked about school settings earlier; here it is appropriate again to mention teachers. A teacher can ask the following questions to create a more accepting classroom environment: (1) Do I make **heterosexist** (characterized by the belief that heterosexuality is the privileged and powerful norm) assumptions? (2) Do I ignore homophobic remarks? (3) Do I blame my audience for their own misinformation?

> **heterosexist**
> An attitude that reinforces heterosexuality as the privileged and powerful norm.

(4) Do I use educational materials that assume that all my students are heterosexual?

Coming Out

The lifestyle of a gay person is greatly influenced by the extent to which he or she decides to remain in the closet—to keep his or her sexual orientation a secret—or to **come out**—accepting that orientation and making it public. Each choice can be made in varying degrees.

> **come out**
> Accept and make homosexual orientation public.

The decision to come out involves several stages: (1) acknowledging, (2) accepting, and (3) openly expressing one's homosexuality. Some homosexuals never acknowledge their sexual orientation, even to themselves. The first step in coming out is usually to realize that one does not fit the heterosexual model. The second step is acceptance, a step that sometimes requires that the individual overcome a learned negative view of homosexuality that becomes a negative view of himself or herself.

Even when a homosexual or bisexual reaches the acceptance stage, he or she can still decide to remain in the closet. It is generally easier to pass as a heterosexual than to take the final step toward openness. However, a person who can live publicly within his or her true sexual orientation generally has a better chance of living a happier life than one who remains secretive. In some situations, however, such as being a parent, the pain of coming out may far outweigh that of staying in the closet.

Telling the family—whether parents, siblings, spouses, or children—can also be extremely difficult, and many people who would prefer an open homosexual life choose not to face this ordeal. In fact, parents are often the last to know if their son or daughter is a homosexual. D'Augelli et al. (2005) conducted an interesting study about parents' awareness of youths' sexual orientation. They found that earlier awareness and disclosure of same-gender attractions and less internalized homophobia were characteristic of youths whose parents were aware of the youths' sexual orientation. However, youths with aware parents reported more past verbal victimization on the basis of sexual orientation from parents, yet more current family support and less fear of future parental victimization on the basis of their sexual orientation.

It is no surprise that family support is an important factor when gays, lesbians, and bisexuals decide to come out. Gays, lesbians, and bisexual young adults with higher levels of family rejection during adolescence are 8.4 times more likely to attempt suicide, 5.9 times more likely to report high levels of depression, 3.4 times more likely to use illegal drugs, and 3.4 times more likely to engage in unprotected sexual intercourse compared with peers from families with no or low levels of family rejection. There is a clear link between parental and caregiver rejecting behaviors and negative health problems for young lesbian, gay, and bisexual adults. Family support is crucial for reducing risk and increasing well-being for these people (Ryan et al., 2009).

For most people, the process of deciding to come out begins during their school years. As students, few homosexuals choose to disclose their sexual orientation to principals, teachers, counselors, or friends. Reasons cited for nondisclosure include fear of the consequences and not wanting others to know. Most of those who do disclose their sexual orientation receive positive feedback for doing so, but both positive and negative consequences of coming out have been reported.

It is not possible to predict others' response to disclosure. This move can result in a student's experiencing everything from lack of support, isolation, rejection, and ostracism to unfair discipline, taunting, harassment, verbal slurs, persistent random acts of violence, and outright vicious beatings. Students must carefully consider the pros and cons of coming out and examine *why* they want to come out.

Cloud (2005) reported that the Point Foundation is one of the fastest-growing gay groups in the nation. It gives scholarships to gay students. Young

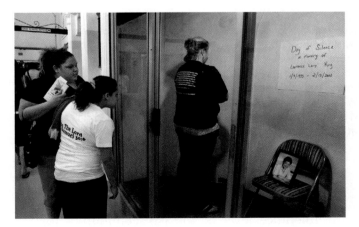

In February 2008, Lawrence "Larry" King, a gay 15-year-old student from Oxnard, California, was shot and killed by fellow student Brandon McInerney. King had reportedly asked McInerney to be his Valentine. McInerney has been charged as an adult with premeditated murder and a hate crime, and faces a maximum sentence of life in prison. The incident received nationwide attention; one news outlet described it as the most high-profile gay-bias crime since the murder of Matthew Shepard in 1998.

people are disclosing their homosexuality with unprecedented regularly—and they are doing so at much younger ages. The average gay person comes out just before or after graduating from high school. In 1997 there were about 100 gay–straight alliances on U.S. high school campuses, but there are now more than 3,000. Nearly one in 10 high schools has one. Also, gay kids can now watch fictional and real teens who are out on shows like *Desperate Housewives*, the dating show *Next* on MTV, and *Degrassi*, a high school drama on the N network. Simon & Schuster Publishers released over a dozen novels about gay adolescents in a recent year. Gay kids can subscribe to *YGA Magazine* (YGA stands for "young gay America"). Gay men today recall first desiring other males at an average age of 10. The average age for lesbians is 12. At many schools around the country, it is now profoundly uncool to be seen as anti-gay.

In 2005 Sheryl Swoopes, the three-time most valuable player of the Women's National Basketball Association, announced she was gay. She said she felt as if a burden had been lifted. It appeared that her announcement did not have an impact on her opportunities for endorsements or on other aspects of her career (Robbins, 2005).

Recently the Internet has played a key role in the stages of coming out. Many young men initially come out into a virtual gay community, with online observation and connection with other gay or questioning people, well before making actual contact in the real world. This virtual coming out involves being able to watch and learn about the culture, language, and norms of gayness before actually moving into this new world. The Internet can serve as an important tool for psychological adaptation for homosexual youth, especially those who are geographically or psychologically isolated (Ross, 2007).

Unfortunately, it is difficult if not impossible to know what the reactions of people will be when a person comes out. For many reasons, the decision to come out remains difficult for most homosexuals.

The Gay Rights Movement

Gay and lesbian organizations can help gays deal with the stresses experienced as a result of their sexual orientation. There are many different organizations that can provide the social support needed to manage such potentially stressful life situations as coming out or staying in the closet. The support of people who understand what you are experiencing and who can offer advice can be invaluable.

The gay rights movement has progressed, largely because of these homophile organizations and their ability to mobilize their membership to march, to

Communication
DIMENSIONS

Coming Out Each of us may be in a position to communicate with someone who is thinking about coming out. A few facts and a few communication suggestions may be helpful. First, the facts:

1. Coming out can be important as an affirmation of one's sexual orientation.
2. Coming out can jeopardize some relationships.
3. Coming out can promote a sense of pride in one's sexual orientation and, in the long run, actually improve relationships with both gay and straight people.
4. Coming out is usually a two-part process—first, coming out to oneself; second, coming out to others.
5. Coming out to oneself may involve gradually dealing with denial, putting matters into focus, and even dealing with personal homophobia.
6. Coming out to others probably involves stages—first involving a few very close friends or relatives, later more relatives, and then a larger public, such as employers, fellow students, and coworkers.
7. Some gays may be out only to a certain degree. For example, only families and very close friends may know about their sexual orientation.

Here are a few communication suggestions from professional counselors (Black & Underwood, 1998) that can be helpful to all of us:

1. Coming out should be postponed until the person has a reasonably high sense of self-worth and a support network.
2. The person should be secure in his or her identity before coming out to others.
3. The person should be helped to weigh the pros and cons of coming out and to examine why he or she wants to come out.
4. People who are planning to come out, or who are coming out, usually need a great deal of support and encouragement from others.
5. It is not our responsibility to "make" the person straight or gay. It is our responsibility to help provide a supportive environment.
6. It is important to be ourselves and be sincere.
7. Confidentiality must be respected.
8. Communication should be done in a helpful way but not in a forceful way.
9. Use words that do not assume that everyone is or should be heterosexual. For example, substitute terms such as *partner* or *significant other* for *boyfriend* or *girlfriend*.
10. Role playing can be used to help someone who is going to come out to be prepared to handle a variety of situations.

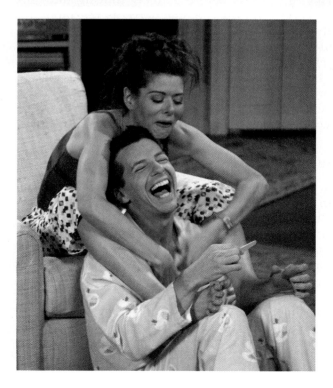

Just a few years ago, featuring a homosexual character on a television sitcom would most likely result in a show's cancellation. Later, one of television's most popular comedies proudly and overtly addressed the topic of homosexuality. *Will & Grace*, which focused on the unique relationship between Will, who was gay, and his best friend, Grace, who was straight, won three Emmys in 2000. Through the experiences of Will and Grace and their friends Jack and Karen, the show frankly and hilariously explored the universal subjects of friendship, sex, relationships, and love, whether heterosexual or homosexual.

vote, and to boycott when necessary. The movement began in earnest after a raid by the New York City police on the Stonewall gay bar in June 1969. That raid led to a 2-day riot that forever changed the tolerance level of the gay community toward societal prejudice based on sexual orientation. As a result, gays have presented a united front in voting for political candidates who are willing to sponsor their causes. In cities such as San Francisco and Washington, D.C., where there are significant numbers of homosexual citizens (voters), politicians are particularly sensitive to gay rights issues. In these cities, gays have made a difference in those elected to public office.

There is no way to know whether social activities, such as the gay rights movement, have influenced other aspects of society or whether aspects of society have influenced gay rights. There is no question that there is more openness about homosexuality in today's society. A prime example of this was Ellen DeGeneres's decision to come out on her TV show in 1998. Another example is the way that homosexual films have moved into the mainstream. In movies, homosexuals were first ignored, then scorned. By the early 1990s, with the AIDS epidemic, homosexuals began to be pitied in films. Films about them tended to be about their homosexuality and not about their overall lives. There are now more movies about homosexuals than ever, but these movies deal with overall issues and not just people's homosexuality and generally appeal to viewers of all sexual orientations.

In 2000, a Gallup poll showed that Americans were evenly divided over the morality of homosexual relations, with 48% considering them morally acceptable and 48% saying they are morally wrong. Despite the divided reaction on a moral basis, the majority believed homosexual relations should be legal (55%) and accepted as an alternative lifestyle (57%). The belief that homosexuals should have equal rights in terms of job opportunities was strongly supported (89%). Giving the same legal sanction to same-gender marriage as the law does to traditional marriage was supported by 40% of Americans and opposed by 56%. During the past quarter-century, there have been important changes in public attitudes about homosexuality and gay rights. Americans have shifted from frowning on homosexuality as an alternative lifestyle and being divided over whether it should be legal, to now supporting gay rights on both fronts. Even so, support for legalizing gay marriage lagged far behind the less culturally sensitive matter of gays having equal job rights (Saad, 2008).

In 2011 a Gallup poll found that, for the first time, a majority of Americans (53%) believed same-gender marriage should be legal, with the same rights as other marriages (Newport, 2011). That year's 9-percentage-point increase in support for same-gender marriage was the largest year-to-year shift yet measured. The increase came exclusively among political independents and Democrats. Republicans' views did not change. Support for gay marriage is greater among college freshmen than Americans at large. Lipka (2010) reported that 65% of college freshmen supported same-gender marriage.

Legal Rights

Marriage in the United States is more than a public recognition of love. It is also a legally binding contract, providing the married couple with myriad tax and legal support benefits, from which gay relationships are usually excluded.

Gays have long argued that marriage is not a requirement for a strong family unit. In 1989, Mayor Ed Koch of New York City agreed (Koch grants benefits for domestic partners, 1989). He issued an order recognizing domestic partnerships of gays. Not merely symbolic, Koch's declaration meant that gay city employees who had live-in companions could be eligible for death benefits. It also allowed labor unions to negotiate for health benefits for such families.

Not all of New York City's politicians agreed with Koch. One argued, "I think that Koch's executive order undermines one of society's most essential institutions: marriage." Koch responded, "Over time, society changes. So must the government that serves it. Practices or policies that might have seemed unacceptable to our grandparents or unusual to our parents seem equitable, indeed necessary, to our generation. We honor the past, but we cannot be held captive to it."

Following are some of the legal benefits for married couples.

- *Income taxes*—In many instances, married couples receive a lower tax rate than would two individuals filing separately. (An exception to this, known as the "marriage penalty," occurs when both spouses earn relatively equal high incomes and consequently pay a higher rate than they would as individuals.) At any rate, any income tax benefits for married couples do not include gay couples.

- *Adoption*—Many states do not allow gay couples to adopt children. Even states that do allow it generally put married couples first in line.

- *Estate taxes*—Married couples do not have to pay any federal estate taxes (and usually only a limited amount of state estate tax) on the death of a first spouse. State laws provide (for people without wills) that property moves directly to the spouse (or spouse and children, depending on the state). Unless a gay couple has an updated will (and most people in the United States do not), the biological family of the deceased can claim all possessions.

- *Employment benefits*—Married couples share a variety of benefits from work (health, dental, and life insurance, to name some) that gay partners do not. Many *Fortune* 500 companies have instituted policies in recent years to allow gay partners such rights, but

Multicultural DIMENSIONS

The Chinese Lawyer Who Is Out

A young Chinese lawyer named Zhou Dan started writing about being gay on Chinese websites in 2001. He hoped his honesty would help combat prejudice. Homosexuality was, and still is, very much in the closet in China. In 2001, officials in Beijing took it off the country's official list of mental disorders. However, gay people still face discrimination and social pressures. In May 2005, Peking University authorities banned a gay-and-lesbian film festival before it was to open on campus.

Zhou's entries, signed with his own name, had an unintended consequence. Gay men from around China who had faced workplace discrimination, blackmail, and even prison time started to seek his legal counsel. Zhou helped start a hotline for sexual minorities in Shanghai in 2003. He taught China's first graduate class on homosexuality and social science at Fudan University. Some claim he is China's leading voice for gay rights.

Interestingly, the first undergraduate course on gay studies ever offered at a Chinese university was also given at Fudan University in the fall of 2005 (Mooney, 2005). It drew far more applicants than the 100 available seats. The class focused on health, legal, and social issues related to homosexuality in China. The instructor said the new course's popularity stemmed from ignorance about gay issues in China. The students didn't know much about homosexuality and wanted to learn more.

Sources: Data from The lawyer who is out. *Time, 165, no. 26* (June 27, 2005), 42–43; Mooney, P. Chinese students line up for first undergraduate gay- studies course. *Chronicle of Higher Education, Today's News.* August 23, 2005. Available: http://chronicle.com/daily/2005/08/2005082305n.htm.

there is no law requiring this. Companies like Disney and Apple offer these benefits to recruit and retain high-quality talent. Whereas many large companies can afford to do this, many smaller companies are not so inclined.

- *Social Security survivorship benefits and pensions*—At death, the law provides that the surviving spouse receive continued benefits. Not so for gays.

- *Disability decision making*—If a married person becomes seriously injured and needs medical care decisions made for him or her, the law provides that spouses can make those decisions. But in cases in which parents or siblings of a disabled gay person do not approve of his or her relationship, they can—and often do—challenge the domestic partner's decisions in court.

Related to many of these legal rights are financial issues. Bernard (2011) profiled a lesbian couple to determine how their costs compared to a similar heterosexual married couple. Using a couple who made $140,000 per year, which is about average for a college-educated couple in the three states with the highest estimated gay populations—New York, California, and Florida—she estimated that in a worst-case scenario the lifetime cost of being gay was over $467,000. In the best case for a couple with significantly better health insurance, plus lower taxes and other costs, it was about $42,000.

You can see from this list that there are many problems related to legal rights of gay couples. There is much to be done to ensure equal rights for all married couples.

In 2012 the Secretary of the Department of Health and Human Services indicated that the Affordable Care Act would give LGBT Americans improved access to health coverage. Insurers would no longer

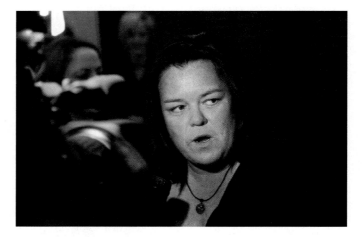

Increasingly, gay men and lesbians are choosing in vitro fertilization or adoption to start their own families. The issue of gay and lesbian adoption was widely discussed in the media after former talk-show host Rosie O'Donnell publicly criticized President George W. Bush's opposition to gay adoption. O'Donnell, who is openly gay, has three adopted children and says that her own experiences as a mother make her certain that gay people should have the right to be parents.

¿? Ethical DIMENSIONS

Should Gay Marriages Be Legal?

Given the many legal benefits for married couples, there seems to be increasing pressure to legalize gay marriages. Those who feel gay marriages are not proper, for whatever reasons, would argue that we should not make gay marriages legal. Those who feel we have an ethical responsibility to treat all people equally, and to recognize the rights of various groups, would argue that gay marriages should be legal.

In recent years there have been measures considered in some states to recognize the legal rights of people involved in same-gender partnerships. The question of whether it is ethical to provide or not to provide legal sanction to these partnerships fosters interesting debates.

---

be able to turn someone away just because he or she was lesbian, gay, bisexual, or transgender.

In 2000 Vermont became the first state to approve same-gender unions. Although the term *marriage* was not used, this bill provided homosexual couples with essentially the same rights as heterosexual couples (Drummond, 2000). In 2004 Massachusetts began granting the first-ever marriage licenses to same- gender couples. The state's highest court had ruled that gays and lesbians had a constitutional right to marry. In 2005 Connecticut joined Vermont in approving gay civil unions (Schweitzer, 2005). Also in 2005, a federal judge struck down Nebraska's ban on same-gender marriage, saying the measure interfered not only with the rights of gay couples but also with those of foster parents, adopted children, and people in a variety of other living arrangements. The amendment to the state's constitution, which defined marriage as a union between a man and a woman, had passed overwhelmingly by voters in 2000 (Judge voids same-sex marriage ban in Nebraska, 2005).

In 2010 a federal judge found that a law barring the federal government from recognizing same-gender marriage is unconstitutional, ruling that gay and lesbian couples deserve the same federal benefits as heterosexual couples (Goodnough & Schwartz, 2010). Many issues related to gay marriages continue to be debated.

As of 2011, according to the National Gay and Lesbian Task Force (Relationship recognition for same-sex couples in the U.S., 2011), states with full marriage equality were Massachusetts, Connecticut, Iowa, Vermont, New Hampshire, and New York. The nation's capital, Washington, D.C., also had full marriage equality. States with broad relationship recognition laws included Vermont, New Jersey, Illinois, Delaware, and Hawaii, which recognized civil unions, and California, Oregon, Washington, and Nevada, which recognized domestic partnerships. States with limited relationship recognition law were Colorado, Rhode Island, Maine, Maryland, and Wisconsin. States that recognized same-gender marriage performed in other states were Rhode Island, Maryland, New Mexico, and Illinois. On the flip side, a number of states had passed constitutional amendments banning same-gender marriages, whereas others had passed statewide laws recognizing marriage as occurring only between a man and a woman.

Should same-gender couples be allowed to marry legally? Some people feel that same-gender couples should have the same human rights as others. They argue that when people work, pay taxes, enter into lifetime commitments, and raise children, there is no reason they should not be afforded the same social and legal benefits and status as heterosexual couples—including legal marriage. In opposition to this idea, the 1996 federal Defense of Marriage Act says that "Marriage in the United States shall consist only of the union of a man and a woman." There are still quite varied opinions about the topic of same-gender marriage.

Herdt and Kertzner (2006) argue that depriving lesbians and gays of the right to marry restricts their citizenship and hinders their health and well-being. Even though research confirms the capacity of gays and lesbians to form committed relationships and parent successfully, marriage denial continues to perpetuate an opportunity structure that disenfranchises gays and lesbians in the sociocultural, legal, economic, and political aspects of their lives. Herdt and Kertzmer point out that denial of marriage is an act of discrimination against both gays and lesbians.

In 2001 the Belgian government approved a bill to legalize same-gender weddings. It made Belgium the second country in the world to recognize gay marriages, after its northern neighbor, the Netherlands (Ames, 2001). In 2005 the Canadian government passed legislation granting same-gender couples the same legal rights as those in traditional unions between a man and a woman. According to most polls, a majority of Canadians support the right for gays and lesbians to marry in spite of the fact that the Roman Catholic Church, the predominant denomination in Canada, vigorously opposes the legislation (Duff-Bell, 2005).

As of 2011, seven countries issued marriage licenses to same-gender couples. They were Belgium, Canada, the Netherlands, Norway, South Africa, Spain, and Sweden. An additional 19 countries granted same-gender couples some rights and domestic partner protection (International policies on same-sex marriage, 2011).

In 2011 the U.S. Census Bureau reported that there were 131,729 same-gender married couple households and 514,753 same-gender unmarried partner households in the United States. The census tally is higher than the actual number of legal marriages, but this may be because respondents answered based upon their perception instead of a legal definition.

Some people believe that gay marriage bans have inspired a new wave of activists. For example, in 2008 a group planned "A Day Without a Gay." The event organizers asked gay-rights supporters to avoid going to work by "calling in gay" and volunteering for the gay-rights movement instead. The burst of energy drew some comparisons to demonstrations during the early days of the AIDS crisis in the 1980s. Many activists were also motivated by the film *Milk*, which chronicled the fight by a member of the San Francisco Board of Supervisors, Harvey Milk, to beat back a 1978 ballot measure that would have barred gay teachers from California's public schools (McKinley, 2008).

In 2012 it was found that a majority of Americans (54%) said that same sex marriage should be legally recognized, while 42% were opposed. There was a sharp partisan divide, with 70% of Democrats and 60% of independent voters saying it should be legal, but 72% of Republicans were opposed to same-sex marriage (Pruitt 2012).

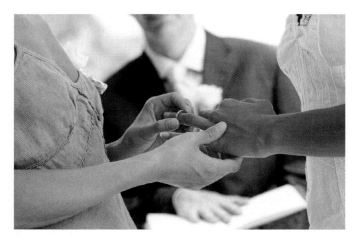

People disagree about the rights of homosexual couples.

In 2003 the U.S. Supreme Court struck down state sodomy laws as demeaning to homosexuals, and said the government has no authority to regulate the sexual behavior of "consenting adults acting in private" (Murphy, 2003). Many people felt that this decision would have far-reaching implications for the popular discussion about gay rights. For example, some said that by essentially acknowledging gay relationships as legitimate, the Supreme Court justices gave the gay-rights movement a new credibility in debates about marriage, partner benefits, adoption, and parental rights.

Two interesting, but unrelated, legal rulings about homosexual rights were made in 2005. In one, the Hillsborough County Commission in Florida approved a policy directing county government to "abstain from acknowledging, promoting, or participating" in gay-pride recognition or events. It was approved after a Gay and Lesbian Pride Month display at a library upset some library patrons. Community leaders feared that the policy would damage efforts to promote the Tampa region as being multicultural and diverse (Waddell, 2005). In a second situation, the California Supreme Court ruled that country clubs must offer gay members who register as domestic partners the same discounts given to married ones. If the clubs did not do this, the court said it would be "impermissible marital status discrimination" (Leff, 2005).

Should lesbian and gay couples be allowed to adopt children? Some people start with the premise that homosexuality is wrong and believe that such a relationship is an inappropriate context in which to raise children. Because they fear that sexual orientation and behaviors can be learned, they fear that a child raised by a lesbian or gay couple would be more likely to become a lesbian or gay man. Others do not believe that sexual orientation determines one's ability to parent. They feel the most important requirements are the abilities to love, support, and care for a child. Most lesbians and gays were raised by heterosexual parents. Therefore, they believe being raised by a lesbian or gay couple will not create lesbian or gay children any more than being raised by a heterosexual married couple would guarantee heterosexuality (Should lesbian and gay couples be allowed to adopt?, 2003). Interestingly, researchers in developmental psychology have concluded that no significant differences exist between children raised by lesbians and gay men and those raised by heterosexuals (Zanghellini, 2007).

As lawmakers and courts expend the legal definition of the American family, some same-sex couples feel the same what-about-children pressure that heterosexual couples have long felt. Many gay men had resigned themselves to the idea that they would never be accepted by society as good and loving parents and assumed that they would never have children. However, parenting among same-sex couples is now more common and there can be pressure for same-sex couples to have childern. This raises related issues about whether to adopt or use a surrogate. At the same time, many people are uncomfortable with the idea of same-sex couples being parents. A Pew Research Center survey found that for the first time a majority of people (52%) said that gay men and lesbians should be allowed to adopt children, up from 46% in 2008 and 38% in 1999 (Swarns, 2012).

In 2005 the California Supreme Court, stepping into largely uncharted territory, ruled that both members of a lesbian couple who plan for and raise a child born to either of them should be considered the child's mothers even after their relationship ends. This meant that the law could require former members of such couples to assume parental rights and obligations. Those supporting such rights and requirements were very happy with the decision. Lawyers for groups defending what they called traditional values were troubled by the decision (Liptak, 2005).

Finally, freshmen entering college have their own ideas about legality and homosexuality. Thirty-one percent of men and 18% of women think it is important to have laws prohibiting homosexual relationships. Fifty-nine percent of men and 72% of women think same-gender couples should have the right to legal marital status (Hoover, 2009).

Overall, 77% thought gays and lesbians should have the legal right to adopt a child (A profile of this year's freshmen, 2011).

Exploring the Dimensions of Human Sexuality

Our feelings, attitudes, and beliefs regarding sexuality are influenced by our internal and external environments. Go to go.jblearning.com/dimensions5e to learn more about the biological, psychological, and sociological factors that affect your sexuality.

Go to go.jblearning.com/dimensions5e

Case Study

No single scientific theory about the biological causes of sexual orientation has been substantiated; neither have any psychological theories. It is likely that the biological, psychological, and sociocultural factors interact to influence our sexual orientation. Because the dimensions change over time, an individual's sexual orientation may change over time as well.

Culturally, not all societies view homosexuality in the same manner. In areas of the Pacific such as Papua New Guinea, boys regularly participate in homosexual activities until they reach the age of marriage (19 years). In Mexico, only a male who plays the receptive role in anal intercourse is considered homosexual.

Socially, gays and lesbians in the United States can feel stigmatized and socially isolated as a result of fear of disclosure. Those who disclose their orientation ("come out") face discrimination and possibly even violence. Further, family and friends may reject them.

Biological Factors

- Research into genetic factors affecting homosexuality has been inconclusive. No specific gene has been identified. Any genetic link would be only part of the picture for determining sexual orientation.
- Research into hormonal imbalances (either prenatal or postnatal) as a factor driving homosexuality has proved inconclusive. No specific hormonal factors have been identified. Any hormonal link would be only one aspect of determining sexual orientation.

Sociocultural Factors

- Homosexual students often feel isolated and stigmatized.
- Family life can be disrupted by disclosure of homosexuality.
- Different cultures view homosexuality in different terms.
- Some states have laws making homosexual sexual activities illegal. Further, gay marriages generally do not have legal standing for state or federal benefits. Many large corporations have begun to offer employee benefits for domestic partners.

Psychological Factors

- Most theories suggesting that the influence of mothers or early sexual experiences lead to changes in sexual orientation have been discounted.
- Most homosexuals lead lives as fulfilling and satisfying as those of most heterosexuals.

Summary

- Sexual orientation can be viewed on a continuum, which Kinsey described as having seven points.

- Sexual orientations include heterosexuality, homosexuality, bisexuality, pansexuality, and asexuality.

- There are many theories about what determines sexual orientation, including biological, psychological, and integrated theories. None of the theories is generally agreed upon.

- Both homosexual and heterosexual youths and adolescents face the same challenges related to growth and development, but gays, lesbians, and bisexuals face additional issues related to their acceptance.

- There are many examples of discrimination against people who have a sexual orientation other than heterosexual.

- In the United States, the homosexual subculture centers on private clubs, bars, and homophile organizations. These groups are designed to protect homosexuals, promote their rights, promote a positive image of homosexual lifestyles, and help the general public better understand homosexuality.

- Social issues related to sexual orientation include military policies, discrimination based on sexual orientation, and general understanding and support for people of various sexual orientations.

- There are many points of view about sexual orientation based on religion and morality.

- The gay-rights movement has helped many people better understand homosexuals and have more positive attitudes about homosexuality in general.

- Many legal issues remain related to sexual orientation, including the legal status of same-gender relationships of various types, the right of homosexual and bisexual individuals to be parents, and legal rights concerning issues such as inheritance, health insurance coverage, income taxes, and employment benefits.

Discussion Questions

1. What defines a person's sexual orientation? Is sexual orientation constant throughout life, or can it change over time?

2. Describe the theories of the causes of sexual orientation, and indicate whether research supports their theoretical claims.

3. Compare and contrast the homosexual lifestyle with the heterosexual lifestyle.

4. What are the social issues surrounding homosexuality? How do such issues adversely affect homosexuals?

Application Questions

Reread the chapter-opening story and answer the following questions.

1. Explain why Brad was dating and engaging in sexual activities with Peggy if he thought he was gay.

2. Discuss the social and psychological effects on people who are unable to disclose their sexual orientation and introduce a lifetime partner to friends and family.

Critical Thinking Questions

1. If a genetic link were found for homosexuality, how might that affect those found to have the gene? Would society accept homosexuality as an inherited "defect"? Or would homosexuals encounter more discrimination in the workplace, in the military, and so on?

2. Assuming that studies claiming that only a small percentage of the population is gay are correct, why should efforts be made to accommodate such a small minority?

3. The "Don't ask; don't tell" policy of the U.S. military has been repealed. Should sexual orientation make a difference on the battlefield?

4. Given that many states ban same-gender sexual activity, is it ethical to vote admitted homosexuals into public office?

5. If homosexuality had no social stigma, would there be more or fewer people living as homosexuals? Explain your answer.

Critical Thinking Case

When the filmmaker Debra Chasnoff's son started kindergarten, she had more to worry about than the other parents. Her son thought that having two moms was great—but what would the other kids tell him?

From her own experience with school systems, Chasnoff started a film project, *It's Elementary*, which was completed in 1996. She and Helen

Cohen, the film's coproducer, toured the country and filmed teachers in classrooms as they described gay and lesbian lifestyles to children. Their goal was to show that the classroom could be a place where children are taught tolerance and acceptance of lifestyles different from those of their own families.

Originally, the film was used in school systems and colleges to educate teachers about the prejudice that exists among young children regarding homosexuality. But more recently, the film has caused quite a stir on the airwaves. After PBS turned it down for national distribution, San Francisco's KQED agreed to sponsor the film.

During the early summer of 1999, 89 of 347 public stations scheduled it, 17 more were on board, and 53 were considering it. This caused some anger among the Christian Right and other conservative groups who do not believe the film should be broadcast where children might watch it without supervision, although the stations had scheduled it for nighttime airing. They also argued that the film does not take parents' rights into consideration (Ness, 1999).

What do you think? Should teachers be encouraged to educate elementary school children about the topic of homosexuality, or should this responsibility be left to parents? Should films like *It's Elementary* be broadcast on national TV if the goal is to get people talking and thinking about educational issues?

Exploring Personal Dimensions

Take a few moments to measure the strength of your feelings about homosexuality and gender identity by using this values grid.

Place in the appropriate square of the grid the *italicized* key term in the questions following that shows how you feel about the question. Note that you will be identifying the *degree* of your feelings, not whether they are positive or negative. Fill in all 16 squares, placing only one key term in any one square. (You may change your mind as you go along if you discover other key words about which you feel more or less strongly.) After you complete the grid, look it over to see how strong your feelings are. If you can find a willing partner, compare your grids and discuss your responses.

	Very Strongly	Strongly	Mildly	No Reaction
1. How would you feel if your closest *friend* told you he or she was a homosexual?	❑	❑	❑	❑
2. How do you feel about *two girls* who greet each other with a kiss after a long summer vacation?	❑	❑	❑	❑
3. How do you feel about *two boys* greeting each other with a kiss after a long summer vacation?	❑	❑	❑	❑
4. How do you feel about a person who would *beat up* a homosexual for fun?	❑	❑	❑	❑
5. How do you feel about two *girls holding hands* on the way to class?	❑	❑	❑	❑
6. How do you feel about girls wearing *boys' clothes*?	❑	❑	❑	❑
7. How do you feel about boys wearing *girls' clothes*?	❑	❑	❑	❑
8. How do you feel about two *boys holding hands* on the way to class?	❑	❑	❑	❑
9. How do you feel about *boys* who do not like sports?	❑	❑	❑	❑
10. How do you feel about *girls* who do like sports?	❑	❑	❑	❑
11. How do you feel about taking *group showers*?	❑	❑	❑	❑
12. How do you feel about a man taking over the household *chores*?	❑	❑	❑	❑
13. How do you feel about a male *hairdresser*?	❑	❑	❑	❑
14. How do you feel about a woman who becomes a *construction worker*?	❑	❑	❑	❑
15. How do you feel about going out only with persons of the *opposite sex*?	❑	❑	❑	❑
16. How do you feel about going out only with persons of the *same sex*?	❑	❑	❑	❑

How did you feel about these questions? Did any of them bother you for any reason? Why or why not? Do you have strong feelings about homosexuality?

Source: Bruess, C. E., & Greenberg, J. S. *Sexuality education: Theory and practice, 3rd ed.* Sudbury, MA: Jones and Bartlett Publishers, 2014.

Suggested Readings

Barker, J. C., Herdt, G., & deVries, B. Social support in the lives of lesbians and gay men at midlife and later. *Sexuality Research and Social Policy, 3, no. 2* (June 2006), 1–23.

Bily, C. A. *Homosexuality (opposing viewpoints).* Chicago: Greenhaven Press, 2008.

Creating supportive environments for lesbian, gay, bisexual, and transgender youth. *The Prevention Researcher, 17, no. 4* (November, 2010) (Special Issue containing 5 related articles).

Goldfarb, E. A. Lesson on homophobia and teasing. *American Journal of Sexuality Education, 1* (2006), 55–66.

Journal of Bisexuality. Taylor & Francis Online. Available: www.tandfonline.com/toc/wjbi20/current.

Journal of Homosexuality. Taylor & Francis Online. Available: www.tandfonline.com/loi/wjhm20.

Miller, L. The religious case for gay marriage. *Newsweek* (December 15, 2008), 27–36.

Patterson, C. J. Children of gay and lesbian parents. *Current Directions in Psychological Science, 15, no. 5* (October 2006), 241–244.

Peters, J. A. *Keeping you a secret.* New York: Little-Brown, 2005.

Russell, S. T., Ryan, C., Toomey, R. B., Diaz, R. M., & Sanchez, J. Lesbian, gay, bisexual, and transgender adolescent school victimization: Implications for young adult health and adjustment. *Journal of School Health, 81, no. 5* (May, 2011), 223–229.

Tracy, E. C., & Satariano, N. P. Differentiating between gay and heterosexual male speech. *Journal of the Acoustical Society of America, 129, no. 4* (2011), 2421.

Wilson, R. Gay academics find new paths to the top. *The Chronicle of Higher Education, 42, no. 30* (April 1, 2011), A1, A9–A10.

Web Resources

For links to the websites below, visit *go.jblearning.com/dimension5e* and click on Resource Links.

American Civil Liberties Union: Lesbian Gay Bisexual Transgender Project
www.aclu.org/lgbt-rights

Documentation of the ACLU's actions to fight discrimination and educate the public regarding LGBT rights.

American Psychological Association
www.apa.org/topics/sexuality/sorientation.pdf

Provides answers to questions about sexual orientation and homosexuality.

Hartford Institute for Religion Research: Homosexuality and Religion
http://hirr.hartsem.edu/research/homosexuality_religion.html

Articles and research on the topic of homosexuality and religion.

Lambda Legal
www.lambdalegal.org

Contains information about many legal issues including laws related to sexual orientation.

National Organization for Women: Information on Same Sex Marriages
www.now.org/issues/lgbi/marr-rep.html

Information on NOW's work on lesbian rights including support of same-gender unions.

References

Airing it out. *Time, 160, no. 19* (November 4, 2002), 84.

Ames, P. Belgian cabinet OKs gay marriages. *The Birmingham News* (June 24, 2001), 11A.

Archibald, G. Pro-gay group seeks support at PTA convention. *The Washington Times* (June 28, 2005).

Bailey, H. M., & Pillard, R. C., A genetic study of male sexual orientation. *Archives of General Psychiatry, 48* (1991), 1089–1086.

Bailey, J. M., Dunne, M. P., & Martin, N. G. Genetic and environmental influences on sexual orientation and its correlates in an Australian twin sample. *Journal of Personality & Social Psychology, 78, no. 3* (2000), 524–536.

Banerjee, N. Lutherans recommend tolerance on gay policy. *The New York Times* (January 14, 2005).

Barnes, S. Individuals who don't follow the standard script of sex and romance find they are not alone. *Albany Times Union* (May 29, 2005), G1.

Bell, A. P., Weinberg, M. S., & Hammersmith, S. K. *Sexual preference: Its development in men and women.* Bloomington: Indiana University Press, 1981.

Bernard, T. S. The financial hurdles gay couples face. *The New York Times* (March 26, 2011). Available: http://bucks.blogs.nytimes.com/2011/03/26/the-financial-hurdles-gay-couples-face/.

Bieber, I., Dain, H., Dince, P., Drellich, M., Grand, H., Gundlach, R., Kremer, M., Rifkin, A., Wilbur, C., & Bieber, T. *Homosexuality: A psychoanalytic perspective.* New York: Basic Books, 1962.

Bishop, G. Three straights and you're out in gay softball league. *The New York Times* (June 29, 2011). Available: http://www.nytimes.com/2011/06/30/sports/softball-case-raises-question-who-qualifies-as-gay.html.

Black journalists criticize media coverage of "down low" phenomenon, say articles wrongly link behavior to blacks, increase in AIDS cases. *Kaiser Daily HIV/ AIDS Report*, August 9, 2005. Available: http://www.kaisernetwork.org.

Burri, A., Cherkas, L., Spector, T., & Rahman, Q. Genetic and environmental influences on female sexual orientation, childhood gender typicality and adult gender identity. *PLoS ONE 6, no. 7* (2011), e21982. doi:10.1371/journal.pone.0021982.

Calefati, J. Gay high schools offer a haven from bullies. *U.S. News & World Report* (January 2, 2009). Available: http://www.usnews.com/articles/education/2008/12/31/gay-high-schools-offer-a-haven-from-bullies.

Census Bureau releases estimates of same-sex married couples. United States Census Bureau Newsroom (September 27, 2011). Available: http://www.census.gov/newsroom/releases/archives/2010_census/cb11-cn181.html.

Census shows nearly 600,000 same-sex couple homes in most comprehensive count yet of gays and lesbians. Harvard Medical School's *Consumer Health Information* (August 21, 2001). Available: http://www.intellihealth.com.

Clark, T., & Epstein, R. Self-concept and expectancy for social reinforcement in noninstitutionalized male homosexuals. *Proceedings of the 77th Annual Convention of the American Psycho-analytical Association, 4* (1969), 575.

Cloud, J. The battle over gay teens. *Time, 166, no. 15* (October 10, 2005), 42–51.

D'Augelli, A. R., Grossman, A. H., & Starks, M. T. Parents' awareness of lesbian, gay, and bisexual youths' sexual orientation, *Journal of Marriage and Family, 67, no. 2* (May 2005), 474–482.

Davies, M. Correlates of negative attitudes toward gay men: Sexism, male role norms, and male sexuality. *Journal of Sex Research, 42, no. 3* (August, 2004), 259–266.

Dawood, K., Pillard, R. C., Horvath, C., Revelle, W., & Bailey, J. M. Familial aspects of male homosexuality. *Archives of Sexual Behavior, 29, no. 2* (2000), 155–163.

Demir, E., & Dickson, B. J. Fruitless splicing specifies male courtship behavior in Drosophila. *Cell, 121* (June 3, 2005), 785–794.

DeQuine, J. Out of the closet and on to fraternity row. *Time, 161, no. 11* (March 17, 2003), 8.

Dew, M. The effects of attitudes on inferences of homosexuality and perceived physical attractiveness in women. *Sex Roles, 12* (1985), 143–155.

Dewan, S. United Church of Christ backs gay marriage. *The Birmingham News* (July 5, 2005), p. A1.

Doell, R. G. Sexuality in the brain. *Journal of Homosexuality, 28, nos. 3–4* (1995), 345–354.

Dolance, S. A whole stadium full: Lesbian community at Women's National Basketball Association games. *Journal of Sex Research, 42, no. 1* (February 2005), 74–83.

Dorner, G. Hormonal induction and prevention of female homosexuality. *Journal of Endocrinology, 42* (1968), 162–163.

Dorner, G., Rohde, W., Stahl, F., Krell, L., & Masius, W. A neuroendocrine predisposition for homosexuality in men, *Archives of Sexual Behavior, 4* (1975), 1–8.

Drummond, T. A win for gays. *Time, 155, no. 12* (March 27, 2000), 38.

Duff-Bell, B. Same-sex marriage bill passes in Canada's House. *The Birmingham News* (June 29, 2005), 14A.

Ehrhardt, A. A., Evers, K., & Money, J. Influence of androgen and some aspects of sexual dimorphic behavior in women with the late-treated adreno-genital syndrome. *Johns Hopkins Medical Journal, 123* (1968), 115–122.

Ehrhardt, A. A., Myer-Bahlburg, H. F. L., Rosen, L. R., Feldman, J. F., Veridiano, J. F., Zimmerman, N. P., & McEwen, B. S. Sexual orientation after exposure to exogenous estrogen. *Archives of Sexual Behavior, 14, no. 1* (1985), 57–77.

Ellingson, L. Lesbian health issues: A 10-year review. *Health Education Monograph Series, 19, no. 1* (2002), 40–45.

Fontaine, J. H. Experiencing a need: School counselors' experiences with gay and lesbian students. *Professional School Counseling, 1, no. 3* (February 1998), 9–14.

Frankowski, B. L. American Academy of Pediatrics Clinical Report: Guidance for the clinician in rendering pediatric care. *Pediatrics, 113* (June 2004), 1827–1832.

Gay, lesbian, and bisexual adolescents. SIECUS fact sheet, 1998. Available: www.siecus.org/pubs/fact/fact0013.html.

Gladue, R., Green, R., & Hellman, R. Neuroendocrine response to estrogen and sexual orientation. *Science, 225* (1983), 1496–1499.

Goodnough, A., & Schwartz, J. Judge topples U.S. rejection of gay unions. *The New York Times* (July 8, 2010). Available: http://www.nytimes.com/2010/07/09/us/09marriage.html.

Goodstein, L. Presbyterians approve ordination of gay people. *The New York Times* (May 10, 2011). Available: http://www.nytimes.com/2011/05/11/us/11presbyterian.html.

Herdt, G. H., & Kertzner, R. I do, but I can't: The impact of marriage denial on the mental health and sexual citizenship of lesbians and gay men in the United States. *Sexuality Research & Social Policy, 3,* no. 1 (March 2006), 33–44.

Hoffman, R. M. Conceptualizing heterosexual identity development: Issues and challenges. *Journal of Counseling and Development, 82* (2004), 375–380.

Hoover, E. Freshmen's views: Politics, admissions, and marijuana. *Chronicle of Higher Education, 45, 21* (January 20, 2009), A18–A19.

Horvath, K. J., Beadnell, B., & Bowen, A. M. Sensation seeking as a moderator of Internet use on sexual risk taking among men who have sex with men. *Sexual Research and Social Policy, 3, 4* (2006), 77–90.

Hutchinson, J. B., ed. *Biological determinants of sexual behavior.* New York: John Wiley & Sons (1978).

International policies on same-sex marriage. Infoplease, 2011. Available: http://www.infoplease.com/world/countries/international-policies-same-sex-marriage.html.

Jacobson, J. Rice U. football coach chastised for comments on gay athletes. *Chronicle of Higher Education, 49, no. 11* (November 18, 2002b), A32.

Jacobson, J. The loneliest athletes. *Chronicle of Higher Education, 49, no. 10* (November 1, 2002a), A36–A38.

Judge voids same-sex marriage ban in Nebraska. *The New York Times* (May 13, 2005).

Just the facts about sexual orientation and youth. Washington, DC: American Psychological Association, 2000.

Kallman, F. J. Comparative twin study on the genetic aspects of male homosexuality. *Journal of Nervous and Mental Disease, 115* (1952), 283–298.

Kann, L., Olsen, E. O., McManus, T., Kinchen, S., Chyen, D., Harris, W. A., & Wechsler, H. Sexual identity, sex of sexual contacts, and health-risk behaviors among students in grades 9–12—Youth Risk Behavior Surveillance, selected sites, United States, 2001–2009. *Morbidity and Mortality Weekly, 60/ss07* (June 10, 2011), 1–133.

Kendler, K. S., Thornton, L. M., Gilman, S. E., & Kessler, R. C. Sexual orientation in a U.S. national sample of twin and nontwin sibling pairs. *American Journal of Psychiatry, 157* (2000), 1843–1846.

Klach, D. *Woman plus woman: Attitudes toward lesbianism.* New York: Simon & Schuster, 1974.

Koch grants benefits for domestic partners. *Washington Post* (August 8, 1989), A6.

Laumann, E. O., Gagnon, J. H., Michael, R. T., & Michaels, S. *The social organization of sexuality: Sexual practices in the United States.* Chicago: University of Chicago Press, 1994.

Leff, L. Court rules country club treated lesbians unfairly. *The Birmingham News* (August 2, 2005), 4A.

LeVay, S. A difference in hypothalmic structure between heterosexual and homosexual men. *Science, 253* (1991), 1034–1037.

Lipka, S. Colleges court gay students with e-mail and dance parties. *Chronicle of Higher Education 57, no. 35* (May 6, 2011), A11–A12.

Lipka, S. Support for gay marriage is greater among college freshmen than Americans at large. *Chronicle of Higher Education 56, no. 28* (March 16, 2010), A14–A15.

Liptak, A. California ruling expands same-sex parental rights. *The New York Times* (August 23, 2005). Available: http://www.nytimes.com/2005/08/23/national/23gay.html.

Martin, D., & Lyon, P. *Lesbian-woman.* New York: Bantam (1972).

McKinley, J. Gay marriage ban inspires new wave of activists. *The New York Times* (December 10, 2008).

Money, J. Sin, sickness, or status: Homosexual gender identity and psychoneuroendocrinology. *American Psychologist, 42* (1987), 384–399.

Money, J., & Ehrhardt, A. E. *Man and woman, boy and girl.* Baltimore: Johns Hopkins Press, 1972.

Money, J., & Schwartz, M. Dating, romantic and nonromantic friendships and sexuality in 17 early-treated androgenital females, aged 16–25, in *Congenital adrenal hyperplasia,* Lee, P. A., et al., eds. Baltimore: University Park Press, 1977.

MTV launches new gay cable TV channel. *ABC News* (June 28, 2005). Available: http://abcnews.go.com.

Murphy, D. E. Gays celebrate, and plan for broader rights. *The New York Times* (June 27, 2003). Available: www.nytimes.com.

Ness, C. PBS shies from show. *San Francisco Examiner* (June 6, 1999).

Newport, F. For first time, majority of Americans favor legal gay marriage. Gallup, May 20, 2011. Available: http://www.gallup.com/poll/147662/first-time-majority-americans-favor-legal-gay-marriage.aspx.

Ontario Consultants on Religious Tolerance. Brief descriptions of the sex belief systems, 2009. Available: http://www.religioustolerance.org/hom6beli1.htm.

Ontario Consultants on Religious Tolerance. Homosexuality and bisexuality: All sides to the issue (2005). Available: http://www.religioustolerance.org/homosexu.htm.

An open letter to religious leaders on marriage equality. Religious Institute on Sexual Morality, Justice, and Healing 2004. Available: http://www.religiousinstitute.org.

Padgett, T. A welcome mat for gays? *Time, 165, no. 23* (June 6, 2005), 20.

Presgraves, D. 2009 National School Climate Survey: Nearly 9 out of 10 LGBT students experience harassment in school. Gay, Lesbian and Straight Education Network (September 14, 2010). Available: http://www.glsen.org/cgi-bin/iowa/all/news/record/2624.html.

A profile of this year's freshmen. *Chronicle of Higher Education*, January 27, 2011. Available:http://chronicle.com/article/A-Profile-of-This-Years/126067/.

Pruitt, P. Majority of Americans support legalizing same-sex marriage, poll shows. *ABC News* (June 6, 2012). Available: http://abcnews.go.com/Politics/OTUS/majority-americans-support-legalizing-sex-marriage-poll-shows/story?id=16505633#.UCwBDVZlS2X.

Relationship recognition for same-sex couples in the U.S. National Gay and Lesbian Task Force, 2011. Available: http://www.thetaskforce.org/reports_and_research/relationship_recognition.

Robbins, L. Swoopes says she is gay, and exhales. *The New York Times* (October 27, 2005).

Ross, M. W. Situating sexuality electronically: The Internet and sexual expression. *Sexuality Research & Public Policy, 4, 2* (June 2007), 1–4.

Ruscombe-King, R. Homophobia, prejudice and attitudes to gay men and lesbians. AVERT (an international AIDS charity), 2009. Available: http://avert.org/homophobia.htm.

Russell, S. T. LGBTQ youth are at risk in U.S. school environment. *SIECUS Report, 29, no. 4* (April/May 2001), 19–22.

Russell, S. T., Ryan, C., Toomey, R. B., Diaz, R. M., & Sanchez, J. Lesbian, gay, bisexual, and transgender adolescent school victimization: Implications for young adult health and adjustment. *Journal of School Health 81, no. 5* (May, 2011), 223–229.

Ryan, C., & Futterman, D. Social and developmental challenges for lesbian, gay, and bisexual youth. *SIECUS Report, 29, no. 4* (April/May 2001), 5–18.

Ryan, C., Huebner, D., Diaz, R. M., & Sanchez, J. Family rejection as a predictor of negative health outcomes in white and Latino lesbian, gay, and bisexual young adults. *Pediatrics, 123, 1* (January 2009), 346–352.

Saad, L. Abortion views hold steady over past year: Public makes sharp distinction about abortion circumstances. *Gallup News Service* (June 2, 2003). Available: http://www.gallup.com/poll/content/default.aspx?ci=8521.

Sadowski, M. Sexuality minority students benefit from school-based support—where it exists. *Harvard Education Letter, Research Online* (September/October, 2001). Available: http://www.edletter.org/current/.

Saewyc, E. M., Homma, Y., Skay, C. L., Bearinger, L. H., Resnick, M. D., & Reis, E. Protective factors in the lives of bisexual adolescents in North America. *American Journal of Public Health, 99, 1* (January 2009), 110–117.

Saewyc, E. M., Taylor, D., Homma, Y., & Ogilvie, G. Trends in sexual health and risk behaviours among adolescents students in British Columbia. *Canadian Journal of Human Sexuality, 17, 1–2* (2008), 1–13.

Savic, I., Berglund, H., & Lindstrom, P. Brain response to putative pheromones in homosexual men. *Proceedings of the National Academy of Sciences, 102, no. 20* (May 17, 2005), 7356–7361.

Schuklenk, U., & Ristow, M. The ethics of research into the cause(s) of homosexuality. *Journal of Homosexuality 31, no. 3* (1996), 5–30.

Schweitzer, S. Connecticut approves gay civil unions. *The Boston Globe* (April 21, 2005).

Should lesbian and gay couples be allowed to adopt? In *Taking sides: Issues in family and personal relationships*, Schroeder, E., ed. Guilford, CT: McGraw-Hill/Dushkin, 2003.

SIECUS Policy and Advocacy. A portrait of sexuality education and abstinence-only-until-marriage programs in the states (fiscal year 2008 edition), 2008. Available: http://www.siecus.org/index.cfm?fuseaction=Page.ViewPage&PageID=1164.

SIECUS position statements on sexuality issues, 2012. Available: http://www.siecus.org.

Smith, G. ... the only openly gay male athlete. *Sports Illustrated* (May 3, 2010), 56–62.

Staley, M., Hussey, W., Roe, K., Harcourt, J., & Roe, K. In the shadow of the rainbow: Identifying and addressing health disparities in the lesbian, gay, bisexual, and transgender population—a research and practice challenge. *Health Promotion Practice, 2, no. 3* (July 2001) 207–211.

Statement by Secretary Kathleen Sebelius on LGBT Health Awareness Week 2012. March 26, 2012. Available: http://www.hhs.gov/news/press/2012pres/03/20120326a.html.

Student sexuality: How can and should schools respond? *Alabama School Boards, 25, no. 3* (September–October 2004), 6–7+.

Suicide Prevention Resource Center. Suicide risk and prevention for lesbian, gay, bisexual, and transgender youth. Newton, MA: Education Development Center, 2008.

Swarns, R. L. Male couples face pressure to fill cradles. *The New York Times* (August 9, 2012). Available: http://www.nytimes.com/2012/08/10/us/gay-couples-face-pressure-to-have-children.html?pagewanted=all.

Thomas, K. College team teaches a lesson in acceptance. *The New York Times* (May 7, 2010). Available: http://www.nytimes.com/2010/05/09/sports/09oneonta.html.

Trebay, G. The secret power of lesbian style. *The New York Times* (June 27, 2004).

UNAIDS. HIV prevention hampered by homophobia, 2009. Available: http://www.unaids.org/en/KnowledgeCentre/Resources/FeatureStories/archive/2009/20090113_MSMLATAM.asp.

Vo, K. Universities reach out to gay, lesbian students. *San Jose Mercury News* (May 25, 2003), A7.

Waddell, L. Florida county ending official support of gay events. *The New York Times* (June 26, 2005), sect 1, p. 15.

Wallick, M. M. Homophobia and heterosexism: Out of the medical school closet. *North Carolina Medical Journal, 58, no. 2* (March–April 1997), 123–125.

Weinstein, N., Ryan, W. S., DeHaan, C. R., Przybylski, A. K., Legate, N., & Ryan, R. M. Parental autonomy support and discrepancies between implicit and explicit sexual identities: dynamics of self-acceptance and defense. *Journal of Personality and Social Psychology, 102, no. 4* (April 2012), 815–832.

Whitman, F., & Diamond, M. *A preliminary report on the sexual orientation of homosexual twins.* Paper presented at the Western Region Annual Conference of the Society for the Scientific Study of Sex, Scottsdale, AZ, January 1986.

Why it's important to talk about sexual orientation. *Families Are Talking 3, no. 2* (2004), 1–3.

Worthington, R. L., Savoy, H. B., Dillon, F. R., & Vernaglia, E. R. Heterosexual identity development: A multidimensional model of individual and social identity. *The Counseling Psychologist, 30,* (2002), 496–531.

Young, J. R. Gay student is forced out of a campus leadership post at an Iowa college. *Chronicle of Higher Education, 49, no. 13* (November 22, 2002), A58.

Zanghellini, A. Scientific positivism and the controversy over research into lesbian and gay parenting. *Sexuality Research & Social Policy, 4, 3* (September 2007), 100–114.

CHAPTER 11

Sexuality in Childhood and Adolescence

FEATURES

Communication Dimensions
Tips for Discussing Sexual Messages and Scandals on TV with Children

Communication Dimensions
Resources for Becoming Askable

Ethical Dimensions
Is It Ethical to Ignore Your Child's Developing Sexuality?

Gender Dimensions
How Gender Stereotypes Affect Sexuality

Multicultural Dimensions
Racial and Ethnic Differences in Sexual Behaviors

Global Dimensions
Teenagers and Sexuality Around the World

CHAPTER OBJECTIVES

1 Explain why an infant is a sexual being; include the role that touch plays in development.

2 Explain the sexual development of children from preschool through the early elementary years.

3 Describe the differences in puberty for boys and girls.

4 Identify the three developmental stages of adolescence.

5 Compare the findings of various surveys concerning adolescent sexual behaviors and attitudes.

6 Discuss the prevalence of sexual abuse and sexual harassment of children and adolescents.

go.jblearning.com/dimensions5e

Sexual Development During Preschool and Early Elementary Years
The Media as Sexuality Educator of Children
Late Adolescence

INTRODUCTION

Shawna is a precocious 5-year-old who already reads. She's been eating lunch at a nice restaurant with her mother after a morning of shopping. In the restroom before heading for home, she notices a vending machine mounted on the wall and asks, "Mama, why are they selling napkins in the bathroom when they already give them to everyone when they're eating?" Mama, visibly flustered, says, "We'll talk about it later, after we get home." Shawna feels as if she has asked something she shouldn't have mentioned and never brings it up again. Neither does her mother.

A few years later, still a precocious child, she reaches menarche just as she enters fifth grade, before she turns 10. Shawna has used the dictionary to learn all the "facts of life" she can find. She knows what is happening to her body, but is afraid to tell her mother. She privately rejoices at this sign of her physical maturity. Finally, some stained panties in the laundry disclose her secret. Then she and her mother have "the talk" about menstruation. Shawna's mother shares that when she was growing up, she was expected to announce when every period came at the breakfast table. That was very embarrassing to her, and she doesn't want Shawna to feel the same way. So she suggests, "Just let me know if there is anything you need or if something doesn't seem right." Looking back, that assurance was both positive and comforting. Shawna hopes someday she will be able to treat her own daughter with that kind of respect. But she will have "the talk" sooner and will try to answer questions candidly whenever they come up.

Now as a young mother, Shawna is in a public restroom with both her daughters, aged 3 and 5. Her 5-year-old, Samantha, asks, "Mom, how come they sell 'tampads' in here?" Remembering her own early questions, Shawna *decides to respond on the spot in front of both girls and anyone else that happens to be listening. She says, "The pads are for women or older girls who are having a menstrual period. It's a natural and healthy thing that happens every month. A period helps a girl's body to be able to have babies."*

As you read this chapter, you may want to think about your own life and ask yourself, "How did I become who I am today?" "Which experiences helped promote my sexual health?" "What happened to me that I must overcome as I move into sexual adulthood?"

Learning the sexual values of parents and caregivers happens through observation and nonverbal cues, along with the "talks" that may or may not have helped move one over the speed bumps that happen as children grow up. Reflect on past experience; think about how situations might have been handled differently. Perhaps questions could have been answered more honestly. Puzzling dilemmas might have been discussed more openly.

Today, honest answers, balanced discussion, and decision-making options are more available than ever before. Reliable websites, well-informed educators, and parental resources abound. (See suggestions in Communication Dimensions: Resources for Becoming Askable.) Yet, this open discussion leads to more emphasis on sexuality in the media. Parents are understandably confused about how to answer their children's questions about the most recent scandal related to sexuality.

How much should they tell their children? Should they answer their children's questions directly? Should they try to shield their children from the news?

Sexual Development of Infants and Toddlers

Sexuality education begins in the delivery room. Of course, we are not talking about giving newborn babies facts about reproduction or sexual behaviors. But think for a minute: What is the first or second question parents ask after the birth of a child? They ask, "Is it a boy or a girl?" And sexuality education about gender roles begins.

Newborn babies develop sexually. In some ways, the first 18 months of life is one of the most important times for learning about love and touch and developing a sense of trust in the world. It is during their infancy that babies learn they are loved

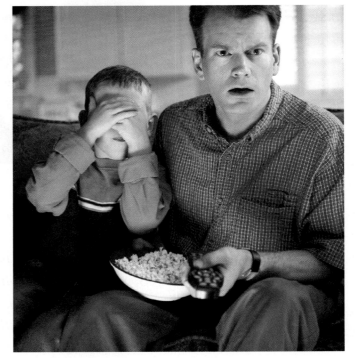

Many parents find it hard to discuss sexual relationships that are sensationalized in the media. However, it is important to realize that parents teach their children about sexuality with what they say—as well as by what they do not say. By *not* saying anything about the latest incidents in the news, parents may be inadvertently telling their children not to ask questions about sexuality.

Communication
DIMENSIONS

Tips for Discussing Sexual Messages and Scandals on TV with Children

If a sexuality scandal of a high public official or a popular entertainer makes headlines, most likely any child in school will hear about it. Many parents wonder whether they need to discuss these scandals at all. The question parents need to ask is, Who do I want to tell my children about this sad situation? Another child on the playground? An acquaintance on the school bus?

Here are some tips for discussing scandals with your children:

1. Think about values as they relate to the current situation. What are your family values about sexual behavior outside marriage, fidelity, telling the truth?
2. Find out what the children already know. Do not wait for them to ask questions. That may never happen. You can start by saying, "Tell me what you've heard about ...." You may be surprised how much they know.
3. Ask them to tell you what certain words mean to them. For example, a child may say that a celebrity had "oral sex" and think that means kissing.
4. Clarify the facts. Give short, age-appropriate answers. A short answer on "oral sex" for a child below the age of 10 years is, "Adults kiss, hug, or touch each other in special ways to show caring and share sexual pleasure. Oral sex is one way." Ask preteens or teenagers for their definition. Then correct any misinformation.
5. Help your children understand the larger issues surrounding sexuality scandals. These issues will affect the families of those involved, careers, and possibly the welfare of the nation.
6. You do not have to answer questions about your personal life. The answer to "Do you and Daddy do that?" is "Daddy's and my sex life is personal. When you are an adult, you will decide what sexual behaviors are comfortable for you."

Television has become a primary part of most children's sexuality education. Rather than viewing media as an adversary in efforts to educate, it can become an ally. Suit the conversation to the developmental level of the child.

Age 3–6: Focus on varied family configurations and non-normative sex roles to help little ones learn about different grown-up possibilities.

Age 7–10: Identify concerns about racial and ethnic differences, body image, clothing, and hairstyles, especially unwarranted stereotyping and advertising.

Age 11–13: Programs featuring hidden feelings and deceptions make good lessons as emotions and hormones escalate. Discuss how feelings are expressed and directed.

Age 14–17: Major adolescent concerns involve sexual behaviors and their consequences. Use viewing to discuss issues; muse aloud.

Source: Data from Garrity, J. *Tuning in to TV sex: Using television for dialogue with your children.* Santa Monica, CA. Center for Media Literacy, 2002. Retrieved June 5, 2009, from http://medialit.org/reading_room/pdf/24_TVsex_teachable.pdf.

and learn how to love when parents kiss them, hug them, and talk to them. Babies also learn whether care providers will meet their needs or whether they will have to tough it out. They learn quickly whether they can count on their care providers to respond to their basic needs.

Actually, biological sexual development begins during pregnancy. Prenatal ultrasound technology has verified that the sexual response system begins to develop in males during the middle stages of gestation. Erectile response begins to appear at around 16 weeks; respiratory function does not begin until almost 12 weeks later. And, although sexual response in female fetuses is not readily observable, it is assumed that the capacity for lubrication begins at this time as well.

During the first few months of life, **infants**, babies from birth to 1 year, begin to discover their bodies. By 7 or 8 months, they discover their hands and toes. About the same time, boys discover their penis. Girls, on average, seem to discover their vulva about 2 months later. Infants love to put their fingers and toes into their mouths, and they love to touch their genitals. Baby boys have erections regularly throughout the day and during sleep, as many as three or more times a night. Infant boys may become erect simply by crying, coughing, stretching, or urinating. Baby girls' vaginas are believed to lubricate about just as often, although

infants
Babies from birth to 1 year old.

this is not easily observable, and studies on this topic have not been done.

Psychosexual Development

Cuddling and stroking babies help them learn that their bodies feel good when they are touched and also help cement the parent–child bond. In fact, research shows that parents should hold their babies as much as possible. Touch is one of the first ways that a baby learns he or she is loved. Some psychologists theorize that a loving touch helps set the stage for adult intimacy. Touching and holding infants teach them how parents feel about them. When I am crying, will I be picked up? Can I count on you to show me that you love me? Responding to infants' needs teaches them that the world is a predictable, safe place. It boosts their self-confidence and their ability to believe that when they need help and support, they will get it. When parents and caregivers convey love and delight when they hold their infants, the infants learn they are loved.

Bonding, based on this love, begins at birth when mother and newborn are brought together. It continues during feeding, diapering, smiling, talking, and acknowledging the infant. As an active and comfortable participant in parenting, the father also bonds with the infant through touch. This fosters trust that all needs will be fulfilled and the infant is **thriving**. Developing a sense of trust in the world is an important foundation for adult mental health, including sexual health. The developmental psychologist Erik H. Erikson wrote that the first psychosocial crisis in life is to resolve "basic trust versus basic mistrust." According to Erikson, between birth and 18 months of age, children learn whether their needs will be met and whether they can trust the people and the world around them. If their needs are met, they develop the ability for intimacy and a sense of hope. Erikson wrote that feeding is the primary way that an infant resolves these issues (Erikson, 1950).

In the early 1960s, two researchers did an important experiment with rhesus monkeys. They separated some monkeys from their mothers at birth and offered them surrogate wire mothers to hold. Some of the surrogates were only wire frames; others were covered with soft fabric. The monkeys would cling to a dummy covered with soft fabric but rejected one made up just of wire, even when it had a bottle of milk attached. In other words, the baby monkeys preferred a soft touch to being fed. The baby monkeys denied touch grew up to be troubled adult monkeys. They were more likely to bite and scratch; the males did not approach females sexually; and the females were mostly infertile (Bullough & Bullough, 1994). Some psychologists believe that such studies show that a lack of touch in infancy can affect future adult sexual and intimate relationships.

Teaching Body Parts

Bath time and diaper changes are wonderful times to start teaching a child about body parts—*all* the parts of his or her body. Many parents play this game to teach body parts with their 5- or 6-month-old children: "Here is your nose, here's your tummy, here are your knees, here are your toes." In addition to teaching the names of these body parts, these parents may be inadvertently conveying an early message about their willingness to address sexual issues. These parents may be communicating to their child that many (one-third) of the body's parts have no names and that they are different from all the other parts of the body. How much more sex-positive it would be if parents could learn to say, calmly and without flinching, "Here's your nose, here's your tummy, here's your penis (or vulva), here are your knees, here are your toes." Thus all the parts of the body that the baby is exploring have names, and parents can speak about all of them.

Parents should treat all body parts equally. When parents use euphemisms only for the genitals, they give their child a message that these parts of the body are shameful or different. They may, without meaning to or realizing it, even introduce a sense of guilt about certain parts of the body. These feelings sometimes persist into adulthood, making it difficult for grown men and women to be comfortable with their bodies and sexual feelings. They may also affect a child's ability to tell about sexually abusive incidents accurately.

Infant Genital Touching

Babies begin to explore their genitals during diaper changes. This usually happens at about 7 to 10 months, a little after they discover that they have fingers and toes. And they experience for themselves that it feels good to touch all the parts of their bodies.

Many parents are uncomfortable when they see their babies touch their genitals. They wonder what, if anything, they should do. They wonder whether their child is masturbating or is becoming obsessed with this behavior. This type of genital exploration is not the same as masturbation; it is generally not purposeful and not directed at orgasm. It is about exploring and learning more about the body.

psychosexual development
The blending of sexual aspects of one's development with other psychological factors.

bonding
A process of developing a close physical and psychological relationship with one's caregiver.

thriving
Normal physical and psychological pattern of weight gain, neuromuscular development, and other developmental attributes of infants.

Communication
DIMENSIONS

Resources for Becoming Askable

Here are some guidelines for becoming askable—10 healthy hints—as well as examples of questions and answers.

1. Start early, using body language and nonverbal behaviors to convey messages of approachability.
2. Giving "too much" information should not be a concern. Observe reactions to gauge how much is needed.
3. Communicate openly, even acknowledging discomfort.
4. Admit ignorance and offer to find out—together if possible.
5. Concise, simple answers are better than long lectures.
6. Too much technical information won't hurt; it allows children to sort it out and honors their ability to understand.
7. Mistakes will happen; admit them, correct them if possible, and handle them as you would other mistakes.
8. Share your values about sexual matters; children want to know what you believe.
9. Encourage laughing and learning by using a sense of humor.
10. Use books as a springboard for discussion; they are lasting and can be referred to over and over (Blonna & Levitan, 2006).

Having resources at hand is helpful when talking to children about sexuality issues in the home. See the suggested reading list at the end of the chapter to begin a resource library at home.

Sexuality education often begins with a child's curiosity about his or her body. Let the child set the pace with his or her questions.

If your child points to a body part, simply tell him or her what it is. This is also a good time to talk about which parts of the body are private.

Expect self-stimulation. Teach your child that masturbation is a normal—but private—activity. If it happens in public, try distraction. If that fails, take your child aside for a reminder about the importance of privacy.

Curiosity about others—examining another child's sex organs—is usually normal exploration and far removed from adult sexual activity. It's harmless when only young children are involved, but as a family matter, you may want to set limits on such exploration.

Take advantage of everyday opportunities. Consider these examples:

- **How do babies get inside mommy?** You might say, "A mom and a dad make a baby by holding each other in a special way."
- **How are babies born?** It might be enough to say, "Doctors and nurses help babies who are ready to be born." If your child wants more details, you might say, "Usually a mom pushes the baby out of her vagina."
- **Why doesn't everyone have a penis?** Try a simple explanation such as, "Boys' and girls' bodies are made differently."
- **Why do you have hair down there?** Simplicity often works here, too. You might say, "Our bodies change as we get older." If your child wants more details, add, "Boys grow hair near their penises, and girls grow hair near their vaginas."

Answer specific questions using correct terminology. Even if you're uncomfortable, forge ahead. Remember—you're setting the stage for open, honest discussions in the years to come.

Source: Reproduced from Mayo Clinic, 2009. Retrieved June 5, 2009, from www.mayoclinic.com/health/sex-education/HQ00547.

Self-exploration lays the foundation for development of a broad range of sexual feelings and behaviors. Parental reaction also impacts development. Consider the effect of punishment—yelling, pushing the hand away, and admonishing the behavior as dirty. Conveying a strong negative message about behavior that is pleasurable creates confusion—ultimately leading to feelings of shame and fear about sexuality.

Some responses that encourage healthy sexual development include viewing exploratory behavior as normal learning, socializing for privacy rather than forbidding, using natural opportunities to provide basic information, and becoming more "askable."

Gender During the Early Years

Many experts believe that there are some innate differences between boy babies and girl babies. In general, boy babies seem to be more active than girl babies. Girl babies may develop faster. This is often shown by girls sitting up, reaching for objects, and talking earlier than boys. However, there can be a wide variation of timing in both boys and girls, so we cannot say that all boy babies or all girl babies follow exact timing.

The expectations of parents for their babies can also influence gender development. For example, today many people going through a pregnancy know the gender of their baby well before the baby is born. Some experts believe that these parents start talking differently to their unborn babies and act differently towards them once they know the gender of the baby. This same behavior often occurs after the baby is born. Many parents speak differently to boy infants and girl infants. They may touch and hold them differently as well. They may even react differently to the needs of the baby depending upon its gender.

During the first 18 months of life, children are beginning to learn the differences between males and females (that is, **gender identity**). As they approach 3 years old, most boys and girls can identify dolls and photographs as male or female. They can also tell an adult whether they are a girl or a boy.

In their early years, children encounter many **gender stereotypes**. They identify certain behaviors as male or female. They

> **gender identity**
> Having an internal sense of self as male or female; part of one's self-image.
>
> **gender stereotypes**
> Beliefs about how each gender should behave, which may be over-generalized or rigidly held.

might think male things and female things are supposed to be different colors. Children learn from the world around them. In their homes they might see (or be told) that males do certain things and females do other things. They might learn that opportunities and behaviors are supposed to be very different for males and females. Children are also influenced by what they see in the media related to gender stereotypes. Perhaps most important, what adults say and do around children can have a big impact on what these children believe about gender and the amount of gender stereotypes they believe in their own lives.

■ Sexual Development During Preschool and Early Elementary Years

During the years from age 3 years to age 5 years, children begin to develop a strong sense of gender and what that means to them and the people around them. They are finishing with toilet training, and if they are in school or a day care center, they have probably observed other children and learned for themselves that boys and girls have different body parts. At this time the child realizes that he or she will not normally change over the life span. This concept is known as **gender constancy**. Children of this age are very curious about their own and other people's bodies. This is the age when a child is first likely to ask, "Where did I come from?"

> **gender constancy**
> Recognition by a child that he or she will remain the same gender throughout life.

Preschool Genital Touching

Three- and 4-year-olds delight in their own bodies. And just as they learn it feels good when they run, jump, and cuddle, they are also discovering that it feels good when they touch their own genitals. Most professionals believe that preschool children touch their genitals as a natural part of child development. In a study of mothers of 2- to 5-year-olds, mothers reported that 25% of their sons and 15% of their daughters touched their genitals in public. Sixteen percent of both preschool boys and girls had been observed masturbating with their hands (Delamater & Friedrich, 2002).

Toddlers and preschoolers touch their genitals in a much less purposeful way than older children and adolescents, and many do so without embarrassment or anxiety. In fact, it is not unusual in a preschool to have several of the boys touching their penis unconsciously throughout the day. Little girls find it pleasurable to touch their vulva and clitoris as well.

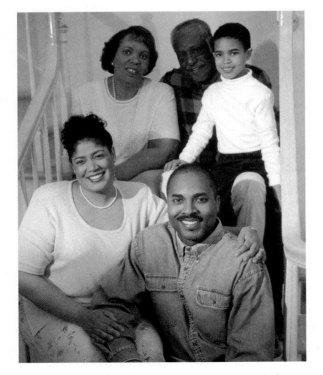

The affection displayed by parents sets an example for their children. Parents who are violent or abusive to each other around a child also set an example for the child to follow.

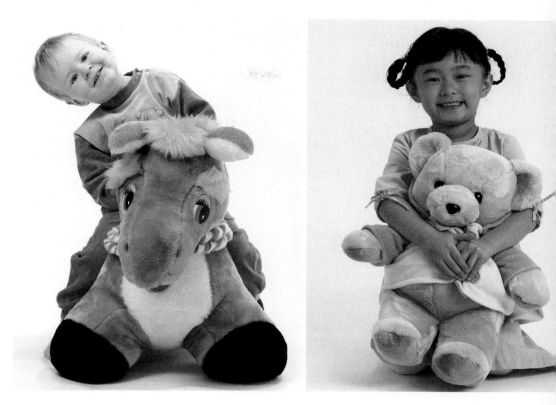

Not only do parents treat boys and girls differently, but children themselves learn gender differences in voices, levels of aggression, and even the colors of toys.

Many children appear not even to be aware that they are touching their genitals in this way. Some children do discover that this activity helps them calm down. Many children touch their genitals right before naps or bedtimes to help them fall asleep. (Just as for adults, some children never touch their genitals at all. It is normal for a preschooler to touch the genitals and it is normal for him or her not to.)

Attraction to Parents

Sigmund Freud felt that 3- to 5-year-old boys develop fantasies of possessing their mother sexually and become jealous of their father. He named it the **Oedipus complex** after the Greek tragedy in which Oedipus unknowingly kills his father and then marries his mother. According to Freud's theory, this period is accompanied by castration anxiety; boys fear that their father will retaliate against their interest in their mother by cutting off their penis. Freud also theorized that girls develop an **Electra complex**; they develop "penis envy" and want to take their father away from their mother. Girls, he said, reject their mother because they blame her for their lack of a penis. Freud named

Oedipus complex
Libidinal feelings of a child toward the parent of the opposite sex and hostile or jealous feelings toward the parent of the same sex.

Electra complex
Freud's theory that 3- to 5-year-old girls want to take their father away from their mother.

this "complex" the Electra complex after the Greek tragedy in which a princess helps kill her mother.

Most modern psychologists debunk these ideas. Feminist psychologists critique Freud's views as extremely sexist, and anthropologists point out that these "complexes" are not found in all cultures. Still, it is not uncommon for preschool children to prefer the parent of the opposite gender at this time.

Preschool children love their parents intensely and may be confused about whether all love is expressed romantically. Many children try to kiss their parents romantically. Some even try to imitate adults they have seen in person or on TV or in the movies by putting their tongue into their parents' mouths.

Preschool children sometimes may even seem jealous when their parents show affection to each other. In one study, 13% of mothers of 2- to 5-year-olds reported that their children became upset when they saw adults kiss (Delamater & Friedrich, 2002).

Preschoolers and Sex Play

Many adults remember playing "doctor" or "house" with other children. Playing doctor, including undressing each other and examining each other's genitals, is quite common. Most child development experts see this type of sex play as expected and natural childhood sexual curiosity. If the children are of the same age and stage of development, experts do not believe that it is harmful. And studies of adults show that engaging

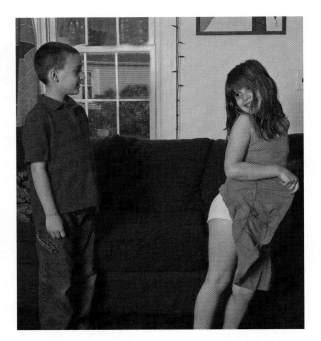

In early childhood, availability of playmates influences interaction. Games that provide opportunities for sex play and exploration such as "doctor" or "nurse" are responses to natural curiosity. According to Erickson's developmental stages (Erikson, 1950), these children need to accomplish autonomy and initiative rather than shame, doubt, or guilt.

in childhood sexual play does not seem to have any effect, either positive or negative, on adult sexuality.

Besides concern about childhood sex play among peers, exposure to nudity or parental sexual intercourse has been studied. The researchers concluded that such exposure is not detrimental to the mental health of children. Characterizing exposure as harmful or even a subtle form of abuse might better be conceptualized as myth (Okami et al., 1998). Another concern, that of erections among young boys as evidence of romantic interest, is also a myth. Erections come and go, rise and fall, among babies and young boys, even sleeping and waking adults, with odd timing (Schwartz & Rutter, 2000). Another study examined the impact of noncoercive sexual contact with similarly aged individuals. Researchers found that adult adjustment problems were no different from those who had no sexual abuse experience. Among those who had been abused, problems escalated according to the amount of coercion reported (Friedrich, Whiteside, & Talley, 2004).

That said, there is a big difference between normally harmless child sexual play and play that is exploitative or abusive. Children do not normally engage in painful sexual behavior, oral–genital contact, or simulated or real intercourse or penetration with fingers or objects with another child, and they do not engage in normal sexual play with children more than a few years older than they are. These behaviors may indicate a child who *may* have been sexually abused. (They could also indicate exposure to inappropriate TV or videos.) Table 11.1 provides some guidelines on distinguishing between harmless play and exploitative, inappropriate behaviors.

Questions About Reproduction

Some time between the ages of 2½ and 5 years, children ask, "Where did I come from?" Children at this age are often very curious about pregnancy and birth. According to psychologists, at around the age of 4 years, children understand that babies do not just spontaneously appear and that something must have happened for this process to begin.

The psychologist Anne C. Bernstein did research with small children about how they understand reproduction (Bernstein, 1994). She labels the preschooler asking about reproduction a "geographer." The emphasis really is on the *where*: They want to know *where* the baby comes from and *where* it was before it was born. Preschoolers can be offered a very simple answer: "You grew in a special place inside Mom called a uterus. You began from a tiny egg (the size of a pencil dot) from Mom and an even tinier sperm from Dad." This will satisfy most preschoolers. If they ask, "But how did I get into the uterus?" they can be given a very simple definition of sexual intercourse:

When two grown-ups love each other, they like to kiss and hug and touch each other in ways that feel good. Sometimes, the man and woman place the man's penis into the woman's vagina. The man's penis releases sperm into the woman and sometimes a baby begins.

TABLE 11.1 **A Quick Way to Assess Whether Childhood Sex Play Is Likely to Be Harmless or Whether Parents Should Be Concerned**

	Expected	Problematic
Age of children	Similar	More than 3 years apart
Children seem	Giggly, curious, happy	Aggressive, angry, fearful, withdrawn
Activities	Undressing, playing doctor ("You show me yours I'll show you mine")	Oral, anal, or vaginal intercourse; penetration with fingers, objects
After parental Intervention	Behavior stops	Behavior continues

Elementary School Years

The early elementary school years (kindergarten to grade 3) are years of tremendous growth and change. Naps and playtime give way to homework and tests. Preschool teacher hugs may be replaced by neutral hellos. The class of 12 now has 20 children, and individual attention is no longer the rule. Children begin to learn about sexuality issues from other children on the bus or the playground.

Freud wrote that the period from 5 to 11 years of age was the **latency period**. Although some blame Freud for mistakenly characterizing this as a period of sexual *dis*interest, Bullough describes it differently. He credits Freud with breaking the taboo on full discussions of sexuality, recognizing it as a prime factor in human development. Rather than *dis*interest, Freud expected active sexual exploration and information seeking, the prepubescent hormone surge and accompanying growth of internal and external sexual organs (Bullough, 2004).

latency period
Outdated Freudian theory that children aged 6–12 years old have no sexual feelings or interest.

Five- to 8-year-olds continue to be very interested in sexual issues; it is just that their interest is no longer as apparent to the adults in their lives as it used to be. In a 1998 study of more than 11,000 children aged 2 to 12 years, mothers reported that they had observed sexual behaviors in children at all of these ages. For example, 14% of 6- to 9-year-old boys were still touching their genitals in public, 40% did so at home, 20% tried to look at people nude, 8% wanted to watch nudity on TV, and 14% were very interested in girls. Girls this age exhibited similar sexual behaviors that were observed by their mothers (Friedrich et al., 1998).

As mentioned, 5- to 8-year-olds continue to develop as sexual persons, and they are very curious about pregnancy and birth. They develop strong friendships, and most boys and girls show a strong preference for playing with children of the same gender. They become even more aware of socially defined gender roles. They may continue to engage in sex play with children of both genders. And in private, their exploration of their genitals may become more purposeful.

Developing Empathy

Some sexologists believe that the period from age 5 years to age 8 years is critical in sexual development. They believe that the elementary school years are the most important time for people to develop as moral thinkers, and that development is important to adult sexual health. While they are preschoolers,

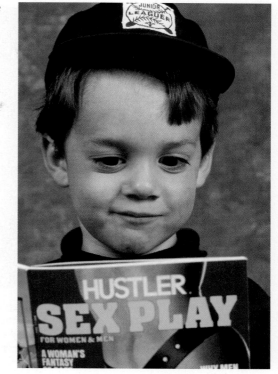

Children are naturally curious about sexuality.

children believe that their way of thinking is the only way possible. But in early elementary school, children begin to understand that there may be other points of view and ways to consider a situation. They can begin to understand the "golden rule": Treat others with the same respect you would want for yourself.

Developing an ability to empathize and make good decisions is part of the foundation for adult sexual health. A sexually healthy adult is able, for example, to make decisions about his or her sexuality that are consistent with his or her own values.

The Media as Sexuality Educator of Children

The media—television, movies, magazines, even the news—are among many children's most prominent sexuality educators. On average, children ages 2 to 5 years spend 32 hours a week in front of a TV—watching television, DVDs, DVR, and videos and using a game console. Children ages 6 to 11 years spend about 28 hours a week in front of the TV. TV can be entertaining and help children learn about different cultures and gain exposure to ideas they may never encounter in their own community. However, children can also learn things from TV that may affect their health, behavior, and family life in negative ways. For example, children may learn to accept the stereotypes presented on TV. Research indicates that what children see on TV does affect how they see

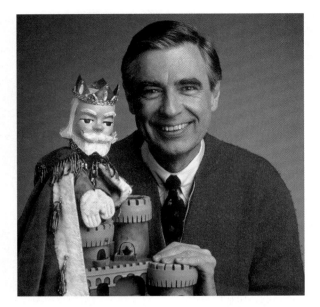

Although it was clearly intended for preschoolers, the second largest audience for *Mister Rogers' Neighborhood* was preadolescents, who want to hear that they are special and that they are OK just as they are. What other media programs offer positive self-esteem messages to preadolescents?

male and female roles in society. In addition, children can get lots of information about sexuality from TV. Sexual content is a real presence on TV. The number of sex scenes on TV has nearly doubled since 1998. Some researchers are concerned that watching sexual content on TV will influence children to make poor decisions about their own sexual activity (Television and children, 2011).

In addition to television, movies, music videos, video games, print, and the Internet are pervasive forms of media in today's world. According to the *Surgeon General's Call to Action to Promote Sexual Health and Responsible Sexual Behavior* (Satcher, 2001), sexual talk and behavior are increasingly explicit and frequent. Much of the content in videos and films portrays sexual eroticism, and more than half of television programming has sexual content. Thus the media do have potential for providing sexuality information and education. In a national survey, more than half the students said they learned about topics such as birth control, contraception, and preventing pregnancy from television and magazines. Yet the impact of media on actual behavior is controversial and research is indecisive (Weinstein & Rosen, 2006).

Focusing on media literacy rather than potential harm may be a way of enhancing the benefits of media as a source of useful information. More and more schools are embracing the notion that learning how information is assembled and edited will help students read, hear, and view media more critically

(Goldstein, 2005). An analytical perspective can help young people entering puberty as they view media norms that present a narrow cultural definition of physical perfection. The goal is to foster an internal **locus of control** in which one's sense of identity is personally defined and not dependent on the scripts of others. An example of such an educational approach for girls in grades 4–8 is called *Full of Ourselves: A Wellness Program to Advance Girl Power, Health, and Leadership* (Steiner-Adair & Sjostrom, 2006). It is a primary prevention program aimed at helping girls decrease their vulnerability to body preoccupation and eating disorders. One of the units focuses on media literacy, particularly advertising strategies. Both parents and schools are encouraged to create a supportive environment for students entering puberty.

> **locus of control**
> Refers to an individual's perception of the main causes of events in life. More simply, is life's destiny controlled by the self (*internal locus*) or by external forces such as fate or other people (*external locus*)?

■ Sexual Development During Puberty

Puberty, teenager, and *adolescence* are not interchangeable words. *Puberty* is the stage of maturation when a human being becomes capable of sexual reproduction. *Teenager* is defined chronologically: A teenager is a young person between the ages of 13 and 19 years. *Adolescence* is actually a relatively new concept: It is the period of development that extends from puberty (or the end of childhood) through the attainment of full adult status. Before 1900, and still today in many developing societies, children marry shortly after puberty and begin their adult responsibilities. Today, as more American young people stretch their college and graduate school education through their 20s and even 30s—and then return to live in their parents' homes—some have wondered when contemporary U.S. adolescence ends: At 30 years? When you buy your own home? Have your own children? Before your midlife crisis?

Preparing for Puberty

Young people, at some time between the ages of 8 and 16 years, go through a predictable process of biological development called *puberty*. Normal pubertal changes, indicated by the development of **secondary sexual characteristics** such as breast buds and pubic hair, may begin

> **secondary sexual characteristics**
> Changes occurring during adolescence—such as growth of pubic hair, breast development, and testes and penile development.

as early as age 8 years for girls and as early as age 9 years for boys, but some teens may not begin these changes until they are 15 or 16 years old. The median age for puberty to begin for boys is between 11 and 12 years; for girls, it is between 10 and 11 years. Still, *average* means that half of young people begin this process earlier, and half begin it later. The process of puberty from the first physical changes to obtaining a fully adult body and full reproductive potential may last 4 or 5 years. On average, boys begin and end puberty about 1 year to 2 years later than girls do.

Many young women in college human sexuality classes say they were not prepared adequately for pubertal changes. Some received little or no education in school. Many who did have some education report that it was poorly done and contained little helpful information. Fortunately, there are some who report good educational programs related to puberty, but they seem to be in a relatively small minority. Other college women report that they received only scant information from their mother or father or older siblings or friends.

Puberty for Girls

The first noticeable sign of puberty in girls is generally the development of **breast buds**; the breast begins to elevate as a small mound. Later, the breast and the nipple get bigger. Light, sparse pubic and underarm hair begins to appear about 6 months later. Girls begin to experience a growth spurt, often growing as much as several inches in a year. Their genital and underarm areas begin to produce sweat glands, and body odor may result. Most girls begin menstrual periods about 2 years after breast budding begins, but some girls have completed breast development before their first

breast budding
First stage of breast development in females, whereby breast tissue elevates as a small mound.

period, and some girls' breasts continue to develop for many years after.

Girls today are experiencing first menstruation at earlier ages than girls growing up three or four decades ago. The average age for first menstruation, **menarche** (pronounced "men-ar-key"), in the United States is now 12½ years. That means that many girls have their first period before the end of seventh grade, and many begin as early as fourth or fifth grade. It also means that many girls will at least be in the eighth grade before their first period, and some may be seniors in high school before they get a period. All of these situations are normal.

menarche
First menstruation for girls.

Tanner scale
Scale developed by Dr. John Tanner for measuring pubertal development in boys and girls.

Many pediatricians use a measurement called a **Tanner scale** to rate physical sexual development in both boys and girls (see Table 11.2).

Puberty for Boys

Puberty in boys begins on average during the sixth or seventh grade, but in some boys it begins at 9 years, and in others puberty does not begin until they are almost 14 years old. Boys experience many of the same changes as girls do. The first physical sign is usually an increase in the size of the testes; unlike breast budding in girls, this is unlikely to be observed by parents. During puberty, they too develop light, sparse pubic and underarm hair, and their sweat glands become activated. Between the ages of 12 and 14 years, their penis and scrotum begin to enlarge. At first, the testes become larger, and the skin on the scrotum reddens and coarsens. As boys mature, their penis starts to grow longer. Pubic hair slowly becomes darker, and it starts to curl. During puberty, the penis doubles in size.

By Tanner stage 3 (see Table 11.3), ejaculation has usually occurred, and there may be some production of sperm. In fact, some sexologists call this **semenarche**, to correspond to the first period of girls (menarche). Most often, a boy experiences this as nocturnal emissions, or wet dreams. By Tanner stage 4, males are fertile and able to cause a pregnancy. The average length of time for a

semenarche
First ejaculation of semen for boys.

TABLE 11.2 Tanner Scale for Girls

Tanner Stage	Pubic Hair	Breasts
1	None	None
2	Sparse	Small breast buds
3	Darker, begins to curl	Breasts and nipples enlarged
4	Coarse, less curly than adult	Continued breast development
5	Adult triangle	Mature; nipple projects

Source: Data from Marshall, W. A., & Tanner, J. M. (June 1969). Variations in pattern of pubertal changes in girls. *Archives of Disease in Childhood, 44,* no. 235, 291–303.

TABLE 11.3 Tanner Scale for Boys

Tanner Stage	Pubic Hair	Penis/Scrotum
1	None	Childlike
2	Sparse	Scrotum: reddened, thinner, larger Penis childlike
3	Darker, begins to curl	Penis length increases Scrotum continues to enlarge and darken
4	Coarse, less curly than adult	Penis increases in length and circumference
5	Adult	Adult

Source: Data from Marshall, W. A., & Tanner, J. M. (February 1970). Variations in the pattern of pubertal changes in boys. *Archives of Disease in Childhood, 45, no. 239,* 13–23.

boy to go through puberty is 3 years, but it can vary from 2 to 5 years.

Significant numbers of boys are troubled by a condition called **gynecomastia**. During puberty, they begin to develop an increase in the glandular tissue around their breasts; in fact, these boys sometimes are very worried and fearful that they are growing breasts or turning into a girl. Nearly one in five 10-year-olds will have this kind of tissue development. In rare cases, gynecomastia may be the result of diseases that are rare in young people: liver disease, **hypogonadism**, **hyperthyroidism**, or **hypothyroidism**. It could also be a sign of drug use. However, most of the time it is just a variation of male pubertal development, and it usually resolves itself within 1 year to 1½ years. It continues longer than 2 years in fewer than 1 in 10 boys.

gynecomastia
Glandular tissue development in the breasts of boys.

hypogonadism
Decreased activity of the gonads that may result in retardation of growth and sexual development.

hyperthyroidism
Excessive functional activity of the thyroid gland.

hypothyroidism
A deficiency of thyroid activity.

Early and Late Developers

Although the majority of young people finish puberty a few years after the start of their teen years, some begin puberty much earlier and some go through it much later. Both early and late developers face special challenges.

Early-developing girls have special problems. Because they look more mature, adults often expect them to act more mature. A third- or fourth-grade girl with developing breasts may feel awkward and want to hide her body. She may be relentlessly teased by her male and female classmates. She may indeed feel that she is not normal. Conversely, late development in boys may be more of a problem than early development. A 15- or 16-year-old boy who is still short, has no facial hair, and has a high voice may be relentlessly teased.

Some children begin puberty much earlier than age 9 or 10 years. Some children even enter what is called **precocious puberty** in the first year of life. Interestingly, this seems to be largely the result of genetic coding in girls, and most often there is no underlying disease. Conversely, precocious puberty in boys is much more likely to be an indication that something is wrong. If parents observe pubertal changes in a boy younger than 7 years old, they should see a health practitioner for a medical evaluation and possible interventions.

What Is Normal?

Early, late, and average developers *all* share a common concern: *Am I normal?* Rapid body changes can be very confusing. Nine- to 12-year-olds can become obsessed with their appearance. In fact, psychologists say preteens have an **imaginary audience**: They think that everyone is looking at them. Getting dressed and preparing their hair and faces can take hours. They need adult reassurance that they are attractive, and they need to understand that it is not true that everyone is looking at them.

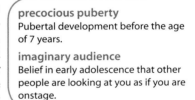

precocious puberty
Pubertal development before the age of 7 years.

imaginary audience
Belief in early adolescence that other people are looking at you as if you are onstage.

They are concerned about their height and breast size or penis size, and they wonder whether they are too developed or too underdeveloped. They wonder whether their feelings, which sometimes fluctuate immensely, are normal. It is important to reassure preadolescents that they are developing according to their own personal genetically predetermined clock. When they ask questions like "How come I don't have my period yet?" or "Why am I the shortest boy in the class?" the question behind the question is almost always "Am I normal?"

The reality is that during preadolescence and the years following it, conflicts with parents peak. Yet, it is important to know that only about one in six teenagers and parents experience a severe disruption in their parent–child relationship (Grunbaum et al., 2004). Preadolescents are just beginning to separate

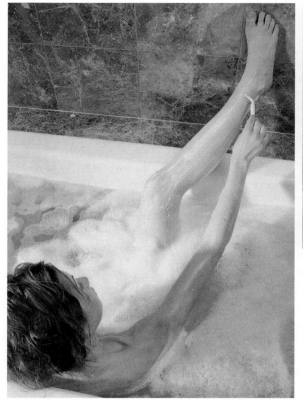

Development of body hair in both boys and girls and facial hair in boys results in shaving, viewed by some as a rite of passage indicating sexual maturity.

from their parents, but they are also still looking to their parents for guidance and support.

Children learn about many aspects of sexuality and relationships from their parents—much of it by astute observation rather than through discussion. Yet, the value of parental involvement and maintaining open lines of communication is well documented as a deterrent to a variety of risky behaviors. Parents can enhance their children's sense of self-worth with assurances of affection and acceptance in spite of the many changes adolescence brings (Strong et al., 2005).

Emotional Changes in Preadolescence

The rapid physical changes of puberty we have described initiate many psychosocial changes. Preadolescents are beginning to move toward independence and are often very self-conscious of their bodies. They may even be embarrassed by parents. Children at this age also need to test parental authority and sometimes the authority of teachers and other adult figures in their lives. This may include trying out values that are different from their parents'. The research literature demonstrates that most teenagers go through a period of seeming to reject their parents' values; yet, by the time they reach adulthood, almost all of them adopt values similar to their parents'.

Friends become very important during the preadolescent years. Being popular is of utmost importance. The good news is that needing to be just like friends, known by psychologists as **conformity with peers**, peaks in early adolescence and then starts to decline. The bad news for parents is that peer pressure can be intense during this period and usually dictates the type of clothes that are acceptable. It also can lead to experimentation with cigarettes, alcohol, and sexual activity.

> **conformity with peers**
> Desire to be like everyone else.

Cliques often emerge during this period. Preadolescents may for the first time feel pressure to engage in certain activities to be part of a group, and, for some young people, that means experimenting with smoking, shoplifting, or cheating on tests.

Preadolescents are also beginning to develop a sense of identity. Their ability to think abstractly has just begun. They frequently daydream and turn inward and imagine acting out different roles. Daydreaming is normal and actually quite healthy. Giving a child a diary or journal and then respecting his or her right to keep it private can be an effective way to encourage a new adolescent to think about and explore his or her feelings. Children at this age can seem very dramatic. They often feel that they are continuously onstage. They may become convinced that their problems are unique and no one understands them.

Masturbation

During puberty, many boys and girls begin to masturbate for sexual pleasure. In addition to providing relief from sexual tension, masturbation has several physical and mental health benefits (Yudt, 2004).

These include relief from migraine headaches and menstrual cramps, and self-knowledge about sexual functioning that can be shared with a partner. In spite of these positive aspects, along with its relative safety—no chance of pregnancy or infection—masturbation creates anxiety. Again, questions arise about what is normal because masturbation is one of the most widely practiced forms of sexual behavior but the least discussed (Weinstein & Rosen, 2006). Data indicate that a majority of boys begin masturbating between the ages of 13 and 15, whereas the onset among girls is more gradual (Bancroft, Herbenick, & Reynolds, 2003). Frequency is also a concern, but is highly individual. Some adults masturbate every day; some, once a year. Some people never masturbate. In fact, teenagers need to know that although many pre-teens, teens, and adults masturbate, some never do.

■ Sexuality in Adolescence

There is public and professional consensus about what is sexually unhealthy for teenagers. Professionals, politicians, and parents across the political spectrum share a deep concern about unplanned adolescent pregnancy; out-of-wedlock childbearing; STIs, including AIDS; sexual abuse; date rape; and the potential negative emotional consequences of premature sexual behaviors.

However, there is little public, professional, or political consensus about what is sexually healthy for teenagers. The public debate about adolescent sexuality has often focused on which sexual behaviors are appropriate for adolescents and ignored the complex dimensions of sexuality.

Some groups support the "Just say no" approach to adolescent sexuality. They believe that the only healthy adolescent sexuality is abstinence from all sexual behaviors until marriage and that adults should work to eliminate teen sexual experimentation. Another approach could be described as "Just say not now." This philosophy encourages young people to abstain until they are more mature but, given the high rates of teenage sexual involvement in intercourse, recommends that it is important to provide young people with access to contraception and condoms regardless of whether adults approve of their behavior. This approach might also be labeled "If you can't say no, protect yourself!" Other adults adopt a "Don't ask; don't tell" posture and simply pretend that adolescent sexuality and sexual behavior do not exist (Grunbaum et al., 2004).

Sexuality Education

It is important for parents and educators to approach sexuality education in a positive way and handle topics as positively as possible. Sources of sexual

Myth **vs** Fact

Myth: People become sexual at puberty.
Fact: People are sexual from birth to death. Although people sexually mature at puberty and become capable of reproduction, infants and children experience sensual feelings and identify themselves as boys and girls.

Myth: Dressing boys in blue and girls in pink teaches them about their gender.
Fact: By the time they are 3 years old, almost all boys and girls identify themselves by gender. They know that they will have that gender throughout their lifetime (the concept known as gender constancy). Clothes' colors do not make a difference.

Myth: Children in elementary school go through a latency period about sexual issues.
Fact: Elementary school children remain very interested in sexuality-related issues, and many continue to be involved in sex play with friends or genital self-pleasuring. They have just learned to hide this behavior from adults.

Myth: The average age of first intercourse has plummeted in the past 5 years.
Fact: The biggest change in adolescent sexual behavior occurred in the 1970s. The average age of first intercourse has decreased by 1 year since 1971.

Myth: Most teenagers have had sexual intercourse.
Fact: Only about half of teenagers aged 15–19 years have had sexual intercourse.

Myth: Masturbating more than once a week is harmful.
Fact: There is no "standard" for frequency of masturbation. Once is too often if you do not like it. Frequency is highly individual, and it is not harmful as long as it does not interfere with school, work, or relationships.

information can exert strong influence on adolescents' sexual behavior. Rosengard et al., (2012) reported that many 15 to 18-year-olds identified the family as sexual health information sources. Their primary messages recalled were risks of sexual behavior, protection, and relationship advice. Many portrayed their learning experiences as negative, cautionary, lacking detail, and not always balanced with positive messages. The authors concluded that sexual health messages should be tailored to adolescents' needs for practical and sex-positive guidance regarding mechanics of sex and formation of healthy relationships, and balanced with cautions regarding negative consequences.

The Sexuality Information and Education Council of the United States (SIECUS) publishes the *Guidelines for Comprehensive Sexuality Education: Kindergarten–12th Grade*, third edition, compiled by the National Guidelines Task Force. The following sections are adapted with permission. "The primary goal of sexuality education is to promote adult sexual health. It should assist young people in developing a positive view of sexuality, provide them with information they need to take care of their sexual health, and help them acquire skills to make decisions now

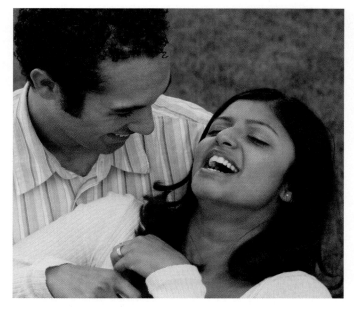

Many adults become concerned when their adolescent children begin to explore their emerging sexuality. But honest communication between an adult and a child can help him or her develop into a sexually healthy adult.

and in the future. Life behaviors of a sexually healthy adult are essentially outcomes of instruction. The following lists reflect the actions students will be able to take after having applied the information and skills.

Human Development Life Behaviors:
Having applied the human development subconcepts at the appropriate age, the learner will be able to:

- Appreciate one's own body.

- Seek further information about reproduction as needed.

- Affirm that human development includes sexual development, which may or may not include reproduction or sexual experience.

- Interact with all genders in respectful and appropriate ways.

- Affirm one's own sexual orientation and respect the sexual orientations of others.

- Affirm one's own gender identities and respect the gender identities of others.

Relationship Life Behaviors:
Having applied the relationships subconcepts at the appropriate age, the learner will be able to:

- Express love and intimacy in appropriate ways.

- Develop and maintain meaningful relationships.

- Avoid exploitative or manipulative relationships.

- Make informed choices about family options and relationships.

- Exhibit skills that enhance personal relationships.

Personal Skills Life Behaviors:
Having applied the personal skills subconcepts at the appropriate age, the learner will be able to:

- Identify and live according to one's own values.

- Take responsibility for one's own behavior.

- Practice effective decision making.

- Develop critical-thinking skills.

- Communicate effectively with family, peers, and romantic partners.

Sexual Behavior Life Behaviors:
Having applied the sexual behavior subconcepts at the appropriate age, the learner will be able to:

- Enjoy and express one's sexuality throughout life.

- Express one's sexuality in ways that are congruent with one's values.

- Enjoy sexual feelings without necessarily acting on them.

- Discriminate between life-enhancing sexual behaviors and those that are harmful to self and/or others.

- Express one's sexuality while respecting the rights of others.

- Seek new information to enhance one's sexuality.

- Engage in sexual relationships that are consensual, nonexploitative, honest, pleasurable, and protected.

Sexual Health Life Behaviors:
Having applied the sexual health subconcepts at the appropriate age, the learner will be able to:

- Practice health-promoting behaviors, such as regular check-ups, breast and testicular self-exam, and early identification of potential problems.

- Use contraception effectively to avoid unintended pregnancy.

- Avoid contracting or transmitting an STI, including HIV.

- Act consistently with one's own values when dealing with an unintended pregnancy.

- Seek early prenatal care.

- Help prevent sexual abuse.

¿? Ethical DIMENSIONS

Is It Ethical to Ignore Your Child's Developing Sexuality?

One of us once attended a presentation with a group of Swedish sexuality educators who were talking about the difference in sexual mores between Sweden and the United States. One of the Swedish women told us a story about her first sexual experience. She was 17 years old and very much in love. She and her boyfriend told her parents that they were ready to have sexual intercourse, and they asked to make love in her bedroom at home. The next morning, her parents served them breakfast in bed to celebrate this passage! The American educators were stunned.

Whether parents in America would openly accommodate their teens' first experience of sexual intercourse at home or not, it *is* happening. Almost half (46%) of all high school students reported in 2010 they have had sexual intercourse, and sexual activity increased with grade level, while condom use decreased (Eaton et al., 2010). When asked the location, 68% of 16- to 18-year-olds reported their first sexual intercourse occurred in their family home (22%), their partner's family home (34%), or a friend's house (12%) (Child Trends, 2003).

The boundaries between parents and their teen children about sexuality are often difficult to negotiate and raise many moral and ethical issues. Is it ethical to ignore a teen's developing sexuality? Is it ethical to withhold information about contraception and condoms? Does talking about condoms and contraception encourage teens to experiment with sexual behaviors? Should parents help a teen obtain contraception, or is a teen who is old enough to be having intercourse old enough to go to a clinic or a drug store unassisted? And if you know your teen child is having intercourse, should you allow him or her to do so in your home? While you are out? Overnight? And what is your responsibility to the other child's parent?

How did your parents handle these issues? How do you think you will handle them when you are a parent? Which issues do you need to think about in answering these questions?

Society and Culture Life Behaviors:
Having applied the society and culture subconcepts at the appropriate age, the learner will be able to:

- Demonstrate respect for people with different sexual values.

- Exercise democratic responsibility to influence legislation dealing with sexual issues.

- Assess the impact of family, cultural, media, and societal messages on one's thoughts, feelings, values, and behaviors related to sexuality.

- Critically examine the world around them for biases based on gender, sexual orientation, culture, ethnicity, and race.

- Promote the rights of all people to accurate sexuality information.

- Avoid behaviors that exhibit prejudice and bigotry.

- Reject stereotypes about the sexuality of different populations.

- Educate others about sexuality.

The following four areas contribute to an educational experience that will encourage achievement of the life behaviors listed above.

Information: Sexuality education seeks to provide accurate information about human sexuality, including growth and development, human reproduction, anatomy, physiology, masturbation, family life, pregnancy, childbirth, parenthood, sexual response, sexual orientation, gender identity, contraception, abortion, sexual abuse, HIV/AIDS, and other STIs.

Attitudes, Values, and Insights: Sexuality education seeks to provide an opportunity for young people to question, explore, and assess their own and their community's attitudes about society, gender, and sexuality. This can help young people understand their family's values, develop their own values, improve critical thinking skills, increase self-esteem and self-efficacy, and develop insights concerning relationships with family members, individuals of all genders, sexual partners, and society at large. Sexuality education can help young people understand their obligations and responsibilities to their families and society.

Relationships and Interpersonal Skills: Sexuality education seeks to help young people develop interpersonal skills, including communication, decision making, assertiveness, and peer refusal skills, as well as the ability to create reciprocal and satisfying relationships. Sexuality education programs should

? Did You Know . . .

A number of interesting comparisons can be made between comprehensive sexuality education programs and abstinence-only-until-marriage programs. They include:

Comprehensive Sexuality Education Programs	Abstinence-Only-Until-Marriage Programs
Teaches that sexuality is a natural, normal, healthy part of life.	Teaches that sexual activity outside of marriage will have harmful social, psychological, and physical consequences.
Provides values-based education and offers students the opportunity to explore and define their individual values as well as the values of their families and communities.	Teaches one set of values as morally correct for all students.
Includes accurate, factual information about abortion, masturbation, and sexual orientation.	Either omits or contains biased information about topics such as abortion, masturbation, and sexual orientation.
Teaches that consistent use of contraception can greatly reduce a couple's risk of unintended pregnancy.	Discusses contraception only in terms of failure rates; often exaggerates contraceptive failure rates.
Teaches that religious values can play an important role in an individual's decisions about sexual behavior; offers students the opportunity to explore their own and their family's religious values.	Often promotes specific religious beliefs.

Source: Modified from Comparing comprehensive sexuality education with abstinence-only-until-marriage programs. SIECUS Community Action Kit, 2008. Available: www.communityactionkit.org/index.cfm?pageId=889&printview=true.

prepare students to understand sexuality effectively and creatively in adult roles. This includes helping young people develop the capacity for caring, supportive, noncoercive, and mutually pleasurable intimate and sexual relationships.

Responsibility: Sexuality education seeks to help young people exercise responsibility regarding sexual relationships by addressing such issues as abstinence, how to resist pressures to become involved in unwanted early sexual intercourse, and the use of contraception and other sexual health measures" (National Guidelines Task Force, 2004).

Linking Research and Programs

While the content and goals of a comprehensive sexuality education program are presented as the ideal, the research literature identifies antecedents of risky sexual behavior and pregnancy that provide implications for program delivery. Five sets of associated factors need to be considered: race and ethnicity; socioeconomic status; social influences; attitudes toward contraception, condoms, and pregnancy; and safer sex behavioral skills. The following is a list of eight programmatic implications designed to reduce high-risk behaviors among adolescents.

- Programs should begin earlier and target younger adolescents.

- New program models for minority teens need to be developed.

- Risk reduction programs need to be systematically linked to other youth programs that directly address socioeconomic disadvantage.

- Professionals need to understand that many youth lack the skills to practice safer sex. A variety of behavioral skills are necessary for condom use; these include communication, negotiation and refusal skills, and technical condom use skills.

- Programs need to effectively address the influence of peer groups, social norms, and pressures to have sex.

- Professionals working with adolescents should not assume that sexual behavior is always freely chosen.

- Professionals should not assume that sexual activity among teens is limited to vaginal sex.

- Professionals cannot assume that teens are unambivalent about preventing pregnancy.

There are also impediments to program success with adolescents. These include learning disabilities and cognitive immaturity, insufficient male involvement, very early sexual activity of males (as yet largely unexplored by research), and single program opportunities due to one-time clinic visits (Kalmus et al., 2003). Another researcher, Dr. Douglas Kirby, has investigated a range of school-based sexuality and HIV education programs over many years to determine program outcomes (Kirby, 2002b). He has found that the more comprehensive programs do not increase sexual intercourse or the number of sexual partners, and some delay the onset of sexual intercourse, decrease the frequency of intercourse, and increase the use of condoms and other contraceptives. In contrast, there are methodological flaws in the evaluation of abstinence-only sexuality education programs. Therefore, Kirby concludes that evidence is lacking to support claims made for the effectiveness of these programs.

Risk and Protective Factors

Kirby has contributed to a summary of risk and protective factors affecting teen sexual behavior, pregnancy, childbearing, and STI. More than 400 research studies were analyzed to determine which factors influence adolescents' decisions about sexual behavior and which of these factors can be altered. The likelihood that a teen will have sexual activity, become pregnant or cause a pregnancy, or contract an STI increases as the number of risk factors in a teen's life increases and/or the number of protective factors decreases. These risk and protective factors are as follows: (1) individual biological factors such as age, physical maturity, and gender; (2) disadvantage, disorganization, and dysfunction in the lives of teens, including violence, substance abuse, divorce, and low levels of education; (3) sexual values, attitudes, and modeled behaviors as expressed by teens themselves and by parents, peers, and romantic partners; and (4) connection to adults and organizations that discourage sexual activity, unprotected sex, or early childbearing, such as parents and adults in schools and places of worship (Kirby, Lepore, & Ryan, 2005).

Although more research is certainly warranted, most professionals agree that age-appropriate and targeted sexuality education is one of the best preventive means available for reducing risks and enhancing sexual health. Parents can guide, schools can inform, and other community support can be provided so that adolescents will have the knowledge and self-confidence to make informed decisions regarding their own sexual outcomes.

The Three Stages of Adolescence

Developmental psychologists and health professionals have categorized adolescence into three developmental stages: early adolescence, middle adolescence, and late adolescence. These stages are key to understanding adolescents' behavioral decisions and adolescent sexuality. Table 11.4 summarizes these stages.

While reading this section, it is important to remember that there is no such thing as an "average adolescent." Individual adolescents vary widely in the pace of their development. Adolescent sexuality emerges from cultural identities mediated by ethnicity, gender, sexual orientation, class, and

---

TABLE 11.4 Highlights of Adolescent Developmental Stages

Early Adolescence

Females ages 9–13; males ages 11–15

- Puberty as hallmark
- Adjusting to pubertal changes such as secondary sexual characteristics
- Concern with body image
- Beginning of separation from family, increased parent–child conflict
- Presence of social group cliques
- Identification in reputation-based groups
- Concentration on relationships with peers
- Concrete thinking but beginning of exploration of new ability to think abstractly

Middle Adolescence

Females ages 13–16; males ages 14–17

- Increased independence from family
- Increased importance of peer group
- Experimentation with relationships and sexual behaviors
- Increased abstract thinking ability

Late Adolescence

Females ages 16 and older; males ages 17 and older

- Autonomy nearly secured
- Body image and gender-role definition nearly secured
- Empathetic relationships
- Attainment of abstract thinking
- Defining of adult roles
- Transition to adult roles
- Greater intimacy skills
- Sexual orientation nearly secured

Source: Reprinted with permission from Haffner, D. *Facing facts: Sexual health for America's adolescents.* New York: SIECUS, 1995.

physical and emotional capacity. Adolescent development is affected by parents, other family members, and other adults, as well as schools and the peer group.

early adolescence
First stage of adolescence, defined by pubertal changes—usually ages 9–13 years for females and ages 11–15 years for males.

Early Adolescence
The **early adolescent** (females aged 9–13 years, males aged 11–15 years) experiences body changes more rapidly than at any time since infancy—secondary sexual characteristics begin to appear; growth accelerates; and physical changes require psychological and social adjustments of the adolescent, family, and other adults. These young people are often concrete thinkers and therefore have difficulty projecting themselves into the future. This phenomenon creates problems when young people are asked to modify their behaviors and delay gratification to achieve a distant future goal. The young adolescent is beginning to separate from the family but usually values parental guidance on important issues. Peer norms, especially identification with a particular group or set of groups, assume increasing importance.

Experimenting with some sexual behaviors is common, but sexual intercourse of any kind is usually limited. Males may initiate intercourse during this stage but most often delay regular sexual activity until middle or late adolescence. Adolescent girls are much less likely to begin having sexual intercourse at this age. Of those who do, many are in relationships with much older males.

Young adolescents seek to develop a sense of identity, connection, power, and joy. For many adolescents in communities that do not support the development of personal identity in other ways, drugs and sexual experimentation may provide a way to achieve it. Early sexual involvement is one way that disadvantaged youth may meet developmental needs for power, identity, connection, and pleasure. Involvement in sexual behaviors may not be motivated by sexual pleasure but rather may reflect peer norms, boredom, conflicts with adults, low self-esteem, and poor ability to control impulsivity.

middle adolescence
The typical "teenage years," usually ages 13–16 years for females and ages 14–17 years for males.

Middle Adolescence
Middle adolescence (females aged 13–16 years, males aged 14–17 years) is the stage that most typifies the stereotype of "teenager." The transitions in this stage are so dramatic that they seem to occur overnight. The secondary sexual characteristics become fully established, and, for girls, the growth rate decelerates. Abstract thought patterns begin to develop in significant proportions of middle adolescents.

Middle adolescents are sometimes described as feeling omniscient, omnipotent, and invincible. These feelings provide young people with the support to develop increased autonomy but may also put them at risk. In a study of ninth graders, their early sexual decision-making processes highlighted active consideration of health and social risks and benefits, as well as generating options, setting boundaries and limits, and evaluating sexual experiences (Michels et al., 2005).

As adolescents continue the process of separation from the family, they cling more tightly to the peer group that they defined for themselves in early adolescence. The peer group begins to define the rules of behavior. Parents generally place more value on long-term issues such as the importance of education and career preparation than peers do. The desire to be accepted by the peer group often influences experimentation with drugs or sex. By its acceptance or rejection, the peer group influences the adolescent's self-image.

Middle adolescents often focus on themselves and assume others will, too. Many middle adolescents choose to show off their new bodies with revealing clothes. Although adults may define these styles as sexually provocative, that may not be the intent of the middle adolescent.

Middle adolescents often fall in love for the first time. Again, because they are self-centered, their love object may serve as a mirror and reflect characteristics that they admire; that is, they may not love an individual for himself or herself. Sexual experimentation is common, and many adolescents first have intercourse in middle adolescence.

Late Adolescence
Teenagers in **late adolescence** (females aged 16 years and older; males aged 17 years and older) are explicitly moving toward adult roles and

late adolescence
Period of transition to adulthood, beginning usually at age 16 years for females and age 17 years for males.

responsibilities. Some are beginning full-time jobs; others are beginning families. Many are preparing for these adult roles. The late adolescent completes the process of physical maturation. Many young people at this stage achieve the ability to understand abstract concepts, and they become more aware of what their limitations are and how their past will affect their future. They understand the consequences of their actions and behaviors, and they grapple with the complexities of identity, values, and ethical principles. Within the family, they move to a more adult relationship with their parents. The peer group recedes in importance as a determinant of behavior, and sexuality may become closely tied to commitment and planning for the future.

Adolescent Developmental Tasks

Developmental psychologists have identified six key developmental tasks for adolescents. Becoming a sexually healthy adult depends on the completion of these key developmental tasks (Grunbaum et al., 2004). The six key tasks are as follows:

1. *Physical and sexual maturation:* Adolescents mature biologically into adults, a process that occurs at an earlier chronological age than it did in the past.

2. *Independence:* Adolescents develop autonomy within the structure that gave them nurture and support during their childhood. This is usually the family but may include some similar surrogate structure. The parent–child relationship is transformed during adolescence, as the young person obtains the skills to maintain satisfying relationships.

3. *Conceptual identity:* Adolescents establish and place themselves within the religious, cultural, ethnic, moral, and political constructs of their environments.

4. *Functional identity:* Adolescents begin to prepare themselves for adult roles in society. By identifying their competencies, they discover how they will support themselves and contribute to their own families and society.

5. *Cognitive development:* Children and young adolescents are concrete thinkers and focus on real objects, present actions, and immediate benefits. During adolescence they develop a greater ability to think abstractly, plan for their future, and understand the effect of their current actions on their future lives and other people.

6. *Sexual self-concept:* During adolescence, young people tend to experience their first adult-like erotic feelings, experiment with sexual behaviors, and develop a strong sense of their own gender identity and sexual orientation.

conceptual identity
Who am I in my world?

functional identity
What adult roles will I play in the world?

cognitive development
Explains the ability to think concretely or abstractly.

sexual self-concept
Who am I as a sexual being?

The pursuit of these developmental tasks answers three psychosocial questions that adolescents ask themselves: Am I normal? Am I competent? Am I lovable and loving? Many adolescent behaviors can be attributed to the search for affirmative answers to these questions.

Physical and Sexual Maturation

As noted in the section on puberty, sexual maturation differs significantly among young men and young women. On average, young girls begin pubertal events 1 to 2 years before boys. The adolescent female completes the process of puberty in 3 to 5 years, whereas for males, the process lasts 4 to 6 years. Adjusting to the biological changes of puberty is a major task of early adolescence, and society does not adequately prepare or support young people during these changes.

Sexual cognitions of girls appear to change prior to sexual experiences such as breast fondling and genital contact. Because most research focuses on intercourse as a key marker or pivotal event, the importance of attitudes, perceptions, and sexual self-esteem may have been overlooked as an important aspect of sexual development (O'Sullivan & Brooks-Gunn, 2005). The discrepancy between maturation among young women and young men is one factor that may contribute to some young women's seeking partners older than they are. This difference in age places young women at considerable risk for sexual exploitation.

sexual cognitions
Attitudes, expectations, beliefs, and values framing one's sexual experiences

Cognitive Development

During adolescence, young people develop a range of intellectual characteristics that increase the probability that they will be able to become sexually healthy adults. Ideally, this includes developing the ability to reason abstractly, to foresee consequences of actions, and to understand the social context of behaviors. Adolescents develop an increased ability to control impulsivity, to identify the future implications of their actions, and to obtain control of their future plans.

Although the study of child development from 0 to 3 years of age has recognized the importance of brain development, study of adolescents has tended to focus more on psychological and social factors rather than on physiological ones. Recent imaging advances have allowed neuroscience—the scientific study of the biology of the brain—to demonstrate brain growth patterns. These studies in teens reveal remarkable changes during the second decade of life (Weinberger, Elvevåg, & Giedd, 2005). Of particular interest is the frontal cortex area, which governs impulse control, judgment, and decision making; that portion does not fully mature until around the age of 25. That means that teenagers, though very capable of huge intellectual and creative endeavors, are limited in strategies, organizing, and recognizing potential consequences. Conversely, the teen brain is adept at learning by example. Thus, modeling behavior to be emulated could be a good tactic for both parents and teachers (Giedd, 2005).

Developmental age and general level of cognitive and emotional development may influence adolescent sexual decisions, contraceptive use, and safer sex practices. An adolescent's degree of cognitive maturity may place limits on his or her ability to plan for sexual relationships, clearly articulate personal values, negotiate with a partner, and obtain contraception and condoms. Further, the adolescent's ability to form empathetic relationships is dependent on **social cognition**: the capacity to see a situation from another person's perspective. Social cognition is one aspect of cognitive development. Understanding one's feelings and the feelings of others is central to emotional growth.

social cognition
Ability to see a situation from another person's point of view.

Sexual Self-Concept

Sexual self-concept, an individual's evaluation of his or her sexual feelings and actions, develops during adolescence. Young people develop an increasing sense of gender identity as men and women. An understanding of one's sexual orientation also develops during adolescence: Young people become more aware of their sexual attractions and love interests, and adultlike erotic feelings emerge. Sexual experimentation is common among all groups of adolescents.

Gender Identity

During adolescence, young people solidify their gender identification by observing the gender roles of their parents and other adults. Gender identification includes understanding that one is male or female, as well as understanding the roles, values, duties, and responsibilities of being a man or a woman. Most young people have a firm sense of their maleness or femaleness before adolescence, but in adolescence, clear identification with adult masculine and feminine models emerges. The markers of masculinity and femininity vary by culture and are adopted to a greater or lesser extent by adolescents. *Gender-role behavior, expression,* and *conformity* are all current terms used to describe sex-typed attributes. Differences that have been studied include peer affiliation preference, aggression, and activity level (Zucker & Bradley, 2005).

Sexual Orientation

One's erotic attraction to others is discovered as one matures sexually. Sexual orientation, whatever it may be, does not seem to be something one chooses. Gay, lesbian, and bisexual people are not seduced, recruited, or taught to become homosexual. Rather, one's sexual orientation often emerges in adolescence.

In retrospective studies, many gay and lesbian adults identify adolescence as a period of confusion about their sexual orientation. Although a majority of adult gay men recall feeling different as children, most did not self-identify as gay until their late teenage years.

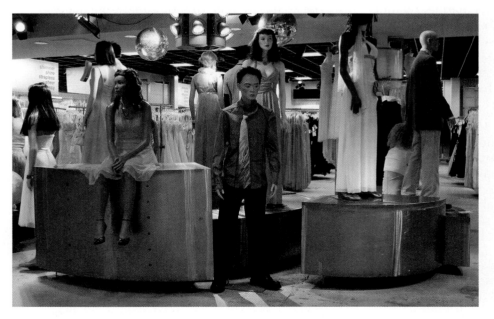

Adolescents express sexual cognitions, social cognitions, peer affiliations, and various aspects of gender identity such as gender role expression, behavior, and conformity as they participate in proms, graduation events, and other social activities that mark passages throughout the teen years.

♂♀ Gender
DIMENSIONS

How Gender Stereotypes Affect Sexuality

Gender-role stereotypes impede both young men and young women in attaining sexual health. Young women may learn that "It is better to be cute and popular than smart," "Girls have few sexual feelings," and "Girls who carry condoms are bad." Boys may learn that "Real men are always ready for sex" and that "Guys should never act like girls." In an online article for teens written by a 17-year-old male staff writer for Sex, Etc., women clearly are short-changed. He says, guys get to enjoy sex but girls are told by society they can't. Females faking orgasm is a laughing matter. Another problem is that many people, especially teens, are focused on sexual intercourse (where the "goal" is for the male to have an orgasm). Other ways of experiencing pleasure are less valued or ignored. Or, as one concerned male suggests, men are afraid they don't know how to please their partner, so they're reluctant to try. Regarding masturbation, there is silence and disdain for women but with men, it's common conversation. The suggested solution is T-A-L-K. When discussing safer sex, pleasure should be included, too. Since communication is the key to better relationships, maybe the real payoff *and* the best pleasure of all is an enhanced sexual connection (Dalal, 2005).

Although patterns of sexual involvement are increasingly similar for boys and girls, persistent gender stereotypes mean that expectations regarding sexual pleasure for young women are still quite different from those for young men.

Why do these different standards continue to exist? Will they ever change?

Adolescent Sexual Behavior

Regardless of one's sexual orientation, almost all American adolescents engage in some type of sexual behavior (Table 11.5). Although policy debates have tended to focus on sexual intercourse and its negative consequences, young people explore dating, relationships, and intimacy from a much wider framework. Sexual behavior is almost universal among American adolescents.

The majority of adolescents move from kissing to other more intimate sexual behaviors during their teenage years.

- Just over half of teens (aged 15 to 19) have had oral sex, and it is now more common than sexual intercourse. About one in four teens who have *not* had sexual intercourse report they have had oral sex. Among teen boys who have not had sexual intercourse, the proportion of those who say they have had oral sex did *not* increase between 1995 and 2002, but for those who have had sexual intercourse, the proportion saying they have had oral sex increased from 82% in 1995 to 88% in 2002 (Teens and oral sex, 2005).

- Copen et al. (2012) reported on the first time young people were surveyed about the timing of oral sex relative to intercourse. It was about equally likely for oral sex to happen before intercourse as after. Among females aged 15 to 24, 26% had first oral sex before first intercourse, and 27% after first intercourse. Among males aged 15 to 24, 24% had first oral sex before first intercourse and 24% had first oral sex after first intercourse.

- Between 5% and 10% of adolescent males report having sexual experiences with someone of the same gender, compared with 6% of adolescent females (Bancoft, Herbenick, & Reynolds, 2003). These adolescents usually report their first experience was with another adolescent (DeLamater & Friedrich, 2002).

When data are collected about teen sexual behavior, the focus becomes *what, when,* and *how often,* but rarely *with what emotional intent.* Thus it is difficult to pin down aspects of sexual experience that are nuanced. Much has been written recently about changes in relationship patterns, particularly the phenomenon of "friends with benefits" and hooking up (a euphemism for a sexual encounter, particularly oral sex, without emotional involvement). Much of the discussion is anecdotal and involves use of the Internet to post personal profiles, chat online, and arrange meetings. Whether such interaction is viewed as healthy or harmful may depend on one's age and experience. Most of the experts cited in a recent feature article in the popular press indicate that females may have less to gain than males and the ultimate risk may be increased chance of STIs.

TABLE 11.5 Trends in the Prevalence of Sexual Behaviors— National YRBS: 1991–2009

The national Youth Risk Behavior Survey (YRBS) monitors priority health risk behaviors that contribute to the leading causes of death, disability, and social problems among youth and adults in the United States. The national YRBS is conducted every 2 years during the spring semester and provides data representative of ninth- through twelfth-grade students in public and private schools throughout the United States.

	1991	1993	1995	1997	1999	2001	2003	2005	2007	2009	Changes from 1991–2009[1]	Change from 2007–2009[2]
Ever had sexual intercourse												
	54.1	53.0	53.1	48.4	49.9	45.6	46.7	46.8	47.8	46.0	Decreased, 1991–2009	No change
	(50.5–57.8)[3]	(50.2–55.8)	(48.4–57.7)	(45.2–51.6)	(46.1–53.7)	(43.2–48.1)	(44.0–49.4)	(43.4–50.2)	(45.1–50.6)	(42.9–49.2)		
Had sexual intercourse with four or more persons during their life												
	18.7	18.7	17.8	16.0	16.2	14.2	14.4	14.3	14.9	13.8	Decreased, 1991–2009	No change
	(16.6–21.0)	(16.8–20.9)	(15.2–20.7)	(14.6–17.5)	(13.7–19.0)	(13.0–15.6)	(12.9–16.1)	(12.8–15.8)	(13.4–16.5)	(12.4–15.4)		
Currently sexually active (Had sexual intercourse with at least one person during the 3 months before the survey.)												
	37.5	37.5	37.9	34.8	36.3	33.4	34.3	33.9	35.0	34.2	Decreased, 1991–2009	No change
	(34.3–40.7)	(35.4–39.7)	(34.4–41.5)	(32.6–37.2)	(32.7–40.0)	(31.3–35.5)	(32.1–36.5)	(31.4–36.6)	(32.8–37.2)	(31.9–36.5)		
Used a condom during last sexual intercourse (Among students who were currently sexually active.)												
	46.2	52.8	54.4	56.8	58.0	57.9	63.0	62.8	61.5	61.1	Increased, 1991–2003 No change, 2003–2009	No change
	(42.8–49.6)	(50.0–55.6)	(50.7–58.0)	(55.2–58.4)	(53.6–62.3)	(55.6–60.1)	(60.5–65.5)	(60.6–64.9)	(59.4–63.6)	(59.0–63.1)		
Used birth control pills or Depo-Provera before last sexual intercourse (To prevent pregnancy, among students who were currently sexually active.)												
	N/A	N/A	N/A	N/A	19.5	23.6	20.7	20.5	18.8	22.9	No change, 1999–2009	Increased
	N/A	N/A	N/A	N/A	(16.5–22.9)	(20.8–24.5)	(18.1–23.6)	(17.9–23.5)	(16.6–21.1)	(20.3–25.7)		
Drank alcohol or used drugs before last sexual intercourse (Among students who were currently sexually active.)												
	21.6	21.3	24.8	24.7	24.8	25.6	25.4	23.3	22.5	21.6	Increased, 1991–2001 Decreased, 2001–2009	No change
	(18.7–24.8)	(19.3–23.5)	(22.1–27.8)	(22.9–26.7)	(21.8–28.0)	(23.8–27.4)	(23.2–27.8)	(21.1–25.6)	(20.7–24.5)	(20.0–23.3)		
Were ever taught in school about AIDS or HIV infection												
	83.3	86.1	86.3	91.5	90.6	89.0	87.9	87.9	89.5	87	Increased, 1991–1997 Decreased, 1997–2009	No change
	(80.1–86.0)	(83.4–88.4)	(79.0–91.3)	(90.3–92.5)	(89.1–91.9)	(87.6–90.3)	(85.8–89.7)	(85.8–89.7)	(88.1–90.7)	(85.7–88.3)		

[1] Based on trend analyses using a logistic regression model controlling for sex, race/ethnicity, and grade.
[2] Based on t-test analyses, $p < .05$.
[3] 95% confidence interval.

Source: Reproduced from Centers for Disease Control and Prevention. Trends in the Prevalence of Selected Risk Behaviors and HIV Testing National YRBS: 1991–2011, Youth Risk Behavior Survey. Available at http://www.cdc.gov/healthyyouth/yrbs/pdf/us_sexual_trend_yrbs.pdf.

The role of commitment and dating seems to be changing, perhaps due to the expectation that marriage and romantic relationships won't happen until later in life (Denizet-Lewis, 2004).

Clearly, research is needed to measure more than numbers. Detailed studies might discover whether friends with benefits are truly a widespread and long-term change in relationship patterns or a minor blip in reaction to new technology that will be reversed when another trend appears. Some data suggest that the progression from kissing to noncoital behaviors to intercourse differs among different groups of adolescents. Many teenagers move through a progression of intimate behaviors; lower-income teenagers are less likely to follow this progression, moving more rapidly from kissing directly to sexual intercourse (Brooks-Gunn & Furstenberg, 1990).

Sexting and Sexual Behavior

Temple et al. (2012) found that adolescents who engaged in sexting behaviors were more likely to have begun dating and to have had sexual intercourse than those who did not sext. For girls, sexting was also associated with risky sexual behaviors.

Dake et al. (2012) found statistically significant correlations between sexting and sexual behaviors. Of those who had anal sex, 71% had sexted; of those who had 4 or more sexual partners, 65% had sexted; of those who did not use contraceptives at last intercourse, 65% had sexted; of those who had oral sex, 54% had sexted; and of those who had ever had sexual intercourse, 47% had sexted.

Teenagers Who Have Intercourse

Substantial changes in adolescent sexual behavior have occurred in the past five decades. From the late 1960s until 1988 the proportion of teens who had had sexual intercourse increased. Then the trend reversed, and from 1991 to 2001 the proportion of teens reporting having had sexual intercourse dropped from 54.1% to 45.6%. However, since 2001 the proportion of students who had ever had sexual intercourse has stayed about the same (Eaton et al., 2010) (see Table 11.5).

Contraceptive use among teens has also undergone remarkable change. In the 1970s, the most commonly used method was the birth control pill, followed by condom use and withdrawal. In the 1980s, condom use increased and the use of birth control pills declined. This trend continued into the 1990s, and now condom use among high school students has stabilized at 63% with no significant change from 2003 to 2009 (Eaton et al., 2010).

Rates of teen pregnancy, including births and abortions, have changed dramatically. A record high (96 births per 1,000 teen girls aged 15–19) was reached in 1957, followed by a steady decline to the mid-1980s. Then the birth rate increased again by 24% by 1991. Then there was a decrease of more than 33% in the birth rate, to a low of 41 births per 1,000 teen girls in 2004 (Santelli et al., 2004). After 14 years of decline, the birth rate for teens *increased* by 3% in 2006 and by 1% in 2007 (CDC, 2009). However, it declined 8% from 2007 through 2009, reaching a historic low at 39.1 births per 1,000 teens. Rates fell significantly for teenagers in all age groups and for all racial and ethnic groups (Ventura & Hamilton, 2011). Abortion rates for teens rose in the 1970s, were mostly stable in the 1980s, and have declined steadily since 1991 (Santelli et al., 2004).

Data from the Youth Risk Behavior Surveys (YRBS) for estimates of sexual activity and contraceptive use were combined with data from National Surveys of Family Growth (NSFG) for method-specific contraceptive failure rates and from the National Vital Statistics System for pregnancy rates. These data suggest that both delayed initiation of sexual intercourse and improved contraceptive practice contributed equally to declines in the pregnancy rates among high school-aged teens during the 1990s. Specifically, decreased sexual experience accounted for 53% of the pregnancy rate decline and better contraception accounted for 47%. There was an increase in condom use from 40% to 51%, a decrease in use of withdrawal from 20% to 13%, and decline in use of no method from 17% to 13% (Santelli et al., 2004).

Although the data do not suggest a dramatic turnabout in either sexual activity or contraceptive use, they do indicate a loss of momentum when compared to the steady improvements in the 1990s. Moreover, the U.S. teen birth rate remains much higher than the rates in other developed nations. Research is lacking, but hypotheses abound, including those related to changes in the economy, attitudes, anxiety, schooling, public policy, programs and services, families, and media messages. In addition, prevention fatigue and the need for new strategies to reach teens who have not been reached by existing approaches have been suggested as critical factors (Moore, 2008).

While more teens are doing the right thing, adults debate whether the reduction in unintended pregnancies is the result of promoting abstinence or promoting better contraceptive protection. Speculation must suffice because the surveys provide little information to explain the shift in behaviors. The important point is to support teens in each decision by providing accurate information, encouragement, and validation, whether their concern is initiating sex, limiting activity or partners, or choosing to use contraception (Sonenstein, 2004).

Early Sexual Activity

- Female adolescents who first had sexual intercourse prior to the age of 14 had more sexual partners than females who first had it at age 15 or older, thus increasing their risk of STI or pregnancy.

- One in ten young women who first had sexual intercourse before the age of 15 described it as nonvoluntary and many more said it was unwanted.

- Survey data indicate that younger teen girls who are sexually experienced are more likely than older teens to say they "wish they'd waited."

- Relationships between a young adolescent (aged 12–14) and an older partner (by 2 or more years) compared to a partner only slightly older, the same age, or younger, is more likely to include sexual intercourse.

- More than half the girls and two-thirds of the boys aged 12–14 say they used some form of contraception the most recent time they had sexual intercourse. (This is a higher percentage than among 15- to 19-year-olds.)

- Approximately one in five adolescents has had sexual intercourse before his or her 15th birthday (Sexual behavior of young adolescents, 2003).

- High school boys are more likely than girls to have four or more partners (17% versus 11%). This pattern is the same across grades and racial/ethnic groups.

- Young boys (aged 12–14) are slightly more likely than older boys (aged 15–19) to think it is embarrassing to say they are virgins. Boys in general are more embarrassed than girls the same age to say they are virgins.

- Boys are slightly more likely than girls the same age to report feeling pressured to have sex (82% versus 79%). Girls say romantic partners cause pressure, while boys say pressure is most likely to come from friends (Sexual attitudes and behavior of male teens, 2003).

Figure 11.1 shows teen birth rate data from 1940 to 2009. The United States has the highest rates of teen pregnancy and births in the Western industrialized world. Thirty-four percent of young women become pregnant at least once before they reach the age of 20. Eight in ten of these pregnancies are unintended. Although the teen birth rate has steadily declined since 1991, Hispanic teens have the highest teenage birth rate. The rate for African American teens declined the most but remains higher than other groups except Hispanic teens. Prior to 1980, most teen mothers were married, whereas today most are unmarried.

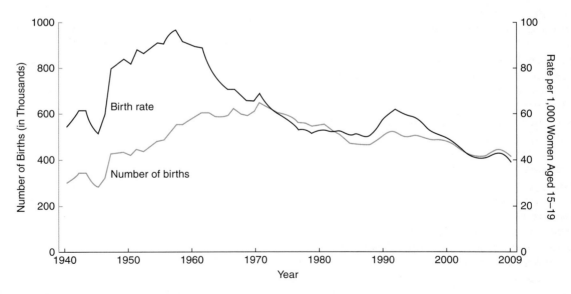

FIGURE 11.1 Teen Birth Rates in the United States, 1940–2009
From 1940 to 1957, the teen birth rate increased to a record high. It dropped fairly steadily from the end of the 1950s through the mid 1980s, but then increased between 1986 and 1991. Between 1991 and 2009, the teen birth rate decreased to a record low of 39.1 per 1,000 teens in 2009. The teen birth rate in 2009 was 59% lower than the historic high in 1957. The following chart reflects births per 1,000 teen girls aged 15–19 in the United States and is the most recent national data available.
Note: Data for 2009 are preliminary.

Source: Reproduced from Ventura, S. J., Hamilton, B. E. U.S. teenage birth rate resumes decline. *NCHS Data Brief, no 58.* Hyattsville, MD: National Center for Health Statistics, 2011. Available at http://www.cdc.gov/nchs/data/databriefs/db58.htm.

Kost and Henshaw (2012) provided some related information. For example, in 2008 about 7% of U.S. teens became pregnant. This was a 42% decline from the peak in 1990. The teen birthrate declined 35% between 1991 and 2008, and the abortion rate declined 59% from its 1988 peak. The authors concluded that teens appear to be making the decision to be more effective contraceptive users, and their actions are paying off in lower pregnancy, birth, and abortion rates.

Kann et al. (2012) reported that the rate of all teenagers engaging in risky sexual behavior declined slightly since 1991. The number of high school students who reported ever having sexual intercourse dropped from 54% in 1991 to 47% in 2011. Of those who had sexual intercourse, about 15% reported having had four or more sexual partners compared with 19% in 1991. The number of teens who reported using a condom the last time they had sexual intercourse increased from 46% in 1991 to 60% in 2011—but the 2011 rate was lower than the high of 63% reached in 2003.

Parents are rated by most teens as trustworthy and a preferred source of birth control information. About 6 out of 10 teens find it easy to talk to their parents about relationships. Still, about 1 in 4 teens say it's difficult (National Campaign to Prevent Teen and Unplanned Pregnancy, 2007). Teens raised by two parents (biological or adoptive) from birth have a lower probability of having sex than teens growing up in any other family situation. Eight in 10 girls and 6 in 10 boys say they wish they had waited to have sexual intercourse until they were older (National Campaign to Prevent Teen Pregnancy, 2005).

The self-assessment exercise at the end of this chapter raises many of the questions that a young person—indeed, an adult—needs to consider to determine his or her readiness for a sexual relationship.

■ Sexual Abuse of Children and Adolescents

Sexual abuse occurs in all types of homes. It happens hundreds of times a day in the United States. The real prevalence of child and adolescent sexual abuse is not known because so many victims do not disclose or report their abuse. There also can be differences in how child sexual abuse is defined in various studies as well as the time periods over which studies are conducted. Thus, estimates range from 1.2 victims per 1,000 and 1.9 victims per 1,000 in studies focusing on occurrences

sexual abuse
The psychological exploitation or infliction of unwanted sexual contact on one person.

Myth vs Fact

Kiss and Tell: What Teens Say About Love, Trust, and Other Relationship Stuff

It's a relationship world. Seven in 10 teens say their friends are in romantic relationships.

Relationships

The good news is that most teens (68%) say that their friends are in "healthy" romantic relationships. The proportion saying this is almost identical for teen boys and teen girls.

The not-so-good news is that one in five teens (19%) aged 15–17 say that most of their friends are in *unhealthy* relationships—those without love, trust, mutual respect, and honesty.

Trust and Honesty Rule. When it comes to relationships, teens say it's all about trust—40% of guys and 48% of gals say that *trust* is the most important part of a healthy relationship. Teens say that *honesty* is the second most important factor. Surprisingly, 10% of teen boys say that *compatibility* is most important; yet only 3% of teen girls agree. Fewer than 3% of teens say *looks* or *popularity* matters most.

Pressure

More good news is that most teens (84% of guys and 85% of gals) say they have never felt pressure to be in a romantic relationship before they were ready.

Fast Fact. Teens who are in relationships with someone who is 3 years older are far more likely to say that sex was unwanted.

Role Models

Teens in focus groups indicated that they can learn a lot about what to avoid from seeing unhealthy relationships.

Almost one in five (17%) teens say they don't know *anyone* who serves as an example of a healthy relationship.

Fast Fact. Most teens aged 15–17 say they enjoy spending time with their mother (79%) and father (76%).

Source: Data from Kiss and tell: What teens say about love, trust, and other relationship stuff survey results. National Campaign to Prevent Teen and Unplanned Pregnancy. 2007. Retrieved June 5, 2012, from www.thenationalcampaign.org/resources/pdf/pubs/kiss_tell.pdf.

in 1 year. At the upper end, between 90 and 280 per 1,000 victims have been found in a survey of adults who experienced some sexual abuse or assault in their childhood. It seems that females are more at risk than males. Also, children from low-income families are more at-risk as are children who have been victims of other forms of crime, violence, and abuse. With regard to the perpetrators, men perpetrate most sexual abuse and sex crimes. Sex offenders against children tend to be juveniles or young adults younger than age 30. Most sexual abuse is committed by people who know the victims, followed by family members (Sexual abuse, 2011).

Sexual Abuse of Children

Most parents teach their children not to talk to strangers, accept candy from people they do not know, or ever get into a car with a stranger. Indeed, many

Multicultural DIMENSIONS

Racial and Ethnic Differences in Sexual Behaviors

The likelihood of having several sexual partners varies by race and ethnicity, as does condom use. The percentages of high school students who have had four or more sexual partners by race/ethnicity as well as high school students who used condoms (either they or their partner) during their last sexual intercourse are shown below.

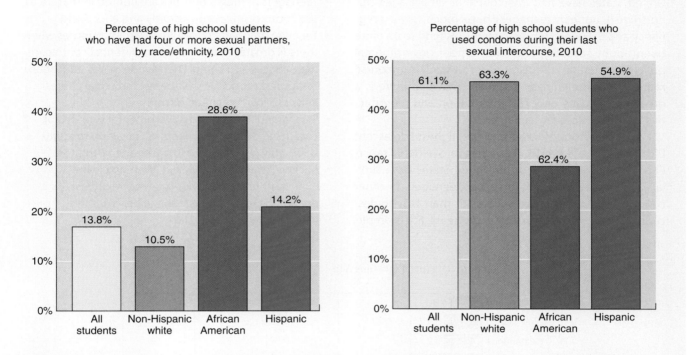

Percentage of high school students who have had four or more sexual partners, by race/ethnicity, 2010

Percentage of high school students who used condoms during their last sexual intercourse, 2010

Source: Data from Youth risk behavior surveillance—United States, 2009. *Morbidity and Mortality Weekly Report, 59, no. SS-5* (June 4, 2010). A-142.

preschools and kindergartens offer "stranger danger programs." However, the reality is that, in 90% of the cases, the assailant was someone in the child's family or someone close to the family.

Children can also be sexually abused by other children. This is different from the sex play described earlier in this chapter. In sex play, children are usually of the same age, they are engaging in light-hearted exploration, and they appear to be enjoying themselves—at least until they realize they have been "discovered" by an adult. And, in general, once they are told by an adult that they should stop, they do.

Some children, however, engage in inappropriate behaviors and become sexually abusive to other, usually younger, children. This may include engaging in oral or genital sex with other children, with or without their consent. Many of these children have been

sexually abused themselves, and many of them have inappropriately been exposed to sexually explicit materials or adult erotic behavior. Most of the males and females who sexually abuse children have earlier been molested themselves.

Family and Acquaintance Sexual Abuse Using the Internet

The Internet and related technologies have transformed many aspects of communication. It is realistic to assume it will have an effect on child mistreatment as well. So far, concern has focused on online meeting crimes in which adult strangers have used the Internet to meet and develop abusive relationships with vulnerable youth. However, just as most face-to-face sexual abuse involves family members and acquaintances of the victim, so it is realistic to

Global
DIMENSIONS

Teenagers and Sexuality Around the World

Young people around the world experiment with sexual behaviors. Young people in northern European countries and the United States have first intercourse at similar ages, but northern European teenagers have much lower pregnancy and STI rates. European countries tend to be more open about sexuality, and their official governmental policies focus on reducing unprotected intercourse rather than on eliminating sexual behaviors. There is a greater availability of sexual information and reproductive health services for teenagers.

The United States has one of the highest adolescent birth rates in the world. Teenagers in Sweden, France, Canada, Great Britain, and the United States have similar levels of sexual intercourse, but teenagers in other countries are much more successful than U.S. adolescents at preventing pregnancy and disease. For example,

Sweden has one-third the U.S. rate of teenage pregnancies, despite similar levels of teenage sexual intercourse.

Reasons for these birthrate differences may include the following factors:

- Teenagers in these countries are not too immature to use contraceptives consistently and effectively.
- Teenage pregnancy rates are lower in countries where there is greater availability of confidential contraceptive services and comprehensive sexuality education.
- Social and economic well-being and equality are linked to lower teenage birthrates.
- Strong and widespread governmental support for parents and for young people's transition to adulthood may contribute to low teenage birthrates.
- Positive attitudes about sexuality and clear expectations for behavior in sexual relationships encourage responsible teenage behavior (Guttmacher Institute, 2001).

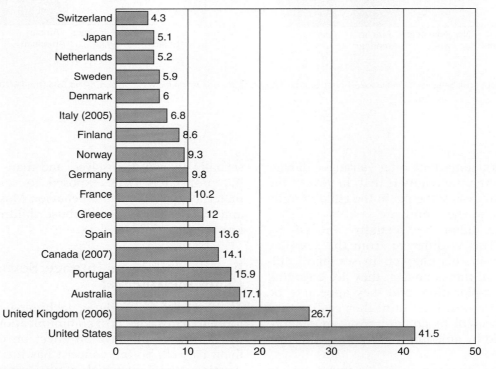

Teen Birth Rate (per 1,000 Girls Age 15–19) by Country, 2008*

Country	Rate
Switzerland	4.3
Japan	5.1
Netherlands	5.2
Sweden	5.9
Denmark	6
Italy (2005)	6.8
Finland	8.6
Norway	9.3
Germany	9.8
France	10.2
Greece	12
Spain	13.6
Canada (2007)	14.1
Portugal	15.9
Australia	17.1
United Kingdom (2006)	26.7
United States	41.5

Note: *All birth rates are for 2008 unless otherwise noted.

Source: Data from United Nations Statistics Division. (2008). Demographic Yearbook 2008. New York: United Nations. Available at http://unstats.un.org/unsd/demographic/products/dyb/dyb2008/Table10.pdf.

CHAPTER 11 **Sexuality in Childhood and Adolescence** **435**

Global DIMENSIONS

Teenagers and Sexuality Around the World—cont'd

Teen Pregnancy, United States, France, Germany

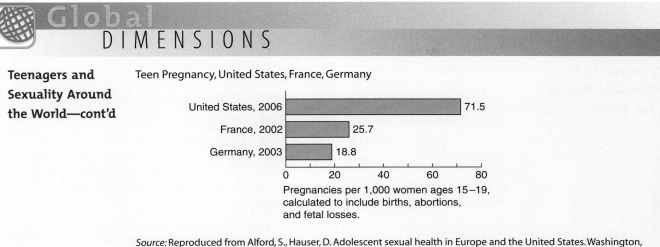

Pregnancies per 1,000 women ages 15–19, calculated to include births, abortions, and fetal losses.

Source: Reproduced from Alford, S., Hauser, D. Adolescent sexual health in Europe and the United States. Washington, DC: Advocates for Youth, 2011. Available: http://www.advocatesforyouth.org/publications/419?task=view.

Teen Pregnancy, United States and the Netherlands

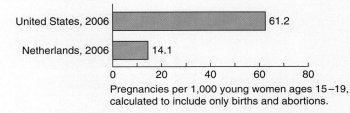

Pregnancies per 1,000 young women ages 15–19, calculated to include only births and abortions.

Source: Reproduced from Alford, S., Hauser, D. Adolescent sexual health in Europe and the United States. Washington, DC: Advocates for Youth, 2011. Available: http://www.advocatesforyouth.org/publications/419?task=view.

Teen Birth

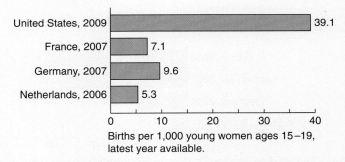

Births per 1,000 young women ages 15–19, latest year available.

Source: Reproduced from Alford, S., Hauser, D. Adolescent sexual health in Europe and the United States. Washington, DC: Advocates for Youth, 2011. Available: http://www.advocatesforyouth.org/publications/419?task=view.

Abortion

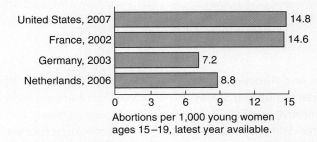

Abortions per 1,000 young women ages 15–19, latest year available.

Source: Reproduced from Alford, S., Hauser, D. Adolescent sexual health in Europe and the United States. Washington, DC: Advocates for Youth, 2011. Available: http://www.advocatesforyouth.org/publications/419?task=view.

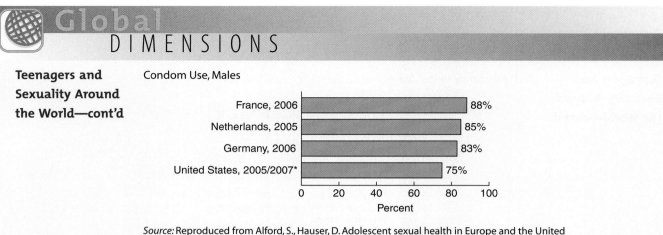

Teenagers and Sexuality Around the World—cont'd

Condom Use, Males

Source: Reproduced from Alford, S., Hauser, D. Adolescent sexual health in Europe and the United States. Washington, DC: Advocates for Youth, 2011. Available: http://www.advocatesforyouth.org/publications/419?task=view.

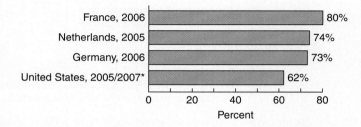

Condom Use, Females

Source: Reproduced from Alford, S., Hauser, D. Adolescent sexual health in Europe and the United States. Washington, DC: Advocates for Youth, 2011. Available: http://www.advocatesforyouth.org/publications/419?task=view.

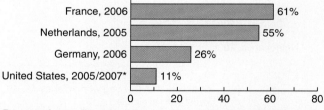

Contraceptive Pill Use, Females

Percent of sexually active 15-year-olds reporting use of contraception at most recent sex. Graphs depict averaged date for U.S. 15-year-olds generated from the 2005 and 2007 Youth Risk Behavior Surveillance.

Source: Reproduced from Alford, S., Hauser, D. Adolescent sexual health in Europe and the United States. Washington, DC: Advocates for Youth, 2011. Available: http://www.advocatesforyouth.org/publications/419?task=view.

Adolescent Pregnancy, Birth, and Abortion Rates in Europe Are Lower than those in the United States*

There is no one best way to improve adolescent sexual health, but leaders in the United States can learn from efforts in some other countries. In many instances these efforts are designed to promote the idea that sexuality is a normal and healthy part of being human and being an adolescent. Here are some examples:

- In France, Germany, and the Netherlands, adults respect adolescents and expect them to act responsibly. Sexuality education for youth is strongly supported by governments.

Global DIMENSIONS

Teenagers and Sexuality Around the World—cont'd

- Public health policies to reduce unintended pregnancies, abortions, and STIs, including HIV, are based on research and not the whims of political and religious interest groups.
- Easy access to condoms and other contraceptive methods, consistent and effective sexuality education, and widespread public education campaigns support the desire to improve adolescent sexual health.
- Long-term government-supported public education campaigns are provided through the Internet, television, films, radio, billboards, discos, pharmacies, and healthcare providers. Campaigns are direct and humorous and focus on both safety and pleasure.
- Youth have convenient access to free or low-cost contraception through national health insurance.

- Sexuality education is usually integrated across school subjects and at all grade levels. It is based on accurate and complete information in response to students' questions.
- Families support educators and healthcare providers' efforts to make sexual health information and services available to teens. Families also have open and honest discussions with adolescents about sexuality.
- Sexual relationships are viewed as normal and natural for older adolescents, a positive component of emotionally healthy maturation. Also, young people believe it is 'stupid and irresponsible' to have sexual activity without protection.
- The values of responsibility, respect, tolerance, and equity are included in ethical views of sexual behavior.

Source: Adapted from Alford, S., & Hauser, D. Adolescent Sexual Health in Europe and the United States. Advocates for Youth, 2011. Available: www.advocatesforyouth.org/publications/419?task=view.

---

assume that Internet sexual abuse would also involve nonstranger sex offenders.

Internet technology provides a number of ways for this to happen. Digital photography has made online production and distribution of child pornography a more frequent component of abuse. Availability and ease of online communication may allow acquaintance and family member offenders a means of bypassing parents and other caregivers so as to develop abusive relationships with potential victims. The Internet may provide opportunities for family and acquaintance offenders to seduce children and adolescents by bringing up sexual topics and exposing potential victims to sexual images and materials.

In response to this concern, child sexual abuse researcher David Finkelhor and others designed a National Juvenile Online Victimization (N-JOV) Study. They examined information provided by law enforcement agencies on almost 800 cases of online sex crimes and found that approximately half of all the arrests involved family and acquaintance offenders. Offender demographics showed that all but 1% were male, most (87%) were over 26 years of age, and 95% were non-Hispanic whites. Almost all victims of family member abuse were female (93%) and younger than 12 (82%), whereas victims of acquaintance offenders were nearly half (49%) male and most (71%) were teenagers.

Crimes were committed in five primary ways: seduction and grooming, child pornography production, arranging meetings and other communication, rewarding victims, and advertising or selling victims. Implications from this study for law enforcement must be to expand the notion of Internet crime to include family and acquaintance offenders. For mental health professionals, Internet involvement should be an inquiry topic for victims and offenders. Both prevention messages and investigation approaches should be revised to incorporate this potential form of sexual abuse (Mitchell, Finkelhor, & Wolak, 2005).

Sexual Harassment

Sexual harassment is a fact of life in most middle and high schools. *Sexual harassment in school* is defined as "unwanted and unwelcome sexual behavior that interferes with the student's life." Sexual harassment includes unwanted sexual comments, jokes, and gestures; receiving from another student sexual pictures, photographs, and notes; sexual graffiti about a specific student in the bathroom or locker room; spreading of sexual rumors; flashing or mooning; touching, grabbing, or pinching in a sexual way; brushing against another student in a sexual way; pulling

sexual harassment
Unwanted sexual behavior that interferes with the student's life.

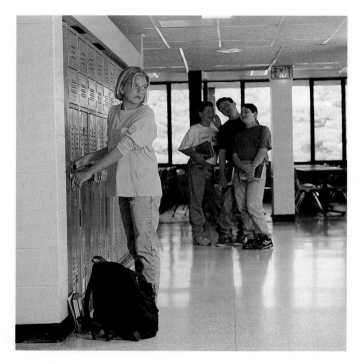

Sexual harassment in schools is common. What type of program could be instituted to help stop such harassment?

clothes off; blocking another student in a sexual way; and forcing kissing and other sexual behaviors.

Statistics about sexual harassment in schools vary by study. One study done in middle and high schools in Memphis, Tennessee, found that over 90% of students reported being sexually harassed at least once while in their current school. The pattern held in both public and private schools, with 91.3% of public school students and 85.5% of private school students reporting being sexually harassed. Students of all racial and ethnic backgrounds reported similar experiences with sexual harassment. Girls were more likely than boys to have been sexually harassed by a student, although the majority of both girls and boys had experienced sexual harassment in their current school. Most students did not report the sexual harassment when it happened. Only 16% said they had ever reported an incident of sexual harassment to school authorities. Sexual harassment has a negative impact on students' mental health, sense of being safe at school, body image, self-esteem, and school participation (Nowhere to hide, 2009).

Most sexual harassment in schools occurs openly in classrooms and hallways, rather than in secluded areas. Students are usually harassed by other students, but occasionally they are harassed by adult employees.

Schools are supposed to protect students against sexual harassment. Schools need to have sexual harassment policies, with clear penalties for perpetrators, which should be communicated to students and parents. A clear procedure for handling complaints of sexual harassment should be established.

Recognizing a Sexually Healthy Relationship

Although sexual abuse and harassment are critical concepts to define and avoid, the components of a **sexually healthy relationship** are less often discussed. This is unfortunate because development of self-identity, particularly in personal and intimate relationships, is a key developmental task of young adults. Being skilled at recognizing a positive relationship provides protection from being exploited, misled, or victimized.

> **sexually healthy relationship**
> Consensual, non-exploitative, honest, mutually pleasurable, safe and protected from unwanted pregnancy, STIs, and other harm (National Guidelines Task Force, 2004).

Here the focus is on health rather than harm. To distinguish between potentially healthy and harmful sexual relationships, the following list provides a tool for assessing relationships by applying the defining characteristics to one's own personal relationships or those of others (Conklin & Peters, 2004).

Who is your partner? What is your relationship with this person? Sexual activity often involves many feelings and emotions that can be confusing. How will you and your partner handle these feelings if they come up? How will sex change your relationship with this person?

Do you feel safe? Consider your partner, the situation, the location … Do you feel safe and taken care of? Do you feel respected by your partner? Do you respect your partner? Can you talk and listen to him or her? Are you worried that someone might walk in?

Is it consensual? No one has the right to be sexual with another person without that person's explicit permission. Have you talked about which behaviors you give permission for and have permission to start? Have you talked about where you will stop? Do you feel like your partner respects your decisions? Do you respect your partner's decisions?

What is your motivation? Why are you thinking of doing this? People can have many reasons for having sex, like to become closer, to feel loved, to express love, to feel good, to satisfy curiosity, to gain popularity, to get someone to like them, to fit in, or to rebel. Let's face it, some of these aren't very good reasons for getting sexually involved with someone else. Be honest with yourself, what are your reasons?

Is it non-exploitative? Exploitation is when one person uses someone else for selfish reasons.

Exploitation should not be part of sexual relationships. Partners should be interested in each other's well-being as well as their own. Are you and your partner looking out for each other?

Are you being honest? Have you talked to your partner about your feelings, what you want to do, and what you don't want to do? Were you truthful in these conversations? Being honest with yourself and your partner can help you have a better relationship.

Is it pleasurable? One reason that many people participate in various sexual activities is because these behaviors provide physical, emotional, and psychological pleasure. Does the sexual activity you are considering or engaging in feel good?

Is it protected? Most sexual behaviors carry some risk of STIs or pregnancy. It's important to protect yourself from these risks—either by avoiding behaviors and eliminating the risk or by using effective protection and reducing the risk. Do you understand the risk involved in each behavior you are considering? Do you understand the benefits of abstaining from some or all risky behaviors? Do you understand how condoms or birth control can reduce your risk? Do you know how to use condoms or birth control correctly?

What does your gut instinct say? A lot of people talk about listening to their inner voice or gut to let them know whether they are making the right decision. Whatever the decision is—if it feels wrong, it is wrong for you. And remember, you can always change your mind. You and your partner always have the right, the ability, and the responsibility to stop if either one of you changes your mind (Kemper & Rodriguez, 2005).

Questions courtesy of SIECUS, www.siecus.org.

Exploring the Dimensions of Human Sexuality

Our feelings, attitudes, and beliefs regarding sexuality are influenced by our internal and external environments. Go to go.jblearning.com/dimensions5e to learn more about the biological, psychological, and sociological factors that affect your sexuality.

Case Study

Sexual maturation is a time of constant physical and psychological changes. At the same time, deeply rooted sociocultural influences, once able to provide a sense of comfort, now may cause confusion.

Many adolescents feel they have almost no control over physiological changes and the accompanying mood swings. In an attempt to preserve the child's body they once had, some girls attempt to control their food intake. But a girl with a bad self-image may develop an obsession with food intake that leads to an eating disorder.

Boys also feel out of control, experiencing erections and hormonal surges at almost any stimulus.

A cultural double standard does not help. Boys who do not want to be permissive feel out of place, as do girls who want to experience sexual behaviors. Such confusion can lead to sexual experimentation—usually in the form of unsafe sexual practices.

Biological Factors

- Puberty changes boys and girls into men and women.
- Genetic coding affects the onset of puberty and general overall appearance.
- Reproduction becomes possible after menarche and semenarche.
- Sexual arousal and response become important issues in an adolescent's life.
- Physical appearance changes dramatically during puberty, affecting body image.
- Growth and development, in terms of physical and mental maturity, greatly affect a person's self-concept.

Sociocultural Factors

- Socioeconomic status affects sexual behaviors. Lower-economic status youths have sexual intercourse earlier than teens who are more well off, and they experience a higher rate of STIs and births.
- Religion and ethnic heritage affect beliefs about sexuality and permissiveness.
- Many cultures' double standard expects boys to be sexually aggressive and girls to remain sexually passive.
- Media and ad information often convey information to adolescents about sexuality and sexual behavior.
- Friends often convey false information about sexual behaviors to adolescents.
- Use of the Internet can provide access to reliable sexuality information but can also lead to sexually abusive situations (Common Sense Media, 2009).

Psychological Factors

- Emotions are dramatically affected by hormones, which cause dramatic mood swings for adolescents.
- Early or late developers may have issues with securing their body image.
- Sexual experience used to be gained slowly, starting with kissing games, moving to petting, then intercourse. Today's teens often move directly from kissing to intercourse.
- Self-concept is influenced by social status and peers.
- Learned attitudes and behaviors are put to the test as the body goes through constant physical changes.

Summary

- Biological sexual development begins during pregnancy. Infants develop a sense of trust based on loving touch and reliable need fulfillment.

- Healthy sexual development of infants and toddlers is fostered by teaching correct names of all body parts and responding non-punitively to self-stimulation and curiosity about genitals.

- Gender is assigned at birth, usually based on genital appearance. By age 3, a child recognizes gender differences; by age 5, a child has an internal sense of being male or female (gender identity) and knows his or her gender will not change (gender constancy).

- Preschoolers develop autonomy and intiative rather than shame or guilt when curiosity-based sex play is expected as normal behavior and questions about reproduction are answered truthfully.

- Parents can use the media as an effective teaching tool, encouraging elementary-school-age children to develop empathy and to critically examine what they see and hear for sexism, gender role stereotypes, and other prejudices.

- Puberty—the predictable process of biological sexual development—usually occurs between the ages of 8 and 17; the median age is 10–11 years for girls and 11–12 years for boys. Physical changes during puberty include emergence of secondary sexual characteristics such as body and facial hair, glandular changes, growth spurt in height and weight, and reproductive maturity indicated by menarche (first menstrual period for girls) and semenarche (first ejaculation for boys).

- The goal of comprehensive sexuality education is to promote adult sexual health. Key concepts include human development, relationships, personal skills, sexual behavior, sexual health, and sexual aspects of society and culture. These concepts are learned through obtaining accurate information, exploring attitudes and values, developing interpersonal skills including communication, and exercising responsibility.

- Adolescence—the period of development from puberty to adulthood—consists of three stages during which thinking, emotions, relationship skills, autonomy, body image, gender-role definition, and sexual self-concept become mature.

- Teen sexual behavior is often examined through the lens of risk behaviors, STIs, and teen birthrates. After 14 years of birth-rate decline, attributed to decreased sexual intercourse and increased use of condoms, the birthrate among U.S. teens increased 4% from 2005 to 2007. However, it decreased again and reached a record low in 2009. It remains the highest in the Western industrialized world.

- Sexual abuse and harassment can occur online via the Internet—that is, electronically as well as directly.

- A sexually healthy relationship can be recognized as one that is safe, consensual, non-exploitative, honest, pleasurable, and protected.

Discussion Questions

1. Discuss how touch, including genital touching, differs for infants and toddlers versus adolescents.

2. Describe the roles that parents, peers, and the media play in teaching preschoolers and early elementary students about sexuality.

3. Compare and contrast puberty in boys and girls, both physiologically and emotionally.

4. Identify and describe the three stages of adolescence, including the development of sexual self-concept.

5. Describe how trends in sexual behaviors, attitudes, and birthrates have changed since the first YRBS was administered in 1991.

6. Distinguish between expected childhood sex play and behaviors that could be abusive.

Application Questions

Reread the chapter-opening story and answer the following questions.

1. On *Mister Rogers' Neighborhood*, Fred Rogers sings a song that says, "Boys are special on the outside/Girls are special on the inside." Is there any reason to tell a young child more than that?

2. Some parents choose to teach their young children about sexual intercourse and reproduction; many other parents do not want their children learning such information. Given that children repeat what they know, is it important to respect the rights of those who—for religious or

cultural reasons—want such information withheld from their children?

3. Given that children do hear explicit sexual references on the national news at some point, how should the mass media handle this content with adequate discretion? If you were a reporter *and* a parent, how would you balance the responsibility to report the news but protect young children?

Critical Thinking Questions

1. You are the parent of a 4-year-old and have just received a phone call from a parent who has a child the same age. It seems the two children were in the garage "examining" each other. The other parent is furious, accusing your child of initiating the "perversities." What do you say to the parent? What do you say to your child?

   You have 10 minutes before your child arrives home, time enough to check out the SIECUS website. Which information will help you talk to your child?

2. Some pressures of adolescence are the result of society's double standard—that it is OK for men but wrong for women to be interested in engaging in sexual behaviors. Given what the chapter says about normal sexual feelings, what pressures does a double standard place on women? On men?

   Is it possible for society to eliminate the double standard and emphasize equality? If so, would society choose that both men and women have an equal right to say yes or no to sexual experiences? Explain your answer.

3. Refer to the Multicultural Dimensions feature when answering these questions. What is the influence of race and ethnicity on condom use? What might account for these differences? What is the influence of race and ethnicity on the number of sexual partners? Why might these differences exist? How might cultural differences influence partner impregnation? How can young people who choose to engage in sexual intercourse be encouraged to use condoms consistently?

Critical Thinking Case

Adolescents have a hard enough time coming to grips with their sexuality even if they receive proper information and support. But few do. In addition, some school-based sexuality education programs have a "fear-based" component. The aim of many fear-based programs is abstinence outside marriage. There is

nothing wrong with teaching abstinence; however, many fear-based programs tend to distort information and use incorrect information to make their point.

The SIECUS website features a large section on fear-based programs, with general information and critiques of seven fear-based programs.

Choose one fear-based program and prepare a critique. What are the strong points and weak points of the program? How could it be improved? Would the fear techniques used in the program have prevented you from engaging in sexual activity?

Exploring Personal Dimensions

Readiness for a Sexual Relationship

Teenagers and young adults often wonder, "How do I know if I am ready for sex?" The following checklist may help them assess their readiness for mature sexual relationships.

This checklist may help adolescents *and* adults evaluate whether they are ready for a mature sexual relationship with a partner. Ideally, these criteria would be met *before* a young person or an adult engaged in intimate sexual behaviors, including any type of intercourse. Think about your own decisions or the decisions of people you know. Do they meet these criteria?

Are you and your partner

_____ Physically mature?
_____ Patient and understanding?
_____ Knowledgeable about sexuality and sexual response?
_____ Empathetic and able to be vulnerable?
_____ Committed to preventing unintended pregnancies?
_____ Able to handle responsibility for positive consequences?
_____ Able to handle responsibility for potential negative consequences?
_____ Honestly approving of your behavior?

Is your relationship

_____ Committed, mutually kind, and understanding?
_____ Do you trust and admire each other?
_____ Have you experimented with and found pleasure in nonpenetrative behaviors?
_____ Have you talked about sexual behaviors before they occur?
_____ Is your motivation for a sexual relationship pleasure and intimacy?
_____ Do you have a place for the sexual relationship that is safe and comfortable?

Source: Haffner, 1995.

Suggested Readings

Albert, B. *With one voice 2010: America's adults and teens sound off about teen pregnancy.* Washington, D.C.: The National Campaign to Prevent Teen and Unplanned Pregnancy, 2010. Available: www.thenationalcampaign.org/resources/pdf/pubs/wov_2010.pdf.

Chandra, A., Mosher, W. D., Copen, C., & Sionean, C. Sexual behavior, sexual attraction, and sexual identity in the United States: Data from the 2006–2008 National Survey of Family Growth. *National Health Statistics Report, 36* (March 3, 2011), 1–36. Available: www.cdc.gov/nchs/data/nhsr/nhsr036.pdf.

Goldman, L. *Coming out, coming in: Nurturing the well-being and inclusion of gay youth in mainstream society.* New York: Routledge Press, 2007.

Haffner, D. W. *Beyond the big talk: A parent's guide to raising sexually healthy teens, revised and updated edition.* New York: Newmarket Press, 2008.

Haffner, D. W. *From diapers to dating: A parent's guide to raising sexually healthy children,* revised 2nd Ed. New York: Newmarket Press, 2008.

Harris, R. H., & Emberley, M. *A family library: It's not the stork! A book about girls, boys, babies, bodies, families and friends.* Cambridge, MA: Candlewick Press, 2006.

It's perfectly normal. Cambridge, MA: Candlewick Press, 2009.

It's so amazing! A book about eggs, sperm, birth, babies, and families. Cambridge, MA: Candlewick Press, 2009.

Sonfield, A., Kost, K., Gold, R. B., & Finer, L. B. The public costs of births resulting from unintended pregnancies: National and state-level estimates. *Perspectives on Sexual and Reproductive Health, 43, no. 3* (June 2011), 94–102.

Web Resources

For links to the websites below, visit *go.jblearning.com/dimension5e* and click on Resource Links.

Answer/Sex, Etc.
www.sexetc.org

Sex, Etc. is part of the Teen-to-Teen Sexuality Education Project developed by Answer. Answer—part of the Center for Applied Psychology at Rutgers University—is a national organization dedicated to providing and promoting comprehensive sexuality education to young people and the adults who teach them.

Sexuality Information and Education Council of the United States
www.siecus.org

SIECUS has been a national voice for sexuality education, sexual health, and sexual rights for more than 40 years. It provides information, education, public policy, and media outreach to educators, healthcare providers, parents, journalists, policy makers, religious leaders, community members, and young people.

National Campaign to Prevent Teen and Unplanned Pregnancy
www.thenationalcampaign.org

Founded in 1996, this nonprofit, nonpartisan initiative is supported almost entirely by private donations. Its mission is to improve the well-being of children, youth, and families by reducing the nation's teen and unplanned pregnancy rates. It offers a host of research-based resources for teens, parents, faith leaders, researchers, and professionals.

Planned Parenthood Federation of America
www.plannedparenthood.org/teen-talk

Teen-Talk is the official teen outreach website of Planned Parenthood. It provides honest and nonjudgmental information about sexuality in language teens can understand. The goal of this site is for teens to use this knowledge to reduce their risk of unintended pregnancy and sexually transmitted infections.

References

Bancroft, J., Herbenick, D., & Reynolds, M. Masturbation as a marker of sexual development, in *Sexual Development in Childhood*, J. Bancroft, ed. Bloomington, IN: Indiana University Press (2003), 438.

Berk, L. *Exploring lifespan development.* Boston: Allyn & Bacon, 2011.

Bernstein, A. C. *Flight of the stork.* Indiana: Perspectives Press, 1994.

Brooks-Gunn, J., & Furstenberg, F. F. Coming of age in the era of AIDS: Puberty, sexuality, and contraception. *The Millbank Quarterly, 68, suppl. 1* (1990).

Bullough, V. L. Children and adolescents as sexual beings: A historical overview. *Child and Adolescent Psychiatric Clinics of North America, 13, no. 3* (2004), 447–459.

Bullough, V. L., & Bullough, B. *Human sexuality: An encyclopedia.* New York: Garland Press, 1994.

Centers for Disease Control and Prevention. *HIV and AIDS in the United States: A picture of today's epidemic.* Atlanta, GA: Author, 2009. Available: http://www.cdc.gov/hiv/topics/surveillance/united_states.htm.

Child Trends. Science says: Where and when teens first have sex. *Science Says, 1* (June 2003).

Common Sense Media. *Talking about "sexting,"* 2009. Available: http://www.commonsensemedia.org/talking-about-sexting.

Copen, C. E., Chandra, A., & Martinez, G. Prevalence and timing of oral sex with opposite-sex partners among females and males aged 15–24 years: United States, 2007-2010. *National Health Statistics Reports, no. 56,* (August 16, 2012), 1–14.

Dake, J. A., Price, J. H., & Ward, B. Prevalence and correlates of sexting behavior in adolescents. *American Journal of Sexuality Education, 7, no. 1,* (January–March 2012), 1–15.

Dalal, A. Sexual stereotypes stop females from feeling pleasure. *Sex, Etc.* (2005).

DeLamater, J. D., & Friedrich, W. N. Human sexual development. *The Journal of Sex Research, 39* (2002), 10–14.

Denizet-Lewis, B. Friends, friends with benefits and the benefits of the local mall. *The New York Times* (May 30, 2004).

Eaton, D. K., Kann, L., Kinchen, S., Shanklin, S., Ross, J., Hawkins, J., Harris, W. A., Lowry, R., McManus, T., Chuyen, D., Lim, C., Whittle, L., Brenner, N. D., & Wechsler, H. Youth Risk Behavior Surveillance—United States, 2009. *Morbidity and Mortality Weekly Report 59, no. SS-5* (June 4, 2010): A–146.

Erickson, E. H. *Childhood and society.* New York: Norton, 1950.

Friedrich, W. N., Fisher, J., Broughton, D., Houston, M., & Shafran, C. R. Normative sexual behavior in children: A contemporary sample. *Pediatrics, 101, no. r* (April 1998), e9.

Friedrich, W. N., Whiteside, S. P., & Talley, N. J. Noncoercive sexual contact with similarly aged individuals: What is the impact? *Journal of Interpersonal Violence, 19, no. 9* (September 2004), 1075–1084.

Giedd, J. Teen brains: Still under construction. Parents play important role. *NIH News in Health* (September 2005). Available: http://newsinhealth.nih.gov.

Goldstein, H. Making movies, mastering the media. *Teenwire .com,* (November 18, 2005).

Grunbaum, J., et. al. Youth Risk Behavior Surveillance—United States, 2003. *Surveillance Summaries, Morbidity and Mortality Weekly Report, 53.SS-2* (May 21, 2004), 1–95. Available: http://www.cdc.gov/nccdphp/dash/yrbs/.

Guttmacher Institute. Can more progress be made? Teenage sexual and reproductive health behaviors in developed countries. In *Executive summary.* New York: Author, 2001, 1–6.

Haffner, D. ed. *Facing facts: Sexual health for America's adolescents.* New York: Sexuality Information and Education Council of the United States, 1995.

Kalmus, D., Davidson, A., Cohall, A., Laraque, D., & Cassell, C. Preventing sexual risk behaviors and pregnancy among teenagers: Linking research and programs. *Perspectives on Sexual and Reproductive Health, 35, no. 2* (March/April 2003).

Kann, L., Lowry, R., Eaton, D., & Wechsler, H. Trends in HIV-related risk behaviors among high school students—United States, 1991–2011. *Morbidity and Mortality Report, 61, no. 29* (July 27, 2012), 556–560.

Kemper, M., & Rodriguez, M. Talk about sex. SIECUS, 2005. Available: http://www.siecus.org/_data/global/images/TalkAboutSex.pdf.

Kirby, D. *Do abstinence-only programs delay the initiation of sex among young people and reduce teen pregnancy?* Washington, DC: National Campaign to Prevent Teen Pregnancy, 2002a.

Kirby, D. Effective approaches to reducing adolescent unprotected sex, pregnancy, and childbearing. *Journal of Sex Research, 39, no. 7* (2002b), 51–58.

Kirby, D., Lepore, G., & Ryan, J. Executive summary: Sexual risk and protective factors, in *Putting what works to work,* ETR Associates (September 2005).

Kost, K., & Henshaw, S. U.S. teenage pregnancies, births and abortions, 2008: National trends by age, race and ethnicity. New York. The Guttmacher Institute. Available: http://www.guttmacher.org/pubs/USTPtrends08.pdf.

Michels, T. M., Kropp, R. Y., Eyre, S. L., & Halpern-Felsher, B. L. Initiating sexual experiences: How do young adolescents make decisions regarding early sexual activity? *Journal of Research on Adolescence, 15* (2005), 583–607.

Mitchell, K. J., Finkelhor, D., & Wolak, J. The Internet and family and acquaintance sexual abuse. *Child Maltreatment, 10, no. 1* (February 2005), 49–60.

Moore, K. A. *Teen births: Examining the recent increase.* National Campaign to Prevent Teen and Unplanned Pregnancies, October 2008.

National Campaign to Prevent Teen Pregnancy. The general facts and stats. *teenpregnancy.org* (May 2005).

National Guidelines Task Force. *Guidelines for comprehensive sexuality education: Kindergarten–12th grade,* 3rd ed. New York: Sexuality Information and Education Council of the United States, 2004.

Nowhere to hide. Center for Research on Women, University of Memphis, 2009. Available: http://www.memphis.edu/crow/sexualharassment.php.

O'Sullivan, L. F., & Brooks-Gunn, J. The timing of changes in girls' sexual cognitions and behaviors in early adolescence: A prospective, cohort study. *Journal of Adolescent Health, 37, no.3* (2005), 211–219.

Okami, P., Olmstead, R., Abrahamson, P. R., & Pendleton, L. Early childhood exposure to parental nudity and scenes of parental sexuality ("primal scenes"): An 18-year longitudinal study of outcome. *Archives of Sexual Behavior, 27, no. 2* (1998), 361–384.

Rosengard, C., Tannis, C., Dove, D. C., van den Berg, J. J., Lopez, R., Stein, L. A. R., & Morrow, K. M. Family sources of sexual health information, primary messages, and sexual behavior of at-risk, urban adolescents. *American Journal of Health Education, 43, no. 2* (March/April 2012), 83–87.

Santelli, J. S., Abma, J., Ventura, S., Lindberg, L., Morrow, B., Anderson, J. E., Lyss, S., & Hamilton, B. Can changes in sexual behaviors among high school students explain the decline in teen pregnancy rates in the 1990s? *Journal of Adolescent Health, 35* (2004), 80–90.

Satcher, D. *Surgeon General's call to action to promote sexual health and responsible sexual behavior.* United States Department of Health and Human Services, July 9, 2001.

Schwartz, P., & Rutter, V. *The gender of sexuality.* Walnut Creek, CA: AltaMira Press, 2000.

Sexual abuse. Crimes Against Children Research Center, 2011. Available: http://www.unh.edu/ccrc/sexual-abuse/.

Sexual attitudes and behavior of male teens. *Science Says, 6,* (Oct. 2003).

Sexual behavior of young adolescents. *Science Says, 3* (Sep. 2003).

Sonenstein, F. What teenagers are doing right: Changes in sexual behavior over the past decade. *Journal of Adolescent Health, 35* (2004), 77–78.

Steiner-Adair, C., & Sjostrom, L. *Full of ourselves: A wellness program to advance girl power, health, and leadership.* New York: Teachers College Press, 2006.

Strong, B., DeVault, C., Sayad, B. W., & Yarber, W. L. *Human sexuality: Diversity in contemporary America,* 5th ed. New York: McGraw-Hill, 2005.

Teens and oral sex. *Science Says, 17* (September 2005).

Television and children. University of Michigan Health System, 2011. Available: http://www.med.umich.edu/yourchild/topics/tv.htm.

Temple, J. R., Paul, J. A., van den Berg, P., Le, V. D., McElhany, A., & Temple, B. W. Teen sexting and its association with sexual behaviors. *Archives of Pediatrics & Adolescent Medicine,* (2012), 1–6. doi: 10,1001/archpediatrics.2012.835.

Ventura, S. J., & Hamilton, B. E. U.S. teenage birth rate resumes decline. *NCHS Data Brief, no 58.* Huntsville, MD: National Center for Health Statistics, 2011.

Weinberger, D. R., Elvevåg, B., & Giedd, J. N. *The adolescent brain: A work in progress.* National Campaign to Prevent Teen Pregnancy, June 2005. Available: http://www.teenpregnancy.org/resources/reading/pdf/BRAIN.pdf.

Weinstein, E., & Rosen, E. *Teaching about human sexuality and family: A skills-based approach.* Belmont, CA: Thomson Wadsworth, 2006.

Yudt, S. Masturbation myths. *Teenwire.com.* Planned Parenthood Federation of America (November 9, 2004).

Zucker, K. J., & Bradley, S. J. Gender identity and psychosexual disorders. *American Psychiatric Association Focus, 3* (2005), 598–617.

CHAPTER 12

Sexuality in Adulthood

FEATURES

Global Dimensions
Young People, Unprotected Sexual Activity, and Trustworthy Information

Multicultural Dimensions
The Jefferson–Hemings Affair

Communication Dimensions
Tempted by Digital Dalliances

Global Dimensions
Single-Parent Households in Various Countries

Multicultural Dimensions
The Boomer Sandwich

Ethical Dimensions
Should Donor Eggs Be Used to Let Women Older Than 50 Years Produce Viable Babies?

Gender Dimensions
Coming to Terms: Masculinity and Physical Challenges

CHAPTER OBJECTIVES

1 Discuss the major theories of love and sexuality.

2 Describe the typical college relationship, including sexual activities.

3 Cite the factors that have led to the increase in the number of single people and the postponement of marriage.

4 Evaluate the advantages and disadvantages of cohabitation.

5 Describe the characteristics of a happy marriage.

6 Discuss the reasons for the high number of divorces.

7 Describe changes that occur during the aging process.

8 Discuss the sexuality challenges for the disabled and ill, as well as how to overcome them.

go.jblearning.com/dimensions5e

Cohabitation
Multicultural Dimensions: The Jefferson–Hemings Affair
Types of Marriage
Divorce

INTRODUCTION

*L*ynn and Chris first met in a small town's only junior high when they were 12 years old. By high school, they had become friends and had their first date at the homecoming dance their sophomore year. After a couple of years of dating, they lost their virginity together at age 16 years. Throughout high school, they stayed together and began planning for college and a life together.

They applied to the same colleges and entered the college where they were both accepted. The struggles of college produced many changes, but they made a conscious effort to change together. As they grew up together, they did things they perceived to be more grown-up: traveling, saving up for an apartment, and the like. During their junior year, they got an off-campus apartment in the heart of the local city.

Although they had been together for more than 5 years and were engaged, they were surprised at their parents' reactions—shock and dismay—to their living together. After all, it was the late 1970s, and both families had had other relatives who had lived together. Lynn and Chris saw living together as a "next step" toward marriage. Why, they thought, was society so backward?

Surviving college made them more determined to pursue their dream of life together, with children and good jobs. At age 24 years, they married. Four years later, a first child was born; 3 years later, a second child. With each change, they managed to adapt. But slowly—almost imperceptibly—they realized that they were not always changing in the same ways.

As they hit full stride in their careers in their mid-30s, and their children reached school age, decisions had to be made. Holding a high-level management position that requires long hours and travel also requires support at home—with children and housework. The old saying

"Behind every great man, there's a great woman" today would be phrased as "A successful person has family support."

Lynn supported the family by working from a home office and taking care of the children—schools, homework, sick days, vacation days, doctor and dentist appointments, play dates, sports, and extracurricular activities. Chris rarely returned home from work before 7:30 P.M., worked many weekends, and traveled around the world. Conflicts developed over what was important in their lives, and, because Chris made more money than Lynn, issues concerning how to spend also arose. Chris's lack of time at home increased tensions. Eventually, Lynn discovered that Chris was having an affair with a business associate.

After considering the possibility of divorce for several years, Lynn and Chris finally proceeded—after 14 years of marriage and almost 25 years together. The children stayed with Lynn, and Chris was ordered to pay child support and alimony. Both Lynn and Chris expressed a feeling of relief after the divorce was finalized.

Lynn and Chris had a great deal of positive support from friends, many of whom had been divorced themselves. It seemed that society had begun to accept divorce. But once again, they were surprised by the reaction of their parents, who felt that they should stay together and try to work out their problems. Some things never change!

In this chapter we explore how people fall in love, then we follow the life cycle from singlehood, through cohabitation, marriage, and divorce. Finally, we take a look at sexuality and the elderly.

▓ Love and Sexuality

What is love? How do you know when and whether you are in love, whether you are loved, or whether you love another person? These questions have been asked through the ages by young people just beginning to long for and seek intimacy outside their parental families. And through the ages love has never grown any easier to define. There are many types of love—love of one's parents, of a friend, of a pet. Perhaps the most difficult sort of love to describe is love of a person with whom one could potentially share a sexual relationship.

Theories About Love

Love may take a variety of forms, as Greek philosophers long ago demonstrated: *eros*, passionate and/or erotic love; *agape*, a selfless, giving love; *storge*, affectionate love, usually of the type parents have for their children; *ludus*, playful love (partners keep the relationship at a distance by keeping love at a game level); and *mania*, a love consumed by emotional extremes such as misery, possessiveness, and jealousy.

Erich Fromm presented his ideas about love in *The Art of Loving* (1956). He distinguishes brotherly love, motherly love, erotic love, and self-love.

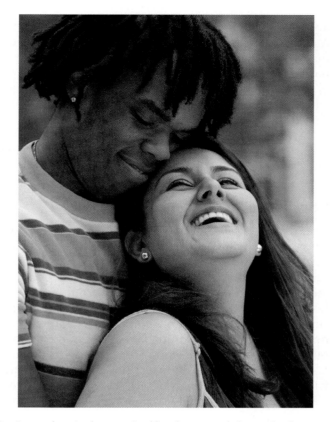

Passionate love is characterized by almost total absorption in another person.

He believes that loving is an art—something that must be learned and practiced. Fromm indicated that immature love is characterized by a dependent relationship between two people, and mature love is characterized by care, responsibility, respect, and knowledge of the loved person. He defines erotic love as a craving for total union with another person that is exclusive and enduring.

Abraham Maslow distinguished between B-love and D-love (1968). Those who experience B-love (short for *Being* love) are unselfish in their love for another; those who experience D-love (short for *Deficiency* love) are selfish and have a strong need for love.

Rempel and Burris (2005) suggested that love is a motive based on the valuing of the other person, and is associated with the goal of preserving or promoting the other's well-being. They said that intense, powerful emotions may serve as eliciting experiences for different types of love. Benefitting the other person can be an ultimate goal for the various forms of love.

Types of Love

Love takes many forms and can be distinguished as romantic love or conscious love. Romantic love, also known as passionate love, is characterized by almost total absorption in another, with strong feelings of elation, sexual desire, anxiety, and arousal. This form of love is often accompanied by physiological reactions—perspiration, stomach churning, blushing, and increased pulse rate.

Intense, passionate love is most likely to occur early in a relationship. At this point people often overlook faults, avoid conflicts, and ignore logic and reasoned consideration. Conscious love, in contrast, is a more realistic view of another person. We see both the strengths and weaknesses of the loved one and do not depend completely on him or her to fulfill our needs and give us what we ourselves lack. The sexual activity in conscious love may be more rewarding than in romantic love because the sexual behavior communicates and expresses loving feelings. People who have an honest view of each other can enjoy giving as well as receiving. People who feel romantic (passionate) love are often intent on receiving pleasure and fulfilling their desires, rather than on giving and taking equally.

In addition to being romantic or conscious, love can take various forms—erotic, friendship, devotional, parental, or altruistic. In erotic love there is a type of biological "chemistry" that binds lovers together and leads them to form a binding relationship (Lee, 1988). Individuals experiencing erotic love are preoccupied with their love and constantly think about their partner. Erotic love becomes less intense as time goes on, but even at a lower level it can be a positive part of a relationship.

Friendship involves deep and intimate feelings, but these are not physical. The Greek term for this type of friendship or liking is *philia*. Although there are many similar attitudes and feelings among lovers as well as friends, lovers tend to differ from friends in sexual intimacy, exclusiveness, and fascination (Davis, 1985). Men and women can be friends without becoming sexually involved.

Devotional love does not involve physical contact and is a very specific kind of love. This type of love is most likely to be directed to a god, a country, an ethnic group, or other significant groups or institutions.

Parental love can be intense, but the feelings are different from other forms of love. Infants and children learn this type of love through holding and touching—even very early in life. For some people, parental love represents the most intense form of love they will ever feel.

Altruistic love is a generous giving of the self. Some say this is a special form of parental love; it is seen in people who spend great amounts of time doing church work, volunteering in hospitals, and

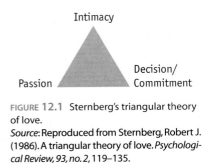

FIGURE **12.1** Sternberg's triangular theory of love.

Source: Reproduced from Sternberg, Robert J. (1986). A triangular theory of love. *Psychological Review, 93, no. 2,* 119–135.

assisting others in a variety of ways. Some people who work in helping professions—for example, as therapists or teachers—might find they have a great capacity for altruistic love.

Sternberg (1986) has proposed a triangular theory of love suggesting that there are three components of love: intimacy, passion, and decision/commitment. These components can be visualized as points on a triangle (Figure 12.1); the triangle metaphor is used to show how a couple can be matched or mismatched in the love they have for each other. The top of the triangle is intimacy, which is the emotional component of love, according to Sternberg. Here are feelings of mutual understanding, bondedness, willingness to share, giving of emotional support, and valuing of the other person as part of your life. Passion is the motivational drive of love that includes physical attraction, sexual relations, and romance. Passion can usually differentiate romantic love from love in a friendship or of a family member. This component is usually first in a relationship but is also the first to fade. Passion and intimacy are interwoven and one may precede the other, depending on how the relationship begins. Decision/commitment is the cognitive component of the triangle, as one makes the decision to love the other person and then makes the long-term commitment to maintain the relationship.

Perfectly matched involvements of partners exist when the vertexes of the triangles are equally matched and are at the same level. Closely matched couples may be slightly off on one of the components, and this is usually not a perilous situation. Moderately mismatched partners exhibit mismatching at one or two of the vertexes and the partners are at different levels within those components. For example, they may be equally matched on the passion vertex, but one partner is slightly more committed

and has greater feelings of intimacy than the other. A severely mismatched couple is one whose partners may be equally committed but are very disparate in the passion and intimacy components.

This theory of love may help partners determine whether they are on the right track in their relationship and may help diagnose any problems.

Sternberg (1988) has outlined eight types, or phases, of love based on his triangular model. They are listed in Table 12.1.

Characteristics of Romantic Love

Because we are focusing on human relationships and sexuality in this text, it is appropriate to consider briefly the characteristics of romantic love—companionship, intimacy, caring, commitment, sexual activity, and romance. Companionship involves sharing experiences and receiving emotional support from each other. At first this characteristic might not seem as exciting as some of the others, but over time it can be enduring and very necessary.

Intimacy involves sharing thoughts and feelings with a person who is considered very special. Whereas traditionally women and not men revealed their innermost thoughts, in recent years there is a tendency for both genders to disclose highly personal feelings within a relationship (Hatfield, 1988; Pearson, 1985).

Caring is the desire to do things for another person without expecting anything in return. As in most other aspects of a relationship, balance is important. For example, it is possible to think of situations in which there is so much caring that the relationship is completely one-sided.

TABLE 12.1 **Sternberg's Types (Phases) of Love**

1. **Nonlove:** All three components of love are absent. Most personal relationships are of this type.

2. **Liking:** Intimacy is present, but passion and commitment are not.

3. **Infatuation:** There are passionate desires, but intimacy and commitment are not present. This is a kind of "love at first sight."

4. **Empty love:** Commitment exists, but passion and intimacy are missing. Relationships that once had passion and intimacy can become stagnant.

5. **Romantic love:** There is no commitment, but there is passion and intimacy.

6. **Companionate love:** A combination of intimacy and commitment exists, but passionate attraction has died down. The relationship becomes a kind of committed friendship.

7. **Fatuous love:** Passion and commitment are present, but intimacy is not. This type is associated with whirlwind romances and "quickie marriages."

8. **Consummate love:** This is the complete measure of love involving passion, intimacy, and commitment. It can be very hard to achieve this type of love, and even harder to maintain it.

Source: Data from Sternberg, Robert J. (1986). A triangular theory of love. *Psychological Review, 93, no. 2,* 119–135.

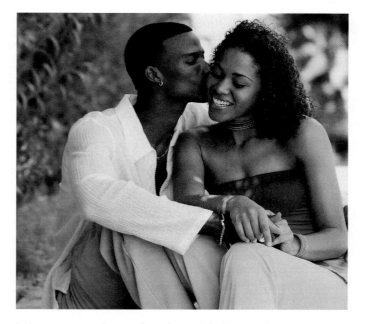

Intimacy means sharing thoughts and feelings with someone we consider very special.

Commitment means pressing on with a relationship even during difficult times. When conflict or problems exist, commitment is needed to give other aspects of love a chance to grow.

Sexual activity sometimes seems to be the major part of romantic love; however, there are many couples who love each other but have a minimal amount of sexual activity. Sexual activity alone, even when highly pleasurable, is not enough to maintain a poor relationship (Blumstein & Schwartz, 1983). There does seem to be a connection between sexual activity and positive relationships, but a good relationship probably has a positive influence on sexual activity, rather than the converse.

The decision to participate in sexual activity can be very simple for some people, and very complicated for others. Sexual activity can have different meanings for different people. It can be a validation of deep intimacy in a relationship, it can be a way to help get to know another person, it can be done to promote reproduction, it can reduce sexual tension, it can produce excitement and risk, and for some it can be a form of recreation.

For many college students it is helpful to base decisions about sexual activity on their values. Some students may have clear guidelines based upon what they have learned from their family, their religion, or their peers; others may not have such guidelines. In either case it may be wise to consider personal values in life and relationships before getting sexually involved. This can mean thinking about the role of relationships and sexual activity in life at

that time, which norms are most highly valued and why, and what should be done for protection against unwanted pregnancy and sexually transmitted infections (STIs) if a decision is made to participate in intimate sexual activity. Communication about these decisions with a potential partner is especially important.

The nature of love typically changes as a relationship develops. For example, the passionate or romantic love of an early stage might evolve into a companionship type of love. This does not mean that passion and romance have evaporated, nor does it mean that the relationship is not as good as before. It simply means that there are common stages of relationships, and they can all be of high quality. Relationships can be thought of as having different phases of growth. At any stage there are ways to promote better relationships.

Aron et al. (2005) reported interesting research about romantic love and related changes as relationships develop. They used MRI brain scans and studied 17 college students who were intensely "in love" from 1 to 17 months. Participants alternately viewed a photograph of their beloved and a photograph of a familiar individual. The MRI detected increases or decreases of blood flow to the brain, which reflected changes in neural activity. Based on brain activity, they found that romantic love is a biological urge distinct from sexual arousal. It is close to the neural profile of drives like hunger and drug craving. In its early stages, love can be very intoxicating and the drive for romantic love can be stronger than the will to live. With time, however, the intoxication mellows and brain scans show different findings. The scans show that different parts of the brain are stimulated later in a relationship as compared to the earlier stages. The researchers indicated that, among other processes, new love involves psychologically internalizing a lover, absorbing elements of the other person's opinions, hobbies, expressions, and character, as well as sharing one's own. The expansion of the self happens very rapidly, and it is one of the most exhilarating experiences there is.

Many have traditionally believed that romantic love fades over time and evolves into warm feelings. However, Acevedo and Aron (2009) found that long-term relationships do not necessarily kill the romance. Their research indicates long-term romantic love (with intensity, sexual interest, and engagement, but without the obsessive element common in new relationships) appears to be real and is associated with marital satisfaction, mental health, and overall well-being.

The relationship between love styles and lifetime number of sexual partners has also been explored among college students. Hans (2008) found that the number of sexual partners was positively correlated with age, romantic lovers, and game-playing lovers (who typically value fun and self-indulgence over commitment and emotional involvement), and was negatively correlated with religiosity.

Hormonal and Chemical Aspects of Love

The characteristics and types of love presented so far have been mainly based upon emotional, psychological, and spiritual kinds of feelings. Some experts argue that hormonal and chemical factors are also involved in love. One reason may be related to brain chemistry. Another relates to pheromones, which are chemical substances secreted by some animals that supposedly affect the reproductive behavior of another same-species animal.

Related to brain chemistry, during the intense passion of a developing love relationship some people report a natural high, almost as though they were on drugs. Researchers (Liebowitz, 1983; Walsh, 1991) reported that this "high" results from surging levels of three brain chemicals that allow brain cells to communicate with each other. They are similar to amphetamine drugs and cause effects such as giddiness, euphoria, and elation. As with use of amphetamines, the "high" typically does not last—perhaps because the body develops a tolerance for the chemicals just as it does for amphetamines, or perhaps because the intensity of the relationship decreases.

The same researchers also point out that there are brain chemicals that help explain why some relationships develop into long-term loving relationships. These substances, called endorphins, are morphine-like chemicals that help cause a sense of security, tranquility, and peace. The researchers suggest that these chemicals help explain why abandoned lovers may feel such a loss: They are not getting their doses of feel-good chemicals.

The topic of pheromones has received greater attention in recent years. For more than a hundred years scientists have documented the effects of pheromones on mating behavior in insects and animals. The big question has been, Do pheromones have the same effects on humans?

In 1986 Dr. Winnifred Cutler began to document the effects of human pheromones (Link & Copeland, 2001). Those who believe in human pheromones claim they send signals that are picked up by organs inside the nose. We cannot smell them, but they supposedly can have a major impact on sex drive, increase in fertility, and regulation of women's menstrual cycles. Behaviors that are reported to increase as a result of pheromones include making conversation, expressing an interest in another person, being responsive to another person, paying unsolicited compliments,

overtly flirting, brushing up against another person, and becoming sexually excited.

On the basis of the concept that there are natural human pheromones, entrepreneurs developed numerous products designed to mimic the alleged effects of pheromones. These include towelettes with pheromones as well as creams and oils that are supposed to help with sexual attraction. It is too early to tell whether such products are effective—and even the basic effects of pheromones are not agreed upon by experts.

The overall biology of love is still a mystery. However, many people report that biological factors and changes seem to influence their strong feelings for another person. Obvious things like increased heart rate, slight sweating, and hormonal changes do seem to occur. For example, levels of glucocorticoids and norephinephrine can increase in the bloodstream very quickly when seeing a very attractive person. These reactions, along with the potential influence of pheromones, result in biological impacts on potential love relationships (Gonzales, 2005).

At the 2009 annual meeting of the Advancing Science, Serving Society (AASA), several researchers talked about the biology of romantic love (Borenstein, 2009). Among other points, they indicated that parts of the brain respond strongly when people are around those they love romantically, brain cells make chemicals and send them to different brain regions, and love works chemically in the brain like a drug addiction.

Love Problems

With all its positive aspects, love can also create problems. Perhaps the most obvious ones are rejection, jealousy, and falling out of love. Being turned down by another person (rejection) can be difficult to experience. This can happen at various stages of a relationship, and fear of rejection is natural. Of course, as with so many other aspects of life, obtaining the many positive benefits of a relationship always entails a gamble (such as the possibility of rejection). Dealing with rejection can be difficult for some, but often it simply involves trying again. If a strong relationship already exists, it might be wise to use good communication skills and talk about the rejection with the other person. Couples counseling can help single and married couples. At any rate, rejection can also be used as a learning experience to help in future relationships.

Some jealous feelings are probably natural, but jealousy is also a bothersome feeling that can get in the way of good love relationships. It can be helpful to understand why jealous feelings occur, to use good communication skills to talk about jealousy within a relationship, and to avoid doing things that might contribute to a partner's jealous feelings. For some, effective means of coping with jealousy are thinking about one's positive qualities, selectively ignoring some activities that might be upsetting, and simply containing feelings of jealousy. It might be wise to recognize jealous feelings and accept and deal with them as part of an overall relationship.

Related to love problems, Amber Vennum studied couples in cyclical relationships—the term used for a couple who breaks up and then gets back together. She said that with college-age people, about 40% are currently in a relationship where they have broken up and gotten back together. Generally, the results of getting back together were less than desirable. Couples in a cyclical relationship tended to be more impulsive about major relationship transitions—like moving in together, buying a pet together or having a child together. As a result, they tended to be less satisfied with their partner, had worse communication, made more decisions that negatively affected the relationship, had lower self-esteem, and had a higher uncertainty about their future together. Couples often said they had gotten back together because they believed their partner had changed for the better or that communication had improved, but the results indicated otherwise. She said many studies show that when our relationships are poor, we don't function well. In most cases it does not make sense to get back together (Why Couples Who Have Broken Up Should Not Get Get Back Together: Relationships Expert, 2012).

What Causes Attraction?

Many factors contribute to attraction and falling in love. Unlike in the fairy tale in which the prince marries the commoner, in real life we are usually attracted to someone we consider attainable. This attraction differs from adolescent crushes on movie stars, sports stars, politicians, or teachers. In adulthood, we seek intimate relationships with someone who can love us in return.

Most North Americans marry someone who has the same sociocultural dimensions, someone whose race and ethnicity, religion, age, and social class are similar to their own (Henslin, 1995). Why do we like

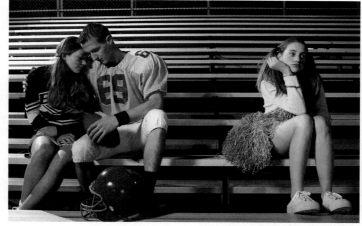

It may be hard to deal with feelings if you are attracted to someone who is in a relationship with another person.

people who are like us? One explanation is that doing so provides us with validation for our personality characteristics and beliefs (Baron, 1998). Similarity is a very powerful determinant of attraction.

Gender also plays a role in mate selection. Researchers interviewed more than 9,000 young adults (males and females), all in their 20s, who lived in 33 countries. Subjects were given a list of 18 traits and asked to rank them in terms of most (1) to least (18) desirable in a potential mate (Buss et al., 1990). The results are listed in Table 12.2.

Buss and associates found a gender difference as well: Males in all cultures in the study placed an emphasis on youthfulness and attractiveness. Data showed that at the time of marriage, the average male was 2 to 5 years older than his partner. Women, however, placed an emphasis on mates who were somewhat older, had better prospects for financial

TABLE 12.2 Ranking of Desirable Traits in a Partner (Male and Female Combined)

1. Mutual attraction (love)
2. Dependable character
3. Emotional stability and maturity
4. Pleasing disposition
5. Good health
6. Education and intelligence
7. Sociability
8. Desire for home and children
9. Refinement, neatness
10. Good looks (ranked higher by males)
11. Ambitious and industrious
12. Good cook and housekeeper
13. Good financial prospects (ranked higher by females)
14. Similar education
15. Favorable social status or rating
16. Chastity (ranked higher by males)
17. Similar religious background
18. Similar political background

security, and were industrious. Buss explains the difference in terms of evolutionary needs: Males select younger, physically attractive women because such characteristics are viewed as good indicators of reproductive success. Women select older, more established males because such characteristics are viewed as good indicators of security for their offspring (Buss, 1994).

Attraction, then, can be caused by many characteristics. Features such as height, eye color and size, size of body parts, skin characteristics, musculature, and body symmetry can all play a role for some people. Related to all of this is the waist-to-hip ratio. It is determined by dividing your waist measurement by your hip measurement. For example, a ratio of 0.7 might be considered desirable for a female, while a ratio of 0.9 might be desirable for a male. The hips are measured at the widest part of the buttocks, and the waist is measured at the smaller circumference of the natural waist, usually just above the belly button. Research indicates that people with "apple-shaped" bodies (with more weight around the waist) face more health risks than those with "pear-shaped" bodies who carry more weight around the hips. It has also been found that in most cultures waist-to-hip ratio is viewed as a measure of attractiveness and health for men and women (Singh, 2002).

Whatever causes attraction, it is interesting that many of us have a "love-is-blind bias" (a tendency to perceive romantic partners as more attractive than the self). For example, Swami (2009) found that both gay men and lesbians rated their partners as significantly more attractive than themselves. The author called this a "robust positive illusion in self–partner perceptions."

■ Sexuality During the College Years

Before the late 1960s, there were strict rules on campuses about men's and women's socializing. Older readers may remember the "one foot on the floor" rule: Women were allowed to have men in their college dorm room only with the door open and only with each person's having one foot on the floor. Curfews were common. Coed dorms were nonexistent. Today, most campuses have long given up these types of rules.

Since 2000, the American College Health Association (2011) has conducted the National College Health Assessment every fall and spring term. Some of the questions relate to sexual behavior, and more than 30,000 college students respond each term. Here are highlights from the most recent findings:

- 22.9% of respondents had ever been tested for HIV infection.

- 16.9% of sexually active women had used emergency contraception within the past school year.

- 2.0% of females and 2.5% of males who had vaginal intercourse within the past school year had become pregnant unintentionally or had gotten someone else pregnant unintentionally.

- 41.7% of students had oral sexual activity in the past 30 days.

- 45.4% of students had vaginal intercourse in the past 30 days.

- 4.7% had anal intercourse in the past 30 days.

- 34.2% had no sexual partner, 41% had one sexual partner, 10.3% had two sexual partners, 5.7% had three sexual partners, and 8.8% had four or more sexual partners in the past 12 months.

- Using a condom within the last 30 days (mostly or always) was reported by 59.5% of those who had vaginal intercourse and 29.4% of those who had anal intercourse. Approximately the same percentage of students used a condom the last time they had sexual intercourse of either type.

- The most common forms of birth control used by students or their partners the last time they had vaginal intercourse were male condoms (63.6%), birth control pills (59.4%), and withdrawal (28.8%).

It is interesting that in general respondents thought that their college peers were participating in much more sexual activity than they actually were. This reminds us that perceptions of other people's sexual behavior are often not accurate.

Late high school and early college years are a time of transition to sexual activity for males. Fewer than 25% are sexually experienced by age 15, but more than 90% have intercourse before their 20th birthday. Slightly more than 20% of sexually experienced men have had only one partner by their late teens, and about 30% have had six or more (In their own right, 2002).

Seventeen Magazine and the National Campaign to Prevent Teen and Unwanted Pregnancy (That's what he said, 2010) surveyed 1,200 boys and men ages 15–22. The results were surprising to some people. For example, many commonly accepted stereotypes about males (that they're all in a rush to have sexual activity, that relationships don't matter, and that they don't care what girls or their parents think) were not supported by the survey. However, other stereotypes (the double standard between the genders when it comes to sexual activity and that guys lie a lot about sexual activity) were supported. Thirty percent of the college-age males lied about the number of sexual partners they had had, and 35% of those who lied about sexual activity said they did so to appear "cooler."

Although there can be many motivations to participate in sexual activity, Oswalt (2010) surveyed 422 college students to determine their main motivations. She found that physical gratification was the most constant reason for them to engage in sexual activity.

Types of Relationships

The Institute for American Values (Mulhauser, 2001) interviewed 1,000 college women and reported that dating among college students is all but dead. Apparently, college students either participate in random hookups or are in a very serious relationship. For many, there is nothing in between. Hooking up does not have to mean having sexual intercourse. In fact, 39% of the respondents were virgins. Dating, however, was not reported to be very common. One-third of the women said they had been asked on two or fewer dates. Of the seniors interviewed, only 50% said they had been asked on six or more dates since college started. Because few people are asking for dates, what is left is an informal hookup.

Previously, noncollege singles in their 20s were almost entirely overlooked in research about sexual

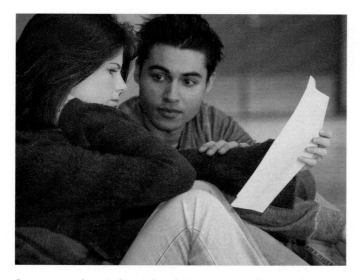

Some researchers indicate that dating among college students is almost dead. Many seem to participate in random hookups or very serious relationships instead.

behavior and attitudes. Popenoe and Whitehead (2001) found that this group aspire to marriage and expect their marriage to last a lifetime. However, many are first looking to get ahead on their own. Both men and women are committed to making it on their own and getting a place of their own before marriage. The mating culture is described as "sex without strings and relationships without rings." Sexual activity is viewed as being for fun. Casual sexual activity is an expected part of the dating scene. The threat of HIV and AIDS looms large over the dating scene. However, although both men and women fear AIDS, it is mainly the women who take the initiative and responsibility for protection. Both men and women see the club scene as a place for drinking, fun, and casual sexual hookups. In seeking a high-quality relationship, these men and women say you should look for a partner through church, friends, or school. Entering a relationship usually means postponing sexual activity until you get to know each other. Before becoming seriously involved, couples often are tested for HIV and AIDS. Once a couple can prove to each other that they have recently tested negative, they are less vigilant about using condoms.

Overall there has been an increase in "casual" sexual relationships among high school and college students (Surveys show change in attitudes toward sex among high school and college students, 2003). Thirteen hundred Ohio seventh- to eleventh-grade students were interviewed about dating, relationships, and sexual activity. About 55% had engaged in intercourse and one-third of those had engaged in intercourse with "someone whose attachment went no further than friendship." The study also reported a significant shift in attitudes toward oral sexual activity, noting that respondents consider it "an acceptable alternative" to intercourse and different from sexual intercourse. The proportion of young adults who have engaged in oral sexual activity has risen; one-third of 15- to 17-year-olds and two-thirds of 18- to 24-year-olds have engaged in oral sexual activity.

Some people have wondered whether relationships that begin as "hookups," "friends with benefits," or casual dating are less satisfying and rewarding than serious sexual involvements. Paik (2010) found that couples who start a relationship based on physical interaction may be less satisfied in the long run than those who delay sexual activity. However, he also pointed out there are people who are mainly interested in sexual activity and people who are mainly interested in long-term relationships. Perhaps this is the reason that the people who delay sexual activity also have more relationship satisfaction. In other words, it might have been the type of people selecting certain relationships and not the timing of

? Did You Know . . .

Dr. Joe McIlhaney, Jr., founder of the Medical Institute for Sexual Health in Austin, Texas, feels that the pressure on college students to practice unhealthy behavior is much more intense than most adults realize. He feels that parents, university personnel, and others who care about the well-being of college students have to act. His ideas include a return to single-sex dorms and bathrooms, more abstinence and pro-marriage messages, and parent-led "inspector committees" to track high-risk health behaviors on all campuses. He is concerned that college personnel turn a blind eye to sexual behavior, while campus groups boldly advertise sex-toy sales, "fetish" fairs, and other sexually oriented activities. Dr. McIlhaney thinks parents should be more involved on campus, while other experts do not feel this is needed.

Another expert advocates a return to dating. He says it is healthier than the casual sexual activity that comes through hookups or "friends with benefits."

How do you feel about this? Is there "sexual chaos" on college campuses?

Source: Data from Wetzstein, C. "Sexual chaos" at college. *The Washington Times* (August 9, 2005), 9B.

the sexual activity that made a difference in relationship satisfaction.

The term "hooking up" can be very vague. In your authors' human sexuality classes we often ask students in the class to define the term. There is never much agreement about what the term means. Some have said it can be anything from kissing on the dance floor to going to someone's room and having various sexual activities and spending the night. It is interesting that the term is used so commonly with little consensus about its meaning. It is also interesting that studies of young adults in the United States have indicated a rise in casual relationships based on sexual activities, but at the same time other studies have shown an increase in the number of young adults who say they are virgins (Studies show shifting paradigm of sexual relationships among young adults, 2011).

Some relationships develop over the Internet. The Internet can be a useful technology for meeting potential partners and even carrying out cyber-relationships. It can even be a unique site for sexual experimentation. However, these relationships may make it difficult to be safe when pursuing personal contact with those met via the Internet. Safety strategies include seeking reliability of a person's responses by repeated questioning, conducting Google searches on the person, setting boundaries and limits on sexual activity before the in-person meeting, and relying on intuition and gut feelings. Strategies for achieving safety during in-person encounters include meeting a person by day and in public, making safe calls during the date, using personal transportation, having a friend in the area, and carrying a cell phone. Despite all these precautions, one study showed that one-third of Internet daters had sexual activity on the first personal encounter, and nearly 80% did not use a condom or question the new partner about STIs. Perhaps this was because of "accelerated intimacy" as a result of developing the relationships via the Internet (Ross, 2007).

Safer Sexual Activities and College Students

Most studies of condom use among college students date from the early 1990s; the results then indicated that condom use was relatively rare. Studies found that between 15% and 41% of students reported that they always used condoms, and the more partners a person had, the lower the rate of condom use (Lewis et al., 1997). A 1998 telephone survey of college students was much more encouraging; 54% reported that they always or almost always use condoms, and 24% said that they sometimes did. Still, one in five respondents reported that he or she almost never

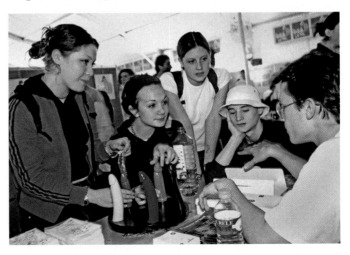

College students need to know about contraception and prevention of HIV and AIDS.

Global DIMENSIONS

Young People, Unprotected Sexual Activity, and Trustworthy Information

As you might expect, there are a number of differences in various countries related to both obtaining sexual information and participating in sexual activity. Here are some examples:

1. It is not possible to know the quality of the education received, but it seems that about 55% of young people in Europe receive sexuality education in school. In the United States the number is 74% as compared to 78% of young people in Latin America and 76% in Asia Pacific.

2. About 20% of the respondents said that their school does not provide an environment that is comfortable for questions and discussions about sexuality and intimacy.

3. Forty-two percent of respondents in Asia Pacific and 28% in Europe said they could not get contraception when they needed it because they were too embarrassed to ask a healthcare professional.

4. In recent years the number of people having sexual intercourse without contraception with a new partner has increased by 111% in France (from 19% to 40%), 39% in the United States (from 38% to 53%), and 19% in Great Britain (from 36% to 43%).

5. In Egypt a little more than one-third of men and women think that bathing or showering after sexual intercourse is an effective form of contraception.

6. More than a quarter of people in Thailand and India think that having sexual intercourse during menstruation is an effective way to prevent a pregnancy.

Source: Data from The "Clueless or Clued Up: Your Rights to be Informed About Contraception" Survey, 2011. Bayer Healthcare Pharmaceuticals. Available: http://multivu.prnewswire.com/mnr/prne/bayergroup/52124/.

---

used condoms (Survey USA, 1998). As a result, one in five males and nearly one in three college-age females have been infected with an STI (Reinisch et al., 1995).

Relatedly, it is interesting to note that 6 in 10 pregnancies involving teenage fathers end in a birth; 4 in 10 end in an abortion. Thirteen percent of abortions each year involve teenage men. Also, most males use a condom the first time they have intercourse, but condom use subsequently declines and reliance on female methods increases. Condom use is more common among males who are not in a union than among those who are cohabiting or married (In their own right, 2002).

In 2004 it was found that 84% of adults between the ages of 18 and 35 said they take "necessary" steps to protect themselves against STIs, but their actions did not support their claims. Although 63% of respondents said they were "well informed" about the risks associated with sexual activity, 82% said they never use protection against STIs during oral sexual activity, 64% did not use protection during anal sexual activity, and 47% did not use protection during vaginal sexual activity. In addition, although 93% said they believed their current sexual partners did not have STIs, 33% said they had never discussed the issue with their partners. About 53% said their partners had undergone screening for STIs (Survey finds gaps between safe-sex claims, behavior among

U.S. adults, 2004). Sixty-eight percent of respondents said that STI tests should be part of a routine health exam, but only 51% had ever spoken to a healthcare provider about STIs. Also, 68% did not feel concerned about contracting an STI.

Communication is the key to an honest and protected sexual relationship. Yet, most studies indicate that college students do not talk before they have sexual activity.

Planned Parenthood (2009) indicates that these are the most important ways to practice safer sexual activities:

- Understand and be honest about the risks you take.

- Keep your blood, pre-cum, semen, or vaginal fluids out of each other's bodies.

- Always use latex male or female condoms for anal or vaginal intercourse.

- Don't have sex play when you have a sore caused by an STI.

- Find ways to make safer sex as pleasurable as possible.

In addition, be aware of your body and your partner's body. Cuts, sores, or bleeding gums may all increase the risk of spreading STIs. Lubricants can increase sexual stimulation, and they also reduce the chance that condoms or other barriers will break. Of course, abstinence is totally safe. Sexual activity with just one partner is also safe as long as neither of you is infected and neither of you ever has sexual activity or shared needles with anyone else (Safer sex guidelines, 2009).

■ Singlehood

For most heterosexual young adults—male and female—singlehood is a temporary status. The vast majority of people eventually marry, but they are delaying marriage longer than in the past. In 1970, the median age for first marriage was 20.6 years for women and 22.5 years for men (Renzetti & Curran, 1998); by 1997, it had reached 25 years for women and 26.8 years for men (Schmid, 1998). According to the U.S. Census Bureau, it is now about 26.1 years for women and 28.2 years for men.

While there can be variation from person to person, singles seem to delay or avoid marriage for a number of common reasons. These can include improved social attitudes toward being single, increased caution because of perceived high divorce rates, increased availability of better contraceptives, an enjoyment of freedom from unnecessary commitments, opportunities to meet new people and develop new relationships, and the desire to have a varied sex life free of guilt. Economic constraints probably also contribute to longer periods of singlehood. For

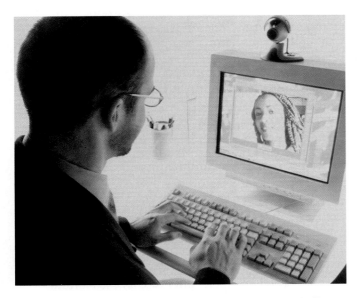

Add the Internet to the places to meet singles. On singles bulletin boards, singles can read extended personal ads, complete with photos. In chat rooms, singles have the opportunity to "meet" and "talk" to prospective dates in a safe environment. But be wary— experts warn that a first encounter with someone met on the Internet should be in a public place, perhaps among other friends.

example, housing prices have increased significantly at the same time that good jobs are harder to find. In addition, many who have graduated from college might have large debts as a result of college expenses.

This group has been labeled the "twixters." They aren't kids anymore, but they're not adults either. They are a new breed of young people who won't or can't settle down. The percentage of 26-year-olds living with their parents has nearly doubled since 1970, from 11% to 20% (Grossman, 2005). Instead of moving from adolescence to adulthood, some experts feel there is a new, intermediate phase of development for the twixters. They are called this because they are betwixt and between. Some who study this new life phase see it as a good thing—a chance for young people to savor the pleasures of irresponsibility and search their souls for new life paths. Others are worried that twixters aren't growing up because they can't. They feel that the cultural machinery that used to turn kids into grown-ups has broken down. They fear that society no longer provides young people with the moral backbone and the financial means to take their rightful places in the adult world. They point out that growing up may be harder than it used to be.

The number of people who never marry has increased since 1970. This is true for both males and females and for every age group. In the United States, approximately 29% of females and 35.4% of males 15 years and older have never married. In addition, 51.2% of the population 15 years and older is not currently married. This includes 49.5% of males and 52.9% of females. There are also about 15 million families with a female householder with no husband present and about 5.4 million families with a male householder with no wife present (American Fact Finder, 2011).

Some people feel that living alone is the new norm. In 1950 people living alone made up only 9% of households. But, in 2011 that number was 28%. People living alone were tied with childless couples as the most prominent residential type, more common than the nuclear family. Some people feel that living alone helps us pursue sacred modern values—individual freedom, personal control, and self-realization. It may mean that living alone is exactly what we need to reconnect (Klinenberg, 2012).

Of course, some people who are single would like to get married. "The majority of people still want to get married, but they see it sort of as dessert now, something that's desirable rather than necessary," said the executive director of the Albany, New York– based Alternatives to Marriage Project, which aims to fight discrimination based on marital status and to seek equality and fairness for unmarried people. He feels that people want to be sure that they don't make a marriage mistake. Also, societal pressures to marry before having children have decreased. About 41% of births are to unmarried women (Births to unmarried women, 2011).

Online dating, once viewed as a refuge for the socially inept and as a faintly disrespectable way to meet other people, is quickly becoming a fixture of single life for adults of all ages, backgrounds, and interests. Some people feel that the traditional means for getting people together are not working as well as they did previously, and that there is a need for something new. As more people choose to marry later in life, few social institutions have arisen to replace the role that local communities, families, and schools once played. The Internet is filling that need. For many, there is a disconnect between who people say they are online and what they really are like. However, many people have found success through Internet dating and feel that online dating may be making it more acceptable to openly signal what they want.

A Match.com study (2010) found that more than twice as many couples who married in a recent year met through online dating services than in bars, at clubs, and other social events combined. Seventeen percent of those who married in a recent 3-year period met online, making it the third most frequent method of introduction, behind meeting through a mutual acquaintance or at work or school. In addition, 1 out of 5 single people have dated someone they met on an online dating site.

Matchmaking has become a serious and fast-growing business. Real-life matchmakers with names like Great Expectations and It's Just Lunch are popping up around the country. The Matchmaking Institute, which offered the nation's first certification course, opened in October 2004. It describes itself as a school of matchmaking and relationship sciences and offers 22 hours of intensive training. The modern matchmaker offers much more than a dating service. It may involve acting as a pal, coach, mom, and concierge (Cullen, 2004). As an example of such a service, It's Just Lunch promises its clients low-pressure introductions on their lunch breaks or over post-work drinks. Various formats are used to help participants get to know as many other potential dating partners as possible. For $1,000 to $1,500, clients join for a year and are guaranteed a minimum of 14 dates. If a spark is ignited, they can put their memberships on hold for up to a year. Some clients indicate that a short date with no commitment set up by someone else builds self-confidence, because the whole fear of rejection is minimized (Brooks, 2004).

Even newer dating tools have been established in the past few years (Rosenbloom, 2010). For example, Cheek'd had its debut in 2010. Users receive calling cards to dole out to alluring strangers they see in their everyday lives. Recipients of the cards can use the ID code on them to log into Cheekd.com and send a message to their admirer. A pack of 50 cards and a month's subscription to Cheek'd, where users can receive messages and post information about themselves, is $25. There is no fee for those who receive cards to communicate with an admirer through the site. Each card has a sassy phrase like "I am totally cooler than your date" or "I'm hitting on you." Another company integrating calling cards and the Internet is FlipMe! which was founded in 2010. On each FlipMe! card is an explanation for the recipient: "I've said 'what if' too many times … not this time." Many card users feel that companies such as FlipMe! and Cheek'd allow them to approach people who might otherwise have been missed connections. It also reverses the online dating process—observe someone in person first, then send an electronic message.

Other companies are helping singles connect through location-based technology on their mobile phones. Websites and applications such as Grindr, Are You Interested?, and Urban Signals have swelled. One of the most popular is the free iPhone application Skout. It uses a cell phone's global positioning system (GPS) to help users find like-minded people within a walkable radius of one another. For safety reasons, Skout does not identify a user's precise location. Those who sign up for the application create basic profiles with photos and then use an instant message feature to communicate when they are within range of each other. Then, they can arrange a mutual meeting spot (Rosenbloom, 2010).

Cohabitation

Cohabitation is the situation in which people who live together and share a sexual relationship are not married. Just a generation or two ago people who lived together were said to be "living in sin"— a remark meant as religious scorn, not humor. Today cohabitation is not regarded as negatively as it used to be.

One reason for the increased acceptance of cohabitation is the vast increase in the number who cohabitate—from 439,000 in 1960 to more than 6.66 million in 2010. About a quarter of unmarried women age 25–39 are currently living with a partner of the other gender, and an additional quarter has lived with a partner of the other gender in the past. More than 60% of first marriages are now preceded by living together, as

cohabitation
Situation in which people who live together and share a sexual relationship are not married.

compared with virtually none 50 years ago. For many, cohabitation is a prelude to marriage. For others, it is simply better than living alone. For a small but growing number it is considered an alternative to marriage (Wilcox & Marquardt, 2010).

Cohabitation is more common among those of lower educational and income levels. It is also more common among those who are less religious than their peers, those who have been divorced, and those who have experienced parental divorce, fatherlessness, or high levels of marital discord during childhood. A growing number of cohabiting-couple households, now over 40%, contain children. Although many people believe that cohabitation is a good way to avoid a bad marriage and an eventual divorce, a substantial body of evidence indicates that those who live together before marriage are more likely to break up after marriage (Wilcox & Marquardt, 2010).

However, some research disputes the idea that those who cohabit are more likely to get a divorce. One study showed that among women who married since the mid-1990s, cohabitation is not tied to increased risk of divorce. Also, nearly two-thirds of adults who have ever cohabited thought about it as a step toward marriage. Also, public acceptance of cohabiting couples has been increasing through the years. Most Americans now say the rise in unmarried couples living together either makes no difference to society (46%) or is good for society (9%) (Cohn, 2011).

Reasons for Cohabitation

Some people feel that cohabitation has become more acceptable because of the increasing numbers who cohabitate. Another reason for increased acceptance is that some major companies have extended "domestic partner benefits" to both homosexual and heterosexual cohabitors. A further reason is the availability of effective contraceptives that reduce the fear of pregnancy for those who want to live together but not start families.

Traditionally, many reasons have been given for living together. They include finding out more about the habits and character of a partner, wanting to test compatibility, avoiding the risks of being trapped in an unhappy marriage, working on personal issues before deciding to marry, and saving money.

Popenoe (2008) pointed out additional reasons why people cohabit. He suggests that the "sexual revolution" of the 1960s gave premarital sexual activity more of a stamp of approval. Traditional norms were challenged, and relatively reliable birth control for women became available. Some men pulled back from marriage and from having children and simply lived with their sexual partners in cohabitation. Women had gained more equality in many ways and got married many years later, on average. Childbearing was also delayed, and cohabitation was a natural outcome. Also, as the number of divorces increased, people became worried about marriages going wrong. Cohabitation—rather than marriage—became increasingly popular.

Some argue that there are economic benefits to cohabitation. But it seems to play a different role in the lives of adults with or without college degrees. For the most educated, living as an unmarried couple usually is an economically positive way to combine two incomes and is a step towards marriage and having children. But for adults without college degrees, cohabitation is more likely to be a parallel household arrangement to marriage—complete with children—but at a lower economic level than married adults enjoy (Fry & Cohn, 2011).

Disadvantages to Cohabitation

Unmarried couples may experience discrimination in housing, insurance, taxes, child custody, and other areas. They may also face pressure to marry from parents and friends—who may have social and religious backgrounds different from the cohabitors'.

Some people, especially divorced people, become cohabitors because they do not want the legal and economic "entanglements" of another marriage should the relationship end. In reality, though, the legal "entanglements" of marriage can also prove to be legal "entitlements." When cohabitors break up, one partner may lose financially because of inability to prove that assets were jointly purchased. Also, if one partner dies without a will, property would pass to surviving family members—not to the intended surviving partner. For example, in Massachusetts, the property would go half to parents, half to siblings, and none to the partner. Further, if a partner is disabled or hospitalized, the cohabitor has no rights to make medical decisions and can even be legally barred from hospital visits.

After dissolution of a cohabiting relationship, formerly cohabiting men's economic standing declines moderately. However, formerly cohabiting women's economic standing declines a great deal, leaving a substantial proportion of women in poverty. This is particularly true for African American and Hispanic women (Avellar, 2005).

Are Cohabitations Successful?

Do cohabiting couples have a higher rate of success if they marry later than do married couples who did not live together first? A critical look at the body of research fails to prove whether prior cohabitors have better marriages.

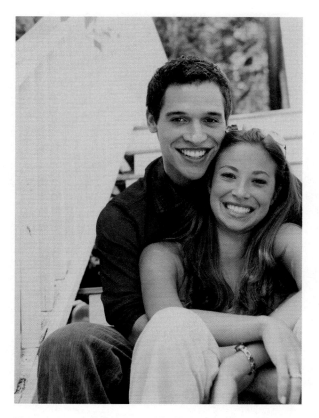

There is contradictory research about the effects of cohabitation.

In some ways, cohabitation is replacing dating. There also seems to be an increase in "serial cohabitation," or living with one partner for a time and then another. It is interesting that women seem to perceive cohabitation as a step before marriage to that partner, whereas men tend to see cohabitation as something to do before you make a commitment. Men who live with women they eventually marry don't seem to be as committed to the union as those who didn't live with their mates before getting married (Smock et al., 2005).

There is also a growing number of older Americans living together. The reasons vary, but for many it is a combination of bad experiences in previous marriages, the desire to keep their finances separate, and for some, loss of benefits if they remarry. According to U.S. Census Bureau figures, cohabitation numbers for people 65 and older tripled from 193,000 in 2000 to 575,000 in 2010.

Cohabitation seems to differ for older and younger adults. Older cohabitors report significantly higher levels of relationship quality and stability than younger cohabitors, although they are less likely to have plans to marry their partners. Reasons for cohabitation are similar, but assessing compatibility is a more important reason for younger cohabitors. Older cohabitors are more likely to view their relationship as an alternative to marriage, whereas younger cohabitors are more likely to view their relationship as a prelude to it (King, 2005).

A comparison of gay and lesbian cohabiting couples with heterosexual married couples showed that in many respects they do not differ. However, it seems that gay or lesbian partners function better in their relationships than heterosexual partners (Kurdek, 2004). According to the U.S. Census Bureau, there are almost 515,000 same-gender unmarried-partner households in the United States (Census Bureau releases estimates of same-sex married couples, 2011).

So, is cohabitation a positive or a negative thing? There are different opinions among different people. For example, some reports indicate that marriages of people who have cohabited and later marry are significantly more likely to end in divorce (Living together before marriage may hurt—not help—chances of successful match, 2002). Some people feel this is partly because people who choose to live together tend to be younger, to be less religious, or to have other qualities that put them at risk for divorce. Seventy percent of those who lived together for at least 5 years did eventually marry, but after 10 years 40% had broken up, as compared to 32% who did not live together first. Others argue that marriage is too great a commitment and prefer cohabitation (Should people not cohabit before getting married?, 2003). They feel that the emphasis should be on the commitment between two people and that the quality of the relationship is the most important consideration. They indicate that society discriminates against people who wish to commit themselves to another person and remain unmarried.

? Did You Know . . .

Sweden leads the Western nations in the degree to which nonmarital cohabitation has replaced marriage. The United States, by comparison, has a lower rate of nonmarital cohabitation than all but the Catholic nations of southern Europe.

About 28% of all couples in Sweden are cohabiting versus 8% of all American couples. In Sweden, virtually all couples live together before marriage, compared to approximately two-thirds of couples in America (Popenoe & Whitehead, 2005).

Marriage

Marriage has changed over the years, but in many respects it has remained the same. June is still the most popular time to marry, more adults marry than never marry, and marriage is still a legal entity. It involves a fee to the county, a marriage license, and a marriage ceremony—either civil or religious. Although there is no legal requirement that a wife take the husband's last name, she usually does. Most Americans spend most of their lives within a marital relationship.

Although most people marry, the marriage rate has fluctuated. The highest marriage rate (the number of marriages per 1,000 unmarried women age 15 and older) in relatively recent decades was 76.5 in 1970. It has steadily declined since then and was 36 per 1,000 in 2010. The median age at first marriage went from 20 years for females and 23 years for males in 1960 to about 26 and 28 years, respectively, in 2010 (Wilcox & Marquardt, 2010).

Popenoe and Whitehead (2001) reported that although older age at first marriage seems detrimental to marriage as an institution, it may have a strongly positive effect. This is because it appears to be by far the most important factor for a leveling off of divorce rates. Nevertheless, there can be disadvantages to the trend for postponing marriage to much older ages. For example, it can result in increased exposure to the hazards of nonmarital sexual activity and childbearing, sexual exploitation, loneliness, and lack of social integration. The question of the optimal age at which to marry, then, is still open. It seems best to wait until the early 20s, but how much beyond that cannot be answered definitively.

There are many statistics available about marriage, and many articles are written about it. For example, we already mentioned that age at first marriage has been steadily increasing. Interestingly,

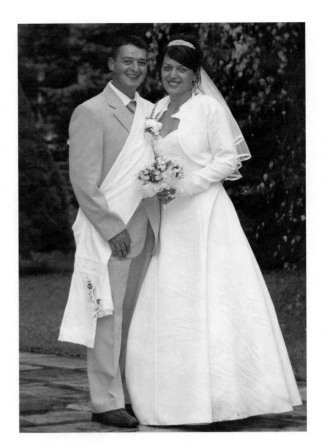

Marriage customs vary in different cultures.

the age at remarriage after a divorce has also been increasing. In addition, the number of interracial marriages has increased.

Although 9.2% of males and 11.8% of females 15 years and older in the United States were divorced as of 2010, 69.3% of males and 60.7% of females were married (Wilcox & Marquardt, 2010). Because it is clear that a majority of people choose to be married, it is appropriate to consider the attraction of marriage and marriage partners.

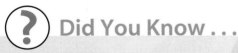

? Did You Know . . .

Key Findings About Cohabitation from Cross-Cultural Investigation

- Cohabitation has become a permanent part of the life-course. A great majority of people in many countries cohabit sometime during their lives.
- Cohabitation has decreased the desire of many couples to move to marriage.
- Cohabiting couples break up at a much higher rate than married couples.
- Couples who cohabit before marriage have a higher risk of divorce when they do marry.

- In most countries, cohabiting couples tend to have fewer children than married couples.
- Cohabitation has been a major contributor to the rise of unwed births and single-parent families.
- Cohabitation has negative effects on child well-being. Children in these relationships have 5 times the risk of experiencing their parents' separation and higher rates of child abuse, family violence, and lower incomes.

Source: Data from Popenoe, D. Cohabitation, marriage and child well-being. National Marriage Project, 2008. Available: http://marriage.rutgers.edu/Publications/2008cohabreport.html.

The Attraction of Marriage

The attraction to marriage is the result of several factors:

1. *Marriage provides companionship.* It is nice to have someone committed to spending time with you and sharing important occasions in your life.

2. *Marriage provides for emotional security.* The intimate nature of the marital relationship can help alleviate the anxieties, fears, and insecurities you experience in today's society.

3. *Marriage provides for a sexual outlet.* The knowledge that your sexual needs will be satisfied in a loving, caring relationship can be quite appealing.

4. *Marriage can improve your self-esteem.* Just knowing that you are worthy enough for someone else to marry can make you believe you are an attractive, appealing, valuable person.

5. *Marriage can provide financial security.* The addition of another wage earner, or someone who can earn money while you contribute to the partnership by doing chores that would cost money to pay someone else to do, can make you more financially able to live the life you desire.

6. *Marriage can legitimize reproduction.* If you want children and believe they will do best in a socially sanctioned family—a marriage— you may want to be married.

Kempner (2005) summarized the ways that marriages benefit couples. She pointed out that the benefits include legal and financial benefits ranging from family leave, health care, and parenthood to those involving taxes, property rights, and inheritance. Marriage seems to also provide a wealth-generation bonus. Married people are more likely to save money and become more economically productive. Marriage can also provide couples with an economy of scale (two can live as cheaply as one), and act as a small insurance pool against life's uncertainties such as illness or job loss. In addition, research indicates that married people are not only wealthier but happier, healthier, and having better sex lives. Married people also take fewer risks, have better health habits, and enjoy a wider social support network.

Related to the association between marriage and well-being, Musick and Bumpass (2012) examined the persistence of changes in well-being as marriages and cohabitations progress (and sometimes dissolve)

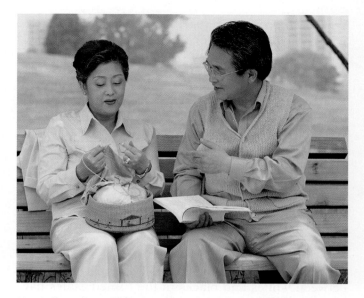

Married people can enjoy a wide variety of activities together throughout their marriage.

over time. The effects of marriage and cohabitation were found to be similar across a range of measures looking at psychological well-being, health, and social ties. They found that while married couples experienced health gains—likely linked to the formal benefits of marriage such as shared healthcare plans—cohabiting couples experienced greater gains in happiness and self-esteem.

Obviously, marriage has numerous attractions that have made it the predominant family lifestyle. However, not all these attractions are present in all marriages, and, depending on the expectations before the marriage and on other important considerations—such as the personality traits of the partners and their love for each other—the resultant disappointments either are overlooked or are deemed important enough to cause divorce.

It is interesting that, in general, American women are waiting to begin families. For women who earn a 4-year college degree or better, the age at first marriage is close to 30. After marriage, women are waiting longer before they have their first child than they did several decades ago. As a result of these trends, the years of life before children have expanded, as have the years of life after children are no longer living in the home. The years of life with children represent a shrinking share of women's life course (Whitehead & Popenoe, 2008).

Choosing a Life Partner

Interestingly, when and if you choose another person with whom to form a lifelong commitment, that person will most likely be similar to you in many ways. Most people choose others of similar religion, age, social class, race, and education (Baron, 1998).

When two people join together after 20 or 30 or more years of living independently of each other, they have all the problems of adjustment you can imagine. They may have to learn to eat the same foods, wake and go to sleep at the same times, and put up with each other's myriad idiosyncrasies. In other words, they have enough problems without adding still others that occur when they have different religions, social classes, educational backgrounds, and so on. It would be unfair, however, to overlook the relationships that work in spite of the partners' dissimilarities. That elusive concept, love, can do wonders with problems. However, the odds against partners of dissimilar backgrounds are greater than those for similar partners.

Although similar characteristics are important to many people when choosing a life partner, marriages between whites and blacks in the United States have increased. Thirty years ago just 5% of black men were married to a white woman, but that figure has risen almost threefold to 14%. The proportion of black women marrying white partners has increased from 1% to 6% during the same time (Qian & Lichter, 2011).

Over the last several decades, the American public has grown increasingly accepting of interracial dating and marriage. About 85% of millennials (those age 18–29 years) say they would be fine with a family member's marriage to a person from another racial group. The amount of support drops to about 73% among those 30–49 years, 55% among those 50–64 years, and 39% among those ages 65 and older (Almost all millennials accept interracial dating and marriage, 2010).

Many factors come into play when choosing a person for a relationship. For example, research has found that women who believed the men liked them a lot were more attracted to the men than women who thought the men liked them only an average amount. However, women who found the men most attractive were the ones who were not sure whether those men were into them or not. Perhaps keeping people in the dark about now much we like them will increase how much they think about us and will pique their interest (Whitchurch et al., 2011).

A "premarital inventory" developed at the University of Minnesota could be helpful for those contemplating marriage. It is an example of how researchers have studied divorced couples to see which questions they wish they had asked before taking the leap. Sample items include the following: We have some important disagreements that never seem to get resolved, and I am satisfied with the way we have decided to share household duties. It is available at www.lifeinnovations.com (September 2009).

Multicultural DIMENSIONS

The Jefferson–Hemings Affair

If you think some current scandals go on for a long time, consider the case of Thomas Jefferson. In 1801, the newly elected Jefferson was first accused of having children with a young black slave named Sally Hemings. But it was not until the fall of 1998 that DNA tests proved that descendants of the Hemings family were indeed related to Jefferson. Sally Hemings's youngest son, Eston, was fathered by either Thomas Jefferson or his brother.

The DNA findings do more than put to rest a question of paternity; they also lay the foundation for all the Jefferson descendants—African American and white—to join together as one openly biracial family. For the first time, descendants of Jefferson's slave were welcomed at the annual gathering of the Monticello Association (the organization of descendants of Jefferson's white daughters) at Monticello on May 15, 1999.

"It's not just our story—it resonates for the whole country," said Dr. Michelle Cooley-Quille, a Hemings descendant and a clinical psychologist at Johns Hopkins University, who attended the event. Her father was denied entry into the Monticello Association and denied burial at Monticello, a privilege accorded to all members, when he died in 1997. "It's symbolic of what we've been denied but where we belong."

Indeed, the Jefferson clan has followed the multicultural path of many Americans. The number of official interracial marriages was 1,264,000 in 1997, almost double the 651,000 in 1980. However, as the Jefferson story suggests, there have been many unrecorded interracial relationships during the history of the United States. The growing acceptance of contemporary interracial marriages—as well as the acceptance of our past—is a positive step in the direction of racial harmony.

Sources: Data from Reed, D. Jefferson reunion adds slave's kin, AP/AOL (May 6, 1999); Edwards, T. M. Family reunion, *Time, 125, 21* (November 23, 1998); Cawthorne, N. *Sex lives of the presidents.* New York: St. Martin's, 1998; U.S. Bureau of the Census. *Statistical abstract of the United States 1998.* Washington, DC: U.S. Government Printing Office, 1998.

Promoting a Happy Lifelong Commitment
Advice from many sources tells you how to be happy in a relationship. For example, Wallerstein (1996) lists nine "psychological tasks" that are the pillars on which good lifelong relationships rest:

1. To separate emotionally from the family of one's childhood so as to invest fully in the relationship.

2. To build togetherness based on mutual identification, shared intimacy, and an expanded conscience that includes both partners and protects each partner's autonomy.

3. To establish a rich and pleasurable sexual relationship.

4. For couples with children, while protecting their own privacy, to embrace the roles of parenthood and to absorb the effect of a baby's entrance into the marriage.

5. To confront and master the inevitable crises of life.

6. To maintain the strength of the relationship in the face of adversity. It should be a safe haven in which partners are able to express their differences, anger, and conflict.

7. To use humor and laughter to keep things in perspective.

8. To nurture and comfort each other, satisfying each partner's needs for dependency and offering continuing encouragement and support.

9. To keep alive the early romantic, idealized images of falling in love while facing the sober realities of the changes wrought by time.

Many other factors can relate to the quality of marriage. For example, Kiecolt-Glaser (2009) reported that couples whose disagreements were nastier or hostile showed large increases in stress hormones during and after an argument. Among other potential problems, it was found that women who were unhappy in their marriages had higher risks of heart and circulatory problems. This gives medical support for the need to follow the advice given previously for promoting a happy lifelong commitment.

Also, the increase in "boomerangers" can be stressful on marriages. These are people who are young adults or even in their 30s or 40s who move back in with their parents. This practice commonly occurs for economic reasons, and it can cause tensions for both the older and younger generations. Suggestions for dealing with this situation include talking about

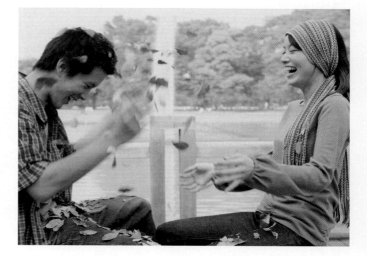

It is wise to learn a lot about a potential marriage partner before getting married.

expectations, building in privacy for all concerned, sharing household expenses, realizing that the house is the property of the parents (grandparents?), and being realistic about expectations (Koss-Feder, 2009).

A nationwide survey by the Pew Research Center revealed some interesting things about marriage (The decline of marriage and rise of new families, 2010). While declining among all groups, marriage remains the norm for adults with a college education and good income, but is markedly less prevalent on the lower rungs of the socioeconomic ladder. There is a gap of 16 percentage points between marriage rates of college graduates (64%) and of those with a high school diploma or less (48%). In 1960 this gap was just 4 percentage points (76% versus 72%). Also, the young are much more inclined than their elders to view cohabitation without marriage and other family forms—such as same-gender marriage and interracial marriage—in a positive light. In addition, almost 40% of the survey respondents felt that marriage is becoming obsolete.

The same survey also found other feelings about marriage. Seven in 10 (69%) said the trend toward more single women having children is bad for society, and 61% said that a child needs both a mother and father to grow up happily. On the more accepting side, only a minority said the trends toward more cohabitation without marriage (43%), more unmarried couples raising children (43%), more gay couples raising children (43%), and more people of different races marring (14%) are bad for society. Relatively few said that any of these trends are good for society, but many said they make little difference. In addition, the young are more accepting than the old of the emerging arrangements, the secular are more accepting than the religious, liberals are more accepting than conservatives, the unmarried are more accepting than the married, and in general blacks are more accepting than whites. Finally, women have reached near parity with men as a share of the workforce and have begun to outpace men in educational attainment. About 60% of wives work today, nearly double the share in 1960. More than 62% of survey respondents endorsed the modern marriage in which both partners work and both take care of the household and children. Even so, the public has not entirely discarded the traditional male-breadwinner role in marriage. Sixty-seven percent of respondents said that to be ready for marriage it is very important for a man to be able to support his family financially; just 33% said the same about a woman.

Types of Marriage

In some states heterosexual couples who have lived together for a specified period and who have represented themselves as married are recognized as legally married. These associations are called **common-law marriages**.

A **nuclear family** is usually defined as a father and mother and their children. According to the U.S. Census Bureau, there were 1.3 million fewer nuclear families in the United States in 2010 than in 2000. Not all parts of the country changed in the same ways. Two-thirds of the decline came in only eight states, seven of which are in the Northeast and Midwest. Nuclear families account for about one-fifth of all households (Francese, 2011).

Peer marriages are relationships in which couples have worked out at least a 60–40 split on child rearing, housework, and control of discretionary funds and consider themselves equal. Most partners in peer marriages work outside the home. Partners in peer marriages require lots of honesty, a dedication to fair play, flexibility, generosity, and maturity.

Related to peer marriages, Orecklin (2004) pointed out that the past 30 years have seen the emergence of the working mom, the supermom, the soccer mom, and—because full-time motherhood is often considered a choice rather than a given—the stay-at-home mom. The title of "dad" has rarely been linked to a modifier. However, the majority of men today are vastly more involved in the rearing of children and maintenance of households than their fathers ever were. In straining to manage

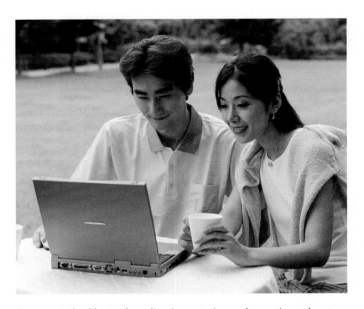

Some couples like to do online inventories and questions about relationships to learn more about themselves and each other.

responsibilities at work and at home, many men say they don't feel an adequate sense of control in either realm. As with women of a generation ago, men are experiencing the notion of a second shift, and they are doing so in a shaky economy. They must contend with buyouts, layoffs, mergers, and a need to keep up with changing job skills. There is sometimes also uncertainty in men's roles at home.

According to the American Time Use Survey done by the Bureau of Labor Statistics, on an average day in all types of marriages combined 84% of women and 67% of men spent some time doing household activities such as housework, cooking, lawn care, or financial and other household management. On the days they did household activities, women spent an average of 2.6 hours on such activities and men spent 2.1 hours. On an average day, 20% of men did housework, such as cleaning or doing laundry, compared with 49% of women. Forty-one percent of men did food preparation or cleanup, compared with 68% of women. However, married men and women with full-time jobs have almost equal total workloads, with or without children younger than age 18 (American Time Use Survey, 2011).

About 20% of American women end their childbearing years without having a child, compared with about 10% in the 1970s. Childlessness has risen for all racial and ethnic groups and most education levels. It has fallen for women with advanced degrees. Various reasons have been given for an increase in childlessness. They include decreased social pressure to bear children and more recognition of the decision to have children as an individual choice. Also, improved job opportunities for women and improved

common-law marriage
The recognition by some states that heterosexual couples who have lived together for a specified period and have represented themselves as married are in fact legally married.

nuclear family
A father and mother and their children.

peer marriage
Relationship in which partners have equal status.

? Did You Know . . .

Popenoe and Whitehead (2005) listed 10 important research findings on marriage and choosing a marriage partner. While several overlap points already made, the list taken as a whole provides helpful facts for young adults and older adults about marriage. The research findings are:

1. Marrying as a teenager is the highest known risk factor for divorce.
2. The most likely way to find a future marriage partner is through an introduction by family, friends, or acquaintances.
3. The more similar people are in their values, backgrounds, and life goals, the more likely they are to have a successful marriage.
4. Women have a significantly better chance of marrying if they do not become single parents before marrying.

5. Both women and men who are college educated are more likely to marry, and less likely to divorce, than people with lower levels of education.
6. Living together before marriage has not proved useful as a "trial marriage."
7. Marriage helps people to generate income and wealth.
8. People who are married are more likely to have emotionally and physically satisfying sex lives than single people or those who just live together.
9. People who grow up in a family broken by divorce are slightly less likely to marry, and much more likely to divorce when they do marry.
10. For large segments of the population, the risk of divorce is far below 50%.

---

contraceptive methods have created alternatives for women who choose not to have children (Livingston & Cohn, 2010)

An increasing number of children live in a **stepfamily**. Stepfamilies can be more complex than the families of first marriages, but, contrary to myth, stepfamilies have a high rate of success in raising healthy children. Stepkids seem to be very resilient. Their major source of problems is parental conflict left over from a first marriage. Stepfamilies experience most of their troubles in the first 2 years; after 5 years, stepfamilies are more stable than first-marriage families, because second marriages are generally happier than first marriages. Stepfamilies are not just make-do households limping along after loss. All members experience real gains, notably the opportunity to thrive in a happier relationship.

Some people choose a **same-gender marriage**. Because of differences in laws and opinions related to same-gender marriage, it is difficult to get accurate information about such relationships. However, the U.S. Census Bureau indicated that there are almost 132,000 same-gender married couple households and about 515,000 same-gender unmarried partner households in the United States (Census Bureau releases estimates of same-sex married couples, 2011). For the first time, in 2011 a CNN poll found that just over one-half of all Americans believe that marriages between gay or lesbian couples should be legally valid. However, there is a generation and gender gap on this issue. Sixty percent of Americans younger than age 50 support same-gender marriage, but only 40% of those older than 50 feel the same. More than half of men are against legalizing same-gender marriage, but 57% of women are in favor of it (Poll: More Americans favor same-sex marriage, 2011).

One researcher indicates that there are seven basic types of relationships—three of them happy and four of them unhappy (An arrangement of marriages, 1993). The four unhappy ones make up about 75% of marriages and are labeled *devitalized, financially focused, conflicted*, and *traditional*. These relationships hinge on external elements, leisure activities, religious attitudes, financial management, children, family, and friends—and distress dominates. The three happy ones make up 25% of relationships and are labeled *balanced, harmonious*, and *vitalized*. In these relationships the partners are held together by smooth working of most or all factors intrinsic to relationships—personality compatibility, communication, conflict resolution, and sexuality.

With many new marriages in the United States destined to end in divorce, an increasing number of couples are turning to prenuptial agreements to protect their assets in the event of a marital breakup. Most such agreements simply state how assets will be divided in case of divorce or death. Some people argue that prenuptial agreements contribute to marital happiness; others believe they contribute to distrust and overemphasize personal assets.

In some states, it is legal to back up marriage laws with tougher, individually designed and legally

stepfamily
A family with children that is formed as a result of remarriage.

same-gender marriage
A marriage between two people who perceive themselves to be of the same gender.

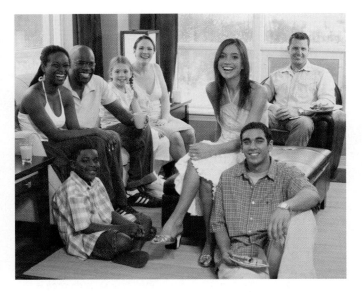

Blended families come in many sizes and can look very different from each other.

mandated divorce standards. This is called a *covenant marriage*. In this marriage style, the option of walking out is eliminated. For example, Louisiana's covenant marriage requires premarital counseling and, for divorce, 2 years of living apart plus mandated marital counseling. The goal is to make marriage more committed.

So, how does the American public feel about the changes in the structure of the family and marriage relationships that have occurred over the past 50 years? The Pew Research Center surveyed a nationally representative sample of almost 2,700 adults to answer this question. Respondents were asked whether they considered the following seven trends to be good, bad, or of no consequence to society: more unmarried couples raising children, more gay and lesbian couples raising children, more single women having children without a male partner to help raise them, more people living together without getting married, more mothers of young children working outside the home, more people of different races marrying each other, and more women not ever having children. Although views can vary on different trends, overall about a third (31%) of the subjects were "accepters," indicating that these trends make no difference to society. A similar share of the public (32%) rejected virtually every trend that the acceptors endorsed. The third group, the "skeptics" (37%) generally shared most of the tolerant views of the accepters, but expressed concern about the potential impact of the trends on society (Morin, 2011).

Building a good relationship obviously takes a lot of effort. There are sources of help for couples desiring to use them. For example, the Association for Couples in Marriage Enrichment is an organization designed to preserve and strengthen relationships.

Sexual Behavior in Marriage

Nonmarital sexual behavior has received more attention than marital sexual behavior from researchers for many decades. It still does today. While the information about marital sexual behavior is comparatively limited, it is still appropriate to consider what is known.

Today's married couples have sexual intercourse more often, experience more sexual pleasure, and engage in a greater variety of sexual activities and techniques than the people surveyed in the 1950s. There is now more precoital activity and it tends to last longer than in earlier years. Oral stimulation of the breasts and manual stimulation of the genitals have increased, as has oral–genital contact (Clements, 1994; Laumann et al., 1994).

We can ascribe these changes to a loosening up of society in general and to the fact that even heterosexual sexual activity has come out of the closet. It is now permissible to talk about sexual behavior freely with one's partner and with others. Thus, communication between partners has become more open and honest and certainly has had an effect on their lovemaking. Women have become more aware of their capacity for and their right to sexual satisfaction through orgasm. As a result they have been assuming an active role in lovemaking and in communicating what turns them on. When their partners have responded positively, one result has been that partners spend more time exploring each other sexually, attending to each other's bodies, and experimenting with various coital positions that may better satisfy women's needs.

Many married people also masturbate. Hunt's survey (1974) found that 72% of young married males and 68% of young married females masturbated. The frequency rates were higher for husbands (once or twice a month) than for wives (less than once a month). The reasons married people cite for masturbating vary. Some people masturbate when they are separated from their partner. Some do so as a variation on their sexual experience. Also some couples like to watch each other masturbate as part of their mutual sexual activity. Others masturbate because they do not achieve satisfaction with their partner and are unwilling to forgo it altogether.

The National Opinion Research Center (NORC) study found that frequency of sexual interactions is a factor of age, relationship duration, and marital status. In general, married couples engage in sexual activities more frequently than singles; cohabiting couples engage in sexual activities more often than married couples (Laumann et al., 1994). Nearly 40% of married couples engage in sexual activities twice a week, compared with 25% of singles (Elmer-Dewitt, 1994).

Some people wonder whether their sex life is "normal." Statistics on sexual behavior can be misleading. For example, if a couple heard that the average married couple had sexual intercourse three times a week, they may not realize that the average includes a wide range. The frequency of intercourse might range from zero for some to 15 to 20 times a week for others. So, even if their frequency of intercourse is more or less than three times a week, their behavior is within the range of normal human experience. The most important consideration isn't whether their frequency and pattern of sexual activity matches some numerical average, but whether each partner is satisfied and comfortable with the sexual relationship. There should be a feeling of overall satisfaction, relaxation, and enjoyment following sexual activity (Osborne, 2004).

As with other research, the data about frequency of marital sexual activity will vary in different research studies. However, it is generally agreed that the frequency of sexual intercourse in marriage tends to decrease the longer a couple is married. For example, for newly married couples the average rate of sexual intercourse is about three times per week. In early middle age, the average rate is about one-and-a-half to two times a week. After age 50 years the rate is about once a week or less. This does not mean that sexual activity is not important or that the marriage is no longer satisfactory. The decrease may be the result of biological aging, fatigue, and a decrease in sex drive (Call, Sprecher, & Schwartz, 1995). Higher levels of sexual satisfaction and pleasure are found in marriage than in extramarital relationships or in singlehood (Laumann et al., 1994).

The decline of marital sexual activity is explained by several factors. First, the "honeymoon effect" leads to the highest rates among the recently married, and those recently married tend to be younger.

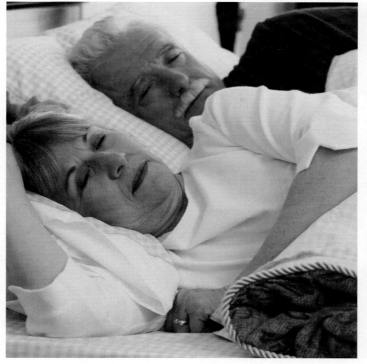

Today's married couples experience much more sexual pleasure than those of past decades.

Second, biological aging reduces hormonal output, and poor health in general and sexual arousal problems increase with age. As a result, even among couples who consider their marriages to be very happy and say they are still in love, frequency of intercourse goes down with age. Third, some research indicates that the quality of sexual activity declines with marital duration and that might reduce frequency. Among married people, intercourse is more frequent among those who have happier marriages (Smith, 2003).

Related to the above, data from the National Survey of Sexual Health and Behavior (2010) also indicated that the frequency of heterosexual intercourse for married men and women tends to decline with age. For example, for 18- to 24-year-olds 83% of men and 73% of women reported vaginal intercourse at least a few times per month. However, comparable numbers for older married couples were 89% for males and 85% for females age 25–29, 80% for males and 77% for females age 30–39, 75% for males and 70% for females age 40–49, 54% for both males and females age 50–59, 45% for males and 42% for females age 60–69, and 22% for males and 21% for females age 70 and older.

Are married couples generally satisfied with their sex life? According to Hunt's data, a majority of married people—60% to 66%—are satisfied. Two-thirds of the men in the sample rated their marital coitus as very pleasurable, whereas about 60% of the women said the same. Most women who said they found coitus very pleasurable were 35 to 44 years old; the men so reporting were younger. It appears, then, that as women mature and gain sexual experience, they enjoy their experiences more than at a younger age, and men experience more of their pleasure when they are young.

Stritof and Stritof (2010) reported that 44% of married couples are fully satisfied with their sex lives. They also reported twice as many men (64%) as women regularly have orgasms and that those older

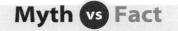

Myth vs Fact

Myth: Single adults have more sexual activity than married adults.
Fact: The 1994 national survey of adults 18 to 59 years old found that married adults had more sexual activity than single adults.

Myth: Liberals enjoy sex more than conservatives.
Fact: In the same study, marriage was a great equalizer. Married couples, regardless of religious or political background or past sexual history, have roughly the same amount of sexual activity. And conservative women report more frequent orgasm than liberal women.

Myth: Almost all married couples have affairs.
Fact: Only 25% of men and 15% of women report that they have had an extramarital affair.

Myth: People lose interest in sexual activity as they get older, and, by their 60s, few people are having sexual relationships.
Fact: People can have a satisfying sexual life as they age. Sexual relationships may change as a couple ages, but many couples in their 60s, 70s, and 80s report pleasurable, exciting sexual relationships.

than age 65 are still having sexual intercourse more than once a week. Mutual respect plays a vital role in a satisfying sex life, with 82% of those who are sexually satisfied saying they feel respected by their partner.

Also, Baron (2010) indicated that midlifers seem to be the ones most dissatisfied with their sex lives. Nearly half of 44- to 55-year-old men reported dissatisfaction with their sex lives. Just 28% of adult men younger than age 45 felt that way, as did 17% of the 66-plus seniors. Perhaps age, expectations, and quality of the relationship can all influence satisfaction with one's sex life.

In general, husbands and wives closely agree on the frequency of intercourse (Smith, 2003). Married women seem to be less satisfied with sexual activity in marriage than married men. This may be because they report a lower rate of orgasm compared to that of men (Liu, 2003).

It seems that both married men and married women tend to believe that sexual activity is integral to a good marriage, and that men may be more interested in sexual activity than women. Sometimes husbands and wives experience conflict related to sexual activity and need to work emotionally to manage their own and their spouse's feelings about sexual activity (Elliott & Umberson, 2008).

One factor that can contribute to problems in marital sexual activities is timing—particularly in the years when couples are both raising children and working hard at their jobs. Married people often have sexual activities late in the evening after a long day and just before sleep. The presence of children in the family can make it hard for parents to find time to be alone. Because many people feel that a quiet and private time is necessary for sexual activities, there may be pressure to "work sex in" during the short evening.

Extramarital Relationships

Despite all the media hype over the past few years about extramarital sexual activity by government officials, the reality is that most people are faithful to their spouses. In the NORC study, a relatively large number of adults reported that they have been completely monogamous during the course of their marriage. Only 10% of women and 25% of men reported that they had had an extramarital sexual relationship (Laumann et al., 1994)—far below the 50% of men and 25% of women reported by Kinsey back in 1948 and 1953.

A NORC researcher (Smith, 2003) pointed out that there are probably more scientifically worthless "facts" on extramarital relations than on any other facet of human behavior. He said that extramarital relations are less prevalent than pop and pseudo-scientific accounts contend. The best estimates are that 3% to 4% of currently married people have a sexual partner other than their spouse in a given year. About 15% to 18% of people have had a sexual partner other than their spouse while married. It does not seem that levels have changed much in the past 20 years. The rates of extramarital relations are about twice as high among husbands as among wives. They are also more common among African Americans, those with lower incomes, those who attend church less frequently, those who have been separated or divorced, and those who are unhappy with their marriage.

Wilcox and Marquardt (2010) indicated that marital infidelity is more common among the lower educated than among the highly educated. For example, 21% of the least educated, 19% of the moderately educated, and 13% of the highly educated had sexual intercourse with someone other than their spouse while married during the 2000s.

Because husbands are more involved in extramarital sexual relations than wives are, presumably without their spouses' knowledge, more women may be at risk of STIs than has been thought. Research is not available on what proportion of husbands have same-gender relationships outside their marriage. However, married men and women who perceive themselves to be at no (or low) risk of STIs and HIV may, in fact, be at risk because of their partner's extramarital sexual activities (Laumann et al., 1994).

Extramarital sexual activity can take place in two different contexts: one in which the partners have no agreement (nonconsensual context) and one in which the partners agree to have sexual relations with someone else (consensual context).

Nonconsensual Extramarital Sexual Activity

Married people engage in **nonconsensual**—and therefore usually secret—extramarital relationships for many and complex reasons. On a practical level, one's spouse may be unable to have sexual intercourse because of illness, or a couple may be separated for a long period. Thus the person deciding on an extramarital relationship does so to have sexual relations at all. But in other situations an individual might search for someone outside the marriage simply to add excitement or variety to life. Another might feel dissatisfied sexually with his or her partner and look for a more satisfactory emotional and physical relationship while maintaining the marriage. Or a person might feel drawn to someone outside the marriage by sexual attraction alone and choose to act on that attraction.

> **nonconsensual**
> In this context, a married person's engaging in sexual intercourse without the consent of the spouse.

A number of forces tend to restrain or increase extramarital sexual activity:

1. Because religiously devout people tend to have lower rates of extramarital sexual activity, rising rates can be predicted from the decline in traditional religious activity.

2. Those who participate in nonmarital sexual intercourse are more likely to participate in extramarital activity, too.

3. Because women are more aware of their right to sexual satisfaction than in years past, some females are more likely to now seek sexual pleasures outside marriage.

4. The more money a person has, the greater is the opportunity for extramarital sexual activity.

5. The changing role of women in the labor force is also a factor; women who work outside the home have a greater opportunity for extramarital activity than women who do not.

Although there are cultures in which it is expected that married people will have affairs, most people in the United States say they believe in monogamy and want it in their marriage. However, two of three married couples experience an affair during their marriage, and 17% of divorces are caused by infidelity. Traditionally, more men than women take part in affairs, but women are catching up. Affairs are a sign that the wandering spouse is dissatisfied in the

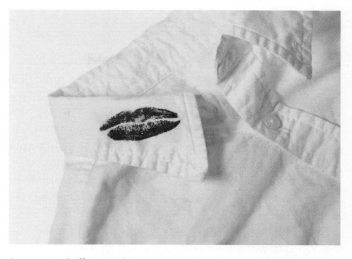

Extramarital affairs are less common than the media might lead us to believe.

marriage. They can be a way of expressing pain and confusion that the person cannot verbally articulate. However, an affair does not necessarily mean that he or she wants to end the marriage. An affair can be a way of expressing that there are problems that need to be resolved (Stanton, 2001).

What are the effects of extramarital sexual relationships on a marriage? Initially, many people who learn their spouse has been having affairs feel both betrayed and emotionally devastated, especially if they believe their spouse to be honest, loyal, and loving. When they learn of the affair, there is a chance that the marriage will fall apart quickly. However, if the couple can talk about the situation, taking the opportunity to improve their communication and assess their own relationship, the marriage does not necessarily dissolve.

Sometimes the type of extramarital relationship has a great effect on the eventual outcome. When a spouse has engaged in a one-night stand, the other spouse might be likely to forgive and forget. If the extramarital affair was intimate, was long-lasting, and involved a strong emotional commitment, however, the other spouse may find it difficult to get over the unfaithfulness.

Consensual Extramarital Sexual Activity

There are many types of **consensual** activities; we discuss the two major ones—open marriage and swinging. **Open marriage** became publicized with the appearance of George and Nena O'Neill's book, *Open Marriage*, in 1972. The O'Neills believed that traditional marriage was too confining and limiting for the partners and that one partner could not fulfill all the intimate needs and expectations of the other. They described an open marriage as one in which the partners allow each other to have intimate

Global DIMENSIONS

Tempted by Digital Dalliances

Internet infidelity is a topic that would not have been mentioned too many years ago. Not all people see Internet infidelity as a real act of betrayal, but in one study the majority did see this as not only real infidelity but as also having as serious an impact on the couple as a traditional offline affair. Emotional infidelity was given as much attention as sexual infidelity was (Whitty, 2005).

The Internet's anonymity, convenience, and ready access to potential partners make it easy to participate in cyber-sex with other people. Cyber-infidelity occurs when a partner in a committed relationship uses a computer to violate agreements of sexual exclusivity. Internet affairs often go through progressive steps: non-sexually explicit flirting, sexual innuendo and explicit repartee, scheduling sex-laced chats, discussing sexual preferences and fantasies, simultaneous masturbation online, and planning or (in fewer cases) conducting face-to-face meetings and physical contact. Women are as likely to engage in cyber-affairs as men. For therapists, treating Internet affairs is no different than treating other affairs (Schnarch & Morehouse, 2002).

and emotional relationships—sexual or nonsexual—with others. For instance, the married couple might decide that each partner is entitled to one night a week alone to engage in another intimate relationship. The idea is that this arrangement allows the married couple to grow and contribute more to the marriage. Another aspect of the open marriage is the renewable contract. The partners formally agree that extramarital relationships are permitted in the marriage and might even foster support, loyalty, and trust between partners but that the partners may change their contract regarding extramarital activity as they continue to grow. The idea here is that the agreement is flexible and renewable so that neither partner is forced to stand by a commitment that he or she no longer feels.

Swinging is the exchange of partners among married couples. (This phenomenon used to be called *wife-swapping*, but the term lost favor with the rise of the women's movement because of its suggestion that wives were property and that men made the decisions.) All those involved participate willingly, and both partners in a marriage usually engage in it simultaneously.

Swingers object to calling this type of activity extramarital, because they view it as part of the marriage relationship. Most swingers do not want emotional involvements outside the marriage. Most often swingers find one another by advertising in tabloids or in special magazines devoted to swinging. People who engage in swinging are apparently very ordinary outside their sexual life.

Like other aspects of society, some for-profit ventures have developed related to extramarital sexual activity. For example, in 2002 the Ashley Madison Agency launched its website to the public. It is designed to promote social networking. As it says on the website, the agency deals with "risqué business." Its purpose is to cater to people who are already in relationships, but still want to date. In its first 3 years the agency signed up more than 500,000 members, with about 8.5 men signing up for every 1.5 women. In July 2011 Ashley Madison hit 10 million members, ensuring that it is the most popular and successful website for heterosexual married dating services. Ashley Madison Down Low has also had enormous success in breaking into the same-sex market for bisexual married men who want to have an affair with another man (Ashley Madison News, 2011).

consensual
In this context, a married person's engaging in extra-marital sexual activity with the knowl-edge and permission of the spouse.

open marriage
A marriage in which partners allow each other to have intimate and emotional relationships with others.

swinging
Swapping of mates for sexual activities.

■ Divorce

There are many reasons that marriages break up. Among these are greater economic independence of women, greater ease of getting a divorce, decreased stigma attached to divorce, unrealistic expectations for marriage, communication difficulties, infidelity, and feelings of incompatibility (Center for Families in Transition, 2003).

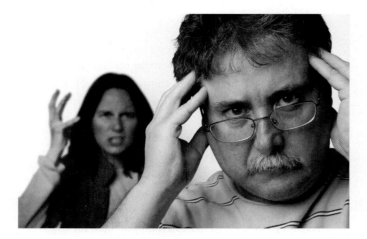

Communication difficulties are one of the major reasons for divorce.

The current U.S. divorce rate (16.4 per 1,000 married women) is much higher than that of 1960 (9.2 per 1,000 married women), but has declined significantly since hitting its highest peak during the 1980s (22.6 per 1,000 married women). Two probable reasons for the decline in the divorce rate are an increase in the age at which people marry for the first time and a higher educational level of those marrying, both of which are associated with greater marital stability (Wilcox & Marquardt, 2010).

Trail and Karney (2012) wanted to separate myth from reality related to divorces among various groups. They found that people with lower incomes value the institution of marriage just as much as those with higher incomes and have similar romantic standards for marriage. However, low-income respondents were more likely than more affluent couples to say that their romantic relationships were negatively affected by economic and social issues such as money problems, drinking, and drug use. They concluded that initiatives to strengthen marriage among low-income populations should move beyond promoting the value of marriage and instead focus on the actual problems that low-income couples face.

Most divorced persons eventually marry, but there has been an increase in the percentage of adults who are currently divorced. For example, this percentage, which was only 1.8% for males and 2.6% for females in 1960, was 8.5% for males and 10.8% for females in 2010. There are more divorced women than divorced men mainly because divorced men are more likely to remarry and to do so sooner. One relatively new divorce trend is that the educational divide is increasing: less-educated Americans have a much higher divorce rate than do college-educated Americans. At the same time, teenagers still have much higher divorce rates than those who marry after age 21, and the nonreligious are much more likely to divorce than are the religiously committed (Wilcox & Marquardt, 2010).

The significant effect of divorce on family life cannot be exaggerated. The spouse who maintains custody of the children has to supervise their care, earn enough money to meet their needs, and provide, usually without help, the love and affection all children crave. In addition, the divorced parent must reestablish a social life at the same time the emotional scars from the failed marriage are healing. The children may blame themselves for the divorce and must manage without the constant contact with one parent. Many experts feel that the most important factor in how divorce affects a child's life is how the parents treat each other and their children during and after the divorce.

The question of whether divorce creates long-term negative effects for children has long been debated. Some studies indicate that about twice as many children of divorced parents have emotional problems. In addition, they have greater challenges negotiating relationships once they are older, have a greater chance of choosing the "wrong" partner, and are much more likely to divorce. Critics of this research question these findings. They point out that most of the studies do not involve interviews with the children, but instead are colored by caregivers' views of how a divorce affects children. Some researchers indicate that children of divorce often have a greater sense of responsibility, independence, and maturity than their counterparts whose parents have remained together. In addition, if there has been great discord and constant fighting in the household, a divorce can provide relief to the children who have been living in that highly stressful setting.

Problems with the economy can also contribute to divorce. Money issues can drive a wedge between couples. They can lead couples to either withdraw from each other or attack each other about things that don't have anything to do with financial matters. Financial anxiety can lead spouses to alcohol or substance abuse, gambling, or extramarital affairs. At the same time, however, many couples may be motivated to make their marriages work. People are realizing it is more expensive to break up a family than it is to stay together (Johnston, 2009).

With the share of married adults at an all-time low in the United States, some researchers have

? Did You Know . . .

The Top Ten Myths of Divorce

1. **Half of all marriages end in divorce.** If today's divorce rate continues, the chance that a marriage contracted this year will end in divorce is probably a little higher than 40%.

2. **Second marriages tend to be more successful than first marriages.** The divorce rate of remarriages is higher than that of first marriages.

3. **Living together before marriage is a good way to reduce the chance of divorce.** Those who live together before marriage have a considerably *higher* chance of divorce.

4. **Problems caused for children of divorce are not long-lasting.** Many such problems are long-lasting and become worse in adulthood.

5. **Having a child will improve a marriage and prevent divorce.** The decreased risk is far less than it used to be.

6. **After divorce, the woman's standard of living plummets while the man's greatly improves.** The difference is not as great as previously thought, but the gender gap is real. A woman's loss is about 27% and a man's gain is about 10%.

7. **When parents do not get along, children are better off if their parents divorce.** Only the children in very high-conflict homes benefited from the conflict removal that divorce can effect. In lower-conflict marriages that end in divorce, the situation of the children is often much worse.

8. **Children who grow up in a home broken by divorce have as much success in their own marriages as those from intact homes.** Children of divorce have a much higher rate of divorce than those from intact families.

9. **After divorce, children involved are better off in step-families than in single-parent families.** There seems to be no difference between the two.

10. **Being very unhappy at certain points in a marriage is a good sign that the marriage will end in divorce.** Eighty-six percent of a large national sample who were unhappily married indicated 5 years later that they were happier. Three-fifths of them said they were "very happy" or "quite happy."

One additional myth: It is usually men who initiate divorce proceedings. Two-thirds of all divorces are initiated by women.

Source: Data from Popenoe, D. The top ten myths of divorce. National Marriage Project. Available: http://www.virginia.edu/marriageproject/pdfs/MythsDivorce.pdf.

found that one of the main reasons why couples do not get married is that they fear divorce (Miller et al., 2011). Among cohabiting couples, more than two-thirds had concerns about dealing with the social, legal, emotional, and economic consequences of possible divorce. Middle-class subjects spoke more favorably about marriage and viewed cohabitation as a natural stepping stone to marriage compared to their working-class counterparts. Lower-income women, in particular, disproportionately expressed doubts about the "trap" of marriage, fearing it could be hard to exit if things go wrong or it would lead to additional domestic responsibilities but few benefits. Working-class cohabiting couples were more apt to view marriage as "just a piece of paper," nearly identical to their existing relationship.

When everything is considered, your chances of divorce may be much lower than you think. While it has been said that the national divorce rate is close to 50%, for many people the actual chances of divorce are much less. If you are a reasonably well-educated person with a decent income, come from an intact family, are religious, and marry after age 25 without having a baby first, your chances of divorce are very low indeed (Wilcox & Marquardt, 2010).

Single-Parent Families

Families with a single parent (**single-parent families**) are becoming increasingly prevalent. According to the U.S. Census Bureau, the number of single-parent families has increased greatly. In 1980, for example, 19.5% of all households with children were single-parent households. In 1990 it was 24%, in 2000

single-parent family
For whatever reason, only one parent who is living with a child or children.

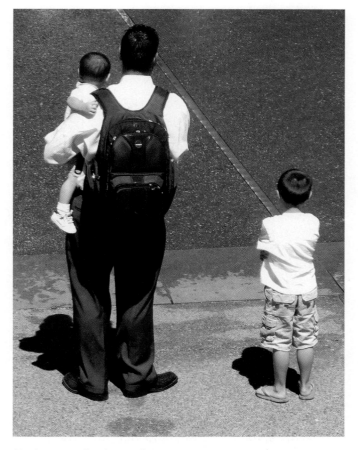

Single-parent families are becoming more common.

of marriage, which means that adults were single for more years; and the growth in divorce among couples with children (Fields, 2004). More than half of births to American women under 30 occur outside of marriage (two-thirds of U.S. children are born to mothers under 30). The fastest growth of this number has occurred in white women in their 20s who have some college education but no four-year degree. In the mid 1990s a third of Americans were born outside marriage. In 2012 the figure was 41% (DeParle and Tavernise 2012). Usually when we think of single-parent families, we think of them as being headed by women. However, the number of households headed by single fathers has been growing significantly.

Father-headed single-parent families often place the father in a new role. We say "often" because now-adays men in two-parent families more and more are helping with what were heretofore considered to be the wife's household chores and responsibilities. For these husbands the adjustment to heading a single-parent family will be less difficult because they are accustomed to cooking, cleaning, nurturing, and changing diapers. For the more traditional husband, the adoption of these necessary chores and responsibilities, added to the financial and emotional burdens of divorce, means that a more significant adjustment is required.

Life in a single-parent family can be stressful for the adult and the children. Members may unrealistically expect that the family can function as a two-parent family does and may feel that something is wrong if it cannot. The single parent may feel overwhelmed by the responsibility of caring for the children, maintaining a job, and keeping up with the bills and household chores. Typically, the family's finances and resources are drastically reduced by the parents' breakup.

it was 27%, and in 2010 it was 34%. This meant that over 24 million children were living in single-parent households in 2010 (U.S. Bureau of Labor Statistics, 2011; Kids Count Data Center, 2011).

Reasons for the increase in the number of children living with single parents include a larger proportion of births occurring to unmarried women; the delay

Global DIMENSIONS

Single-Parent Households in Various Countries

Although we don't know the reasons for these differences, it is interesting to look at the percent of single-parent households in other countries. Here they are in declining order:

1. United Kingdom   25.0%
2. Canada   24.6%
3. Ireland   22.6%
4. Denmark   21.7%
5. Germany   21.7%
6. France   19.8%
7. Sweden   18.7%
8. Netherlands   16.0%
9. Japan   10.2%

Source: Data from Section 30—International Statistics, Statistical Abstract of the United States. U.S. Census Bureau, 2012.

Single-parent families deal with pressures and potential problem areas that the nuclear family does not have to face (Single parenting and today's family, 1998):

- Visitation and custody problems
- The negative effects of continuing conflict between the parents
- Fewer opportunities for parents and children to spend time together
- Negative effects of the breakup on children's school performance and peer relations
- Disruptions of extended family relationships
- Problems caused by parents' dating and entering new relationships

The demand for social services to meet the special needs of single-parent families is growing. Because single-parent families often have financial, psychological, custodial, and other needs that are more acute than those of conventional two-parent families, they need counseling and/or support groups. Many single parents have the added responsibility of providing role models for their other-sex children. Day care, a virtual necessity (as it also is for many two-parent households), solves some problems, yet it may also be a source of anxiety, or at least concern, for financial, educational, psychological, or other reasons.

Although some of these research findings might seem discouraging—or they might seem wrong to readers who come from single-parent families—it is important to remember that these findings refer to trends in groups and have no bearing on particular individuals. Children in single-parent families are often very successful. Our intention here is to suggest that single parenthood does require special care and consideration. Perhaps most of all, the special needs of single-parent families should be understood both by family members themselves and by teachers, employers, and others with whom they interact. To meet this need for understanding, a group called Parents without Partners serves as a sounding board and a source of counsel for single parents.

The need for good parenting skills remains constant regardless of the parent's marital status. However, the situation can be more demanding for both the parents and the children in single-parent households. The following are some suggested guidelines.

1. Be honest with your children about the situation that caused you to become a single parent.

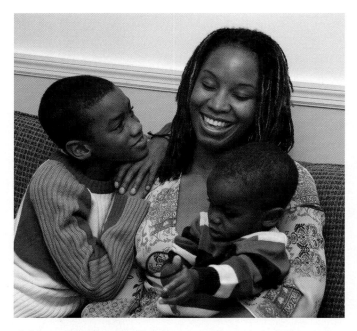

Children in single-parent families can be just as successful as other children.

2. In case of a separation or divorce, assure children that they are not responsible for the breakup of the relationship.

3. Try to maintain as much of the same routine as possible.

4. Do not try to be both mother and father to the children. Establish a family atmosphere of teamwork.

5. In the case of divorce, acknowledge that the relationship between you and your former partner is over, and do not encourage your children to hope for reconciliation.

6. Reassure children that they will continue to be loved and cared for (by both parents, if true).

7. Do not use children to gain bargaining power with a separated or divorced spouse.

8. Encourage relatives to help children maintain a sense of belonging to a continuing family.

Wilcox & Marquardt (2010) have provided helpful information to summarize this section. For example, they indicate that the percentage of children who grow up in fragile—typically fatherless—families has grown enormously over the past five decades. This is mainly due to increases in divorce, out-of-wedlock births, and unmarried cohabitation. Children in such families have negative outcomes at two to three times the rate of children in married two-parent families. In earlier times, most single mothers were divorced or widowed. Today the number of never-married single mothers is higher than that of divorced mothers. A major reason for the increase in number of never-married single mothers is that single motherhood has become a permanent status for many women.

■ Sexuality and Aging

There was a time when it was believed that sexual desire and functioning became unimportant with age. Although a gradual decline in sexual activity occurs around age 50 years and accelerates after age 70 years, sexuality remains an important part of life into old age.

Understanding the sexuality of elders is important because of the rapidly increasing elderly population. The population of U.S. citizens aged 65 years and older grew from 25.5 million in 1980 to 35 million in 2000. It was more than 40.4 million in 2010. It is projected to rise to about 71 million by 2030. This will represent 20% of the total U.S. population (Healthy aging for older adults, 2009; Population 65 years and over in the United States, 2011). As people live longer, it is important to understand how sexuality is affected in later years.

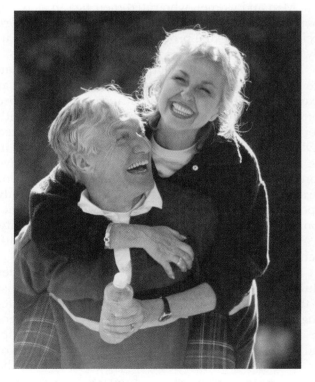

As people get older they can continue to have excellent relationships that include sexual activity.

Many studies have confirmed that people remain sexually active into their 70s and 80s. Bretschneider and McCoy (1988) found that 62% of the men and 30% of the women they studied engaged in intercourse. These people ranged in age from 80 to 102 years. DeBeauvoir (1973) revealed that 70% of those men older than 65 years of age who were listed in *Who's Who* had sexual intercourse on an average of four times a month. Kaplan (1974) found that women tend to want more rather than less sexual activity as they approach their middle and older years.

In 1998, the National Council on the Aging conducted a telephone survey of 1,300 Americans older than the age of 60 years. It found that nearly half engage in sexual activity at least once a month, and 4 in 10 said they would like to engage in sexual activities more frequently than they currently do. Three-quarters of the men and the women said that they are emotionally satisfied or even more satisfied with their sexual activities than they were in their 40s. Forty-three percent said that sexual relations were just as good as or better than they were in their youth, and 43% said they were less satisfying.

Older men were more than twice as likely to report wanting more sexual activity than women, and men were much more likely to be sexually active than women older than 60 years. Nearly two-thirds of senior men are currently sexually active, whereas only 37% of women are currently sexually active. This gap exists partially because women live longer and thus are much more likely to be widowed than men. However, men were much more likely to say that a medical condition prevents them from engaging in sexual activities (51% of men, 12% of women) and that medications are reducing their sexual desire (44% of men, 16% of women).

Jacoby (2005) reported the results of a nationwide study conducted by the American Association of Retired People (AARP). The study focused on sexual attitudes and behavior of adults ages 45 and older. Here are some of the findings:

- The number of men who have tried treatments to improve their sexual functioning doubled from 10% in 1999 to 22% in 2005. Sixty-eight percent of those men said the treatments improved their sexual satisfaction. Women said their own sexual satisfaction was enhanced by their partners' use of drugs and they increased their frequency of sexual activity.

- Phone sex with a spouse or intimate partner was popular among the 45 to 49 age group. Seventeen percent of the men and 18% of the women admitted to talking dirty on the phone, and 22% of men and women said they've penned erotic notes or exchanged sexy email messages.

• Slightly more than 25% of the men and 21% of women confessed to having had sexual relations in a public place, and 11% of both men and women in the 50 to 69 age group also admitted to this behavior.

• Concerning extramarital sexual activities and swinging, an overwhelming 95% said they would not do those things.

• Nearly half the women in the 45 to 49 age group reported masturbating at least once in the last six months. Twenty percent of women age 70 and older said they masturbated. A majority of all women said that self-stimulation is an important part of sexual pleasure at any age.

• About 60% of all men age 45 and older said they masturbated at least once in the last six months. More unmarried men (73%) than married men (51%) masturbated.

• While a majority of all subjects agreed that a satisfying sexual relationship is important to one's quality of life, for most it wasn't the number one priority. Good spirits, good health, close ties with friends and family, financial security, spiritual well-being, and a good relationship with a partner were all rated as more important.

• Men placed a higher value on sexual activity than did women. Sixty-six percent of men, compared to 48% of women, said that satisfying sexual activity is important to their quality of life. This gender split changes with age. In the 45 to 49 age group, men and women place almost equal importance on sexual activity. By age 60, though, 62% of men, but only 27% of women, placed a high priority on a satisfying sexual relationship.

• A majority of men and women with partners described themselves as either "extremely satisfied" or "somewhat satisfied" with their sex lives.

Lindau et al. (2007) reported that the prevalence of sexual activity declines with age (73% among those 57–64 years old, 53% among those 65–74 years old, and 26% among those 75–85 years old). Women were less likely than men at all ages to report sexual activity. About half of those who were sexually active reported at least one bothersome sexual problem. The most

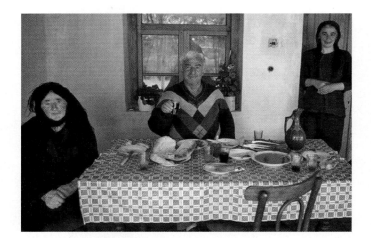

The Abkhasian people of Georgia (a republic of the former Soviet Union) often live to be more than 100 years old. One reason they believe they live so long is their sexual customs. The Abkhasian people believe that sexual energy should be conserved. They do not marry until about age 30 years and do not believe in premarital sexual activity. It is essential that a bride be a virgin. In marriage, sexual activity is considered a pleasure to enjoy, but for the sake of one's health it should not be overdone.

prevalent problems among women were low desire (43%), difficulty with vaginal lubrication (39%), and inability to reach climax (34%). Among men, the most prevalent sexual problems were erectile difficulties (37%). Fourteen percent of men reported using medication or supplements to improve sexual function. Men and women who rated their health as being poor were less likely to be sexually active and more likely to report sexual problems when they were sexually active.

A study of sexually active older women (mean age of 67; 63% were postmenopausal) found that sexual satisfaction increased with age and that those not engaging in sexual activity were satisfied with their sex lives. Half of the respondents who reported having a sexual partner had been sexually active in the last 4 weeks. The majority of the sexually active women (67%) achieved orgasm most of the time or always. The youngest and oldest women in the study reported the highest frequency of orgasm satisfaction. Regardless of partner status or sexual activity, 61% of all women in this study were satisfied with their overall sex life (Trompeter et al., 2012).

Penhollow et al. (2009) studied a sample of older adults age 55–89 (mean age of 68). They found most of the group believed that sexual behavior is a life-long need, that it has beneficial effects in older people, that it is a critical part of a good relationship, and that it is important to their overall quality of life. Twenty-eight percent of the men and 19% of the women were current users of sexual performance-enhancing medications.

Multicultural
DIMENSIONS

The Boomer Sandwich

A study done by the American Association of Retired People on 45- to 55-year-olds (the sandwich generation) showed how different cultures take care of their own (The boomer sandwich, 2001). Compared with other generations, this one is better educated (38% are college graduates compared with 23% of the general population). More of them are married (67%, well above the national average). They are also more economically secure (almost a third earn more than $75,000 per year).

Who helps their aging relatives most? Forty-two percent of Asian Americans provide care for their aging relatives compared with 34% of Hispanics, 28% of African Americans, and 19% of whites. Those born outside the United States are much more likely to care for or support older family members (43%) compared with those who are born in the United States (20%). Overall, 69% do not want their children to have to look after them when they get older.

Prevalent in our society is the performance ethic, which is concerned with the frequency of intercourse and orgasm. As we mature (age, if you will), it becomes apparent that other types of sexual activity become important. These include caressing, hugging, petting, kissing, and sharing of intimacies. People who experience a satisfying sexual life in their early years will most likely continue this pursuit. However, those people who are today 65 years and older lived under very different mores. Your grandparents and possibly your parents led more restricted sexual lives, especially the women. Women were not taught about masturbation, nor were they taught to ask that they be sexually satisfied.

Older people can not only be sexually satisfied by having relationships with others, but can also experience active sexual behaviors by themselves. Masturbation is a viable activity for older people, especially women. If the male loses the capacity to maintain erections, women can masturbate; or men can masturbate to orgasm even after they can no longer become erect. Mutual masturbation becomes popular, once again, as it may have been when they were younger.

Physiological changes are often attributed to changes in sexuality associated with aging. However, onset of menopause for women and declining levels of testosterone for men represent only one factor in sexuality changes. Psychological and sociocultural changes occur as well.

Some sexual dysfunction associated with aging, such as erectile disorder, can now be overcome with pharmacology. Drugs such as Viagra and Cialis can restore the physical ability to have an erection; however, it does not rekindle the psychological or social aspects that make for a loving relationship. These drugs pose special problems to a relationship: A woman may wonder whether the erection is caused by the drug or by attraction to her.

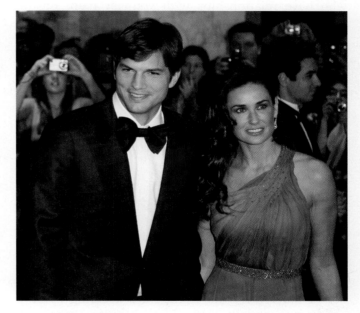

A phenomena in Hollywood, both on- and off-screen, is that of a romantic involvement between a younger man and older woman. Is the pairing, such as occurred from 2003 to 2011 with Demi Moore and Ashton Kutcher the start of a trend?

Psychological changes also occur across the aging process, such as changes in mood. For women, causes may include stress, health problems, menopause, hormone replacement therapy, and other lifestyle changes. For men, they may include a shift in focus from career to increased focus on family, challenge to the traditional male role as leader and protector of the family, increased need for affirmation and acceptance, or irritation and anger with aging (especially the physical changes).

Social factors affecting psychological changes include the fact that socialization of people in their 70s, 80s, or 90s in regard to sexuality is substantially different from that of those in their 30s or 40s. For example, images of sexual attractiveness tend to be youth oriented and may affect the self-esteem of aging women (Sanders, 1999). Ironically, men are sometimes viewed as more attractive as they age. And Hollywood movies often capitalize on this double standard by pairing an older, experienced male actor with a young actress.

It has been common to see older men dating younger women, but a survey showed that 34% of single women ages 40 to 69 were dating younger men (Montenegro, 2003). The main reason given for women dating younger men was energy, refreshing optimism, and sexual stamina. One woman indicated that she liked dating younger guys who keep the romance stirring and their sex lives buzzing.

The term "cougar" is used to refer to older women who have relationships with younger men. Easton et al. (2011) reported that older women have evolved a reproduction-expediting physiological adaptation designed to capitalize on their remaining fertility. These women experience increased sexual motivations and sexual behaviors compared to women not facing a similar fertility decline. Their research showed that women with declining fertility think more about sexual activity, have more frequent and intense sexual fantasies, are more willing to engage in sexual intercourse, and report actually engaging in sexual intercourse more frequently than women in other age groups.

Interestingly, some long-married couples actually experience more sexual satisfaction during their older years. Once their offspring are out of the house and they are retired from working, they can devote more time to each other and have more fulfilling and rewarding lovemaking.

On a related, but different, note, a growing number of older men and women are deciding to have children (Crandell, 2005). The birthrate for women 45 and older more than doubled between 1990 and 2002. Among older women having babies are celebrities like Cheryl Tiegs, Sharon Stone, Joan Lunden, and Susan Sarandon. Many older moms and dads are happy to devote what might have been leisure-filled years to the frenzy of childcare and related responsibilities. People may have to get creative to do this and use cutting-edge techniques like frozen embryos, fertility treatments and drugs, and adoption. Many older parents feel they do a better job of parenting than they would have done while they were younger.

In recent years, more attention has been paid to the needs of the lesbian, gay, bisexual, and transgender (LGBT) people as they get older. Many issues are the same as those for older heterosexuals, but there are also some that are unique to LGBT people. For example, there may be limited access to LGBT-friendly health care. They might experience homophobia, deal with stigmas, and be socially isolated. Denial of hospital and nursing home visitation rights for their partners may also be a problem. In addition, ageism may exist within the gay and lesbian community.

The National Institute on Aging suggests the following ways for women to stay healthy after menopause (Menopause, 2010):

- Don't smoke.

- Eat a healthy diet, low in fat, high in fiber, with plenty of fruits, vegetables, and whole-grain foods, as well as all the important vitamins and minerals.

- Make sure you get enough calcium and vitamin D—either in your diet or with vitamin/mineral supplements.

- Learn what your healthy weight is, and try to stay there.

- Do weight-bearing exercise, such as walking, jogging, or dancing, at least 3 days each week for healthy bones. Also try to be physically active in other ways for your general health.

Menopause

Usually between the ages of 40 and 55 years, women produce progressively less estrogen and progesterone, as an effect of aging on the ovaries. Whereas the pituitary continues to produce follicle-stimulating hormone (FSH) and luteinizing hormone (LH), the ovaries can no longer respond to these pituitary hormones as they once could. This decrease in estrogen and progesterone occurs over approximately a 5- to 10-year period and results in a cessation of menstruation. The period when these changes take place is called the **perimenopause**, or the **climacteric**; when menstruation has not occurred for a year, we call that **menopause**.

> **perimenopause (climacteric)**
> The period just before menopause when the production of estrogen and progesterone is decreasing, usually a 5- to 10-year period.
>
> **menopause**
> The time when a woman's menstrual cycle ceases, usually between 40 and 55 years of age.

Symptoms of Perimenopause and Menopause

Most perimenopausal women report mild symptoms or no symptoms at all; only about 20% report symptoms severe enough to cause them to seek medical attention. The symptoms that perimenopausal and menopausal women experience can vary from headaches, dizziness, palpitations, insomnia, anxiety, depression, and weight gain to hot flashes and vaginal dryness. **Hot flashes**

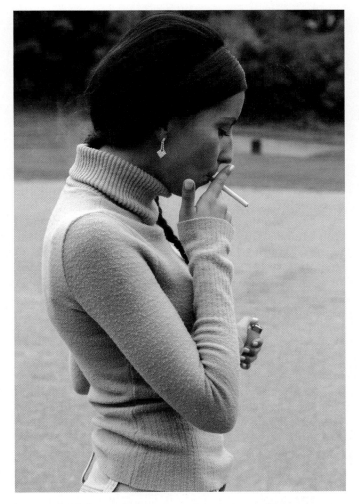

Increased risk factors for osteoporosis include smoking, consumption of alcohol, physical inactivity, being underweight, and having a diet low in calcium.

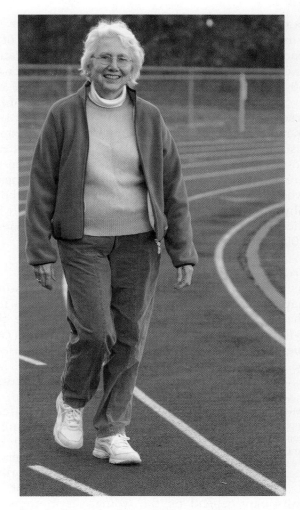

Exercise is one way for women to prevent osteoporosis, the weakening of their bones. Thus exercise, along with proper nutrition, not smoking, and refraining from drinking alcoholic beverages, is helpful in preventing bone fractures.

hot flashes
Intermittent sensations of heat reported by menopausal women, possibly caused by decreased estrogen production.

(sometimes referred to as *hot flashes*) are sudden waves of heat felt throughout the body, often accompanied by reddening and sweating (Menopause, 2010). Some women experience hot flashes infrequently, whereas others may have them every few hours or so. They may last a few seconds or, in severe cases, a full 30 minutes. And some women never have hot flashes. Because hot flashes tend to occur more frequently at night, they often disturb sleep, causing the woman to awaken in a sweat. In particularly bothersome cases, they may contribute to insomnia. Hot flashes appear to be caused by hormonal fluctuations that affect the nerves governing the dilatation or constriction of the blood vessels. When the blood vessels rapidly dilate in response to hormonal secretions, a sense of warmth may result. Generally, hot flashes cease after 2 years, but in some cases they may last longer.

Vaginal dryness results from the lowered amount of estrogen in the vaginal walls, which causes shrinking and thinning and causes the vaginal mucosa to become thinner. The net result is that both the length and the width of the vagina become smaller and the vagina cannot expand during penile insertion as it once could. In addition, there is diminished vaginal lubrication during perimenopause and menopause. These changes can mean painful intercourse as well as an increased risk of vaginal infection (Menopause, 2010). Over-the-counter lubricants can be helpful in these cases.

A significant symptom caused by the decrease in estrogen production is the decalcification of the bones. **Osteoporosis** is the disease that results when enough calcium is lost in the

osteoporosis
A condition of weakened bones resulting from decalcification (loss of calcium) of bone that increases in the absence of estrogen and is of particular concern in postmenopausal women.

bones to make the person susceptible to bone fractures and bending (for example, curvature of the back—sometimes called "dowager's hump" because it is common among older women). Women older than 50 years of age lose about 10% of their bone mass every 10 years; the result is an increased risk of bone fractures. Women older than 60 years of age suffer many more bone fractures than do men (Osteoporosis handout on health, 2011). It seems that osteoporosis occurs more frequently in white women who are fair skinned (especially blonds and redheads), who smoke cigarettes, who drink alcohol, who are physically inactive, who are underweight, and whose diet is low in calcium (National Institutes of Health, 2005). Osteoporosis can develop in men, too.

Treatment for Menopause

As we have mentioned, only a minority of women have menopausal symptoms severe enough to make them seek medical attention. To help relieve these symptoms, some women use hormones. This is called **menopausal hormone therapy (MHT)**. It used to be called *hormone replacement therapy* (HRT). MHT is a more current umbrella term that describes different hormone combinations available in a variety of forms and doses. The form of MHT a doctor suggests may depend on the woman's symptoms. For example, an estrogen patch or pill can relieve hot flashes, night sweats, and vaginal dryness. Other forms—vaginal creams, tablets, or rings—are used

menopausal hormone therapy (MHT)
Replacement of hormones that a woman's ovaries stop making at the time of menopause, easing some of the symptoms of menopause.

mostly for vaginal dryness. The vaginal ring insert might also help some urinary tract symptoms. The dose can also vary, as can the timing of these doses. Some women might even take estrogen or progesterone continuously—every day of the month (Hormones and menopause, 2009).

The use of MHT can be controversial. It is important for a woman to discuss the pros and cons of MHT with her physician and see if the potential benefits are worth the potential risks. For example, research indicates that for some women the use of MHT poses some serious risks, such as increasing the risk for breast cancer, heart disease, stroke, and pulmonary embolism (blood clot in the lung). Women who choose to use MHT should use the lowest dose that helps for the shortest time needed (Womenshealth.gov, 2011).

Other treatments for menopause disorders specific to preventing osteoporosis include sufficient physical exercise to strengthen the bones, a diet rich in calcium to slow bone decalcification, refraining from smoking of cigarettes and drinking of alcohol, and avoidance of carbonated soft drinks that contain high levels of phosphorus, which may contribute to a phosphorus–calcium imbalance associated with osteoporosis. Foods such as milk, sardines and salmon canned with bones, oysters, and dark green vegetables are recommended because they are all high in calcium.

Some physicians may also prescribe tranquilizers for women who have difficulty with the psychological aspects of menopause. It is unclear whether the depression some women report during menopause is a cause of that condition or is caused by other changes that usually occur during that stage of life (for example, children leaving home, aged parents needing more attention, or a woman's life taking a new direction).

Treatment for vaginal dryness can include the use of lubricated creams, vegetable oils, or water-soluble jellies (such as K-Y or Lubifax) and suppositories (Sexual problems overview, 2005). In addition, it appears that regular masturbation or participation in sexual intercourse helps reduce vaginal soreness.

It would be unfortunate to close this section without citing the benefits and positive aspects of menopause. Because women can no longer conceive, the fear of pregnancy is removed, and lovemaking is often more enjoyable as a result. However, a woman who has ceased to menstruate has not necessarily ceased to ovulate. So-called **change-of-life babies** have been known to surprise women just

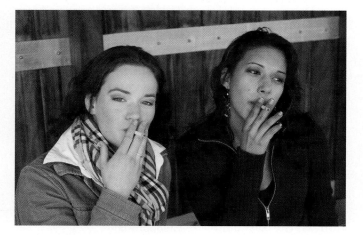
As if smoking weren't enough of a risk of cancer, it has been found that women who replace estrogen after menopause are at an increased risk of contracting breast cancer and ovarian cancer, not to mention the increased risk of stroke and heart disease.

change-of-life baby
A baby born to a menopausal woman who, in spite of not menstruating regularly, ovulated.

entering menopause who thought they could no longer conceive. Especially during perimenopause—when the menses occurs, however infrequently—caution is advised.

The anthropologist Margaret Mead talked of "postmenopausal zest" to describe the excitement, stimulation, and enjoyment that can result from menopause. If viewed in this way, the postmenopausal years can be rich with new opportunities and experiences. If its negative aspects become the focus, menopausal symptoms will probably increase, and psychological discomfort will result. It is up to a woman's friends, relatives, and colleagues at work to help her focus on the positive aspects of menopause rather than its less desirable components. In addition, many women now turn to support groups (for example, The Red Hot Mamas) or online forums to share strategies on ways to manage menopausal symptoms.

Male Climacteric

Do men have an experience analogous to menopause (termed the **male climacteric**)? The answer to this question is not clear. There is evidence that at approximately the same age at which women experience menopause, some men experience what is called a **midlife crisis**. Men wonder about the meaning of their lives thus far and worry about what the future holds for them. They may become more people oriented and less job-and-task oriented. They may grow concerned about a diminishing interest in sexual activity and a reduction of sexual potency. Some men, to reassure themselves about their sexual capabilities, begin to date younger women or initiate extramarital affairs.

male climacteric
Sometimes termed the "male menopause," which occurs at about the same age that women experience menopause, when men experience slightly decreased testosterone production and begin to question the directions in which their lives are headed.

midlife crisis
A time of life, usually between 40 and 50 years of age, during which men question the path their lives have taken and make plans for changing their goals.

The hormonal evidence usually cited for this male climacteric is a decrease in testosterone production at about age 40 to 50 years. However, the decrease in the testosterone level is believed by many experts to be minimal, too insignificant to influence male behavior. Furthermore, middle-aged women face many of the same concerns and fears about the past and the future and put themselves through similarly agonizing self-examinations. In trying to decide what accounts for the midlife crisis, researchers' difficulties in distinguishing the psychological and sociological influences from clearly identifiable physiological and hormonal changes are practically insurmountable. In women, decreased estrogen production and increased FSH production, as well as a lack of menstrual flow, serve as irrefutable evidence of menopause. No similar evidence exists for a male climacteric. Still, most observers admit that males often go through a change of life—whether hormonally, psychologically, or culturally based—that deserves recognition and attention.

Hormone Therapy

Hormone therapy is sometimes administered to men. For instance, testosterone supplements are sometimes administered to treat erectile dysfunction in older men (although testosterone levels are not low in all men who have trouble maintaining erection). Sometimes this treatment for erectile dysfunction is effective; other times it is not. The reason for this inconsistency is unclear; however, it is safe to say that the complex nature of sexuality makes it only partially responsive to hormone treatment. Testosterone supplements may not have much effect when personality, past experiences, the sexual partner, effectiveness in communication, setting, and so on, continue to have negative effects.

Other Aging-Related Physiological Changes

Direct physical changes do occur in men as they age: The testes become smaller, the scrotal skin becomes thinner and less elastic, seminal fluid may become thinner and be produced in lower quantities, and sperm become less lively. Erections occur more slowly and the plateau phase lasts longer. Another important occurrence is that older men do not feel imminent ejaculation—it is less forceful. It is common for the refractory period to become longer as men age. One possible advantage of slower response is the likelihood that middle-aged and older men can prolong sexual activity and actually be better sexual partners. It should be remembered, however, that even elderly men continue to produce sperm and can become fathers if appropriate precautions are not taken.

The capacity to enjoy sexual experiences is not lost in older men, as it is not lost in older women. Masters and Johnson (1966) maintain the importance of continued and frequent sexual experiences for aging males:

> If elevated levels of sexual activity are maintained from earlier years and neither acute nor chronic physical incapacity intervenes, aging males usually are able to continue some form of active sexual expression into the 70- and even 80-year age groups.

Masters and Johnson further indicate that women who do not regularly participate in sexual activity tend to have difficulty accommodating a penis when they do attempt sexual intercourse. Those who can accommodate a penis and have adequate lubrication are likely to have maintained regular sexual response (once or twice a week).

If an older woman has not been sexually active for a long time, it may take a little time and patience to be able to resume sexual activity. For example, it may take longer for the vagina to swell and lubricate. Longer foreplay can be helpful, as can the use of a lubricant, such as K-Y Jelly. For some women, vaginal treatment with estrogen works well. It may also take time to stretch out the vagina so it can accommodate a penis if the woman has not had sexual intercourse for a long time. Touching, cuddling, and good communication between partners help to promote sexual satisfaction (Resuming sexual activity later in life, 2004; Sexuality in later life, 2010).

Influences on Sexual Activity in Later Years

Many older adults say their sex lives improve as they age. Improvements probably require more communication with partners and possible small changes both people can make. Here are a few examples (Intimacy and aging: Tips for sexual health and happiness, 2003):

- *Expand your definition of sex*. It is more than intercourse. Other options for sexual activity might be more comfortable and more fulfilling. Touching, holding, sensual massage, masturbation, and oral sexual activity are all possibilities.

- *Communicate with your partner*. Discuss changes and possible accommodations. Try different positions and activities. Ask your partner about his or her interests and needs and how you can be helpful. Communication itself can be arousing.

- *Make changes to your routine*. Change the time of day to a time when you have the most energy. Take more time to set the stage, such as a romantic dinner or an evening of dancing. Try new sexual activities.

- *Manage your expectations*. Be realistic. For example, if you didn't have much sexual activity when you were younger, you probably won't when you are older.

- *Take care of yourself*. Healthy living habits can help improve sexual activity at any age.

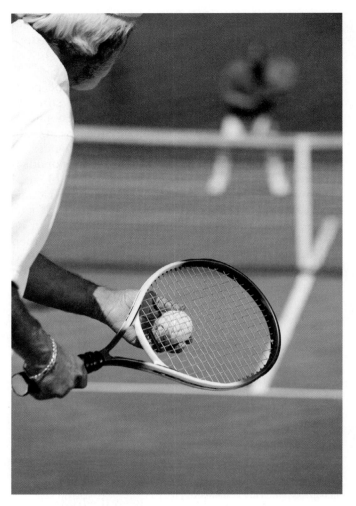

With age, men experience physiological changes that slow their sexual response.

Although health problems can interfere with sexual activity for older people, they need not end all sexual activity. For example, arthritis or lower back pain might require understanding and a variety of sexual positions. Diabetes can result in diminished sexual response, but sexual pleasuring can still provide satisfaction. Stroke victims might lose some control of speech or movements but still be capable of sexual response under appropriate conditions.

Heart attacks are sometimes of particular concern in relation to sexual activity. Some people think that sexual activity may bring about a heart attack, and although in reality this is not a common problem, heart attack victims often hesitate to return to sexual activity. In general, those who have been sexually active before the heart attack will have little, if any, problem being sexually active again. Of course it makes sense to improve personal health as much as possible after a heart attack. Those who have a proper diet, exercise appropriately, and control stress

¿? Ethical DIMENSIONS

Should Donor Eggs Be Used to Let Women Older Than 50 Years Produce Viable Babies?

Women older than 50 years are just as likely to conceive and deliver a baby with donor eggs as younger women are. Many people argue that there is no medical reason why healthy women in their 50s should not have babies with donor eggs. They say that people in their 60s and 70s are much more active than in past years, so they have enough stamina to raise a child. Also, knowing that they can reproduce after age 50 will take the pressure off some women to reproduce when they are younger. They can concentrate more on their marriage and their careers and not worry about child rearing until later in life.

Others feel that it is wrong for a woman older than 50 years to reproduce. They feel that there is a much higher possibility of their offspring's being orphaned at a young age. Even if people are healthy and active, statistics show that many people die in their 60s and 70s. If that happens, relatively young children will be without parents for more of their lives. Also, for healthy people, raising a child takes a lot of energy and it is more likely younger parents will have that energy.

Do you think donor eggs should be used to let women older than 50 years reproduce? At what ages should women be allowed to reproduce?

Source: Data from Rubin, R. Donor eggs can let women over 50 produce viable babies, *USA Today* (November 11, 2002), 9D.

responses are most likely to have satisfactory sexual activity as well.

The availability of partners for the older divorced or widowed person can present severe restrictions on intimacy. How can one have a successful relationship if there are no possible mates? Older women outnumber older men; they tend to live 7 years longer and they generally marry men a few years older than they are. Hence the older woman, who is supposed to have sexual relationships only with her spouse, is alone.

Another problem that exists for older men and women is that their sphere of friendships may be couples—that is, pairs. If one of only a few single people, the person may be omitted from social activities or may appear to be a fifth wheel, and so he or she is not very comfortable with other couples. This indeed limits sexual activity; even more importantly, it may limit intimacy and friendships in later life.

For older people living in nursing homes, there might be additional problems. For example, nursing home personnel sometimes resist sexuality programs. People may be segregated to discourage sexual activities. Medications may be prescribed without considering their effects on sexual functioning; for example, some high blood pressure or arthritis medications can lessen sexual response. Fortunately, attitudes of the staff in nursing homes as well as the families of those in the homes are changing. This is an excellent example of the need to accept people of all ages as sexual beings.

It should be noted that there are times when couples may want to sleep apart, because medication may cause a person to snore loudly, shake violently,

or talk loudly, making it uncomfortable for the other partner. As well as elderly adults, some younger couples choose to sleep in separate bedrooms for similar reasons. It should be remembered that sexual activity can occur in either bedroom and at any time during the day or evening.

Aging and Safer Sexual Activity

STIs and HIV are generally thought of as diseases that the young must worry about. But the number of older Americans with various STIs and HIV is steadily rising. Some of this is related to the fact that more older people are sexually active. However, older adults can also be more vulnerable to HIV infection because the linings of the vagina and anus become more fragile and more susceptible to tears during sexual activity, providing a direct path into the bloodstream for the virus. The immune system also tends to grow weaker with advancing age. To make matters worse, older people are much less likely than younger people to be tested for STIs or HIV. As a result, diseases are typically not diagnosed until a late stage. It is important that older adults take the same precautions to promote safer sexual activity as younger people are encouraged to do.

One problem is that many people may not think to use a condom—after all, pregnancy is not possible among older women. But condom use and safer sexual practices are still needed throughout life to prevent transmission of STIs and HIV, and because an elderly man can impregnate a woman late into his life, safer sexual practices must include contraception.

Because of concern for the overall health of older people, the American Association for Retired People (AARP) surveyed over 2,000 older adults on their sexual attitudes and practices (Fisher, 2010). Results showed that a sort of "sexual revolution" continues in the older population. For example, opposition to sexual activity among those who are not married was down by half over a 10-year period. Also, the belief that there is too much emphasis on sexuality in our culture was also down. However, both the frequency of self-stimulation and sexual thoughts and fantasies did not change. The researchers pointed out that an economic environment that adds to stress and financial anxiety has previously been shown to decrease sexual satisfaction. Men continue to think about sexual activity more than women, see it as more important to their quality of life, engage in sexual activities more often, are less satisfied if without a partner, and are twice as likely as women (21% versus 11%) to admit to sexual activity outside of their relationship.

Homosexuality Among the Aging

Like all sexual beings, homosexuals eventually become old and need to deal with problems caused by aging. The loss of partners and friends may be compounded for older gay men, who saw many of their friends die of AIDS during the 1980s and 1990s. For them, AIDS meant that the good-byes that would have been said as they approached old age were made not only to lifelong friends but also to younger and younger men.

Because they grew up in such a sharply homophobic society, many gays are still cautious about coming out. Many elderly lesbians are still careful about coming out in today's somewhat more accepting society because they have become accustomed to hiding their identity. When older gay men or lesbians do not disclose their sexual identity, they prevent themselves and others from sharing in a comprehensive understanding of their lives.

Many gays may decide to keep their sexual identities secret because of fears of receiving biased or inferior services from doctors, attendants, or nursing homes. Help is available from Senior Action in a Gay Environment (SAGE), an organization concerned with gay, lesbian, bisexual, and transgender elders. It provides social services, individual and group therapy, and home visits for the homebound. It also acts as advocates on behalf of older lesbians and gays.

As people and society in general have become more open and accepting about homosexuality, changes have slowly occurred related to homosexuality and aging as well. One germane example is the opening of retirement communities especially for homosexuals. However, retirement communities for gays and lesbians have experienced some of the same problems as other community developments in recent years. For example, RainbowVision opened its doors in 2006 as one of the first retirement communities in the country to proudly serve gays and lesbians. Its problems were similar to other gay retirement communities, and other new communities in general—a weakened housing market and a deflated economy. These factors make it difficult for anyone to sell a home and move to a new community or perhaps even to have enough money to think about making such a change. A number of communities planned for gay and lesbian retirees never opened because of a lack of finances and a decline in real estate values. As a result, housing options tailored to the estimated 1.5 million elderly people in the United States who are gay are still rather limited. Many are growing older without the support of children or extended family members. Gay and lesbian seniors are twice as likely to live alone (Frosch, 2011).

■ Sexuality for the Physically and Mentally Challenged

In July 2005, the U.S. Surgeon General released a report related to disabilities. More than 54 million Americans, or one in five people, are living with at least one disability. Most Americans will experience a disability some time during the course of their lives. The Surgeon General's report emphasizes that people with disabilities can learn, get married, have

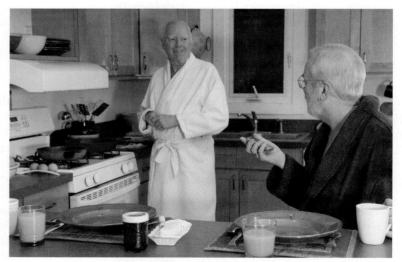

Some elderly gay and lesbian partners recall sanctions applied to homosexuals when they were younger and choose to remain "closeted," whereas others are adamant about expressing their sexuality openly in a more tolerant society.

a family, worship, vote, work, and live long, productive lives. There is a need to treat them as active members of society. In this spirit, the four goals of the Surgeon General's Call to Action to Improve the Health and Wellness of Persons with Disabilities are (U.S. Surgeon General issues first call to action on disability, 2005):

- Increase understanding nationwide that people with disabilities can lead long, healthy, and productive lives.

- Increase knowledge among healthcare professionals and provide them with tools to screen, diagnose, and treat the person with a disability with dignity.

- Increase awareness among people with disabilities regarding the steps they can take to develop and maintain a healthy lifestyle.

- Increase accessible health care and support services to promote independence for people with disabilities.

There are implications related to sexuality for each of the four goals. For example, a healthy lifestyle is important related to sexual interest and activity. It is also important for healthcare professionals to understand the whole person—including his or her sexuality.

Although we think of physical or mental challenges and illness as physical (biological) dimensions of sexuality, psychological and sociocultural dimensions also come into play. Mild depression is common among not only those with a chronic illness but also their caregivers and spouses, and it affects the couple's sexual activities. Further, an illness or disability may force a person to withdraw from normal social activities, thereby removing himself or herself from social support. Those who suffer from a disability also may suffer from body-image or gender-identity problems.

As with any sexual problem, it is not just the ill or disabled spouse who suffers. Both partners have to come to terms with changes in sexuality. Communication becomes a critical tool for acceptance of a new sexuality.

Physical Challenges

Physical challenge can result in any number of specific problems—for example, low energy levels, blindness or limited vision, movement problems, sensory loss, and the need to manage bags or tubes. Nevertheless, the challenged can generally find, or be helped to find, creative ways of overcoming such impediments to physical intimacy. For example,

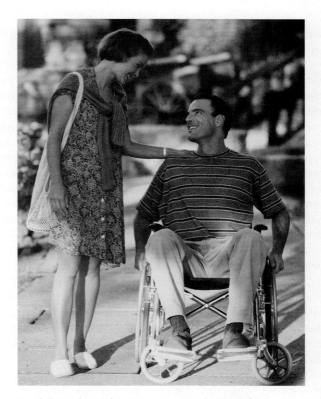

Disabilities do not have to prevent individuals from experiencing all the dimensions of human sexuality.

although most of us tend to focus on stimulating the genital area, in fact, the whole body can be stimulated and aroused. We can achieve sexual satisfaction—and possibly orgasm—without an erect penis or a well-lubricated vagina. With conscious intention and learning, anyone can use any part of the body in an infinite number of ways to achieve sexual satisfaction. For the challenged—as well as for the able-bodied—such learning can lead to a rich sexual life.

Even though sensory challenges, such as blindness and deafness, do not directly influence overall sexual responsiveness, they may affect sexuality. For example, people who have been blind for most or all of their life may have difficulty in understanding a partner's anatomy. Fortunately, educational programs, including learning about sexual anatomy and intercourse positions through the use of models, can be very helpful.

Deaf people may also have special challenges related to sexuality. For example, some of the usual communication routes may be blocked. Deaf people may miss words in lipreading or may be misunderstood when using sign language if others are not familiar with it. As people without such challenges do, those with sensory challenges may feel afraid or embarrassed when attempting to communicate about sexuality. Educational programs are needed for the sensory challenged just as they are needed for people without such challenges.

Cerebral palsy usually does not preclude interest in sexual activity, fertility, or ability to experience orgasm. Depending upon the nature and extent of problems with muscle control, those with cerebral palsy may have difficulty with certain sexual activities or positions. In addition, social rejection or feelings of inadequacy may become problems. Fortunately, education and counseling to help those with cerebral palsy understand their sexuality and learn appropriate social skills can help improve body image and ability to have intimate relationships.

Sometimes challenged people have to adapt their behavior to meet new conditions. For example, a woman with severe arthritis of the hip joints may find she cannot spread her legs wide enough for intercourse in the standard frontal position or that the weight of a partner's body may produce pain. She can employ rear entry or side-by-side coital positions that reduce or eliminate discomfort.

It is important to recognize certain aspects of sexual functioning in paralyzed individuals (Woods, 1979):

1. Some components of the human sexual response cycle (such as erection) are mediated by spinal-cord reflexes. Therefore, it is not necessary to have pathways from the brain to the sex organs. For example, stimuli resulting from pressure or tension in the pelvic organs or from touch excite impulses that can cause erection.

2. The level of the spinal-cord lesion and the degree of interruption of nerve impulses influence the nature of sexual functioning. For example, the local reflexes important in female orgasm are thought to be integrated into the lumbar and sacral regions of the cord.

3. Gratification can be obtained from sexual responses other than those from the sex organs during sexual stimulation. Many physically challenged people develop other areas of stimulation to high levels.

4. Adaptation of previous sexual practices may be needed after spinal-cord injury. Sexual activity may need to take place in different positions, and sexual aids may be helpful.

5. Fertility and the ability to bear children are usually not lost by women with spinal-cord injuries.

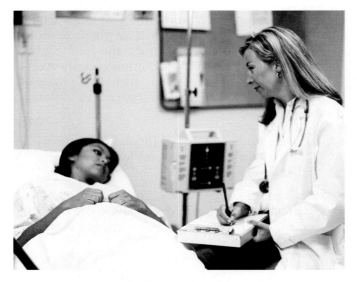

It is important to consider the sexuality of ill people just as we consider the sexuality of all other people.

Sexuality and Illness

The ill are another group whose sexuality has mainly been ignored. In the past both patients and medical personnel avoided any mention of sexual topics, no doubt because both were too embarrassed to discuss them. Now questions about sexual history are often asked in addition to standard questions about medical history. And physicians, patients, and partners are encouraged to discuss, when relevant, the effects of illness or other medical problems on sexual functioning.

Diabetes, neurological disorders, gynecological disorders, inflammation of the male's prostate gland, castration, rectal surgery, and heart attacks usually have a direct (or assumed) effect on sexual functioning. But people with other nonrelated physical medical problems often experience sexual problems caused by psychological factors. Some of us, for example, feel guilty when we get sick and try to determine where the fault lies. Because the topic of sexuality is a leading producer of guilt, we may consciously or unconsciously avoid sexual activity. We may even allow illness to restrict our sexual life, not because restriction is necessary but because we failed to ask medical personnel whether restriction was actually required.

To reduce sexual problems associated with illness, we need to feel that sexuality is appropriate to discuss, and we need to be aware of guilty feelings. And, in all cases of illness, we need to take responsibility for finding out the earliest and safest time to resume normal sexual activity to prevent other detrimental effects on interpersonal relationships,

Gender DIMENSIONS

Coming to Terms: Masculinity and Physical Challenges

Men with physical challenges are marginalized and stigmatized in American society. The image and reality of men with challenges undermine cultural beliefs about men's bodies and physicality. The body is a central foundation of how men define themselves and how they are defined by others. Bodies are vehicles for determining value, which in turn translates into status and prestige. Men's bodies allow them to demonstrate the socially valuable characteristics of toughness, competitiveness, and ability .... Thus, one's body and relationship to it provide a way to comprehend the world and one's place in it. The bodies of men with challenges serve as a continual reminder that they are at odds with the expectations of the dominant culture. As anthropologist Robert Murphy writes of his own experiences with disability:

> *Paralytic disability constitutes emasculation of a more direct and total nature. For the male, the weakening and atrophy of the body threaten all the cultural values of masculinity: strength, activeness, speed, virility, stamina, and fortitude.*

This article seeks to sharpen our understanding of the creation, maintenance, and re-creation of gender identities by men who, by birth, accident, or illness, find themselves dealing with a physical challenge. We examine two sets of social dynamics that converge and clash in the lives of men with physical challenges. On the one side, these men must deal with the presence and pressures of hegemonic masculinity, which demands strength. On the other side, societal members perceive people with disabilities to be weak.

Recently, the literature has shifted toward understanding gender as an interactive process. Thus, it is presumed to be not only an aspect of what one *is*, but more fundamentally it is something that one *does* in interaction with others .... Whereas previously gender was thought to be strictly an individual phenomenon, this new understanding directs our attention to the interpersonal and institutional levels as well. The lives of men with challenges provide an instructive arena in which to study the interactional nature of gender and its effect on individual gender identities.

In *The Body Silent*, Murphy (1990) observes that men with physical challenges experience "embattled identities" because of the conflicting expectations placed on them as men and as people with disabilities. On the one side, contemporary masculinity privileges men who are strong, courageous, aggressive, independent, and self-reliant .... On the other side, people with challenges are perceived to be, and treated as, weak, pitiful, passive, and dependent .... Thus, for men with physical challenges, masculine gender identity and practice are created and maintained at the crossroads of the demands of contemporary masculinity and the stigmatization associated with disability. As such, for men with physical disabilities, being recognized as masculine by others is especially difficult, if not impossible, to accomplish. Yet not being recognized as masculine is untenable because, in our culture, everyone is expected to display an appropriate gender identity.

Source: Data from Kimmel, M. S., & Messner, M. A. *Men's lives.* Needham, MA: Allyn & Bacon, 1998.

as well as on self-concept. For example, after a heart attack it would be helpful to know the following (Sexual activity and heart disease or stroke, 2005):

1. Having heart disease, a heart attack, or undergoing heart surgery does not mean an end to a satisfying sex life.

2. Sexual activity is not really risky for the heart.

3. If a person doesn't get short of breath, have chest pain, or get tired when climbing two

flights of stairs, the heart can meet the demands needed for sexual activity.

4. A person is usually able to resume sexual activity 3 to 4 weeks after a heart attack and 2 to 3 weeks after heart surgery.

5. A decrease in sexual desire after a heart attack or surgery can be expected. This is normal and should only be temporary.

The American Heart Association (2009) recommends that when people who have heart disease engage in sexual activities, they:

? Did You Know . . .

Persons with physical, cognitive, or emotional challenges have a right to sexuality education, sexual health care, and opportunities for socializing and for sexual expression. Family, healthcare workers, and other caregivers should receive training in understanding and supporting sexual development and behavior, comprehensive sexuality education, and related health care for individuals who have these challenges. The policies and procedures of social agencies and healthcare delivery systems should ensure that services and benefits are provided to all persons without discrimination and their caregivers have information and education about ways to minimize the risk of sexual abuse and exploitation.

Source: Modified from Position statement of Sexuality Information and Education Council of the United States, 2011. Available at http://www.siecus.org/index.cfm?fuseaction=Page.viewPage&pageId=494&parentID=472

- Choose a time when they are rested, relaxed, and free of the stressful feelings produced by the day's schedules and responsibilities.

- Wait 1 to 3 hours after eating a full meal, so that digestion can take place.

- Select a familiar, peaceful setting that is free of interruptions.

- Take medicine before sexual relations if prescribed by a physician.

Alzheimer's disease also affects sexuality. Some Alzheimer's sufferers develop a loss of libido, whereas others develop hypersexuality—a constant desire to engage in sexual activities. However, an affected spouse may demand sexual activity but not even recognize his or her own spouse. Caregivers say that the sexual encounter may be emotionless, mechanical, or marred by inappropriate behavior, such as giggling (Pope, 1999).

We also need to realize that sexual problems can be expressed through physical symptoms; a person who asks for an examination of the genital area because of a supposed concern about cancer may actually be seeking an acceptable way to talk about a sexual difficulty. The relationship between illness and sexuality needs to be understood to help reduce the incidence of problems in medical settings and to increase our acceptance of both ourselves and others when illness is present—either in or out of the hospital.

Emotional Challenges

Throughout this text we have emphasized a comprehensive concept of human sexuality. One excellent example of this concept is the influence of emotional states upon sexual responsiveness. Many life problems, such as stress, problems at work, death of a friend or relative, or work overload, may interfere with sexual interest or response. Apprehension about intimacy, fear of pregnancy, or possibly fear of contracting an STI may influence relationships with others. Depression or poor self-esteem can also create problems related to intimate relationships.

Whatever the reason, emotional well-being has a strong influence on overall sexuality and on sexual response. It can be helpful to understand that, at times, lack of interest in sexual activity or even inability to respond can be natural and common. Fortunately, these situations are usually temporary and can be effectively handled through personal understanding or professional counseling if needed.

Sexuality of the Mentally Challenged

For many years, the sexuality of the mentally challenged was dealt with by restricting or preventing

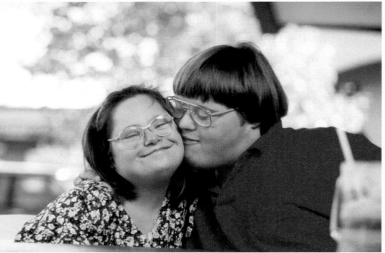

Despite many factors that must be considered, including safe sex and the ability to make proper decisions regarding sexuality, the mentally challenged are certainly capable of participating in sexual relationships. With the support of education and counseling, the mentally challenged can often greatly benefit from the affection and intimacy encountered through a sexual relationship.

sexual behavior; indeed, the mentally challenged were sterilized to prevent any chance of pregnancy. The societal fear was that the mentally challenged would have mentally challenged children and that they would not be able to care for their children properly—thus costly medical care would be needed. A turning point in the rights of the mentally challenged occurred with the election of President John F. Kennedy in 1960. His mentally challenged sister, Rosemary, had a profound effect on him and was a major factor in his proposing of legislation to educate and help the mentally challenged (Wilson et al., 1996).

The American Association on Intellectual and Developmental Disabilities has a position statement (Sexuality and Intellectual Disability, 2012) related to human sexuality. Among other points it says:

1. People with intellectual disabilities have sexuality, regardless of their degree of disability.

2. A person's ability to participate depends upon his or her functional social understanding.

3. Many adults with intellectual disability can develop meaningful, mutual relationships that may include a range of sexual activity and/or marriage.

4. People with intellectual disabilities have the right to be sexually active and the right and responsibility to be educated about sexuality, just like everyone else.

5. Some individuals who exhibit inappropriate sexual behavior do so as the result of limited communication and social skills.

6. Culturally acceptable, personally enjoyable social behaviors are the best safeguards from abuse for people with intellectual disabilities.

Mentally challenged people who are allowed to have sexual relationships can and do build feelings of affection and tenderness that appear to contribute to their happiness and tranquility. In 1970, the United Nations passed a resolution supporting the right of mentally challenged individuals to sexuality education, cohabitation, and marriage. Although the rights of the mentally challenged are indisputable, their ability to make proper decisions regarding sexuality is often disputed.

As everyone else can, the mentally challenged can benefit from sexuality education and counseling. Because being challenged is just one more dimension of human sexuality, it needs to be factored into the decision-making process. For example, a long-term contraceptive might be selected instead of oral contraceptive pills, because contraceptive effectiveness would not depend on remembering to take a pill every day. Through factual knowledge, role playing, and personal experience, the mentally challenged are able to have fulfilling sexual lives.

Personal and Social Support

Society in general continues to deny the sexuality of the ill and the challenged. If this situation is to change, we need to remember that these people are sexual beings in the same way as everyone else. We also need to prevent public service personnel from denying the sexuality of their clientele. Attention must be paid to policy decisions influencing human services; to approaches used to serve the ill and the challenged; and to attitudes of those working with these people, as well as of society in general. Organizations that provide services to the ill and challenged need to teach classes in sexuality, not only for their patients but also for their patients' relatives and those who work with them.

Exploring the Dimensions of Human Sexuality

Our feelings, attitudes, and beliefs regarding sexuality are influenced by our internal and external environments. Go to go.jblearning.com/dimensions5e to learn more about the biological, psychological, and sociological factors that affect your sexuality.

Case Study

The life cycle of sexuality, from high school graduation through aging, offers many opportunities to see the interaction of the dimensions of human sexuality.

Consider the aging process: Biological changes, especially in levels of hormones, can bring about psychological changes, such as in mood. In addition, a psychological shift occurs in men as they shift their attention from career to family. Cultural expectations affect elderly adults' perceptions and expectations of their sexuality.

New advances in pharmacology such as the introduction of Viagra and Cialis may solve a biological problem, but the couple must then solve the psychological and social problems related to reintegrating the ability to have an erection in the relationship. Although medication can solve most erectile disorder issues, an erection is also a function of psychosocial sexual attraction—something that cannot yet be purchased.

Biological Factors

When a sperm with a Y chromosome meets an egg, a male will develop. Biological factors continue to influence development throughout life.

- Genetic coding affects physical appearance, including height; coloration of skin, hair, and eyes; muscularity; and many aspects of health.
- Physiological changes result at puberty from the hormone testosterone, which in turn affects muscle development and body size. Testosterone also increases aggression and leads to increased rates of heart attacks.
- Toward middle age, testosterone levels begin to drop, resulting in decreased muscle mass, increased fat, and a reduced sex drive.

Sociocultural Factors

Sociocultural factors interact with biological factors to influence health.

- Laws affect what health insurers must cover. The Affordable Care Act contains requirements that will influence this.
- Religion may affect the decision as to whether to circumcise the penis.
- The cultural bias allowing men to be sexually permissive can compromise a man's sexual health and wellness.
- Ethnic heritage influences health; for example, African American males tend to have higher levels of stress and heart disease than white men do.
- Media and ads portray the ideal man with extreme muscularity which is achievable only with tremendous work and, in many cases, illegal steroids.
- Family, neighbors, and friends often reinforce gender stereotypes.
- Behavior proscribed by society as illegal can influence health; for instance, a man can compromise his health by taking anabolic steroids.

Psychological Factors

Biological and sociocultural factors combine to influence psychological factors.

- Body image and self-concept is enhanced for many men through exercise and competitive sports.
- Men often suppress their emotions, which can result in increased levels of stress.
- Learned attitudes and behaviors about gender roles can lead to unhealthy lifestyles for men.

Summary

- There are many theories about the types of love.

- It is important to understand sexual development during the college years. Many experiences and relationships with others will lay the foundation for future happiness.

- Although most people eventually marry, many are delaying marriage longer than in the past. Some people decide to remain single throughout life. In the United States, approximately 29% of women and 35.4% of men have never married.

- Cohabitation has drastically increased through the years. Today, some 6.66 million people live in a cohabiting relationship. There are a number of advantages and disadvantages related to cohabitation.

- Marriage is attractive to people for many reasons. More than 60% of males and females older than age 15 are married in the United States.

- There are many types of marriage—including the nuclear family, peer marriages, and step-families.

- Extramarital relationships may be consensual or nonconsensual. Many worthless facts exist about extramarital relationships.

- The divorce rate has declined in the last two decades largely because of people getting married later and being better educated. Approximately 9% of males and 11% of females in the United States are divorced.

- Most older people remain interested in sexual activity and participate in various forms of sexual activity. Some health difficulties associated with aging may impede sexual activities.

- Today there is increased recognition of the sexuality of physically and mentally challenged people.

Discussion Questions

1. Compare and contrast the different theories about love. Which do you agree with? Explain why.

2. Summarize the studies about college relationships and sexual activities.

3. Discuss why increased numbers of people are remaining single.

4. Compare the advantages and disadvantages of cohabitation versus marriage.

5. Discuss why marriage is popular.

6. Discuss the reasons for divorce. What can be done to help protect children?

7. Discuss how and why the aging process affects sexuality.

Application Questions

Reread the chapter-opening story and answer the following questions.

1. The names Lynn and Chris were deliberately used as pseudonyms because they are names used by both genders. When you read the story, who did you think was the male? The female? Explain your answer. Then switch the genders of Lynn and Chris and reread the story. Does it strike you differently now? Why?

2. What advice from the chapter might have helped Lynn and Chris have a better marriage?

Critical Thinking Questions

1. Should mildly mentally challenged people be allowed to have children? Would they be any better or worse than typical parents (who have to learn from the start as well)? If mentally challenged parents are denied reproduction rights, what about those who have diagnosed psychiatric illness (such as depression)?

2. An increasing percentage of the population is remaining permanently single. Discuss whether this trend appears to be long term or just temporary. What are its implications for population growth? The future of Social Security?

3. Because of all the problems that divorce causes, should it be outlawed? What effects would such a law have on families?

4. Write a prenuptial agreement, indicating your expectations and responsibilities in marriage. Be sure to include how financial decisions, household tasks, child-rearing responsibilities, and so on, will be handled. Would such a document help or hinder a marriage?

Critical Thinking Case

Although dual-income families have become very common, equal sharing of work around the house is not as common. It is common for women to be responsible for things like shopping, cooking, and cleaning. It is common for men to more often be responsible for maintenance and repairs around the house.

The fact that many women are responsible for more of the housework has commonly been referred to as the "second shift." The first shift is the paid job outside the home, and the second shift is all the work at home. Putting the two shifts together, women put in much more work time than men.

In addition, many of women's tasks with children involve maintenance activities such as feeding, bathing, taking them to the doctor, and helping with homework. In contrast, men often help out with the more fun activities like going to the movies or playing in the park.

Consider which dimensions of human sexuality influence the continuation of this phenomenon. What could be done to break out of the stereotyped roles and create a more equal home environment? Should there be a more equal home environment?

Exploring Personal Dimensions

Are You Ready for Marriage?

The following quiz, developed by three clinical psychologists and marriage therapists, can help you decide whether marriage is right for you at this point in your life. Respond as honestly as you can to the following statements. Indicate which of the two choices more closely reflects your personal opinions and priorities by placing a check before line "a" or "b." (If you have a mate, you might each fill out the quiz separately, and then compare your answers.)

1. _____ a I wouldn't feel alive unless I were married.

   _____ b Give me liberty or give me death.

2. _____ a My "favorite things to do" are typical of married people.

   _____ b My hobbies and interests are those of a single person.

3. _____ a Being married can give me more of the security I want.

   _____ b Being single can probably give me more of the career opportunities I want.

4. _____ a I'd love to vacation alone somewhere with my spouse.

   _____ b I'd love to vacation with different people at different times.

5. _____ a Married means being sexually content.

   _____ b Single means being sexually content.

6. _____ a I prefer the stability and security of married life.

   _____ b I prefer the self-reliance and adventure of single life.

7. _____ a I want sex and affection from one reliable person.

   _____ b I want a variety of lovers.

8. _____ a Marriage is underrated.

   _____ b Marriage is overrated.

9. _____ a I'm willing to work to make my spouse happy.

   _____ b I don't want to be responsible for my mate's happiness.

10. _____ a It's morally more correct to live a married life.

    _____ b I'd like to do things when I want, without family constraints.

11. _____ a I'm ready to share my life and my credit cards.

    _____ b I'm ready to share good times, but let's not get too serious.

12. _____ a I believe that people should be married.

    _____ b I think people are happier if they are single.

13. _____ a Sex is best with one's spouse.

    _____ b Sex is too delicious to limit it to one person.

14. _____ a My career plans can tolerate or maybe even benefit from my being married.

    _____ b My career plans benefit from my being single.

15. _____ a I prefer the majority of my friends to be married.

    _____ b I prefer the majority of my friends to be single.

16. _____ a A marriage can be a beautiful experience.

    _____ b A marriage can be a trap.

17. _____ a I'd like to know whom I'll be sleeping with for the rest of my life.

    _____ b I don't want to know whom I'll be sleeping with for the rest of my life.

18. _____ a Today's smart people are getting married.

    _____ b Today's smart people are single and enjoying it.

19. _____ a The pleasures of marriage are wonderful.

_____ b The risk of a bad marriage more than offsets any pleasure.

20. _____ a "Love" and "marriage" go together.

_____ b "Love" and "independence" go together.

21. _____ a I don't mind sharing bank accounts and expenses.

_____ b I'm too independent to enjoy sharing my money with a spouse.

22. _____ a I want to pour all my love into a permanent relationship.

_____ b I'm not happy with an exclusive love relationship.

23. _____ a The economic advantages of being married are important to me.

_____ b I like the idea of being single so I can spend my money as I wish.

24. _____ a Being married is important from a moral/religious standpoint.

_____ b Morality and religion have little to do with marital status.

25. _____ a Lovemaking with one's spouse is certainly best.

_____ b The many sexual opportunities of being single are a great advantage.

26. _____ a My greatest chance for personal growth is through marriage.

_____ b My greatest chance for personal growth is through independence.

27. _____ a I'd prefer to share the risks of life with a spouse.

_____ b My privacy is too important for me to enjoy being married.

28. _____ a I want a reliable lifetime relationship in marriage.

_____ b I'd rather live free and easy and singly.

29. _____ a I'd be willing to make major changes, such as moving to another state, to help a spouse.

_____ b I'm not ready to move, or make other major changes, to help a spouse.

30. _____ a Marriages are made in heaven.

_____ b Marriages are too often made in hell.

31. _____ a My recreational interests are family oriented.

_____ b My recreational interests are for singles.

32. _____ a I'd enjoy the security involved in being married.

_____ b I prefer the freedom of being single.

33. _____ a I would love to have children.

_____ b I don't want the responsibility of a family.

34. _____ a Being married offers joint tax returns and other financial benefits.

_____ b I prefer to spend my money the way I want to.

35. _____ a I prefer sex and affection with my spouse for life.

_____ b I prefer love affairs with many people.

36. _____ a I prefer the steady companionship of being married.

_____ b I prefer the excitement of companionship with many lovers.

37. _____ a I'd enjoy spending leisure time with my spouse.

_____ b I like spending my leisure time as I please.

38. _____ a If I have to choose between career advancement and marriage, I choose marriage.

_____ b If I have to choose between career advancement and marriage, I'll take career.

39. _____ a Married people can count on sexual satisfaction from a trusted partner.

_____ b Single people can find lovers from an endless pool of possibilities.

40. _____ a Marriage requires major compromises, and I'm willing to make them.

_____ b Marriage requires major compromises, and I'm not yet ready to make them.

Scoring the Quiz

1. Count the number of your "a" responses and write the total here: _____

2. Compare your number of "a" responses with the following scale to determine your level.

   0–20 = Low readiness

   21–30 = Medium readiness

   31–40 = High readiness

Interpreting Your Score

Low marriage readiness: If you scored here, your values are heavily weighted toward a single lifestyle. Even if you've found a partner who shares your interests and values, the importance you attach to marriage at this time isn't enough to ensure success. Don't marry on the assumption that your values will change. They may not. And you shouldn't marry on the basis of other people's expectations or views about being married. *Yours* are the only ones that really count when it comes to marriage.

Though you may not value married life now, marriage readiness can develop rapidly. You may grow tired of the freedom and lifestyle that characterize being single, or come to appreciate more those elements associated with being married. Continue to review your marriage readiness from time to time, but do NOT marry until your values will support it.

Medium marriage readiness: Your values blend support for both single and married lifestyles, which means there's a certain level of risk if you choose to get married at this time. Probably the most important issue for you to consider is your potential mate's marriage readiness. Someone with a high readiness level can add stability to the relationship, increasing the likelihood of its success. Conversely, someone without it would dramatically reduce your already uncertain potential for a good marriage.

If he/she is less ready for marriage than you, be wary of demands for concessions. For example, he/she may say, in effect, "Do what I want or I'm getting out. I don't really want to be married as much as you do anyway." This is a destructive gambit; don't be pushed into a decision you're not ready to make.

A second major issue for you is the parity "fit" between you and your potential mate—your approximate equality in terms of personality, status, and appearance. Medium marriage readiness provides little cushion against the costs of an unequal match. High parity may lead to a successful marriage even if one or both partners possess only medium marriage readiness. But as the parity levels decrease, the greater the need for both partners to have a strong commitment to their marriage.

High marriage readiness: Your values strongly support married life, and your only challenge will be to find the right match. Be on guard, however, against projecting your own high level of marriage readiness onto a potential mate. The key for you is to realize that although you may be ready, you still need to choose your partner wisely.

Suggested Readings

Fisher, H. The Match.com Single in America study, 2011. Available: http://blog.match.com/singles-study/.

Kim, H. S. Consequences of parental divorce for child development. *American Sociological Review*, 77, no. 30 (2011), 487–511.

Menopausal symptoms and CAM. National Center for Complementary and Alternative Medicine, 2011. Available: http://nccam.nih.gov/health/menopause/menopausesymptoms.htm.

Parker-Pope, T. *For Better: The science of good marriage*. New York: Dutton, 2010.

Schwartz, P., & Young, L. Sexual satisfaction in committed relationships. *Sexuality Research and Social Policy*, 6, no. 1 (March 2009), 1–17.

Sexuality in later life. National Institute on Aging, 2011. Available: www.nia.nih.gov/HealthInformation/Publications/sexuality.htm.

Shildrick, M. Contested pleasures: The sociopolitical economy of disability and sexuality. *Sexuality Research and Social Policy*, 4, no. 1 (March 2007), 53–66.

Wilcox, W. B. & Marquardt, E. The State of Our Unions. The National Marriage Project, The University of Virginia, 2011. Available: http://www.virginia.edu/marriageproject/pdfs/Union_2011.pdf.

Web Resources

For links to the websites below, visit *http://sexuality.jbpub.com/dimensions/5e* and click on Resource Links.

Child Trends Data Bank
www.childtrendsdatabank.org

Information about the well-being of children, family structure, and family trends.

The National Marriage Project
www.virginia.edu/marriageproject/

Information about marriage, divorce, cohabitation, and some international comparisons.

U.S. Census Bureau
www.census.gov

Statistics on marriages, divorces, and various types of families and living arrangements.

Mayo Clinic.com
www.mayoclinic.com

Information on sexual health of various groups of people.

Surgeon General's Call to Action to Improve the Health and Wellness of Persons with Disabilities
www.surgeongeneral.gov/library/disabilities/

Provides a copy of the full call to action along with fact sheets about parts of the call.

References

Acevedo, B. P., & Aron, A. Does a long-term relationship kill romantic love? *Review of General Psychology, 13, 1* (2009), 59–65.

Almost all millennials accept interracial dating and marriage. Pew Research Publications, 2010. Available: http://pewresearch.org/pubs/1480/millennials-accept-iinterracial-dating-marriage-friends-different-race-generations.

American fact finder. U.S. Bureau of the Census, 2011. Available: http://factfinder2.census.gov/.

American Heart Association. *Sexual Activity and Heart Disease or Stroke*, 2009. Available: http://www.americanheart.org/presenter.jhtml?identifier=4714.

American Time Use Survey. U. S. Bureau of Labor Statistics, June 22, 2011. Available: http://www.bls.gov/news.release/pdf/atus.pdf.

An arrangement of marriages. *Psychology Today, 26* (January/February 1993), 22.

Aron, A., Fisher, H. A., Mashek, D. J., Strong, G., Li, H., & Brown, L. L. Reward, motivation and emotion systems associated with early-stage intense romantic love. *Journal of Neurophysiology, 94* (May 31, 2005), 327–337.

Ashley Madison News, 2011. Available: http://www.ashleymadison.com/cheating/news.html.

Avellar, S. The economic consequences of the dissolution of cohabiting unions. *Journal of Marriage and Family 67, no. 2* (May 2005), 315–327.

Baron, K. New poll reveals that we are not happy with our sex lives. Associated Press LifGoesStrong.com poll, 2010. Available: http://www.lifegoesstrong.com/sex-poll.

Baron, R. A. *Psychology*, 4th ed. Needham Heights, MA: Allyn & Bacon, 1998.

Births to unmarried women. Child Trends Data Bank, 2011. Available: http://www.childtrendsdatabank.org/?=node/196.

Blumstein, P., & Schwartz, P. *American couples*. New York: William Morrow, 1983.

The boomer sandwich. *Modern Maturity, 44, no. 5* (September/October 2001), 94.

Borenstein, S. The science of romance: Brains have a love circuit. *ajc.com: The Atlanta Journal Constitution* (February 13, 2009).

Bretschneider, J., & McCoy, N. Sexual interest and behavior in healthy 80–102 year olds. *Archives of Sexual Behavior, 17* (1988), 109–130.

Brooks, S. B. Matchmaking ASAP. *The Birmingham News* (January 11, 2004), 1E & 8E.

Buss, D. *The evolution of desire: Strategies of human mating*. New York: Basic Books, 1994.

Buss, D., et al. International preferences in selecting mates. *Journal of Cross-Cultural Psychology, 21* (1990), 5–47.

Call, V., Sprecher, S., & Schwartz, P. The incidence and frequency of marital sex in a national sample. *Journal of Marriage and the Family 57, no. 3* (August 1995), 639–652.

Census Bureau releases estimates of same-sex married couples. U.S. Census Bureau, 2011. Available: http://2010.census.gov/news/releases/operations/cb11-cn181.html.

Center for Families in Transition, Scottsdale, AZ. 2003. Available: http://www.centerforfamilies.net/index.htm.

Clements, M. Sex in America today. *Parade* (August 7, 1994), 4–6.

Cohn, D. New Facts About Families. Pew Research Center Publications, 2011.

Crandell, S. Oh baby. *AARP The Magazine* (September/October, 2005), 108–117.

Cullen, L. T. Cupid academy. *Time, 163, no. 7* (February 16, 2004), 67–68.

Davis, K. E. Near and dear: Friendship and love compared. *Psychology Today, 22* (February 1985).

DeBeauvoir, S. *The coming of age*. New York: Warner Books, 1973.

The decline of marriage and rise of new families. Pew Research Center Publications, November, 2010. Available: http://pewresearch.org/pubs/1802/decline-marriage-rise-new-families.

DeParle, J., & Tavernise, S. For women under 30, most births occur outside marriage. *The New York Times*, February 17, 2012. Available: http://www.nytimes.com/2012/02/18/us/for-women-under-30-most-births-occur-outside-marriage.html?pagewanted=all.

Easton, J. A., Confer, J. C., Goetz, C. D., & Buss, D. M. Reproduction expediting: Sexual motivations, fantasies, and the ticking biological clock. *Personality and Individual Differences, 49* (2010), 516–520.

Elliott, S., & Umberson, D. The performance of desire: Gender and sexual negotiation in long-term marriages. *Journal of Marriage and Family, 70, 2* (April 2008), 391–406.

Elmer-Dewitt, P. Now for the truth about Americans and sex. *Time* (October 17, 1994), 64.

Fields, J. America's families and living arrangements: 2003. *Current Population Reports*, U.S. Census Bureau, 2004.

Francese, P. Stat of the day: Census finds 1.3 million fewer nuclear families. ADAGESTAT, June 8, 2011. Available: http://adage.com/article/adagestat/census-finds-1-3-million-fewer-nuclear-families/228057/.

Fromm, E. *The art of loving*. New York: Harper and Row, 1956.

Frosch, D. Hard times for gay retirement havens. *The New York Times*, October 28, 2011. Available: http://www.nytimes.com/2011/10/29/us/gay-retirement-communities-struggling-in-the-recession.html?pagewanted=all.

Fry, R., & Cohn, D. Living together: The economics of Cohabitation. Pew Research Center Publications, 2011.

Gonzales, L. The biology of attraction. *Men's Health, 20, no. 6* (September 2005), 186–193.

Hans, J. D. Do love styles predict lifetime number of sex partners? *American Journal of Sexuality Education, 3, 2* (2008), 149–159.

Hatfield, E. Passionate and compassionate love. In *The psychology of love*, Sternberg, R., & Barnes, M., eds. New Haven: Yale University Press, 1988.

Henslin, J. M. *Sociology*, 2nd ed. Needham Heights, MA: Allyn & Bacon, 1995.

Hunt, M. *Sexual behavior in the 1970's*. Chicago: Playboy Press, 1974.

In their own right: Addressing the sexual and reproductive health needs of American men. Alan Guttmacher Institute (2002). Available: http://www.agi-usa.org/pubs/exs_men.html.

Intimacy and aging: Tips for sexual health and happiness. *MayoClinic.com* (November 18, 2003). Available: http://www.mayoclinic.com/invoke.cfm?id=HA00035.

Jacoby, S. Sex in America 2005. *AARP the Magazine, 48, no. 4b* (July/August 2005), 57–62+.

Kaplan, H. S. *The new sex therapy: Active treatment of sexual dysfunction.* New York: Brunner/Mazel, 1974.

Kempner, M. E. Marriage: Institution or relationship? *SIECUS Report, 33, no. 1* (winter 2005), 2–4.

Kids Count Data Center, 2011. Children in Single-Parent Families (Number)-2010; Children in Single-Parent Families (Percent)-2010. Available: http://datacenter.kidscount.org/data/acrossstates/Rankings.aspx?.

Kiecolt-Glaser, J. The risks of marital discord. *U.S. News & World Report* (January 28 2009). Available: http://researchnews.osu.edu/archive/fighting.htm.

King, V. A Comparison of cohabiting relationships among older and younger adults. *Journal of Marriage & Family, 67, no. 2* (January 2005), 271–285.

Klinenberg, E. Living alone is the new norm. *Time, 197, no. 10* (March 12, 2012), 60–62.

Koss-Feder, L. Bunking in with mom and dad. *Time, 173, 8* (March 2, 2009), 537.

Kurdek, L. A. Are gay and lesbian cohabiting couples really different from heterosexual married couples? *Journal of Marriage & Family, 66, no. 4* (November 2004), 880–900.

Laumann, E. O., Gagnon, J. H., Michael, R. T., & Michaels, S. *The social organization of sexuality: Sexual practices in the United States.* Chicago: University of Chicago Press, 1994.

Lee, J. Love-styles, in *The psychology of love*, Sternberg, R., & Barnes, M., eds. New Haven: Yale University Press, 1988.

Lewis, J. E., Malow, R. M., & Ireland, S. J. HIV/AIDS risk in heterosexual college students: A review of a decade of literature. *Journal of American College Health, 45, no. 4* (1997), 147–158.

LGBT older adults in long-term care facilities: Stories from the field. National Senior Citizens Law Center, 2011. Available: http://lgbtlongtermcare.org/.

Liebowitz, M. *The chemistry of love.* Boston: Little, Brown, 1983.

Lindau, S. T., Schumm, L. P., Laumannm, E. O., Levinson, W., O'Muircheartaigh, C. A., & Waite, L. J. A study of sexuality and health among older adults in the United States. *New England Journal of Medicine, 357, 8* (August 23, 2007), 762–774.

Link, A., & Copeland, P. Sexual magnetism: Pheromones—the scent of sex. *Urban Male Magazine* (Winter 2001), 38–39.

Liu, C. Does quality of marital sex decline with duration? *Archives of Sexual Behavior, 32, no. 1* (February 2003), 55–60.

Living together before marriage may hurt—not help—chances of successful match. *InteliHealth* (July 25, 2002). Available: http://www.intelihealth.com.

Livingston, G., & Cohn, D. More women without children. Pew Research Center, June 25, 2010. Available: http://pewresearch.org/pubs/1642/more-women-without-children.

Marriage Project, Rutgers, the State University of New Jersey, 2005. Available: http://marriage.rutgers.edu.

Maslow, A. H. *Toward a psychology of being*, 2nd ed. Princeton, NJ: Van Nostrand, 1968.

Masters, W. H., & Johnson, V. E. *Human sexual response.* Boston: Little, Brown, 1966.

Match.com and Chadwick Martin Bailey 2009–2010 studies: Recent trends: Online dating, 2010. Available: http://cp.match.com/cppp/media/CMB_Study.pdf.

Menopause. National Institute on Aging, 2010. Available: http://www.nia.nih.gov/health/publication/menopause.

Menopause. National Institute on Aging, 2010. Available: http://www.nia.nih.gov/HealthInformation/Publications/menopause.htm.

Miller, A. J., Sassler, S., & Kusi-Appouh, D. The specter of divorce: Views from working-class and middle class cohabitors. *Family Relations, 60* (2011), 602–616.

Montenegro, X. P. Lifestyles, dating and romance: A study of midlife singles. *AARP the Magazine* (September 2003). Available: http://www.aarp.org.

Morin, R. The public renders a split verdict on changes in family structure. Pew Research Center, February 6, 2011. Available: http://pewsocialtrends.org/files/2011/02/Pew-Social-Trends-Changes-In-Family-Structure.pdf.

Mulhauser, D. Dating among college students is all but dead, survey finds. *Chronicle of Higher Education, 47, no. 48* (August 10, 2001), A51.

Musick, K., & Bumpass, L. Reexamining the case for marriage: union formation and changes in well-being. *Journal of Marriage and Family, 74, no. 1* (February 2012), 1–18.

National Council on the Aging. *Half of older Americans report they are sexually active: 4 in 10 want more sex, says new survey.* Press release, September 28, 1998.

National Survey of Sexual Health and Behavior. Indiana University Center for Sexual Health Promotion, 2010. Available: http://www.nationalsexstudy.indiana.edu/.

Orecklin, M. Stress and the superdad. *Time, 164, no. 8* (August 23, 2004), 38–39.

Osborne, D. Sexual health: An interview with a Mayo clinic specialist. Mayo-Clinic.com (December 2004). Available: http://www.mayoclinic.com/invoke.cfm?id=HQ01363.

Osteoporosis Handout on Health. National Institute of Health Osteoporosis and Related Bone Diseases National Resource Center, 2011. Available: http://www.niams.nih.gov/Health_Info/Bone/Osteoporosis/osteoporosis_hoh.asp.

Oswalt, S. B. Beyond risk: Examining college students' sexual decision making. *American Journal of Sexuality Education 5, no. 3* (July–September, 2010), 217–239.

Paik, A. "Hookups," dating, and relationship quality: Does the type of sexual involvement matter? *Social Science Research 39, no. 5* (September, 2010), 739–753.

Pearson, J. C. *Gender and communication.* Dubuque, IA: William C. Brown, 1985.

Penhollow, T. M., Young, M., & Denny, G. Predictors of quality of life, sexual intercourse, and sexual satisfaction among active older adults. *American Journal of Health Education, 40, 1* (January/February 2009), 14–22.

Planned Parenthood Federation. *Thinking about adoption,* 2009. Available: http://www.plannedparenthood.org/health-topics/pregnancy/adoption-21520.htm.

Poll: More Americans Favor Same-Sex Marriage. CNN Political Ticker, April 19, 2011. Available: http://politicalticker.blogs.cnn.com/2011/04/19/poll-more-americans-favor-same-sex-marriage/.

Pope, E. When illness takes sex out of a relationship. *SIECUS Report, 27, no. 3* (February/March 1999), 8–11.

Popenoe, D. Cohabitation, marriage and child wellbeing. National Marriage Project, 2008. Available: http://marriage.rutgers.edu/Publications/2008cohabreport.html.

Popenoe, D., & Whitehead, B. D. The state of our unions 2000. The National Marriage Project. 2001. Available: http://marriage.rutgers.edu/state_of_our_union%202000%20text%20only.htm.

Popenoe, D., & Whitehead, B. D. The state of our unions 2005. The National Population 65 years and older in the United States, 2011. U.S. Census Bureau, American Fact Finder. Available: http://factfinder2.census.gov/faces/tableservices/jsf/pages/productview.xhtml?pid=ACS_10_1YR_S0103&prodType=table.

Qian, Z., & Lichter, D. T. Changing patterns of interracial marriage in a multicultural society. *Journal of Marriage and Family, 73, no. 5* (October, 2011), 1065–1084.

Reinisch, J. M., Hill, C. A., Sanders, S. A., & Zembia-Davis, M. High-risk sexual behavior at a Midwestern university—a confirmation survey. *Family Planning Perspectives, 27, no. 2* (March/April 1995), 79–82.

Rempel, J. K., & Burris, C. T. Let me count the ways: An integrative theory of love and hate. *Personal Relationships, 12, no. 2* (June 2005), 297–313.

Renzetti, C. M., & Curren, D. J. *Living sociology.* Needham Heights, MA: Allyn & Bacon, 1998.

Rosenbloom, S. The new dating tools: A card and a wink. *The New York Times,* July 21, 2010. Available: http://www.nytimes.com/2010/07/22/fashion/22date.html.

Ross, M. W. Situating sexuality electronically: The Internet and sexual expression. *Sexuality Research & Public Policy, 4, 2* (June 2007), 1–4.

Safer sex guidelines. Information. Education. Action (2009). Available: http://www.aids.org/factSheets/151-Safer-Sex-Guidelines.html.

Sanders, S. A. Midlife sexuality: The need to integrate biological, psychological, and social perspectives. *SIECUS Report, 27, no. 3* (February/March 1999), 3–7.

Schmid, R. E. Unmarried couples top 4 million. *AP/AOL* (July 27, 1998).

Schnarch, D., & Morehouse, R. Online sex, dyadic crises, and pitfalls for MFTs. *Family Therapy Magazine, 1, no. 5* (September/October 2002), 14–19.

Sexual activity and heart disease or stroke. American Heart Association, 2005. Available: http://www.americanheart.org/presenter.jhtml?identifier=4714.

Sexual problems overview, 2005. Available: http://www.drkoop.com/ency/93/001951.html

Sexuality and Intellectual Disability. American Association on Intellectual and Developmental Disabilities, 2012. Available: http://www.aamr.org/content_198.cfm.

Should people not cohabit before getting married? In *Taking sides: Issues in family and personal relationships*, Schroeder, E., ed. Guilford, CT: McGraw-Hill/Dushkin, 2003.

Singh, D. Female mate value at a glance: Relationship of waist-to-hip ratio to health, fecundity, and attractiveness. *Human Ethology & Evolutionary Psychology, 23* (December 2002), 81–91.

Single parenting and today's family. American Psychological Association, 1998. Available: http://helping.apa.org/family/single.html.

Smith, T. W. *American sexual behavior: Trends, socio-demographic differences, and risk behavior*. Chicago: National Opinion Research Center, 2003.

Smock, P. J., Bergstrom, C., Huang, P., & Manning, W. Why shack up? Motivations to cohabit among young adults in the U.S. Presented at 37th World Congress of the International Institute of Sociology, Stockholm, Sweden, July 5–9, 2005.

Stanton, A. Affairs, part 2: Understanding what went wrong. Health and age. Novartis Foundation for Gerontology, 2001. Available: http://www.healthandage.com/Home/gid2=1258.

Sternberg, R. A triangular theory of love. *Psychological Review, 93* (1986), 119–135.

Sternberg, R. *The triangle of love: Intimacy, passion, commitment*. New York: Basic Books, 1988.

Stritof, S., & Stritof, B. Marital sex statistics. About.com. Marriage, 2010. Available: http://marriage.about.com/cs/sexualstatistics/a/sexstatistics.htm.

Studies show shifting paradigm of sexual relationships among young adults. National Partnership for Women and Health, April 4, 2011. Available: http://www.nationalpartnership.org/site/News2?abbr=daily2_&page=NewsArticle&id=28190.

Survey finds gaps between safe-sex claims, behavior among U.S. adults. *Kaiser Daily Reproductive Health Report*, (April 7, 2004). Available: http://www.kaisernetwork.org.

Survey USA public opinion poll (1998). Available: http://www.surveyusa.com.

Surveys show change in attitudes toward sex among high school and college students, higher incidences of "casual" and oral sex. *Kaiser Daily Reproductive Health Report* (January 21, 2003). Available: http://www.kaisernetwork.org.

Swami, V. An examination of the love-is-blind bias among gay men and lesbians. *Body Image* (February 3, 2009).

That's what he said. Seventeen Magazine and the National Campaign to Prevent Teen and Unplanned Pregnancy, 2010. Available: http://www.thenationalcampaign.org.

Trail, T. E., & Karney, B. R. What's (not) wrong with low-income marriages. *Journal of Marriage and Family, 74, no. 3* (June 2012), 413–427.

Trompeter, S. E., Bettencourt, R., & Barnett-Connor, E. Sexual activity and satisfaction in health community-dwelling older women. *American Journal of Medicine 125, no. 1* (January 2012), 37–43.

U.S. Bureau of Labor Statistics. Single-parent households by country, September 30, 2011. Updated and Revised from Families and Work in Transition in 12 Countries, 1980–2001, *Monthly Labor Review* (September 2003), with national sources, some of which may be unpublished.

U.S. Surgeon General issues first call to action on disability. United States Department of Health and Human Services, July 26, 2005. Available: http://www.surgeongeneral.gov.

Wallerstein, J. S. *Nine "psychological tasks" needed for a good marriage*. American Psychological Association, 1996.

Walsh, A. *The science of love: Understanding love and its effects on mind and body*. Buffalo, NY: Prometheus, 1991.

Whitchurch, E. R., Wilson, T. D., & Gilbert, D. T. "He loves me, ne loves me not ...", uncertainty can increase romantic attraction. *Psychological Science, 22, no. 2* (February 2011), 172–175.

Whitehead, B. D., & Popenoe, D. Life without children: The social retreat from children and how it is changing America. National Marriage Project, Rutgers, the State University of New Jersey, 2008.

Whitty, M. T. The realness of cybercheating: Men's and women's representations of unfaithful Internet relations. *Social Science Computer Review, 23, no. 1* (Spring 2005), 57–67.

Why couples who have broken up should not get back together: Relationships expert. Health, Medical, and Science Updates. Stone Hearth News, February 20, 2012. Available: http://www.stonehearthnewsletters.com/why-couples-who-have-broken-up-should-not-get-back-together-relationships-expert/relationships/.

Wilcox, W. B., & Marquardt, E. The state of our unions. The National Marriage Project, The University of Virginia, 2010. Available: http://www.virginia.edu/marriageproject/pdfs/Union_11_12_10.pdf.

Wilson, G. T., Nathan, P. E., O'Leary, K. D., & Clark, L. A. *Abnormal psychology: Integrating perspectives*. Needham, MA: Allyn & Bacon, 1996.

Womenshealth.gov. Menopausal Hormone Therapy (MHT), 2011. Available: http://womenshealth.gov/glossary/index.cfm#M.

Woods, N. F. *Human sexuality in health and illness*. St. Louis: Mosby, 1979.

CHAPTER 13

Sexual Techniques and Behavior

FEATURES

Global Dimensions
Global Religious Views on Sexuality

Gender Dimensions
Differences Between Male and Female Sexual Fantasies

Ethical Dimensions
Should People Who Do Not Feel Comfortable with Oral or Anal Sexual Activity Learn to Enjoy These Activities?

Multicultural Dimensions
Does Level of Education Influence Sexuality?

Global Dimensions
Age of First Intercourse

Communication Dimensions
Word Choice Affects Study Results

CHAPTER OBJECTIVES

1 Identify the historical basis for present-day societal, religious, and/or cultural attitudes toward masturbation.

2 Cite the prevalence of sexual fantasy, describe its content and function, and note differences in male and female sexual fantasies.

3 Describe the role of touch, sight, smell, sound, and taste in sexual foreplay. Then list and describe various positions of sexual intercourse, including their advantages and disadvantages.

go.jblearning.com/dimensions5e

The Importance of the Senses
Global Dimensions: Global Religious Views on Sexuality

INTRODUCTION

*O*ne often hears that the 20th century's sexual revolution has led to more promiscuity and sexual freedom. The following excerpt, written before a different sort of revolution—the American Revolution—shows that many sexual techniques have not changed in a long time:

> As I kept hesitating and disconcerted under this soft distraction, Charles, with a fond impatience, took the pains to undress me; and all I can remember amidst the flutter and discomposure of my senses was some flattering exclamations of joy and admiration, more specially at the feel of my breasts now set at liberty from my stays, and which panting and rising in tumultuous throbs, swell'd upon his dear touch, and gave it the welcome pleasure of finding them well form'd, and unfail'd in firmness.

> I was soon laid in bed, and scarce languish'd an instant for the darling partner of it, before he was undress'd and got between the sheets, with his arms clasp'd round me, giving and taking, with gust inexpressible, a kiss of welcome, that my heart rising to my lips stamp'd with its warmest impression, concurring to my bliss, with that delicate and voluptuous emotion which Charles alone had the secret to excite, and which constitutes the very life, the essence of pleasure....

> But as action was now a necessity to desires so much on edge as ours, Charles, after a very short prelusive dalliance, lifting up my linen and his own, laid the broad treasures of his manly chest close to my bosom, both beating with the tenderest alarms: when now, the sense of his glowing body, in naked touch with mine, took all power over my thoughts out of my own disposal, and deliver'd up every faculty of the soul to the sensiblest of joys, that affecting me infinitely more with my distinction of the person than of the sex, now brought my conscious heart deliciously into play: my heart, which eternally constant to Charles, had never taken any part in my occasional sacrifices to the calls of constitution, complaisance, or interest.

The preceding excerpt, from John Cleland's 1749 novel *Fanny Hill, or Letters of a Woman of Pleasure*, shows that erotic literature has detailed sexual liaisons for centuries.

Relatively few people actually set out to learn effective sexual arousal techniques. What learning takes place often occurs through trial and error *(with plenty of both). The results may be total pleasure, or they may be shame and embarrassment, confusion, and perhaps sexual dysfunction. Furthermore, such naivete and ignorance too often result in unwanted pregnancies. We believe that a strong foundation of sexual knowledge includes not only anatomical and physiological facts but also specific information about what people find sexually stimulating. Therefore, this chapter covers nonphysical means of arousal, as well as techniques in beginning play (foreplay), sexual intercourse, and oral–genital sexual activity.*

■ Autoerotic Sexual Behaviors

The two solitary sexual behaviors we discuss in this section are masturbation and fantasy. We should note, however, that although these are usually solitary behaviors, they can also be engaged in with a partner in the form of mutual masturbation or shared sexual fantasizing.

Masturbation

One need not have a partner to be sexually stimulated. **Masturbation** is the stimulation of one's own genitals for sexual pleasure. As Woody Allen said in the movie *Annie Hall*, masturbation is sex with the person you love most.

> **masturbation**
> Self-stimulation of the genitals.

Negative Attitudes: A Matter of History
Many of our attitudes regarding sexual activity are part of our cultural past. Masturbation is a good example of this. Ancient Hebrews believed they were partners of God in replenishing the Earth. In addition, they needed male offspring to maintain the patriarchal system and to supply needed labor. Consequently, laws were enacted to discourage nonprocreative sexual behavior. Any sexual activity that did not potentially lead to conception was devalued.

Many believe this attitude is best represented by the story of Onan in Genesis in the Old Testament. Onan was the brother of Er, whom God slayed because he was "wicked." However, Er had not yet conceived any children with his wife, Tamar. It was Judaic law that the next of kin of the husband must impregnate the widow so that the dead man had an heir. God, therefore, ordered Onan to impregnate Tamar, but Onan, not wanting to sire a child who would not be his, "wasted his seed" on the ground by withdrawing his penis just before ejaculation. The Lord killed Onan for this indiscretion, and, erroneously, masturbation came to be nicknamed *onanism*. Christian mores were influenced greatly by Jewish codes of behavior, and, consequently, masturbation was condemned by Christian law as well.

Global DIMENSIONS

Global Religious Views on Sexuality   Different religions confront sexual behaviors and sexual mores differently. For example, in Judaism, a *mikva* (ritual bath) is prescribed for women who have just finished menstruating to cleanse her physically and spiritually. Muslims and Jews perform circumcisions as part of their religious rituals, although they perform them at different times and for different reasons. Muslim circumcision of men is a rite of passage into manhood and of women is a means to prevent them from being easily sexually aroused and, therefore, potentially unfaithful to their husbands. In Jewish practice, circumcision is performed only on young male infants 8 days old and represents a covenant with God. In Catholicism, abortion is a sin, because the religion teaches that life begins when fertilization occurs; the mother has no more status than does the unborn. In several other religions, abortion is allowed to remain a decision between the pregnant woman and her physician.

If you have a religion, what does it teach about sexuality? Perhaps you will want to interview a member of the clergy to understand better the rules, regulations, rituals, and rationale behind these teachings.

To this day our attitudes toward masturbation are colored by these ancient proscriptions. For example, although Freud believed masturbation to be a normal childhood practice, he feared that if carried into adulthood it would interfere with the formation of healthy sexual relationships. As recently as 1976 the Vatican stated in a *Declaration on Sexual Ethics* that masturbation was an "intrinsically and seriously disordered act." In 1993, Pope John Paul II reaffirmed that masturbation is an immoral act (Religious tolerance, 2008).

The Danger

No physiological harm can be attributed to masturbation. It will not cause insanity, sterility, sexual dysfunction, or any other physical affliction. Nor is there evidence that masturbation leads to an inability to establish meaningful sexual relationships. The primary danger associated with masturbation is within the individual's own mind—the guilt or shame he or she may feel about masturbating. Masturbation is so common that human sexuality experts now consider it a normal sexual act. It is normal to masturbate, and it is normal not to. As all sexual behaviors are, masturbation is a matter of personal choice. Awareness of this current thinking should go a long way toward alleviating a good deal of the guilt and shame people feel about engaging in this behavior.

Prevalence

Sexual research is fraught with limitations. Consequently we can only present data from several different studies and present a composite view about the prevalence of masturbatory behavior. The majority of studies have found that approximately 90% of adult males and slightly more than 60% of adult females report having masturbated (Arafat & Cotton, 1974; Downey, 1980; Hunt, 1974; Kinsey, Pomeroy, & Martin, 1948, 1953). These figures have remained remarkably consistent through the years (Clement, 1990). In fact, studies in the 1990s found that 60% of American men and 40% of American women had masturbated in the past year. Among couples living together, 85% of the men and 45% of the women had masturbated within the past year (Laumann et al., 1994; Michael et al., 1995). More recently, 73% of men and 37% of women reported masturbating in just the prior 4 weeks in one study (Gerressu et al., 2008). A similar study found that 61% of men and 38% of women had masturbated in the prior 4 weeks (Das, 2007). A number of sociodemographic and behavioral factors were associated with their masturbation. Among both men and women, masturbation increased with higher levels of education and social class, and was more common among those reporting sexual function problems. For women, masturbation was more likely among those who had more

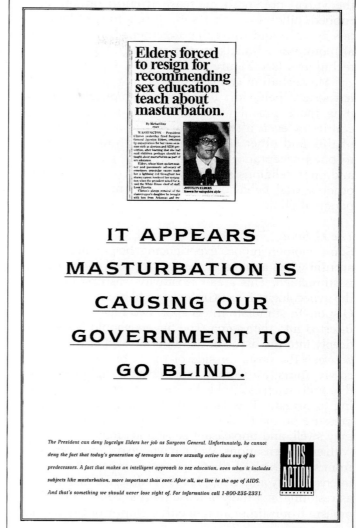

frequent vaginal sex, who had a greater repertoire of sexual activity (such as oral and anal sex), and who had more sexual partners in the past year. In contrast, the prevalence of masturbation was lower among men reporting more frequent vaginal sex. Furthermore, both men and women reporting same-gender partners were more likely to masturbate than heterosexual partners.

Techniques

Males masturbate by stroking the shaft of the penis, often stimulated by erotic literature, films, or the Internet. Some men use gadgets to assist them. Artificial vaginas, furlike clothes, inflatable dolls, and other devices have been reported as masturbatory aids by some men.

Women masturbate by rubbing the vulva—in particular, the clitoris—or inserting an object (a finger, a dildo, a banana, or a similarly shaped object) into the vagina. There are, of course, many variations on this theme, and the use of a vibrator to stimulate the vulva, cream to decrease friction on the area rubbed, pillows or other soft objects to rub the genitals against, and squeezing together of the thighs are all common adjuncts to the standard masturbatory techniques (see Figure 13.1).

Masturbation is a pleasurable, common, and varied sexual behavior; it is devoid of physical harm; it is more prevalent in men than women; and it continues even after marriage. The appropriateness of this and other sexual behaviors, however, relates to one's acceptance of them without guilt or shame and one's religious and moral points of view. As with other sexual behaviors, whether to masturbate is a personal choice.

The G Spot

Some women report experiencing heightened sexual arousal when an area of the interior wall of the vagina is stimulated. This area's sensitivity was first noted by the gynecologist Ernst Grafenberg; hence it is called the G spot. To stimulate the G spot, two fingers should be inserted into the vagina. The fingers should be pressed deeply into the tissue of the anterior wall of the vagina between the posterior side of the pubic bone and the cervix. Initially a woman may report a slight feeling of discomfort, a pleasurable feeling, or a sensation of needing to urinate. This latter reaction is probably due to pressure on the bladder. After a short period the tissue may swell, and unpleasant sensations may be replaced with erotic sensations. Women who experience orgasms from stimulation of the G spot often report them to be intense. Perry and Whipple (1981) describe this orgasm as resulting in a more intense uterine contraction than orgasm from stimulation of either clitoris or the vagina.

Other researchers do not agree that a "uterine orgasm" distinct from other orgasms exists (Pastor, 2010).

Recently evidence has been found that might verify the existence of what appears to be a G spot in some women (Geddes, 2008; Henderson, 2008). Using vaginal ultrasound, researchers compared women who reported experiencing a vaginal orgasm with women who did not (Gravina et al., 2008). They found the tissue in the area thought to contain the G spot to be thicker in women who experienced vaginal orgasm. Still, some experts suggest this might really be a result of the size of the clitoris rather than a distinct G spot. Others wonder if the thicker vaginal wall is a result of women learning to orgasm vaginally, thereby altering their anatomy, much like exercising a muscle makes it grow. With subsequent research, perhaps the existence of the G spot will be either validated or refuted. In the meantime, the controversy continues.

Fantasy

Fantasies are thoughts and images, daydreams, and scenarios. In a sexual context, we call these **sexual fantasies**.

Prevalence of Sexual Fantasies

Sexual fantasies are quite commonplace (Halderman, Zelhart, & Jackson, 1984). One researcher surveyed middle-class women and found that only 7% had never experienced sexual daydreams or

> **sexual fantasies**
> Thoughts, images, and daydreams of a sexual nature.

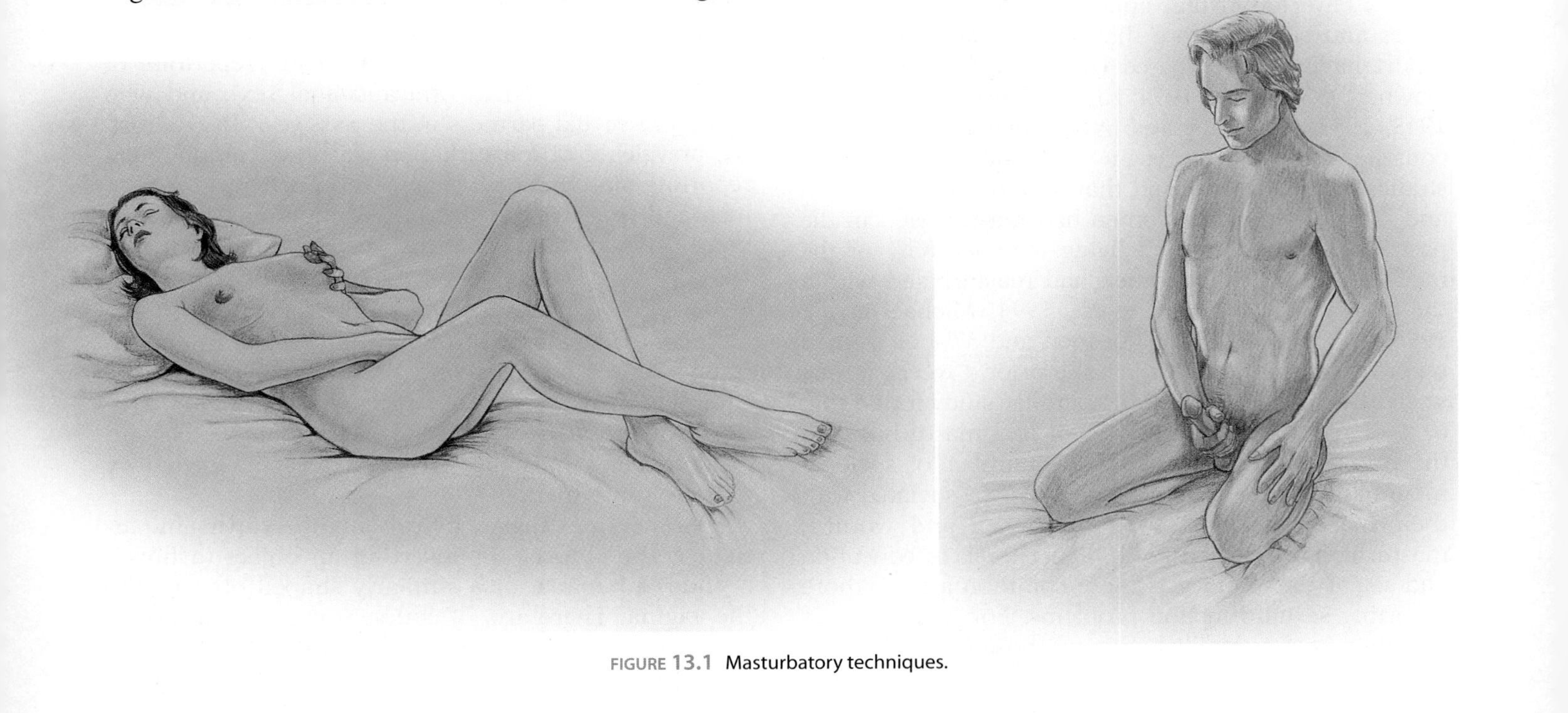

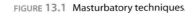

FIGURE **13.1** Masturbatory techniques.

Gender DIMENSIONS

Differences Between Male and Female Sexual Fantasies

In one of the author's college classes, students are asked to write their most erotic fantasy on one side of a sheet of paper. They are then instructed to write the letter *M* or *F* on the back to indicate male or female. Of course, students can opt out of this exercise regarding what males and females find erotic, but they seldom do. The papers are collected and placed face up on a long table. Students read the fantasies, one at a time, and try to determine whether a male or a female wrote each. When all the fantasies are read, the males meet in one room and the females in another and generalize about what the opposite sex seems to find erotic. The following are typical observations:

1. In both male and female fantasies, the males were active and the females passive. In other words, males were doing "it" (whatever "it" happened to be) to the females.

2. The female fantasies involved more of a relationship between the sexual partners than did the male fantasies. For example, many females described sexual activity after a walk on the beach, dinner, or long conversation. Many female fantasies involved people with whom the writer actually had had a long-term relationship, whereas the male fantasies included more quick sex. For instance, some male fantasies involved picking up a hitchhiker and doing "it" in the back seat of the car. Others described encounters with strangers in elevators, shopping malls, or locker rooms.

3. The male fantasies were more likely to include more than one opposite-sex partner; for example, "I walked into my apartment and there were the Dallas Cowboy Cheerleaders. Boy did we get it on!" The female fantasies seldom included more than one sexual partner, but when they did, they were more likely to include both opposite-sex and same-sex partners.

4. Female fantasies included a more detailed description of the setting than did male fantasies. Females described the colors in the room, the music in the background, the candles flickering, or the bright sun-filled, leafy knoll of grass. If males described anything, it was the sexy clothing the objects of their fantasies were in the process of shedding.

The findings from our sexuality class are similar to those reported by other sexuality experts. For example, Hicks and Leitenberg (2001) studied university students and found a larger proportion of males have sexual fantasies involving someone other than their current partner than do females. They cite other studies that found "women's sexual fantasies are more likely to involve an emotional connection with a particular partner, whereas men's fantasies are more focused on explicit sexual imagery, often without romantic or emotional context" (Leitenberg & Henning, 1995, 48). Christensen (1990) puts it this way—more men than women imagine doing something to a partner, whereas more women imagine something sexual being done to them. In a review of the differences between male and female sexual fantasies, Masters, Johnson, and Kolodny (1985, 350) conclude, "Several studies have shown that the sex fantasies of women tend to be more passive than those of men (women tend to visualize their role in the fantasy as having something done to them by someone else, rather than being the active 'doer')." Obviously, there are many exceptions to these findings. Some men include romantic elements in their fantasies and some women do not. Some women include explicit, active sexual behavior by them and some men do not. However, as a generalization, it appears the findings of our students are valid.

---

fantasies (Hariton, 1973). Earlier, Kinsey had found that 84% of men and 67% of women had sexual fantasies. Other researchers have also found sexual fantasies prevalent; for example, when studying college students, Sue (1979) found that 60% of men and women fantasized during sexual intercourse; Crepault and associates (1977) reported that 94% of their sample of women engaged in sexual fantasies; Zimmer and colleagues (1983) found that 71% of men and 72% of women fantasized about sex to become more sexually aroused; and Masters, Johnson, and Kolodny (1985) reported that 86% of the women they studied fantasized abut sex. More recently, in a study of university students and employees, 98% of men and 80% of women reported having sexual fantasies about someone other than their current partners during the past 2 months (Hicks & Leitenberg, 2001). Studies have consistently shown males have more frequent sexual fantasies than females (Leitenberg & Henning, 1995; Hicks & Leitenberg, 2001; Ellis & Symons, 1990).

Fantasies also come in many varieties. A recent study, for example, evaluated the rape fantasies of female undergraduates and found 62% of women have had a rape fantasy, which is somewhat higher than previous estimates (Bivona & Critelli, 2008).

In a study of gay and straight men, both groups' most arousing sexual fantasies involved oral sex (Keating & Over, 1990). Heterosexual men next found the following to be most arousing (presented in order of arousal): vaginal intercourse, undressing a woman, woman manually caressing penis, and being undressed by a woman. After oral sex, homosexual men found the following to be most arousing (presented in order of arousal): man manually caresses penis, anal intercourse, and kissing a man on the lips.

Most people realize that it is permissible to have sexual fantasies. A *New York Times* poll (The way we live now, 2000) found that 55% of people younger than 30 years of age think it is okay to fantasize about having sex with someone other than their partners. Even many older people believed that—27% of those older than 70 thought it okay to fantasize about sex with someone other than their partners. One of the benefits of these fantasies is being able to imagine whatever one wishes unencumbered by "social convention, practical and legal barriers, or by fears of embarrassment, criticism, or rejection" (Wilson, 1997, 43). Research has demonstrated that sexual fantasizing can be healthy for both men and women (Strassberg & Lockerd, 1998; Chick & Gold, 1987–1988; Davidson, 1985; Knafo & Jaffe, 1984).

Sexual fantasies may be triggered externally, such as by a movie or by photographs. Or, they may be triggered by internal stimuli, such as thoughts of another person or a sexual situation. Alternatively, fantasies may be generated by a combination of external and internal triggers (Jones & Barlow, 1990). In addition, sexual experience appears related to sexual fantasies. For example, in two studies, women with more coital experience reported more sexual fantasies than women who were virgins or had less sexual experience (Hicks & Leitenberg, 2001; Knafo & Jaffe, 1984).

Another source of fantasy images is the Internet. Although fraught with limitations (Are students being truthful?), several studies have explored the prevalence of college students' use of the Internet to view sexually explicit material. In one study of 506 college students, 44% reported accessing sexually explicit material online (Goodson, McCormick, & Evans, 2001). In another study of 985 university students, 38% reported they used the Internet to view sexually explicit images (Rumbough, 2001). Others have reported that 64% of male and 18% of female college students spend some time viewing Internet porn (Leahy, 2009). More specifically, 51% percent of male students and 16% of female students spend less than 5 hours per week viewing Internet porn, whereas 11% of male students and 1% of female students spend 5 to 20 hours per week at online porn sites.

Content of Sexual Fantasies

The content of sexual fantasies is both similar and dissimilar when gender is the variable. Interestingly, when males and females are by themselves they tend to fantasize about engaging in sexual activities with their usual partners; however, when they are engaged in sex with their usual partners, they fantasize about sex with someone else (for example, a movie star or a model) (Leitenberg & Henning, 1995). Although quite a diversity in the content of sexual fantasies exists, other prevalent fantasies are having oral–genital sex, being found sexually irresistible by others, and having sex forced upon oneself. The most prevalent female sexual fantasies include having sex in a secluded setting, engaging in sexual activity in a different place than usual (such as a hotel), and having thoughts about an imaginary lover (Strassberg & Lockerd, 1998). Table 13.1 presents favorite male sexual fantasies. Table 13.2 lists favorite sexual fantasies of gays and lesbians. Sexual fantasies may also include group sex, sex with celebrities, voyeuristic activities (peeping or watching others engaged in sex), sadomasochism, or experimentation with other partners or other activities. In a 1995 study that reviewed more than 200 other studies of sexual fantasies, the researchers concluded that women's fantasies tended to include sex with a new male partner, sex with a celebrity, seduction of a younger man or boy, and sex with an older man. Men's favorite fantasies included seeing women nude and having sex with a new female partner, multiple sex partners, and the power to drive women wild (Leitenberg & Henning, 1995).

Functions of Sexual Fantasies

Sexual fantasies serve several purposes. They are a source of pleasure, and, as such, they enhance sexual

TABLE 13.1 Men's Favorite Sexual Fantasies

- Seeing woman nude
- Having sex with a new partner
- Having sex with multiple partners at the same time
- Having the power to drive women "wild"

Source: Reproduced from Leitenberg, H., & Henning, K. Sexual fantasy. *Psychological Bulletin, 117* (1995), 469–496.

TABLE 13.2 Gays' and Lesbians' Favorite Sexual Fantasies

Gays' Fantasies

- Unspecified sexual activity with another man
- Performing oral sex
- Having partner perform oral sex
- Participating in anal sexual intercourse
- Sex with another man not previously involved with

Lesbians' Fantasies

- Unspecified sexual activity with another woman
- Having partner perform oral sex
- Performing oral sex
- Anticipating sexual activity with a partner
- Being held and touched

Source: Reproduced from Price, J. H., & Miller, P. A. Sexual fantasies of black and white college students. *Psychological Reports, 54* (1984), 1007–1014. © *Psychological Reports* 1984.

arousal. Furthermore, sexual fantasies allow people to test and rehearse various sexual activities if they are concerned about being judged by their partners. In this way the activity is tested in a nonthreatening setting and no one knows whether it works out. And sexual fantasies allow people to acknowledge sexual feelings without acting on them.

There is also research to indicate that sexual fantasies may be helpful in overcoming sexual anxiety (Coen, 1978; Leitenberg & Henning, 1995; Hicks & Leitenberg, 2001). Consequently, many sexual therapists encourage fantasies in counseling clients with sexual dysfunctions. In fact, low sexual desire in women has been found to be associated with a lack of sexual fantasizing (Nutter & Condron, 1983).

In addition, sexual fantasies allow us to be "better" than we really are—that is, better lovers, more confident, more experienced, more risky, and more desirable. They also provide us with a safe means of engaging in sexual activities in which we may never wish to participate. For example, though some women fantasize about being forced to have sex, few would actually want that fantasy to come true. It is hypothesized that the frequency with which a woman reports this forced-sex fantasy is a function of her desire to be risqué in her sexual behavior but not accountable for it, because our society generally frowns on sexually adventurous women. Another interpretation of this forced-sex fantasy is that women seek greater power rather than less, so they fantasize that they are so desirable that the man cannot resist (Hawley & Hensley, 2009; Critelli & Bivona, 2008). Although Hunt (1974) found twice

as many women had this fantasy as men, he did find 10% of men also had submission fantasies.

Sexual fantasies also provide us with a means of fulfilling our every desire while not hurting ourselves or those we love. It is a private and safe way of doing anything we want. It is a means of acting out our wildest dreams while never acting improperly. For example, we may wonder what sex with an animal would be like, or what the experience of sex with our lover's friend would feel like. By fantasizing about these situations we do not harm ourselves, our lovers, or our pets, yet we can experience the situation vicariously. Fantasies of this kind are safe as long as they do not become obsessive. If they do, therapy may be indicated.

There are those who argue that sexual fantasies are unhealthy. For example, Apfelbaum (1980) believes fantasizing during sex with a partner can decrease the degree of trust and intimacy in the relationship. Others have taken a similar point of view (Hollender, 1970; Shainess & Greenwald, 1971).

Maltz and Boss (2001) provide a list of nine questions to ask to determine whether, and to what extent, a sexual fantasy may be causing problems:

- Does the fantasy lead to risky or dangerous behavior?
- Does the fantasy feel out of control or compulsive?
- Is the content of the fantasy disturbing or repulsive?
- Does the fantasy hinder recovery or personal growth?
- Does the fantasy lower my self-esteem or block self-acceptance?
- Does the fantasy distance me from my real-life partner?
- Does the fantasy harm my intimate partner or anyone else?
- Does the fantasy cause sexual problems?
- Does the fantasy really belong to someone else?

The predominant view is that sexual fantasizing can enhance sexual relationships as long as it does not become obsessive and as long as there is no compulsion to act out the fantasy. Some fantasies may be acted out with the consent of the sexual partner, but if one person feels uncomfortable, problems may arise. Guilt or shame may lead to other psychological and/or sexual problems. With the willing consent of both partners, however, acting out sexual fantasies can actually enhance sexual satisfaction and improve the relationship. It appears, though, that most sexual fantasizers do not intend to act out their fantasies, and, if they do, they may be disappointed. Nancy Friday (1975) reports that most individuals who have acted out their sexual fantasies were disappointed. It seems that reality seldom matches fantasy.

Sexual Behavior with Others

foreplay
Physical contact preceding sexual intercourse.

Foreplay is the physical contact that usually precedes coitus or oral–genital sexual activity. Generally foreplay includes touching, kissing, biting, and genital fondling. The word *foreplay* is really a misnomer, because this behavior can be enjoyed for itself and need not be a prelude (*fore-*) to anything. All such activity is meant to express love, sensuousness, desire, or all these feelings. We might more appropriately term this activity *pleasuring each other*. However, foreplay does also serve to prepare

Myth vs Fact

Myth: Sexual fantasies mean a person is fixating on sex and needs either to get professional help or to work hard to stop fantasizing.
Fact: Sexual fantasizing is prevalent and is not indicative of a sexual problem. Many males and females fantasize both before and during sexual intercourse, even if engaged in sexual intercourse with their usual partner.

Myth: Women who fantasize about being raped are "sick" and, if raped, get what they deserve.
Fact: First of all, no one "deserves" to be forced to engage in any sexual activity against his or her will. Second, having a fantasy does not indicate that someone actually wants the fantasy to come true. Rape fantasies may even indicate a woman's wish to be so desirable that men cannot resist her rather than a desire to give up control to a male.

Myth: Masturbation is normal for young people but can interfere

with the healthy sexual relationship of older people, especially if they are married.
Fact: There is no evidence that masturbation is harmful either physically or psychologically. In fact, there are some times when a sexual partner is unavailable and masturbation can serve as a healthy sexual outlet. Furthermore, many married people with regular sexual intercourse still enjoy masturbating.

Myth: It is unfortunate, but people with disabilities cannot have a meaningful sex life because of the restrictions placed on them by their disabilities.
Fact: Certainly some disabilities place restrictions on sexual positions or sexual stamina. Still, there are many accommodations that can be made so that people who have heart disease, who are physically disabled, or who are ill can achieve and maintain meaningful sexual lives.

the participants, both psychologically and physically, for coitus.

The importance of foreplay to sexual enjoyment has been widely acknowledged. Data (Hunt, 1974) show that unmarried people younger than 25 years of age spend an average of 15 minutes in foreplay and another 15 minutes in intercourse, whereas Kinsey's 1948 data showed that a majority of males reached orgasm just 2 minutes after penile insertion. Michael and colleagues (1994) found that for 69% of men and 71% of women, intercourse took from 15 minutes to 1 hour. Because women need more time to be vaginally lubricated sufficiently for intercourse than men do to achieve erection and be ready (Masters & Johnson, 1966), perhaps this acknowledgment represents an increased understanding of women's needs to be sexually stimulated for a longer period than men before coitus.

Interestingly, some men are fearful of foreplay. They worry about losing their erection or ejaculating before intercourse (Elder, 2009). This is unfortunate because foreplay is the perfect time for communicating with your partner to find out what he or she likes (Srovney, 2009). To rush through it is to lose this opportunity.

The Importance of the Senses

Sexual stimulation in foreplay, intercourse, or any other activity involves the imagination and all of the senses: touch, sight, smell, hearing, and taste.

Touch

Sensual touching is central to sexual stimulation. Although the skin is not a sexual organ as such, stroking the skin on any part of the body can contribute to and even initiate sexual arousal. The gentle stroking of a partner's face, ear, or neck can be both exciting and effective at communicating affection. Furthermore, each manner and intensity of body contact carries its own kind of stimulation. Gentle touching, where the fingers barely make contact with the skin and perhaps focus on one part of the body, can be tantalizing. Caressing—gentle stroking or rubbing—is firmer than gentle touching and communicates affection or appreciation. Firmer touches, too, can be sexually arousing. Hugs, embraces, and squeezes are all expressions of caring. Some might consider a full-body massage the ultimate expression of the sensual touch.

So sensual touching is not necessarily focused on the genitals. But once the body and emotions are primed for sexual activity, touching in and around specific areas of the body is intensely stimulating. The breast (especially the nipple), the inner thighs, the clitoris, the penis, the neck, the ears, and the navel are particularly receptive to sensual touching because of an abundance of nerve endings. However, touching of some of the sensitive genital areas (for example, the vulva or the glans) can result in irritation unless some kind of lubricant is used. Of course, the best lubricant is that produced vaginally by the woman herself. However, any lotion, such as hydroxyethyl cellulose (K-Y) jelly, that does not contain alcohol is also safe and useful for this purpose (unless you are using a condom, in which case Vaseline should not be used). Touching on all parts of the body can be of a teasing nature: moving here, then there, but not there (though almost), then back here. Genital touching should be done in a gentle manner, because rough handling (for example, of a testicle) could result in injury.

We should not overlook the use of touching for sexual self-stimulation. Masturbation is often the method by which people learn which body areas and which types of touching are most stimulating for them. Vibrators have become popular both for masturbating and for sexually stimulating partners. Many couples masturbate each other to orgasm and find this form of sexual activity very exciting and a safe alternative to intercourse.

As with other sexual behaviors, good communication is important for guiding partners in touching each other effectively. Such phrases as "I like that," "That hurts," and "Keep doing that, but just a little more gently (or more firmly)" will help your partner use touching on the specific areas and in the particular ways most stimulating to you. If you are the toucher and do not get this feedback, ask for it.

Sight

The power of visual images is clear everywhere in modern society—for example, in advertising, in films, and in television. These images sometimes work on us without our notice, but it is possible to use sexual imagery consciously for sexual stimulation. Sexual partners sometimes use sexual imagery in books, magazines, films, and photographs to become aroused together. Clothing can also serve this purpose. Men and women often dress in a manner termed sexy, not only to attract others but to add to their partners' or their own sexual excitement. Some people are excited by the sight of hair, eyes, legs, or other body parts. Partners can learn to make use of each other's particular visual stimulants to initiate or enhance sexual arousal.

Smell

The popularity of perfumes and colognes is probably attributable to their potential for arousing

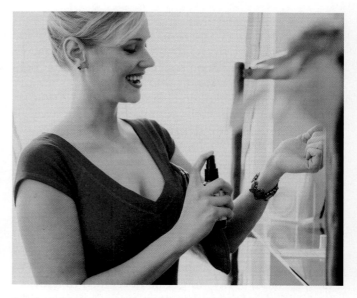

Smell can be sexually stimulating. Research with both animals and humans demonstrates the sexually arousing nature of certain smells. Perfume manufacturers have long recognized this fact.

sexual interest. It is no small wonder that the old-time bordello is associated with highly perfumed and painted women (even though

pheromones
Substances that when secreted have a specific scent found to be sexually arousing.

these ladies might have been a far sight raunchier than their counterparts in the modern media). Animal studies have identified smell as being more important in many species than sight or sound in attracting a mate (Bhutta, 2007). Substances called **pheromones** are secreted by some female animals to attract male sexual partners. Conversely, unpleasant smells such as bad breath can interfere with sexual arousal. Attention to normal body hygiene can prevent these problems.

Although it has long been suspected that humans produce pheromones, it was only in the late 1980s that scientists verified this. Human pheromones do not actually serve as sexual attractants, but they do alter the timing of women's menstrual cycles. The Monell Chemical Studies Center and the University of Pennsylvania Medical School (Cutler et al., 1986) studied this issue for several years and found that women who experience coitus weekly are more likely to have normal menstrual cycles, fewer infertility problems, and milder menopauses than women who either are celibate or have sexual intercourse only sporadically (Rensberger, 1986). It seems that male aromatic chemicals secreted from sweat glands in the armpits, nipples, and genitalia are transmitted to their sexual partners by smell and skin absorption. Once transmitted, these chemicals affect the woman's reproductive system.

Women also produce a pheromone that affects other women's menstrual cycles. For years anecdotal reports indicated that women who live together or who work together seem to have synchronous menstrual cycles. These reports now have evidence both to support and to explain them (Preti et al., 1986).

The manner in which human pheromones work is not fully understood. The suspicion is that molecules of the substances reach receptors of the nervous and endocrine systems and act on them to stimulate signals transmitted in the brain (Keverne, 2004). These brain signals influence the endocrine system's secretion of hormones, and these hormones influence the woman's reproductive system (Lanuza et al., 2008; Spors & Sobel, 2007).

There are several potential practical applications of this knowledge regarding human pheromones. For example, nasal sprays might be developed to alleviate certain kinds of infertility problems, to regulate the menstrual cycle (for instance, to make the rhythm method of birth control more effective), or to effect the onset of menopause or minimize its effects.

Hearing

Have you ever heard the expression "Whisper sweet nothings in my ear"? Well, those murmurings are not just nothings! Words and sounds before and during coitus can be sexually stimulating, as can music that contributes to an erotic atmosphere. Sexual talk can take many forms. Some people are aroused by "dirty words," and others are completely turned off by them. Similarly, some people find moaning during sexual activity to be exciting, whereas others are unimpressed with such guttural goings-on. Furthermore, some people report that saying or hearing "I love you" after orgasm can be one of the most exciting and romantic experiences in the world (Haffner & Schwartz, 1998). Once again, communication between sexual partners is the key.

Taste

The use of the mouth can be quite sexually arousing. Kissing, when both partners attend to it, can be intensely stimulating, whatever the variation: open mouth, closed mouth, a nibble here, a nibble there, a tongue darting from spot to spot, and lips or teeth closing gently on a sensitive body part. Kissing with tongues touching (soul kissing, French kissing, deep kissing) can also take various forms. More on the use of the mouth, tongue, and teeth is discussed in the section on oral–genital sexual behavior. As with the other senses, taste can also be a turnoff. Obviously French kissing someone who has bad breath or licking a smelly body can be anything but arousing. Proper body hygiene and

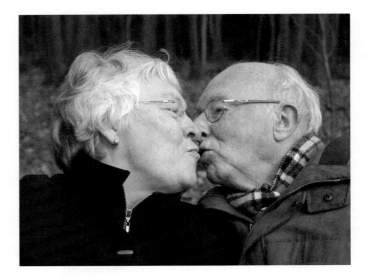

Kissing can be a very erotic, sensual activity in and of itself.

communication on such simple matters between sexual partners can go a long way toward improving sexual relations.

In the following sections, we discuss specific sexual behaviors and provide guidance for enhancing sexual satisfaction through the use of these activities.

Oral–Genital Sexual Behavior

Oral–genital sexual behavior involves contact between the mouth, lips, and tongue of one partner and the genitals of another. When a female's genitals are orally stimulated, the act is called **cunnilingus** (meaning in Latin "one who licks the vulva"). When the penis is taken into the partner's mouth, the act

> **cunnilingus**
> The stimulation of the female genitalia by the mouth, lips, and/or tongue of the sexual partner.
>
> **fellatio**
> Oral contact with a male's penis.

is called **fellatio** (from the Latin *fellare*, meaning "to suck"). As with most sexual acts, some find oral–genital sexual contact sexually arousing; others are indifferent to it or find it repulsive. It is generally agreed, however, that oral–genital activity is quite common. Hunt's (1974) study, for example, indicated that 90% of married couples younger than age 25 years had experienced oral–genital sexual stimulation. The most recent large-scale study of oral sex was conducted by Michael and associates (1994), who found that 77% of men and 68% of women reported having given oral sex *to* a partner, and 79% of men and 73% of women had received oral sex *from* a partner.

Many of the techniques described as foreplay are applicable to oral–genital sexual activity. Thus a teasing approach, gentle in nature and varied in form, involving the mouth, lips, and tongue is particularly stimulating. Some women report especially enjoying the licking or sucking of the clitoris and labia minora or a thrusting of the tongue into the vagina. Men are often aroused when their partners lick the underside of the penile shaft and the glans or lick or lightly hold a testicle in the mouth. Again, the testicles and clitoris are very sensitive and should be treated gently. And, of course, attention to personal hygiene is important to maximal—and even minimal—pleasure.

Sexual partners need to discuss whether ejaculation should occur in the mouth during fellatio. Contrary to rumor, the ejaculate is not fattening when swallowed; however, it does have a unique taste. Some like or are indifferent to the taste; others dislike it. One word of caution here, though: Because the ejaculate can contain HIV if the male is infected, unless the relationship has been monogamous for some time and both partners are known to be HIV-free, the ejaculate should not be swallowed. In any case, whether the ejaculate is swallowed does not need to diminish the pleasure of either partner.

When couples orally stimulate one another simultaneously, the act is referred to as **69** (because their bodies in position resemble the numbers 6 and 9 (Figure 13.2). Couples can perform 69 side by side or with one partner on top of the other, depending on which position they consider more comfortable and stimulating.

69
Two partners' simultaneous stimulation of each other's genitalia orally. The numerals 6 and 9 visually describe the body positions.

Some couples prefer to stimulate one another simultaneously, whereas others find they cannot concentrate on their own pleasurable sensations while concentrating on pleasuring someone else.

Partners also need to discuss the need for a male to wear a condom and a female to wear a dental dam during oral–genital contact. These behaviors decrease, although they do not eliminate, the possibility of contracting HIV, as well as other STIs. That is why they are called "safer sex" behaviors. To be "safer," partners should consider agreeing to engage in these behaviors.

Anal Stimulation

Some people enjoy becoming sexually aroused anally, because there are numerous nerve endings in that area. Partners can stimulate each other by inserting a finger into the anus, stroking the anal opening, or licking the area. However, licking the anus, termed **analingus**—also commonly referred to as "rimming"—is risky to one's health. Intestinal infections, such as *Escherichia coli*, can be spread through analingus, as can hepatitis and STIs. This threat exists even though the anus may be carefully washed. In addition, minute tears that occur in the anus during **anal intercourse** provide easy entry into the body for organisms that cause STIs. This is especially likely if a condom is not used. Penile penetration of the anus is also possible, for both heterosexual and homosexual couples. **Dildos** (fake penises)

analingus
Licking of the anus.

anal intercourse
Insertion of the penis into the anus.

dildos
Artificial penises.

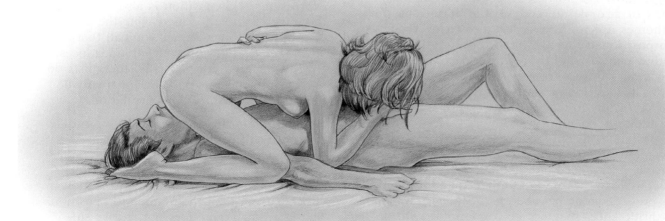

FIGURE **13.2** Simultaneous oral–genital stimulation.

¿? Ethical DIMENSIONS

Should People Who Do Not Feel Comfortable with Oral or Anal Sexual Activity Learn to Enjoy These Activities?

Some people believe that the more sexual acts one experiences, the more sexually satisfied one will be, and that to enhance our sexual lives, we need a variety of sexual expressions and sexual excitation. They feel that those who are not comfortable with oral–genital sexual activity or anal intercourse ought to be instructed in how to engage in these activities and given counseling to relieve any shame, guilt, or anxiety associated with them. People with this viewpoint argue that to ignore this discomfort is to forever accept a less satisfying sexual life than is possible; and when sexual partners have different desires related to oral and anal sexual activity, there is a threat to the relationship itself.

Others believe that sexual expression can occur in many forms and that no one person need accept all forms for himself or herself. If some sexual activities are uncomfortable, these people argue, choose other activities to include in your sexual repertoire. People should not be coerced into behaviors that they find repulsive; that is not fair. Furthermore, if one partner desires oral or anal sexual activity and the other does not, a good relationship will result if the one who does want these activities understands and accepts the other's feelings. Anything short of that and the relationship is probably not worthwhile anyhow.

What do you believe a couple who disagrees on this issue should do?

can also be used for anal insertion. Because of the nature of the anus, one should take care not to tear the surrounding tissue (a lubricant should be used), and to prevent infection the penis should be thoroughly cleansed immediately after anal insertion. Because anal intercourse is one of the risk behaviors for HIV, a condom should be used whenever this sexual activity is performed.

Sexual Intercourse

Variety may truly be the spice of life, at least relative to coital (penile–vaginal intercourse) positions. Although most authorities recognize four basic positions of sexual intercourse, the variations on these themes are infinite. A leg thrown over here, an arm positioned there, a hand fondling this, lips doing that can all slightly alter the sexual experience so that it differs from past experiences. Consequently this section can serve only as a guide, not the last word, on coital positions.

In addition to the desire for variety, other situations—such as pregnancy, obesity, or poor health—may dictate certain modifications. For example, it is more comfortable for a pregnant or obese woman to be on top rather than have her partner press down on her abdomen. Similarly, a man with arthritic knees may not be comfortable with his knees bent in the on-top position. In addition, some coital positions may influence the effectiveness of a condom—male or female. As an example, when the

man lies on his back with the woman on top, there may be some seepage of semen from the condom, especially if it is not placed on the penis correctly. When the man is on top, this is not as likely.

1. *Man on top*. The man-on-top position (Figure 13.3) is sometimes called the "missionary position" or the male superior position. The position has a lot going for it: It allows full frontal body contact, which is usually pleasurable; because the couple is lying down, their hands are free to roam; and because they are facing each other, partners can kiss, talk, and watch each other's expressions. This position is also considered the most effective for increasing the chances of pregnancy, but whether you call that an advantage depends on your circumstances. On the negative side, sexuality therapists do not recommend this position for men who have difficulty controlling ejaculation.

2. *Woman on top*. In the woman-on-top position, also called the female superior position (Figure 13.4), the woman can be either prone or on her knees. In either case this position permits more clitoral stimulation by either partner than the man-on-top position. Thus a woman who does not receive sufficient clitoral stimulation to achieve orgasm through coitus alone can reach orgasm through manual stimulation in this position

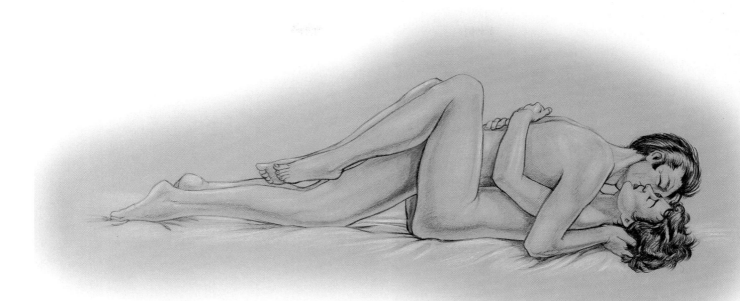

FIGURE **13.3** Man-on-top position.

Sex can be enjoyable at any age. Studies have found that the elderly engage in sex well into their 70s and 80s. For example, Lindau (2007) found that many older adults are sexually active, but that about half of the men and women surveyed reported at least one sexual problem and about a third reported at least two problems. Specifically:

1. *In general, older adults are sexually active.* A large portion of respondents said they were sexually active in the preceding 12 months, but the percentage declined with age—from 73% of those age 57–64 to 53% of those age 65–74, to 26% of those age 75–85. Older women, however, were significantly less likely to report sexual activity than older men and less likely to be in intimate relationships, due in part to women's status as widows and the earlier mortality, on average, of men.

2. *Healthier people are more likely to report being sexually active.* Eighty-one percent of men and 51% of women reporting excellent or very good health said they had been sexually active in the past 12 months. Of those in fair or poor health, a considerably lower percentage (47% of men and 26% of women) reported activity in the previous year. Diabetes and hypertension were strongly associated with some sexual concerns.

3. *About half of sexually active older adults report at least one "bothersome" sexual problem.* Thirty-seven percent of sexually active men said they had erectile difficulties. Women most often reported low desire (43%), difficulty with vaginal lubrication (39%), and inability to climax (34%).

while her partner's penis is inside her vagina. In this way she can experience the pleasure of orgasm around an erect penis while the man has the pleasure of feeling her orgasmic contractions on his penis. In addition, the woman is free to move rather than being pinned under her partner. This is a good posi-

tion for men who are attempting to control their orgasms; the squeeze technique is easy to use because the penis is relatively accessible. Another advantage is that both partners' hands are free, allowing them to caress each other. The one disadvantage of this position is that the effort by the man necessary for

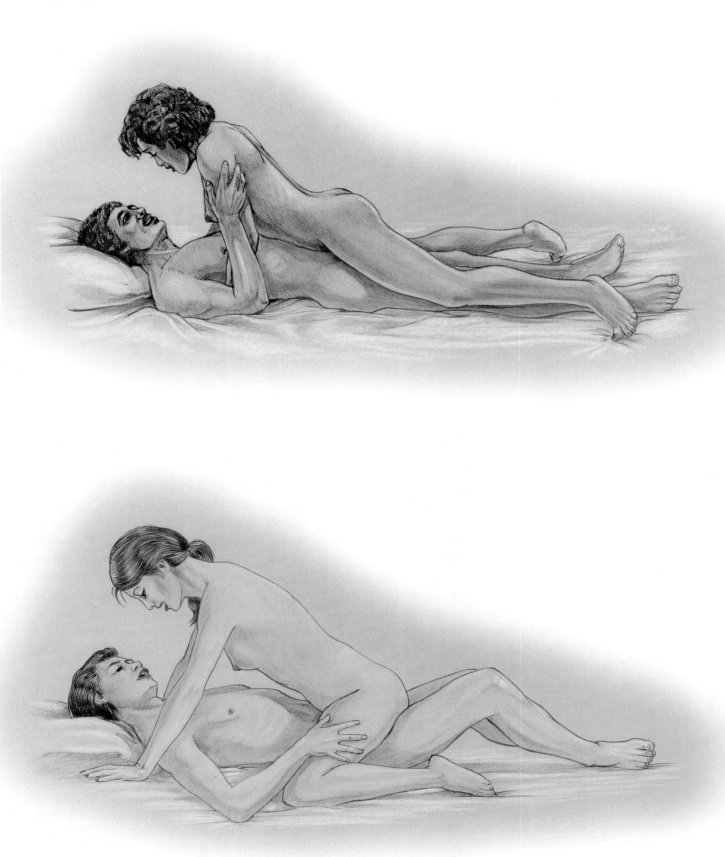

FIGURE 13.4 Woman-on-top position.

Multicultural DIMENSIONS

Does Level of Education Influence Sexuality?

Sexual practices vary greatly from person to person and from couple to couple. Yet, these practices seem to be influenced by education. Laumann and colleagues (1994) found that sex and education were related in the following ways.

1. Whereas 72% of men with any college education reported their last sexual encounter took between 15 minutes and 1 hour, only 61% of men with less than a high school education reported it took that long. With women, the results were comparable. Seventy-four percent of women with any college education reported their last sexual encounter took between 15 minutes and 1 hour, whereas only 60% of women with less than a high school education reported it took that long.

2. Although 81% of men and 78% of women with some college education reported having ever performed oral sex on a partner, only 59% of men and 41% of women with less than a high school education reported having ever performed oral sex on a partner. And although 84% of men and 82% of women with some college education reported ever having oral sex performed on them, only 61% of men and 50% of women with less than a high school education reported ever having oral sex performed on them.

3. In terms of anal intercourse, 28% of college educated men and 24% of college-educated women reported ever having that experience, whereas only 21% of men and 13% of women with less than a high school education reported experiencing anal intercourse.

It appears that being educated results in being less conservative sexually. Why do you think that is the case?

---

thrusting his penis can be tiring because the woman's weight is bearing down on his pelvis. Consequently women might do more of the movement in this position than in some others.

3. *Side-by-side.* In the side-by-side position (Figure 13.5), neither person is bearing the weight of the other. This is a relaxing position, because pelvic thrusts do not meet as much resistance as with the woman or man on top. However, because arms and legs may be pinned under other arms and legs, blood circulation can be temporarily cut off, making periodic switching or adjustment necessary for comfort. The side-by-side position also allows for kissing and face watching, and it too frees the hands for stroking and caressing. However, it is sometimes difficult to keep the penis in the vagina in this position, and even vigorous thrusting can result in little or no clitoral contact. Still, hands work well here too, as in the woman-on-top position.

4. *Rear entry.* The rear-entry position (Figure 13.6) can be performed in two ways: with both people lying down, either side-by-side or with the woman atop the man, or with the partners kneeling (called

the "dog position" for reasons clear to anyone who has seen dogs copulating). In either case the male's hands are free to fondle his partner's breasts and stimulate her clitoris. The disadvantages of this position include the lack of face-to-face contact and the feeling of some people that they are being animal-like (others find this position sexually stimulating for this very reason). People who try the rear-entry position for the first time may be surprised by the sound effects: Air may enter the vagina and produce noises when it leaves (some sexologists have termed this sound a "vart").

Once again we should say that the variety of coital positions is limited only by your imagination. Coitus, or any other sexual activity, can be pleasurable and exciting when the technique is pleasurable and exciting and when partners follow their inclinations. However, sexual techniques alone may not always be satisfying. The bond between sex makers that sometimes turns them into lovemakers can be as important as technique. A loving relationship of responsible people can add much to the pleasure obtained from sexual activity. Still, the very nature of sexual expression is pleasing, and it is obvious that sexual behavior can be enjoyed by people who are not in love but still care for each other.

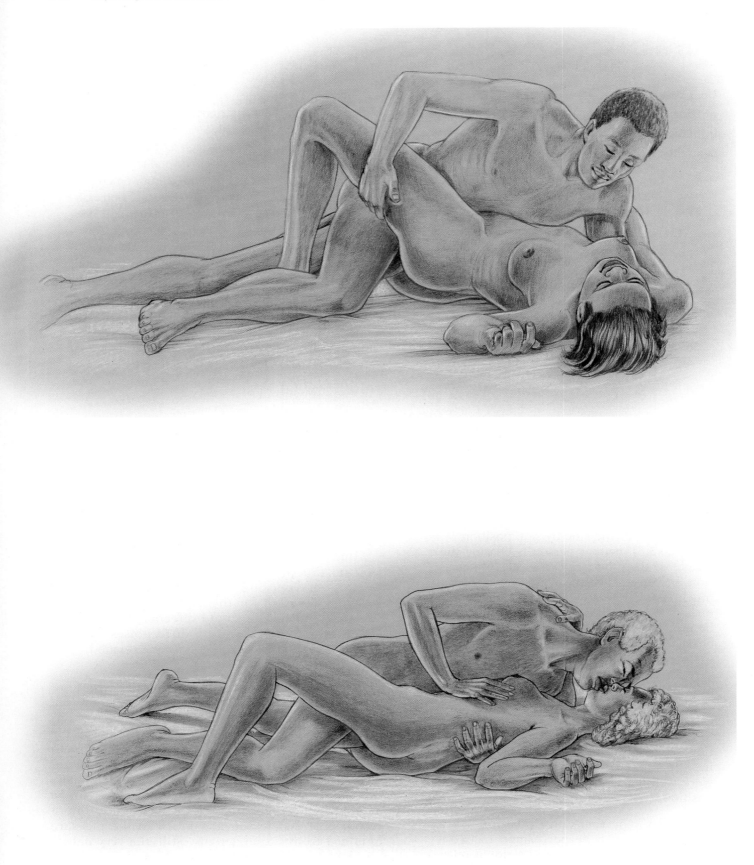

FIGURE **13.5**   The side-by-side position. Note the subtle variations that are possible.

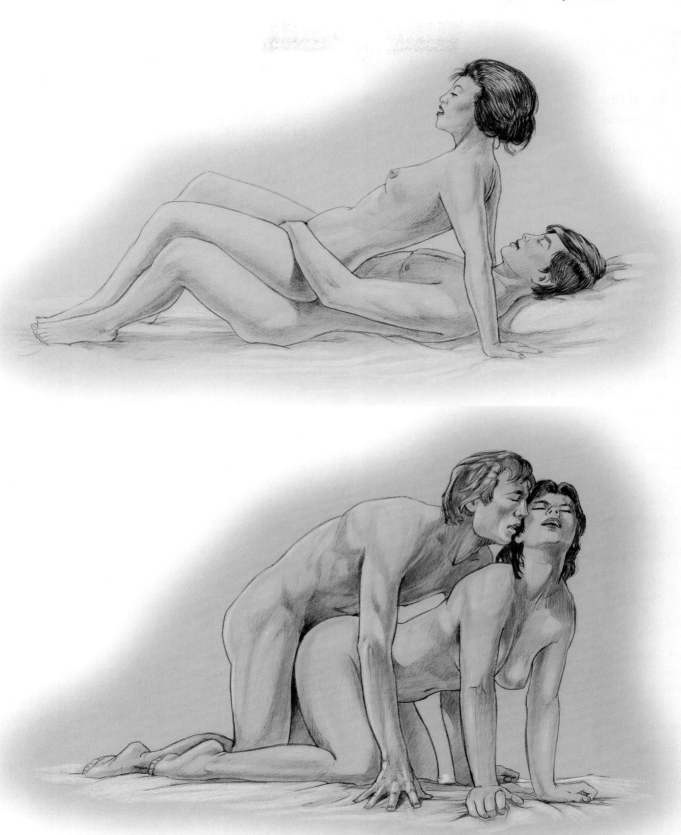

FIGURE **13.6** The rear-entry position.

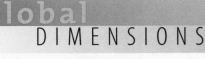

DIMENSIONS

Age of First Intercourse
The age of first intercourse differs by gender, region of the world, and country within a particular regions. For example, the median age of first intercourse for women in the United States is 17.2 years, whereas it is 19.6 years in Peru and 15.8 years in Mali. The median age of first intercourse for men in the United States is 16.1 years, whereas it is 19.0 years in Thailand and 15.4 years in Jamaica.

Median Age in Years of First Intercourse, by Country and Gender

Region/Country	Female	Male
Sub-Saharan Africa		
Ghana	16.9	18.4
Mali	15.8	18.7
Tanzania	17.4	17.8
Zimbabwe	18.8	18.7
Asia		
Philippines	na	na
Thailand	na	19.0
Latin America and Caribbean		
Brazil	18.6	16.2
Costa Rica	19.4	17.4
Dominican Republic	18.7	17.1
Haiti	18.7	17.8
Jamaica	16.9	15.4
Peru	19.6	17.4
Developed Countries		
Great Britain	17.4	17.2
United States	17.2	16.1

Source: Data from Singh, S., Wulf, D., Samara, R., & Cuca, Y. P. Gender differences in the timing of first intercourse: Data from 14 countries. *International Family Planning Perspectives, 26* (2000), 21–28, 43.

Whether such sexual behavior is moral or legal, however, is another issue, which depends on your ethics and society's.

Sexual Behavior of Homosexuals

Although study findings vary, approximately 12.5% of U.S. females have engaged in sex with same-gender partners, as have 5.2% of males. Over 9% of females and 5% of males have engaged in oral sex with a same-gender partner, and 2.9% of males have engaged in anal sex with a same-gender partner (Chandra et al., 2011). With regard to the sexual activity of homosexuals, they enjoy most of the same activities as heterosexuals (Figures 13.7 and 13.8). One difference that has been noted, however (Tripp, 1976), is that intimacy and closeness seem to be more important than what is specifically done by the partners. Yet, more recently it has been reported that more gay men who have been living with a partner for 2 to 10 years have sex with someone other than their partner (79%) than do heterosexual males living with a partner 2 to 10 years (11%). In addition, gays tend to have more sexual partners than do lesbians (Peplau & Cochran, 1990; Blumstein & Schwartz, 1990). People seem to have stereotyped ideas of specific sexual acts in which homosexuals participate (Spalding & Peplau, 1997). In contrast to these myths, both male and female homosexuals appear to take their time and make sexual activity last longer. They seem to prolong the pleasure rather than rush to orgasm (Masters & Johnson, 1979). Perhaps this is due to

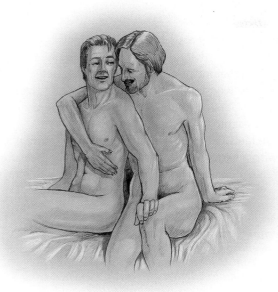

FIGURE **13.7** Gay men engage in varied sexual activities.

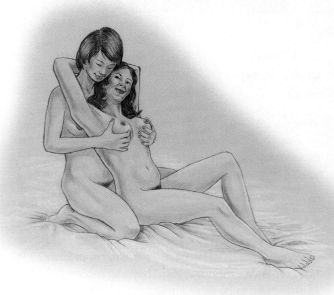

FIGURE **13.8** Oral and manual stimulation, and touching, are some of the sexual activities enjoyed by lesbians.

the fact that a person stimulating another person of the same sex can better understand what that person enjoys. Contrary to popular belief, male homosexuals do not generally have a preference to receive or insert the penis (Rathus, Nevid, & Fichner-Rathus, 2008, 300–301). Some people are under the misconception that one man plays the male and the other plays the female. This is not the case.

Masters and Johnson (1979), on the basis of their study of homosexuality, have reported a number of findings about the specific sexual behavior of homosexual men and women.

1. There are no major differences between the fantasy patterns of homosexuals and heterosexuals.

2. Homosexuality is learned and is definable only by overt behavior.

3. Homosexuality is a pattern of sexual interaction that a person can move into or out of at any time in life.

4. Physiologically homosexuals respond exactly as heterosexuals do to the same sexual stimuli— no sexual stimulus is unique to homosexuals.

5. Homosexuals are as amenable to treatment (with partners of their own choice) for sexual inadequacy as are heterosexuals.

6. Among established couples, homosexuals get more pleasure from lovemaking, even without intercourse, than do heterosexuals.

From a developmental standpoint, it is common for male and female homosexuals and bisexuals to have a history of sexual activity with the same and opposite genders, and to become sexually active during their early teens. No significant gender differences are found in lifetime prevalence rates or ages at initiating homosexual practices, but females tend to become sexually active at an older age than males and engage in more heterosexual activity. Sexual practices follow an initiation sequence beginning with manual sexual activity during their early teens and leading to further sexual activities during the middle and late teens (Rosaria, 1996).

Lesbian Sexual Activities

In lesbian lovemaking, oral sexual activities are common, as are manual stimulation and tribadism. **Tribadism** is the rubbing of genitals against someone's body or genital area. Touching, caressing, and hugging—the emotional components of lovemaking— play a large role in lesbian lovemaking. Vaginal penetration with dildos is rare. In fact, lesbians tend

tribadism
Rubbing genitals against someone's body or genital area.

Communication
DIMENSIONS

Word Choice Affects Study Results

Some years ago Blumstein and Schwartz (1983) conducted a study of couples and how often they "have sex." Lesbian, male homosexual, heterosexual nonmarried couples, and heterosexual married couples participated. They reported that lesbian couples "have sex" far less frequently than any other type of couple and that lesbian couples are less "sexual" as couples and as individuals than anyone else. In their sample, only about one-third of the lesbians in relationships of 2 years or longer "had sex" once a week or more; 47% of lesbians in long-term relationships "had sex" once a month or less, and among heterosexual married couples only 15% "had sex" once a month or less. They also reported that lesbians seemed to be more limited in the range of their "sexual" techniques than did other couples.

In commenting on the Blumstein and Schwartz study, Frye (1997) points out that what 85% of heterosexual married couples are doing more than once a month and what 47% of lesbian couples are doing less than once a month is not the same thing. She indicates that the comparison is not accurate because the focus

has been on sexual activity whereby a penis is inserted. When the only activity that counts as "doing it" involves interactions that include some sort of penile activity, she says, it is "no wonder [lesbians] discover [themselves] to 'do it' rather less often than do pairs with one or more penises present."

Frye feels that we would get a clearer picture if we start with a wide field of passions and bodily pleasures and create meanings that weave a web across it. She says:

> *I suggest that we begin the creation of a vocabulary that can encode and expand our meanings by adopting a very wide and general concept of "doing it." Let it be an open, generous, commodious concept encompassing all the acts and activities by which we generate with each other pleasure and thrills, tenderness, and ecstasy, passages of passionate carnality of whatever duration or profundity.... Our vocabulary will arise among us as we explain and explore and define the pleasures and our preferences across this field, teaching each other what the possibilities are and how to make them real.*

to do more overall genital stimulation, rather than direct clitoral stimulation, as is often the case in heterosexual relationships (Masters & Johnson, 1979).

Gay Sexual Activities

Homosexual men engage in foreplay activities similar to those of heterosexuals, such as hugging, kissing, petting, and nipple stimulation. Anal intercourse is actually the least frequent male homosexual activity. More often, gay men participate in mutual masturbation or fellatio (oral sex). Laboratory studies by Masters and Johnson (1979) showed that gay men were likely to pay more attention to the area of the penis on the lower side than heterosexual couples.

Keeping It Going

College-age students sometimes wonder how long-term partners can maintain monogamous sexual relationships over many years. Doesn't it get stale after a while? Certainly, for some couples, it does. For many others, sex remains exciting and fulfilling. This must be the case if so many older people are still sexually active. For example, one study found

that 60% of women ages 42 to 52 reported having regular sexual intercourse and 24% experienced oral sex on a regular basis (Cain et al., 2003). Another study conducted by the American Association of Retired Persons found that 19% of men 75 years of age or older have sexual intercourse at least once a week (AARP, 1999).

Although the frequency of sexual activity may decrease with age due to physical changes, such as taking longer to achieve an erection or vaginal lubrication, accommodations can be made to account for these changes. Foreplay may have to be extended, and the goal may have to be changed from achieving orgasm to intimacy and sexual pleasure.

In addition, as we've stated elsewhere in this text, variety can be vital in maintaining a satisfying sexual relationship over time. Some couples use sexual aids such as vibrators, others make use of pornographic materials to spice up their sex lives, and still others use sexual fantasy or role playing. In addition, long-term partners have learned what is sexually stimulating for each other, and the level of intimacy they develop over time goes a long way toward their still finding sex exciting.

Exploring the Dimensions of Human Sexuality

Our feelings, attitudes, and beliefs regarding sexuality are influenced by our internal and external environments. Go to go.jblearning.com/dimensions5e *to learn more about the biological, psychological, and sociological factors that affect your sexuality.*

Many factors influence what we find sexually arousing. Biologically, a physical disability may limit some sexual activities; however, it may also lead to other activities that are equally stimulating for a partner.

Psychologically, emotional attachment lends itself to sexual pleasuring. The greater the emotional attachment to someone we feel, often the greater the sexual pleasuring.

Schools play a broad role in developing our sense of what is acceptable or unacceptable. Community standards have an influence on what is taught, and that in turn influences student perceptions. Some fundamentalist religions ask young people to sign a public pledge to abstain from premarital sexual activity.

Communication is an important dimension. You and your partner need to be able to communicate which techniques you find sexually arousing. In addition, you must be able to communicate your love.

Family and friends influence sexual opinions as well. For example, comments by family and friends about Tiger Woods' affair may have influenced your perception of extramarital activity.

Biological Factors

- Sexual stimulation involves all five senses—touching, seeing, hearing, smelling, and tasting.
- Physical characteristics can enhance or inhibit sexual activities. For example, varying positions of intercourse offer varying degrees of comfort, depending on weight, physical stamina, or physical limitations.
- Foreplay allows for vaginal lubrication and erection before penile insertion.
- Physical disabilities may limit some sexual activities.
- Safer sexual activities decrease the risk of STI or HIV transmission.

Sociocultural Factors

- Sexual experience plays a role in what you find arousing.
- Sodomy laws prohibited certain sexual activities; however, these laws have been largely overturned.
- People who have more education tend to be less conservative sexually.
- Many religions prohibit certain sexual activities, such as premarital sex and masturbation. Pope John Paul II reaffirmed masturbation as an immoral act in 1993.
- School sexuality education programs often reflect community standards about what is perceived to be acceptable sexual behaviors. Parent and peer reactions to sexual information affect your perception of sexual activities.

Psychological Factors

- Emotional involvement with a partner plays a role in sexual pleasuring.
- Sexual fantasies are common among males and females.

Summary

- Two autoerotic, or solitary, sexual behaviors are *masturbation* and *sexual fantasy*. These activities are considered normal with a majority of people engaging in them at one time or another. There are usually no negative physical or psychological effects of either.

- Some women report experiencing heightened sexual arousal when an area of the interior wall of the vagina is stimulated. This area is known as the *G spot*, named after Ernst Grafenberg who first discovered it. Although recent evidence has been found that might verify the presence of the G spot, experts still disagree as to its existence.

- *Foreplay* is usually the name given to the physical contact preceding coitus or oral sex. Foreplay includes touching, kissing, biting, and genital fondling. However, the term foreplay is a misnomer since it may not precede any other sexual activity but might be engaged in just for its own pleasure.

- Sexual stimulation involves all the senses: touch, sight, smell, hearing, and taste. Among these senses, the secretion of *pheromones*—substances that attract sexual partners—has long been recognized to be produced by animals. In the late 1980s, scientists verified the secretion of pheromones in humans as well.

- Oral–genital sexual behavior includes three activities. *Cunnilingus* is the oral stimulation of the female genitalia. *Fellatio* is the oral stimulation of the male genitalia. *Analingus*—commonly referred to as *rimming*—is the oral stimulation of the female or male anus.

- Sexual intercourse can include many different positions. Among the most prevalent of these are the man on top, the woman on top, side-by-side, and the rear entry positions.

- Homosexuals enjoy many of the same sexual activities as heterosexuals. Lesbian sexual activities often involve rubbing the genitals against someone's body or genital area. This is called *tribadism*.

- One of the challenges faced by long-term sexual partners is to remain monogamous over many years. Although the frequency of sexual activity may decrease with age due to physical changes, accommodations can be made to account for these changes. Foreplay may be extended, and a variety of sexual behaviors may be engaged in to spice up the relationship.

Discussion Questions

1. Discuss the many dimensions that shape current attitudes toward masturbation and fantasies. How do male and female fantasies differ?

2. Explore the role of the senses, oral–genital contact, and various intercourse positions and sexual stimulation. Describe how sexual contact with another person can be made safer.

Application Questions

Reread the chapter-opening story and answer the following questions.

1. Many people are surprised to find that such an erotic novel dates back to the mid-18th century. Given that your ancestors reproduced (if they had not, you would not be reading this text), why is it widely believed that sexuality in the 1700s was inferior to today's sexuality?

2. One major change in sexual techniques since the novel was written is the more common prevalence of oral–genital sex. What might have prompted such a change?

3. This novel, as well as *Lady Chatterly's Lover* and many others, was banned in Boston, meaning that the book was not allowed to be sold in the city. The ban was finally rendered legally useless by the mid-20th century. How do current efforts to ban or limit the distribution of sexually explicit materials differ from the efforts of our ancestors?

Critical Thinking Questions

1. If you are in a sexual relationship, is it inappropriate to masturbate? Some people believe to do so is to risk fantasizing about someone else, which is tantamount to infidelity; that it uses sexual energy that is better directed toward one's partner; and that it is an expression of dissatisfaction with one's partner,

thereby insulting him or her. Others argue that masturbation has no effect on the sexual relationship; it is merely another means of sexual expression. They also believe that fantasizing about having sex with someone else is perfectly acceptable, as long as one doesn't act on that fantasy. Lastly, fantasizing can lead to uncovering new and exciting sexual activities that can be shared with one's partner. What do you think?

2. Is it better to do what is natural during sexual activity with a partner or to act according to what is learned in books such as this one?

Critical Thinking Case

The author Susan Minot, in her short story "Lust," mentions sexual technique: "I lay back with my eyes closed, luxuriating because he knew all sorts of expert angles, his hands never fumbling, going over my whole body, pressing the hair up and off the back of my head, giving an extra hip shove, as if to say *There*" (p. 15). But Minot continues the description as though the "expert" was very cold and unloving in his sexual activities.

Critics of sexuality education argue that knowing of the existence of the Grafenberg spot, erogenous zones, and the like makes sexual relationships too mechanistic. Each partner is trying so hard to recall what is stimulating and how to stimulate it that the spontaneity that makes sexual relationships so enjoyable is lost. People would be better off just "flying by the seat of their pants." Is that not the way sex has been conducted for eons? Have we not done all right with that system for generation after generation? Why add science to a nonscientific experience? Just lie back and enjoy yourself.

Others agree that sexual relationships have been adequate in the face of little knowledge of sexual arousal and response. However, they argue, adequate is not good enough. With knowledge of how the body is organized—for example, where nerve endings are accumulated—and how to achieve increased sexual excitement, sexual relationships could be enhanced. Further, there is nothing wrong with consciously, even during a highly emotional sexual encounter, thinking of how best

to please your partner, because that means that your partner will be thinking of how best to please you. The result will be a more sexually satisfying relationship.

What do you think? Spontaneous sexual experiences or mechanistic ones? Thoughtless sexual experiences or thoughtful ones?

Exploring Personal Dimensions

Assessing Your Sexual Fantasies
Are your sexual fantasies similar or dissimilar to other people's sexual fantasies? In what ways are they similar? In what ways are they dissimilar? To find out, answer the following questions. A discussion follows.

1. Do you fantasize about sex? How often?

2. What do you fantasize about when you fantasize about sex?

3. Do your sexual fantasies when you are with your partner differ from those when you are alone? If so, describe the difference.

4. Do you discuss your sexual fantasies with anyone else? If so, why? If not, why not?

Discussion
In a summary of research on sexual fantasies that reviewed more than 200 studies, the *Washington Post* reported the following information. Compare your responses to the typical responses of other adults.

1. Men average seven sexual fantasies a day, five of these triggered by outside stimuli such as watching a beautiful woman and two by inner thoughts. Women average five sexual fantasies a day, three from outside stimuli and two from their internal selves.

2. Women's favorite sexual fantasies involve a new sexual partner, sex with a celebrity, and sex with either a younger man or boy or an older "gent." Men's sexual fantasies include observing women nude and having sex with a new partner, sex with multiple partners at the same time, and having the sexual prowess to "drive women wild."

3. When men and women are alone, their sexual fantasies tend to be of their usual sexual partner, if they have one. Ironically, though,

when they are actually engaged in sexual activity with their usual sexual partner, they tend to fantasize about sex with someone else. Often, this fantasy involves a celebrity.

4. Because many men and women feel guilty about fantasizing about someone else while being engaged in sexual activity with their usual partner they do not discuss their sexual fantasies with their partner. A mere 26% of men and only 32% of women tell their sexual partner about their fantasies.

Well, how do you compare with the average adult female or male? Is there anything about your sexual fantasies that you will work to change?

Source: Tasker, F. X marks the fantasy, *The Washington Post* (July 27, 1995), D5.

Suggested Readings

Bakos, S. C. *The little book of the big orgasm: More techniques and games for amazing orgasms than you could possibly imagine trying.* Beverly, MA: Quiver, 2010.

Bakos, S. C. *The orgasm bible: The latest research and techniques for reaching more powerful climaxes more often.* Beverly, MA: Quiver, 2008.

Bakos, S. C. *The sex bible: the complete guide to sexual love.* Beverly, MA: Quiver, 2008.

Castleman, M. *Great sex: A man's guide to the secret principles of total-body sex.* Emmaus, PA: Rodale Press, 2004.

Davis, P. *The passion parties guide to great sex: Secrets and techniques to keep your relationship red hot.* Bel Air, CA: Broadway, 2007.

Deida, D. *The enlightened sex manual: Sexual skills for the superior lover.* Louisville, CO: Sounds True, 2007.

Foley, S. *Sex and love for grownups: A no-nonsense guide to a life of passion.* New York: Sterling, 2005.

Hooper, A. J., & Razazan, D. *Great sex games.* New York: DK Publishing, 2001.

Hutchins, D. C., & Sinclair, A. *The sensuous couple's (flip over) guide to seismic oral sex.* Philadelphia, PA: JPS, 2008.

Newman, F. *The whole lesbian sex book: A passionate guide for all of us.* San Francisco, CA: Cleis Press, 2004.

Paget, L. *The great lover playbook: 365 sexual tips and techniques to keep the fires burning all year long.* Bel Air, CA: Gotham, 2005.

Schell, J. *Lesbian sex: 101 lovemaking positions.* Berkeley, CA: Celestial Arts, 2008.

Spurr, P. *Naughty tricks and sexy tips: A couple's guide to uninhibited erotic pleasure.* Berkeley, CA: Amorata Press, 2007.

Vatsyayana. Translated by Burton, Richard F. and Arbuthnot, F. F. *The illustrated Kama Sutra: Ananga-Ranga and Perfumed Garden—the classic Eastern love texts.* South Paris, ME: Park Street Press, 1991.

Westheimer, R. K. *Sex for dummies.* New York: Wiley, John & Sons, 2001.

Web Resources

For links to the websites below, visit *go.jblearning.com/dimensions5e* and click on Resource Links.

Good Vibrations
www.goodvibes.com

A website that provides links related to sexual techniques and behaviors. Included are links to sex toys, sex education, erotic and informative books, adult DVDs, and other sexual-related materials. Products may be purchased at this website.

AllSex Guide
www.allsexguide.com

Offers links on matters pertaining to sex. Information made available in the form of guides on various topics, including couples sex, solo sex, kinky sex, safe sex, how to, and sex toys.

Sex Information Associates: Sex Positions and Techniques
www.sex-techniques-and-positions.com

A guide to a variety of sexual positions and techniques to enhance sexual pleasure. The guide includes photographs of people demonstrating the sexual positions. Also offers videos of sexual positions and sexual techniques.

AllSex Guide
www.allsexguide.com

Offers links to matters pertaining to sex. Links include a guide to sex positions, learn to talk dirty, guide to having an orgasm—for women, lesbian sex, communication, erotic massage, and others.

SexualHealthConnection.com: Sex Tips and Advice
www.healthcentral.com/sexual-health/sextechniques
.html

Recommendations for enhancing one's sex life. Among the topics included are speaking up for better sex, salvaging so-so sex, tantric sex, multiple orgasms, 5 steps to a healthy sex life, and 10 sexy gifts to give your partner.

References

AARP. *American Association of Retired Persons/Modern Maturity sexuality study*. Washington, DC: Author, 1999.

Apfelbaum, B. Why we should not accept sexual fantasies, in *Expanding the boundaries of sex therapy*. Berkeley, CA: Berkeley Sex Therapy Group, 1980.

Arafat, I., & Cotton, W. L. Masturbation practices of males and females. *Journal of Sex Research, 10* (1974), 293–307.

Bhutta, M. F. Sex and the nose: Human pheromonal response. *Journal of the Royal Society of Medicine, 100* (2007), 268–274.

Bivona, J., & Critelli, J. The nature of women's rape fantasies: An analysis of prevalence, frequency, and contents. *Journal of Sex Research, 45* (2008), 1–13.

Blumstein, P., & Schwartz, P. *American couples*. New York: William Morrow, 1983.

Blumstein, P., & Schwartz, P. Intimate relationships and the creation of sexuality. In *Homosexuality/heterosexuality: Concepts of sexual orientation*, McWhirter, D. P., Sanders, S. A., & Reinisch, J. M., eds. New York: Oxford Press, 1990, pp. 307–320.

Cain, V. S., Johannes, C. B., Avis, N. E., Mohr, B., Schocken, M., Skurnick, J., & Ory, M. Sexual functioning and practices in a multi-ethnic study of midlife women: Baseline results from SWAN. *Journal of Sex Research, 40* (2003), 266–276.

Chandra, A., Mosher, W. D., Copen, C., & Sionean, C. Sexual behavior, sexual attraction, and sexual identity in the United States: Data from the 2006–2008 National Survey of Family Growth. *National Health Statistics Reports, 36* (March 3, 2011).

Chick, D., & Gold, S. R. A review of influences on sexual fantasy: Attitudes, experiences, guilt and gender. *Imagination and Cognitive Personality, 7* (1987–1988), 61–76.

Christensen, F. M. *Pornography: The other side*. New York: Praeger, 1990.

Clement, U. Surveys of heterosexual behavior, in *Annual Review of Sex Research, Vol. 1*, Bancroft, J., Davis, C. M., & Weinstein, D., eds. New York: Society for the Scientific Study of Sex Research, 1990, 45–74.

Coen, S. Sexual interviewing, evaluation, and therapy: Psychoanalytic emphasis on the use of sexual fantasy. *Archives of Sexual Behavior, 7* (1978), 229–41.

Crepault, C. C., et al. Erotic imagery in women, in *Progress in sexuality*. Gemme, R., & C. C. Wheeler, ed. New York: Plenum, 1977.

Critelli, J. W., & Bivona, J. M. Women's erotic rape fantasies: An evaluation of theory and research. *Journal of Sex Research, 45* (2008), 57–70.

Cutler, W., Berg, G. P., Krieger, A., Huggins, G. R., Garcia, C. R., & Lawley, H. J. Human axillary secretions influence women's menstrual cycles: The role of donor extract from men. *Hormones and Behavior, 20* (1986), 463–473.

Das, A. Masturbaton in the United States. *Journal of Sex and Marital Therapy, 33* (2007), 301–317.

Davidson, J. K. The utilization of sexual fantasies by sexually experienced university students. *Journal of American College Health, 34* (1985), 24–32.

Downey, L. International change in sex behavior: A belated look at Kinsey's males. *Archives of Sexual Behavior, 9* (1980), 267–317.

Elder, S. Sexual foreplay: What's in it for men? *WebMD*, 2009. Available: http://men.webmd.com/guide/sexual-foreplay-whats-for-men.

Ellis, B. J., & Symons, D. Sex differences in sexual fantasy: An evolutionary psychological approach. *Journal of Sex Research, 27* (1990), 527–555.

Friday, N. *Forbidden flowers*. New York: Pocket Books, 1975.

Frye, M. Lesbian sex, in *Through the prism of difference: Readings on sex and gender*, Zinn, M. B., Hondagneu-Sotelo, P., & Messner, M. A., eds. Boston: Allyn & Bacon, 1997.

Geddes, L. Ultrasound nails location of the elusive G spot. *Independent* (February 20, 2008). Available: http://www.sensualism.com/sex/g-spot.html.

Gerressu, M., Mercer, C. H., Graham, C. A., Wellings, K., & Johnson, A. M. Prevalence of masturbation and associated factors in a British national probability survey. *Archives of Sexual Behavior, 37* (2008), 266–278.

Goodson, P., McCormick, D., & Evans, A. Searching for sexually explicit materials on the Internet: An exploratory study of college students' behavior and attitudes. *Archives of Sexual Behavior, 30* (2001), 101–118.

Gravina, G. L., Brandetti, F., Martini, P., Carosa, E., Di Stasi, S. M., Morano, S., Lenzi, A., & Jannini, E. A. Measurement of the thickness of the urethrovaginal space in women with or without vaginal orgasm. *Journal of Sexual Medicine, 5* (2008), 610–618.

Haffner, D. W., & Schwartz, P. *What I've learned about sex*. New York: Perigee Books, 1998.

Halderman, B. L., Zelhart, P. F., & Jackson, T. T. The study of fantasy: Determinants of fantasy function and content. *Journal of Clinical Psychology, 41* (1984), 325–330.

Hariton, B. E. The sexual fantasies of women. In *Psychology Today* (editors). *The female experience*. Del Mar, CA: Communications/Research/Machines, 1973.

Hawley, P. H., & Hensley, W. A. Social dominance and forceful submission fantasies: Feminine pathology or power? *Journal of Sex Research, 46* (2009), 568–585.

Henderson, M. Scientist may be first man to find the female G-spot. *The Times* (February 21, 2008). Available: http://www.timesonline.co.uk/tol/news/uk/science/article3406113.ece.

Hicks, T., & Leitenberg, H. Sexual fantasies about one's partner versus someone else: Gender differences in incidence and frequency. *Journal of Sex Research, 38* (2001), 43–50.

Hollender, M. H. Women's wish to be held: Sexual and nonsexual aspects. *Medical Aspects of Human Sexuality*, (October 1970), 12–26.

Hunt, M. *Sexual behavior in the 1970's*. Chicago: Playboy Press, 1974.

Jones, J. C., & Barlow, D. H. Self-reported frequency of sexual urges, fantasies, and masturbatory fantasies in heterosexual males and females. *Archives of Sexual Behavior, 19* (1990), 269–279.

Keating, J., & Over, R. Sexual fantasies of heterosexual and homosexual men. *Archives of Sexual Behavior, 19* (1990), 461–475.

Keverne, E. B. Importance of olfactory and vomeronasal systems for male sexual function. *Physiology and Behavior, 83* (2004), 177–187.

Kinsey, A. C., Pomeroy, W. B., & Martin, C. E. *Sexual behavior in the human female*. Philadelphia: Saunders, 1953.

Kinsey, A. C., Pomeroy, W. B., & Martin, C. E. *Sexual behavior in the human male*. Philadelphia: Saunders, 1948.

Knafo, G., & Jaffe, Y. Sexual fantasizing in males and females. *Journal of Research in Personality, 19* (1984), 451–462.

Lanuza, E., Novejarque, A., Martinez-Hernandez, J., Agustin-Pavon, C., & Martinez-Garcia, F. Sexual pheromones and the evolution of the reward system of the brain: The chemosensory function of the amygdala. *Brain Research Bulletin, 75* (2008), 460–466.

Laumann, E. O., Gagnon, J. H., Michael, R. T., & Michaels, S. *The social organization of sexuality: Sexual practices in the United States*. Chicago: University of Chicago Press, 1994.

Leahy, M. *Porn university: What college students are really saying about sex on campus*. Chicago: Northfield Publishers, 2009.

Leitenberg, H., & Henning, K. Sexual fantasy. *Psychological Bulletin, 117* (1995), 469–496.

Maltz, W., & Boss, S. *Private thoughts*. Novalo, CA: New World Library, 2001.

Masters, W. H., & Johnson, V. E. *Homosexuality in perspective*. Boston: Little, Brown, 1979.

Masters, W. H., & Johnson, V. E. *Human sexual response*. Boston: Little, Brown, 1966.

Masters, W. H., Johnson, V. E., & Kolodny, R. C. *Human sexuality*, 2nd ed. Boston: Little, Brown, 1985.

Michael, R. T., Gagnon, J. H., Laumann, E. O., & Kolata, G. *Sex in America: A definitive survey*. New York: Warner Books, 1995.

Michael, R., Gagnon, J., Laumann, E., & Kolata, G. *Sex in America*. Boston: Little, Brown, 1994.

Nutter, D., & Condron, M. Sexual fantasy and activity patterns of females with inhibited sexual desire versus normal controls. *Journal of Sex and Marital Therapy, 9* (1983), 276–282.

Pastor, Z. [G spot—myths and reality.] *Ceska Gynekologie, 75* (2010), 211–217.

Peplau, L. A., & Cochran, S. D. A relationship perspective on homosexuality, in *Homosexuality/heterosexuality: Concepts of sexual orientation*, McWhirter, D. P., Sanders, S. A., & Reinisch, J. M., eds. New York: Oxford Press, 1990, pp. 321–349.

Perry, J. D., & Whipple, B. Pelvic muscle strength of female ejaculators: Evidence in support of a new theory of orgasm. *Journal of Sex Research, 17* (1981), 22–39.

Preti, G., Winnifred, C., Celso, R., Garcia, G. Huggins, R., & Lawley, H. J. Human axillary secretions influence women's menstrual cycles: The role of donor extract of females. *Hormones and Behavior, 20* (1986), 474–482.

Rathus, S. A., Nevid, J. S., & Fichner-Rathus, L. *Human sexuality in a world of diversity*. Boston, MA: Pearson, 2008.

Religious tolerance. About Masturbation: Diversity of Beliefs within the Roman Catholic Church, 2008. Available: http://www.religoustolerance.org/masturba10.htm.

Rensberger, R. Pheromones discovered in humans: Substances help regulate female reproductive cycle. *Washington Post* (November 1986) A1, A7.

Rosaria, M. The psychosexual development of urban lesbian, gay, and bisexual youth. *Journal of Sex Research, 33, no. 2* (1996), 113–126.

Rumbough, T. B. *Controversial uses of the Internet by college students*, 2001. Available: http://www.eucuase.edu/ir/library/pdf/C5D1618.pdf.

Shainess, N., & Greenwald, H. Debate: Are fantasies during sexual relations a sign of difficulty? *Sexual Behavior, 1* (1971), 38–54.

Spalding, L. R., & Peplau, L. A. The unfaithful lover: Heterosexuals' perceptions of bisexuals and their relationships. *Psychology of Women Quarterly, 21* (1997), 611–625.

Spors, H., & Sobel, N. Male behavior by knockout. *Neuron, 55* (2007), 689–693.

Strassberg, D. S., & Lockerd, L. K. Force in women's sexual fantasies. *Journal of Sexual Behavior, 27* (1998), 403–414.

Strovny, D. The importance of foreplay. *AskMen.com*, 2009. Available: http://www.askmen.com/dating/love_tip/sextip18.html.

Sue, D. Erotic fantasies of college students during coitus. *Journal of Sex Research, 15* (1979), 299–305.

Tripp, C. A. *The homosexual matrix*. New York: New American Library, 1976.

The way we live now. *New York Times* (May 7, 2000), p. 18.

Wilson, G. D. Gender differences in sexual fantasy: An evolutionary analysis. *Personality and Individual Differences, 22* (1997): 27–31.

Zimmer, D. E., Borchardt, E., & Fischle, C. Sexual fantasies of sexually distressed and nondistressed men and women: An empirical comparison. *Journal of Sex and Marital Therapy, 9* (1983), 38–50.

Alternative Sexual Behavior

FEATURES

Communication Dimensions
Communicating Accurately

Multicultural Dimensions
Paraphilias Across Cultures

Gender Dimensions
Paraphilias and Gender Differences

Ethical Dimensions
The Ethics of Chemical Treatment for Paraphilias

CHAPTER OBJECTIVES

1 Discuss how some alternative sexual behaviors exist on a continuum of sexual activity.

2 Describe the most common paraphilias.

3 Name and define paraphilias other than the most common ones.

4 Explain what can be done to treat paraphilias.

5 Summarize what is known about sexual addiction.

go.jblearning.com/dimensions5e

The Most Common Paraphilias
Sexual Addiction

INTRODUCTION

*V*arieties of sexual behaviors have been around a long time, as have many opinions about them. Many people were surprised when a well-known sportscaster was indicted on charges of assault and sodomy. His accuser, a 41-year-old female friend whom he had known for 10 years, claimed that he viciously bit her several times on the back during an argument in his hotel room.

The woman claimed that her partner became enraged when she refused to join in a "three-way" with him and another man and that he threw her on the bed and bit her on the back 10 to 15 times. Then, according to court documents, he forced her to perform oral sexual activity. After the woman sought treatment at a local hospital, the police were notified.

To many, the charges against the sportscaster seemed very much out of character. For example, one of his producers said that on both a professional and a personal level he was a joy to be around. The executive producer of the network sports said he was "in total shock" about the charges.

As the allegations were investigated, additional stories came out about the sportscaster's sexual behavior, including his alleged fondness for wearing women's underwear and participating in threesomes. As a result, he was removed from sportscasting and taken off network shows. About 3 years later, he returned to broadcasting as the radio voice of a pro sports team.

Stories like this one cause people to wonder about varieties of sexual behavior and talk more about them. Although many varieties of sexual behavior are relatively uncommon, it can be important to know more about them.

Common Versus Atypical Sexual Behaviors

A few points about atypical sexual behavior in general should be noted before we consider specific behaviors. First, in many instances there are gradations of a sexual behavior existing on a continuum. For example, most people enjoy looking at other people. However, if someone spends many hours each day just looking at others, we would probably assume that person has a problem. There would be spots on the continuum between these two extremes that might be hard to judge. Is the behavior common or is it atypical? Is it acceptable or unacceptable? It is up to each individual, and society, to decide where on the continuum of sexual behavior activities become unacceptable. For instance, when is behavior obsessive (that is, the individual does not freely choose the behavior); when is it associated with emotional distress or with the inability to interact satisfactorily with other people; when is it forced on another person; when is it illegal?

Because many behaviors vary in degree, it is not surprising that many of us may recognize some degree of atypical behaviors or feelings in ourselves—perhaps only in private fantasies. In most instances, such behaviors or feelings should be accepted as natural—as long as they do not interfere with our optimal functioning or with the rights of others.

It is also common for us not to know a great deal about atypical sexual behaviors. Because in most cases such behavior is not common, and in most cases it is performed in private, it is difficult to study. Therefore, as we consider atypical sexual behaviors, many questions will be left unanswered.

It is also interesting that atypical sexual behaviors often occur in combination. For example, one well-known celebrity apparently did some cross-dressing along with participating in group sexual activity and violence.

Some people wonder about causes of paraphilias. Not a great deal is known about this topic, but theories can be grouped into psychoanalytical, behavioral, and sociobiological (Brannon & Carroll, 2008). Psychoanalytical theory centers on possible distortion of courtship phases. Some people are unable to adhere to socially acceptable norms and develop deviant or unconventional sexual practices. Behavioral theory attributes the development of certain paraphilias to the process of conditioning. For example, if nonsexual objects are frequently associated with a pleasurable sexual activity, the objects can become sexually arousing. In some cases, the constant threat of discovery may be as arousing as the act itself. Sociobiological theory includes the idea that even atypical sexual behavior relates to survival of the species. For example, different paraphilias may be responsible for enhancing society's level of sexual excitation. In turn, this increases the likelihood of people engaging in sexual acts that would ultimately lead to procreation.

Within this minichapter, we briefly discuss some of the most common atypical sexual behaviors.

The Most Common Paraphilias

Unusual or problematic sexual behaviors are scientifically known as paraphilias. **Paraphilia** means love (*philia*) beyond the usual (*para*). There are about 50 different paraphilias, and each exists in fantasy and in reality. It is generally accepted that the prevalence and variety of paraphilias are greater in males than in females, but as indicated previously, in most instances little is known about them.

Paraphilic behaviors are unconventional sexual behaviors that are obsessive and compulsive. They can interfere with love relationships and intimacy. Paraphilias are defined as recurrent, intense sexually arousing fantasies, sexual urges, or behaviors involving (1) nonhuman objects, (2) the suffering or humiliation of oneself or one's partner, or (3) children or other nonconsenting persons. Also, the behavior, urges, or fantasies cause significant

> **paraphilia**
> Literally meaning "love (*philia*) beyond the usual (*para*)," this term refers to various sexual behaviors previously referred to as deviant.

? Did You Know ...

One theory suggests that paraphilias may be related to erotic target location errors (ETLEs), involving the erroneous location of erotic targets. For example, ETLEs may be responsible for people with preferred erotic targets such as children, amputees, plush animals, and real animals, to name a few.

Source: Data from Lawrence, A. A. Erotic target location errors: An underappreciated paraphiliac dimension. *Journal of Sex Research 46,* nos. 2 & 3 (March 2009), 194–215.

stress in social, occupational, or other important areas of functioning. Some behaviors, such as sadomasochism, when they are consensual and do not impair life functioning, are not considered to be a paraphilia because they do not meet all of the diagnostic criteria (Coleman, 2005).

Paraphilias include sexual behaviors that many people view as distasteful, unusual, or abnormal and that they subsequently reject. In descending order, the most common are pedophilia, exhibitionism, voyeurism, and frotteurism. Far less common are fetishism, sexual masochism, sexual sadism, and transvestism (Paraphilias, 2005).

Exhibitionism

Exhibitionism (commonly called *flashing* or *indecent exposure*) occurs when an individual achieves sexual gratification by exhibiting the genitals to observers. The American Psychiatric Association (2005) has

> **exhibitionism**
> Achievement of sexual gratification by exhibiting the genitals to observers.

officially defined exhibitionism as "over a period of at least six months, recurrent, intense sexually arousing fantasies, sexual urges, or behaviors involving the exposure of one's genitals to an unsuspecting stranger." Though exhibitionism is a good example of a sexual behavior that is difficult to classify as one that causes problems, we would probably agree that if someone's primary motivation in life is exhibitionism, that person has a problem. At what point does the behavior become abnormal?

There are three key features of true exhibitionism: (1) There is sexual arousal directly related to the shock; (2) the victim is unwilling; and (3) no further sexual contact is desired (Exhibitionism, 2005).

A few facts about exhibitionists might help to put this behavior into perspective. The exhibitionist receives sexual gratification through the victim's (observer's) response. Exhibitionists might achieve orgasm by the very act of exposure, but more likely they will masturbate either while exhibiting or later. Exhibitionists feel inadequate, they are afraid of rejection, they are shy, and commonly they have had unsatisfactory sexual relationships. They may be looking for attention or affirmation of their masculinity (most exhibitionists are male) or attempting to frighten others.

Although people often think exhibitionists are violent and aggressive, they usually are not. It is extremely rare for exhibitionists to do more than display the genitals. They do not want contact with a person. Punishment and imprisonment do not seem to prevent the recurrence of exhibitionism. Although it may be difficult, generally the best response is to ignore an exhibitionist and continue usual activities. In this way the exhibitionistic behavior is not reinforced.

The incidence of exhibitionism in the general population is difficult to estimate because, as with most other paraphilias, persons with this disorder do not usually seek counseling by their own free will. Exhibitionism is one of the three most common sexual offenses in police records. The other two are voyeurism and pedophilia (Exhibitionism, 2011).

Voyeurism

In a very general sense, the term **voyeurism** (or **scopophilia**, "love of viewing") means obtaining sexual pleasure from observing unsuspecting individuals who are naked, in the process of undressing, or engaging in sexual acts. The person being observed is usually a stranger to the

> **voyeurism (scopophilia)**
> Obtaining pleasure from watching people who are undressing or engaging in sexual behavior.

observer. The act of looking is done for the purpose of achieving sexual excitement. The observer generally does not seek to have sexual contact or activity with the person being observed. If orgasm is sought it is generally achieved through masturbation. This may occur during the act of observation or later,

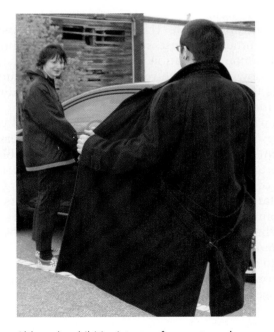

Although exhibitionists are often portrayed comically, in real life the phenomenon is quite different. Exhibitionists gain sexual pleasure from eliciting a harsh reaction to their unprovoked actions. It is best to ignore one if you are ever flashed.

relying on the memory of the act that was observed (Voyeurism, 2011). A "peeping Tom" is a voyeur. The voyeur learns from experience where to find people to watch. His erotic excitement lies in the forbidden act of looking at the person.

The fantasies, sexual urges, or behaviors cause clinically significant distress or impairment in social, occupational, or other important areas of functioning. Voyeurs derive sexual gratification from seeing sex organs and sexual acts (Brannon & Carroll, 2008).

Voyeurs, who are often shy and lonely and lack social skills, commonly fantasize about having sexual relations with the people they are watching and often masturbate while fantasizing. Voyeurs derive satisfaction from the fear of being caught, the anonymity of the person being watched, and the fact that the person does not know he or she is being watched. Generally voyeurs are not violent and, in fact, are fearful of any contact with the people they observe.

Some degree of voyeurism probably exists in everyone. Society even condones some forms of voyeurism; for example, some magazines are designed to satisfy peoples' voyeuristic tendencies, and the popularity of sexually explicit movies and websites is due to voyeurism.

Obscene Communication

The most common and traditional form of obscene communication has been obscene telephone calls; through the years there have also been many examples of obscene letter writing. In more recent years obscene emails have appeared as well.

Erotic telephone calling is a form of erotic distancing. As do the exhibitionist and the voyeur, the obscene caller or writer obtains sexual pleasure from a distance and not from direct contact with another person. Telephone callers receive sexual gratification from making obscene remarks over the telephone, usually suggesting that the person meet them to have sexual relations (even though they would probably never go through with this act). The recipient may be a stranger or a consenting listener. Professional consenting listeners, trained to take part in erotic telephone fantasies, charge for playing this role.

It seems that the vast majority of females receive obscene messages at some time in their life. The typical communicator is an adult male unknown to the victim. Such communications can affect the person receiving them emotionally, and a common response is fear.

Obscene telephone callers have counterparts in those whose primary turn-on is not genital sexual activity with a partner but erotic narrations or readings. The obscene letter writer or the obscene

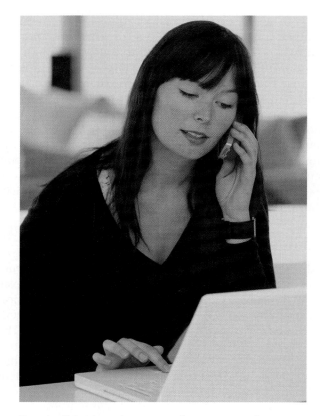

Females living in major metropolitan areas are the most likely victims of obscene communication.

computer message sender is hoping for sexual gratification as well.

According to the U.S. Department of Justice, "Any comment, request, suggestion, proposal, image, or other communication which is obscene or indecent, knowing that the recipient of the communication is under 18 years of age" is illegal. In addition, "any indecent communication for commercial purposes which is available to any person under 18 years of age or to any other person without that person's consent" is illegal. These offenses are punishable by a fine up to $50,000 for each violation or imprisonment of up to 6 months or both (United States Code Annotated Title 47, 2003). Note that this covers any telecommunication device, including computers.

What should someone who receives an obscene communication do? Above all, people are advised to remain calm and not reveal shock or fright: These reactions can reinforce the message sender and increase the likelihood of repeated contact. The recommended response is to say nothing and end the communication. Most people who send obscene messages are not dangerous, and most do not make repeat contacts with the same person. In the case of obscene phone calls, it might be helpful to get an unlisted phone number, obtain caller ID capabilities, and/or contact the police about threatening or repeated calls.

Communication
DIMENSIONS

Communicating Accurately

With any sexual behavior, the concept of consent is crucial. For example, if a partner wants to be tied up, that might be fine; however, prior communication about the goal is important. A student once confessed (under the influence of alcohol) to a group of people that she wanted to be tied up. Another time, though, she said that her fantasy really involved being tied down with silk ribbons to a luxurious four-poster bed. Still later she said that what she really wanted was a partner who would initiate sexual activity with her. Thus she did not always like being the aggressor, and her fantasy was really about having her lover "take charge." But in respect to her original assertions, that underlying desire would not have been known to a partner, nor would her desire for an initiating partner be fulfilled when she engaged in nonbondage activities. As always, effective communication is a must.

First, it is crucial to explain desires and intentions clearly in such situations. The student in our example was not clear, and this could have led to behavior or attempts at behavior that were not desired. This, in turn, could have caused overall relationship problems. Second, as with any form of sexual behavior, it is important to obtain consent. It is not enough to assume that you know what your partner meant or that consent is implicit because you have a good relationship. Without consent, sexual behavior is forcible. With consent, it can be enjoyable for everyone and contribute to a positive relationship.

Masochism and Sadism

The American Psychiatric Association (2005) defines sexual masochism as "over a period of at least six months, recurrent, intense sexually arousing fantasies, sexual urges, or behaviors involving the act (real, not simulated) of being humiliated, beaten, bound, or otherwise made to suffer." It defines sexual sadism as "over a period of at least six months, recurrent, intense sexually arousing fantasies, sexual urges, or behaviors involving acts (real, not simulated) in which the psychological or physical suffering (including humiliation) of the victim is sexually exciting to the person."

Sexual masochism, therefore, is sexual gratification that results from experiencing pain. This might include scratching, biting, beating, and the use of various devices. The pain involved must be planned as a part of an overall experience; accidentally hitting a finger with a hammer is not the kind of experience the masochist wants. **Sexual sadism** occurs when an individual gets sexual gratification from inflicting pain on another person—the hallmark of sadism is intentional torture of the victim to sexually arouse the offender. Sadists have persistent fantasies in which sexual excitement results from inflicting psychological or physical suffering (including humiliation and

sexual masochism
Sexual gratification that results from experiencing pain.

sexual sadism
Sexual gratification that results from inflicting pain on another person.

terror) on a sexual partner. At its most extreme, sadism involves illegal activities such as rape, torture, and even murder, in which case the death of the victim produces sexual excitement (Paraphilias, 2009). Sadists obviously make good partners for masochists, but sadomasochistic partner matching is difficult to achieve because it requires that the fantasies of the two people match completely. There is one sadistic scenario, however, that requires an unsuspecting partner or a stranger to be subjected to abuse. Sadism does not seem to be as common as masochism.

Domination and degradation are important to both the sadist and the masochist. Some psychiatrists feel that sadism is an expression of anger and hostility. Masochism, in contrast, is sometimes thought to result from a belief that sexual activity is dirty and evil; therefore, the activity could be viewed as just punishment for sexual sins. It is difficult to understand the true psychology of these behaviors.

Sadomasochism is a paraphilia that combines both sadistic and masochistic sexual behavior. The main characteristic is the eroticizing of pain. What appears to the outsider to be painful is experienced as somewhat painful but mostly pleasurable and very sexually arousing to the sadomasochist. Sadomasochistic sexual encounters usually occur in the context of scripted scenes that simulate interactions between master and slave, employer and servant, and parent and child. Sadomasochists tend to alternate between masochistic and sadistic roles. In milder forms, dominance and submissive behaviors may be found in many relationships or may be an element of fantasy life (Sadomasochism, 2001).

There is more information available on masochism and sadism than on most other paraphilias, and a brief chronological review of a few studies will help to shed some light on these two behaviors.

bondage perversion
Getting sexual pleasure from being bound, tied up, or otherwise restricted.

transvestite
A person who achieves sexual satisfaction from wearing clothes usually worn by the other gender.

Baumeister (1997) pointed out that masochism fosters temporary escape from the stressful awareness of one's ordinary identity. Litman (1997) suggested that sexual masochism is more widespread and can be more dangerous than current literature indicates. Danger can arise from being humiliated, endangered, and enslaved and being physically bound, restrained, and rendered helpless to the degree that life is threatened. He indicates that **bondage perversion** (deriving pleasure from being bound, tied up, or otherwise restricted) can be fatal—a mix of suicide and accident.

Sexual masochism is more common in males, but the incidence in females is on the rise. Masochists often seek partners to tie up, humiliate, blindfold, or hurt. They may enjoy being whipped, beaten, shocked, or cut. Verbal abuse is common. Some masochists require pain or humiliation to function sexually (Masochism, 2001). Some sadists also require the pain or humiliation of a partner to function sexually. As long as it occurs with a consenting partner, sadism is not considered a psychological disorder. It is considered a disorder when it causes the person unhappiness or causes problems with work, social setting, or family. If the other person is not willing, sadism can be a severe and even criminal disorder. Sadism is much more common in males (Sadism, 2001). People who engage in masochism and sadism must be especially careful about diseases transmitted by body fluids, such as hepatitis and HIV.

Masochism can range from mild to extreme versions. Examples of mild versions might include bondage (being tied up for the purpose of sexual arousal), or being spanked or overpowered by physical force. The crucial point is that they are mainly symbolic enactments done under carefully controlled conditions with a trusted partner. At the opposite end of the spectrum are genuinely painful and harmful activities (Discovery Health: Paraphilia, 2005).

Sadism can also be a consensual activity in milder forms. For example, it might involve role-playing with dominant and submissive roles such as master and slave. Like masochism, however, it is important to have controlled conditions with a trusted partner

to avoid unplanned injuries. Sadism is commonly found in association with other paraphilias—particularly masochism, fetishism, and transvestism (Sexual sadism, 2005).

Sadism and masochism are good examples of sexual behaviors in which we need to differentiate between fantasy and behavior. For example, many more people have reported sexual fantasies involving masochism and sadism than have actually participated in such behavior. It is possible to enjoy a sexual fantasy without needing to act it out in real life.

Transvestism

Transvestism is sometimes confused with transsexualism and homosexuality. A **transvestite** takes pleasure in wearing clothing of the other gender and is likely to achieve sexual gratification from doing so but has no interest in having a sex-change operation or in relating sexually to members of the same gender. While transvestites may be male or female, they typically are heterosexual married males (Brannon & Carroll, 2008).

Transvestism is also known as cross-dressing or dressing in drag. Some homosexual men dress in drag for fun. Some people with a gender identity disorder

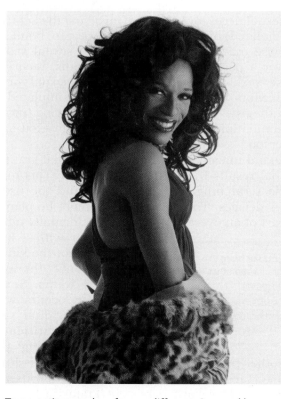

Transvestites can be of many different sizes and have various appearances.

dress in clothes of the other gender to try to pass as the other gender or because they simply feel that is their proper gender. Transvestites, however, generally cross-dress for sexual arousal. Most are male and do not wish to be mistaken for women. Transvestism is considered to be a psychological disorder only when the person meets the following conditions (Transvestism, 2005). He:

- Is heterosexual, or straight.
- Has intense sexual fantasies, urges, or behaviors involving dressing in women's clothing.
- Is distressed by these fantasies, urges, or behaviors and they cause problems in his life.

Some transvestites cross-dress only periodically, and the use of female clothes (most transvestites are males) may approximate a fetish. Others may wear female clothing under their male clothes. No one knows for sure why some people are transvestites, and it is interesting to note that most transvestites have quite normal heterosexual relationships.

Most transvestites begin to experiment with cross-dressing when they are children or adolescents. Some feel guilty and uncomfortable about this preference; others do not. Many are happily married to people who understand their behaviors. Others have had relationships ruined by cross-dressing. There are numerous support groups for transvestites and their partners (Transvestism, 2001).

It is common for transvestism to be classified as a fetish. It is usually done in private, although undergarments can also be worn in public under regular street clothes. Transvestites will often masturbate while wearing female clothing and/or make-up while fondling specific items. Transvestism, by itself, is usually not associated with criminal behavior, although it could be combined with other fetishes or disorders that result in criminal behavior (Transvestic fetishism, 2005).

Fetishism

Fetishism is a paraphilia in which an inanimate object elicits sexual arousal. Articles of clothing and materials made of rubber, silk, fur, or leather are common fetishistic objects. The American Psychiatric Association (2005) defines the symptoms of fetishism as "over a period of at least six months, recurrent, intense sexually arousing fantasies, sexual urges, or behaviors involving the use of nonliving objects. The fantasies, sexual urges, or behaviors cause clinically significant distress or impairment in social, occupational, or other important areas of functioning."

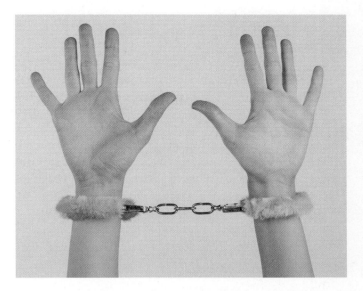

Various items, articles of clothing, and materials can be fetishistic objects.

The fetishist may masturbate while engaging in fetishistic behavior or may just enjoy stimulation from the objects. In a related paraphilia, **partialism**, people are aroused by a particular body part (breasts, muscular chests, feet, and so on). Most fetishes are practiced in private or with a willing partner.

> **fetishism**
> Paraphilia in which an inanimate object elicits sexual arousal.
>
> **partialism**
> Paraphilia in which sexual arousal is associated with a particular body part.

Generally, a person who has fetishism must have the fetish present to become sexually excited. It usually begins in childhood or adolescence and is most common among males. Although many people are aroused by undergarments or other items, this is not considered fetishism except when a person cannot perform sexually unless the partner is wearing the items (Fetishism, 2001).

The fetish may replace sexual activity with a partner or may be integrated into sexual activity with a willing partner. When the fetish becomes the sole object of sexual desire, sexual relationships often are avoided (Paraphilias, 2009). Most fetishes and partialisms are harmless. However, occasionally someone may commit burglary to obtain the fetish object.

Inanimate object fetishes can be categorized into two types: form fetishes and media fetishes. In a form fetish, it is the object and its shape that are important, such as with high-heeled shoes. In a media fetish, it is the material from which the object is made that is important, such as silk or leather. Although the list of objects that fetishists can use for sexual gratification is inexhaustible, among the more common

Multicultural DIMENSIONS

Paraphilias Across Cultures

The amount of paraphilias seems to vary across cultures. Also, not all cultures appear to manifest certain paraphilic practices or to view them as an issue. For example, paraphilias may be more common in egocentric and sex-positive cultures where sexual intercourse is mainly practiced for pleasure and arousal is a predominant theme. In contrast, societies that emphasize sexual activity for reproduction (sex-negative cultures) may have rates of paraphilia

different from sex-positive cultures. Also, in societies that stress egocentric or individualistic values, social mores are more likely to be constrained by legal factors than by norms, thereby making paraphilias seem more common because they are more likely to be reported to and seen by clinicians. Culture does seem to influence paraphilias, including their understanding and identification.

Source: Data from Bhugra, D., Popelyuk, D., & McMullen, I. Paraphilias across cultures: Contexts and controversies. *Journal of Sex Research, 47, no. 2–3* (March 2010), 242–256.

---

inanimate objects are panties, bras, slips, stockings or panty hose, negligees, shoes, boots, and gloves. Common media objects include leather, rubber, silk, and fur. In most cases, the person with a fetish is no danger to others and pursues the use of the fetish objects in private, usually through masturbation. The causes of fetishism are not clearly understood. Some experts believe that it develops from early childhood experiences, in which an object was associated with a particularly powerful form of sexual arousal or gratification (Fetishism, 2005).

■ Other Paraphilias

Bestiality

Bestiality (or **zoophilia**) is sexual contact with animals. In Kinsey's research (1948, 1953), about 8% of males and 4% of females reported having had sexual experiences with animals at some time. The frequency of bestiality was higher (17% for males) for those raised in rural areas. Men most often had sexual contact with farm animals; women most often had sexual contact with household pets.

bestiality
Sexual contact with animals—also called *zoophilia*.

zoophilia
Sexual contact with animals—also called *bestiality*.

Human sexual relationships with animals have been an interesting topic for some people for hundreds of years. Stories of human–animal contact are found throughout ancient folklore. For example, Zeus, in the form of a swan, had sexual intercourse with Leda, the queen of Sparta. Greek and Roman mythology portrayed females having sexual

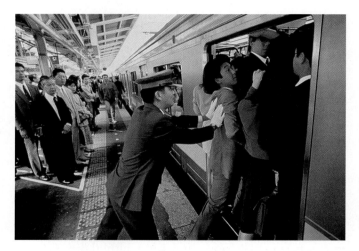

The overcrowding of subways in Tokyo and other Japanese cities lends itself to frottage, or deriving sexual pleasure from rubbing up against a nonconsenting person. The situation is exacerbated by the male-dominated Japanese culture, which prevents police from dealing with the problem.

relationships with bears, apes, bulls, goats, horses, wolves, snakes, and crocodiles. Historically, taboos against human–animal contact have been severe. The laws in many states treated bestiality as a felony. In eight states, the maximal penalty was life imprisonment. Many such laws remain on the books today (Bestiality, 2003).

Sexual experience with animals is usually only a transitory experience for young people who do not have acceptable sexual partners. It most likely occurs during adolescence, and most people move on to more common adult sexual relations with humans. It is generally agreed that a condition is really zoophilia only if someone prefers sexual contact with animals even if other forms of sexual activity are available.

There has been very little research on bestiality. Even though it has been present throughout history, addressing the subject often seems to evoke prejudices and emotional reactions rather than objective reflection. A large part of the information on bestiality stems from criminological reports, and this is a very limited sampling (Beetz, 2004).

Frottage

Frottage is the act of obtaining sexual pleasure from rubbing or pressing against a nonconsenting person. The American Psychiatric Association's official definition (2000) is "over a period of at least six months, recurrent, intense sexually arousing fantasies, sexual urges, or behaviors involving touching and rubbing against a nonconsenting person." It is likely to occur in crowds, on elevators, and in buses and subways. It is even possible that the frotteur will achieve orgasm. Women and girls, the usual recipients, generally find this behavior offensive. Normally no additional contact or other form of behavior follows.

Necrophilia

Necrophilia is a rather rare behavior in which a person receives sexual pleasure from viewing or having sexual relations with a dead person. Sometimes necrophiliacs (almost all of whom are men) pay women to pretend to be dead so as to provide sexual pleasure. This might even include dressing in a certain way, using white powder to look very pale, and lying very still. In this way the participants are simulated corpses.

> **frottage**
> Obtaining of sexual pleasure from rubbing or pressing against another person.
>
> **necrophilia**
> Sexual relations with a dead person.

Necrophiliacs are usually severely emotionally disturbed, sexually and socially inept, and hate and fear women. Although local newspapers do not report instances, law enforcement officers indicate that bodies are sometimes stolen for this purpose.

It is interesting to note that necrophilia was depicted within the range of normal expression in the television program, *Buffy the Vampire Slayer*. The sexual encounter of Buffy with Angel, two characters in the show, was presented as the natural culmination of their love for each other. The fact that Buffy was technically making love to a corpse was overlooked entirely by the audience. Over the years, a staple of the show was Buffy's relationship with vampire lovers—first Angel and then Spike. The connection between love and death and the acceptance of the undead or necrophilic lover was presented (Spaise, 2005).

Troilism

Troilism is having sexual relations with another person while a third person watches. In one respect, troilism combines elements of exhibitionism and voyeurism. In another respect, it represents an illusion of prostitution, because there are elaborate ruses and pretenses of prostitution. An example might be a husband's inviting another man to have intercourse with his wife. The husband watches and is able to get an erection. He then achieves penetration and orgasm, which are not possible unless his wife plays the role of a prostitute.

Troilism clearly does not qualify as a safe sexual activity. Because multiple partners are involved, this is a high-risk activity.

Asphyxiophilia

Asphyxiophilia is the desire for a state of oxygen deficiency to enhance sexual excitement and orgasm. It has also been called *erotic* or *autoerotic suicide, sexual suicide, autoerotic strangulation, autoerotic asphyxiation, hypoxophilia,* and *autoerotic accident.* Most information about asphyxiophilia is found in reports from police or doctors of forensic medicine who examine people who have died during this behavior (Innala & Ernulf, 1989).

> **troilism**
> Having sexual relations with another person while a third person watches.
>
> **asphyxiophilia**
> Desire for a state of oxygen deficiency to enhance sexual excitement.

Self-induced oxygen deficiency is used to produce sexual euphoria, increased excitement, or heightened orgasm during masturbatory activities. Reduced supply of oxygen to the brain results in giddiness, lightheadedness, or exhilaration that is reported to enhance sexual climax.

Oxygen deficiency can be induced in many ways. Because the circumstances and features of autoerotic deaths are not commonly known, they are often misinterpreted as suicides or homicides. And death can easily result, because cutting off the flow of blood to the brain can produce unconsciousness in as little as 5 to 10 seconds. Although the person probably did not intend to die, death results when an escape mechanism fails or the person cannot recover from self-induced oxygen deprivation.

Because of the nature of asphyxiophilia and the fact that it is often covered up, it is difficult to get accurate statistics about it. However, Jenkins (2000) indicated that cases are often reported as intentional suicide; conservative estimates place it at 6.5% of all adolescent suicides and at least 31% of all adolescent hangings. The deceased victims are most often white, middle-class unmarried males. Although it might seem that practitioners of this dangerous behavior suffer mental illness, this is usually not the case. The victims are usually well-adjusted, nondepressed, high achievers.

Asphyxiophilia is really a subcategory of sexual masochism. Although not unheard of for it to be practiced with a partner, it is usually done as a solitary act. The practice is intended to produce sexual pleasure, but practitioners are well aware of the inherent risk element. Because of that, they use some kind of safety mechanism to prevent accidental death in the event of unconsciousness. There is no evidence that deaths from asphyxiophilia are a form of disguised suicide. Such deaths are a complete surprise to family and friends. Nearly all reported deaths have been males, and most under 40 years of age. However, the practice can begin at puberty for some. There are no known signs of predisposition to this behavior or the existence of the paraphilia. In many cases of death from asphyxiophilia, the cause of death has been attributed to suicide even though that is not what happened (Hypoxyphilia/auto-erotic asphyxia, 2005).

Klismaphilia

In **klismaphilia** sexual arousal is obtained from enema use. Klismaphiles most often prefer the receiving role, but less commonly erotic arousal may be associated with administering an enema. The background of many individuals who show klismaphilia often indicates that as infants or young children they were frequently given enemas by concerned and loving mothers. This association with loving attention, or perhaps even sexual pleasure, learned early in life may eroticize the experience for some people, so they show a need to receive an enema for sexual satisfaction as adults. Because klismaphilia involves anal contact, it is not a safe sexual activity unless latex gloves are used and there is great attention to cleanliness.

> **klismaphilia**
> Sexual arousal produced by the use of enemas.

Coprophilia

In **coprophilia**, sexual pleasure is associated with feces. People who show coprophilia reach high levels of sexual excitement by watching someone defecate or by defecating on someone. The connection of feces with sexual arousal may also go back to childhood. Some children seem to enjoy holding back on a bowel movement and then

> **coprophilia**
> Sexual pleasure associated with feces.

carefully expelling the feces. It could also be that the connection between changing of soiled diapers and sexual stimulation during infancy eroticizes feces. Because it appears that HIV can be present in any body tissue or fluids, coprophilia is not a safe sexual activity.

Urophilia

In **urophilia**, sexual pleasure is associated with urine. Similarly to coprophilia, the person may want to urinate on someone or be urinated on. Again, as with coprophilia, there may be childhood beginnings for urophilia. For example, stimulation of the urethra during urination may become associated with pleasure, or there may have been stimulation from the changing of wet diapers. Urophilia has been referred to as "golden showers" or "water sports." Urophilia is not a safe sexual activity because HIV and other STIs can be transmitted through urine.

> **urophilia**
> Sexual pleasure associated with urine.

■ Treatment for Paraphilias

A number of issues surface when one considers treatment for paraphilias. For example, people with paraphilias often do not want treatment. Also, they often feel they cannot control their urges, so they cannot accept personal responsibility for their actions. However, personal responsibility is usually a prerequisite for successful behavior change. In addition, some helping professionals think it is not their responsibility to provide treatment for paraphilias—they believe it is the responsibility of the criminal justice system. In spite of these issues, it is appropriate to consider what might be done to help those with paraphilias. Possible treatments fall into three categories: (1) psychotherapy, (2) behavior therapy, and (3) pharmacological approaches (drug therapy).

Psychotherapy

Not much information is available about successful treatment of paraphilias by psychotherapy. The purpose of psychoanalysis is to discover unconscious conflicts that are believed to originate in childhood. If conflicts can be drawn to the surface and resolved, the hope is that the particular behavior can be changed.

Group therapy involves breaking through the denial so commonly found in people with paraphilias by surrounding them with others who share their condition. Once they begin to admit that they have

Gender DIMENSIONS

Paraphilias and Gender Differences

Because it is hard to find accurate statistics about the incidence of paraphilias, it is also difficult to find a great deal of information about paraphilias and gender differences. Although we know that the majority of paraphilias occur among men, here is a brief summary of what is found in the literature on this topic.

1. Janus and Janus (1993) reported that
   a. Eleven percent of both men and women have had experience with bondage.
   b. Six percent of men and 4% of women have participated in urophilia.
   c. Eleven percent of men and 6% of women have engaged in fetishistic behaviors.
   d. Six percent of men and 3% of women report cross-dressing.
2. Regarding voyeurism, Person and associates (1989) reported that

   a. Among college students, 23% of women and 38% of men have watched their partners masturbate.
   b. Eleven percent of women and 18% of men have performed sexual acts in front of mirrors.
   c. Five percent of women and 4% of men have watched others engage in sexual intercourse.
3. How common are paraphilias in general? (How common are paraphilias?, 2011)
   a. Most are rare.
   b. Most are more common among males than females by about 20 to 1.
   c. The reason for the disparity between males and females is not clear.
   d. Several paraphilias are associated with aggressive behavior.
   e. Most paraphilias are not considered aggressive or harmful.

a sexual divergence, the therapist begins to address individual issues such as past sexual abuse or other problems that may have led to the sexual disorder. When these issues have been identified, individual therapy may be used to help patients get past the guilt and shame that might be associated with their particular paraphilia (Brannon & Carroll, 2008).

Behavior Therapy

Behavior therapy applies learning principles to help people change their behavior. Many techniques have been used to help change paraphilic behavior. For example, in systematic desensitization the therapist tries to break the link between a sexual stimulus (such as leather for a fetishist) and the inappropriate response (sexual stimulation). The client is taught to relax muscle groups so that relaxation replaces sexual arousal in response to the stimulus.

In **aversion therapy** the undesirable behavior (such as masturbation for a voyeur) is paired repeatedly with a negative stimulus, such as a painful (but harmless) electric shock. The objective is that negative reactions to the paraphilic behavior will develop.

In **social training** the individual is helped to improve his or her social skills. It is hoped that if the person can better relate to people, he or she will be able to develop sexual relationships that would be considered more typical.

In **orgasmic reconditioning** the goal is to increase sexual arousal by socially appropriate stimuli. For example, if the person becomes sexually aroused by masturbating, as he or she approaches orgasm, "socially appropriate imagery" such as pictures of attractive people would be used. The hope is that orgasm will then be connected with these images and not the paraphilic ones.

Drug Therapy

Although no drug can eliminate paraphilic behavior, some chemicals can sometimes be helpful in reducing the intensity of sexual drives and establishing an environment for more successful treatment using one of the other approaches. For example, Prozac, which is commonly used for treating depression,

behavior therapy
Applying learning principles to help people change behavior.

aversion therapy
Pairing an undesirable sexual behavior with a painful response.

social training
Improving a person's social skills.

orgasmic reconditioning
Increasing sexual arousal to socially appropriate stimuli.

¿? Ethical DIMENSIONS

The Ethics of Chemical Treatment for Paraphilias

Is it ethical to force paraphilic sex offenders to take hormones or tranquilizers to reduce their drives for paraphilic behaviors? Although in some cases Depo-Provera reduces the paraphilic sex drive to a level that allows the person to have a more normal sex drive, in others it causes a complete elimination of the sex drive—meaning that the individual has almost no interest in any sexual behavior.

One difficulty is that some paraphilics enjoy their behavior. Therefore, they do not want treatment because they do not view their behavior as a problem.

Some experts would argue that chemical treatment for paraphilic offenders should be required to protect other people from them. Others feel that such treatments should be required only for people who have paraphilias that violate the rights of others or harm them.

When faced with the possibility of arrest or imprisonment, paraphilic sex offenders could waive their right of informed consent and sign up for treatment just to avoid legal action. It can be difficult to balance the right of society to be protected from harm against the right of a person to avoid being given chemicals that may have undesired side effects.

---

antiandrogen drugs
Chemicals that reduce the sex drive by lowering the testosterone level in the bloodstream.

has been used to help some people reduce obsessions and compulsions. Also, **antiandrogen drugs**, chemicals that reduce the sex drive by lowering the testosterone level in the bloodstream, can reduce sexual desire and erections in males. Such a drug is Depo-Provera, which must be injected weekly to be effective. However, even Depo-Provera does not change the nature of sexual stimuli for people; it only reduces the intensity of their reactions.

The International Association for the Treatment of Sexual Offenders was founded in 1998. It is committed to advocate for humane, dignified, compassionate, ethical, and effective treatment of sexual offenders. It also is interested in furthering knowledge about individual and social conditions that lead to sexual offenses, and in improving treatment methods. Members of the organization are convinced that punishment is not a sufficient deterrent for sexual crimes, and that treatment will result in the reduction of sexual crimes and is a human right (Pfafflin & Eher, 2003).

■ Sexual Addiction

In 1998 President Clinton's sexual activity stirred up the debate over "sexual addiction." The idea that some people might have very strong, or even insatiable, sexual needs has been around a long time. The term **nymphomania** refers to an excessive,

nymphomania
An excessive, insatiable sexual drive in women.

satyriasis
An excessive, insatiable sexual drive in men—also called *Don Juanism*.

insatiable sexual drive in women. The same condition in men is referred to as **satyriasis**, or **Don Juanism**. Many professionals have argued about the appropriateness of these labels for years. They contend that the labels should not be used at all because judgments about how much sexual behavior is "normal" or "excessive" are subjective.

Some experts believe that sexual addiction is mainly a male abnormality caused by childhood trauma that usually requires intense psychotherapy. Many others say this is nonsense because there is no such thing as too much sexual behavior, unless it is with the wrong partner. They say that some people who have the symptoms do not experience conflict and are not really troubled by it. Still others are concerned that use of the label *sexual addiction* may help people inappropriately excuse their behavior.

Experts are not in agreement with regard to the causes of sexual addiction. Some experts blame biological factors such as mood disorders (such as bipolar disorders) (Kaplan & Krueger, 2010) or brain differences such as frontal lobe dysfunction or temporal lobe abnormalities (Chughtai et al., 2010). Other experts blame psychological factors such as negative early childhood experiences (Birchard, 2011).

Obviously, most people engage in various forms of sexual activity without it becoming disruptive related to other behaviors. Some experts argue that some people become addicts because of changes in the chemistry of the brain. Other experts believe that this view is not correct, and the question of whether addicts experience differences in the way their brains work is still hotly debated (Bodo, 2008).

Dodge et al. (2004) found that college students who are sexually compulsive are more likely to participate in sexual behaviors that are high risk in terms of HIV and STI infections. Bancroft and Vukadinovic (2004) reported that out-of-control sexual behavior seems to result from a variety of mechanisms. They also said that sexual addicts tend to experience increased sexual interest when they are depressed or anxious about something.

A more clinical name for sexual addiction is *hypersexual disorder*. Hypersexual disorder is characterized by recurrent and intense sexual fantasies, sexual urges, or sexual behaviors. The behavior has some of the following characteristics: (1) interferes with other goals and obligations, (2) is used as a distraction from negative moods or stressful life events, (3) is engaged in without regard for physical or emotional safety, and (4) repeated attempts to stop or limit behavior have been unsuccessful (Kafka, 2010). Other popular nonclinical terms for sexual addiction are *out-of-control sexual behavior* and *sexual compulsivity*.

Sexual addiction can involve a wide variety of practices. They can include compulsive masturbation, multiple affairs, multiple or anonymous sexual partners and/or one-night stands, consistent use of pornography, unsafe sexual behaviors, phone or computer sex, prostitution or use of prostitutes, exhibitionism, obsessive dating through personal ads, voyeurism, sexual harassment, and molestation/rape (Sexual addiction, 2009.) Sometimes an addict has trouble with just one unwanted behavior, sometimes with many. As in other addictions, the sexual addict experiences powerlessness over a compulsive behavior. The addict may wish to stop but repeatedly fails to do so. The consequences can be loss of relationships, difficulties with work, arrests, financial troubles, a loss of interest in matters not sexual, low self-esteem, and despair (What is sexual addiction?, 2003).

Among the writings about sexual addiction have been several books by Patrick Carnes, who outlines 10 practical and useful indicators of compulsive sexual behavior.

1. A pattern of out-of-control behavior
2. Severe consequences caused by sexual behavior
3. Inability to stop despite adverse consequences
4. Persistent pursuit of self-destructive or high-risk behavior
5. Ongoing desire or effort to limit sexual behavior, usually at a partner's insistence
6. Sexual obsession and fantasy as a primary coping strategy
7. Increasing amounts of sexual experience because the current level of activity is no longer sufficient

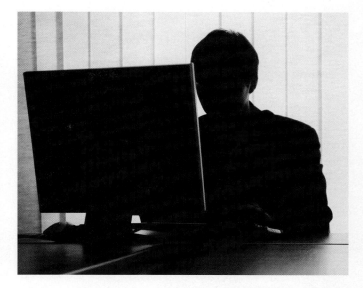

Cybersex addiction has become more common in recent years.

8. Severe mood changes related to sexual activity
9. Inordinate amounts of time spent in obtaining sexual activity, being sexual, and/or recovering from sexual experience
10. Neglect of important social, occupational, and/or recreational activities caused by behavior

The main way to identify any addictive behavior is to consider whether it is causing negative or unwelcome problems and yet the person continues it anyway. Sexual addicts are often unable to make and keep commitments to themselves and others about stopping or changing particular sexual behaviors over the long term, and most have problems with real intimacy.

In more recent years, one form of sexual addiction is cybersex addiction. There may be many symptoms of cybersex addiction; common symptoms are (1) spending increasing amounts of online time focused on sexual or romantic intrigue or involvement, (2) failed attempts to cut back on frequency of online sexual involvement, (3) online use that interferes with work and personal life, (4) secretiveness or lying about the amount of time spent on online sexual activity, and (5) a primary focus of sexual activity related to computer activity (Cybersex addiction checklist, 2001).

Most addicts live in denial of their addiction. Success in treating addiction depends on the person accepting and admitting that he or she has a problem. In many cases, like with other addictions, it takes a significant event—such as the loss of a job, the breakup of a marriage, or an arrest—to force the addict to admit his her or her problem (Sexual addiction, 2009).

? Did You Know . . .

Sexual Addiction Recovery Resources

Email Groups

Sex/Porn Addiction: *S-panon@ontos.usa.com*

Addiction research and treatment: *Addict-L@listserv.kent.edu*

Internet addiction support group: *listserv@netcom.com*

Open self-help discussion: *solution@sjuvm.stjohns.edu*

Resource and Recovery Sites

www.kicksexaddiction.com

www.themeadows.com

www.sexualrecovery.com

www.gentlepath.com

National Resources

Sex Addicts Anonymous (SAA)

www.sexaa.org

(713) 869-4902

PO Box 70949

Houston, TX 77270

Sex and Love Addicts Anonymous (SLAA)

www.slaafws.org

(210) 828-7900

1550 NE Loop 410, Suite 118

San Antonio, TX 78209

Sexual Compulsives Anonymous (SCA)

www.sca-recovery.org

(212) 606-3778

1-800-977-HEAL

PO Box 1585, Old Chelsea Station

New York, NY 10011

email: *info@sca-recovery.org*

Source: Data from Sex Addiction Help. Available: www.sexaddicthelp.com/Links/index.htm.

Even though there is no agreement about how to deal with compulsive sexual activity—if it can be done at all—organizations have been formed to help people deal with their activities if they feel there is a problem; for example, there is a 12-step program modeled after Alcoholics Anonymous called Sex and Love Addicts Anonymous (Branon & Carroll, 2008). Other such groups are called Sex Addicts Anonymous, Sexaholics Anonymous, and Sexual Compulsives Anonymous.

Finally, many issues remain unresolved with regard to sexual addiction. For example, some argue over whether it is a real disease or an excuse for people to cheat and spend hours watching porn and participating in other ways to sexually stimulate themselves. If it is a disease, should insurance companies have to pay for sex addiction treatment?

Summary

- Because many sexual behaviors vary in degree, it is not surprising that many of us recognize some amount of atypical behaviors or feelings in ourselves.

- There is not a great deal known about atypical sexual behaviors.

- The most common paraphilias are exhibitionism, voyeurism, obscene communication, masochism and sadism, transvestism, and fetishism.

- Other paraphilias include bestiality, frottage, necrophilia, troilism, asphyxiophilia, klismaphilia, coprophilia, and urophilia.

- Possible treatments for paraphilias fall into three categories: psychotherapy, behavior therapy, and drug therapy.

- Some people have very strong, or even insatiable, sexual needs and may be sex addicts. Most treatment programs for sexual addiction resemble treatment programs for people addicted to other behaviors.

Discussion Questions

1. Describe how sexual feelings or behaviors vary from common to atypical along a continuum.

2. What are the most common forms of paraphilia? Describe the type of person who might practice them.

3. What are the less common forms of paraphilia? Discuss why someone would practice them.

4. Describe the major types of treatment programs for paraphilias, including the ways they work and their effectiveness.

5. Is "sexual addiction" a true disorder? Explain your answer.

Application Questions

Reread the chapter-opening story and answer the following questions:

1. In spite of his well-publicized sexual behavior, the sportscaster's fiancée married him. Would you have advised her to go through with the wedding? Explain your answer.

2. Discuss the issues of safer sex surrounding the sexual acts engaged in by the sportscaster.

3. In addition to causing immense embarrassment, the sportscaster's sexual habits cost him his job (and probably some friends as well). What might have caused him to take such risks?

Which therapies are available to help him with his atypical behaviors?

Critical Thinking Questions

1. Look over the American Psychiatric Association's definitions for the varied paraphilias supplied throughout the chapter. What are the common elements? On the basis of that information, how would you define "atypical sexual behavior"?

2. Given that the pornography industry takes in about $2 billion per year, are we a nation of voyeurs? What differentiates a diagnosed voyeur from someone who views porn? Explain your answers.

Critical Thinking Case

Bill and Anne, college juniors, were in a monogamous relationship for about 5 months when Bill said that he wanted to add some "variety" to their sex life. Anne's immediate reaction was to feel that she was not giving Bill enough sexual satisfaction, so she did not respond to his suggestion. As much as she loved Bill, she felt unsure about his request for variety.

After he broached the subject several more times, she finally asked him what he wanted. He said that a former girlfriend had enjoyed having another girl join them from time to time. Anne was initially aghast at the idea of including a third person, especially a girl. But a few months later, Anne and a female friend had a brief sexual encounter after drinking heavily. Anne did not enjoy it. When she told Bill what had happened, he reacted sharply: What was she doing with another sexual partner?

Why did Bill react as he did? What did Bill really want from the encounter—another girl for his girlfriend or a threesome for himself? Why was it important for him to communicate correctly what he wanted?

You want something your partner does not want. How do you approach it? How do you make sure you are comfortable?

Exploring Personal Dimensions

Respond about only your sexual activity. If you do not participate in any sexual activity, skip this assessment. Check the following items that apply to you.

_____ 1. I tell my partner what feels good.

_____ 2. I tell my partner what hurts, if anything.

_____ 3. I avoid frequent sexual encounters because I do not like them.

_____ 4. I let myself just go with my feelings and behave the way I want to act during sexual encounters.

_____ 5. My partner and I have talked about and resolved how often to have sexual activity.

_____ 6. Sexual activity is a problem for me and my partner.

_____ 7. I have told my partner what I want during sexual activity.

_____ 8. My partner and I enjoy holding hands, kissing, and just talking as much as we do having sexual activity.

_____ 9. It is important that each time we express love or go on a date that it culminate in sexual intercourse to be a really meaningful experience.

Scoring

Give yourself the following points for the items you check, and total your score.

1. 2	4. 2	7. 2
2. 2	5. 2	8. 2
3. –2	6. –2	9. –2

Interpretation

This exercise indicates whether you have healthy communication in your sexual relationship. Interpret your score as follows:

6–10 = Your communication is healthy.
0–5 = Your communication is moderately healthy.
–1 – –6 = You need to improve your communication skills.

Source: Bruess, C., & Richardson, G. _Decisions for health._ Madison, WI: Brown & Benchmark, 1995.

Suggested Readings

Accordina, M. P., & Hewes, R. L. Investigation of Internet use, sexual and nonconsensual sensation seeking, and sexual compulsivity among college students. _Sexual Addiction and Compulsivity: The Journal of Treatment and Prevention, 14, no. 4_ (December 2007), 321–335.

Cloud, J. The truth about sex addiction. _Time, 177, no. 8_ (February 28, 2011), 42–50.

Kaplan, M. S., & Krueger, R. B. Diagnosis, assessment, and treatment of hypersexuality. _Journal of Sex Research, 47, no. 2–3_ (March 2010), 181–198.

McBride, K. R., Reece, M., & Sanders, S. A. Using the Sexual Compulsivity Scale to predict outcomes of sexual behavior in young adults. _Sexual Addiction and Compulsivity: The Journal of Treatment and Prevention, 15, no. 2_ (2008), 97–115.

Paraphilias. Encyclopedia of Mental Disorders, 2011. Available: http://www.minddisorders.com/Ob-Ps/Paraphilias.html.

Paraphilias. Sexual Conditions Health Center. _WebMD,_ 2011. Available: http://www.webmd.com/sexual-conditions/paraphilias-overview.

Web Resources

For links to the websites below, visit _go.jblearning.com/dimensions/5e_ and click on Resource Links.

BDSM Backroom
www.bcwsd.com/backroom

Contains information about bondage, dominance, sadism, and masochism for those who are curious about what BDSM is and want to learn more about it.

The Fetish Information Exchange
www.fetishexchange.org

Provides knowledge about a number of fetishes. Contains many additional sources of information including websites about fetishes.

Society for the Scientific Study of Sexuality: What Sexual Scientists Know About Compulsive Sexual Behavior
www.sexscience.org/dashboard/articleImages/SSSS-CompulsiveSexualBehavior.pdf

Summarizes scientific information about compulsive sexual behavior.

The Society of Janus
www.soj.org

The Society of Janus is a support and educational group for people interested in learning about BDSM. It emphasizes safe, consensual, and nonexploitative activities.

Discovery Health: Paraphilia
healthguide.howstuffworks.com/paraphilia-dictionary3.html

Contains information about many forms of atypical sexual behavior.

Psychology Today: Paraphilias
www.psychologytoday.com/search/query?keys=paraphilias

Contains information from _Psychology Today_ about various paraphilias and their treatment.

References

American Psychiatric Association. *Diagnostic and Statistical Manual of Mental Disorders, Fourth Edition, Text Revision.* Washington, DC: American Psychiatric Association, 2000.

American Psychiatric Association. *Diagnostic and statistical manual of mental disorders.* Washington, DC: Author, 2005.

Bancroft, J., & Vukadinovic, Z. Sexual addiction, sexual compulsivity, sexual impulsivity, or what? Toward a theoretical model. *Journal of Sex Research, 42, no. 3* (Aug. 2004), 225–234.

Baumeister, R. F. The enigmatic appeal of sexual masochism: Why people desire pain, bondage, and humiliation in sex. *Journal of Social and Clinical Psychology, 16, no. 2* (1997), 133–150.

Beetz, A. M. Bestiality/zoophilia: A scarcely investigated phenomenon between crime, paraphilia, and love. *Journal of Forensic Psychology Practice, 4, no. 2* (2004), 1–36.

Bestiality, Go ask Alice. Columbia University, 2003. Available: http://www.goaskalice.columbia.edu/0707.html.

Birchard, T. Sexual addiction and paraphilias. *Sexual Addiction and Compulsivity: The Journal of Treatment and Prevention, 18, no. 3* (2011), 157–187.

Bodo, C. Addicted to love. National Sexuality Resource Center, 2008. Available: http://nsrc.sfsu.edu/print/2835.

Brannon, G. E., & Carroll, K. S. Paraphilias. *eMedicine Specialties—Psychiatry,* February 14, 2008. Available: http://emedicine.medscape.com/article/291419-print.

Chughtai, B., Sciullo, D., Khan, S. A., Rehman, H., Mohan, E., & Rehman, J. Etiology, diagnosis and management of hypersexuality: A review. *Internet Journal of Urology, 6, no. 2* (2010). Available: http://www.ispub.com/journal/the-internet-journal-of-urology/volume-6-number-2/etiology-diagnosis-amp-management-of-hypersexuality-a-review.html.

Coleman, E. What sexual scientists know …: About compulsive sexual behavior. *Society for the Scientific Study of Sexuality* (2005). Available: http://www.sexscience.org.

Cybersex addiction checklist. Sexual Recovery Institute, 2001. Available: http://www.sexualrecovery.com.

Discovery Health. Paraphilia 2005. Available: http://health.discovery.com/centers/sex/sexpedia/paraphilia_print.html.

Dodge, B., Reece, M., Cole, S. L., & Sandfort, T. G. Sexual compulsivity among heterosexual college students. *Journal of Sex Research, 41, no. 4* (November 2004), 343–350.

Exhibitionism. Encyclopedia of Mental Disorders, 2011. Available: http://www.minddisorders.com/Del-Fi/Exhibitionism.html.

Exhibitionism. Psychology Today's Conditions Center (2005). Available: http://cms.psychologytoday.com/conditions/index.php?term=exhibitionism&print=1.

Fetishism. Discovery Health, 2005. Available: http://health.discovery.com/centers/sex/sexpedia/fetishism_print.html

Fetishism. Sinclair Intimacy Institute, 2001. Available: http://www.intimacyinstitute.com.

How common are paraphilias? WebMD, 2011. Available: http://www.webmd.com/sexual-conditions/paraphilias?page=3.

Hypoxyphilia/auto-erotic asphyxia. PsychDirect, 2005. Available: http://www.psychdirect.com/forensic/Criminology/para/aea.htm.

Innala, S. M., & Ernulf, K. E. Asphyxi-ophilia in Scandinavia. *Archives of Sexual Behavior, 18* (1989), 181–189.

Janus, S., & Janus, C. *The Janus report on sexual behavior.* New York: John Wiley & Sons, 1993.

Jenkins, A. P. When self-pleasuring becomes self-destruction: Autoerotic asphyxiation paraphilia. *International Electronic Journal of Health Education, 3, no. 3* (2000), 208–216.

Kafka, M. P. Hypersexual disorder: A proposed diagnosis for DSM-V. *Archives of Sexual Behavior, 39* (2010), 377–400.

Kaplan, M. S., & Krueger, R. B. Diagnosis, assessment, and treatment of hypersexuality. *Journal of Sex Research, 47* (2010), 181–198.

Kinsey, A. C., Pomeroy, W. B., & Martin, C. E. *Sexual behavior in the human female.* Philadelphia: Saunders, 1953.

Kinsey, A. C., Pomeroy, W. B., & Martin, C. E. *Sexual behavior in the human male.* Philadelphia: Saunders, 1948.

Litman, R. E. Bondage and sadomasochism, in *Sexual dynamics of anti-social behavior,* 2nd ed., Schlesinger, L. B. & Revitch, E., eds. Springfield, IL: Charles C. Thomas, 1997.

Masochism. University of Iowa Health Care, 2001. Available: www.uihealthcare.com/topics/mentalemotionalhealth/ment3155.html.

Paraphilias. *MedicineNet.com,* 2009. Available: http://www.medicinenet.com/paraphilia/article.htm.

Paraphilias. *Psychology Today's* Conditions Center, 2005. Available: http://cms.psychologytoday.com/conditions/index.php?term=paraphilias&print=1.

Person, E. S., Terestman, N., Myers, W. A., & Goldberg, E. L. Gender differences in sexual behaviors and fantasies in a college population. *Journal of Sex and Marital Therapy, 15, no. 3* (1989), 187–214.

Pfafflin, F., & Eher, R. What to do with sexual offenders? *International Journal of Offender Therapy and Comparative Criminology, 47, no. 4* (2003), 361–365.

Sadism. University of Iowa Health Care, 2001. Available: http://www.uihealthcare.com/topics/mentalemotionalhealth/ment3168.html.

Sadomasochism. Sinclair Intimacy Institute (2001). Available: http://www.intimacyinstitute.com.

Sexual addiction. *MedicineNet.com,* 2009. Available: http://www.medicinenet.com/sexual_addiction/article.htm.

Sexual sadism. PsychDirect, 2005. Available: http://www.psychdirect.com/forensic/Criminology/para/sadism.htm.

Spaise, T. L. Necrophilia and SM: The deviant side of *Buffy the Vampire Slayer. Journal of Popular Culture, 38, 4* (May 2005), 744–762.

Transvestic fetishism. *PsychDirect,* 2005. Available: http://www.psychdirect.com/forensic/Criminology/para/transfetishism.htm.

Transvestism. University of Iowa Health Care, 2001. Available: http://www.uihealthcare.com/topics/mentalemotionalhealth/ment3174.html.

Transvestism. University of Iowa Health Care, 2005. Available: http://www.uihealthcare.com.

United States Code Annotated Title 47. U.S. Department of Justice (March 3, 2003). Available: www.usdoj.gov/criminal/cybercrime/47usc223NEW.htm.

Voyeurism. Encyclopedia of Mental Disorders, 2011. Available: http://www.minddisorders.com/Py-Z/Voyeurism.html.

What is sexual addiction? Sex Addicts Anonymous, 2003. Available: http://www.sexaa.org/addict.htm.

CHAPTER 14

Forcible Sexual Behaviors

CHAPTER OBJECTIVES

1 Differentiate among rape, statutory rape, stranger rape, and date (acquaintance) rape. Discuss what makes someone rape. Discuss the myths surrounding rape.

2 Discuss pedophilia, including the profile of the pedophiliac, incidence and effects of pedophilia, and prevention.

3 Describe the incidence of incest and the typical effects on incest victims.

4 Summarize important information about violence in marriage, including marital rape and domestic abuse.

5 Discuss sexual harassment in the workplace, in schools, on campus, and in the military, and indicate what can be done to prevent and deal with it.

go.jblearning.com/dimensions5e

Social Responses to Rape
Incidence of Pedophilia
Domestic Violence
Sexual Harassment

INTRODUCTION

*A*fter a discussion about forcible sexual behavior in my sexuality class, a female student who was in her late 20s asked to go to my office to talk for a few minutes. When we got there, she said that she had found the information and the discussion on forcible sexual behavior interesting and enlightening. She also said she was feeling personally troubled because it reminded her of something that had happened to her. She then told me about it.

She remembered when she was 15 years old. She said she was a typical middle-class high school girl. Although her parents and her teachers did not say a lot about sexuality, she had heard quite a bit about rape on TV and seen stories about it in magazines and newspapers. Her parents, as had many of her friends, warned her about being careful and about not trusting strangers. She dated Ed, a neighbor who lived just a block away. Ed's parents and her parents sometimes got together socially, and they had been friends for at least 10 years. Ed's parents had always been friendly to her too, and she probably saw them at least two or three times each week.

Ed was 2 years older and a star basketball player. He was an excellent student and considered a leader and one of the most popular boys at school. She remembered that he had always seemed to be one of the best athletes as they were growing up. After a few dates, they had started to become intimate. She enjoyed the closeness with him and found him very attractive. She had some tears in her eyes when she said that on one date, after an exciting basketball game, he had intercourse with her while she was crying and asking him not to do it. Although he was a little forceful, he did not raise his voice and he did not hit her. He just paid no attention to what she was saying.

At the time she said she did not realize it was rape. She asked him why he was doing this to her, but he did not answer. Afterward she did not want to date him anymore, and her parents wondered why. Her friends thought she was crazy not to want to go out with him. She said she had not told anyone about this before, but that she just had to get it out. When we talked about forcible sexual behavior in class, all the memories rushed back to her.

Many readers of this chapter are probably survivors of forcible sexual behavior—whether it was rape, child sexual abuse, sexual harassment, or another form of forcible sexual behavior. Sometimes it can be difficult and painful to think about these topics. However, most people, such as the student in our story, find it helpful to learn more about such topics and to deal more directly with their feelings about them.

Many sexual behaviors exist and various factors contribute to these behaviors. Most often people voluntarily choose a particular behavior, but some sexual behaviors are not voluntary. In this chapter we focus on rape and child sexual abuse because of their seriousness. By no means, however, are these the only forcible sexual behaviors. Other representative forcible sexual behaviors are also considered. A characteristic of all these behaviors is that we know very little about them because of their obvious secretive and private nature. Although knowledge about forcible sexual behavior has rapidly increased, a great need for continued study and research is evident.

■ Sexual Violence

Sexual violence is a serious problem that affects millions of people each year. The victims of sexual violence are at increased risk of being abused again. Sexual violence perpetrators are also at increased risk of perpetrating again. Statistics about sexual violence are given throughout this chapter. It is important to remember, however, that statistics about sexual violence vary due to differences in definition and how data are collected. Such data usually come from police, clinical settings, nongovernmental organizations, and survey research.

For more than 25 years, researchers have noted that sexual violence is a relatively common experience. For example, at least 20% of all females in the United States will be victims of sexual violence during their lives. It is a life-altering experience for many who experience sexual violence. The effects are often experienced long after the event, with many psychological, physical, and behavioral consequences such as STIs,

chronic pain disorders and other physical ailments, as well as anxiety, depression, substance use, sexual problems, and interpersonal difficulties being documented in survivors of sexual violence. Even though much is known, there is a need for continued work related to research, public policy, providing treatment and prevention services, and educating the public about sexual violence. For example, it is known that childhood sexual abuse is one of the best predictors of sexual victimization in adulthood (Marx, 2005). Knowing this and other important facts will help people better understand and deal with sexual violence.

Sexual assault and abuse is any nonconsensual sexual activity, including:

- Inappropriate touching

- Vaginal, anal, or oral penetration

- Sexual intercourse after you say no

- Rape

- Attempted rape

- Child molestation

Sexual assault can be verbal, visual, or anything that forces a person to join in unwanted sexual contact or attention (What is sexual assault?, 2005).

Each year the American College Health Association surveys more than 100,000 college students about a variety of behaviors related to their health. In a recent year, 3.1% of males and 7.4% of females were sexually touched against their will. Eight-tenths of one percent of males and 3.2% of females said sexual penetration (vaginal, oral, or anal) was attempted against their will. Six-tenths of one percent of males and 1.9% of females said they were sexually penetrated (vaginal, oral, or anal) without their consent. Of the males, 7.3% reported an emotionally abusive intimate relationship, as did 11% of the females. A sexually abusive intimate relationship was reported by 0.9% of the males and 1.9% of the females (American College Health Association, 2011).

As can be seen from these numbers, both males and females can be victims of sexual violence. It is true that females are victims far more often than males, and males are perpetrators of sexual violence much more often than females. Nevertheless, it is estimated that 1 out of every 6 boys will be sexually assaulted by age 16. Adult men are also victims of sexual violence. The experience of sexual assault can be very confusing for men because our society and culture often associate sexual assault with women (Porche, 2008).

In 2011 the Centers for Disease Control reported on its first look at national rates of intimate partner and sexual violence in over 10 years (Black et al., 2011). Researchers surveyed over 9,000 women and about 7,500 men on topics including rape and other types of sexual violence. The survey defined rape as completed forced penetration, forced penetration facilitated by drugs or alcohol, or attempted forced penetration. According to the study, 18.3% of U.S. women have been raped, including about 1.3 million in the year before the study. About half of rapes involved women's intimate partners, and 1 in 4 women said they were violently attacked by an intimate partner. About 1.4% of U.S. men reported being raped at some point in their lives, more than half of them by an acquaintance. Nearly 80% of rapes of females occurred before age 25, and more than 25% of men were first raped at age 10 or younger. Researchers found that rape and sexual violence often have negative health-related repercussions, such as higher incidences of asthma, irritable bowel syndrome, and diabetes in victims. Victims of sexual violence were also more likely to report symptoms of post-traumatic stress disorder, frequent headaches, chronic pain, and difficulty sleeping.

■ Rape

Rape is a forcible act. Legal definitions of rape and law enforcement procedures for handling rape cases are changing, and they differ from state to state. However, a practical definition of **rape** is "forcible sexual intercourse." This can include forced oral sexual activity, penile–vaginal sexual activity, and anal sexual activity. Penetration may be made by a body part or an object. If a person is forced to do any of these things when

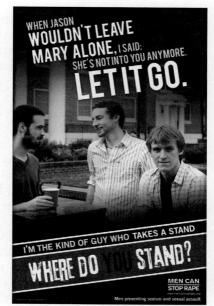

As a female, what can you do to improve your odds of preventing rape? As a male, what can you do to make sure you never are involved in forced sexual activity?

he or she does not want to, that is rape. In 2012 the U.S. Attorney General announced changes to the Uniform Crime Report's definition of rape (Siegelbaum, 2012). The Justice Department stated that the new definition would better reflect state criminal codes and focus on the various forms of sexual penetration understood to be rape. It was also felt that these long-overdue updates to the definition of rape would also help ensure justice for those whose lives have been devastated by sexual violence. The Uniform Crime Report's previous definition of rape, first adopted in 1929, was limited only to forcible penetration of a vagina. The new definition of rape is: "The penetration, no matter how slight, of the vagina or anus with any body part or object, or oral penetration by a sex organ of another person, without the consent of the victim." The revised definition includes "any gender of victim or perpetrator, and includes instances in which the victim is incapable of giving consent because of temporary or permanent mental or physical incapacity, including due to the influence of drugs or alcohol or because of age."

Rape victims may be forced through threats or physical means. In about 8 out of 10 rapes, no weapon is used other than physical force. Anyone may be a victim of rape: women, men, or children, straight or gay (Was I raped?, 2011).

Sexual assault is unwanted sexual contact that stops short of rape or attempted rape. This includes sexual touching and fondling. This terminology can be confusing because some states use this term interchangeably with rape.

Some people wonder how to determine if what happened was rape. There are three main considerations in judging whether a sexual act is consensual (that is, both people are old enough to consent, have the capacity to consent, and agreed to the sexual contact) or it is a crime. Laws vary from state to state, but here are some examples related to these three considerations (Was I raped?, 2011).

Are the participants old enough to consent? Each state has an "age of consent" that varies from age 14 to 18. Commonly it is 16 or 18. It might also vary according to the age difference between the participants. It is not enough to assume that someone is old enough to legally participate. It is up to both participants to be sure that each is old enough.

Do both people have the capacity to consent? States also define who has the mental and legal capacity to consent. Those with diminished capacity, such as people with disabilities, some elderly people, and those who have been drugged or unconscious, may not have the legal ability to agree to have sexual activity.

Did both participants agree to take part? Using physical force or threats means that it is rape. Also, it does not matter if you think your partner means yes, or if you have already started intimate behavior, "no" means "stop." If you proceed despite your partner's expressed instruction to stop, you have not only violated basic codes of morality and decency, you may have also committed a crime.

Within the category of rape, there are several types. For example, **statutory rape** is intercourse with a person who is younger than the age of consent (ranging from 14 to 18 years from state to state). Even with consent, statutory rape is considered to have occurred if one of the participants is not of legal age. **Stranger rape** is rape of a person by an unknown assailant. If a rape is committed by someone known to the victim, it is **acquaintance rape**, or **date rape**, both of which are discussed later in this chapter.

> **rape**
> Forcible sexual intercourse with a person who does not give consent.
>
> **sexual assault**
> Unwanted sexual contact that stops short of rape or attempted rape.
>
> **statutory rape**
> Intercourse with a person younger than the legal age of consent.
>
> **stranger rape**
> Rape of a person by an unknown person.
>
> **acquaintance rape**
> Rape by a friend, acquaintance, or date; also known as *date rape.*

Rape Myths

In spite of the increased attention given to the topic of rape in recent years, rape myths remain prevalent (see Myth vs. Fact on page 556). It is important for people to know the facts about rape to help reduce some related problems. For example, some of the more prevalent rape myths include that women lead men on and therefore deserve to be raped, women often make false accusations of rape, no woman can be raped against her will, and most rapists are strangers. *All of these statements are false!* We know that men tend to believe rape myths more than women, that those who believe rape myths are more likely to assign blame to the victim, and that those who believe rape myths are more tolerant of the rapist and less tolerant of the victims (Notice to readers: Sexual Assault Awareness Month, 2005).

Society and Rape

Some people have wondered whether particular characteristics of a given society help promote rape. Even after many years of research, we don't have a definitive answer to this question. The United States has the highest rape rate among Western countries, but the reasons for this are not clear. Some people feel that the reasons may relate to the relative roles of males and females, the presence of pornography that endorses and legitimizes rape, and the fact that rape is a crime of violence in an already violent society. Others feel that these characteristics have nothing to do with the issue.

Rape is one of the most underreported crimes. This makes it difficult to accurately count the number of cases. Some researchers believe that as many as 84% of victims do not report sexual assault to the police. A primary reason given for the underreporting is cultural norms that stigmatize and blame victims for their assaults (Notice to readers: Sexual Assault Awareness Month, 2005).

Victims of rape are generally viewed more sympathetically by females than by males, and by whites more than by African Americans. However, the effect of race disappears when socioeconomic variables are controlled. Younger people and those with higher education levels are also more likely to view sexual assault victims more sympathetically (Nagel et al., 2005).

Although experts agree that statistics regarding rape and other sexual assault are not totally accurate because many cases are not reported, it is important to consider some statistics to get a clearer view of the overall situation. For example, 15% of sexual assault and rape victims are younger than age 12, 44% are younger than 18, and 80% are younger than 30. One out of every 6 American women has been the victim of an attempted or completed rape, which is a total of 17.7 million women. One out of every 6 American women has been the victim of an attempted rape in her lifetime (14.8% completed rape; 2.8 % attempted rape), and about 3% of men have also experienced an attempted or completed rape. Each year there are about 213,000 victims of sexual assault, which is about one every 2 minutes. Sixty percent are not reported to the police, and 15 of 16 rapists will never spend a day in jail. Fortunately, the incidence of sexual assault has fallen more than 60% in recent years. Victims of sexual assault are 3 times more likely to suffer from depression, 6 times more likely to suffer from post-traumatic stress disorder, 13 times more likely to abuse alcohol, 26 times more likely to abuse drugs, and 4 times more likely to contemplate suicide (Statistics, 2011).

Related to information already discussed about rape myths, those who score higher on a rape myth acceptance scale blame the victims of sexual assault more and are less likely to believe rape did occur (Mason & Riger, 2004). In addition, there are different responses to a marital rape scenario where the victim was dressed somberly or seductively. In one study, males rated the victim more deserving of the attack than did females. The suggestively dressed victim was rated more responsible and deserving than the somberly dressed victim. Also, those holding more traditional attitudes toward marriage assigned more victim responsibility and deservingness than those with more egalitarian attitudes (Whatley. 2005).

In Australia, the declining rate of convictions for sexual assault is attributed to the fact that juries are reluctant to convict in situations where victims know their attackers. Particularly problematic is the issue of whether there was consent. At least some of the blame for this is placed on romance novels. Traditionally, although not as common today, heroines typically rejected sexual advances, only to be overcome and later admit that they had really welcomed the advances (Philadelphoff-Puren, 2005).

Although sexual assault against women has received increasing attention over the past decades, the sexual assault of the elderly has not been well addressed. Print media and the Internet regularly report on these cases and the crises and trauma that follow for the victim and their families. Elderly victims of sexual violence represent a vulnerable and poorly understood population. They may be sexually assaulted in their homes or communities, in an assisted living facility, or in a nursing home environment. Offenders can be strangers, domestic partners, family members, nursing home residents, or caregivers. There is a need for education about sexual abuse of the elderly (Burgess & Morgenbesser, 2005).

Apparently, steps need to be taken to reduce the cultural acceptance of violence and to restructure male and female sex roles to specify equality, warmth, and supportiveness. In the past, male dominance, toughness, and violence have often been emphasized. A restructuring of the relationships between genders might reduce the high incidence of rape in American society. Steps to reduce your personal risk of sexual assault are found in Table 14.1.

The Rapist

The topics of rape and rapists are hot-button issues in American society. Some theorists argue that rape is an act of uncontrolled passion or the result of a lack of sexual partners; others suggest that it is an extreme expression of male power and violence. For others, rape is a biologically driven phenomenon whereby men forcefully try to maximize the number of women with whom they procreate.

Most rapists rape to be aggressive, to wield their power, or to degrade the victim. In most instances their motivations and satisfactions are not sexual. In fact, it is unlikely that they achieve any sexual satisfaction from the act of rape.

Many experts have developed theories about why people commit rape. For example, some believe that rape occurs to enhance the offender's sense of masculinity and power, while others believe that the rapist is angry toward women or men and wants to hurt, humiliate, or degrade someone. Still others believe that sadistic rapists may be sexually aroused in response to assault and violence, or that, for some

TABLE 14.1	**How Can I Protect Myself from Being Sexually Assaulted?**

There are things you can do to reduce your chances of being sexually assaulted. Here are some tips from the National Crime Prevention Council (*www.ncpc.org*):

- Be aware of your surroundings—who's out there and what's going on.
- Walk with confidence. The more confident you look, the stronger you appear.
- Don't let drugs or alcohol cloud your judgment.
- Be assertive—don't let anyone violate your space.
- Trust your instincts. If you feel uncomfortable in your surroundings, leave.
- Don't prop open self-locking doors.
- Lock your doors and your windows, even if you leave for just a few minutes.
- Watch your keys. Don't lend them. Don't leave them. Don't lose them. And don't put your name and address on the key ring.
- Watch out for unwanted visitors. Know who's on the other side of the door before you open it.
- Be wary of isolated spots, like underground garages, offices after business hours, and apartment laundry rooms.
- Avoid walking or jogging alone, especially at night. Vary your route. Stay in well-traveled, well-lit areas.
- Have your key ready to use before you reach the door—home, car, or work.
- Park in well-lit areas and lock the car, even if you'll be gone only a few minutes.
- Drive on well-traveled streets, with doors and windows locked.
- Never hitchhike or pick up a hitchhiker.
- Keep your car in good shape with plenty of gas in the tank.
- In case of car trouble, call for help on your cellular phone. If you don't have a phone, put the hood up, lock the doors, and put a banner in the rear mirror that says, "Help. Call police."

rapists, sexual offenses may be only one component of an extensive criminal history.

It is also possible that the reasons for a rape might vary depending on the situation. For example, perhaps with separated couples, the rape might be used to punish the victim. Or, in a dating situation, the rape might occur as part of a feeling of conquest. The reason an individual commits rape can be difficult to determine in each particular instance.

According to McCabe and Wauchope (2005), there are four main types of rapists: the anger rapist, the power exploitative rapist, the power reassurance rapist, and the sadistic rapist. The anger rapist displays his anger in overt ways, such as by using a knife, using force, displaying overwhelming anger, and projecting a macho image. Even though in general rapists do not seriously harm their victims, this type can inflict serious injury, and their rage is not related to sexual satisfaction. Their anger may also be expressed as a way to humiliate victims and put them in their place.

The power exploitative rapist seems to be motivated by a desire to display hostility and power over victims by assaulting them because of his own inadequacies, particularly a sexual dysfunction or a physical deformity. The motivation seems to be domination and control of the victim sexually even though he likely has difficulties with sexual performance. This rapist gains power by targeting one of the victim's most vulnerable points. This results in dominance and control of the victim.

The behavior of the power reassurance rapist may be very similar to that of the power exploitative rapist. The main difference is that the motivation of the power reassurance is reassurance of his own status and abilities.

The sadistic rapist is motivated to assault because of sexual and aggressive fantasies. He may make excessive use of anger, force, and restraints. This rapist wants to live out personal fantasies on an unwilling victim. Except for their sadism and their greater amount of planning, these rapists can be very similar to anger rapists.

McCabe and Wauchope (2005) also point out that there is an overlap of characteristics among types of rapists, making the picture very complex.

Rapists commonly give excuses for their behavior. Some justify their actions in various ways. Others point out that sexual assault is not their fault because it is beyond their control. Some excuse their behavior because of the presence of alcohol or drugs. Still others feel their behavior was appropriate in the situation. Finally, some feel that their victims "got what they deserved."

There are three categories of stranger rape (Stranger rape, 2012). The first is blitz sexual assault, where the perpetrator rapidly and brutally assaults the victim with no prior contact. Blitz assaults usually occur at night in a public place. The second is contact sexual assault, where the suspect contacts the victim and tries to gain her or his trust and confidence before the assault. Contact perpetrators pick their victims in bars, lure them into their cars, or otherwise try to coerce them into a situation of sexual assault. The third is home-invasion assault, where a

(?) Did You Know . . .

What should you do if you've been sexually assaulted? Take these steps right away:

- Get away from the attacker to a safe place as fast as you can. Then call 911 or the police.
- Call a friend or family member you trust. You can also call a crisis center or hotline to talk with a counselor—for example, the National Sexual Assault Hotline at 800-656-HOPE (4673) or the National Domestic Violence Hotline at 800-799-SAFE (7233). It is important to get help from a trusted professional.
- Do not wash, comb, or clean any part of your body. Do not change clothes if possible, so the hospital staff can collect evidence. Do not touch or change anything at the scene of the assault.

- Go to the nearest hospital emergency room as soon as possible. You need to be examined, treated for any injuries, and screened for possible STIs or pregnancy.
- You or the hospital staff can call the police from the emergency room to file a report.
- Ask the hospital staff about possible support groups you can attend right away.

How can you help someone who has been sexually assaulted? Listen and offer comfort. Go with her or him to the police, the hospital, or counseling. Reinforce the message that she or he is not at fault and that it is natural to feel angry and ashamed.

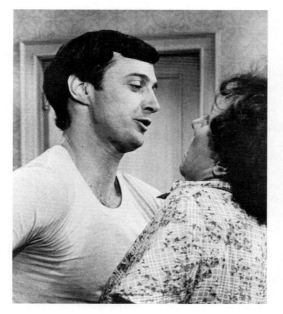

Public awareness of rape and its accompanying trauma has been raised in media depiction. An early appearance of a true-to-life rape situation appeared in the sitcom *All in the Family*. During the episode, which was written and developed by rape counselors, Edith Bunker is raped in her own home. The show, plus the publicity it created, helped many real-world victims to step forward.

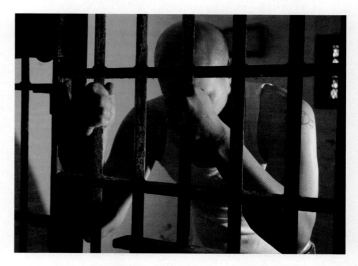

Most rapists rape to demonstrate power and not to obtain sexual satisfaction.

stranger breaks into the victim's home to commit the assault.

However, in most cases the rapist isn't a stranger. About two-thirds of rapes and 73% of sexual assaults are committed by someone known to the victim.

Thirty-eight percent of rapists are a friend or acquaintance, and 28% are an intimate. In addition, more than 50% of rapes and sexual assaults occur in the victim's home or within a mile of their home (The offenders, 2012).

Date Rape

Date rape, or acquaintance rape, is much more common than most people realize, although because of its nature gathering reliable data on this topic is difficult. It is suspected that some incidents of date rape might be a result of poor communication, because many people still have a difficult time talking about sexuality.

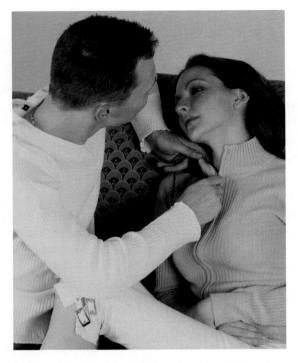

In cases of rape on college campuses, about 80% are committed by an acquaintance.

At any rate, it might help those dating to realize the following: Spending money on a date does not justify expecting sexual favors; a person who participates in other forms of sexual behavior does not necessarily find intercourse acceptable; and if a date uses sexual behavior as a means of proving masculinity or femininity, it might be better to date other people.

Unfortunately, forced sexual contact has always happened between dating partners. Women often blamed themselves for "leading a date on." It was not until the mid-1970s that the term *date rape* was coined and women had legal rights to go after assailants they had dated.

Some statistics related to date rape are included in the periodic Youth Risk Behavior Surveillance (YRBS; Eaton et al., 2010). With regard to dating violence, during the 12 months preceding the survey, approximately 10% of students in grades 9 through 12 had been hit, slapped, or physically hurt on purpose by their boyfriend or girlfriend. Overall, the prevalence of dating violence was higher among

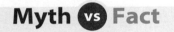

Myth vs Fact

Myth: Rape is an impulsive act of passion—meaning that men cannot control their sex drive.
Fact: Rapists themselves do not see rape as compulsive sexual behavior. The objective for rape is not usually sexual pleasure; it is to have power and to commit violence. Sexual activity is used to carry out nonsexual needs.

Myth: Women want to be raped—meaning that women have fantasies that reflect their desire to be raped.
Fact: Rape is an act of violent aggression. No healthy individual desires to be dehumanized and violated.

Myth: Women ask to be raped—meaning they tempt the man. "She should have worn a bra," "Hitchhikers get what they deserve," and "She shouldn't have been out so late at night" are examples of this thinking.
Fact: The blame and responsibility for a criminal assault are the assailant's, not the victim's.

Myth: A woman can run faster with her skirt up than a man can with his pants down—meaning a woman cannot be raped against her will.
Fact: Rape is an aggression committed under force or the threat of force on an unconsenting person. A knife, gun, or even verbal threat is often understandably stronger than a person's will.

Myth: You cannot blame a man for trying—meaning the responsibility for stopping a man is the woman's; therefore, it is her fault if matters get out of hand.
Fact: A criminal, not a victim, is responsible for criminal acts. Rape is not an impulsive act of passion. It is done for power and control.

Myth: The rapist is usually of a different race from the victim—meaning rape usually reflects ethnic or racial hatred.
Fact: In most instances the rapist and the victim are of the same race.

Myth vs Fact

Myth: If a woman is going to be raped, she might as well relax and enjoy it—meaning it is just sexual activity.
Fact: Rape victims experience intense psychological and physical trauma. Rape is a violent, dehumanizing, and intimate invasion of a woman's privacy and integrity as a human being. The motive for rape is power; it is not sexual enjoyment. Rape is anything but enjoyable!

Myth: Most rapes are committed by strangers—meaning we are safe with people we know.
Fact: It is common for the rapist and the victim to know each other, to have been acquainted, or at least to have seen each other on the street, in the grocery store, in the student union, and so on.

Myth: It's not sexual assault if it happens after drinking or taking drugs.
Fact: A person under the influence of drugs or alcohol does not cause others to assault him or her. Many state laws say that a person who is impaired due to the influence of drugs or alcohol is not able to consent to sexual activity.

Myth: A person who has really been sexually assaulted will be hysterical.
Fact: Victims of sexual violence can show a wide variety of responses, including calm, hysteria, withdrawal, anger, apathy, denial, and shock. Reactions and the length of time needed to work through the experience vary.

Myth: Only young, attractive people are assaulted.
Fact: Sexual assault is a crime of power and control, and offenders often choose people they view as vulnerable to attack or over whom they believe they can assert power. Victims come from all walks of life and represent all ages—including males, females, and persons with disabilities.

Myth: Men can't be raped.
Fact: About 92,700 men are raped each year in the United States

Myth: I don't know anyone who's ever been raped.
Fact: Rape victims are doctors, lawyers, nurses, military personnel, cooks, accountants, or anyone. Fewer than one-third of sexual assaults are reported to the police.

African American students (14%) than among Hispanic (11%) and white (8%) students. Nationwide, 8% of students had ever been physically forced to have sexual intercourse when they did not want to participate. Overall, the prevalence of having been forced to have sexual intercourse was higher among female (11%) than male (5%) students, and higher among African American (10%) and Hispanic (8%) than white (6%) students.

While experts do not understand a great deal about date rape, many researchers have studied the topic. Because of the relationship of date rape to overall dating violence, information about the two topics is often put together in research studies. From these studies we know that the vast majority of rapes on college campuses are committed by someone with whom the victim is acquainted. Many are committed on dates, and drinking alcohol and date rape often go together. Many women who are date raped do not report the assault to authorities because of feelings of self-blame and embarrassment.

Like other forms of sexual assault, acquaintance assault is motivated by a need to control, to humiliate, and to harm. It is important to remember that a prior or current relationship or previous acts of intimacy are insufficient indicators of consent. Also, verbal consent must be obtained both in each instance of sexual intimacy and as the level of sexual intimacy increases (for example, moving from kissing to petting, from petting to oral sexual activity, from oral activity to intercourse or anal activity, etc.) (Acquaintance rape, 2012).

McEwan et al. (2005) studied the relationship between date rape, ego-identity achievement, and locus of control. They found that, compared to women who had not been assaulted, date rape survivors reported lower ego-identity achievement and greater beliefs that the outcomes of their lives were controlled by luck, chance, or powerful others.

Rempala and Bernien (2005) studied the effect of target information disparity on judgments of guilt. Merely adding trivial information, such as the victim's age, college major, and city of residence, to the rape trial vignette decreased judgments of guilt for the alleged rapist. However, adding such information about the alleged rapist increased judgments of his guilt.

Lee et al. (2005) compared attitudes toward rape of Asian and Caucasian college students. Their findings suggest that Asian students are more likely than Caucasian students to believe women should be held responsible for preventing rape and to view sexual pleasure as the primary motivation for rape. Asians also had stronger beliefs than Caucasians that victims cause the rape and that most rapists are strangers and not acquaintances.

Humphreys (2007) had college students read several vignettes in which consent for sexual intercourse was ambiguous. As the degree of intimacy between the couple increased, perceptions of consent and acceptability increased. Also, men, more than women, perceived the scenarios as more consensual, acceptable, and clear regardless of relationship experience.

Marelich et al. (2008) studied the use of deception in association with sexual encounters. The three components of sexual deception used were blatant lying, self-serving lying, and avoiding confrontation. Those persons who used any of these deceptions reported more sexual partners and one-night stands. Those telling blatant lies to have sexual activity were more likely to report greater needs for sexual activity, while those using self-serving lies or having sexual intercourse to avoid confrontation experienced greater worry about partner loss. Men were more likely to use blatant lies to have sexual activity, while women were more likely to have sexual activity to avoid confrontation.

Ways to Help Prevent Acquaintance Rape

Because of the magnitude of date rape, many steps have been taken to help deal with and reduce the problem. Awareness is the first step, and materials have been developed to help college students understand date rape and how to prevent it. The American College Health Association (2008) has developed a pamphlet titled *Sexual Violence: What Everyone Should Know*, which contains suggestions for both men and women.

For example, the pamphlet indicates that alcohol and other drugs can inhibit clear thinking, make talking and listening more difficult, and make it harder to assess risk. Consenting sexual activity doesn't just happen. It requires sober, verbal communication without intimidation or threats. Many states' laws recognize that someone must be sober to give true consent. Also, being drunk or high is never an excuse for raping someone.

The pamphlet also has a section titled "What You Can Do," which indicates that you can think about how to respond to social pressures and ask yourself:

- How does sex fit into my definition of being a man or a woman?

- What role do I want sex to play in my life?

- How does alcohol affect my sexual decision-making?

- How do I learn someone's desires and limits?

- How do I express my own desires and limits?

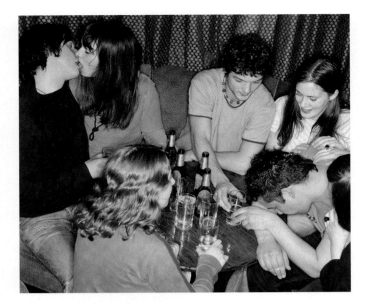

Alcohol can play a role in acquaintance rape.

The pamphlet emphasizes the need to communicate effectively. It suggests expressing your limits clearly, listening carefully to what the other person is saying, asking rather than assuming, trusting your instincts, and remembering that effective and assertive communication may not always work. Sometimes people simply don't listen. However, no one ever *deserves* to be raped!

The Antioch College policy requiring verbal consent to sexual behavior is shown in Table 14.2. It has been the subject of many articles in which varying opinions have been expressed.

The Mentors in Violence Prevention (MVP) Program was founded at Northeastern University in 1993 and is still functioning (www.northeastern.edu/sportinsociety/leadership/mentors/index.html). It is a leadership program that motivates student-athletes and other student leaders to play a central role in helping to solve problems that have been traditionally considered "women's issues": rape, battering, and sexual harassment. The program has four main goals: (1) to raise awareness of the level of men's verbal, emotional, physical, and sexual abuse of women; (2) to challenge thinking by countering mainstream messages about gender, sexual behavior, and violence; (3) to open a dialogue by creating a safe environment for men and women to share opinions and experiences; and (4) to inspire leadership by empowering participants with concrete options to effect change in their communities. Today the MVP program is used on a number of other campuses.

One effective, but controversial, way to prevent date rape or other rapes came from a South African inventor (South African anti-rape condom could reduce risk of pregnancy, HIV, STIs, 2005). It is called Rapex, is worn inside a woman's body like a tampon, and hooks onto a man's penis during intercourse. It is made of latex and attaches to the penis by shafts of sharp barbs. The device can be removed by surgery and is so painful that it would disable rapists immediately, allowing women to escape. It would not cause any long-term physical damage to the rapist, and could not accidentally injure the women. Some people are concerned that the device would provoke rapists and increase violence against women. They also feel that the device puts the burden on women to address the problem, instead of focusing on societal issues as motivating factors of rape. Others point out that the problem is so severe that women need protection now.

TABLE 14.2 The Antioch College Policy Requiring Verbal Consent for Each Level of Sexual Behavior

As part of community governance, Antioch College students developed a policy requiring students to obtain verbal consent for each level of sexual behavior. Here are the 10 reasons given to obtain verbal approval for sexual activities:

1. Because many partners find it sexy to be asked, as sexual behavior progresses, if it's okay.
2. Because sexual activity is better when each partner enjoys what is happening and no one is being forced to do something he or she doesn't want to do.
3. Because if your partner is having a good time and is not forced to do something against his or her will, he or she may be more likely to want to see you again. Mutual respect is the best basis for friendship and intimacy.
4. Because forcing sexual activity on another person can violate state and federal laws and your school's policy. In most instances, unwanted touching and fondling is sexual assault.
5. Because it prevents misunderstandings (silence is not a "yes").
6. Because you won't be accused of rape.
7. Because you won't go to jail or be expelled.
8. Because it's better to be safe than sorry.
9. Because if you want to impose your sexual will on someone, your behavior has more to do with dominating the person than with enjoying sexuality and an intimate relationship.
10. Why would you want to have sexual behavior with someone who doesn't like what you are doing?

Source: Reproduced from Antioch College. Ten reasons to obtain a verbal consent for sex. *About women on campus, 2* (Winter 1994).

Situational Model of Sexual Coercion

One way to comprehend better and perhaps reduce the problem of date rape is to understand a situational model of sexual coercion (Snyder & Ickes, 1985) (Figure 14.1). The model includes individual personality characteristics, situational components, cognitive processes, and behavioral effects of participants in a social situation (Craig, 1990). In other words, people introduce certain traits or dispositions to a dating situation, but they also use manipulation to express their dispositions.

In the first step of the model, the dispositions and history of the male lead him to select situations in which he can act in a particular way. Relatedly, there seems to be a common set of characteristics that distinguish between sexually coercive and noncoercive men (Craig, 1990). Coercive males tend to be more aggressive, to believe that relationships with women are basically adversarial, and to support rape myths and sex-role stereotypes. Peer approval also seems important, and sexual behavior is emphasized as a status symbol.

In the second step of the model, coercive males use selective exposure to choose situations that are likely to match their dispositions and characteristics. They tend to select certain types of women, dating situations, and relationships. For example, although there is not total agreement among researchers, it seems that women who are selected as victims by coercive males are more sexually experienced, more sexually passive, and less likely to use methods of avoidance such as running away or screaming.

Regarding the dating situation, sexual coercion seems more likely to occur when the male initiated the date, paid expenses, and drove; when there was miscommunication about sexual behavior; when an isolated location was used; when there was some consensual sexual contact; and when both persons were moderately or extremely intoxicated. In terms of the dating relationship, coercion seems more likely when there is an established relationship between the partners. Also, sexual violence seems more likely when there are differences between partners in age, intelligence, and social status.

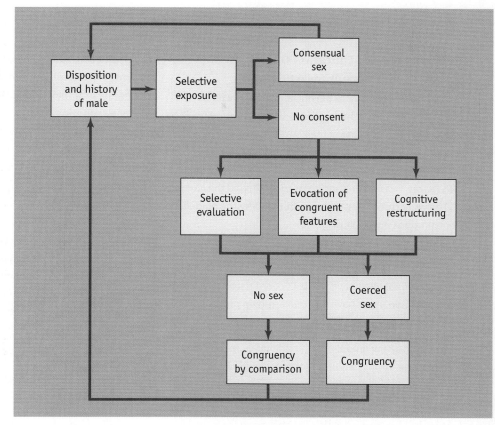

FIGURE 14.1 The situational model of coercive sexual behavior.
Source: Reproduced from Craig, M. E. (1990). Coercive sexuality in dating relationships: A situational model. *Clinical Psychology Review, 10, no. 4,* 395–423, with permission from Elsevier.

If the factors suggested do not result in consensual sexual activity, there are additional components of the model. Through selective evaluation the male may place major importance on situational aspects that he believes encourage him to make sexual advances. For example, the female's friendliness, appearance, or behavior might cause a male's misperception of the situation.

Even after setting up a situation that increases his likelihood of engaging in sexual activity—and paying attention only to the cues that would seem to encourage sexual advances—the coercive male may still encounter resistance. He may then try to lower the woman's resistance by using alcohol or drugs or by making false statements or promises.

Cognitive restructuring is changing one's interpretations to better fit one's self-image. In relation to coercive sexual behavior, this could include use of alcohol, victim blaming (it was really her fault), and rationalization (perceiving aggressive behavior as appropriate or perceiving aggressive actions as acceptable to women).

Up to this point in the model, the goal for the male has been to make the features of the situation congruent with his self-concept. If that still has not happened, or if sexual activity still has not occurred, he may feel a need to externalize blame for his "failure."

? Did You Know . . .

U.S. Department of Education Guidelines for Colleges' Sexual-Assault Investigations

In 2011 the U.S. Department of Education announced a set of thorough guidelines for how colleges should respond to allegations of sexual assault. One of the key recommendations lowers the burden of proof for finding someone guilty of sexual assault from "clear and convincing" evidence to "more likely than not," which makes it easier for institutions to reprimand the harasser.

There are three key provisions outlined by the guidelines that institutions must follow:

1. Every school must have and distribute a policy against sex discrimination
2. Every school must have a Title IX coordinator
3. Every school must have and make known procedures for students to file complaints of sex discrimination.

Under the new guidelines, the grievance procedures may include voluntary informal methods (e.g., mediation) for resolving some types of sexual harassment complaints. However, the complainant must be notified of the right to end the informal process at any time and begin the formal stage of the complaint process. In cases involving allegations of sexual assault, mediation is not appropriate. In addition, the person who filed the complaint has the right to be notified, in writing, of the outcome. Schools must also disclose to them information about the sanction imposed on the harasser when the sanction directly relates to the harassed student.

If a school knows or reasonably should know about sexual harassment or sexual violence that creates a hostile environment, the school must take immediate action to eliminate the sexual harassment or sexual violence, prevent its recurrence, and address its effects.

Source: Modified from Know Your Rights: Title IX Prohibits Sexual Harassment and Sexual Violence Where You Go to School. Office for Civil Rights, U.S. Department of Education. (2011).

For example, he may indicate she was just cold or that they did not really have the opportunity.

The situational model can be helpful to understanding coercive sexual behavior in dating situations. It can also help us understand why misperceptions occur so frequently. Perhaps most importantly, it can be used in a positive way—particularly to encourage better communication at all levels of a relationship and to recognize prevention or promotion of behaviors that help prevent coercion.

Date-Rape Drugs

In the early 1990s the topic of date rape was further complicated by the availability of **date-rape drugs**. These drugs are sometimes used to assist a sexual assault. They are powerful and dangerous. They can be slipped into your drink when you are not looking. The drugs often have no color, smell, or taste, so you can't tell if you are being drugged. They can make you become weak and confused— or even pass out—so that you are unable to refuse sexual activity or defend yourself. If you are drugged, you might not remember what happened while you were drugged. Date-rape drugs are used on both females and males (Date rape drugs, 2008).

date-rape drugs
Sedative hypnotic drugs used to incapacitate victims who are then sexually molested or raped.

One early date-rape drug was flunitrazepam (Rohypnol). It is a prescription drug marketed legally in many countries around the world. It is used as a sedative hypnotic and as a preanesthetic medication in those countries. However, it is not approved for medical use in the United States. Because of its sedative hypnotic action and amnesialike effect, it is ideal for use in date-rape situations. Rohypnol can be administered without consent to produce disinhibition and to obtain sexual activity. It has no taste or odor when mixed with alcohol. People drugged with Rohypnol may remember nothing about what happened or have only a very sketchy memory. They are often unsure that they have been raped, except that they may wake the next morning feeling genital discomfort or finding themselves undressed. Assailants typically claim the victims consented to sexual activity, and there is no way to know for sure. The effects of Rohypnol can be felt within 30 minutes and can last for several hours (Date rape drugs, 2008).

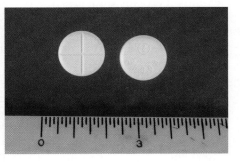

Date rape drugs have no taste and no odor. They are undetectable if added to a drink.

Another date-rape drug is gammahydroxybutyrate (GHB). It can be used by sexual predators to render their victims almost instantly helpless and to leave them with little or no memory of the attack. It is similar to the drug Rohypnol. GHB has no approved medical use, and it can cause depression, seizures, coma, and death. Kits can be purchased to make the drug at home for less than $100. Many argue that GHB should be an illegal substance.

A third drug being used as a date-rape drug is ketamine hydrochloride. It is used medically as an anesthetic for diagnostic and surgical purposes. It produces anesthesia within 40 seconds of intravenous administration and within 8 minutes of intramuscular administration. It is currently widely used by veterinarians. In the United States the popular method of use involves heating of the liquid until it turns into a white powder, which is then smoked or snorted. Full effects of ketamine occur in about 5 to 10 minutes and last up to 1 hour (Date rape drugs, 2008).

Other date rape drugs include gamma-butyrolactone (GBL), benzodiazepines, and Ecstasy (Drug facilitated sexual assault, 2012). GBL, a GHB-like product, is often sold under the guise of a dietary supplement or an industrial cleaner. When the body metabolizes GBL, it becomes twice as potent as GHB. It now comes in flavors and, once ingested, it takes about 30 to 45 minutes to take effect. Benzodiazepines are legal substances commonly prescribed as antianxiety and sleeping medications in the United States. They can be put into an alcoholic drink or soft drink in power or liquid form. They can markedly impair and even abolish functions that normally enable a person to resist, or even want to resist, sexual aggression or assault. Ecstasy is a toxic hallucinogenic and stimulant that has psychedelic effects. It is illegal to sell or produce it in the United States. Ecstasy causes individuals to feel extreme relaxation and positivity towards others and increases sensitivity to touch. Under its influence, individuals are less likely to be able to sense danger, making it difficult to protect themselves from attack.

In 1996 President Clinton signed a bill outlawing Rohypnol and other date-rape drugs and adding 20 years to the sentence of a rapist who uses these drugs on a victim. The law also included increased penalties for illegal manufacturing, distribution, dispensing, or possession of the drugs. It was the first time that using a drug as a weapon was classified as a crime in the United States.

Although the term "date rape" is commonly used, many experts prefer the term "drug-facilitated sexual assault" when referring to these drugs. The drugs can affect a person very quickly, and the length of time that the effect lasts varies, depending on how much is taken and whether it is mixed with other substances such as alcohol. Alcohol can worsen the drug's effects. Here are some ways to protect yourself from being a victim of "drug-facilitated sexual assault" (Date rape drugs, 2005):

- Don't accept drinks from other people.

- Open containers yourself.

- Keep your drink with you at all times, even when you go into the bathroom.

- Don't share drinks.

- Don't drink from punch bowls or other large, common, open containers. They may already have drugs in them.

- Don't drink anything that tastes or smells strange. Sometimes GHB tastes salty.

- Have a nondrinking friend with you to make sure nothing happens.

- If you think you have been drugged and raped:

  - Go to the police station or hospital right away.

  - Get a urine test as soon as possible. The drugs leave your system quickly.

  - Don't urinate before getting help.

  - Don't douche, bathe, or change clothes before getting help. These actions eliminate evidence of the rape.

- Call the National Domestic Violence Hotline at 800-799-SAFE or 800-787-3224 (TTY).

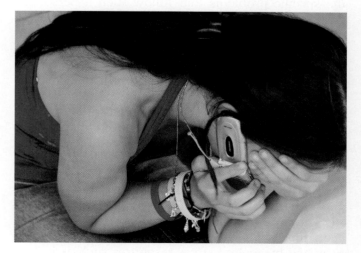

It is important to get help if sexual assault does occur.

Multicultural DIMENSIONS

Sexual Violence Sexual violence may be viewed and handled differently in various cultures. For example, sexual violence against Norwegian women is common but rarely reported. Despite being known for its progressive stance on gender equality, Norway has rates of sexual violence on par with much more unequal societies. According to Norway's largest shelter organization, 1 in 10 Norwegian women older than age 15 has been raped. Of these cases, at least 80% are never brought to official attention and only 10% of those that are end in a conviction. Also, Norway is one of 127 countries in the world that do not explicitly criminalize rape within marriage. Every county in Norway has a rape assault center and a medical facility where rape survivors are offered no-cost counseling and medical care and examined for forensic evidence. Yet, most rape survivors do not go to the hospital for forensic exams or press charges. Even when cases are reported to the police, they don't always pick up the evidence that was collected.

Hate crimes can also be viewed as relating to various cultures. By definition, they are victimization of an individual based on that individual's race, religion, national origin, ethnic identification, gender, or sexual orientation. While any group can experience rape and sexual assault as a form of hate crime, two groups are often noted for being victims of this form of hate crime—women and people in the LGBT community.

Many believe that all violence against women, including rape and sexual assault, is a hate crime because it is not simply a violent act, but that it is "an act of misogyny, or hatred of women." Members of the LGBT community are often targets of hate crimes, many of which include rape or sexual assault. In one study of almost 2,000 lesbian and gay individuals, about one-fifth of the women and one-fourth of the men had been victimized at some point during the past 5 years.

Sources: Data from Sexual violence against Norwegian women common but rarely reported. Women's Health Policy Report. National Partnership for Women & Families, October 29, 2011. Available: http://www.natianalpartnership.ors/site/News21abbr-daily4 &page-News-Article& id- 30801; modified from Hate crimes. Rape, Abuse, & Incest National Network, 2012. Available: www.rainn.org/get-information/types-of-sexual-assault/hate-crimes.

Consequences of Rape

The survivor of a rape, friends, family, and spouse or lover usually respond to the crime's sexual aspects, instead of the violent aspects. Rape survivors and their loved ones need the same kinds of help to get through this difficult time as survivors of other violent acts. And beyond that, they need assistance with the specific problems that follow such a personally destructive attack.

Traumatic events, such as war, accidents, natural disasters, and sexual violence can result in serious stress and detrimental consequences for survivors and their families. Although most individuals will be able to absorb the trauma over time, many survivors will experience long-lasting problems. About 8% of survivors of traumatic events develop post-traumatic stress disorder (PTSD). PTSD symptoms include nightmares, insomnia, somatic disturbances, difficulty with intimate relationships, fear, anxiety, anger, shame, aggression, suicidal behaviors, loss of trust, and isolation (Facts about trauma, 2005).

The **rape trauma syndrome** has two phases. The acute phase can last from days to weeks, and is characterized by general stress responses such as lack of sleep, irritability, and difficulty in thinking clearly.

The long-term phase can last several years and the symptoms are similar to those described for PTSD. Some experts believe that the long-term phase of the rape trauma syndrome is actually a subset of PTSD.

> **rape trauma syndrome**
> A two-phase reaction to rape. An acute phase involves intense emotional responses for several weeks. The long-term phase may last several years and involves reorganization and establishment of control.

In addition to the psychological consequences mentioned previously, physical consequences of rape include the possibility of a pregnancy and/or an STI. Other physical consequences could be chronic pelvic pain, gastrointestinal disorders, migraines and other frequent headaches, back pain, and facial pain. Social consequences include strained family relations, less frequent contact with friends and relatives, and less emotional support from friends and family (Sexual violence: Fact sheet, 2005).

As many as 38% of women engage in more sexually risky behaviors after experiencing a sexual assault than they did before the attack, while 48% significantly reduce their risky behavior (Campbell, Sefl, & Alvon, 2004). About half of the 48% began abstaining from sexual activity after their assault. Sexually risky behavior can include sexual activity with multiple partners, without contraception, and while under the influence of alcohol or other drugs. Rape survivors who had negative interactions with police and medical professionals, and reported experiencing blame for their assault from these sources, tended to fall into the group of women who increased their sexually risky behaviors.

It is clear that individuals who are victims of sexual violence are more likely to experience depression, anxiety, and traumatic symptoms compared to nonvictims. However, the impact of sexual violence is not limited to the act itself. Instead, so-called secondary victimization may result from negative experiences within one's social group or with authorities who may hold negative attitudes toward victims of rape (Nagel et al., 2005).

Adult rape survivors experience a shattering effect on their personal stability and adjustment. Many do not wish to confide in another person and try to hold in their feelings. Some are hesitant to participate in their usual sexual relations. Personal feelings of privacy, dignity, and trust are undermined, and feelings of vulnerability are common. Many women feel they live in a world filled with threats. Anger, rage, shame, and fear profoundly influence the recovery of rape survivors. It is not unusual for this anger to be expressed toward men in general. Although some women suffer physical trauma from rape, requiring surgical repair of the perineum, vulva, or urethra, it is emotional scars that take longest to heal.

In summary, victims of sexual assault are 3 times more likely to suffer from depression, 6 times more likely to suffer from PTSD, and 13 times more likely to abuse alcohol. In addition, they are 26 times more likely to abuse drugs, and 4 times more likely to contemplate suicide (Who are the victims?, 2009).

Many survivors of sexual assault do heal and do just fine in their lives. They probably do not forget, but they do move on. There is a great deal of hope today for such survivors.

Rape of Males

Almost all the information on rape presented so far has focused on rapes of females. This is appropriate because the vast majority of survivors are females. However, in recent years there has been an increased recognition that males can be sexually assaulted, too. Even the rape laws in many states now recognize the existence of male rape. Generally, male rape falls into one of three categories: male rape in prison, male rape by other males outside prison, and male rape by females.

After more than four decades of research, it is still unknown how much rape and sexually violent activity occur in prisons and jails. What is clear is

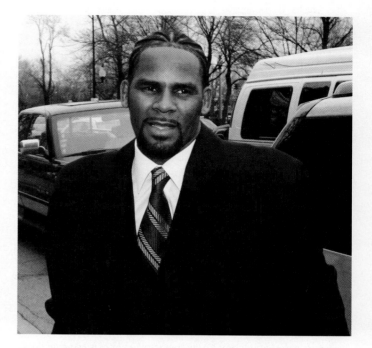

Rap and R & B superstar R. Kelly was charged with 21 counts of child pornography stemming from a videotape that allegedly shows him having sexual activity with a 13-year-old girl. Kelly's CD in 2003 debuted at number one and the first single from the album, "Ignition," peaked at number two on the Billboard's singles chart and enjoyed consistent radio and television play, all while he faced serious charges of a sexual encounter with a minor. Does this send the message that the rap and R & B community condones such behavior?

that, as with rape in free society, prison rape goes largely unreported. It is very difficult to estimate the extent of the problem. The limited information available suggests that from 2% to 13% of all inmates have been raped (Prison rape, 2007). Even though research about prison rape is not conclusive, many people believe that the likelihood of being raped in prison is so great that a judge who sentences a young man to prison passes a sentence of male rape on him as surely as the prison sentence. It appears that male prison rape is an act of heterosexuals rather than homosexuals. This may sound strange at first, but in a prison situation rape is viewed as validation of masculinity and a violent act of conquest.

As one sign of concern about prison rape, in 2003 Congress passed the Prison Rape Elimination Act. This legislation calls for all correction systems to have a zero-tolerance policy regarding prison rape. It requires standards for detection, prevention, reduction, and punishment of prison rape. It standardizes collection and dissemination of information on the incidence of prison rape, and awards grants to implement the act's provisions (About the Prison Rape Elimination Act of 2003, 2007).

? Did You Know . . .

Stalking

The exact definition of stalking can vary by state, but generally it refers to a "course of conduct directed at a specific person that involves repeated visual or physical proximity, nonconsensual communication, or verbal, written, or implied threats, or a combination thereof, that would cause a reasonable person fear." Examples of stalking include:

1. Repeated undesired contact (phone calls, emails, letters, showing up unexpectedly, etc.).
2. Following or laying in wait for the individual.
3. Making threats to the individual or her/his family.
4. Any other behavior used to contact, harass, track, or threaten the individual.

Each year about 3.4 million people in the United States are victims of stalking. The majority of victims are 18 to 24 years old. Most victims know their stalker. About 1 in 4 victims experience some form of cyberstalking.

If you are ever stalked, you should consider:

1. Avoiding all contact with the stalker.
2. Informing family, friends, supervisors, and coworkers of what is going on.
3. Reporting the stalking to the local police.
4. Keeping an accurate journal or log of all incidents connected to the stalking.
5. Keeping all evidence received from the stalker, such as letters, packages, taped phone messages, etc.

All 50 states and Washington D.C. have antistalking laws. The impact of stalking can be life altering. Those who are stalked often change many of their behaviors and can have strong emotional responses, including anxiety, fear, depression, nervousness, and isolation. Many resources are available to help people prevent and deal with stalking.

Source: Modified from Stalking. Rape, Abuse, & Incest National Network, 2012. Available: www.rainn.org/newsroom/sexual-assault-issues/stalking.

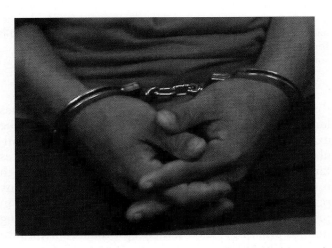

Prison rape is usually the act of heterosexuals rather than homosexuals.

Even outside prison, it is probable that most rapes of males are committed by heterosexual men. This is perhaps more understandable when we consider that violence and power, rather than sexual satisfaction, are the primary motivations for rape. Statistics on the frequency of male rape are almost impossible to obtain. Perhaps this is because of the lack of research on the subject combined with the hesitation of male victims to report an attack. In addition to the reasons females hesitate to report a rape, males often feel they are supposed to be strong and "macho." To report being raped would not be consistent with this image.

A male being raped by a female is hard for many people to imagine. This is because of traditional feelings about sexuality—particularly the ideas that all males are "at the ready" for sexual activity and that males cannot be forced into submission. Although the first attitude is open to question (often based on incorrect logic), the second relates to physiological functioning. People seem to think that a male could not respond sexually while being threatened because he could not achieve a penile erection. It has been found, however, that such emotions as anger, fright, and pain can cause a sexual response, including all the usual physiological changes. This, of course, can be quite upsetting to the victim because it might be interpreted as indicating willingness. Guilt and other negative feelings can occur as well. Consequently, the responses of male rape survivors are very similar to those of female rape survivors.

Walker et al. (2005) investigated the effects of rape on a sample of 40 men recruited by media advertising. They found that most assaults had been carried out using physical or violent force, in a variety of circumstances. All victims reported some form of psychological disturbance as a result of being raped. Long-term effects included anxiety, depression, increased feelings of anger and vulnerability, loss of self-image, emotional distancing, self-blame, and self-harming behaviors.

Stermac et al. (2004) examined victim and assault characteristics among adult male victims of sexual assaults. They found that male victims presenting to an urban sexual assault care center were young, often single adults with significant vulnerabilities (living on the street or in a shelter, unemployed, and with physical disabilities). These same characteristics were not so common with female victims. Males overall were more likely to be victims of an anal and/or fellatio assault. Male stranger assailant victims were also more likely to be attacked by multiple assailants than were female victims, and more likely to be assaulted outdoors. In contrast, male acquaintance assailant victims were more likely to be assaulted in an institutional setting. Male stranger assault victims were more likely to experience assaults involving weapons. Acquaintance male assaults, however, were more likely to involve victims' alcohol use.

As with rape of females, there are many stereotypes and myths about rape of males. Many of these impact the male survivor's ability to face the sexual assault. Some of these myths are that: (1) men are immune to victimization; (2) men should be able to fight off attacks; (3) men should not express emotion; (4) men enjoy all sexual activity, so they must have enjoyed the assault; and (5) male survivors are more likely to become sexual predators. Of course, all of these statements are false. These stereotypes and myths can lead to certain results for male victims of sexual abuse, including dramatic loss of self-esteem; loss of belief in their masculinity; self-blame; feelings of shame, guilt, and anger; feelings of powerlessness, apprehension, withdrawal, and embarrassment; fears that they will not be able to protect and support their families; sexual difficulties; self-destructive behavior (such as drinking, drug use, and aggression); intimacy issues; and questioning of sexual identity (Male sexual assault, 2011).

Most of what was discussed regarding rape trauma syndrome and post-traumatic stress disorder for female victims of sexual violence also applies to male victims. In addition, a male victim often feels that he has totally lost control over the insides of his own body, resulting in feelings of vulnerability and powerlessness. Men are often brought up to defend themselves against attack, and may consider total helplessness incompatible with masculinity. They may feel that their gender identity as a male was compromised or even demolished and reversed (Rape trauma syndrome—What everyone should know, 2005).

Social Responses to Rape

In many communities, sexual assault crisis centers, workshops dealing with prevention of sexual assault, and improved methods of helping survivors have become priorities. Shelters for survivors of assault have been provided so they have a place to receive help. In general, there is a better understanding of the problems in communities and the need for more support.

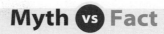

Myth vs Fact

Myths About Male Rape

Myth: Men can't be sexually assaulted.
Fact: Men are sexually assaulted—regardless of size, strength, appearance, or sexual orientation.

Myth: Only gay men are sexually assaulted.
Fact: Heterosexual, gay, and bisexual men are equally likely to be sexually assaulted.

Myth: Only gay men sexually assault other men.
Fact: Most men who sexually assault other men are heterosexuals.

Myth: Men can't be sexually assaulted by women.
Fact: Although most perpetrators are men, women can also sexually assault men.

Myth: Erection or ejaculation during sexual assault means you "really wanted it" or consented to it.
Fact: Erection and ejaculation are physiological responses that may result from mere physical contact or even extreme stress. These responses do not imply that you wanted or enjoyed the sexual assault.

Source: Modified from Myths about male rape. South Eastern Centre Against Sexual Assault 2009. Available: www.secasa.com.au.

On many college campuses there are laudable attempts to deal with sexual assault. An effective program (1) defines and demystifies sexual assault, (2) offers educational programs, (3) empowers women to be assertive, (4) exposes the link between alcohol abuse and unwanted sexual behavior, (5) conducts institutional surveys, and (6) identifies a specific individual on campus to coordinate efforts and clinical services (Meilman, Riggs, & Turco, 1990). There is also greater recognition on college campuses of the need for more attention to the problem of sexual assault. Lighting and security on campuses have improved; courses in sexual assault prevention and self-defense are offered; and escort services are available so women need not be alone on campus, particularly after dark.

There have also been major changes in laws related to rape in the past few decades. Many of the newer rape laws (1) establish "degrees" of rape to describe types of sexual assault more accurately; (2) are gender neutral and do not apply only to attacks by men on women; (3) eliminate requirements that victims prove they resisted by "fighting back" and that corroborating evidence be presented; (4) shield victims from inquiries into past sexual experience; and (5) allow a husband to be charged with raping his wife. In fact, in many states the term *forced sex* or *sexual assault* has replaced the word *rape*. The convicted rapist can often be sentenced to life in prison.

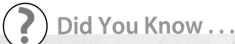

Did You Know . . .

Where to Find Help

The following numbers can be helpful if you want to find out more about reporting abuse or if you want more information about abuse:

Child abuse: (800) 4-A-CHILD (422-4453)

Elder abuse: (800) 677-1116

Sexual assault: (800) 656-4673

Domestic violence: (800) 799-7233

Changes have also been made in relation to law enforcement personnel. Training has been designed to help them become more sensitive to the problem of sexual assault. More female officers are used, and there is improved cooperation between law enforcement personnel and medical and support personnel. Guidelines for handling survivors of sexual assault have also been established.

Women who have been assaulted have begun to fight back in civil court as well. For example, a Seattle woman was awarded $300,000 from three men who raped her and a fourth who prevented her escape; a Vermont woman received $450,000 even after a defendant was acquitted of rape charges; and a Minnesota woman received $21,500 from a physician (who had been her lover) for rape.

But even with the increased emphasis on prevention, a great deal must be done. Major priorities include more changes in legislation, law enforcement policies and practices, educational intervention, and media strategies. The codification of women's equality and rights is an important part of a strategy for preventing assault. Skills training, which includes avoidance strategies, appropriate resistance, and self-defense training, is also needed.

Pedophilia

The term **pedophilia** denotes feelings of adult sexual attraction to children. Even though physical force may not be used, an adult who performs a sexual act with a child is forcing himself or herself on a helpless minor in the eyes of the law. Pedophiliacs may expose their genitals to a child or fondle and even penetrate a child. There are countless ways a

pedophilia
Sexual behavior in which a child is the sexual object.

child might be molested; most often the term *child molestation* refers to pedophilia. For all practical purposes the terms are used interchangeably.

The Pedophiliac

According to the American Psychiatric Association Statement on Diagnostic Criteria for Pedophilia (2003), the criteria for pedophilia are as follows:

1. Over a period of at least 6 months, recurrent, intense sexually arousing fantasies, sexual urges, or behaviors involving sexual activity with a prepubescent child or children (generally age 13 years or younger).

2. The person has acted on these sexual urges, or the sexual urges or fantasies cause marked distress or interpersonal difficulty.

3. The person is at least 16 years of age and at least 5 years older than the child or children in Criterion 1.

Pedophilia is one of the few psychiatric disorders for which the symptoms constitute a criminal act. There has not been a great deal of research on pedophilia. Child molesters are not identical to pedophiles. For example, a child molester can be anyone who has sexually molested a child. However, pedophilia involves a sexual disorder and ongoing sexual desires, urges, fantasies, and possibly, but not necessarily, behavior. Pedophilia is extremely difficult to treat and effective treatment needs to be intensive, long-term, and comprehensive, possibly with lifetime follow-up (Cohen & Galynker, 2002).

A man or a woman can be a pedophiliac, but most commonly we hear about males being the offenders. The objects of their desires may be boys, girls, or both. Their preferences with respect to practices vary from exhibition to penetration. Some have fleeting contacts with a series of children, while others look for long-term relationships, which may be sort of caring or manipulative. Many are considerate in their behavior toward children; others use force. Only a few use violent means. There are instances of consensual sexual activity between adults and children, but this raises the question: Can there ever be sexual consensus between adults and children? Also, there are many cases of nonconsensual sexual contacts between adults and children that are not traumatic for the child, although they do indeed violate the child's right of self-determination. Sexual contacts between adults and children pose a risk of lasting trauma for the latter even when they do not involve violence or the use of force (Schmidt, 2002).

Ethical DIMENSIONS

Should the Media Reveal the Names of Rape Survivors?

The names of rape survivors traditionally have been withheld by the news media to "protect" them. Does this special treatment do rape survivors a disservice by separating them from other survivors of violent crimes? Should the privacy of rape survivors be protected more than the privacy of survivors of other violent crimes? This issue has often been debated, and it arose again when two California teenagers were kidnapped. Their names and pictures were widely distributed to help locate them. When, after their rescue, a sheriff said they had been raped during the abduction, "What should be done now?" asked many journalists. Some media representatives stuck to their own rule and did not refer to the teenagers by name. Others called them by name, reasoning that their names had already been released.

Some people believe that the bright lights of publicity may harm the innocent in crimes of rape. They assert that rape survivors are unwillingly thrust into the limelight, their right to choose is once again removed, and their feeling of powerlessness is perpetuated. They argue that publicly identifying rape survivors without their consent compounds the trauma of rape and may discourage future survivors from reporting crimes.

Others point out that in most states it is legal to publish the names of rape survivors, and, in fact, their names should be published just as the names of people who are victims of other violent crimes are. They point out that it is discriminatory to publish the names of alleged assailants, but not the alleged survivors. They also indicate that not naming the survivors contributes to the perception that rape is a different type of crime and helps to perpetuate the notion that there is some blame or disgrace attached. It is also argued that special treatment by the news media inhibits society from treating rape as a violent crime.

Do you think it is ethical, and the best thing to do, for the media to give the names of rape survivors?

Van Wijk et al. (2005) studied characteristics of sex offenders as compared to non-sex offenders. They found that juvenile sex offenders were significantly younger than other juvenile offenders at the time of their initial offense, that a larger proportion of sex offenders attended special education schools, and that violent offenders were more extroverted and impulsive and showed higher scores on lack of conscience than other offenders. Also, child molesters had significantly higher scores on neuroticism and scored worse on contact with peers. They were socially isolated because of their poorly developed social skills—and had less or no normal contact with peers.

Tardif and Van Gijseghem (2005) researched the gender identity of pedophiles. They found no differences in gender identity among pedophiles who abused male victims, pedophiles who abused female victims, or nonsexual offenders.

Most victims of child sexual abuse do not become pedophiles. However, particular experiences and patterns of childhood behavior are associated with an increased risk of victims becoming abusers in later life. These include neglect, lack of supervision, sexual abuse by a female person, being cruel to animals, and witnessing serious intrafamilial violence (Salter et al., 2003).

Although there are many biological and psychological theories, no one really knows how pedophilia develops (Pedophilia: Who are the men who "love" children in intolerable ways, 2004). The tendency may be established early in life, perhaps genetically or before birth. Hormones may be involved, but consistent hormonal abnormalities are not found in pedophiles. Some experts think that brain function may have something to do with the development of pedophilia, but no one knows for sure. Risk factors for pedophilia—and sexual offenses of all kinds—include childhood emotional abuse, family conflict, childhood behavior problems, substance abuse, and personality disorders—particularly antisocial personality. According to one theory, pedophiles compensate for feelings of powerlessness by engaging in a type of sexual activity that provides them more control than adult relationships permit. Another theory indicates that pedophilia results from a diversion of sexual development that allows immature forms of desire to persist into adulthood. Another common view is that child molestation creates pedophiles. However, as pointed out earlier in another context, most child sex abusers are not pedophiles.

Multicultural
DIMENSIONS

Sexual Contact in Various Cultures

Sexual contact between children and adults may be viewed differently in various cultures. The people following these practices are not pedophiles, but are following cultural or religious tradition. Here are some examples:

- Among the Siwans in North Africa, all men and boys engage in anal intercourse. Males are singled out as peculiar if they do not do so. Prominent Siwan men lend their sons to each other for this purpose.
- Among the Aranda in Central Australia, a man who is not yet married takes a 10- to 12-year-old boy as his wife for several years, until the older man marries.

- In the eighteenth century in Hawaii, copulation in public between an adult male and a young girl was not considered to be indecent or improper. Sexual interactions between an adult and a child were seen as benefiting the child, rather than as gratifying the adult.
- Among the Etoro of New Guinea, from about age 10, boys would have regular oral sexual activity with older men, swallowing their semen to facilitate growth.

Source: Data from Green, R. Is pedophilia a mental disorder? *Archives of Sexual Behavior, 31, no. 6* (December 2002), 467–471.

Incidence of Pedophilia

As with other sexual offenses, it is difficult to know for sure how often pedophilia occurs. It is even more complicated because statistics do not differentiate between pedophilia and **child sexual abuse**. However, it is still germane to consider overall statistics regarding adult sexual contact with children.

child sexual abuse
Any sexual abuse involving fondling, erotic kissing, oral sexual activity, or genital penetration between an adult and a child, including pedophilia and incest.

According to statistics from the Rape, Abuse, and Incest National Network (Who are the victims?, 2012), approximately 44% of sexual assault and rape victims are younger than the age of 18 years. Fifteen percent are younger than age 12. Seven percent of girls in grades 5–8 and 12% of girls in grades 9–12 say they have been sexually abused. Three percent of boys in grades 5–8 and 5% of boys in grades 9–12 say they have been sexually abused. Ninety-three percent of juvenile sexual assault victims knew their attacker (34% of attackers were family members, 59% were acquaintances, and only 7% were strangers to the victim). About 75% of the sexual abuse victims are girls. Nearly 30% of child victims are between the ages of 4 and 7 years.

Overall, 7% of all victims of sexual assault reported to law enforcement agencies are younger than the age of 18; 34% of all victims are younger than the age of 12 years. One out of every six victims of sexual assault reported to law enforcement agencies is younger than the age of 6 years (Sexual assault of young children as reported to law enforcement, 2005).

Regarding males, about one-sixth of men report having had unwanted sexual contact with an older person by the age of 16. On average, boys first experience sexual abuse at age 10. The age range at which boys are first abused, however, is from infancy to later adolescence. Boys are most often abused by males (between 50% and 75%). However, it is hard to estimate the extent of abuse by females, because abuse by women is often covert. Also, a boy may consider it a "sexual initiation" and deny that it was abusive even though he may suffer significant trauma from the experience. A smaller proportion of sexually abused boys than sexually abused girls reports sexual abuse to authorities. While a majority of perpetrators (about 80%) were themselves abused, the vast majority of sexually abused boys (about 80%) never become adult perpetrators. Boys often feel physical sexual arousal during abuse even if they are repulsed by what is happening (Overcoming sexual victimization of boys and men, 2005).

People often think of child sexual abuse only as having sexual activity with a child. However, it includes a variety of possibilities, including fondling, obscene phone calls, exhibitionism, masturbation, intercourse, oral or anal sexual activity, prostitution, pornography, and any other sexual conduct that is harmful to a child's mental, emotional, or physical welfare. It may consist of a single incident or many acts over a long period of time. It often escalates over time, especially if the abuser is a family member (Child sexual abuse, 2012).

The absence of force or coercion does not diminish the abusive nature of the conduct, but it may cause the child to feel responsible for what happened. Physical signs of child abuse may include difficulty walking or sitting; bloody, torn, or stained under-clothes; bleeding, itching, or burning in the genital area; and frequent urinary or yeast infections. Common reactions of the child being abused can include withdrawal, depression, sleeping or eating disorders, school problems, anxiety, guilt, and possibly other reactions as well (Child sexual abuse, 2012).

In 2011 many people were shocked by the unaddressed child sexual abuse at Penn State University. Many questions arose, but one major one was: "What is it about the nature of intimate sexual violence that stops so many bystanders from taking action?" One lesson learned from the Penn State situation was that if you hear or witness sexual abuse or harassment it is important to speak up against it. When abuse happens, it is never a time to keep silent, but always a time to speak and report the abuse. Also, it is important to "abuse-proof" children. For example, the programs they attend should have strong policies on keeping children safe, including screening and background checks for volunteers and employees and ensuring that they are never alone with children. Children need to know that most people would never hurt them, but an older, bigger, stronger person should never touch a child's genitals. Adults do not ask children to be their friends or to keep secrets, and if someone makes them feel bad, funny, or uncomfortable with their touch or their words, they should tell a parent or other trusted adult. Children should realize that their body is wonderful, it belongs to them, and they can say no to unwanted touch. If someone does touch them inappropriately, they need to tell the parent or other trusted adult (Haffner, 2011).

Online Pedophilia

As the Internet has developed, so have opportunities for Internet-related crimes such as pedophilia. Children are particularly vulnerable to sexual predators, such as pedophiles, on the Internet. Pedophiles have been known to use the Internet in at least two different ways. One is a trust-based seductive model in which the pedophile tries to build up trust with the child and then attempts to plan a meeting with the child. The other is a direct sexual model in which the pedophile hopes to make contact with the child (Deirmenjian, 2002).

Wolak et al. (2004) reported on a national sample of online sex abuse cases from a national sample of law enforcement agencies. They indicated that most offenders did not deceive victims about the fact that they were adults interested in sexual relationships. The victims, mainly 13 to 15 years of age, met and had sexual relations with the adults on more than one occasion. Half of the victims were described as being

in love with or feeling close bonds with the offenders. Few offenders abducted or used force to sexually abuse their victims. Offenders targeted adolescents and not younger children. Ninety-nine percent were 13 to 17 years of age and none were younger than 12 years old. Victims and offenders had typically communicated, both online and by telephone, for more than a month prior to meeting in person.

Wolak et al. (2009) reported additional information related to online predators. There has been dramatic growth nationwide in the number of arrests of online predators who solicited law enforcement investigators posing online as juveniles. The numbers nearly quintupled from 644 in 2000 to 3,100 in 2006. While online predator arrests were increasing, overall sex offenses against children and adolescents were declining. Arrests of online predators constituted only 1% of all arrests for sex crimes committed against children and youth. These researchers also found that victims were adolescents and not younger children. Most offenders were open about their sexual motives in their online communications with youth. Few crimes (5%) involved violence.

In 2011 police smashed the world's largest online pedophilia ring. They rescued 230 children from abuse and arrested 184 suspects—including teachers and police officers. The 3-year investigation, code named Operation Rescue, uncovered 670 suspects and identified and safeguarded children in more than 30 countries by arresting people accused of abusing them. The ring was centered on an Amsterdam-based online forum called boylover.net. It was intended as a discussion forum where pedophiles could share their sexual interest in young boys (Foundation to Abolish Child Sex Abuse, 2011).

Guidelines for Internet safety related to online pedophilia are similar to more general guidelines for Internet safety. For example, children need to know not to reveal personal information or information about accounts or passwords online. Emails from unknown sources should be deleted, and mean, threatening, or off-color comments made online should be reported to parents. In addition, children need to remember that nothing they write on the Web is completely private. Parents should help their children learn the difference between credible sources of information and those that are not, establish rules for ordering products or participating in Internet discussions, and tell them to end online experiences when they feel uncomfortable (Internet safety, 2011).

Effects of Pedophilia

As with rape survivors, there can be a tendency to blame survivors of pedophilia. This blame can have psychological effects on the young people involved.

Communication
DIMENSIONS

Helping Survivors of Rape and Sexual Abuse

Even if you are not a trained counselor, if someone who has been raped or sexually abused talks with you about what has happened, you can be helpful by remembering the following points:

1. Listen in a supportive and nonjudgmental way, showing sympathy and concern. Ask questions and do not argue.
2. Encourage the person to express his or her feelings about the incident(s).
3. Control your own emotions. Do not react strongly and do not question the judgment of the survivor.
4. Indicate that you believe the account of what happened.
5. Let the survivor know that it was not his or her fault and that he or she is not to blame.
6. Give comfort and support.
7. Help the person focus on actions that might be needed, such as seeking medical treatment or reporting to police.
8. Try not to interrupt or ask a lot of questions.
9. Do not tell others what happened without your friend's permission.
10. The survivor must decide what to do; you cannot force him or her or make any decision you've determined.
11. Help the person find professional follow-up services—professional counseling, crisis center or domestic violence center guidance, legal assistance, medical follow-up—and accompany the person if that is appropriate and if the person desires it.
12. Survivors of rape and/or sexual abuse can respond in almost any way. They may be hysterical, amazingly calm, or anything in between. Almost any (or no) reaction is "normal."
13. Let the person know you are available to help or give support in the future.
14. Check as often as necessary to see how the person is progressing toward full recovery.

Source: Adapted from Bruess, C, & Richardson, G. *Decisions for health.* Madison, WI: Brown & Benchmark, 1995; Rape and sexual assault: Information for victims and friends. West Virginia Foundation for Rape Information and Services, 2005. Available: www.fris.org/Pages/Rape9020Info/RapeInfo.html.

There has been a great deal of debate about the effects of pedophilia and sexual abuse of children. Some studies connect sexual abuse to many future problems, while others show little or no indication of negative effects of sexual victimization. In fact, a percentage of both men and women reported the experience as positive.

Obviously all children do not react the same way to child abuse. Some research has identified effects of child abuse that include sleeping and eating disturbances, anger, withdrawal, and guilt. Or there might be sexual preoccupation (excessive masturbation and an unusual interest in sexual organs and nudity) and a host of physical complaints such as rashes, vomiting, and headaches without medical explanation. Other common symptoms include shame, poor body image, self-destructive behavior, nightmares, relational and/or sexual dysfunction, and compulsive behaviors like drug addiction, gambling, or overeating (Overcoming sexual victimization of boys and men, 2005). Other related effects could include depression, phobias, psychosomatic symptoms (such as stomachaches or headaches), school problems, poor hygiene or excessive bathing, anxiety, and regressive behaviors (thumb-sucking, etc.) (Child sexual abuse, 2012).

Hillis and coworkers (2001) indicated that physical abuse and sexual abuse are related to subsequent unintended pregnancies and STI. In a study of more than 5,000 females, they found such abuse resulted in increased risk of intercourse by age 15 years and in sexual activity with multiple partners.

Although not a lot of information is available on the topic, the effects among homosexuals and heterosexuals seem to be very similar. For example, Arreola et al. (2008) studied the effects of forced, consensual, and no childhood sexual experiences on health outcomes among a sample of adult men who have sexual activity with men. They found that the forced-sex group had the highest levels of psychological distress, substance use, and HIV risk.

Often, sexual assault experiences are less traumatic for the child than for the parents. It is important that adults understand children's feelings and reactions, because a child often suffers no lasting trauma if parents can control their reactions.

Prevention

Preventing child sexual abuse demands attention. Fortunately, in recent years programs have been

Global DIMENSIONS

Examples of Coercive Sexual Behaviors in Other Countries

In Japan, rape is described as having sexual intercourse with a woman through force or against her will, but there is no clear legal definition. However, the victim or her parent or legal guardian must file a complaint for the rape to be recognized as a criminal act. Fewer than 2,000 cases are reported annually throughout the country.

Protection against sexual harassment in Japan lags far behind American and European standards. The Japanese Labor Ministry has specifically forbidden sexual harassment; however, much remains to be done.

There seems to be a tolerance of violence in Japan's male-dominated society. There is a long history of violence's being condoned as a symbol of manliness. As a result, in comic books, general sexual content has been curbed but portrayals of sexual violence are common. There are even "ladies' comic books" that seem to glorify sexual violence and rape. These are not a fringe phenomenon—the leading one claims annual sales of 400,000 copies.

Late in 2005, the Supreme Court of Mexico ruled that rape within marriage is a crime. This brought Mexican laws into line with much of the world, and removed one of the many obstacles Mexican women face in reporting rape. This ended a legal battle fought since 1994 when the Supreme Court ruled that because the purpose of marriage was procreation, forced sexual relations by a spouse was not rape but "an undue exercise of conjugal rights." Many women's advocates said that there are still deep-rooted opinions that women should be subservient. They warned that entrenched attitudes still make it very difficult for women to report rape. It is thought that 9 of 10 sexual assaults go unreported in Mexico and that 18% of victims were not aware that it was a crime. Only a few countries in the world do not recognize rape within marriage as a crime. India and Malaysia are the most prominent examples.

Sources: Data from Hatano, Y., & Shimazaki, T. Japan, in *The international encyclopedia of sexuality*, vol. 2. R. T. Francoeur, ed. New York: Continuum Publishing, 1999; Malkin, E., & Thompson, G. Mexican court says sex attack by a husband is still a rape. *The New York Times* (November 17, 2005).

---

designed to educate children and adults to distinguish between appropriate and inappropriate touch, to say no to unwanted or uncomfortable touch, to tell a trusted adult if inappropriate touch occurs, and to identify their family and community support systems. In addition, adolescents have been encouraged to consider the risks related to certain behaviors, the selection of a mate who will not abuse their children, and ways in which they will protect children from sexual abuse.

Developing children's competence is essential, with the objective of helping children to recognize abusive situations and disclose victimization. In addition, parents can help children learn about sexual abuse in appropriate ways. They can also help children know some basic ways to help prevent sexual abuse such as (Pedophilia: Who are the men who "love" children in intolerable ways?, 2005):

- Never disclose personal information, such as your address, to strangers online.

- Never meet privately in person with anyone you have met online.

- Never get close to a car if a stranger stops and asks for directions.

- Never accept a ride from, or go anywhere alone with, an adult you don't know.

- No adult should touch you or ask you to touch him or her in any way that is confusing or frightening. If this happens, refuse and tell your parent immediately.

- No adult should ever ask you to keep a touch or a kiss secret. If this happens, tell your parent immediately.

- If any of these things happen, you will not be punished even if you have broken a rule.

A major challenge for prevention is the population of young teens who are willing to enter into voluntary sexual relationships with adults whom they meet online. People are often reluctant to confront these situations, but effective prevention requires public and private recognition of what actually happens in these cases. Teens may benefit from being told directly about why such relationships are a bad idea and made to understand that adults who care about their well-being would not propose sexual relationships or involve them in risky encounters. Efforts should be focused on the most vulnerable teens, such

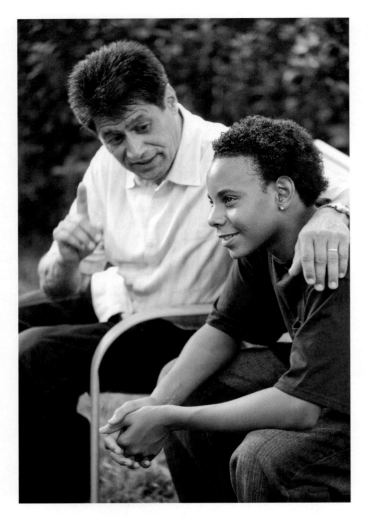

It is important to communicate about sexual abuse and how to prevent it.

interviewing to cooperate with investigators (Wolak et al., 2004).

Educators, parents, and other adults need to learn to recognize physical and behavioral signs of sexual abuse and pay attention to indirectly related comments made by a child. Physical signs may include irritation, pain, or injury in the genital area. Behavioral signs may include nervous, aggressive, hostile, or disruptive behavior toward adults, especially parents. It is wise to remember that one sign alone may not be a positive indication, but if a number of signs are present, the possibility of sexual abuse should be considered. One should believe the child, remain calm, avoid blaming the child, avoid leading questions such as "You did that a lot?" and know where to seek help for counseling services. Adults also need to help children learn that they do not have to agree to demands for physical closeness; that touching can be good, bad, or confusing; that some secrets should not be kept; that at times adults make mistakes and do things they should not; and that there are times to ask for help and to give help when asked for help by a friend.

Another way to help prevent sexual abuse is to carefully screen professionals who work with children. For example, in many states it is necessary for teachers and other school personnel to have a background check before they can assume their responsibilities. This is usually done by requiring fingerprinting of such professionals before they are hired.

A vivid example of the need to screen individuals working with children carefully was seen in 2002 when a Boston church scandal started a chain reaction (Kasindorf, Bayles, & Grossman, 2002). In January 2002, Boston's Cardinal Bernard Law acknowledged that he had moved a priest from parish to parish despite evidence that he had molested children. Soon afterward, church files revealed that another priest had abused children and advocated sexual activities between men and boys but still received the archdiocese's support. Before the year was over, thousands of adults filed lawsuits over abuse they said occurred when they were boys and girls—some as long as

as those who have poor relationships with their parents, those who are lonely or depressed, or gay teens or those who are questioning their sexual orientation and turn to others on the Internet for support or information. Training is also needed for law enforcement personnel because teens may not initially see themselves as victims and may require sensitive

❓ Did You Know...

Law enforcement personnel are recognizing the need for special training to handle child sexual abuse cases. Without proper training, innocent people can be falsely charged, valid cases may have to be dismissed, and children and others involved may not be treated as well as possible.

Training includes the dynamics of child sexual abuse, the science of interviewing children, and approaches to verifying and corroborating allegations. Understanding the psychological needs of the victim, recognizing the sometimes vague symptoms of abuse, and knowing how to elicit sensitive information about sexual behavior from children are essential skills for law enforcement personnel.

50 years earlier. Five U.S. bishops, including Cardinal Law, resigned for reasons related to sexual abuse of children. Although he was not personally accused of abuse, Law resigned because of his failure to deal effectively with abusers who were priests. Interestingly, Law then abruptly moved to Rome and took up a series of positions in the Vatican. He was appointed archpriest of the Basilica di Santa Maria Maggiore, and also took full part in a conclave that selected the successor to Pope John Paul II (Hitchens, 2008). This certainly sent mixed signals regarding the Vatican's feelings about Law's actions.

As a result of this scandal, Roman Catholic bishops adopted a new policy for handling priests accused of sexual abuse. If a priest is found guilty by a board composed mostly of lay Catholics and at least one priest, he cannot wear a collar or give Communion, and he may be stripped of his status. In addition, most priests indicated they will tell the police about sexual abuse allegations in the future (Michaels, 2002). A set of guidelines called the Charter for the Protection of Children and Young People was also developed and adopted by the nation's Roman Catholic Bishops in 2002. In 2011 they voted overwhelmingly to maintain those church policies on the sexual abuse of children. This was a controversial move, because many victims' advocates felt the policies are weak and unenforceable and have not stopped child sexual abuse by Catholic church leaders (Burke, 2011).

In recent years, all 50 states have passed laws requiring sex offenders to alert the community to their presence. Many states run Internet sites listing such criminals. In some states judges have ordered offenders to post signs outside their homes, mandated bumper stickers, and even required temporary placards for traveling in someone else's car. Some people argue these laws are appropriate to help protect society from sex offenders; others consider it inappropriate to brand people and even punish their families. A Washington state study found that such policies did not prevent sex offenders from committing more crimes, but they did help police find and arrest repeat offenders more quickly (Thomas, 2001).

In many states there is a law requiring rapists and child molesters to register each year for inclusion in a database of sex offenders. Failure to register is usually a felony and can result in more jail time. Even so, the state of California lost track of more than 33,000 sex offenders, or 44% of the total number of registered offenders. They simply vanished after registering. Nationally, 52% of rapists are arrested for new crimes within 3 years of leaving prison, according to the U.S. Justice Department (Curtis, 2003).

In 2006, the Adam Walsh Child Protection and Safety Act was passed by the U.S. Congress. It requires all states to adopt strict standards for registering sex offenders and is meant to prevent offenders from eluding authorities, especially when they move out of state. The act made it a federal crime (a felony) to fail to reregister as a sex offender, after moving to another state and requires states to toughen their penalties for failing to register at all; currently, many states treat such failure as a misdemeanor. An estimated 100,000 sex offenders are not living where they are registered. A number of controversial points have been raised in relation to the act. State officials complain about the law's cost, may believe they have more effective laws than the federal one, and say the federal requirements violate the states' right to set their own policies. In addition, some sex offenders and civil liberties groups have argued that juvenile sex offenders should not have to be on public registries for life and note that the law does not take into account the individual circumstances of each sex offender (Goodnough & Davey, 2009).

College officials have to decide how to best deal with the Campus Sex Crimes Prevention Act, a federal law that requires sex offenders, when they register with the state, to indicate whether and where they are enrolled, employed, or volunteering on a college campus. As of October 1, 2003, college officials must tell students, faculty, and administrators where information on registered sex offenders can be obtained. Most have chosen to make the registry available for perusal in the campus police department and made its existence known either through the college's website or by mailing of pamphlets that direct students and others to its location (Boslett, 2003).

In many states treatment for those convicted of sexual abuse of children is required by law. It is hoped that such treatment will help prevent future sexual abuse, but much remains to be learned about effective treatment. Many treatment methods have been tried. For example, aversion therapy is used to associate a pedophilic fantasy or desire with an unpleasant sensation such as nausea or an electric shock. Behavior therapy is also used to help offenders exercise self-control by changing their beliefs and attitudes as well as their behavior. Many other psychological techniques have been tried, such as externalization where the offender learns how his or her actions look and feel to the child. A number of medications have also been tried with the hope of diminishing sexual desire. It is difficult to tell for sure just how effective various treatments have been. Research results about treatments have not been conclusive (Pedophilia: Who are the men who "love" children in intolerable ways?, 2005).

¿? Ethical DIMENSIONS

Is It Ethical to Publicly Identify Sexual Offenders?

Named after Megan Kanka, a 7-year-old New Jersey child who was raped and murdered by a convicted sex offender who lived across the street from her, "Megan's Law" requires that authorities and the community be notified when a convicted sex offender is released or moves into their neighborhood. Variations of Megan's Law are found in a number of states. For example, Alabama's Megan's Law also forbids a convicted offender to live near a school, day care center, or past victim.

Some people want a law requiring that the identity of convicted child molesters be made known to community members. This means that if a convicted child molester moved into your community, you and all your neighbors would be informed that he or she was there and that he or she had been a child molester. Many people support such a law because they feel they have a right to protect their children.

Other people think it is a violation of individual rights and personal privacy if a convicted child molester's identity is made public. They believe that the molester, as has any other person convicted of a crime, has paid for the crime through a prison sentence and in other possible ways, and it is not ethical to reveal his or her identity to the public. The person has a right to live privately and to start a new life if he or she desires. On the basis of these arguments, there have been legal challenges to Megan's Law in New Jersey, and similar laws have been found unconstitutional in other states.

In Virginia, state police developed a website that lists the names of violent sex offenders. They guessed that 5,000 people would log on on the first day. In fact, in the first 12 hours, it was visited more than 45,000 times. By the second day, the site was so jammed that many people could not get through because the site can handle only six "hits" per second. Some people express the point of view that we should not be concerned about former sex offenders being harassed, because "If they don't want their names in the paper, they shouldn't commit the crime." Others question the ethics of this website and feel it treats sex offenders unfairly.

Do you think it is ethical to require that identities of sexual offenders be made public?

Incest

Incest is sexual behavior between relatives who are too closely related to be legally married. Much of what has been said about child sexual abuse also applies to incest. However, it is helpful to consider incest separately because it is rapidly changing from a private subject to a public one.

Most contemporary research studies related to incest seem to focus on the offenders, family relationships, and possible treatments. There is not much new information about incest statistics. Because of that, there are very few reliable statistics about how often incest occurs.

The most commonly reported form of incest is father–daughter, but in practice brother–sister incest probably happens more often. Mother–child incest has traditionally been thought to be virtually nonexistent, but today many experts feel that the amount of sexual abuse of children by women has been underestimated.

> **incest**
> Sexual behavior between relatives who are too closely related to be married.

It is hard to know how many people are affected by incest because many incest situations never get reported. The victim might not report the abuse for a variety of reasons. For example:

1. The victim has been told that what is happening is normal and doesn't realize that it is a form of abuse.

2. The victim may not know that help is available or who he or she can talk to.

3. The victim may be afraid of what will happen if he or she tells someone. (The abuser may have threatened the victim, the victim may be afraid of what will happen, or the victim may care about the abuser and be afraid of what might happen to the abuser.)

4. The victim may be concerned about how many people might react when they hear about the abuse. (Maybe no one will believe him or her, maybe someone will tell the abuser, maybe people will say that she or he did something wrong) (Incest, 2012).

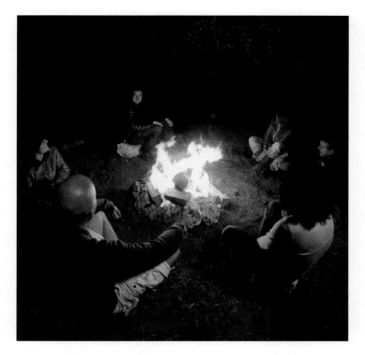

Incest victims look and act like anyone else. However, they may suffer from long-term psychological consequences.

Guilt and shame also play a big part in a child's decision not to ask for help after incest has occurred. This is especially true if the child was raised in a home where sexual behavior is considered dirty or sinful. Also, the child may be uncertain what to think about the experience. With this uncertainty, he/she may decide it is safer not to say anything (Larsen, 2005a).

Those who commit incest usually appear to be very nice people. The vast majority of offenders (often estimated at 95%) are probably male, and there is often a patriarchal family structure. Contrary to what many think, stepfathers do not seem to be involved in incest any more often than biological fathers. When confronted, most offenders are truly sorry for their actions, but the vast majority do not believe they have done anything particularly wrong. Many believe they have a right to educate their children about sexual behavior and to use their children to meet their own sexual needs. Many refuse to believe that they really hurt their children.

The incest taboo seems universal in human culture. Anthropologists often consider it to be the foundation of all kinship structures and even the basis of human social order. Nevertheless, incest occurs in all social classes, in all geographic areas, and among all ethnic and racial groups.

Many of the reactions to and effects from incest are similar to those related to sexual abuse of children in general. However, incest can be especially damaging because it disrupts the child's primary support system, the family. When the abuser is someone in the family, the family may not be able to provide support or a sense of security. Because children often have limited resources outside the family, it can be hard for them to recover from incest. Incest can damage a child's ability to trust, because the people who were supposed to protect and care for them abused them. It can also be very damaging for a child if a nonabusing parent is aware of the abuse and chooses—for whatever reason—not to take action to stop it. This might happen because the nonabusing parent feels dependent on the abuser for financial support, is afraid of losing the partner, thinks incest is normal in families, or feels that the child was "asking for it" or blames the child for some other reason (Incest, 2012).

The possible behavioral signs of incest are also similar to those of sexual abuse in general. They can include eating disorders or loss of appetite, extreme changes in behavioral patterns, lack of self-confidence, unexplained fear of a particular person, unusual knowledge of sexual matters, regressing to infantile behavior, poor interpersonal relationships, or attempts to run away (Larsen, 2005b). Obviously, some of the symptoms of incest can also be normal adolescent problems, but parents and teachers need to at least be aware of the possibility that incest has occurred.

Sexual abuse experts say some victims of incest use overeating to escape inner turmoil and downplay their femininity. They might gain weight so their bodies do not look so good. They might also avoid unwanted attention to their bodies by wearing baggy clothes along with gaining too much weight (McGee, 2007).

Various community organizations offer help for incest survivors and their families—for example, child-protection agencies, rape crisis centers, women's centers, and organizations that offer help for parents who are under extreme stress or are frightened about their feelings toward their children. The best strategy for preventing incest is to provide information to children as well as to parents. This means providing sexuality education at the elementary school level and above, including specific information about incest. For example, children should be taught that Uncle Charlie or Aunt Mary does not automatically have the right to touch them all over. In addition, information about pedophilia and other sexual practices should be provided at the appropriate level of understanding.

The initial focus of crisis intervention should be on stopping the sexual abuse and establishing a safe environment in the family. Once the incest is reported, it is controversial whether the child should be temporarily removed from the home. This might be destructive to the child because she may feel that she has done something wrong, that she is being punished, or that both parents are against her. It is also difficult to find an appropriate place to put the child; however, removal from the home may be the only way to ensure the child's safety.

There is also a nationwide group called Survivors of Incest Anonymous that works very much like Alcoholics Anonymous. It is a self-help group of women and men, 18 years and older, who are guided by a set of 12 Suggested Steps and 12 Traditions. The only requirement for membership is that you are a victim of child sexual abuse, and that you are not abusing any child. More information about Survivors of Incest Anonymous can be found at www.siawso.org.

■ Relationship Abuse

As we have seen, the topics of childhood sexual abuse and incest overlap. The same is true of various aspects of relationship abuse. For example, the abuse may take the form of forced sexual activity, use of violence without sexual activity, or both. Today it is recognized that males and females can both be victims of relationship abuse. In fact, both males and females engage in frequent minor assaults. However, females are more often the victims of severe partner assault and injury, not necessarily because males strike more often but because males strike harder. Because the number of *reported* cases of abuse of wives far exceeds the number of *reported* cases of the abuse of husbands, because physical danger to wives is usually far greater, and because most of the studies available on this topic deal with females, most of the information here is about females as well.

Violence in relationships seems to start well before adult years. For example, in the 12 months prior to one survey, about 9% of students in grades 9 to 12 had been hit, slapped, or physically hurt on purpose by their boyfriend or girlfriend (Grunbaum et al., 2004). Overall, the prevalence of dating violence was higher among African American (13.9%) and Hispanic (9.3%) students than among white (7%) students.

Dating violence is dangerous in many ways, but one of these ways relates to the prevalence of STI, including HIV. Compared with nonabused girls, girls in grades 9 to 12 who experienced both physical and sexual dating violence were three times more likely to have been tested for STI and HIV, and 2.6 times more likely to report an STI diagnosis (Decker, Silverman, & Raj, 2005).

Regardless of the type of relationship or its stage, there are important signs of relationship abuse. When these appear, it is wise to take steps to deal with them

effectively or get out of the relationship. They are (1) isolation, (2) jealousy, (3) possessiveness, (4) double standards, (5) name-calling, (6) controlling behavior, (7) threats of self-harm, (8) playing rough, (9) nonconsensual sexual activity, and (10) violence (Ten signs of relationship abuse, 2008).

Marital Rape

Until the late 1970s, most states did not consider spousal rape to be a crime. In most cases, spouses were exempted from the sexual assault laws. For example, until 1993 North Carolina law stated that "a person may not be prosecuted under this article if the victim is the person's legal spouse at the time of the commission of the alleged rape or sexual offense unless the parties are living separate and apart." These laws date all the way back to the seventeenth century, when it was said that "for by their mutual matrimonial consent and contract the wife hath given up herself in this kind unto the husband which she cannot retract." In the late 1970s, feminists began efforts to change these laws. Currently, rape of a spouse is a crime in all 50 states and the District of Columbia (Spousal rape laws: 20 years later, 2004).

For obvious reasons, it is difficult to obtain accurate information on the frequency of spousal rape. Based on various studies, an estimated 14% of married women report they were raped by their spouse. This percentage probably underestimates the true prevalence of marital rape. Of reporting women, 23% reported rape and sexual assault as the only abuse in the marriage. Also, 10% of all sexual assault cases reported by women involved a husband or ex-husband attacker (Marital rape, 2000).

Why spouses are raped is a question that has not been greatly explored. The few existing studies summarize common reasons as (1) entitlement to sex (thinking that the marriage contract includes the right to sexual intercourse on demand), (2) sexual jealousy, (3) rape as punishment for some "wrong" behavior, and (4) rape as a form of control (asserting of power and control) (Bergen, 1998).

A number of factors contribute to the underreporting of spousal rape and women's reluctance to discuss such experiences. They include the following:

1. Loyalty to husband/privacy of family

2. Unwillingness to accept their own victimization

3. Reluctance to label the experience as "rape"

4. Misunderstandings about a woman's role in marriage and marital responsibilities

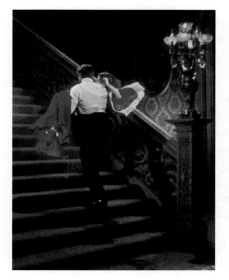

In the movie *Gone with the Wind*, the husband, Rhett Butler (played by Clark Gable), carries his wife, Scarlett O'Hara (Vivien Leigh), kicking and screaming up a staircase, implying sexual activity is to follow. Portrayed as sensual more than 60 years ago, could it be considered spousal rape by today's standards?

5. Sexual inexperience and uncertainty about what constitute "normal" and "forced" sexual relations (Mahoney & Williams, 1998)

Victims of rape by a husband are different from other rape victims because they are violated by someone with whom they share their homes, lives, and maybe children. They are faced with a betrayal of trust and intimacy. Wife rape victims are more likely to be raped multiple times than stranger and acquaintance rape victims. Women who experience wife rape suffer long-lasting physical and psychological injuries that are as severe as or more severe than those of stranger rape victims (Bergen, 2009).

Why would a woman stay with a man who raped her? The answers are usually very complicated but include such reasons as the following:

1. Many women believe it is part of their "duty" to have sexual intercourse with their husband, even if it is violent and against their will.

2. Many women cannot leave because they do not have the financial resources to do so.

3. Women may fear what the offender may do to them or the children.

4. Some women may not leave because of love and loyalty to the husband, which can override their own pain and suffering (Mahoney & Williams, 1998).

It seems that women raped by a spouse are more likely to experience long-term effects than are women raped by an acquaintance or a stranger. Possible long-term effects include (1) negative feelings toward men; (2) low self-esteem; (3) fear; (4) anxiety; (5) guilt; (6) embarrassment; (7) outrage; (8) changes in behaviors, including an increase in drinking and refusal to consider remarriage; and (9) depression (Peacock, 1998).

Basile (2002a) examined national attitudes toward wife rape. She found that older, nonwhite respondents were less likely to believe wife rape occurs. Males and the less educated were less likely to believe it occurs frequently. Older and less-educated respondents were less likely to believe forced sexual scenarios between a husband and wife constitute wife rape. Among women, nonvictims were significantly less likely than current victims to believe that wife rape occurs.

Basile (2002b) looked at the amount of reported wife rape and other types of sexual coercion based upon statistics from other studies. She estimated that 34% of women were victims of some type of sexual coercion with a husband or partner in their lifetime. Of these women, 10% experienced rape by a current partner. This rate increased to 13% when only rape by a current husband was included. Other findings indicated that women had sexual activity with a current spouse or partner in return for a partner's spending money on them (24%), after the partner begged and pleaded with them (26%), and after their partner said things to bully them (9%).

There are several types of marital rape. *Battering rape* is when beatings and rape are combined. Some may experience physical abuse during the sexual assault. Others may experience sexual assault after a physical assault as an attempt to "make up." *Force-only rape* is motivated by a need to demonstrate power and maintain control. Therefore, the perpetrator asserts his or her feelings or entitlement over the partner in the form of forced sexual contact. *Obsessive/sadistic rape* involves torture and perverse sexual acts. It is characteristically violent and often leads to physical injury. Survivors of partner rape are more likely to be raped multiple times when compared to stranger and acquaintance rape survivors. As such, partner rape survivors are more likely to suffer severe and long-lasting physical and psychological injuries (Partner rape, 2012).

Intimate-Partner Violence

Domestic violence is a significant health and social problem in the United States and many other industrialized societies. In some industrialized societies, however, it is considered to be almost nonexistent. The reasons for the variability from culture to culture have not been established. Intimate-partner violence occurs for many reasons. It can be an indication of manhood, a means of personal control, a reflection of personal animosity, and an expression of social jealousy. Women who are victims of violence are often unable or afraid to seek health care, and violence also has serious consequences for maternal mortality and child survival. Here are some related statistics about international gender-based violence (The facts on international gender-based violence, 2005):

- Intimate partners commit 40% to 70% of homicides of women worldwide.

- Around the world, 1 in 3 women have been beaten, coerced into sexual activity, and otherwise abused in their lifetime. Most often, the abuser is a family member.

- There is a strong relationship between intimate-partner violence and the spread of HIV/AIDS in the developing world. Violence and poverty force many women to remain in dangerous relationships where they are often subject to rape and HIV infection by their partners.

- Between 4% and 20% of women in developing countries experience violence during pregnancy. They then run twice the risk of miscarriage and have four times the risk of having a baby that is below average weight.

- In Nicaragua, research has shown that children of women who are abused are six times more likely to die before the age of 5 than other children.

- A study in India showed that intimate-partner violence was the cause of 16% of maternal deaths during pregnancy.

- In the United States, healthcare costs of intimate-partner violence against women amount to approximately $5.8 billion each year.

It is a difficult task to estimate rates of intimate-partner violence. Many factors inhibit people from reporting these crimes. The private nature of the event, the perceived stigma, and the belief that no purpose would be served by reporting the crime prevent an unknown percentage of survivors from talking about the event. Therefore, available statistics are at best estimates.

Estimates range from 960,000 incidents of violence against a current or former spouse, boyfriend, or girlfriend per year to 3 million women who are physically abused by their husband or boyfriend each year. Nearly one-third of American women report being physically or sexually abused by a husband or boyfriend at some point in their lives. Intimate-partner violence is primarily a crime against women. Women are about 85% of the victims, and men make up the remaining 15%. Women are less likely than men to be victims of crime overall; however, they are five to eight times more likely than men to be victimized by an intimate partner. Women of all races are

about equally vulnerable to violence by an intimate (Prevalence of domestic violence, 2005).

In a recent year, 1,247 women were killed by an intimate partner, as were 440 men. Intimate-partner homicides account for about 33% of the murders of women, but less than 4% of the murders of men. Pregnant and recently pregnant women are more likely to be victims of homicide than to die of any other cause. Thirty-seven percent of women who sought treatment in emergency rooms for violence-related injuries were injured by a current or former spouse, boyfriend, or girlfriend (Domestic homicides, 2005).

Children are also involved in intimate-partner violence. Fifty percent of men who frequently abuse their wives also frequently abuse their children. Slightly more than half of female victims of intimate-partner violence live in households with children younger than the age of 12. Between 3.3 and 10 million children witness some form of domestic violence annually (Domestic violence and children, 2005).

Direct physical attack is the most common abuse, but a woman is also abused when she is repeatedly placed in physical danger or controlled by the use

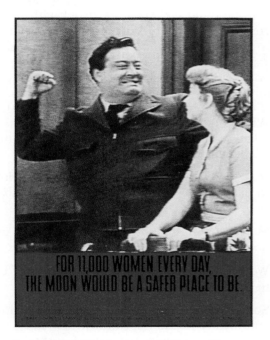

Back in the 1950s, the popular TV show *The Honeymooners* portrayed the blue-collar husband Ralph (Jackie Gleason) as getting mad at his wife and threatening, "One of these days, Alice … Pow … Right to the moon!" The line provoked uproarious laughter. (He never did harm her.) But there is nothing funny about intimate-partner violence. According to the National Coalition Against Domestic Abuse, 4 million U.S. women are victims of assaults by their partners each year.

of threats to hurt her, her children, friends, family, or pets. Physical abuse can also be sexual. A marital or live-in relationship does not give a man the right to force sexual relations or practices that are unwanted, uncomfortable, or degrading. Battered women often have low self-esteem and feel humiliated and ashamed of their body. For the battering man, daily tensions seem to lead to abusive behaviors and violent explosions. Afterward, the man most likely makes excuses, apologizes, and promises it will not happen again. He may even make a special effort to smooth things over by trying to be nice. Because his wife wants to believe him, they often make up and she tries to forget. As time passes, tensions can build again for the abuser. Then, the violence recurs as part of a cycle of violence. This cycle has several steps. The first is "walking on eggs," where everyone is trying to be very careful within the relationship. The second step is when tensions build and violence occurs again. The third step is a time of regret and "I love you"—saying it will never happen again. Then, the cycle repeats itself.

The physical abuse associated with intimate-partner violence is probably heard about most often; such violence, however, is not limited to physical abuse. The National Resource Center on Domestic Violence (*Help end domestic violence*, n.d.) defines it as a "pattern of abusive and controlling behaviors that some individuals use against their intimate partners or former partners." In addition to physical abuse such as hitting, punching, kicking, or using weapons, it can include

- *Sexual abuse:* forcing a partner to engage in unwanted sexual behaviors.

- *Emotional abuse:* name calling and put-downs; stalking; treating a partner as inferior; using threatening looks, actions, or gestures; threatening children or pets.

- *Property/economic abuse:* stealing or destroying property and money; refusing the partner food or medical attention; or interfering with a partner's work or education.

In addition, annually in the United States, more than 503,000 women are stalked by an intimate partner. Seventy-eight percent of stalking victims are women. Eighty percent of women who are stalked by former husbands are physically assaulted by that partner, and 30% are sexually assaulted by that partner (Stalking, 2005).

Those who are battered may stay with a batterer for a number of reasons, including financial dependence, lack of social support (the batterer may have controlled the victim's contact with other people), fear of severe physical attack, self-blame (believing the abuse is a result of the victim's real or imagined offenses), or belief that the violence is temporary or caused by unusual circumstances. Many battered women believe the abuse will stop when "things return to normal" (Dating and domestic violence, 2009).

Intimate-partner violence doesn't stay home while its victims go to work. It also affects employees while they are at the workplace. For example, 74% of employed battered women were harassed by their partner while they were at work. On average, 1.7 million violent victimizations per year are committed against persons while at work. Homicide is the second leading cause of death on the job for women. More than 29,000 acts of rape or sexual assault are perpetrated against women at work each year. Many women report missing work as a result of stalking. In addition, 24% of women who experienced intimate-partner violence said that the abuse caused them to arrive late for work or miss days of work (The facts on the workplace and domestic violence, 2005).

There has been increased awareness of the problem of violence against women in the military. Women in the military are particularly vulnerable to abuse due to geographical isolation from family and friends, and the potential for social isolation within the military culture. The victim of intimate-partner violence in the military is mainly the female, civilian spouse of active-duty personnel. Victims normally have children and more than half have been married 2 years or less. Abused women in military communities are often fearful of reporting incidents due to the lack of confidentiality and privacy as well as limited victim services (The facts on the military and violence against women, 2005).

We have been slow to recognize the problem of intimate-partner violence. In the past, laws and common practice encouraged husbands to discipline their wives by force if they saw fit. But conditions are changing. Family violence research has made it clear that the problem of battering is too widespread to ignore or to explain away by blaming the victim. Many new resources are available. Battered women's shelters are particularly helpful in providing services for battered women and their children and in continuing efforts to educate people about intimate-partner violence.

Most of the research discussed so far has been about heterosexual couples. It has been only in the last 20 years or so that literature about same- gender domestic violence started to appear. Conducting research with this population about a sensitive topic like intimate-partner violence remains difficult. However, existing studies show that the prevalence as well as the types of abuse and the dynamics of abuse are very similar between heterosexual and homosexual couples (McLennen, 2005).

Multicultural DIMENSIONS

Examples of Female Abuse in Other Countries

Don't Talk to Strangers is a 23-part TV series that ran on Chinese networks and has been marketed abroad. The series was credited with putting the uncomfortable subject of spousal abuse in the open in China. This was surprising to many because traditional Chinese culture teaches that family problems should stay within the family. Many were surprised when the show made it past Communist Party propaganda officials, who generally frown on negative portrayals of Chinese society.

Some viewers found the show too violent, too gloomy, and too hopeless. Others consider it important to get the problem out into the open. Activists say spousal abuse occurs in one in three Chinese families compared to one in four in the United States.

In China, the marriage law of 2001 gives victims the right to protection and orders abusers punished. In divorce cases, victims of abuse can also sue for damages. However, willingness to enforce the law varies widely across the country. China's first battered women's shelters were forced to close because of lack of money or authorities' unwillingness to offer protection. Some people consider it normal for couples to fight, and it is difficult to get people to see that as violence.

In 2002, there was a well-publicized example of "honor rape" in Pakistan. Mukhtar Maj, then about 30 years old and from a lower caste, was gang-raped on the orders of the village council as a punishment because her 12-year-old brother was said to have had sexual relations with a woman from a higher caste. She did not commit suicide, as expected, but she founded two schools for children in her village and spoke out against "honor killings" and other outrages against women in her country. In 2005 she was invited to come to the United States to tell her story. The Pakistani government barred her from traveling abroad, but later lifted its travel restrictions (Pakistan lifts travel ban on raped woman, 2005).

In Kyrgyzstan, after 3 months of dating, Melis Aliyev turned to a practice that is a tradition in Kyrgyzstan, but a crime in the rest of the world. The woman he had been dating, Ainur Tairova, was kidnapped and kept in Aliyev's house for 2 days. Many friends and relatives repeatedly tried to force onto her head a white scarf signifying her acquiescence to the marriage. She eventually gave in to the man, who is still her husband 4 years later. Kidnapping to coerce a woman into marriage is on the books as a crime in Kyrgyzstan, but it is so ingrained in the country's male-dominated society that it is rarely prosecuted. In some cases, women who steadfastly refuse are raped by their captor, a crime men know likely will go unreported because filing a case with the police would brand the victim and her family with scandal (Rodriguez, 2005).

In Lagos, Nigeria, after a typical husband–wife argument, a husband followed his wife out the door. Then he beat her unconscious, and left her lying in the street near their apartment. The woman had defied her husband, and many men and women throughout sub-Saharan Africa consider that ample justification for a beating. One in three Nigerian women report having been physically abused by a male partner. In one case, a woman's husband beat her incessantly because she watched television movies. Many men feel that women are inferior and that men can do whatever they want to them. Intimate-partner violence accounts for more than 6 of 10 murder cases in court. Yet, most women remain silent about the abuse. Many men and women say that husbands have a right to beat wives who argue with them, burn the dinner, go out without the husband's permission, neglect the children, or refuse sexual activity. Nigeria's penal code specifically allows husbands to discipline their wives (LaFraniere, 2005).

Source: Data from Bodeen, C. TV show about wife abuse grips China, *The Seattle Times* (February 3, 2003), A18.

There are ways we can combat intimate-partner violence. Here are some possibilities (101 ways to combat domestic violence, 2003):

1. Make violence unacceptable in your life.
2. Contact your local school board and ask its members to address dating violence.
3. Contact your local media representatives and remind them that October is Domestic Violence Awareness Month. Ask them what they plan to do. Tell them about the National Domestic Violence Hotline (800-799-SAFE), and ask them to publicize it.
4. Contact community businesses and agencies, and ask them to display the number of the National Domestic Violence Hotline in prominent places.

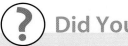 Did You Know . . .

Violence by women received little attention until the mid-1970s. Now we know that women in relationships engage in violent acts as often as men. In about half of violent relationships, the violence is mutual. When there is a sole perpetrator, it is just as likely to be a female as a male. However, female use of violence, even when intended to cause harm, is mainly self-defensive.

Men tend to inflict more severe damage on women than the converse. Reasons given for this are that women tend to cease violent behaviors before causing serious injury and that men are usually physically larger and stronger than women.

The needs of battered men are somewhat different from those of battered women. Abused women have varied needs, including safety for themselves and often for their children; abused men's needs are more limited. Because they usually have the necessary resources to leave the relationship, their primary needs are legal assistance and psychological counseling.

Sources: Data from Flynn, C. P. Relationship violence by women: Issues and implications, *Family Relations, 38, no. 2* (April 1990), 194–198; Morse, B. J. Beyond the conflict tactics scale: Assessing gender differences in partner violence, *Violence and Victims, 10, no. 4* (winter 1995), 251–272.

5. Contact local schools and colleges and let students know about resources available on the Internet concerning intimate-partner violence.

6. Ask the local police department to be sure officers are trained in handling intimate-partner violence.

7. Ask your priest, pastor, rabbi, or other religious leader to have a special service devoted to intimate-partner violence.

8. Do not let jokes about violent behavior go unchallenged.

9. Work with day care centers to make information about intimate-partner violence available to their customers.

10. Learn more about policies and facilities related to intimate-partner violence in your community.

Services for survivors of intimate-partner violence have been improved through the years, but more and better services are still needed. In 1994, the Violence Against Women Act was passed by Congress; it was extended in 2000. Its purpose was to broaden the range of services and counseling available to women victims of abuse. In 2005, the act was reauthorized, and it increased funding for new rape crisis centers and increased grant money to organizations working on intimate-partner violence issues (Feminist Wire Daily Newsbriefs, 2005).

Also, the Office for Victims of Crime of the U.S. Department of Justice provided funding in 1997 to develop Sexual Assault Nurse Examiner (SANE) programs designed to improve the community response to sexual assault victims. There are now hundreds of

these programs around the country, and new ones are started every month. The goal is to see that every victim receives fundamental justice and needed services (Little, 2005).

■ Sexual Harassment

Since the mid-1970s, courts, popular and professional periodicals, newspapers, and books have focused on **sexual harassment**. Hundreds of articles have appeared in print, increasing the national attention paid to the subject. It is not easy to define sexual harassment. Sometimes it is hard to draw the line between harassment and other behaviors, but it can include touching, verbal abuse, demanding of sexual favors, or use of threatening tones.

> **sexual harassment**
> Unwelcome verbal, physical, or sexual conduct that has the effect of creating an intimidating, hostile, or offensive environment

The U.S. Equal Employment Opportunity Commission (EEOC) says that sexual harassment is a form of sex discrimination that violates Title VII of the Civil Rights Act of 1964. It defines sexual harassment as unwelcome sexual advances, requests for sexual favors, and other verbal or physical conduct of a sexual nature when this conduct explicitly or implicitly affects an individual's employment, unreasonably interferes with an individual's work performance, or creates an intimidating, hostile, or offensive work environment (Sexual harassment, 2005). The EEOC also says that sexual harassment can occur in a variety of circumstances, including but not limited to the following:

• The victim as well as the harasser may be a woman or a man. The victim does not have to be of the other gender.

- The harasser can be the victim's supervisor, an agent of the employer, a supervisor in another area, a coworker, or a non-employee.

- The victim does not have to be the person harassed but could be anyone affected by the offensive conduct.

- Unlawful sexual harassment may occur without economic injury to or discharge of the victim.

- The harasser's conduct must be unwelcome.

The Commission further says that it is helpful for the victim to inform the harasser directly that the conduct is unwelcome and must stop. The victim should use any employer complaint mechanism or grievance system available.

Sexual harassment may include verbal abuse; sexist remarks regarding a person's clothing or body; patting, pinching, or brushing up against a person's body; leering or ogling; demand for sexual favors in return for hiring, promotion, or tenure; physical assault; and rape. Two categories of sexual harassment have been described. In the first, something is to be exchanged. Perhaps a boss offers a person a job opportunity in exchange for sexual favors or threatens loss of a job opportunity if the person does not comply. In the second, there is no promise or threat; however, there are sexual remarks, touching/stroking, or lewd looks.

Legally speaking, then, there are two kinds of sexual harassment. The first is quid pro quo (Latin for "something for something"): Something is to be exchanged. For example, a perpetrator might make conditions of employment contingent on the victim providing sexual favors. The second is a hostile environment. This is when unwelcome severe and persistent sexual conduct by the perpetrator creates an uncomfortable and hostile environment (for example, jokes, lewd postures, leering, inappropriate touching, etc.). This type of harassment constitutes up to 95% of all sexual harassment cases (Sexual harassment, 2012).

In 1991 Anita Hill's testimony at confirmation hearings for Supreme Court Justice Clarence Thomas brought into the open the problem of sexual harassment. Previously, it had been an issue that millions of victims privately recognized but rarely discussed before Hill told her story. Since that time, many employers started training programs to deter sexual harassment, but it is thought that even today only a small proportion of sexual harassment victims risk stigma and potential job losses to pursue claims.

The EEOC has kept statistics related to sexual harassment since 1997. The number of charges filed with the EEOC each year has remained relatively

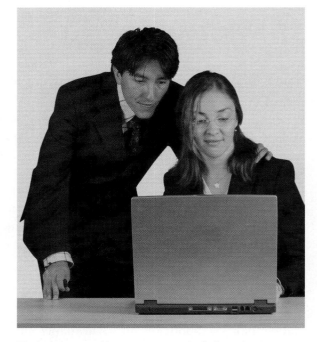

Workplace sexual harassment can include various behaviors. Coworkers need to indicate when behavior is inappropriate and unwanted.

consistent, but has decreased somewhat over the years. For example, there were almost 16,000 charges in 1997, almost 14,000 in 2008, and about 11,700 in 2010. The percentage of charges filed by males increased from 11.6% in 1997 to 16.4% in 2010 (Sexual harassment charges, 2011).

In 2009, the U.S. Supreme Court ruled that workers who cooperate with an internal investigation and report uncouth behavior by a supervisor are protected from retaliation under civil rights laws (Sexual harassment, 2009). This ruling further strengthened laws against sexual harassment in the workplace.

Efforts to end sexual harassment that rely mainly on target reporting are unlikely to be successful because most targets do not report their experiences. They tend to deny the harassment, avoid the harasser, or treat the harassment as a joke rather than confronting the harasser or reporting the behavior. It seems that the targets don't report the offenses because they want to avoid reprisal by the harasser and maintain their reputation and status in the workgroup. For this reason, some experts feel that one way for progress to be made against sexual harassment is for those who observe the harassment to be the ones who report it (Bowes-Sperry & O'Leary, 2005).

In addition to being upsetting and distracting, workplace sexual harassment can even be hazardous to health. For example, Rospenda et al. (2005) found that exposure to workplace harassment increases risk for illness, injury, or assault. Thus harassment may be hazardous not only to targets' health, but also to

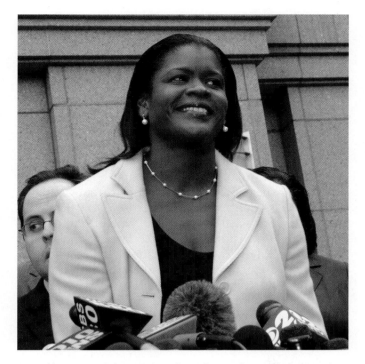

Sexual harassment lawsuits can have far-reaching effects. Anucha Browne Sanders, an executive for the New York Knicks basketball team, accused coach Isiah Thomas of sexual harassment in 2006. The lawsuit also accused team owner James Dolan of firing her in retaliation for her initial harassment complaint. The exposure in the news media led to concerns about the team's leadership and had a negative effect on the team's reputation. Browne Sanders won the lawsuit, but her job was not reinstated; it took her more than a year to find a new job. Thomas was replaced as coach in 2008. Dolan was found liable and was ordered to pay Browne Sanders $3 million, in addition to the $8.6 million ordered to be paid to her by Madison Square Garden. The total punitive damages of $11.6 million was one of the largest sexual harassment judgments in history.

the bottom line of the organization in the form of costly worker's compensation claims.

One interesting multicultural aspect related to sexual harassment is that in 2005 China's parliament amended the Law on the Protection of the Rights and Interests of Women (A woman's right to sue, 2005). Amendments were then passed that made sexual harassment of women unlawful, stipulating that equality between men and women is a basic state policy. It will be interesting to see how many Chinese women take advantage of the opportunity to complain about harassment to their employers and to the "relevant department" in the government, and to bring civil suits against their tormentors.

As use of the Internet has grown, so has sexual harassment on the Internet. While it is impossible to know the extent of sexual harassment on the Internet, it seems that most victims are women (Barak, 2005). The three general types of offline sexual harassment

also exist online: (1) gender harassment—unwelcome comments that insult individuals because of their gender or that use stimuli intended to provoke negative emotions; (2) unwanted sexual attention—uninvited behaviors that communicate sexual desires or intentions toward another individual; and (3) sexual coercion—putting pressure on a person to elicit sexual cooperation. Online sexual coercion might even become actual coercion if a perpetrator uses technical knowledge to break into a person's computer and cause damage or threaten to do so. Sending frightening emails, sending viruses, and flooding an email box are just a few examples of actual sexual coercion. Sending erotic and pornographic pictures and videos are examples of gender harassment. With Internet harassment, a harasser can take advantage of being unidentifiable, anonymous, and invisible, in addition to having immediate, easy-to-execute, almost untraceable escape routes.

Sexual Harassment in Schools

Initial concerns about sexual harassment focused on the workplace; however, more attention has also been given to schools and colleges. Verbal and physical sexual harassment often begin in elementary school. Four out of five girls, and almost as many boys, experience some form of sexual harassment (Sadker & Zittleman, 2005).

The American Association of University Women conducted a national survey on sexual harassment in public schools in 1993 and again in 2001 (Hostile hallways: Bullying, teasing, and sexual harassment in schools, 2001). It found that students in 2001 were much more likely to say that their schools had sexual harassment policies and distribute literature on sexual harassment. As in 1993, in 2001 80% of students experienced some form of sexual harassment at some time during their school life. There was a striking increase (from 18% to 24%) in the number of boys who often experienced sexual harassment in school. In addition, 56% of boys said they experienced sexual harassment occasionally. Girls were more likely than boys to experience sexual harassment ever (83% versus 79%). Students who experienced sexual harassment were most likely to react by avoiding the person who bothered or harassed them (40%), talking less in class (24%), wanting not to go to school (22%), changing their seat in class to get farther away from someone (21%), and finding it hard to pay attention in school (20%).

Using a nationally representative survey of 1,965 students in grades 7–12, the American Association of University Women reported on student experiences with sexual harassment during the past school year (Crossing the line: Sexual harassment at school,

2011). Nearly half (48%) of the students experienced some form of sexual harassment, and 87% of them said it had a negative effect on them. Verbal harassment made up the bulk of the incidents, but physical harassment was also common. Sexual harassment by text, email, Facebook, or other electronic means affected nearly one-third of students. Many students who were sexually harassed through cyberspace were also sexually harassed in person. Girls were more likely than boys to be sexually harassed (56% versus 40%). This was true both in person (52% versus 35%) and electronically (36% versus 24%). The girls' experiences tended to be more physical and intrusive than the boys' experiences. Being called gay or lesbian in a negative way was reported equally (18%) by both genders. Witnessing sexual harassment at school was also common (33% of girls and 24% of boys), and 56% of these students witnessed sexual harassment more than once during the school year. Among those who were sexually harassed, 12% of girls and 5% of boys reported the incident to an adult at school. About one-quarter said they talked about it with parents or family members, and 23% spoke with friends. Boys were more likely than girls to say they sexually harassed other students (18% versus 14%). Almost one-third of students who experienced sexual harassment also identified themselves as harassers. Many who admitted to sexually harassing others did not think of it as a big deal, and many were trying to be funny.

As mentioned, the number of court cases related to sexual harassment in schools is increasing. Although there have been some conflicting decisions, the Supreme Court issued a major decision in 1998 in its ruling that school districts cannot be liable for damages in a private lawsuit about teacher–student sexual harassment unless an official in a position to take corrective action knew of the harassment and was "deliberately indifferent" to it. At the same time Richard W. Riley, Secretary of Education, indicated, "Any sexual harassment of a student—particularly sexual abuse by a teacher—is a basic breach of trust between the school and the student and the family" (Walsh, 1998).

The question of whether schools should be held liable when students sexually harass their peers is extremely sensitive. Some people argue that schools should be responsible only for taking reasonable action rather than for ensuring that the behavior ends—although it can be hard to determine the definition of "reasonable." Others feel school personnel have a responsibility to take strong actions to prevent behaviors often associated with typical child growth and development—such as sexual comments, touching, and jeering. It is a real challenge to design appropriate policies and procedures related to students' sexually harassing their peers.

It is important to talk about sexual harassment with children in appropriate ways and at the appropriate level. For example, elementary school children should know that sexual harassment is unwanted and uninvited sexual attention such as teasing, touching, or taunting; sexual harassment is against the law; and they should be taught their school's sexual harassment policy. In addition, students aged 12 to 15 should know that sexual harassment can occur in a variety of settings including schools, the workplace, and extracurricular programs. They should also know where they can call for information about sexual harassment. Students aged 15 to 18 should also know that whether to report sexual harassment is a personal decision that can be hard to make, and that people who experience sexual harassment may need help and support to deal with the situation (Keeping kids sexually safe, 2004).

Sexual Harassment on Campus

Sexual harassment exists on all types of university campuses. In many cases it is unreported—and is often ignored altogether. In general, women are more likely to define behaviors as harassing and men are more likely to believe victims have contributed to their own problem. There are costs to individuals and to the institution. Victims tend to sacrifice self-confidence, academic and work opportunities, letters of recommendation, and grades. The student's professional development is hindered, and the university acquires a negative image.

Nearly two-thirds of college students experience some type of sexual harassment. Yet, less than 10% tell a college or university employee about it, and an even smaller fraction officially report the harasser to a Title IX officer. These, and other interesting facts, are part of a major report from the American Association of University Women (Sexual harassment on campus: Drawing the line, 2005). Key research findings in the report are highlighted here:

- Sexual harassment is common on college campuses. More than one-third of college students encounter sexual harassment during their first year on campus.

- Men and women are equally likely to be harassed, but in different ways and with different responses. Females are more likely to be the target of sexual jokes, comments, gestures, or looks. Males are more likely to be called gay or a homophobic name. Females are more likely to be upset and to feel embarrassed, angry, less confident, afraid, confused, and disappointed in their college experience.

Gender DIMENSIONS

Same-Gender Sexual Harassment

Sexual harassment is obviously a problem for women in the workplace—and sometimes for men. Most often, the instances we hear about involve other-gender situations. However, more and more same-gender harassment cases have been filed, and lower courts have been inconsistent in their findings. One judge allowed a case to proceed only because the supervisor, accused of harassing, was admittedly gay.

The Equal Employment Opportunity Commission has for years taken the position that Title VII of the Civil Rights Act does not care which genders are involved. In 1998 the Supreme Court allowed a case to proceed in which a man working on an oil rig charged two male co

workers with making taunting comments and threatening rape.

Men and women often deal with sexual harassment differently. Whereas a woman may be more inclined to report harassing conduct, the traditional inclination of many men is just to "deal with it." This attitude has possibly led to less frequent reporting of male same-gender harassment.

Same-gender harassment cases will probably receive heavy media coverage. Treatment in the press will likely have a strong influence on whether men (or women in same-gender harassment situations) will keep harassment complaints to themselves or report them in the future.

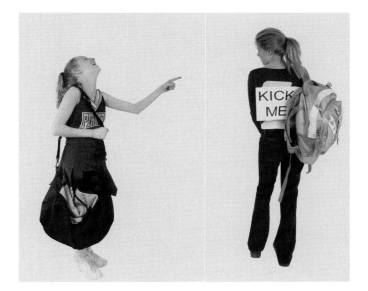

Bullying, teasing, and sexual harassment can be common in schools.

- Lesbian, gay, bisexual, and transgender students are more likely to be harassed.

- Different racial and ethnic groups experience sexual harassment in similar, but not identical ways. Generally, white, African American, and Hispanic students perceive and react to sexual harassment in similar ways.

- Men are more likely than women to harass. Both males and females are more likely to be harassed by a male.

- More than half of harassers think their actions are funny.

- Most victims don't report sexual harassment.

Osman (2004) examined perceptions of sexual harassment based on a vignette in which physical or verbal harassment and the victim's facial expression were varied. She found perceptions of sexual harassment were stronger for physical harassment than verbal harassment except when the target smiled. Overall, women had stronger perceptions of harassment than did men. Also, a stronger belief that women should at least give token resistance to sex was associated with weaker perceptions of sexual harassment even when a victim verbally resisted.

Some university officials feel there should be a general statement of the university's position on sexual harassment because it is not possible to cover specific situations adequately. Others feel that the specifics should be clearly spelled out to prevent potential confusion. Some officials feel policies should prohibit even consensual sexual relationships between students and faculty members. They argue that although such relationships may appear to be consensual, they are not because of the faculty member's position of authority. Others feel that consensual relationships are not the business of the university.

As part of the emphasis on sexual harassment on campuses, many colleges and universities have developed various types of educational programs for students and faculty. It is important to understand and protect the rights of both complainants and accusers and to avoid either sensationalizing or minimizing allegations. It is also crucial for all concerned to understand the institution's policies against harassment and its procedures for handling complaints.

Sexual Harassment/Assault and the Military

It is important to understand the difference between sexual harassment and sexual assault. These terms are defined as part of current SHARP (Sexual Harassment/Assault Response and Prevention) training at all U.S. military installations. The Department of Defense (1995) defines sexual harassment as a form of sex discrimination involving unwelcomed verbal, nonverbal and/or physical behaviors of a sexual nature. It defines sexual assault as sexual contact characterized by use of force when the victim does not or cannot consent (Department of Defense, 2012). It is also important to understand that these are two related issues, as, according to SHARP training statistics, approximately one-third of all reported sexual assaults within the Army are preceded by sexual harassment (U.S. Military Academy, 2011).

In 2003 the National Organization for Women (NOW) reported instances of rape and sexual harassment at the U.S. Air Force Academy. It also indicated that a 1994 Congressional report found that 78% of the 90 female cadets in attendance at the Academy at that time reported either sexual assaults or unwanted sexual advances (NOW staff, 2003).

About the same time, Sadler et al. (2003) reported that 79% of 558 female military veterans reported experiencing sexual harassment during their military service. Thirty percent of the women reported an attempted or completed rape. The report indicated findings consistent with research in civilian populations showing that younger women entering male-dominated work groups at lower levels of authority are those most likely to be harassed. Findings also indicated that military women working with superiors who made sexually demeaning comments or allowed such behavior were found to have a nearly fourfold risk of rape.

Cohen (2005) reported that women in the Israeli Defense Force reported hundreds of incidents of sexual harassment and rape, yet harassers often went unpunished. Some felt that the hierarchal structure encouraged males to misuse their power. Under Israeli law, those found guilty of harassment can be sentenced for up to 3 years of imprisonment. In reality, senior military officers accused of sexual harassment are rarely sent to jail.

Tyson (2005) wrote about a Department of Veterans Affairs report indicating that 60% of women and 27% of men in the military reserves and the National Guard suffered sexual assault or harassment during their service. Eleven percent of women experienced rape or attempted rape, compared with 1.2% of males. More than half of the incidents took place at a military worksite and during duty hours, and in most cases military personnel were the offenders. Fewer than 19% said that they received any help for the trauma.

Boghosian (2005) described how the National Lawyers Guild launched a Women's Military Rights Project to challenge the long-term problem of sexual harassment and abuse within the military system through a combined program of education, legal assistance and litigation, and support for political action. This was a result of many events through the years—particularly the Navy Tailhook Association convention in 1991, the court martial of the most senior enlisted man in the U.S. Army for sexual harassment in 1997, the accusation of the Army's most senior enlisted man in Europe of sexual harassment in 1999, the accusing of Major General Larry G. Smith of sexual harassment by the highest-ranking woman in Army history in 2000, and the Air Force Academy scandal in 2003, which erupted when 142 cadets made sexual assault charges that resulted in zero convictions. In addition, the Miles Foundation reported that from August 2002 through March 2005 there were 316 cases of sexual assault in Iraq, Afghanistan, and Kuwait.

As a result of these incidents, new educational training and awareness programs have been developed to help military personnel recognize potential harassment and assault behaviors, apply intervention techniques, provide victim assistance and counseling, and hold offenders accountable (Department of the Army, 2011a). For example, the Army has instituted the "I. A.M. STRONG" campaign, the purpose of which is to educate all soldiers that assault prevention is a total team effort. The Army (Department of the Army, 2011b) has developed a four-phase strategy for this program, consisting of the following:

Phase I: A committed Army leadership that aggressively condemns sexual harassment/assault.

Phase II: Army-wide ownership of sexual assault prevention strategies to stop them before they occur.

Phase III: Change the culture, whereby Army values are inculcated, and assaults are eliminated within the ranks.

Phase IV: Sustain, refine and share best practices, as well as lessons learned.

Notwithstanding this campaign, the Women's Rights Project and the Service Woman's Action

? Did You Know . . .

Addressing Sexual Harassment in the Military

A climate that negatively affects teamwork within a military unit impacts mission effectiveness. Consequently, the Department of Defense has specific policies and programs that support a zero-tolerance philosophy toward sexual harassment in the armed forces. Because a diverse and talented workforce is essential to mission accomplishment, this is an issue that is addressed at every level of every military unit.

As gender-related incidents are investigated, they have been accompanied by a concerted effort on the part of the Department of Defense to prevent future recurrences. This has been demonstrated by the development and continual reevaluation of programs designed to educate service members as to what constitutes sexual harassment, how to deal with it, and how to report incidents without fear of reprisal.

In an appearance before the Senate Armed Services Committee in 1997, Edwin Dorn, the Undersecretary of Defense for Personnel and Readiness, underscored the importance of military units' functioning as a team. He mentioned trust, loyalty, and self-sacrifice, issues not often found in large organizations. According to Dorn, a climate of discrimination and harassment will erode these elements that are essential for unit effectiveness.

Nevertheless, a policy can only be as strong as the program it supports. According to Sheila Widnall, former Secretary of the Air Force, an Equal Opportunity program to support a zero-tolerance policy on harassment needs to be based on the following five principles:

1. A commander's personal commitment
2. The establishment of goals, principles, and standards of performance
3. Clear, concise written policies
4. Continual training throughout a military member's career
5. Complaint systems that are prompt, thorough, fair, and allow for resolution, support, reprisal prevention, and sanctions.

The military leadership has taken the initiative for monitoring the climate within the services. Programs have been developed to improve the climate through training, prevention, and resolution. These programs have been evaluated using instruments such as command climate surveys, sensing sessions, and other internal review processes. They have also been examined by the media, congressional inquiry, and watchdog organizations. In 2000, an assessment of four key Department of Defense human relations programs that had been fielded or modified since 1997—the Command Climate Survey, The Army Values Program, the Consideration of Others Program, and Equal Opportunity (EO) Training Programs—was conducted. The purpose of this reassessment was to see if the establishment or revision of these programs had improved human relations in the Army. A total of 24,000 Army leaders and soldiers were surveyed and interviewed. Among the findings were indications that although the Army provides a generally effective human relations environment, many service members did not yet consider human relations an important component of combat readiness.

Since the 2000 survey, focus has shifted to the issue of sexual assault in the military. A total of 26,505 active duty members responded to a survey entitled "2010 Workplace and Gender Relations Survey of Active Duty Members, Overview Report on Sexual Assault." A summary of the results indicated that despite efforts to educate service members annually concerning prevention and response to sexual harassment and assault, these incidents still occur. Additional findings indicated that not all service members are aware of resources available, many incidents remain unreported, and incidents of sexual harassment or stalking occurred either before or after an assault incident.

In January 2012, Defense Secretary Leon Panetta said that although 3,200 sexual assaults were reported across all active duty services in 2011, he felt that the number was realistically closer to 19,000, knowing that most crimes go unreported. Commenting on a report on sexual harassment and violence across all U.S. service academies, he reinforced the fact that this was a leadership issue and that further initiatives will be prepared to eliminate such behavior.

Commanders are constantly working toward achieving zero tolerance for sexual harassment; they still have a way to go. The process for reporting incidents has been improved, thus increasing the prospect of investigation and resolution. This sends a clear message that members of the various armed services must be willing to report and be vigilant, and that these behaviors are not tolerated.

Susan M. Tendy, EdD, Director of Assessment, Department of Physical Education, United States Military Academy.

Sources: Data from Dorn, E. DoD committed to zero tolerance of sexual harassment. *Defense Issues*, 12, *no.* 9 (1997), 1–4; Widnall, S., Dorn, E. To stop harassment, leaders must lead. *Defense Issues*. 10, *no.*64 (1995), 1–5; Johnson, E., Harris, B. Special report 46: Human relations update 2000 executive summary (March 2001); Rock, L., Lipari, R., Cook, P., Hale, A. *2010 Workplace and Gender Relations Survey of Active Duty Members, Overview Report on Sexual Assault.* Arlington, VA: Defense Manpower Data Center; March 2011; 2010–2025; Elliott, D. No simple explanation in AF academy sex crime data. *Denver Post* (January 22, 2012). Available: www.denverpost.com/dontmiss/ci_19795071.

Network have joined forces in challenging the alleged lack of oversight of sexual abuse and harassment on the part of the U.S. military by continuing to seek detailed records from the Departments of Defense and Veterans Affairs regarding their response to sexual assault, sexual harassment, and domestic violence in the military. These records are being sought, despite the annual release by the Department of Defense of statistics on the prevalence of sexual assault within each branch (Park & Natelson, 2012).

In 2012 Defense Secretary Leon Panetta announced new policies to reduce sexual assault in the military. The plan's central provision required all sexual assault cases to be handled by senior officers rather than unit officials, which he said will lead to more prosecutions. The plan created new units within each branch of the military to investigate sexual assault cases, required that all incoming service members be briefed on sexual assault policies within two weeks of reporting for duty, required that records be kept on all disciplinary actions related to sexual assault cases, and allowed National Guard and reserve troops who filed complaints to remain on active duty while their cases are investigated (Defense Sec. Panetta Announces Initiative to Address Sexual Assault in the Military, 2012).

In 2012 the Navy adopted new strategies for addressing sexual assault among sailors, including a skit-based program that urges troops to help protect each other. The program teaches troops not to stand by if another person is attacked by a sexual predator. According to Navy data, 2,485 sailors and 1,453 Marines were sexually assaulted in 2011. Internal surveys suggested that sexual assaults among sailors and Marines declined after the program was implemented (Navy Expands Training to Address Sexual Assaults Among Sailors, 2012).

Sexual harassment has consistently negative consequences for working women, including changes in job attitudes (for example, lower satisfaction) and behaviors (for example, increased work withdrawal). Sims et al. (2005) sampled over 11,500 military servicewomen and found that experiences of harassment led to increased turnover. These findings have important implications not only for individual women, but also for organizations.

Kimerling et al. (2010) examined military-related sexual trauma among deployed Operation Enduring Freedom and Operation Iraqi Freedom veterans. Of almost 126,000 veterans, 15.1% of the women and 0.7% of the men reported military sexual trauma. This trauma was associated with increased chance of a mental disorder diagnosis, including post-traumatic stress disorder, other anxiety disorders, depression, and substance abuse disorders.

There has been debate about how the military investigates and prosecutes sexual assault cases. For example, in 2011 a bill was introduced to remove sexual assault crimes from the typical military chain of command and to place them under jurisdiction of a new Sexual Assault Oversight and Response Office within the Department of Defense. Some people feel that such a procedure is a better way to investigate such claims.

Reactions to Sexual Harassment

Reactions to sexual harassment are influenced by individual characteristics and the severity of the harassing behavior. Gender, attitudes toward both women and men, religiosity, and confidence all influence the way people might react to sexual harassment. Responses can range from avoidance or defusion to negotiation or confrontation. Avoidance (ignoring the harassment or doing nothing) is quite common. Defusion (which includes responses such as going along, stalling, or making a joke of it) is a more active way to minimize the impact of conflict. Negotiation is a more assertive response and involves a direct request to the harasser to stop. This shifts the focus of the interaction to the victim's needs and priorities in the relationship. Confrontation, the most assertive response on this continuum, has two components: aggressive personal responses (such as telling the harasser to stop rather than simply asking) and use of the organizational power structure (such as making a formal complaint through channels).

A person being harassed usually has several options—personal action, grievance to an employer (if applicable), union grievance (if applicable), and legal action. Each situation influences the best way to handle the harassment. There are two objectives for personal action: Attempt to stop the harassment and, if that fails, document it. If this fails and there is a grievance procedure, a complaint can be filed through prescribed channels. If none of these routes works, it may be necessary to pursue legal action.

Here are some suggestions for dealing with sexual harassment (About SSSS, 2005):

- Trust your gut. If you feel uneasy or uncomfortable, this is an important cue that something is amiss.

- If you feel as if someone is sexually harassing you, you could either walk away or say that his or her comments or sexual attention are unwanted. Generally, the most effective response is to ask the person to stop his or her unwanted sexual behavior in a firm but cordial and non-angry way.

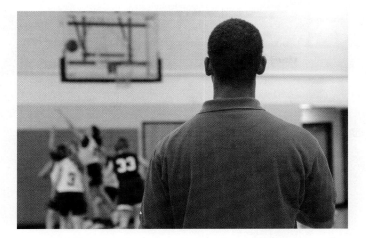

The sexual harasser is often a person who has authority or power over others.

- Use your feelings as permission to either leave the situation or be assertive and provide the other person with good-natured feedback about how you would like to change your interaction. For example, you might say or write: "I really wanted to talk with you, and I imagine you meant well. However, your repeated touches and sexual comments felt inappropriate to me."

- Use an assertive voice and clear body language when you are telling someone else how you would like them to change their behavior. Dissuade them from thinking you are joking by looking them in the eyes and using a serious and businesslike facial expression and tone of voice.

- Try to give the person the benefit of the doubt. Treat the person who upset you as you would want to be treated. Share your concerns and negotiate how to improve future interactions with him or her personally, directly, as soon as possible.

Exploring the Dimensions of Human Sexuality

Our feelings, attitudes, and beliefs regarding sexuality are influenced by our internal and external environments. Go to go.jblearning.com/dimensions5e to learn more about the biological, psychological, and sociological factors that affect your sexuality.

Case Study

Many positive social changes have occurred over the past few decades to help the victims of forcible sexual behaviors. Although child sexual abuse has long occurred—Freud wrote about it almost 100 years ago—it was a hushed, taboo topic. Many victims thought that they were the "only one," or that they had done something wrong. Not anymore.

The media have been a positive force for change by giving coverage to forcible sexual behavior cases. The trial of O. J. Simpson—and the surrounding coverage about battered women—gave many victims the courage to step forward. Many TV shows inform children about what to do in case someone touches them in a way that makes them feel "uncomfortable."

The legal system has made huge strides in recent years, creating and enforcing laws and helping victims of forced sexual behaviors. Police have been trained to take intimate-partner violence calls seriously, and not to let the perpetrator of violence off the hook.

Laws have been passed to help victims of sexual harassment at work or school. And, whereas in 1976 no man could be legally accused of raping his spouse, now marital rape laws have been passed in all 50 states.

Biological Factors

- Alcohol is a factor in 50% of rapes.
- Date-rape drugs produce disinhibition and an amnesia-like effect, so that victims do not remember what happened.
- Younger people commit violent acts more often than older people do.
- Although men and women attack each other at about the same rate (12%), as a result of the usually greater strength of men, women are hurt more often and live in fear of further attacks.

Sociocultural Factors

- Socioeconomic status plays a role in forcible sexual behaviors, as higher levels of aggression are found among lower-income populations. Pedophiles and the children they abuse are members of all socioeconomic and educational groups.
- People who believe in rape myths assign less blame to the perpetrator and more blame to the victim.
- Laws regarding sexual activity of teens vary among countries. Japanese law only prohibits sexual intercourse with someone younger than 12 years old—no other sexual activity, including child pornography, is covered.
- Deliberate interracial rape is uncommon; 88% of victims are the same race as the perpetrator.
- A cultural belief in patriarchy, whereby males have a dominant role over women, can promote abusive behavior.

Psychological Factors

- Sexual abuse in childhood contributes significantly to the risk of development of mental disorders later in life. Adolescent rape survivors have more behavioral problems compared to older survivors. Women with low self-esteem tend not to end an abusive relationship.

Summary

- Millions of people are affected by sexual violence each year. Sexual assault and abuse include inappropriate touching; vaginal, anal, or oral penetration; sexual intercourse after a person says no; rape; attempted rape; and child molestation.

- Rape is one of the most underreported crimes. There are many myths about rape.

- Date rape, also known as acquaintance rape, is much more common than most people realize. There are many ways to help prevent acquaintance rape.

- Pedophilia entails feelings of adult sexual attraction to children. Children are particularly vulnerable to sexual predators, such as pedophiles, on the Internet.

- Preventing sexual abuse demands attention. There is a need to help children and adults distinguish between appropriate and inappropriate touch, say no to unwanted or uncomfortable touch, tell a trusted adult if inappropriate touch occurs, and identify family and community support systems.

- Incest is sexual behavior between relatives who are too closely related to be legally married. The most commonly reported form is father–daughter.

- Intimate-partner abuse is a significant health and social problem in the United States. In addition to physical abuse, it can include sexual abuse, emotional abuse, or property/economic abuse.

- Sexual harassment is unwelcome verbal, physical, or sexual conduct that has the effect of creating an intimidating, hostile, or offensive environment. It is a problem in schools, colleges, and the workplace.

Discussion Questions

1. What are the different categories of rape? Who are the rapists in these categories? What are the effects on the victims?

2. What effects does child abuse have on its survivors?

3. Describe the type of person who commits incest. What drives a seemingly "normal" individual to commit incest?

4. Explain why someone in an abusive marriage stays in the relationship. Can one be absolutely sure when a spouse should leave? Or is every situation different?

5. In what ways is sexual harassment the same and different in the workplace, in schools, in colleges, and in the military? Is the intent of harassment the same in each situation?

Application Questions

Reread the chapter-opening story and answer the following questions.

1. Is date rape a form of miscommunication or a form of sexual violence? Put another way, did Ed simply misinterpret the woman's resistance, assuming that "she wanted to be convinced to have sex"? Even if that were the case, did he have the right to continue sexual activity before she consented?

2. Assume for a moment that you are the woman who has just been date raped. Which actions can and should you take? What might the consequences of those actions be for both you and the rapist?

Critical Thinking Questions

1. In 1991 a Florida federal judge ruled that pictures of naked and scantily clad women displayed in a workplace qualified as sexual harassment under Title VII of the 1964 Civil Rights Act. In his written opinion, the judge said that such a "boys' club" atmosphere is "no less destructive to workplace equality than a sign declaring 'Men Only.'" At the same time, the Florida branch of the American Civil Liberties Union denounced the decision as a possible violation of free speech. Under the federal court ruling, the company involved had to institute an antiharassment policy and take down the photos. In your opinion, what was the right decision in this situation?

2. Several women in an office complained to their human resources department that a male colleague had a photo of a woman in a bikini on his desk and that the photo created a "hostile working environment." When the man was confronted by his supervisor, he stated that the photo was of his wife, and he refused to remove it. What rights does the man have to display a photo of his wife? What rights do the women in the department have to object to the photo?

3. The goal of this question/activity is to increase your awareness of relationship abuse while enabling you to reflect on your own values about what would constitute an abusive romantic or sexual relationship. Read each statement, consider how you feel about it, and discuss your feelings with others in your class to explore the various opinions that might exist in your class.

Is it abuse if ...

1. a man and a woman are arguing when she begins to cry hysterically, and he gives her a light slap to calm her down?

2. a husband takes his wife to work every morning, meets her for lunch every day, and picks her up at the end of each afternoon?

3. a wife tells her husband that he would look better if he lost a few pounds?

4. every time a lesbian couple argues, one of the partners threatens to "out" the other to her family?

5. an 18-year-old has a sexual relationship with a 14-year-old?

6. a woman who wears tight clothing and short skirts walks down the street and men whistle and make sexual comments to her?

7. a man says he wants to have sexual intercourse, his girlfriend says she's not ready, but after talking about it, she gives in and has sexual intercourse with him, even though she doesn't really want to?

Source: Adapted from Schroeder, E. Is it abuse if ...? *American Journal of Sexuality Education, 1, no. 1* (2005), 141–149.

Critical Thinking Cases

Paul Ingram, a deputy in the sheriff's department in Olympia, Washington, suddenly found himself accused of child abuse. His two daughters, aged 18 and 22 years, had just returned from a spiritual retreat when they suddenly recalled that their father had sexually abused them when they were children. During the retreat, a charismatic preacher had said that someone in the audience had been molested as a child—a plausible assumption in any audience given prevalence rates. The more the daughters remembered, the more their stories kept changing. The father was stunned, claiming he remembered no sexual abuse toward his daughters. But he also believed his daughters would never lie. Eventually, he confessed to abusing his daughters. In fact, the more he remembered, the clearer his memories of the events became. A psychologist tried an experiment on Paul, in which false information about abusing his children was told to him. Within days, Paul claimed to "remember" these made-up events. When told that these events had never taken place, Paul tried to retract his other statements from the legal process. Unfortunately, he was too late. Paul was convicted and sentenced to jail for his initial recalled memories (Wilson et al., 1996).

Given this true case study of recovered memories, is it ethical to use them for treatment of a sexual abuse survivor? Is it ethical to use them to charge someone else with sexual assault or sexual abuse many years later?

Explain your answer.

Exploring Personal Dimensions

Date Rape

This exercise is for those who are single and dating. Mark all that apply to you.

_____ 1. When dating, most of the excitement is to see what degree of intimacy I will be able to reach with this person (that is, how far we will go).

_____ 2. I test how far I will go (physical intimacy) with someone by progressive fondling (holding hands, putting arm around waist, rubbing back, chest, or breast and genitals) to see at what point the person will stop me.

_____ 3. When dating, I generally go with others or go somewhere public until I know someone.

_____ 4. I ask around about someone before I go out with her or him.

_____ 5. I make it very clear what my values are about physical intimacy when dating before difficult situations arise.

_____ 6. I have tried to coerce or talk someone into having sexual activity with me.

Scoring

Give yourself the following points for the items you checked, and total your score.

1. 3
2. 3
3. −2
4. −3
5. −3
6. 5

Interpretation

3–11   You are potentially infringing on someone else's right to live within her or his value system and legal rights. You may be "date raping" or attempting date rape.

0–2   You have tendencies to infringe on someone else's right to live within her or his value system.

(–1)–(–3)   You are practicing moderately healthy dating precautions to avoid date rape.

(–4)–(–8)   You are practicing healthy dating precautions to avoid date rape.

Suggested Readings

Acquaintance rape. Rape, Abuse, and Incest National Network, 2012. Available: http://www.rainn.orglget-information/types-of-sexual-assauIt/acquaintance-rape.

Child sexual abuse. Rape, Abuse, and Incest National Network, 2012. Available: http://www.rainn.org/get-information/types-of-sexual-assault/child-sexual-abuse.

Dating and domestic violence. Rape, Abuse, and Incest National Network, 2012. Available: http://www.rainn.org/get-information/types-of-sexual-assault/dating-and-domestic-violence.

Humphreys, T. P., & Brousseau, M. M. The sexual consent scale-revised: Development, reliability, and preliminary validity. *Journal of Sex Research, 47, no. 5* (September 2010), 420–428.

Lorentzen, E., Nilsen, H., & Traeen, B. Will it ever end? The narratives of incest victims on the termination of sexual abuse. *Journal of Sex Research, 45, no. 2* (April 2008), 164–174.

Osman, S. L. Predicting perceptions of sexual harassment based on type of resistance and belief in token resistance. *Journal of Sex Research, 44, no. 4* (October 2007), 340–346.

Reed, E., Silverman, J. G., Raj, A., Rothman, E. F., Decker, M. R., Gottlieb, B. R., Molnar, B. E., & Miller, B. E. Social and environmental contexts of adolescent and young adult male perpetrators of intimate partner violence: A qualitative study. *American Journal of Men's Health, 2, no. 3* (2008), 260–271.

Sexual exploitation by helping professionals. Rape, Abuse, and Incest National Network, 2012. Available: http://www.rainn.org/get-information/types-of-sexual-assault/sexual-exploitation-by-helpingprofessional.

Types of sexual violence. Rape, Abuse, and Incest National Network, 2012. Available: http://www.rainn.org/get-information/types-of-sexual-assault.

Wilson, R. Notoriety yields to tragedy in Iowa sexual-harassment cases. *Chronicle of Higher Education, 55, no. 24* (February 20, 2009), A1, A8–A13.

Web Resources

For links to the websites below, visit *go.jblearning.com/dimensions5e* and click on Resource Links.

MaleSurvivor
www.malesurvivor.org

Provides extensive information about sexual victimization of boys and men designed to help them overcome their sexual victimization experiences.

Men Can Stop Rape
www.mencanstoprape.org

This organization works with male youth to help them be allies with women in preventing rape and other forms of men's violence. Gender equity is promoted along with men's capacity to be strong without being violent.

National Coalition Against Domestic Violence
www.ncadv.org

The mission of the National Coalition Against Domestic Violence (NCADV) is to organize for collective power to end the violence in our lives. NCADV believes violence against women and children results from the use of force or threat to achieve and maintain control over others in intimate relationships. NCADV works for major societal changes necessary to eliminate both personal and societal violence against all women and children.

Violence Against Women—Office of Women's Health
www.womenshealth.gov/violence-against-women/

The Office of Women's Health coordinates the efforts of all of the federal Health and Human Services agencies and offices involved in women's health. Its purpose is to improve the health and well-being of women and girls in the United States through education, programs, and motivating behavior change.

U.S. Department of Justice: Office on Violence Against Women
www.usdoj.gov/ovw

The Office on Violence Against Women handles legal and policy issues regarding violence against women and responds to requests for information regarding violence against women.

Rape, Abuse, and Incest National Network
www.rainn.org

The Rape, Abuse, and Incest National Network is the nation's largest anti-sexual assault organization. RAINN operates the National Sexual Assault Hotline and carries out programs to prevent sexual assault, help victims, and ensure that rapists are brought to justice.

REFERENCES

101 ways to combat domestic violence. Feminists Against Violence Network, 2003. Available: http://www.geocities.com/ Heartland/Meadows/7905/101.htm.

A woman's right to sue. *The Economist, 376, 8442* (September 3, 2005), 38–39.

About SSSS: Mission statement: A special note about Sexual Harassment. Society for the Scientific Study of Sexuality (June 3, 2005). Available: http://www.sexscience.org.

About the Prison Rape Elimination Act of 2003. National Institute of Justice, 2007. Available: http://www.ojp.usdoj.gov/nij/topics/corrections/prison-rape/prea.htm.

Acquaintance rape. Rape, Abuse, & Incest National Network, 2012. Available: http://www.rainn.org/get-information/types-of-sexual-assault/acquaintance-rape.

American College Health Association. American College Health Association-National College Health Assessment II: Reference Group Executive Summary Spring 2011. Hanover, MD: American College Health Association, 2011.

American College Health Association. National College Health Assessment. *Journal of American College Health, 56, 5* (March/April 2008), 469–479.

American Psychiatric Association. Statement: Diagnostic criteria for pedophilia (June 17, 2003).

Arreola, S., Neilands, T., Pollack, L., Paul, J., & Datania, J. Childhood sexual experiences and adult health sequelae among gay and bisexual men: Defining childhood sexual abuse. *Journal of Sex Research, 45, 3* (July 2008), 246–252.

Barak, A. Sexual harassment on the Internet. *Social Science Computer Review 23, no. 1* (Spring 2005), 77–92.

Basile, K. C. Attitudes toward wife rape: Effects of social background and victim status. *Violence and Victims, 17, no. 3* (June 2002a), 341–354.

Basile, K. C. Prevalence of wife rape and other intimate partner sexual coercion in a nationally representative sample of women. *Violence and Victims, 17, no. 5* (October 2002b), 511–524.

Bergen, R. K. Marital rape: New research and directions. National Online Resource Center on Violence Against Women, 2009. Available: http://www.vawnet.org.

Bergen, R. K. The reality of wife rape: Women's experiences of sexual violence in marriage, in *Issues in intimate violence*, Bergen, R. K., ed. Thousand Oaks, CA: Sage, 1998.

Black, M. C., Basile, K. C., Breiding, M. J., Smith, S. G., Walters, M. L., Merrick, M. T., Chen, J., & Stevens, M. R. The National Intimate Partner Sexual Violence Survey (NISVS): 2010 summary report. Atlanta, GA: National Center for Injury Prevention and Control, Centers for Disease Control and Prevention, November 2011.

Boghosian, H. Gauntlet of change. *National Lawyers Guild Foundation: Guild Notes, 30, no. 2* (Summer 2005), 1–14.

Boslett, L. Colleges decide how to comply with new sex-offender law. *The Chronicle of Higher Education, 49, no. 20* (January 24, 2003), A33–34.

Bowes-Sperry, L., & O'Leary, A. M. To act or not act: The dilemma faced by sexual harassment observers. *Academy of Management Review 30, no. 2* (April 1, 2005), 288–306.

Burgess, A. W., & Morgenbesser, L. I. Sexual violence and seniors. *Brief Treatment and Crisis Intervention. 5, no. 2* (2005), 193–202.

Burke, D. Bishops leave sex abuse policies largely intact. Pew Forum on Religion and Public Life, June 16, 2011. Available: http://pewforum,org/Religion-NewsLRNS-Bishops-leave-abuse-policies-Iargely-intact.aspx.

Campbell, R., Sefl, T., & Alvons, C. The impact of rape on women's sexual health risk behaviors. *Health Psychology, 23, no. 1* (Jan. 2004), 67–74.

Child sexual abuse. Rape, Abuse, & Incest National Network, 2012. Available: http://www.rainn.org/get-information/types-of-sexual-assault/child-sexual-abuse.

Cohen, A. Harassment complaints ignored. *Horizons, 19, no. 1* (Summer 2005), 11–12.

Cohen, L. J., & Galynker, H. Clinical features of pedophilia and implications for treatment. *Journal of Psychiatric Practice, 8, no. 5* (September 2002), 276–289.

Craig, M. E. Coercive sexuality in dating relationships: A situational model. *Clinical Psychology Review, 10* (1990), 395–423.

Crossing the line: Sexual harassment at school. Washington, D.C.: American Association of University Women, 2011.

Curtis, K. California loses track of 33,000 sex offenders. *The Birmingham News* (January 8, 2003), 8A.

Date rape drugs. The National Women's Health Information Center, 2005. Available: http://www.4woman.gov.

Date rape drugs. U.S. Department of Health and Human Services, Office on Women's Health, 2008. Available: http://www.womenshealth.gov/faq/date-rape-drugs.cfm.

Dating and domestic violence. Rape, Abuse & Incest National Network, 2009. Available: http://www.rainn.org/get-information/types-of-sexual-assault/dating-and-domestic-violence.

Decker, M. R., Silverman, J. G., & Raj, A. Dating violence and sexually transmitted disease/HIV testing and diagnosis among adolescent females. *Pediatrics, 116, no. 2* (Aug. 2005), 272–276.

Defense Sec. Panetta announces initiative to address sexual assault in the military. Women's Health Policy Report, April 18, 2012. Available: http://www.nationalpartnership.org/site/News2?abbr=daily2_&page=NewsArticle&id=33119.

Deirmenjian, J. M. Pedophilia on the Internet. *Journal of Forensic Sciences, 47, no. 5* (Sep. 2002), 1090–1092.

Department of Defense. Military equal opportunity (MEO) program. In Directive number 1350.2 (p. 19), 1995. Available: http://www.dtic.mil/whs/directives/corres/pdf/135002p.pdf.

Department of Defense. Sexual assault prevention and response program procedures. In Directive NUMBER 6495.01 (p. 17), 2012. Available: http://www.dtic.mil/whs/directives/corres/pdf/649501p.pdf.

Department of the Army. Sexual assault prevention and response program. In AR 600-20, Army Command Policy. Rapid Action Revision (RAR), (pp. 66–77), 2011a. Available: http://www.apd.army.mil/pdffiles/r600_20.pdf.

Department of the Army. Sexual assault prevention strategy goals. In I. A.M. strong: Unit commander's guide, sexual harassment/assault response & prevention (SHARP), (p. 5). Washington, DC: Military OneSource, 2011b.

Diken, B., & Laustsen, C. B. Becoming abject: Rape as a weapon of war. *Body & Society, 11, no. 1* (2005), 111–128.

Domestic homicides. Domestic violence is a serious, widespread social problem in America: The facts 2005. Family Violence Prevention Fund. Available: http://endabuse.org.

Domestic violence and children. Domestic violence is a serious, widespread social problem in America: The facts 2005. Family Violence Prevention Fund. Available: http://endabuse.org.

Eaton, D. K., Kann, L., Kinchen, S., Shanklin, S., Ross, J., Hawkins, J., Harris, W. A., Lowry, R., McManus, T., Chyen, D., Lim, C., Whittle, L., Brener, N. D., & Wechsler, H. Youth Risk Behavior Surveillance—United States, 2009. *Morbidity and Mortality Weekly Report, 59, no. 55–56* (June 4, 2010), 1–143.

Fact sheet. National Center for Injury Prevention and Control, U.S. Centers for Disease Control, 2005. Available: http://www.cdc.gov/ncipc/factsheets/svfacts.htm.

Facts about trauma. APA Online (2005). Available: http://www.apa.org/.

The facts on international gender-based violence. Family Violence Prevention Fund (2005). Available: http://www.endabuse.org.

The facts on the military and violence against women. Family Violence Prevention Fund (2005). Available: http://www.endabuse.org.

Feminist wire daily newsbriefs, September 30, 2005. *Ms. Magazine.* Available: http://www.msmagazine.com/.

Foundation to Abolish Child Sex Abuse. Police smash "world's largest" online pedophilia ring. March 16, 2011. Available: http:// www.abolishsexabuse.org/index.php70ption- com content& view- article& id- 904:policesmash-gworlds-largestg-online-pedophilia-ring&catid- 54:latest-news&ltemid- 179.

Goodnough, A., & Davey, M. Effort to track sex offenders draws resistance. *The New York Times* (February 9, 2009). Available: http://www.nytimes.com/2009/02/09/us/09offender.html?hp.

Grunbaum, J., et. al. Youth Risk Behavior Surveillance—United States, 2003. *Surveillance Summaries, Morbidity and Mortality Weekly Report, 53.SS-2* (May 21, 2004), 1–95. Available: http://www.cdc.gov/nccdphp/dash/yrbs/.

Haffner, D. From the executive director. News from the Religious Institute, The Religious Institute. Westport, CT, November 15, 2011.

Help end domestic violence, National Resource Center on Domestic violence. n.d.

Hillis, S. D., Anda, R. F., Felitti, V. J., & Marchbanks, P. A. Adverse childhood experiences and sexual risk behaviors in women: A retrospective cohort study. *Family Planning Perspectives, 33, no. 5* (September/October 2001), 206–211.

Hitchens, C. Cardinal's law: Two questions for the pope, *Slate,* April 14, 2008. Available: http://www.slate.com/id/2188971.

Hostile hallways: Bullying, teasing, and sexual harassment in school. *American Journal of Health Education, 32, no. 5* (September/October 2001), 307–309.

Humphreys, T. Perceptions of sexual consent: The impact of relationship history and gender. *Journal of Sex Research, 44, 4* (October 2007), 307–315.

Incest. Rape, Abuse, & Incest National Network, 2012. Available: http://www.rainn.org/get-information/types-of-sexual-assault/incest.

Internet safety. Counter Pedophilia Investigative Unit, 2011. Available: http://www.cpiu.us/internet-safety.

Kasindorf, M., Bayles, F., & Grossman, C. L. Boston church scandal starts chain reaction. *USA Today* (December 19, 2002), 13A.

Keeping kids sexually safe. *Families Are Talking 3, no. 3* (2004),1–4.

Kimerling, R., Street, A. E., Pavao, J., Smith, M. W., Cronkite, R. C., Holmes, T. J., & Frayne, S. M. Military related sexual trauma among Veterans Health Administration patients returning from Afghanistan and Iraq. *American Journal of Public Health, 97, no. 8* (June 2010), 1409–1412.

LaFraniere, S. Entrenched epidemic: Wife-beatings in Africa. *The New York Times* (August 11, 2005).

Larsen, D. What are some signs of incest? About incest abuse 2005b. Available: http://incestabuse.about.com/cs/incestrecovery/f/incestafraid_p.htm.

Larsen, D. Why would children be afraid to tell about incest? About incest abuse 2005a. Available: http://incestabuse.about.com/cs/incestrecovery/f/incestafraid_p.htm.

Lee, J., Pomeroy, E. C., Yoo, S. K., & Rheinboldt, K. T. Attitudes toward rape—a comparison between Asian and Caucasian college students. *Violence Against Women, 11, no. 2* (February 2005), 177–196.

Little, K. Sexual assault nurse examiner (SANE) programs: Improving the community response to sexual assault victims. *OVC Bulletin* (2005). Available: http://www.ojp.usdoj.gov/.

Mahoney, P., & Williams, L. M. Sexual assault in marriage: Prevalence, consequences, and treatment of wife rape, in *U.S. Air Force domestic violence literature review,* 1998.

Male sexual assault. Rape, Abuse, and Incest National Network, 2011. Available: http://www.rainn.org/get-information/types-of-sexual-assualt/male-sexualassault.

Marelich, W. D., Lundquist, J., Painter, K., & Mechanic, M. B. Sexual deception as a social exchange process: Development of a behavior-based deception scale. *Journal of Sex Research, 45, 1* (January 2008), 27–35.

Marital rape. Indiana Coalition Against Sexual Assault, 2000. Available: http://www.incasa.org/PDF/Brochures/Marital_Rape.pdf.

Marx, B. P. Lessons learned from the last twenty years of sexual violence research. *Journal of Interpersonal Violence, 20, no. 2* (February 2005), 225–230.

Mason, G. E., & Riger, S. The impact of past sexual experiences on attributions of responsibility for rape, *Journal of Interpersonal Violence, 19, no. 10* (October 2004), 1157–1171.

McCabe, M. P., & Wauchope, M. Behavioral characteristics of men accused of rape: Evidence for different types of rapists. *Archives of Sexual Behavior, 34, no. 2* (April 2005), 241–253.

McEwan, S. L., DeMan, A. F., & Simpson-Housley, P. Acquaintance rape, ego-identity achievement, and locus of control. *Social Behavior and Personality, 33, no. 6* (2005), 587–592.

McGee, R. Don't look at me. National Sexuality Resource Center, April 17, 2007. Available: http://nsrc.sfsu.edu/print/2641.

McLennen, J. C. Domestic violence between same-gender partners: Recent findings and future research. *Journal of Interpersonal Violence, 20, no. 2* (February 2005), 149–154.

Meilman, P. W., Riggs, P., & Turco, J. H. A college health services' response to sexual assault issues. *Journal of American College Health, 39* (1990), 145–147.

Michaels, M. A church plan on sex abuse. *Time, 160, no. 22* (November 25, 2002), 25.

Nagel, B., Matsuo, H., McIntyre, K. P., & Morrison, N. Attitudes toward victims of rape. *Journal of Interpersonal Violence, 20, no. 6* (June 2005), 725–737.

Navy expands training to address sexual assault among sailors. Women's Health Policy Report, August 17, 2012. Available: http://www.nationalpartnership.org/site/News2?news_iv_ctrl=-1&abbr=daily2_&page=NewsArticle&id=34957.

Notice to readers: Sexual Assault Awareness Month—April 2005. U.S. Centers for Disease Control. Available: http://www.cdc.gov/mmwr/preview/mmwrhtml/mm5412a8.htm.

NOW Staff. Military "don't tell" policy hushes up rape and sexual assault. National Organization for Women, 2003. Available: http://www.now.org/issues/military/031103airforce.html.

The offenders. Rape, Abuse, & Incest National Network, 2012. Available: http://www.rainn.orgiget-information/statistics/sexual-assault-offenders.

Osman, S. L. Victim resistance: Theory and data on understanding perceptions of sexual harassment. *Sex Roles: A Journal of Research* (February 2004), 267–275.

Overcoming sexual victimization of boys and men. *Male Survivor* (2005). Available: http://www.malesurvivor.org/10%20Facts.htm.

Pakistan lifts travel ban on raped women. *The Birmingham News* (June 16, 2005), A4.

Park, S., & Natelson, R. Exposing the ugly details of the military sexual violence epidemic. American Civil Liberties Union, 2012. Available: http://www.aclu.org/blog/womens-rights/exposing-ugly-details-military-sexual-violence-epidemic.

Partner rape. Rape, Abuse, & Incest National Network, 2012. Available: http://www.rainn.org/get-information/types-of-sexual-assault/partner-rape.

Peacock, P. Marital rape, in *Issues in intimate violence*, Bergen, R. K., ed. Thousand Oaks, CA: Sage, 1998.

Pedophilia: Who are the men who "love" children in intolerable ways? *Harvard Mental Health Letter, 20, no. 7* (January 2004), 1–4.

Philadelphoff-Puren, N. Contextualising consent: The problem of rape and romance. *Australian Feminist Studies, 20, no. 46* (March 2005), 31–42.

Porche, D. J. Men are victims of sexual violence. *American Journal of Men's Health, 2, 3* (September 2008), 217.

Prevalence of domestic violence. Domestic violence is a serious, widespread social problem in America: The facts 2005. Family Violence Prevention Fund. Available: http://endabuse.org.

Prison rape. National Institute of Justice, 2007. Available: http://www.ojp.usdoj.gov/nij/topics/corrections/prison-rape/welcome.htm.

Rape trauma syndrome—what everyone should know. *Male Survivor, 2005.* Available: http://malesurvivor.org/Professionals/Articles/rts.htm.

Rempala, D. M., & Bernien, F. J. The consideration of rape: The effect of target information disparity on judgments of guilt. *Journal of Applied Social Psychology, 35, no. 3* (March 2005), 536–550.

Rodruguez, A. Kidnapped, forced to wed. *The Chicago Tribune* (July 24, 2005).

Sadker, D., & Zittleman, K. Gender bias lives, for both sexes. *Education Digest, 70, no. 8* (April 2005), 27–30.

Sadler, A., Booth, B., Cook, B., & Doebbeling, B. Factors associated with women's risk of rape in the military environment. *American Journal of Industrial Medicine, 43* (2003), 262–273.

Salter, D., McMillan, D., Richards, M., Talbot, T., Hodges, J., Bentovim, A., Hastings, R., Stevenson, J., & Skuse, D. Development of sexually abusive behavior in sexually victimized males: A longitudinal study. *Lancet, 361, no. 9356* (February 8, 2003), 471–476.

Schmidt, G. The dilemma of the male pedophile. *Archives of Sexual Behavior, 31, no. 6* (Dec. 2002), 473–477.

Sexual assault of young children as reported to law enforcement. U.S. Dept. of Justice (2005). Available: http://www.ojp.usdoj.gov/bjs/abstract/saycrle.htm.

Sexual Harassment Charges. U.S. Equal Employment Opportunity Commission, 2011. Available: http://eeoc.gov/eeoc/statistics/enforcement/sexual_harassment.cfm.

Sexual harassment on campus: Drawing the line. American Association of University Women Educational Foundation, 2005. Available: http://www.aauw.org/research/dtl.cfm.

Sexual harassment. Rape, Abuse, & Incest National Network, 2012. Available: http://www.rainn.org!get-information/types-of-sexual-assauIt/sexual-harassment.

Sexual harassment. U.S. Equal Employment Opportunity Commission, 2009. Available: http://www.eeoc.gov/types/sexual_harassment.html.

Sexual harassment. U.S. Equal Employment Opportunity Commission, 2005. Available: http://www.eeoc.gov/types/sexual_harassment.html.

Siegelbaum, D. Justice expands definition of rape. The Hill.com, January. 6, 2012. Available: http://thehill.com/homenews/administration/202757-department-of-justice-expands-definition-of-rape-to-increase-reporting.

Sims, C. S., Drasgow, F., & Fitzgerald, L. F. The effects of sexual harassment on turnover in the military: time-dependent modeling. *Journal of Applied Psychology 90, no. 6* (November 2005), 1141–1152.

Snyder, M., & Ickes, W. Personality and social behavior, in *The handbook of social psychology*, Lindzey, G., & Aronsen, E., eds. New York: Random House, 1985, 883–937.

South African anti-rape condom could reduce risk of pregnancy, HIV, STDs. *Kaiser Daily HIV/AIDS Report* (September 02, 2005). Available: http://www.kaisernetwork.org.

Spousal rape laws: 20 years later. National Center for Victims of Crime, 2004. Available: http://www.ncvc.org/ncvc/main.aspx?dbName=DocumentViewer&DocumentID=32701.

Stalking: domestic violence is a serious, widespread social problem in America: The facts. Family Violence Prevention Fund, 2005. Available: http://endabuse.org.

Statistics. Rape, abuse, & Incest National Network, 2012. Available: http://www.rainn.org/statistics.

Stermac, L., Del Bove, G., & Addison, M. Stranger and acquaintance sexual assault of adult males. *Journal of Interpersonal Violence, 19, no 8* (Aug. 2004), 901–915.

Stranger rape. Rape, Abuse, & Incest National Network, 2012. Available: http://www.rainn.org!get-information!tvpes-of-sexual-assauIt/stranger-rape.

Ten signs of relationship abuse. Human Relations Media. Mount Kisco, NY, 2008.

Thomas, C. B. A new scarlet letter. *Time, 157, no. 23* (June 11, 2001), 82.

Tyson, A. Sexual abuse is found rife in guard and reserves. *Washington Post* (September 30, 2005), p. A2.

U.S. Military Academy. *SHARP annual training program: Leading the charge against sexual harassment and assault*. West Point, NY: Simon Center for the Professional Military Ethic, 2011.

Van Wijk, A., van Horn, J., Bullens, R., Bijleveld, C., & Doreleijers, T. Juvenile sex offenders: A group on its own? *International Journal of Offender Therapy and Criminology, 49, no. 1* (February 2005), 25–36.

Walker, J., Archer, J., & Davies, M. Effects of rape on men: A descriptive analysis. *Archives of Sexual Behavior 34, no. 1* (February 2005), 69–80.

Walsh, M. Riley restates rules against harassment. *Education Week, 17, no. 4* (July 8, 1998), 1, 30.

Was I raped? Rape, abuse, & Incest National Network, 2012. Available: http://www.rainn.orglget-information/types-of-sexual-assault/was-it-rape.

Whatley, M. A. The effect of participant sex, victim dress, and traditional attitudes on causal judgments for marital rape victims. *Journal of Family Violence 20, no. 3* (June 2005), 191–200.

Who are the victims? Rape, Abuse & Incest National Network, 2009. Available: http://www.rainn.org/get-information/statistics/sexual-assault-victims.

Wilson, G. T., Nathan, P. E., O'Leary, K. D., & Clark, L. A. *Abnormal psychology: Integrating perspectives*. Needham, MA: Allyn & Bacon, 1996.

Wolak, J., Finkelhor, D., & Mitchell, K. *Trends in arrests of "online predators."* Durham, NH. Crimes Against Children Research Center, March 31, 2009.

Wolak, M. A., Finkelhor, D., & Mitchell, K. Online sex abuse cases not characterized by deception, abduction and force, research shows. APA Online, 2004. Available: http://www.apa.org/releases/online_sexabuse.html.

CHAPTER 15

Sexually Transmitted Infections

CHAPTER OBJECTIVES

1 Define STIs and SRDs, describe how are they transmitted, and discuss the reasons for their prevalence.

2 Discuss the bacterially based STIs, including incidence, transmission, symptoms and complications, and diagnosis and treatment.

3 Discuss the virally based STIs, including incidence, transmission, symptoms and complications, and diagnosis and treatment.

4 Discuss the ectoparasitic infestations, including transmission, symptoms and complications, and diagnosis and treatment.

5 Describe ways that STIs and SRDs can be prevented.

go.jblearning.com/dimensions5e

Prevalence of Sexually Transmitted Infections
Bacterial Infections
Viral Infections

INTRODUCTION

*J*essica was enrolled in one of our human sexuality classes. One
day after class, she asked whether she could stop in during office
hours to discuss something "private." Over the years, we have
learned that "private" can mean many things: a student just found out
she is pregnant, is being abused by a romantic partner, or is concerned
about a sexual disorder. In Jessica's case, though, it was a concern that
she might have an STI.

Jessica went on to describe a sexual encounter with Rodney that cul-
minated in penile–vaginal sex. Shortly afterward, Jessica noticed a rash
on her inner thighs and became alarmed. As soon as she described her
concern about having contracted an STI, I knew I would have to refer
Jessica to a clinician at the campus health center for testing and diagnosis. I am an educator, not a medical doctor, and I know my limitations.
Still, I could not refer her immediately for fear that she would think I was
uninterested and be disinclined to discuss with me other concerns she
might have in the future. Consequently, we discussed the reasons for her
concern—the rash appeared, Rodney had not used a condom, they had
not employed any other method of birth control, she met Rodney only
the week before at a party and she did not really know him well—and we
explored any other symptoms she described. Although I did not feel qualified to discuss whether Jessica had an STI, I did take advantage of our
private time together to talk about the wisdom of coitus without the use of
a condom and/or any other method of birth control and explored with her
the decision to engage in coitus with someone she had only recently met.

It turned out that all Jessica had was a rash caused by nylon under-
pants she wore during her weekly jog. The relief on her face said it all, and
I doubt that Jessica forgot that scare the next time she was faced with a

decision regarding whether to engage in sex. That is not to say that she will refrain or become abstinent, although those are certainly possibilities and decisions others have made, but rather that she would understand better that any choice to engage in sexual activity is accompanied by both potentially pleasurable and potentially disturbing consequences. Contracting an STI, one of those disturbing consequences, is always a possibility.

Although Jessica did not have an STI, we have encountered other students who did. Fortunately, most of those students were diagnosed early enough and treated successfully. This chapter describes the more common STIs, ways they can be prevented, and ways they are treated when they are not prevented.

What Are Sexually Transmitted Infections?

The term **sexually transmitted infections (STIs)** describes infections that can be contracted through sexual intimacy. Sexual intimacy includes oral–genital and anal sex, as well as vaginal intercourse. At least 20 STIs have been identified. There are also diseases of the sexual organs referred to as **sexually related diseases (SRDs)**, which are disorders of the reproductive tract that occur in both sexually active and sexually abstinent individuals. These can be caused by organisms that live in the healthy body but under certain conditions, such as stress, diabetes, drug use, and other health-related problems, affect the delicate chemical balance of the body and cause disease conditions of the sexual organs. Some cancers are also considered to be SRDs. A sexually related infection can sometimes be transmitted to a sexual partner, and the conditions under which this occurs are discussed in this chapter.

Whatever the sexual disease, whether contracted during sexual activity or occurring in an abstinent individual, it affects the individual's feelings about his or her sexuality. Some people feel that anyone with a disease of the sexual organs is unclean, evil, and immoral; that a sexual disease is a punishment for sexual intimacy; and that only those of low socioeconomic and low educational status contract these diseases.

sexually transmitted infections (STIs)
Infections that are primarily contracted through sexual contact.

sexually related diseases (SRDs)
Diseases of the reproductive system that can occur in either sexually active or sexually inactive individuals.

There is no truth to these beliefs. Organisms live in our bodies and can multiply when our resistance is low or, as mentioned earlier, when other conditions exist. Pathogenic organisms can sometimes adjust to their habitat, proliferate, and even change in ways that cause symptoms of disease. Not only can they affect the body of an infected individual, but they are also sometimes transferred to another individual through sexual activity.

Prevalence of Sexually Transmitted Infections

STIs have become quite common, even though we have seen a decline in the rates of some particular STIs. There are many reasons for the prevalence of STIs. For example, whereas most states require physicians to report to health departments HIV and AIDS, chlamydia, gonorrhea, and syphilis cases, this was not always the case. Therefore, to compare current STI rates with periods in which reporting was not required would certainly make it appear that there are more cases; in fact, there may not be. In addition, since the 1960s there has been a change in attitudes about sexual behavior. More frequent sex and earlier sex have meant an increase in the number of people subjected to STIs. Other variables include the following:

1. There is considerable social pressure for social and sexual contact, along with widespread ignorance about sexual health and disease transmission.

2. The traditional restraints on sexual behavior are weakening as families and society in general become more loosely knit. Families

Global DIMENSIONS

STIs Around the World

There are wide variations in STIs around the world. Some countries have a high incidence; others have a lower one. The reasons for these differences may at first appear obvious but on further inspection are extremely complex. For example, it is assumed that lack of education is related to STIs, and, in fact, in some countries that is the case. Better educated people have access to information about STIs, their transmission, and their prevention. Furthermore, better educated people are more likely to have better paying jobs, allowing them to act on their STI knowledge (purchase condoms, for example). Yet, this is not always the case. For example, in the early years of the HIV/AIDS epidemic in sub-Saharan Africa, most HIV infections were among more educated people. Speculated causes for this difference included ideas that individuals with more education were wealthier, more

mobile, and had broader networks of sexual partners. However, once educational campaigns were implemented in the region, the HIV rates started to shift, with educated individuals among the first to adopt protective behaviors. This change could be due in part because HIV campaigns were often incorporated into schools, and those who stayed in school longer might have been exposed to more health education messages (Hargreaves & Glynn, 2002). Today, education plays a large role in HIV prevention in Africa, with several studies demonstrating cognitive ability and increased time in school correlated with lower risk levels for HIV (Baker, Collins, & Leon, 2009; Peters et al., 2010).

The reason people contract STIs varies from country to country and even within subpopulations in any one country. The keys to preventing STIs at a policy level are understanding these differences and responding to them systematically.

are more mobile; relocation can threaten the stability of family members as they move away from the support system offered by the extended family and community. Adolescents and young adults are now reared in an atmosphere favoring more personal freedom and less adult supervision. More and more families have two parents in the workforce; adolescent and young adult family members are frequently employed while attending school; and many more adolescents than in the past are unattended during certain times of the day.

3. Adolescence is a time of physical, psychological, and biochemical change and development. There is a wide range in the speed of adolescent development. Physiological maturing occurs at a faster rate than do intellectual, social, and emotional maturing. This places young people in a position of biological readiness for activities that have physical and emotional consequences for which they are not prepared. Often they face sexual decisions that affect their interests and they are not able to judge.

4. Current social values have led to widespread expectations of instant gratification. Learning, growing, and achieving goals require persistence; there seems to be a strong sense of urgency to act now, accompanied by a need for immediate satisfaction.

5. An "everybody does it" attitude undermines convictions about individual responsibility. Thus adolescents who feel stifled by external controls and are eager for independence often take actions, frequently sexual in nature, for which they are unprepared.

6. New modes of contraception have not eliminated unwanted pregnancy, but they have all but eliminated the fear of it. In the past this fear effectively inhibited sexual activity among many people of childbearing age.

One result of the combination of these factors has been an increase in sexual activity among most people—not just the young. This increase, in turn, has led to a rise in the incidence of STIs. There is no doubt that the risk of exposure is greater in people who are sexually active, especially with more than one person, because the chance of contracting an STI increases with the number of sexual contacts.

In spite of these social factors, and because of several other variables such as the fear of HIV infection, the rates of several STIs have decreased dramatically. However, accompanying this decrease in rates for some STIs is an increase in rates for others. The rates, signs, symptoms, potential complications, and means of diagnosing and treating the more prevalent STIs are presented in the following sections.

Bacterial Infections

Some STIs are caused by bacteria. Among these are chlamydia, gonorrhea, nongonococcal urethritis, and syphilis. It is not uncommon for these bacterial infections to be transmitted from one partner to the other, and treatment therefore often requires refraining from sexual activity until the bacteria have been eliminated.

Chlamydia

Incidence

Chlamydial infections, caused by the intracellular parasite **Chlamydia trachomatis**, are the most common reported STIs in the United States today. The Centers for Disease Control and Prevention (CDC) of the Department of Health and Human Services states that because case reporting remains incomplete, estimating the total number of **chlamydia** cases is extremely difficult. However, in 2010 there were more than 1.3 million chlamydial infections reported (Centers for Disease Control and Prevention, 2011a). There are more than three times more chlamydia cases than gonorrhea cases. From 1990 through 2010, reported cases of chlamydia increased from 160 cases per 100,000 persons to 426 cases per 100,000 (see Figure 15.1). This increase reflects increased screening, recognition of the nature of asymptomatic infection (especially in women), as well as actual increases in the disease.

> *Chlamydia trachomatis*
> An intracellular parasite that causes chlamydial infections.
>
> **chlamydia**
> A term that encompasses several major diseases caused by Chlamydia trachomatis, including genitourinary tract infection, a type of conjunctivitis in newborns, a type of pneumonia in infants, lymphogranuloma venereum, and trachoma.

Reported cases of chlamydia in women far exceed reported cases in men (611 cases per 100,000 to 234 per 100,000, respectively). Rates for women are highest in the 15- to 19-year-old age group (3,378 per 100,000 persons) and for 20- to 24-year-olds (3,408 per 100,000) (see Figure 15.2).

Chlamydial infection is an umbrella term that encompasses four major diseases caused by *C. trachomatis*: (1) a genitourinary tract infection in adults, (2) inclusion conjunctivitis (an acute eye infection) in newborns and chlamydial pneumonia in infants, (3) trachoma (a chronic eye infection), and (4) lymphogranuloma venereum. The two diseases of most concern in the United States are adult genitourinary tract infection and infant conjunctivitis and pneumonia.

Symptoms and Complications

Genitourinary tract chlamydial infection has been called "the silent STI." Early symptoms of this infection are often mild and therefore unrecognized. Most infected people are asymptomatic. Symptoms, in those who exhibit them, occur 1 to 3 weeks after exposure. In men the most common symptoms include pain or burning on urination and a white, watery discharge from the penis. Women may note painful urination, a vaginal discharge, and abdominal pain. Individuals who engage in receptive anal sex can become infected with chlamydia in the anus. Symptoms can include rectal pain, discharge, or bleeding. For those performing oral sex on an infected partner, chlamydia can also be transmitted to the throat.

Diagnosis

To diagnose chlamydia, a layer of cells is scraped from the infected area or a urine sample can be tested. The type of laboratory test used depends on the collection method, but nucleic acid amplification tests are

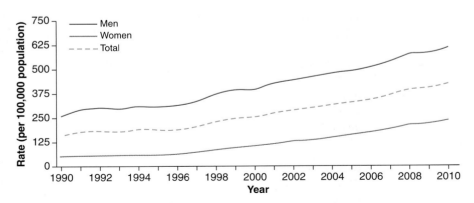

FIGURE 15.1 Chlamydia: rates by sex, United States, 1990–2010.
Source: Reproduced from Centers for Disease Control and Prevention. *Sexually transmitted disease surveillance 2010.* Atlanta: U.S. Department of Health and Human Services, 2011. Available: http://www.cdc.gov/std/stats10/figures/1.htm.

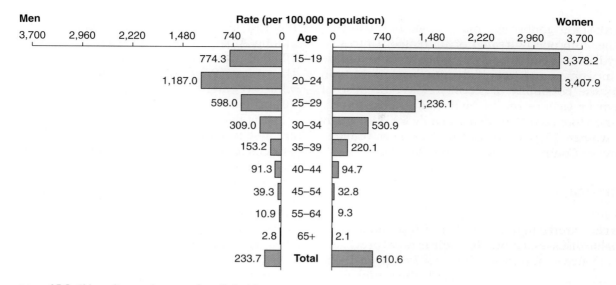

FIGURE 15.2 Chlamydia: rates by age and sex, United States, 2010.
Source: Reproduced from Centers for Disease Control and Prevention. *Sexually transmitted disease surveillance 2010.* Atlanta: U.S. Department of Health and Human Services, 2011. Available: http://www.cdc.gov/std/stats10/figures/5.htm.

the most sensitive tests for endocervical specimens and urethral swab and are FDA-cleared for use with urine. Because of the increased sensitivity, it is less likely that a false negative result will be obtained.

Although most samples are collected by a health-care practitioner, California is trying out a self-service approach in which kiosks allow women to discreetly access testing kits for chlamydia and gonorrhea. One week after the specimens are mailed to the lab, results are available online or via phone with free treatment and follow-up counseling available. The goal of the program is to increase access to testing. On a university campus, a similar program to provide kits for male and female college students to collect a self-obtained sample and then send the kit away to test for chlamydia was unsuccessful. More than 150 individuals were provided with kits, but only 12 returned kits. Another 175 students were directed to an Internet site to request a kit via the mail but only three students internet-requested kits (Jenkins et al., 2012).

Infants born to women with genitourinary chlamydial infections are of risk of acquiring either inclusion conjunctivitis (pink eye) or chlamydial pneumonia during delivery (American Social Health Association, 2012b). In the United States, an estimated 100,000 pregnant women have a chlamydia infection. Because of the magnitude of this health threat, the CDC recommends that all pregnant women be screened for chlamydia at their first prenatal visit, whether or not they exhibit symptoms of infection (Centers for Disease Control and Prevention, 2010c). Additionally, high-risk women should be screened again in their third trimester to prevent complications at birth. Pregnant women should not use doxycycline; erythromycin can be substituted.

Treatment

Chlamydial infections are easily treated in their early stages with antibiotics. The treatment of choice is a single 1-g dosage of azithromycin administered orally or 100 mg of doxycycline administered orally twice a day for 7 days. Alternatively, either erythromycin or ofloxacin may be used. To minimize the risk of reinfection, patients are asked to refer their sexual partners for evaluation, testing, and treatment and to refrain from sexual intercourse with any partners who have not been treated. Reinfection is of prime importance. Many health organizations, including the American Medical Association, the American College of Obstetrics and Gynecologists, the Society for Adolescent Health and Medicine, and the American Academy of Pediatrics, recommend the use of expedited partner therapy (EPT) for chlamydia and gonorrhea in states where the practice is legal. EPT is treating sex partners of patients diagnosed with chlamydia or gonorrhea by providing prescriptions or medications to the patient to take to his or her partner without the healthcare provider first examining the partner. As of August 2012, EPT is permitted in 32 states, and potentially allowable in an additional 11 as well as the District of Columbia and Puerto Rico. The seven remaining states have statutes that prohibit EPT (Centers for Disease Control and Prevention, 2012d). In states where legality is not clear, the American College of Obstetrics and Gynecologists encourages clinicians to advocate for its legality because there is support that this practice can decrease the risk of reinfection (American College of Obstetrics and Gynecologists, 2011).

Unfortunately, because of the asymptomatic nature of the infection and the similarity of symptoms for chlamydia and gonorrhea, many cases of chlamydia are either improperly treated or untreated. Untreated chlamydia can lead to pelvic inflammatory disease (PID) in women and to epididymitis in men. In both genders the possibility of sterility exists. Because of the high prevalence of chlamydia infections, screening is therefore recommended annually for all sexually active women 25 years of age and younger (Centers for Disease Control and Prevention, 2010c).

Gonorrhea

Incidence

Gonorrhea ranks high on the list of reportable communicable diseases. Only chlamydia is more prevalent. The incidence of gonorrhea declined 74% from 1975–1997 after implementation of a national gonorrhea control program. While the decline halted for several years, gonorrhea rates reached their lowest rate—98.1 per 100,000 individuals—in 2009. The rate increased slightly in 2010 to 100.8 per 100,000 individuals, with 309,341 cases reported in the United States. The increase in gonorrhea rates between 2009 and 2010 was observed among men and women and among all racial/ethnic groups (Centers for Disease Control and Prevention, 2011a) (see Figure 15.3).

However, rates of gonorrhea are not equal between these groups. Since 2002, rates of gonorrhea have been higher in women than men. In 2010, the gonorrhea rate was 106.5 cases per 100,000 women and 94.1 per 100,000 men. Regarding ethnicity, the 2010 gonorrhea rates remained highest among blacks (432.5 cases per 100,000), which is over 18 times

> **gonorrhea**
> An STI that commonly starts with inflammation of the mucous membrane lining of the openings of the body (mouth, vagina, etc.).

the rate among whites (23.1 per 100,000). Rates among American Indians/Alaska Natives (105.7 per 100,000) were 4.6 times those of whites. Rates among Hispanics (49.9 per 100,000) were 2.2 times those of whites (Centers for Disease Control and Prevention, 2011a) (see Figure 15.4).

It is believed that many other cases of gonorrhea are not reported because of the social stigma still associated with STIs and the reluctance of Americans to address sexual health in an open manner. Because gonorrhea can result in pelvic inflammatory disease, sterility, ectopic pregnancy, and other serious health conditions, the number of Americans subjected to these risks, in spite of the declining rate of gonorrhea, is still disturbing.

Transmission

Gonorrhea is caused by a bacterium known as *Neisseria gonorrhoeae*, also called *gonococcus*. This bacterium grows in the mucous membrane, the moist protective coat that lines all orifices (openings) of the body. The mucous membranes lining the mouth, throat, vagina, cervix, urethra, and anal canal are all very receptive to gonococcus. When contact occurs between the site of gonococcus in one person and the moist membrane of another—as in all forms of sexual activity—bacteria are transferred. Thus oral–vaginal, oral–anal, penile–anal, oral–penile, oral–oral, and genital–genital contact can result in the transmission of the disease from an infected person to the other partner. Outside the body, however, the gonococcus dies in a few seconds, making it next to impossible to transmit the disease via toilet seats, cups, towels, or other articles used by an infected person. Interestingly

> *Neisseria gonorrhoeae*
> The bacterium that causes gonorrhea; also known as *gonococcus*. Street names include "clap" and "drip."

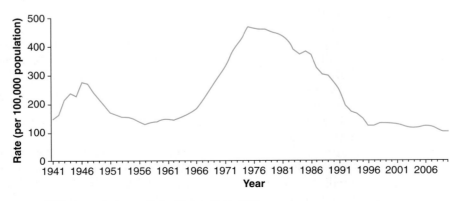

FIGURE 15.3 Gonorrhea: rates, United States, 1941–2010.
Source: Reproduced from Centers for Disease Control and Prevention. *Sexually transmitted disease surveillance 2010.* Atlanta: U.S. Department of Health and Human Services, 2011. Available: http://www.cdc.gov/std/stats10/figures/14.htm.

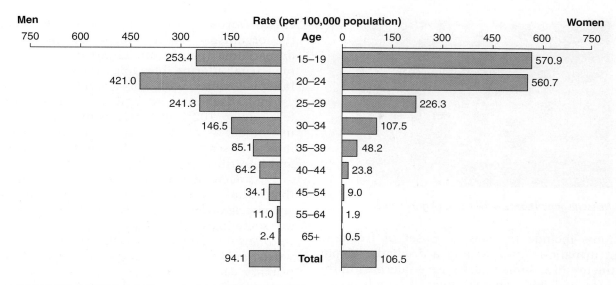

Men		Rate (per 100,000 population)		Women

Men — Rate (per 100,000 population): 750 600 450 300 150 0 **Age** 0 150 300 450 600 750 — **Women**

Men	Age	Women
253.4	15–19	570.9
421.0	20–24	560.7
241.3	25–29	226.3
146.5	30–34	107.5
85.1	35–39	48.2
64.2	40–44	23.8
34.1	45–54	9.0
11.0	55–64	1.9
2.4	65+	0.5
94.1	**Total**	106.5

FIGURE **15.4** Gonorrhea: rates by age and sex, United States, 2010.
Source: Reproduced from Centers for Disease Control and Prevention. *Sexually transmitted disease surveillance 2010.* Atlanta: U.S. Department of Health and Human Services, 2011. Available: http://www.cdc.gov/std/stats10/figures/19.htm.

enough, although bacteria travel from the mucous membrane of the infected partner to that of the uninfected partner, they sometimes die during transfer. Thus exposure does not always result in infection. The risk of transmission from an infected female to a male through vaginal sex is about 20%. This risk increases to 60–80% if there are four or more exposures via vaginal sex. However, for a woman, the risk per episode of vaginal sex for transmission from an infected partner is 50–70%. The difference is because the mucous membrane lining of the vagina, which has a large surface area, is particularly receptive to the bacteria. Any small irritation in the mucous lining can allow the organism rapid entry into the woman's system. Rates of transmission through anal sex have not been quantified, but it appears to be an efficient mode of transmission; pharyngeal gonorrhea (gonorrhea of the throat) is easily acquired when performing oral sex on a male but transmission to someone performing oral sex on a female is less likely (Centers for Disease Control and Prevention, 2012e).

Symptoms and Complications
Males are more likely than females to exhibit symptoms of gonorrhea, and most males will experience symptoms severe enough to seek treatment. It is estimated that 90% to 95% of men infected with gonorrhea have symptoms (Schwebke, 1991a; Smith, Schoonover, Lauver, & Allen, 1990). The males who exhibit symptoms do so within 1 to 14 days after contact; 2 to 5 days is the most likely interval. The primary sites in males are the urethra and the rectum.

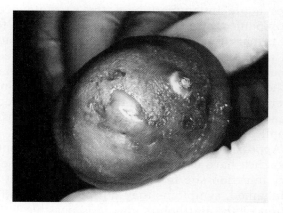

Most males with gonorrhea experience some symptoms, but most females are asymptomatic. For males, the gonorrhea "drip" is a common symptom.

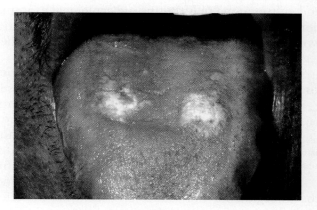

Gonorrhea lesions on the tongue.

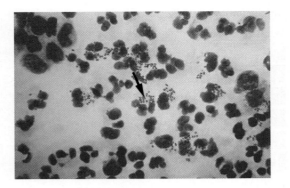

Neisseria gonorrhoeae is the cause of gonorrhea.

Symptoms include the sudden onset of frequent, painful urination (dysuria) and a discharge of pus from the urethra. Some males have tenderness in the groin area and noticeable swelling of lymph nodes. In anal gonorrhea, symptoms include membrane irritation, discharge, and painful defecation.

Complications in the male are seen within 2 to 3 weeks without treatment. Infection spreads up the *genitourinary tract,* the posterior urethra, the prostate, the seminal vesicles, and the epididymis. Sometimes acute inflammation of the prostate occurs, accompanied by pelvic tenderness and pain, fever, and urinary retention. Inflammation of the epididymis may occur; it can be recognized by a feeling of heaviness in the affected testicle, inflammation of the scrotal skin, and sometimes swelling in the lower part of the testicles. If the gonococcal infection spreads to the other testicle, infertility is a possible complication.

Approximately 50% of the females who contract gonorrhea have no symptoms. The cervix is the primary infection site in females, and although it may be inflamed, symptoms may not be evident. Inflammation of the Bartholin's glands is possible but not common. A yellowish discharge may be present but may remain undetected. In actuality most females do not know they have a gonorrheal infection unless the infected partner tells them or they have a smear and culture done in a routine gynecological examination. This fact alone should encourage sexually active women to ask for a gonorrhea test as part of their regular checkups.

A complication of gonorrhea in women is **pelvic inflammatory disease (PID)**. In PID cases, the most common cause is gonorrhea. If the gonorrhea goes untreated in a woman, within 2 months the gonococcal organisms may cause an ascending infection into the internal reproductive organs and pelvic

pelvic inflammatory disease (PID) Infection of the reproductive organs, particularly the uterus and fallopian tubes, and the pelvic cavity.

cavity. During menstruation and immediately after, the organisms travel rapidly. Symptoms include dyspareunia (painful intercourse), occasional non-menstrual uterine bleeding, inflammation of the fallopian tubes with subsequent tubal infection, vaginal discharge, general abdominal pain, and fever up to 102°F. PID is a common complication in women. As the body defenses try to wall off the infection, scarring of the fallopian tubes can occur and infertility can result.

Extragenital complications of gonorrhea (those that occur in areas other than the genitals) include *gonococcal arthritis* and *gonococcal dermatitis.* These are sometimes referred to as *disseminated gonococcal infection.* Gonococcal arthritis affects the hands, wrists, ankles, knees, and elbows. Gonorrhea is the primary cause of arthritis in pregnant women and the most common cause of infectious arthritis in the United States. Gonococcal dermatitis, a rash, is most frequently seen on the hands and lower extremities. White blisters appear and eventually darken, leaving the body without scars. *Gonococcal endocarditis,* inflammation of the heart valves, is a serious but rare gonorrheal complication. Finally, *gonococcal ophthalmic infection* can occur in the newborn; that complication has been reduced by treating the eyes of all babies with silver nitrate tetracycline, or penicillin, at birth.

Diagnosis and Treatment

Diagnosing gonorrhea is usually through a urine sample. In some cases, discharge from body sites will be examined. Throat and rectal cultures are taken if the patient's sexual activity with an infected person involves these body areas. Otherwise, discharge from the urethra in a male and the cervix of a female will be examined. When gonococci are present, approximately 96% of the organism is isolated in these areas.

For many years, the treatment of choice for gonorrhea was penicillin. In 1976, however, a strain of gonococcus resistant to penicillin appeared. This first antibiotic-resistant strain produces a substance that inactivates penicillin. Since then, other antibiotic-resistant strains of gonorrhea have appeared, including those demonstrating resistance to tetracycline and ciprofloxacin. Consequently, only one class of antimicrobials, the cephalosporins, is recommended and available for the treatment of gonorrhea in the United States. Unfortunately, in Japan in 2011 a strain of gonorrhea was found to be resistant to all forms of antibiotics—including all cephalosporin-class drugs (Ohnishi et al., 2011). There are concerns that this gonorrhea strain could spread worldwide in a few decades, especially as the bacteria's susceptibility to cephalosporins has been decreasing rapidly in the United States as well (Bolan, Sparling, & Wasserheit, 2012).

The current treatment of choice for uncomplicated gonorrhea infections of the cervix, urethra, and rectum consists of an intramuscular injection of the drug ceftriaxone or 400 mg orally of cefixime plus an oral dose of either azithromycin or doxycycline (Centers for Disease Control and Prevention, 2012f). This additional medication is recommended because many individuals with gonorrhea infection have a coexisting chlamydial infection (Centers for Disease Control and Prevention, 2010c). As with all drug regimens, special populations, such as pregnant women, require special precautions and alterations.

Nongonococcal Urethritis

Incidence
Nongonococcal urethritis (NGU) and its potential companion, *nongonococcal cervicitis* (in females), are STIs characterized by inflammation of the urethra and cervix, respectively. The signs and symptoms of NGU are similar to those of gonorrhea. If there are indications of urethritis and a laboratory test rules out gonorrhea, NGU is diagnosed.

> **nongonococcal urethritis (NGU)** Inflammation of the urethra caused by *Chlamydia trachomatis,* and *Ureaplasma urealyticum, Mycoplasma hominis, Trichomonas vaginalis,* herpes simplex virus, and unknown organisms.

Before the 1990s this condition was called *nonspecific urethritis* because its causes were unknown. Today, researchers have identified that 15% to 40% of NGU is caused by *Chlamydia trachomatis.* In most cases of nonchlamydial NGU, no pathogen can be detected, though some research shows that *M. genitalium* may account for 15–25% of NGU cases (Centers for Disease Control and Prevention, 2010c). Other potential causes of NGU include *Ureaplasma urealyticum,* adenovirus, *Haemophilus vaginalis, Trichomonas vaginalis* (rare), and herpes simplex virus (rare) (American Social Health Association, 2012c).

Symptoms
NGU symptoms in males include discharge from the penis and a burning sensation during urination. Women who have NGU-related infection sometimes report a mild vaginal irritation, burning, or discharge. At least 70% of infected women, however, are believed to be asymptomatic. Additionally, 10% of infected men may be asymptomatic. NGU is not a reportable communicable disease, so we have no official count of cases in the United States. It is estimated that cases of NGU equal or surpass those of gonorrhea.

Treatment
Treatment consists of either 100 mg of doxycycline taken twice a day for 7 days or a single dosage of 1 g of azithromycin, both administered orally. Alternatively, erythromycin, levofloxacin, or ofloxacin may be used (Centers for Disease Control and Prevention 2010c).

Syphilis

Incidence
After falling to an all-time low in 2000, the syphilis rate in the United States rose for 9 consecutive years before falling again in 2010 (Centers for Disease Control and Prevention, 2011a). In 2010, 13,774 cases of primary and secondary syphilis were reported, a rate of 4.5 cases per 100,000 people (see Figure 15.5).

Outbreaks of syphilis among men who have sex with men (MSM) are believed to be largely responsible for the increasing syphilis rate. High-risk sexual behaviors and HIV co-infection contribute to the rate among MSM. In 2010, 67% of primary and secondary syphilis cases in the 44 states and the District of Columbia that provided information about sex of sex partners were among MSM (Centers for Disease Control and Prevention, 2011a). One analysis of data reported to the CDC showed that co-infection of HIV and syphilis was present in 53% of MSM, compared to 9% of men who reported having sex only with women and 5% among women (Su & Weinstock, 2011).

Wide disparities exist in the rate of syphilis among racial and ethnic groups. While the rate among blacks decreased from 18.4 to 16.8 cases per 100,000 from 2009 to 2010, this rate is eight times higher than the rate for whites (2.1 cases per 100,000). Rates among Hispanics increased between 2009 and 2010 to a rate two times that of whites (4.6 cases per 100,000). Regarding sex, males contract syphilis at a rate seven times higher than females (Centers for Disease Control and Prevention, 2011a) (see Figure 15.6).

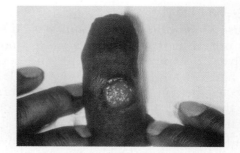

Chancres of primary syphillis on penis.

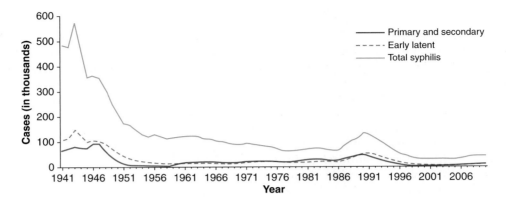

FIGURE 15.5 Syphilis: reported cases by stage of infection, United States, 1941–2010.
Source: Reproduced from Centers for Disease Control and Prevention. *Sexually transmitted disease surveillance 2010.* Atlanta: U.S. Department of Health and Human Services, 2011. Available: http://www.cdc.gov/std/stats10/figures/34.htm.

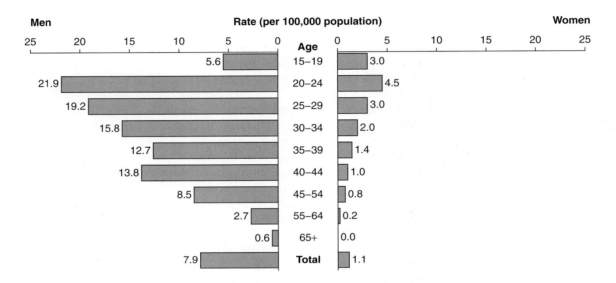

FIGURE 15.6 Primary and secondary syphilis: rates by age and sex, United States, 2010.
Source: Reproduced from Centers for Disease Control and Prevention. *Sexually transmitted disease surveillance 2010.* Atlanta: U.S. Department of Health and Human Services, 2011. Available: http://www.cdc.gov/std/stats10/figures/39.htm.

Congenital syphilis is still a concern in the United States. Rates declined in the 1990s and early 2000s, but demonstrated an increase between 2006 and 2008. Between 2009 and 2010, the rate of congenital syphilis decreased from 9.9 to 8.7 cases per 100,000 live births, with a total of 377 reported cases in 2010 (Centers for Disease Control and Prevention, 2011a).

Transmission

The cause of **syphilis** is *Treponema pallidum,* a spirochete organism that requires a warm, moist area to survive. The **spirochete** is thin and corkscrew-shaped and is transmitted from the open lesions of the infected person to the mucous membranes or cuts in the skin of the other person. The organism can be transmitted by vaginal, anal, or oral–genital contact. Only a few hours after the time of contact, the spirochete reaches the bloodstream of the newly infected person.

The spirochete can also be transmitted by an infected pregnant woman through the placenta to the unborn child. Syphilis bacteria cannot cross the placenta to infect the fetus until after the fourth month of pregnancy because of protection provided by a membrane known as Langhan's layer. Therefore, if the mother is treated before the fourth month of pregnancy, the baby will be free of the disease. Women should be tested early in pregnancy, and if they suspect exposure at any time during pregnancy, they must be retested. Additionally, high-risk women should be retested in the third trimester (Centers for Disease Control and Prevention, 2010c).

> **syphilis**
> An STI caused by the spirochete *Treponema pallidum.*
>
> **spirochete**
> A spiral-shaped bacterium, one of which, *Treponema pallidum,* causes syphilis.

In 1932, the U.S. Public Health Service began a study to determine if syphilis developed differently in African Americans than in whites. The study was conducted in Alabama under the guidance of the Tuskegee Institute, one of the foremost black universities in the United States and, therefore, became known as the Tuskegee Study. The study followed 399 black subjects, all with syphilis—and 201 control subjects who had not contracted the disease—for 40 years.

In 1951, when penicillin became available to treat syphilis, the researchers withheld treatment from the study's subjects because of concern it would interfere with their results. Even in 1966, when the morality of withholding treatment to subjects of the Tuskegee Study was raised with the director of the U.S. Public Health Service's Division of Venereal Disease, a committee specifically organized to decide this issue voted to continue the study and continue to withhold treatment from the study's subjects. Not until a concerned researcher went public in 1972, and another committee chaired by Senator Edward Kennedy in 1973 was formed to study the issue, was a directive ordered to stop the study and treat the remaining subjects. Guidelines were subsequently developed to prevent researchers conducting studies under the aegis of the federal government to ever again behave in such an immoral manner. The remaining subjects of the Tuskegee Study sued the government and eventually settled for $10 million. Unfortunately, a similar study conducted by U.S. researchers in Guatemala in the 1940s was revealed in 2011 in a review of historical documents. In this case, 1,300 Guatemalan patients were intentionally infected with syphilis, gonorrhea, or chancroid (Presidential Commission for the Study of Bioethical Issues, 2011). Because of such incidences, suspicion of researchers, especially among underserved populations, is often prevalent.

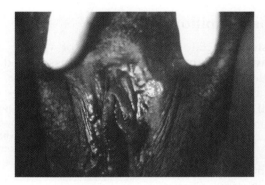

A chancre is symptomatic of the primary stage of syphilis. Often, though, the chancre can appear on hidden parts of the female genital areas, making the disease asymptomatic by appearance. A woman who suspects that her partner has syphilis should request a medical exam or test.

Symptoms and Complications

Syphilis has three stages of development: primary, secondary, and latent. Latent infection lacks any clinical symptoms and can be divided into early latent and late latent. Latent syphilis acquired within the last year is referred to as early latent syphilis. Other cases are referred to as either late latent syphilis or latent syphilis of unknown duration. Syphilis is infectious during the primary, secondary, and early latent stages.

Primary syphilis manifests itself by the appearance of a painless lesion, called a **chancre**. The chancre can appear from 10 to 90 days after exposure; on average, it appears in 21 days. Usually one lesion forms, generally on the glans penis in the male and the cervix in the female; however, the walls of the vagina and the tissues of the labia can also be sites of chancres. Because the lesions occur most frequently on hidden genital areas, they often remain undetected. Lesions can also appear on the nipples, anus, scrotum, or mouth.

Unfortunately the chancre disappears with or without treatment within 3 to 6 weeks. A person who suspects that he or she has been exposed to syphilis should have a blood test and not assume that the disappearance of the lesion means absence of the disease. During the primary stage, however, a blood test result may be negative; thus the test should be repeated. If possible, material exuding from a lesion suspected of being syphilitic should be examined under a microscope in what is called the *darkfield technique*. Sometimes this procedure, too, is repeated.

Secondary syphilis is usually characterized by a generalized rash that appears on the body 6 weeks to several months after initial exposure. The rash does not itch, and it too subsides without treatment. Sometimes in this stage mucous patches are found in the mouth. Other symptoms during secondary syphilis may include fever, swollen lymph glands, sore throat, patchy hair loss, headaches, weight loss, muscle aches, and fatigue (Centers for Disease Control and Prevention, 2012d). This stage usually lasts from 2 to 6 weeks.

primary syphilis
The first stage of syphilis most generally manifested by the appearance of a painless lesion called a *chancre*.

chancre
A painless lesion that is symptomatic of the primary stage of syphilis and appears at the site of contact.

secondary syphilis
The second stage of syphilis, often characterized by a rash.

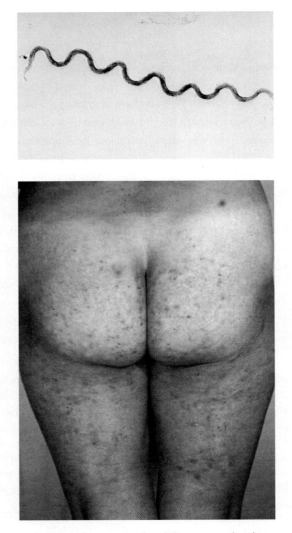

In the secondary stage of syphilis, a generalized rash can appear on the body 6 weeks to several months after initial exposure. Although the rash disappears within a few weeks, medical treatment should be sought for the underlying syphilis bacteria, *Treponema pallidum*.

Latent syphilis has no visible symptoms, and this stage may last for years. The early latent period begins when the secondary symptoms disappear and ends 1 to 4 years later. In the late latent period, the disease may remain asymptomatic or symptoms involving the nervous system or cardiovascular system may appear. The disease can cause blindness, paralysis, crippling, brain damage, and possibly death. In the late latent period, blood tests of untreated persons yield positive findings for the spirochete, although the disease is not infectious at this stage (except to a fetus).

> **latent syphilis**
> A stage of syphilis that may last for years: early latent (about 1 to 4 years in duration) and late latent (may last for years); it may be symptom free or cause degenerative complications.

Diagnosis and Treatment

As noted, early diagnosis is made through a darkfield microscope examination of the material exuding from the chancre or rash, if possible, and through blood testing. Penicillin G is the current method of choice for all stages of syphilis. The preparation used, the dosage, and the length of treatment all depend on the stage and clinical manifestations of the disease (Centers for Disease Control and Prevention, 2010c).

■ Viral Infections

Some STIs are caused by viruses. Among these are genital warts, genital herpes, and hepatitis B. Acquired immunodeficiency syndrome (AIDS) is also caused by a virus, the human immunodeficiency virus (HIV). We discuss HIV/AIDS in the next interchapter. These STIs are among the most difficult to eradicate because the viruses that cause them remain in the body even after symptoms subside. However, as we discuss, there are effective treatments for viral STIs.

Human Papillomavirus

Persistent infection with a group of viruses called **human papillomavirus (HPV)** is associated with the development of cervical cancer and/or genital warts, depending on the type of HPV. Data obtained from the National Health and Nutrition Examination Survey (NHANES) reported overall prevalence of HPV—that associated with cervical cancer and that associated with genital warts—was 42.5% (Centers for Disease Control and Prevention, 2011a). It is estimated that there are more than 20 million people—men and women—who have an HPV infection and that 50% of sexually active individuals will experience an HPV infection at some point in their life. Genital HPV is considered the most common STI in the United States (Centers for Disease Control and Prevention, 2012b).

> **human papillomavirus (HPV)**
> A persistent STI caused by any of a group of viruses associated with the development of cervical cancer and/or genital warts.

Genital Warts

Genital warts occur in most areas of the genitals and anus. In females the warts appear on the labia, in the lower area of the vagina, on the cervix, or around the anus. In males they appear on the glans, foreskin, and shaft of the penis; on the scrotum; and in the anal area as well. Genital warts are growths or bumps that vary in appearance; they may be raised or flat, single or multiple, small or large. Usually, they are flesh-colored

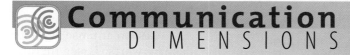

Communication
DIMENSIONS

Talking with a Partner About STI Prevention

Many of our students react incredulously when we suggest they speak with a potential partner about STIs before engaging in sex. "It would ruin the moment," they argue. In frustration, we sometimes respond, "Contract an STI and then let us know about ruining the moment!" If that were all we offer our students, they would be right to be angry. Instead, we also provide them with suggestions to communicate with a potential sexual partner about preventing STIs:

- Begin the conversation before matters are "hot and heavy." Once people are sexually excited, it is more difficult for them to make sensible decisions or to participate in meaningful conversation.
- While many STIs are asymptomatic, examining your partner's genitals can be part of familiarizing yourself for what is normal for your partner. Laughing, soft touch, and expressions of admiration can make the moment enjoyable rather than clinical. Offering to be "examined" first can help reduce your partner's anxiety about the process.
- Discuss your prior sexual history, as it relates to STI risk, with your partner before asking your partner to

share his or her history. Engage in this discussion by disclosing as much detail as you feel comfortable discussing. If expressed in an erotic manner, this discussion can be sexually stimulating as it concurrently accomplishes the purpose of preventing exposure to disease-causing organisms.

- Suggest a "testing" date where you and your partner visit a clinic and get tested together. This can help reduce the pressure or anxiety that you or your partner may feel.
- Demonstrate effective communication skills. Lean forward, nod your head, and look your partner in the eyes to communicate interest. Periodically paraphrase what your partner has said and what you guess he or she is feeling to demonstrate you have been listening. Do not interrupt, raise your voice, or frown in a way that interferes with your partner's communication.

There are ways to make communicating about STIs less embarrassing, less confrontational, and more effective. Discussing STIs with sexual partners is important. Your health, maybe even your life, may depend on it!

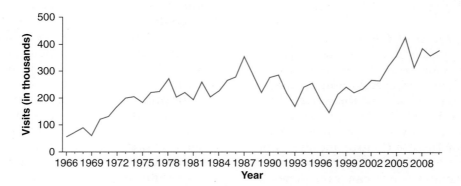

FIGURE 15.7 Genital warts: initial visits to physicians' offices, United States, 1966–2010.
Source: Reproduced from Centers for Disease Control and Prevention. *Sexually transmitted disease surveillance 2010.* Atlanta: U.S. Department of Health and Human Services, 2011. Available: http://www.cdc.gov/std/stats10/figures/50.htm.

or whitish in appearance. Typically, warts do not cause itching, burning, or pain. Warts may appear within several weeks after sex with someone infected with a strain of HPV that causes warts, or it may take several months or years to appear. This extended incubation period makes determining the infection date difficult. It is also possible to transmit the virus to sexual partners when no warts are present; however, it is believed

that HPV is more likely transmitted when warts are present. Most genital warts are caused by HPV 6 and 11 (American Social Health Association, 2012d).

Data based on the initial visit to a physician indicate that the incidence of genital warts may be increasing (Figure 15.7) (Centers for Disease Control and Prevention, 2010c). In a national study, 5.6% of sexually active 18- to 59-year-olds self-reported a

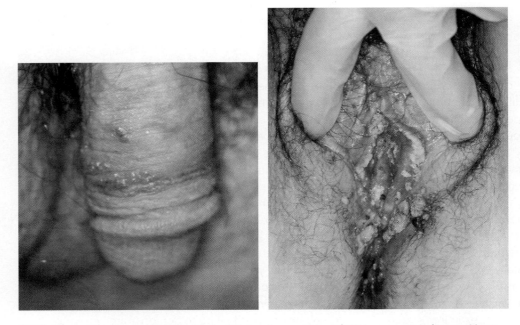

HPV is the most common STI in the United States. Some strains of HPV cause genital warts. Many people who are infected with HPV have a subclinical condition; in other words, the warts are not readily visible. Although the associated symptoms and conditions of HPV are treatable, HPV cannot be cured.

history of genital warts (Dinh et al., 2008), but more recent data collected systematically through clinic diagnoses show ranges for men of up to 12.7%, although results differed based on partner type (men or women) and geographic location (Centers for Disease Control and Prevention, 2010c).

Diagnosis and Treatment of Genital Warts

Genital warts are typically diagnosed through visual exam, although in some cases the warts may be too small to see with the naked eye. A clinician may use acetic acid (vinegar) to "highlight" the warts, because the solution turns warts white. However, because this is not a specific test for HPV, it is not a recommended practice (Centers for Disease Control and Prevention, 2010c).

Treatment of genital warts can vary depending on the size, location, and number of warts; changes in the warts; patient preference; treatment cost; convenience; adverse effects; and a clinician's experience with the treatments. Some methods occur in a clinician's office; others are administered at home by the patient. A number of in-office procedures are available. With cryotherapy, the wart is frozen with liquid nitrogen. The tissue then dies and is replaced with healthy normal tissue. Trichloracetic acid is another chemical applied to the surface of the wart by a doctor or a nurse. The warts can also be cut off, which has the advantage of getting rid of warts in a single office visit. With electrocautery, the warts

are burned off with an electrical current. Laser therapy uses an intense light to destroy warts. Laser therapy usually is reserved for cases with larger wart clusters, especially those that have not responded well to other treatments. Two prescription creams can also be used at home by the patient to treat warts. Podofilox cream or gel may be less expensive than treatment done in a clinic and is easy to use, but it must be used for about 4 weeks. The other cream, imiquimod cream, is also effective and easy to use. Because this cream boosts the immune system to fight HPV, it may reduce the frequency of recurrences (American Social Health Association, 2012d).

HPV, Cervical Changes, and Cancer

HPV can cause normal cells on infected skin to turn abnormal. As previously discussed, some strains of HPV can cause visible changes in the form of genital warts; other strains may cause cell changes that could be precancerous changes in the cervix or other HPV-related cancers such as cancers of the cervix, vulva, vagina, penis, anus, and oropharynx (back of throat including base of tongue and tonsil).

For precancerous changes in the cervix, in many cases the immune system is able to fight off HPV naturally, and the infected cells return to normal. In other cases, the body is not able to fight the virus and persistent infection, and possible complications result. Most HPV-related cancer is caused by HPV 16 and 18. For men who have sex with men, there is an increased risk of anal cancer due to HPV infection.

Risk of either type of HPV infection increases for people who have unprotected sex, especially at a young age, and have many sex partners. Other factors are related to an increased risk of developing cervical cancer. These include smoking, a weakened immune system, chlamydia infection, a diet low in fruits and vegetables, having three or more full-term pregnancies, having a first pregnancy before age 17, low income, and a family history of cervical cancer (American Cancer Society, 2011).

Diagnosis and Treatment of Cervical Changes

HPV is usually diagnosed as part of a gynecological exam. The Pap test looks for abnormal cells in a woman's cervix that may be caused by HPV, but it is not a diagnostic test for HPV. Tests are available for women older than 30 years that look for viral DNA or RNA or capsid proteins related to specific HPV strains. These tests are not recommended for women younger than 20 years of age, men, or as a general test for STIs. For women younger than 21 years of age, the rate of spontaneous clearance of HPV is high; therefore limiting HPV screening reduces the possibility of unnecessary treatment. Unfortunately for men, there is no way to diagnose HPV strains related to these cancers before symptoms develop.

For women who are diagnosed with HPV strains related to cancer, the treatment will vary depending on the woman's age and pregnancy status, the location of the abnormality, and the severity of the cell changes. Because the immune system may be able to combat HPV, in some cases monitoring the cervix and retesting in a few months may be the recommended strategy. In other cases, treatment to remove the affected area may be suggested; this can be done through cryotherapy, Loop Electrosurgical Excision Procedure (LEEP), or a cone biopsy (sometimes called conization) (American Social Health Association, 2012a).

Prevention of HPV

Two vaccines are available in the United States to prevent infection with HPV. Cervarix protects against the two strains of HPV most associated with cervical cancer and has been approved for use in girls and women. Gardasil protects against the four different strains of HPV that are associated with 70% of cervical cancers, 80% of anal cancers (HPV strains 16 and 18), and 90% of genital wart infections (HPV strains 6 and 11). A recent study has shown that Gardasil may provide some protection against anal cancer caused by HPV in MSM (Palefsky et al., 2011). Gardasil has been approved for use in both males and females. Because the vaccine will be most effective when received before becoming sexually active, it is recommended that girls and boys between 11 and 12 years old receive the vaccine (though it can be administered as early as 9 years of age).

Both vaccines are a series of three shots given over a 6-month period, with the second dose 1 to 2 months after the first and the third dose 6 months after the first dose (Centers for Disease Control and Prevention, 2011b). The three doses of the HPV vaccine cost $130 per injection ($390 for the entire series). As a result of the Affordable Care Act, all private insurance must cover the cost of the HPV vaccine. For those without private insurance, the

Vaccines for Children (VFC) program provides federal funds to cover the cost of vaccines in children ages 18 and younger who are either Medicaid-eligible, uninsured, American Indian or Alaska Native, or underinsured. Other support options may be available for those who don't qualify for VFC (Kaiser Family Foundation, 2011).

Whereas health advocates welcome and support the recommendation that all preteens be inoculated, this support is not universal. Some believe that the vaccine encourages sexual behavior, and some parents question the value of vaccinating young children for a sexually transmitted infection. Currently no federal law requires vaccination, and state laws vary regarding requirements of the HPV vaccine for school entry (Kaiser Family Foundation, 2011). In spite of widespread media coverage and financial support, in 2010 only 32% of girls between 13 and 17 received all three doses of an HPV vaccine (Centers for Disease Control and Prevention, 2011e).

Genital Herpes

Incidence

The cause of **genital herpes** is a virus called **herpes simplex virus (HSV)**, which belongs to a family of more than 70 herpesviruses. Humans play host to four herpesviruses:

1. Herpes simplex virus, the agent for fever blisters and genital herpes

2. Cytomegalovirus, a virus that can cause death or retardation if acquired by a fetus

3. Varicella-zoster virus, the agent that causes chickenpox and shingles

4. Epstein-Barr virus, the agent of Burkitt's lymphoma in humans

In 1961, it was found that two types of HSV exist. Type 1 (HSV-1) is seen more frequently in areas of the body above the waist; type 2 (HSV-2) is seen more frequently below the waist. Although most cases of recurrent genital herpes are caused by HSV-2, rates of genital herpes caused by HSV-1 appear to be increasing, especially among younger heterosexual women and men who have sex with men (Ryder et al., 2009). In addition, genital herpes can appear above the waist. For example, when HSV is transmitted through oral–genital sex, a sore may appear on the mouth.

genital herpes
An STI characterized by tiny fluid-filled blisters that appear on the genitals and in the genital tract.

herpes simplex virus (HSV)
The virus that causes oral and genital herpes infections.

Most patients who experience a first episode of HSV-2 infection experience recurrent episodes of genital lesions. However, clinical recurrences are much less frequent for HSV-1 infection than for

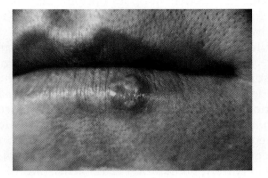

Herpes simplex type 1 can manifest itself as a cold sore.

HSV-2 infection. Therefore, identifying the causative agent has implications for treatment and counseling.

In a nationally representative study, results indicated that about 16.2%, or about 1 in 6, people 14 to 49 years of age has genital HSV-2 infection. Over the past decade, this rate has remained stable. Women are more likely than men to be infected; in opposite-sex sexual experiences, transmission from a male partner to a female partner is more likely than from a female partner to a male partner. There are also racial/ethnic group differences, with black individuals disproportionately at risk for herpes. African Americans have a 39.2% prevalence rate, with black women having a 48.0% prevalence rate (Centers for Disease Control and Prevention, 2010b). Many people—up to 90% of those infected with herpes—do not know they have the virus (American Social Health Association, 2012c). See Figure 15.8 for office visit frequency.

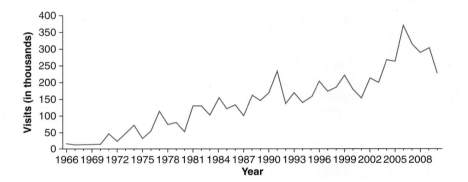

FIGURE 15.8 Genital herpes: initial visits to physicians' offices, United States, 1966–2010.
Source: Reproduced from Centers for Disease Control and Prevention. *Sexually transmitted disease surveillance 2010.* Atlanta: U.S. Department of Health and Human Services, 2011. Available: http://www.cdc.gov/std/stats10/figures/52.htm.

Symptoms and Complications

Primary genital herpes corresponds with the time of actual infection by the herpesvirus and the formation of antibodies. A primary (first occurrence) herpes infection can be very painful but can also be completely symptom free. One recent analysis showed that over 80% of individuals who tested positive for HSV-2 infection were asymptomatic or had symptoms that were unrecognized as herpes (Centers for Disease Control and Prevention, 2010b). For many of these infected individuals, they are carriers of HSV, unaware of their infection and pose a potential risk to sexual partners.

The first outbreak usually occurs within 2 weeks after the initial infection, and the sores typically

primary genital herpes
The first stage of a genital herpes infection; it begins with infection by the herpesvirus and the formation of antibodies. Common symptoms include painful lesions in or around the genital area, a sluggish feeling, fever, and possibly swollen lymph nodes.

heal within 2 to 4 weeks (Centers for Disease Control and Prevention, 2010b). In women the cervix is the main site of infection, although the vagina and vulva may also be involved. Symptoms include painful lesions, a sluggish feeling, and fever, along with possible lymph-node enlargement. Tiny blisters form, filled with a clear fluid in which the virus thrives. The area may become reddened and infected, and when blisters appear the site is in its most infectious state. The open lesions crust over as healing begins. In men, blisters and ulcers appear on the glans penis and the shaft, and urethritis may also develop. In both genders blisters sometimes appear on the thighs and buttocks. Some people experience itching, tingling, or burning sensations where a lesion will appear, known as the **prodrome**.

prodrome
Itching, tingling, or burning sensations that occur where a herpes lesion will appear.

latent genital herpes
The stage of genital herpes characterized by inactivity of the herpesvirus, during which an infected individual is asymptomatic and transmission of the virus is rare.

viral shedding
HSV is excreted from the body even though an infected individual experiences no signs or symptoms.

Once antibodies are formed, the virus enters the **latent genital herpes** stage. Antibodies do not protect against reinfection, but they do tend to make any recurrent infection less severe. During the latent stage the herpesvirus travels up the afferent nerve to the sacral ganglion, where it remains inactive (Figure 15.9). At this point in the infection there are no signs and symptoms.

The virus can become reactivated in the sacral ganglion without producing clinical signs. This occurrence is termed **viral shedding**. During this stage, the virus is excreted from the body even though the infected individual is experiencing no symptoms. HSV is readily transmitted when blisters or ulcers are present. However, the infection can occur through asymptomatic viral shedding.

recurrent genital herpes
The fourth stage of a genital herpes infection, which is characterized by a reactivation of the virus and the appearance of blisters on the skin. Not all people with herpes have recurrences.

Recurrent genital herpes is characterized by reactivation of the virus with clinical manifestations. During this stage the virus travels down the nerve root to the skin, often causing new herpes blisters to erupt. Many individuals experience prodrome symptoms before a recurrence. Symptoms of recurrent infections are usually milder than those of the primary herpes infection and are of shorter duration. The frequency of outbreaks also varies, ranging

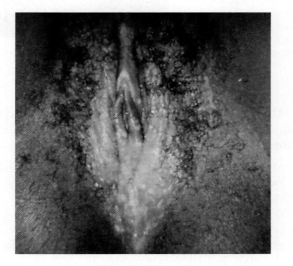

Symptoms of primary genital herpes include painful lesions, a sluggish feeling, and fever, along with lymph-node enlargement.

from one or two recurrences in a lifetime to several outbreaks a month. Researchers have not been able to determine who experiences recurrences or which factors trigger recurrence. It has been suggested that stress, menstruation, or illness may bring on a recurrence; however, more research is needed to clarify the mechanisms at work in the recurrence stage.

Recurrences are not always apparent as blisters may appear inside the genital tract where they cannot be seen, or symptoms may be so mild they are unnoticed. Psychological stress increases for many infected with herpes because they are concerned about recurring symptoms. They are also faced with the difficult decision of how to tell new partners that they have had herpes. They may feel vulnerable to rejection and therefore unwilling to share the information, yet they feel guilty if they are not honest. A variety of local groups across the country help herpes sufferers express their feelings about the infection and work through emotional problems.

Diagnosis and Treatment
Traditionally, HSV was diagnosed visually based on symptoms with a culture taken of fluid from the blisters to confirm the diagnosis. While this method is still preferred if genital ulcers are present, the sensitivity of this method is low, especially for recurrent lesions, and declines rapidly as lesions begin to heal. In addition, because an individual's prognosis and the type of counseling needed depends on whether the genital infection is HSV-1 or HSV-2, clinical diagnosis of genital herpes should be confirmed by laboratory testing that specifies the presence of antibodies for HSV-1 or HSV-2 (Centers for Disease Control and Prevention, 2010c).

Because almost all HSV-2 is sexually transmitted, presence of HSV-2 antibodies implies a genital infection. However, if test results show only HSV-1 antibodies, it is more difficult to interpret. Most persons with HSV-1 antibodies have oral HSV infection acquired during childhood, which might be asymptomatic. At the same time, genital HSV-1 infection appears to be increasing, and genital HSV-1 also can be asymptomatic. Without clinical symptoms, a genital HSV-1 infection may be more difficult to confirm (Centers for Disease Control and Prevention, 2010c).

Treatment for HSV does not remove the virus from the body, but it can help to alleviate symptoms, including outbreaks and viral shedding. Antiviral medication can be used in two primary ways: episodic treatment and suppressive treatment. Episodic treatment is administered during the prodrome or within 1 day of a lesion developing; the goal is to diminish symptom severity and shorten the duration of lesions. Suppressive treatment is usually the treatment option for those with frequent lesion

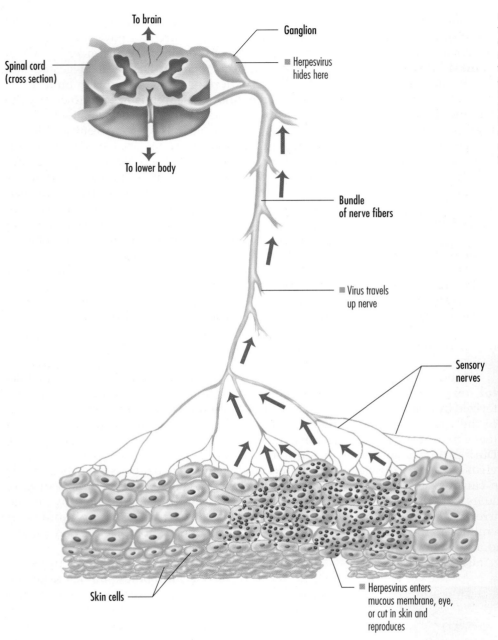

To brain

Ganglion

Spinal cord (cross section)

■ Herpesvirus hides here

To lower body

Bundle of nerve fibers

■ Virus travels up nerve

Sensory nerves

Skin cells

■ Herpesvirus enters mucous membrane, eye, or cut in skin and reproduces

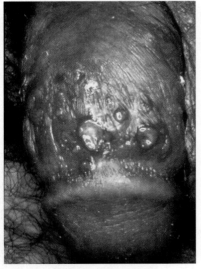

Herpes simplex on penis

FIGURE 15.9 An initial herpes infection takes place when the virus (dots) enters cells of the mucous membranes, eyes, or skin. It reproduces and travels up (arrows) the sensory nerves until it reaches a ganglion (cluster of nerve cell bodies). There it hides, protected from attack by the body's immune system, which overcomes the infection at the place of entry. Though the entry wound soon heals, when conditions allow, the virus may later travel back down the nerve pathway to reinfect skin cells.

recurrences; it requires a daily dosage of antiviral medication. Studies have shown that suppressive therapy reduces the frequency of genital herpes recurrences by 70–80% in patients who have frequent recurrences, and some have reported no symptomatic outbreaks while being on the therapy (Centers for Disease Control and Prevention, 2010c). Suppression therapy with one type of antiviral (valacyclovir) has also been shown to reduce transmission among serodiscordant heterosexual couples (when one individual has HSV and the other does not). Suppression therapy also reduces the risk of viral shedding (Corey et al., 2004).

The best treatment for genital herpes is prevention. Some recommended preventive treatment procedures are as follows:

1. Many cases of genital herpes are transmitted by persons who are unaware that they have the infection or are asymptomatic when transmission occurs. Therefore, condom use is strongly recommended during oral, vaginal, and anal sex. Condoms will not eliminate the risk, but they can reduce it.

2. Persons with genital herpes should refrain from sexual activity when lesions or symptoms

(prodrome) are present and inform their sexual partners that they have herpes.

3. Because there is a risk of transmitting herpes to a fetus neonatally, childbearing-aged women who have genital herpes should inform their healthcare providers, especially those who care for them during a pregnancy, about the infection.

4. Because stress can induce recurrences, it is advisable for persons with genital herpes to learn stress management techniques and employ them on a regular basis. These include relaxation techniques, such as yoga, meditation autogenics, and progressive relaxation, as means of perceiving events as less stressful (Greenberg, 2009).

5. To help prevent infections in other areas, persons with genital herpes should thoroughly wash their hands after touching their genitals.

6. To help speed the healing process, keep the genital (or other infected) area as clean and as dry as possible. Ensuring the area is exposed to air by wearing loose-fitting cotton underwear can also help.

One rare but serious effect of genital herpes is that it can lead to potentially fatal infections in babies. It is important that women avoid contracting herpes during pregnancy because a newly acquired infection during late pregnancy poses a greater risk of transmission to the baby (Centers for Disease Control and Prevention, 2010c). As already noted, the contagious virus is contained within the lesions. If vaginal lesions leak fluid during childbirth, the virus is transmitted to the infant and can result in encephalitis, brain damage, or both. Though less common, HSV can also be transmitted to a fetus through the placenta, thus causing infection before birth.

At this time it is not considered practical or feasible to test all women for herpes during their pregnancies, but women with a history of herpes definitely should be examined weekly from 32 weeks of gestation until delivery to see whether lesions recur. Any primary genital herpes lesions are likely to be detected in the frequent routine prenatal visits. If genital herpes is present at the time of delivery, the infant should be delivered by cesarean section. If laboratory examinations for active herpesvirus yield negative findings at delivery, the infant can be delivered vaginally with little risk of infection.

Hepatitis

There are five hepatitis viruses: A, B, C, D, and E. In the United States, hepatitis D and E are rare. The other three (A, B, and C) can cause similar symptoms but have different modes of transmission and can affect the liver differently. Hepatitis A is usually associated with oral–fecal contamination of water and food, but transmission through oral–anal contact has been increasingly documented, especially among men who have sex with men (MSM). Hepatitis B is transmitted a variety ways, including sexual contact. Transmission of hepatitis C is usually via blood-to-blood contact through needles or other drug paraphernalia. Hepatitis C can also be spread through sexual contact, although it is unclear how frequently this occurs. Having a sexually transmitted disease or HIV, sex with multiple partners, or rough sex appears to increase a person's risk for hepatitis C.

In addition to transmission differences, manifestations of the viruses also differ. Hepatitis A appears only as an acute (self-limited) infection and does not become chronic; people infected with hepatitis A usually improve without treatment. Hepatitis B and hepatitis C can also begin as acute infections, but in some people the virus remains in the body, resulting in chronic disease and long-term liver problems. Vaccines are available to prevent hepatitis A and B; however, there is not one for hepatitis C. Because transmission of the hepatitis B virus (HBV) is often sexual, specifically through blood or blood products, semen, vaginal secretions, and saliva, this discussion will focus on that virus.

Hepatitis B Incidence
In 2009, 3,374 cases of acute hepatitis B in the United States were reported to CDC; the overall incidence of reported acute HBV was 1.5 per 100,000 people, the lowest ever recorded. This low level is due to a

?) Did You Know . . .

Individuals infected with an STI are at a higher risk for becoming infected with HIV, the virus that causes AIDS. Researchers believe that the genital lesions characteristic of STIs—such as the blisters associated with herpes infection—provide HIV with an easy entry point to the body. Thus individuals who engage in unsafe sexual practices while an open lesion exists on the genitals lose an important line of defense against infection—unbroken skin.

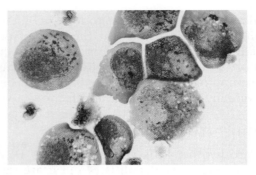

Photomicrograph of cells infected with the herpes simplex virus.

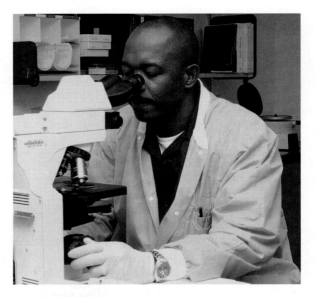

Hepatitis B is diagnosed by a blood test that looks for antibodies or antigens that are present when exposed to the hepatitis B virus.

national effort to eliminate HBV infection, which includes routine vaccination of children born since 1991. However, high-risk adult populations (for example, persons with more than one sex partner in the previous 6 months, MSM, and injecting drug users) are at increased risk (Centers for Disease Control and Prevention, 2012c). In fact, approximately 15–25% of all new HBV infections in the United States are among MSM (Centers for Disease Control and Prevention, 2010c). In the United States, an estimated 800,000 to 1.4 million persons have chronic HBV infection (Centers for Disease Control and Prevention, 2012c).

Hepatitis B Symptoms and Complications

Symptoms of HBV infection vary by age. Most children younger than 5 years and newly infected immune-compromised adults are asymptomatic, whereas 30–50% of persons older than age 5 may experience fever, fatigue, loss of appetite, nausea, vomiting, abdominal pain, dark urine, clay-colored bowel movements, joint pain, or jaundice. Symptoms typically last for several weeks but can persist for up to 6 months (Centers for Disease Control and Prevention, 2012c).

Persons with chronic HBV infection might be asymptomatic, or they may experience more severe conditions such as cirrhosis and liver cancer. In the United States, chronic HBV infection results in 2,000 to 4,000 deaths per year (Centers for Disease Control and Prevention, 2012c).

Hepatitis B Diagnosis, Treatment, and Prevention

Diagnosis of acute or chronic HBV infection requires blood tests for HBV antibodies. Specific antibodies may be present for an acute infection, so clinicians can determine if it is an acute or chronic infection based on the blood tests (Centers for Disease Control and Prevention, 2010c).

No specific therapy is available for persons with acute hepatitis B; treatment is supportive in that it can address any nausea, aches, or other pain. For those with chronic HBV, several antiviral drugs are available. A medical evaluation and regular monitoring should be undertaken to determine whether the disease is progressing and to identify any damage to the liver.

One of the prime methods of HBV prevention is inoculation with the vaccine. If vaccination has not been undertaken, individuals should consider vaccination and, in the meantime, take steps to reduce their risk. HBV is a highly stable virus that can survive outside the body for at least 7 days and still be infectious (Centers for Disease Control and Prevention, 2012c). Likewise, the HBV is 50 to 100 times more infectious than HIV and is easily transmitted during sexual activity (Centers for Disease Control and Prevention, 2010e), so using a condom to reduce risk is essential. Not handling blood or blood products, semen, and vaginal secretions and not sharing items that might contain blood (such as razors or toothbrushes) are also critical strategies to reduce risk.

▌ Vaginal Infections

One category of infection, vaginitises or vaginal infections, occurs in response to changes in an individual's own body and has, therefore, been referred to as a *sexually related disease* (SRD). Two of these vaginitises, trichomoniasis and candidiasis, can also be transmitted from partner to partner and are considered relatively common in women.

Trichomoniasis

Trichomonas vaginalis is a one-celled organism that burrows under the vaginal mucosa to cause **trichomoniasis**, or **trick**. A 2007 study showed the estimated prevalence at 3.1% among women age 15–49, which equals 2.3 million cases (Sutton et al., 2007), although some studies show high-risk populations such as adolescents (Krashin et al., 2010) and women entering prison (Sutcliffe et al., 2010) to have much higher rates. The number of clinician visits is significantly less than the estimated rate, possibly because many women (up to 85%) do not have symptoms (Centers for Disease Control and Prevention, 2011f) (see Figure 15.10).

> **trichomoniasis (trick)**
> A type of vaginitis that can be an STI or an SRD. Symptoms include a foul-smelling, foamy white or yellow-green discharge that irritates the vagina and vulva. Urethritis may also be present.

The common mode of transmission is through sexual contact with an infected partner; vaginal sex, sharing sex toys, and mutual masturbation can all transmit the one-celled protozoan if fluids from one partner are passed to the genitals of the other. For those women who exhibit symptoms, the main ones are an odorous, foamy, white or yellow-green discharge that irritates the vagina and vulva. Frequent and some painful urination can also occur. Men rarely have symptoms, but if they do occur it is usually a discharge from the urethra or frequent and sometimes painful urination.

Trichomoniasis can be passed back and forth between partners; therefore it is important that all sexual partners of an infected individual receive

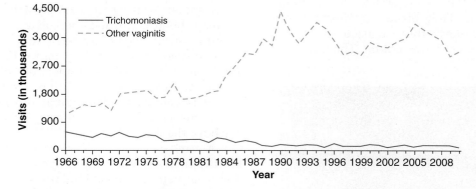

FIGURE **15.10** Trichomoniasis and other vaginal infections: women, initial visits to physicians' offices, United States, 1966–2010.
Source: Reproduced from Centers for Disease Control and Prevention. *Sexually transmitted disease surveillance 2010.* Atlanta: U.S. Department of Health and Human Services, 2011. Available: http://www.cdc.gov/std/stats10/figures/54.htm.

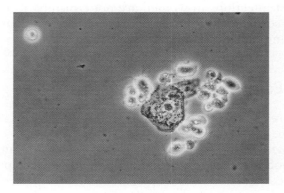

Micrograph of a vaginal discharge revealing the presence of *Trichomonas vaginalis*, a common infection. Prolonged, untreated, or inadequately treated trichomoniasis can result in an increased risk of cancer.

treatment, especially because of the high rates of asymptomatic infections. Metronidazole (trade name Flagyl) is the drug of choice, although tinidazole has also been used as a treatment. Those undergoing treatment should refrain from alcohol use because of undesirable side effects.

Trichomoniasis in pregnant women has been associated with premature rupture of membranes, preterm delivery, and low birth weight. Previous studies identified concerns about treatment during pregnancy, but guidelines today indicate treatment with metronidazole during any stage of pregnancy is acceptable (Centers for Disease Control and Prevention, 2010c). Some studies have shown that infection with trichomoniasis causes an increased risk of HIV infection (McClelland et al., 2007; Van Der Pol et al., 2008).

Candidiasis

The second most common form of vaginitis, **candidiasis**, also called *moniliasis, Monilia,* or *yeast infection,* is caused by the fungus *Candida albicans.* This fungus normally lives and grows in the vagina.

It is also known to be present in the mouth and intestine of many men and women. On occasion when the **lactobacilli**, or *Doderlein bacilli*, that are necessary for a healthy vaginal condition are reduced in number, the yeast multiply and outgrow other vaginal organisms. Women normally have these lactobacilli in the vagina, where they are necessary to maintain a healthy environment. They protect against a variety of infections, particularly those caused by bacteria in the urinary tract and the colon. The protective

candidiasis
A common form of vaginitis, sometimes called a yeast infection, which is caused by the fungus *Candida albicans.*

lactobacilli
Bacteria in the vagina that aid in keeping it healthy; also called *Doderlein bacilli.*

lactobacilli can be reduced by general poor health or lowered resistance, by too frequent douching, and by use of antibiotics (which can kill the lactobacilli as well as the bacteria causing the disease for which the antibiotic is prescribed). When the normally acid environment is changed, the yeast multiply and outgrow other vaginal organisms, resulting in a white and curdy discharge. Examination reveals a whitish plaque around the vagina and on its walls. Itching, frequently associated with a rash or redness of the vulva, is common. In advanced cases intercourse is painful, and burning and discomfort occur during urination.

Women with compromised immune systems, glucose intolerance, or who are receiving antibiotics may be at increased risk for yeast infections. Prolonged exposure to wet, synthetic material, such as bathing suits, prevent air from circulating around the vulva and keep normal discharges in contact with vaginal tissues, contributing to yeast growth. It is important to keep the area around the vulva as dry as possible. Letting towels dry before reuse and not sharing towels can also help. Avoiding panty hose, tight-fitting clothing, and noncotton underwear are other strategies to decrease risk. In addition, if material from the bowel is carried to the vagina, the person becomes more susceptible to moniliasis, because the bowel harbors the *Candida* fungus.

A variety of over-the-counter and prescription intravaginal creams and suppositories are available for treatment of yeast infections. A woman should visit a clinician if she has never been diagnosed with a yeast infection before using any over-the-counter treatment. In addition, the creams and suppositories available are oil-based, so pregnancy prevention methods should be considered because they may weaken latex condoms and diaphragms. Because yeast infections in women are not typically transmitted sexually, no data support the need for partner testing or treatment.

■ Ectoparasitic Infestations

There are two common STIs that are not diseases as such, but rather infestations of parasites. These are pubic lice and scabies. Parasites are found among all socioeconomic classes and are spread by close physical contact.

Pubic Lice

Pubic lice, commonly referred to as crabs, are parasites. Actually there are three different kinds of lice, known as **pediculosis lice**, and each seems to prefer

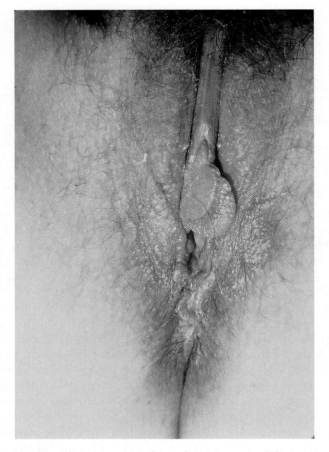

The second most common form of vaginitis is candidiasis, or yeast infection. It can result in white and curdy discharge, as shown here.

Multicultural DIMENSIONS

STIs and Minorities Surveillance data show high rates of STIs for some minority racial or ethnic groups compared with rates for whites. Race and ethnicity in the United States are risk markers that correlate with other more fundamental determinants of health status such as poverty, access to high-quality health care, health-care-seeking behavior, illicit drug use, and residence in communities with high prevalence of STIs.

- In 2010, the chlamydia rate among African Americans was more than 8 times that among whites. The chlamydia rate among African American women was more than 7 times higher than the rate among white women. The chlamydia rate among African American men was almost 11 times higher than the rate among white men.
- In 2010, the chlamydia rate among Hispanics was nearly 3 times higher than the rate among whites. The chlamydia rate among American Indians/Alaska Natives was more than 4 times higher than the rate among whites.
- In 2010, approximately 69% of the total number of reported cases of gonorrhea occurred among African Americans. Overall, the rate of gonorrhea among African Americans in the United States was 19 times greater than that among whites. This disparity was higher for African American men (22.2 times higher) than for African American women (16.2 times higher). Among those aged 20 to 24 years, the gonorrhea rate among African Americans was more than 16 times greater than that among whites (1,881.8 versus 116.5 cases per 100,000 population).

- In 2010, the gonorrhea rate among American Indians/Alaska Natives was 125.7 cases per 100,000 population, which was 4.8 times higher than the rate among whites. The gonorrhea rate among Asians/Pacific Islanders was lower than the rate among whites, and the rate among Hispanics was higher than the rate among whites.
- In 2010, 47.4% of all cases of primary and secondary syphilis occurred in African Americans. Compared to whites, the overall 2010 rate of primary and secondary syphilis among African Americans was 8 times higher.
- Compared to whites, the 2010 primary and secondary syphilis rate among American Indians/Alaska Natives was 1.2 times higher, and the rate among Hispanics was 2.2 times higher.

Reducing the prevalence of many of these STIs in minority populations will require a combination of strategies. Of course, education about prevention is important. Still, education will not have a significant effect in minority populations if it is not combined with strategies to reduce poverty, increase access to good-quality health care, decrease drug abuse and the sharing of drug "works," and create comprehensive sexuality education programs that start in schools at early ages and continue through community agencies into the adult years.

Source: Data from Centers for Disease Control and Prevention. *Sexually transmitted diseases surveillance 2010.* U.S. Department of Health and Human Services, Public Health Service. Atlanta: Centers for Disease Control and Prevention, 2011. Available: http://www.cdc.gov/std/stats10/surv2010.pdf.

---

pubic lice
A parasite, commonly referred to as crabs, a louse that grips the pubic hair and feeds on tiny blood vessels of the skin.

pediculosis lice
Also known as crabs, of three common types: *Pediculus corporis,* a body louse; *Pediculus capitis,* a head louse; and *Pediculus pubis,* a pubic louse.

its own habitat. *Pediculus corporis* is a body louse; *Pediculus capitus* is a head louse; and *Pediculus pubis* is the louse of the pubic area. Pubic lice are usually transmitted from person to person by sexual contact. Infection from infected bedding, clothing, upholstered furniture, and toilet seats is rare. The organism grips the pubic hair and feeds on tiny blood vessels of the skin.

Female crabs live 1 to 2 months and lay up to 10 eggs a day. As they feed on the human skin and blood, they irritate the skin, causing itching and occasionally swelling of glands in the groin. The nits, or eggs, stick to the pubic hair with a thick substance. Aided by body warmth, the eggs hatch and the new lice perpetuate the cycle of feeding on the human before dropping off. They can live for 1 to 2 days off the

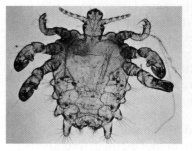

Pubic lice, commonly called "crabs," are usually transmitted from person to person by sexual contact. Direct treatment, plus cleaning of clothes and bedding, eliminate the lice.

body and are visible to the naked eye on clothing and bedsheets. Treatment usually involves a cream rinse applied to the affected area. Reports of resistance to typical treatment methods have been increasing and are widespread. An alternative method is available, though not preferred, because of its strong odor and the longer required application time. And, of course, clothing and bed linen used before treatment should be washed. Fumigation of living areas is not considered necessary.

Scabies

Scabies is caused by a tiny mite that can barely be seen. The organism generally lives for up to 2 months. The female burrows under the skin at night, probably for the warmth of the human host, and the results are intense itching and the formation of pus. There is a characteristic distribution pattern of scabies. It is seen most commonly on the wrists, in the spaces between the fingers, under the breasts, and on the buttocks. Nodular scabies (raised lesions) can last up to 1 year. The mites lay two to three eggs a day, and in 2 or 3 weeks a new cycle begins. Because the incubation period is 4 to 6 weeks for those who have never been infected, one individual can transmit scabies to another before being aware of its existence. Close contact that is usually (but not exclusively) sexual can transmit the mites. Scabies can spread rapidly under crowded conditions where close body and skin contact is frequent. Institutions such as nursing homes, extended-care facilities, and prisons are often sites of scabies outbreaks. Child care facilities also are a common site of scabies infestations.

> **scabies**
> Skin irritation caused by a tiny mite that is transferred from one person to another by close contact, sexual or otherwise.

In addition, a severe form of scabies, called crusted scabies or Norwegian scabies, can occur in persons who are immune-compromised, malnourished, or debilititated. These individuals will have thick crusts of skin that contain large numbers of scabies mites and eggs; they may not show the typical signs and symptoms of scabies and should be considered very contagious.

Diagnosis is usually based on the customary appearance and distribution of the rash and the presence of burrows. However, if possible, the diagnosis should be confirmed by identifying the mite, mite eggs, or mite fecal matter by removing a mite from the end of its burrow using the tip of a needle or by obtaining a skin scraping to examine under a microscope for mites, eggs, or mite fecal matter (Centers for Disease Control and Prevention, 2010a). Typical treatment is application of permethrin cream to all areas of the body (except the head) and washed off after 8 to 14 hours. Lindane (Kwell) is no longer recommended as a primary treatment because of its toxicity; however, if other treatments fail, it can be used under strict guidelines (Centers for Disease Control and Prevention, 2010c). Sexual contacts and those with close personal or household contact within the last month should be examined and treated.

■ Prevention

On the one hand, STIs are often like other diseases in that, for many, there are effective treatments that result in elimination of the disease. On the other hand, for some STIs, even though there are effective treatments, there are no cures (for example, genital herpes). Still other STIs have only recently had potentially effective treatments developed to treat them and, until then, inevitably led to incapacity and death (for example, syphilis). Even when cured, people who have contracted some STIs can be affected for their entire lives—for example, when the disease results in infertility. STIs, therefore, are serious conditions that we would be best advised to prevent. Fortunately, there are actions we can take to prevent contracting an STI or at least minimize the likelihood of contracting one.

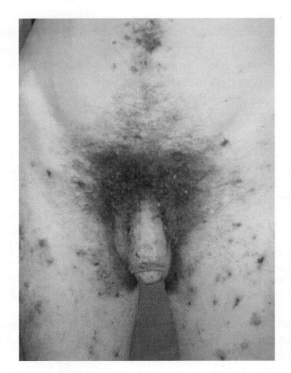

Scabies lesions can last for up to a year and can be transmitted before being aware of its existence.

Ethical
DIMENSIONS

Notifying Partners About STIs

There are many reasons why people with STIs choose not to notify their sexual partner(s) about their infection. They may be embarrassed to do so, they may be in a relationship and have contracted the STI from another partner or they may not want anyone to know about their infection for fear they will not be able to get dates or other sexual partners.

Similarly, there are many reasons people with STIs choose to notify their sexual partners. They may believe that all sexual partners, past and present, should be notified of a sexual partner's STI status. In this way, they can get tested and retested if they are infected. And they can prevent the spread of the infection by refraining from sex with other people until they are disease free.

On the one hand, some people argue that *absent any signs or symptoms,* notifying a sexual partner might do more harm than good. For example, if the infection was contracted during an extramarital affair, notification might result in divorce. Notification might unduly frighten the unsuspecting partner, causing potentially unhealthy consequences associated with stress.

On the other hand, some people argue that to disclose an STI is consistent with the ethical principles of honesty and nonmaleficence (do no harm). Even if the result of the sexual behavior is accompanied by sanctions (such as divorce), they believe it further compounds the violation of trust to withhold information that a loved one can use to protect his or her health.

What do you think is the ethical thing to do? Does the fact that many STIs are asymptomatic affect your decision?

Abstinence

The most certain way to avoid contracting an STI is to abstain from sexual activity. Because STIs can be contracted through oral sex, anal sex, and skin-to-skin contact, refraining from all penetrative behaviors and contact with the genitals is needed to completely eliminate the risk.

Some may choose abstinence until they are married or until they are in a committed relationship. Others may practice abstinence at different points in their lives, such as after a recent divorce. The option of refraining from sexual activity is available to everyone at all times. However, for many people abstinence is not acceptable for a variety of reasons. Perhaps they have an interest in sex and find it so pleasurable that they are not willing to forgo it. They may have no moral or ethical objections to premarital sex. They may have no intention of marrying in the future, or they may be gay or lesbian and live in a state where legal marriage is unavailable to them. For those not willing to remain abstinent, other strategies to reduce the risk of contracting an STI are available.

Monogamy

If a sexual partner is STI free, and he or she is the only person with whom you engage in sexual activity, then you will not contract an STI. Monogamy with an uninfected partner, though, can be problematic. How are you to be sure your partner is uninfected? How are you to be sure that your partner is also monogamous? Without seeing the STI testing results and following your partner everywhere (which is usually not recommended), you can never really be sure that your partner is STI free and monogamous. And in some cases, like the lack of a test for HPV in men or that herpes infections can go unnoticed and be "discovered" years after an infection, even testing and stalking may not prove adequate. For all of these reasons, relying on monogamy with an uninfected partner as protection against contracting an STI can be risky.

 Did You Know . . .

Although it is impossible to determine the exact number of STIs each year, it is agreed that the cost of these diseases is extensive. One estimate is that STI expenditures on direct medical care and related services, as well as the indirect costs associated with the loss of productivity, totaled $15.9 billion in 2008 (Centers for Disease Control and Prevention, 2009). This estimate excludes costs attributed to HIV and AIDS.

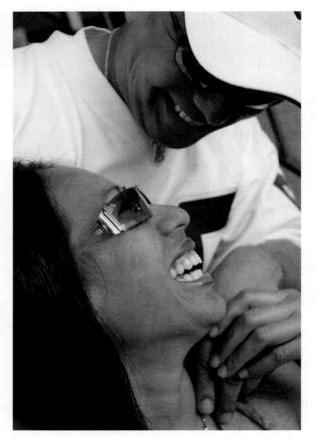

If sexually active, the best way to prevent contracting an STI is by maintaining a monogamous relationship in which both partners are STI free.

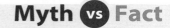

Myth vs Fact

Myth: If you get syphilis, you will know it because a rash will break out.
Fact: A rash may not appear until secondary syphilis has occurred. Furthermore, although a chancre (a sore) may develop early in the course of the disease, it may not be visible or may be dismissed as inconsequential. Also, in women, the early signs of syphilis may not be readily visible on the genitalia.

Myth: Gonorrhea is no more serious than the common cold and can be cured easily.
Fact: Gonorrhea can cause infertility, arthritis, or endocarditis (inflammation of the heart valves). In addition, certain antibiotic-resistant strains of gonorrhea raise concern about the ability to continue to treat this STI with present medications.

Myth: If you get an STI once, you acquire an immunity to it and cannot contract it a second time.
Fact: You do not have immunity to STIs and can contract them anew each time you have contact with the disease-causing organisms.

Myth: STIs occur only in or on the genital organs.
Fact: You can acquire an STI through oral–genital contact, in which case the signs of the disease would occur in the mouth and on the face. Or, you can have contact with an STI-causing organism by touching an infected area with your fingers, in which case the signs of the infection could appear on other body areas (like eyes and mouth) if you touch those areas.

Reduce the Number of Sexual Partners

If a person is unwilling or unable to maintain a monogamous relationship, decreasing the number of sexual partners lessens his or her odds of contracting an STI. The greater number of sexual partners, the greater the likelihood that one of them will be infected.

Refrain from the Use of Alcohol and Other Drugs

Decisions regarding important aspects of your life deserve thoughtful consideration. What more important decision is there than that concerning whether you will engage in an activity that has the potential of causing serious, sometimes life-threatening illness? Alcohol and other drugs can interfere with decision making by decreasing inhibitions and affecting judgment. Therefore, protection against STIs should include abstention from the use of mind-altering drugs.

Discuss STI Concerns with Potential Sexual Partners

Any new sexual partners should discuss concern about STIs before engaging in sexual activity. Whether they know they are infected, the high-risk behaviors they have engaged in and the results of any medical screenings they have had should be shared. This kind of a conversation can lead to concern about a potential sexual partner and a decision to refrain from sex altogether—or at least until a new medical screening can be obtained.

Be Observant

We used to recommend an examination of your own genitals and your partners' genitals for any obvious signs of an STI. However, this is no longer recommended because so many STIs are asymptomatic and the "exam" can give individuals a false sense of security that they are infection-free.

At the same time, being familiar with your own body and examining your genitals for any lesions, blisters, or infected sores can help you identify if something abnormal develops. If so, it is important to refrain from sexual activity until you know the cause. If there is any unusual growth or sore or a foul-smelling odor, you need to see a healthcare provider for an exam and possible testing.

You also want to be observant of your partners' genitals. If you see something that may be a sign of an STI, ask questions and do not continue to engage in any sexual activity until you are certain there is no risk to you. One of us had a student who saw a blister on his partner's vulva, asked her about it and was informed that "it was a pimple." When he later contracted genital herpes, he was devastated and wished he had trusted his instinct that it could be a symptom of an STI.

Use Condoms and Other Barriers

Male condom use is something that is often discussed as a prevention strategy for STIs. For all methods that are intended to reduce the risk of STI transmission, accurately estimating the effectiveness is challenging from a research perspective. Measuring consistent and correct use of the method, whether the infection identified is new or preexisting, and how to ensure that the individuals have exposure to the STI of interest during the study all pose challenges.

The research on male latex condoms demonstrates that they protect well against STIs that are transmitted through genital fluids (for example, pre-ejaculate, semen, vaginal secretions). These STIs include HIV, hepatitis B, gonorrhea, chlamydia, and trichomoniasis. The numerous studies on HIV transmission are the most methodologically strong, but there is epidemiological evidence that support prevention of transmission for the other fluid STIs. In all cases, male latex condoms provide a barrier to particles the size of STI pathogens; no "holes" exist in which HIV or virus could penetrate (Centers for Disease Control and Prevention, 2011c).

For infections that are transmitted by skin-to-skin contact, studies have not shown the same

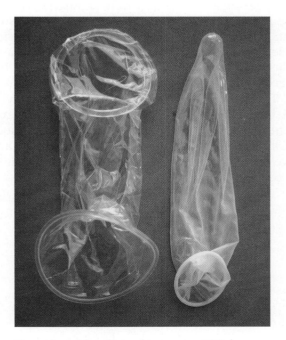

The male and female condoms prevent STIs by establishing a barrier between the infection-causing organism and the body. This barrier prevents the organism from finding a pathway into the body.

level of protection from male condoms. Consistent and correct male condom use can reduce the risk of genital herpes and syphilis only for the covered area. Other studies have shown that condom use may reduce the risk for HPV infection; condom use has also been associated with higher rates of clearance of HPV infection in women and with regression of HPV-lesions on the penis in men. In addition, a few prospective studies have shown condoms as having a protective effect on the acquisition of genital HPV (Centers for Disease Control and Prevention, 2011c).

Research is very limited on female condoms, latex dams (used during oral sex on a female or oral–anal contact), gloves, or other latex-protective barriers and the extent these items protect against STIs. In general, female condoms (Centers for Disease Control and Prevention, 2010c) and latex dams are believed to provide protection from fluid-transmitted STIs and from skin-to-skin STIs on the portion of the body covered. Previously, plastic wrap was recommended as an alternative to latex dams, but there is only one research article that suggested potential protection against herpes during oral sex on a female or oral–anal contact, and there are no data on its effectiveness regarding HIV or other STIs (Centers for Disease Control and Prevention, 2009a).

Avoid High-Risk Behaviors

Because organisms that cause STIs are present in semen and vaginal secretions, the goal is to prevent them from being transmitted from an infected person to a person not infected. Penile–vaginal sex without the use of a condom can result in the depositing of semen that includes infection-causing organisms within a partner's body. So can fellatio without a condom and cunnilingus without a dental dam. Anal sex is a particularly high-risk behavior because the friction creates fissures (tears in the lining) in the anus, allowing easy entrance to infection-causing organisms into the bloodstream. Furthermore, because some organisms that cause STIs reside in the blood, using needles or other products that may contain drops of blood from another person puts one at high risk for disease. Sharing needles is one of the more common ways of contracting HIV in the United States.

Other Protective Measures

Still other behaviors can lessen the likelihood of contracting an STI or increase the likelihood of detecting one at an early stage:

- Wash the genitals before and after sex.
- Obtain regular medical checkups.

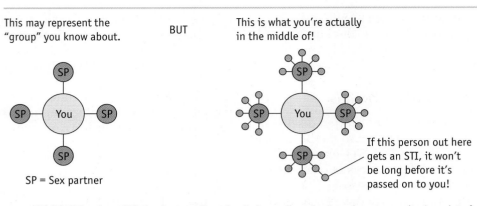

This may represent the "group" you know about.

BUT

This is what you're actually in the middle of!

SP = Sex partner

If this person out here gets an STI, it won't be long before it's passed on to you!

FIGURE **15.11** STIs: a fact of life for the sexually active. By "sexually active," we do not mean having a lot of sex. Instead we are using the term to mean having sex with different people. In general, the fact of life is that, sooner or later, sexually active people will either be exposed to an STI or contract one.

- Inspect the genitalia regularly.
- Do not share razors, hypodermic needles, or scissors.
- Do not handle towels, wet bedding, or undergarments immediately after these have been in contact with another person.

If you suspect you have been exposed to an STI, see a physician or visit a health clinic in your community or on your campus. It is unwise to try to diagnose and treat the condition yourself. It is also extremely important to comply with the treatment regimen, which includes taking all the medication prescribed at the appropriate times and returning for any follow-up visits. Also, if you have an STI, notify your partner(s). Failing to tell a partner of the possibility of infection could result in the spread of the disease, not just to a single individual but possibly to many (see Figure 15.11).

Sexuality Education and STIs

Alarmed at what it called the "hidden epidemic," the Institute of Medicine (IOM) convened a 15-member expert panel in 1994 to strategize ways to address the STI problem. The IOM concluded that society's unwillingness to confront sexual issues is the main barrier to responding to STIs (Eng & Butler, 1996). The IOM report went on to explain that this attitude hinders the dissemination of accurate, straightforward information about STIs in educational programs for adolescents and interferes with communication between parents and their children and between sexual partners. Furthermore, this attitude compromises healthcare professionals' ability to counsel patients, impedes research on sexual behavior, and leads to unbalanced messages being sent via the media. The members of the expert panel noted several studies that found that almost two-thirds of respondents knew little or nothing about STIs other than HIV and AIDS and that most people seriously underestimate their risk of acquiring an STI, as well as its consequences. Not much has changed in the intervening years.

The need for education about STIs is evident, has long been overlooked, and requires the involvement of many different segments of our society, working together to prevent their occurrence and to develop more effective treatments if and when they do occur.

Exploring the Dimensions of Human Sexuality

Our feelings, attitudes, and beliefs regarding sexuality are influenced by our internal and external environments. Go to go.jblearning.com/dimensions5e to learn more about the biological, psychological, and sociological factors that affect your sexuality.

Case Study

Sexually transmitted infections are quite prevalent, especially among young people. Some STIs and SRDs are curable; some are treatable but chronic. Because many cases are asymptomatic or early symptoms are ignored, treatment does not always occur. The STI can then be transmitted further.

Having a curable STI is, at a minimum, embarrassing. Yet having a chronic STI such as genital herpes or genital warts can have a profound psychological impact on a person's life. The STI will affect the individual's sexual activities for an entire lifetime. The fear of rejection after informing a potential sexual partner might cause the individual to say nothing. Self-esteem can diminish.

Socially, race and ethnicity correlate with fundamental determinants of health status such as poverty, access to health care, healthcare-seeking behavior, and residence in areas with a high prevalence of STIs. Thus a higher prevalence of gonorrhea or syphilis among African Americans has social—not biological—underpinnings.

STI risk can be reduced in a number of ways, including abstinence, monogamy, reduction in the number of sexual partners, refraining from alcohol or other drugs, communication with partners, use of latex condoms and other barrier methods, and avoidance of high-risk behaviors. However, if we belong to a community that has high rates of infection, our risk will still be greater unless we practice abstinence from oral sex, vaginal sex, anal sex, and genital contact. Simply engaging in sex with members of our community should not be an increased factor, and society as a whole needs to consider how to address these underlying influences as well as general STI awareness, education, and prevention practices.

Biological Factors

- STIs are contracted primarily through sexual contact.
- SRDs are diseases of the reproductive system that can occur in either sexually active or sexually inactive individuals.
- Individuals with an STI have a higher risk of becoming infected with HIV, possibly because the genital lesions characteristic of STIs give HIV access to the body.
- STIs can be passed to a baby both before and during birth.

Sociocultural Factors

- Society's unwillingness to confront sexual issues is a major barrier in responding to STIs.
- Some ethnic groups have higher rates of STIs than others. Southern states have higher rates of syphilis than the national average.
- Economically, the cost of treating STIs—and the associated lost productivity—exceeds $15 billion per year.

Psychological Factors

Biological and sociocultural factors combine to influence psychological factors.

- Having an STI affects an individual's feelings about his or her sexuality.
- Learning later in life that you became sterile due to an undiagnosed STI can have a devastating psychological effect.
- Psychological stress increases for genital herpes sufferers because they are constantly concerned that symptoms will reappear. They must decide whether to tell new partners of their condition, which can lead to rejection.

Summary

- Sexually transmitted infections (STIs) are infections contracted through sexual activities. There are also diseases of the sexual organs referred to as sexually related diseases (SRDs), which can occur in both sexually active and sexually abstinent individuals.

- Chlamydia is the most prevalently reported STI. More than 1.3 million cases were reported in 2010, more than four times the number of gonorrhea cases reported. Symptoms are often asymptomatic, although men may notice pain or burning during urination and women may notice a vaginal discharge and abdominal pain.

- Gonorrhea is the second most reported STI. In 2010, almost 309,000 cases were reported. Males are more likely to experience symptoms from gonorrhea infection than are females. Males may experience frequent and painful urination and a discharge of pus from the urethra. Females are usually asymptomatic, although some may notice a yellowish discharge.

- Syphilis rates declined in 2010, the first time since 2000. Initial symptoms include the development of a lesion (chancre), which disappears in 2 to 4 weeks. Soon afterward, a rash, fever, and some hair loss can occur. If syphilis goes untreated, blindness, paralysis, brain damage, and death are possible.

- Among viral causes of STIs are human papillomavirus (HPV), which is associated with the development of genital warts and cervical cancer. Vaccines are available, and one of them, Gardasil, can prevent as much as 70% of cervical cancers, 80% of anal cancers, and 90% of genital warts caused by HPV. Other viral causes of STIs include herpes simplex virus (HSV), which is associated with the development of genital herpes, and hepatitis B virus (HBV), which is associated with the development of hepatitis B.

- Sexually related diseases include vaginal infections (such as trichomoniasis and candidiasis) and ectoparasitic infections (such as pubic lice and scabies).

- Among the means of preventing or minimizing the risk of developing an STI are sexual abstinence, maintaining a monogamous sexual relationship, reducing the number of sexual partners, refraining from the use of alcohol or other drugs, and using latex condoms.

Discussion Questions

1. What are STIs, how are they transmitted, and what are the reasons for their prevalence?

2. What are the bacterially based STIs? Include their incidence, transmission, symptoms and complications, and diagnosis and treatment in your answer.

3. What are the virally based STIs? Include their incidence, transmission, symptoms and complications, and diagnosis and treatment in your answer.

4. What are the ectoparasitic infestations? Include their incidence, transmission, symptoms and complications, and diagnosis and treatment in your answer.

5. List the key ways to prevent STIs, evaluating the theoretical and user effectiveness of each in the real world.

Application Questions

Reread the chapter-opening story and answer the following questions.

1. Jessica chose to ask her human sexuality professor about her potential STI. Why didn't she go to the student health clinic or her primary care physician?

2. The author describes several of the "private" conversations students wish to have with human sexuality professors, concerning pregnancy, abuse, sexual disorders, and STIs. Where on your campus (or in your community) could you go for help for each of these problems? Be specific, creating a list with phone numbers.

3. Should professors discuss personal sexuality issues with students? Explain why or why not.

Critical Thinking Questions

1. Applications for marriage licenses in Mississippi require a blood test for syphilis but not for the other STIs. Because many STIs are asymptomatic, should marriage tests require testing for all the major STIs? What difficulties would implementing such a program involve? (Hint: Consider how each disease is diagnosed.)

2. How can undetected STIs affect fetuses and newborns?

3. Criminal laws generally provide that someone who deliberately inflicts harm on another person should be punished. Civil laws allow the victim to seek compensation for harm done. Should people who know they are infected with STIs but who have unprotected sex with others and infect them be prosecuted? Should the people they infect be able to sue for physical and psychological damages?

Critical Thinking Case

Most of us believe that STIs afflict young people. But STIs strike people of all ages—including senior citizens. People who are widowed or divorced do not become asexual; rather, they usually begin dating new people. In fact, 90% of postmenopausal women remain sexually active.

Dr. Peter Leone, medical director of the Wake County, North Carolina, STI Clinic, says: "Women who are past menopause often think they can't get an STI. People link pregnancy and STI risk. But methods to prevent pregnancy aren't the best ones for preventing STIs. On the other hand, some people think, 'Why should I use a condom? I can't get pregnant.'"

Although the STI incidence rates per 100,000 people has remained low for senior citizens, the number of seniors is growing dramatically. So, even if rates remain low, the number will continue to increase. Consequently, in 2009 people 50 years old and older accounted for 22% of the new AIDS cases and 16.5% of the new HIV diagnoses in the United States (Centers for Disease Control and Prevention, 2011d).

Consider your parents or your parents' friends who are divorced or widowed. How could you, as a student in this class, give them information about taking responsibility for their sexual behavior?

Ironically, it seems that senior citizens share the attitude of young people regarding sexual behavior: It cannot happen to me. Explain this attitude. Do young people and seniors have different reasons for their beliefs?

Exploring Personal Dimensionss

Can You Be Assertive When You Need to Be?
To take the necessary actions to prevent contracting an STI, you will have to be assertive: That is, you will need to resist pressure to engage in sexual activity if you choose not to, and you will need to insist on the use of a condom and other safer sex precautions if you decide to engage in sex. Do you have assertiveness skills? To find out, write an assertive response to each of the situations described.

1. You are on a date and your partner insists on engaging in a sexual activity that you decide is not for you at that time. You say:

_____

_____

_____

2. Your partner argues that condoms or latex barriers diminish the sensation. You respond by saying:

_____

_____

_____

3. Your partner states that she or he has been tested for STIs and the test result was negative. Therefore, there are no reasons for using safer sex techniques. You respond by saying:

_____

_____

_____

To be assertive, you need to:

1. Specify the behavior or situation to which the statement refers.

2. Relate your feelings about that situation.

3. Suggest a remedy or what your preference is.

4. Identify the consequences of the change: what will happen if it occurs and what will happen if it does not occur.

Now check your responses and revise them to be consistent with these assertiveness principles.

Suggested Readings

Grimes, J. *Seductive delusions: How everyday people catch STDs.* Baltimore, MD: The Johns Hopkins University Press, 2008.

Handsfield, H. H. *Color atlas & synopsis of sexually transmitted diseases,* 3rd ed. New York: McGraw-Hill Professional, 2011.

Lowy, I. *A woman's disease: The history of cervical cancer.* New York: Oxford University Press, 2011.

Nack, A. *Damaged goods? Women living with incurable sexually transmitted diseases.* Philadelphia, PA: Temple University Press, 2008.

Zenilman, J. M., & Shahmanesh, M. *Sexually transmitted infections: Diagnosis, management, and treatment.* Sudbury, MA: Jones & Bartlett Learning, 2011.

Web Resourcess

For links to the websites below, visit *go.jblearning.com/dimensions5e* and click on Resource Links.

Division of STD Prevention

www.cdc.gov/std

This site provides statistics and reports pertaining to STIs. Among the links are those pertaining to bacterial vaginosis, chlamydia, genital herpes, gonorrhea, hepatitis (viral), HIV/AIDS, human papillomavirus infection, pelvic inflammatory disease, pregnancy and STIs, syphilis, trichomoniasis, and general information about STIs.

American Social Health Association

www.ashastd.org

The American Social Health Association develops and delivers accurate, medically reliable information about STIs. ASHA publishes educational pamphlets and books for clients and students. It helps community-based organizations communicate about risk, transmission, prevention, testing, and treatment of STIs. Links to statistics, prevention tips, and information about particular STIs are included on this website.

National Center for HIV/AIDS, Viral Hepatitis, STD, and TB Prevention

www.cdc.gov/nchhstp/

This division of the CDC is responsible for public health surveillance, prevention research, and programs to prevent and control HIV infection and AIDS, other STIs, viral hepatitis, and tuberculosis. The website offers links to reports that include up-to-date information on the above listed topics.

Navigating HPV

www.arhp.org/hpv-tool

This interactive tool allows both males and females to select information on HPV that is appropriate to their age and circumstances. It also offers information on prevention, treatment, and the HPV vaccines.

STD Wizard

www.stdwizard.org

This interactive tool has visitors provide personal information about their sexual health and then creates recommendations for testing and relevant vaccination based on the details provided. While not a substitute for a visit to a healthcare provider, the results can help identify needs and familiarize someone with the questions a healthcare provider will ask to assess risk and needed medical attention.

References

American Cancer Society. Cervical Cancer Overview, 2011. Available: http://www.cancer.org/acs/groups/cid/documents/webcontent/003042-pdf.pdf.

American College of Obstetrics and Gynecologists. Committee on Adolescent Health Care and Committee on Gynecologic Practice. Committee Opinion No. 506: Expedited partner therapy in the management of gonorrhea and chlamydia by obstetrician-gynecologists. *Obstetrics & Gynecology, 118, no. 3* (2011), 761–766, 2011.

American Social Health Association. Chlamydia, 2012b. Available: http://www.ashastd.org/std-sti/chlamydia.html.

American Social Health Association. Fast Facts, 2012c. Available: http://www.ashastd.org/std-sti/Herpes/learn-about-herpes.html.

American Social Health Association. Genital Warts, 2012d. Available: http://www.ashastd.org/std-sti/hpv/genital-warts .html.

American Social Health Association. Learn about HPV: Cervical dysplasia, 2012a. Available: http://www.ashastd.org/std-sti/hpv/cervical-dysplasia.html.

American Social Health Association. NGU, 2012e. Available: http://www.ashastd.org/std-sti/ngu.html.

Baker, D., Collins, J., & Leon, J. Risk factor or social vaccine? The historical progression of the role of education in HIV/AIDS infection in sub-Saharan Africa. *Prospects: Quarterly Review of Comparative Education, 38, no. 4* (2009), 467–486.

Bolan, G. A., Sparling, P. F., & Wasserheit, J. N. The emerging threat of untreatable gonococcal infection. *New England Journal of Medicine, 366* (2012), 485–487.

Centers for Disease Control and Prevention. *Sexually transmitted diseases surveillance, 2008,* 2009. Available: http://www.cdc.gov/STD/stats08/chlamydia.htm.

Centers for Disease Control and Prevention. Oral sex and HIV risk, 2009a. Available: http://www.cdc.gov/hiv/resources/factsheets/oralsex.htm.

Centers for Disease Control and Prevention. Scabies frequently asked questions, 2010a. Available: http://www.cdc.gov/parasites/scabies/gen_info/faqs.html.

Centers for Disease Control and Prevention. Seroprevalence of herpes simplex virus type 2 among persons aged 14–49 years—United States, 2005–2008. *Morbidity and Mortality Weekly Review, 59, no. 15* (2010b), 456–459.

Centers for Disease Control and Prevention. Sexually transmitted diseases treatment guidelines 2010, 2010c. Available: http://www.cdc.gov/std/stats10/surv2010.pdf.

Centers for Disease Control and Prevention. Syphilis—CDC fact sheet, 2010d. Available: http://www.cdc.gov/std/syphilis/STDFact-Syphilis.htm.

Centers for Disease Control and Prevention. Updated to CDC's Sexually Transmitted Diseases Guidelines, 2010: Oral cephalosporins no longer a recommended treatment for gonococcal infections. *Morbidity and Mortality Weekly Report, 61, 31* (2012f), 590–594.

Centers for Disease Control and Prevention. Viral hepatitis: Information for gay and bisexual men, 2010e. Available: http://www.cdc.gov/hepatitis/Populations/PDFs/HepGay-FactSheet-BW.pdf.

Centers for Disease Control and Prevention. 2010 sexually transmitted diseases surveillance, 2011a. Available: http://www.cdc.gov/std/stats10/surv2010.pdf.

Centers for Disease Control and Prevention. ACIP recommends all 11- to 12-year-old males get vaccinated against HPV: Press Briefing Transcript, 2011b. Available: http://www.cdc.gov/media/releases/2011/t1025_hpv_12yroldvaccine.html.

Centers for Disease Control and Prevention. Condoms and STDs: Fact sheet for public health personnel, 2011c. Available: http://www.cdc.gov/condomeffectiveness/latex.htm.

Centers for Disease Control and Prevention. HIV surveillance report, 2009; vol. 21, 2011d. Available: http://www.cdc.gov/hiv/topics/surveillance/resources/reports/.

Centers for Disease Control and Prevention. National and state vaccination coverage among adolescents aged 13 through 17 years—United States, 2010. *Morbidity and Mortality Weekly Report, 60, no. 33* (2011e), 1117–1123.

Centers for Disease Control and Prevention. Trichomoniasis statistics, 2011f. Available: http://www.cdc.gov/std/trichomonas/stats.htm.

Centers for Disease Control and Prevention. Genital herpes—CDC fact sheet, 2012a. Available: http://www.cdc.gov/std/herpes/STDFact-herpes.htm.

Centers for Disease Control and Prevention. Genital HPV infection—fact sheet, 2012b. Available: http://www.cdc.gov/std/HPV/STDFact-HPV.htm.

Centers for Disease Control and Prevention. Hepatitis B FAQs for health professionals, 2012c. Available: http://www.cdc.gov/hepatitis/HBV/HBVfaq.htm.

Centers for Disease Control and Prevention. Legal status of expedited partner therapy (EPT), 2012d. Available: http://www.cdc.gov/std/ept/legal/default.htm.

Centers for Disease Control and Prevention. Ready-to-use STD curriculum for clinical educators: Gonorrhea module, 2012e. Available: http://www2a.cdc.gov/stdtraining/ready-to-use/Manuals/Gonorrhea/gonorrhea-notes-8-2012.pdf.

Corey, L., Wald, A., & Patel, R., et al. Once-daily valacyclovir to reduce the risk of transmission of genital herpes. *New England Journal of Medicine, 350* (2004), 11–20.

Greenberg, J. S. *Comprehensive stress management,* 11th ed. New York: McGraw-Hill Higher Education, 2009.

Hargreaves, J. R., & Glynn, J. R. Educational attainment and HIV-1 infection in developing countries: A systematic review. *Tropical Medicine and International Health, 7, no. 6* (2002), 489–498.

Jenkins, W. D., Weis, R., Campbell, P., Barnes, M., Barnes, P., & Gaydos, C. Comparative effectiveness of two self-collected sample kit distribution systems for chlamydia screening on a university campus. *Sexually Transmitted Infections, 88* (2012), 363–367. doi: 10.1136/sextrans-2011-050379.

Kaiser Family Foundation. The HPV vaccine: Access and use in the U.S., 2011. Available: http://www.kff.org/womenshealth/upload/7602-03.pdf.

Krashin, J. W., Koumans, E. H., Bradshaw-Sydnor, A. C., Braxton, J. R., Secor, W. E., Sawyer, M. K., & Markowitz, L. E. *Trichomonas vaginalis* prevalence, incidence, risk factors and antibiotic-resistance in an adolescent population. *Sexually Transmitted Diseases, 37, no. 7* (2010), 440–444.

McClelland, R. S., Sangare, L., & Hassan, W. M., et al. Infection with *Trichomonas vaginalis* increases the risk of HIV-1 acquisition. *Journal of Infectious Disease, 195* (2007), 698–702.

Ohnishi, M., Golparian, D., Shimuta, K., Saika, T., Hoshina, S., Iwasaku, K., Nakayama, S., Kitawaki, J., & Unemo, M. Is *Neisseria gonorrhoeae* initiating a future era of untreatable gonorrhea? Detailed characterization of the first strain with high-level resistance to ceftriaxone. *Antimicrobial Agents and Chemotherapy, 55, no. 7* (2011), 3538–3545.

Palefsky, J. M. et al. HPV vaccine against anal HPV infection and anal intraepithelial neoplasia. *New England Journal of Medicine, 365* (2011), 1576–1585.

Peters, E., Baker, D., Deickmann, N., Leon, J., & Collins, J. Explaining the education effect on health: A field-study from Ghana. *Psychological Science, 21, no. 10* (2010), 1369–1376.

Presidential Commission for the Study of Bioethical Issues. "Ethically Impossible": STD research in Guatemala from 1946 to 1948, 2011. Available: http://bioethics.gov/cms/sites/default/files/Ethically-Impossible_PCSBI.pdf.

Ryder, N., Jin, F., & McNulty, A. M., et al. Increasing role of herpes simplex virus type 1 in first-episode anogenital herpes in heterosexual women and younger men who have sex with men, 1992–2006. *Sexually Transmitted Infections, 85* (2009), 416–419.

Su, J. R., & Weinstock, H. S. Epidemiology of co-infection with HIV and syphilis in 34 states, United States, 2009. Paper presented at the August 2011 National HIV Prevention Conference, Atlanta, GA. Available: http://www.2011nhpc.org/archivepdf/2011%20NHPC%20Final%20Abstract%20Book.pdf.

Sutcliffe, S., Newman, S. B., Hardick, A., & Gaydos, C. A. Prevalence and Correlates of *Trichomonas vaginalis* infection among female U.S. federal prison inmates. *Sexually Transmitted Diseases, 37, no. 9* (2010), 585–590.

Sutton, M., Sternberg, M., Koumans, E. H., McQuillan, G., Berman, S., & Markowitz, L. E. The prevalence of *Trichomonas vaginalis* infection among reproductive-age women in the United States, 2001–2004. *Clinical Infectious Diseases, 45, no. 10* (2007), 1319–1326.

Van Der Pol B, Kwok C, Pierre-Louis B, et al. *Trichomonas vaginalis* infection and human immunodeficiency virus acquisition in African women. *Journal of Infectious Disease, 197*:548–54, 2008.

HIV and AIDS

FEATURES

Multicultural Dimensions
AIDS Among Asian Americans

Ethical Dimensions
Should HIV Testing Be Mandatory for Pregnant Women?

Global Dimensions
AIDS in Africa

Gender Dimensions
Women and AIDS

CHAPTER OBJECTIVES

 Describe acquired immunodeficiency syndrome (AIDS), the opportunistic diseases associated with it, and the way in which the human immunodeficiency virus (HIV) invades the body and causes AIDS.

 Discuss different treatments for HIV infection and AIDS, including how the mortality rate has declined as a result of these treatments.

 Cite ways in which HIV infection can be prevented.

go.jblearning.com/dimensions5e

Prevention of HIV Infection and AIDS
Global Dimensions: AIDS in Africa
HIV and College Students
Gender Dimensions: Women and AIDS

INTRODUCTION

Tom applied for a graduate assistantship in our department and, because of his impressive academic record and the nature of his experiences, was awarded one. He was a pleasure to have around, always smiling and willing to help in whatever way he could. Because of his personality and his conscientiousness Tom's graduate assistantship was extended into the next year and several years thereafter.

It was during his fourth year with us that Tom began losing weight and missing some days at school. Attributing it to the flu or a similar condition, no one seemed to take much notice—that is, until Tom started missing even more days and looking emaciated. Before long, the rumor spread that Tom had AIDS and did not have long to live. Unfortunately, the rumor was true and before many more months, Tom died.

With today's new medications and combination of medications, Tom might be alive today. Or at least he would have lived longer with HIV than he did. Of course, that troubles those of us who knew and cared for Tom. However, other issues are also troubling. Until he told us, we did not even know Tom was gay. He contracted HIV through unprotected sex. Why did he feel the need to hide his identity, and how much torment did that hiding create? More to the point, what did we (the department, the faculty, the university, and the society at large) convey to Tom that led him to conclude we would reject him if we knew about his sexual orientation and HIV status? And how many others are in a situation similar to Tom's and are in torment as he was?

We hope that this chapter, by presenting information about HIV and AIDS, will help us all become more understanding of those who are wrestling with not only the physical and psychological effects of HIV infection, but also the social consequences.

■ Acquired Immune Deficiency Syndrome (AIDS)

Acquired immune deficiency syndrome (AIDS), so named because it attacks and slowly destroys the body's immune system, was first identified by American physicians in mid-1981. At that time, physicians noted the unusual occurrence of five cases of *Pneumocystis carinii* pneumonia among previously healthy homosexual men in Los Angeles. Soon thereafter, reports surfaced of a rare form of cancer, Kaposi's sarcoma, also among young homosexual men in New York and California. These observations led to the recognition of AIDS, a disease characterized by **opportunistic diseases** in an immune-compromised individual. Diseases such as *P. carinii* pneumonia and Kaposi's sarcoma are labeled opportunistic because they rarely occur in young healthy individuals, instead relying on the opportunity presented by a depressed immune system. AIDS is considered a syndrome because it is characterized by a range of opportunistic diseases, rather than one particular disease (Table IF4.1).

Research conducted by Robert Gallo at the National Institutes of Health and by Luc Montagnier and colleagues at the Pasteur Institute in Paris led to the discovery of a new virus believed to cause AIDS. Gallo named the virus human T-lymphotropic virus type III (HTLV-III); Montagnier identified it by the name lymphadenopathy-associated virus (LAV). In May 1986 the International Committee on Taxonomy of Viruses announced its recommendation that the virus be consistently identified by the name **human immunodeficiency virus (HIV)** (AIDS virus gets new name amid feuding, 1986). Today we know that HIV is the cause of AIDS.

HIV belongs to a special class of viruses called **retroviruses**. Retroviruses consist of a protein shell surrounding the genetic material ribonucleic acid (RNA) (Figure IF4.1). For HIV to attack a human cell, it must first attach itself to a special receptor on the cell's surface. In humans HIV attaches to CD4 lymphocytes, a type of white blood cell that plays an important role in the immune response to disease. Once attached to the CD4 cell (also called T4), HIV enters the cell and releases its RNA. The RNA is then converted into DNA by an enzyme (reverse transcriptase) also carried by HIV. This HIV DNA combines with the cell's DNA, causing the cell to reproduce HIV (Figure IF4.2). In essence, HIV converts the cells it attacks into factories producing HIV, which then go on to infect other

acquired immune deficiency syndrome (AIDS)
A syndrome caused by the human immunodeficiency virus (HIV), characterized by a depressed immune system and the presence of one or more opportunistic diseases.

opportunistic diseases
A major manifestation of AIDS, diseases that occur in the presence of a suppressed immune system.

human immunodeficiency virus (HIV)
A retrovirus that causes AIDS.

retroviruses
A group of viruses consisting of ribonucleic acid (RNA) surrounded by a protein coat that can convert their RNA into deoxyribonucleic acid (DNA) once they have invaded a living cell, allowing them to take over the cell and reproduce themselves.

TABLE IF4.1 AIDS-Defining Conditions*

Cancers
- Invasive cervical cancer
- Kaposi's sarcoma
- Lymphoma, multiple forms

Fungal Infections
- Candidiasis of bronchi, trachea, esophagus, or lungs
- Cryptococcosis
- Histoplasmosis
- *Pneumocystis carinii* pneumonia

Protozoan, Spore, and Parasite Infections
- Cryptosporidiosis, chronic intestinal (greater than 1 month's duration)
- Coccidioidomycosis
- Isosporiasis, chronic intestinal (greater than 1 month's duration)
- Toxoplasmosis of brain

Viral Infections
- Cytomegalovirus disease (particularly CMV retinitis)
- Herpes simplex: chronic ulcer(s) (greater than 1 month's duration); or bronchitis, pneumonitis, or esophagitis
- Progressive multifocal leukoencephalopathy

Bacterial Infections
- *Mycobacterium avium* complex
- Tuberculosis
- *Salmonella* septicemia, recurrent

Other conditions
- Encephalopathy, HIV-related
- Pneumonia, recurrent
- Wasting syndrome due to HIV

* If someone has HIV and one or more of these opportunistic infections, the person will be diagnosed with AIDS regardless of CD4 count.

Source: Data from Department of Health and Human Services. (2010). Available: http://www.aids.gov/hiv-aids-basics/staying-healthy-with-hiv-aids/potential-related-health-problems/opportunistic-infections/

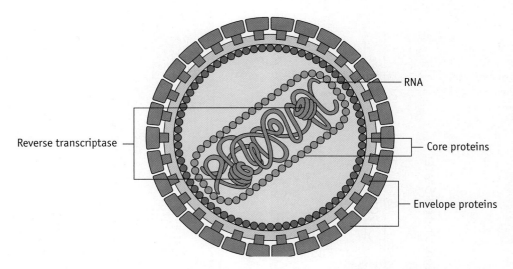

FIGURE IF4.1 HIV consists of an outer shell, or protein envelope, that surrounds a protein core that protects the ribonucleic acid (RNA) and the enzyme reverse transcriptase.
Source: Reproduced from *FDA Consumer* (October 1987), 10.

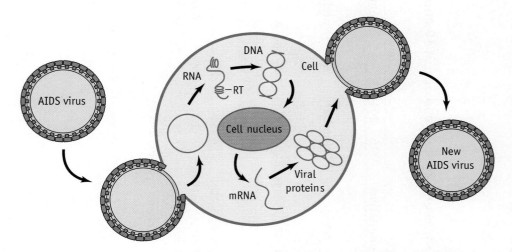

FIGURE IF4.2 HIV infection and replication in a human cell. The virus enters the cell and releases RNA, its genetic material. Using the enzyme reverse transcriptase (RT), the virus converts its RNA into deoxyribonucleic acid (DNA), which enters the cell nucleus and combines with the cell DNA. The cell's altered genetic material then produces messenger RNA (mRNA), which codes for new virus.
Source: Reproduced from *FDA Consumer* (October 1987), 10.

CD4 cells. As this process progresses, CD4 cells are destroyed and the body becomes unable to defend itself against organisms that would normally be no threat to health. Thus the opportunistic diseases that characterize AIDS infect the individual, usually leading to death.

Incidence of HIV and AIDS

As noted in Table IF4.2, through December 2010, more than 1.1 million adults and adolescents had acquired AIDS in the United States (Centers for Disease Control and Prevention, 2012b). HIV infection disproportionately affects African Americans. Despite representing only 14% of the U.S. population in 2010, African Americans accounted for 46% of all new HIV infections that year. Black men accounted for 70% of the estimated new HIV infections among all blacks, which means that the rate of new HIV infection for black men was more than 7 times as high as that of white men and 2.5 times as high as that of Latino men or black women. Most (88%) black women with HIV acquired HIV through heterosexual sex (Centers for Disease Control and Prevention, 2012b).

TABLE IF4.2 Estimated AIDS Cases by Transmission Category and Sex, 2010 and Cumulative, United States

Adult or Adolescent Transmission Category	Males				Females				Total			
	2010		Cumulative		2010		Cumulative		2010		Cumulative	
	Number	%	Number	%	Number	%	Number	%	Number	%	Number	%
Male-to-male sexual contact	16,796	68%	541,330	61%	--	--	--	--	16,796	51%	541,330	48%
Injection drug use	2,745	11%	186,122	21%	1,752	21%	88,400	39%	4,497	14%	274,522	25%
Male-to-male sexual contact and injection drug use	1,446	6%	79,048	9%	--	--	--	--	1,446	4%	79,048	7%
Heterosexual contact	3,629	15%	74,708	8%	6,364	77%	131,904	58%	9,993	30%	20,6612	18%
Other*	133	1%	11,851	1%	127	2%	6,289	3%	260	1%	18,140	2%
Total**	24,749		893,059		8,243		226,593		32,992		1,119,652	

* Includes hemophilia, blood transfusion, perinatal exposure, and risk factor not reported or identified
**Totals may not equal 100% due to rounding

Source: Modified from Centers for Disease Control and Prevention. (2012). HIV Surveillance Report, 2010; vol. 22. Available at: http://www.cdc.gov/hiv/topics/surveillance/resources/reports.

In the United States, HIV affects different age groups at different rates. In 2010, young people between 15 and 29 years of age accounted for 35% of all new HIV infections, but only accounted for 21% of the U.S. population in 2010. In fact, those aged 20–24 had the highest number and rate of HIV diagnoses of any age group (36.9 new HIV diagnoses per 100,000 people) in 2010 (Centers for Disease Control and Prevention, 2012b).

Although the death rate from HIV infection increased steadily from 6 per 100,000 in 1987 to 17 per 100,000 in 1995, it dropped for the first time to 11.1 per 100,000 in 1996. It has continued to decline ever since (see Figure IF4.3). This drop was primarily a result of new treatments, although education campaigns may have played a part. It is in no small part related to the increased funding for HIV and AIDS research, which increased dramatically over the years.

The global issue of HIV has stabilized in recent years. The annual number of new HIV infections has been declining since the late 1990s, and because of increased access to antiretroviral therapy there are fewer AIDS-related deaths. Although the number of new infections has been decreasing, overall, new infection rates are still high and, with the significant reductions in mortality, the number of people living with HIV in the world has increased (Joint United Nations Programme on HIV/AIDS, 2010).

At the end of 2010, an estimated 34 million individuals were living with HIV infection. Most of these are in sub-Saharan Africa (about 22.9 million), with another 4 million in South and Southeast Asia, 1.5 million in Eastern Europe and Central Asia, 1.5 million in Central and South America, and 200,000 in the Caribbean. In North America, there were approximately 1.3 million people living with HIV in 2010. Worldwide, new infections in 2010 were estimated to be 2.7 million, a decrease from the 3.1 million in 2001. Although this decrease is impressive, it still means that over 7,000 new HIV infections occurred every day in 2010. The number of AIDS-related deaths worldwide remained at 1.8 million in 2010 (the same rate as 2001), but there is great variance between regions. Death rates decreased in most areas, while Eastern Europe, Central Asia, and East Asia experienced an increasing number of HIV-related deaths (Joint United Nations Programme on HIV/AIDS, 2011.)

In contrast to the incidence in the United States, where most of the cases of HIV are the result of same-sex sexual contact among men, the majority of HIV infections in other regions of the world are the result of heterosexual contact.

Transmission

HIV is found in large concentrations in two human body fluids: semen and blood. This is related to the large number of white blood cells present in these body fluids. It appears that a concentration of HIV is probably necessary for the transmission of HIV from one individual to another. Thus the most common modes of transmission are those that involve the exchange of semen or blood between individuals. Unprotected penile–vaginal or anal sex with an infected individual is the most common way that infected semen is transmitted. About half of the estimated AIDS cases in the United States involve men who have sex with men (Table IF4.2). While sexual risk—specifically not using a condom during anal sex, and alcohol and drug use that increase this behavior—is the greatest concern, there are other contributing factors. Stigma and homophobia may have a profound impact on the lives of men who have sex with men (MSM) and affect their decision making. Racism, poverty, and lack of access to health care

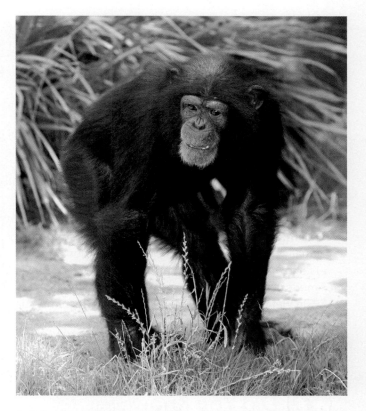

In February 1999, Dr. Beatrice Hahn of the University of Alabama at Birmingham announced that she had tracked HIV's ancestor to a virus that has long infected *Pan troglodytes*, a subspecies of African chimpanzees. In an effort to help human HIV patients, researchers are looking into why the monkeys do not appear to become sick from the virus.

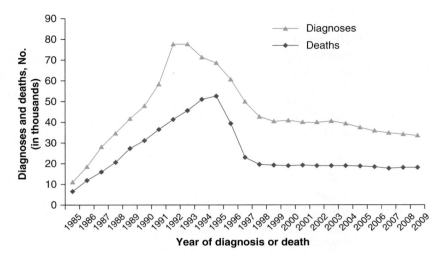

Note: All displayed data have been statistically adjusted to account for reporting delays, but not for incomplete reporting. Deaths of persons with an AIDS diagnosis may be due to any cause.

FIGURE **IF4.3** AIDS diagnoses and deaths of adults and adolescents with AIDS, 1985–2009—United States and dependent areas.
Source: Reproduced from Centers for Disease Control and Prevention. (2012). HIV Surveillance—Epidemiology of HIV Infection (through 2010), Slide 22. Available at: http://www.cdc.gov/hiv/topics/surveillance/resources/slides/general/index.htm

Multicultural DIMENSIONS

AIDS Among Asian Americans

The incidence of AIDS in the Asian American community is assumed to be small. However, there are problems with this assumption. For example, when Asian Americans are grouped together, diverse ethnic and racial subgroups are ignored. There are 28 Asian subgroups and 20 Pacific Islander subgroups. Chinese and Filipinos make up the two largest Asian subgroups, followed by Japanese, Asian Indians, and Koreans. The result is that certain subgroups actually have a high incidence of HIV infection and others a low incidence. For example, in 2002, 16% of Asian Americans with AIDS were born in the Philippines and 7% in Vietnam, whereas only 2% were born in Cambodia and South Korea, and fewer yet (1%) were born in Laos (Zaidi et al., 2005). Grouping Asian American subgroups together conceals the need for intervention in particular subgroups. In addition, shame often prevents Asian Americans who are infected from revealing that fact to their families and friends, thereby falsely lowering the apparent incidence rate. Furthermore, language barriers sometimes prevent Asian Americans from communicating their HIV status to health providers and authorities who maintain health data.

It is estimated that by the year 2050, the Asian American population will have increased to 8% of the total U.S. population (U.S. Census Bureau, 2008). If this projection is accurate, there will be more than 34 million Asian Americans in the United States by the year 2050. It is time that HIV and AIDS in the Asian American community be studied more systematically and interventions adopted as necessary.

? Did You Know . . .

Do mosquitoes transmit HIV? Scientific experiments have shown that HIV does not multiply in insects such as biting flies, mosquitoes, and bedbugs (Centers for Disease Control and Prevention, 2010a). Additionally, it has been noted that the mouths of such insects cannot hold enough blood of one person to be capable of infecting another person. Epidemiological evidence also supports the hypothesis that transmission by insects does not occur.

are barriers to HIV prevention services. A CDC study (2012a) found a strong link between socioeconomic status and HIV among MSM: prevalence increased as education and income decreased. In addition, complacency about HIV among young MSM may affect risk-behavior. Given that young MSM did not experience the severity of the early HIV epidemic, some may falsely believe that HIV is no longer a serious health threat because of treatment advances and decreased mortality (Centers for Disease Control and Prevention, 2012a).

Of the estimated adult/adolescent AIDS cases in 2010, approximately 30% appear to be related to heterosexual transmission. In the United States, this transmission category includes individuals who reported heterosexual contact with a person known to have, or to be at high risk for, HIV infection. Heterosexual transmission is of particular concern to women—for them, 77% of the 2010 estimated cases were transmitted by heterosexual contact compared to only 14.6% of male cases (Centers for Disease Control and Prevention, 2012b). Many women who become infected with HIV through heterosexual contact have partners who are injecting drug users. Women in this category are not necessarily injecting drug users themselves; they become infected through sexual intercourse with partners who are.

The transmission of HIV related to injecting drug use is also of concern. Through December 2010,

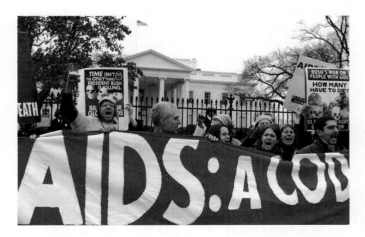

The efforts of the gay community to garner media attention for the HIV and AIDS crisis brought it to the forefront of the U.S. medical agenda during the 1980s. Because of these efforts, HIV and AIDS research and medical funding garnered a far greater percentage of government spending than it would otherwise have, which resulted in a significant reduction of HIV incidence in the mainstream gay community. Unfortunately, within the gay community, gay men are currently experiencing a resurgence of the HIV and AIDS epidemic. Despite the efforts of both the gay and mainstream communities and tremendous scientific advances in treatments for the virus, this crisis is far from averted.

injecting drug use was associated with HIV transmission in 13.6% of the estimated AIDS diagnoses. Infection occurs through the sharing of needles contaminated with HIV. Additionally, these injecting drug users can transmit the virus to their sexual partners through penile–vaginal or anal sex and, in the case of female injecting drug users, to their infants prenatally or postnatally.

Between 1979 and mid-1985, HIV transmission through blood transfusions was of great concern to health professionals and the public. In the spring of 1985 an HIV antibody test was approved by the FDA for the purpose of screening blood donations. **Antibody** tests do an excellent job of protecting the U.S. blood supply from contamination with HIV. There is, however, still a slight risk that the test will miss HIV antibodies (resulting in a false negative test result). Additionally, the test may not detect HIV-infected blood because a person who is infected with HIV may not produce a detectable level of antibodies for up to 3 months after infection. It must be emphasized that this risk is very small. In 1987, the CDC and American Red Cross reported that the risk of contracting HIV through a blood transfusion was 1 in 28,000. Today, more rigorous screening of donors and nucleic acid testing have decreased the risk of contracting HIV through a blood transfusion to 1 in 1.5 million (based on 2007–2008 data) (Zhou et al., 2010). There is no risk of becoming infected with HIV by donating blood.

The risk of contracting HIV (or other infectious diseases, such as hepatitis B or C) is slightly higher for those receiving an organ donation. Nucleic acid testing (NAT) is often performed for procedures that involve a living donor (such as a kidney transplant). In these cases, it is critical to conduct testing as close as possible to the surgery date to ensure the most accurate results for the recipient. However, there is some debate about the risk and the need for NAT in other circumstances because of a possible loss of donor organs. Evidence suggests a higher false positive rate of NAT when performed under the conditions required for organ donation than reported by the blood donation community, and these organs may then not be used when in reality they represent no risk (Ison & Nalesnik, 2011). The transplant community does not recommend universal prospective screening of organ donors for HIV (or hepatitis C and B) using NAT, but the Centers for Disease Control and Prevention does encourage the use of these tests (Humar et al., 2010; Kuehnert, 2011).

antibodies
A class of proteins secreted by the immune system that bonds with antigens. Antibodies fight off disease-causing organisms.

AIDS and the Gay Community

Originally, AIDS was discovered in gay men. Of course, it was soon realized that risky behavior is associated with HIV infection, not one's sexual identity or one's country of origin. (For example, Haitians were targeted with discriminatory immigration regulations because of the relatively high incidence of AIDS in Haiti.) However, given the high incidence of HIV infection among men who have sex with men, much effort has been made to educate gay and bisexual men about safer sex practices. Unfortunately, MSM are still disproportionately affected and infected by HIV. While MSM account for 2% of the population, they accounted for 61% of the estimated new HIV infections in 2010 (Centers for Disease Control and Prevention, 2012b).

Not to be overlooked is the effect of the lobbying efforts by the gay community—males and females—for increased funding for AIDS research and more rapid approval of drugs with the potential for treating HIV infection and AIDS. As more and more people, including celebrities (for example, Rock Hudson, Keith Haring, Freddy Mercury, and Greg Louganis) contracted HIV, the alarm was sounded throughout the gay community and beyond. That alarm led the way to successful local and national lobbying efforts. When compared to that for other diseases, funding for AIDS research far exceeds its ranking in terms of deaths or incidence, a direct result of the gay community's involvement. Imagine what the status of treatment for HIV and AIDS would be today—not to mention the advancements on the horizon—without the gay community's efforts.

Stages of HIV Infection

Once an individual is infected with HIV, the natural course of the infection progresses in three stages. The first stage is **silent infection**. This stage is an asymptomatic period during which the only evidence of infection is the presence of HIV antibodies. The development of antibodies takes at least 2 weeks, and it is often 6 to 8 weeks before antibody levels are high enough to be detected by antibody tests.

> **silent infection**
> A stage of HIV infection characterized by no symptoms other than the presence of HIV antibodies.

Some infected individuals (it is not known how many) progress to the second stage of infection—**symptomatic infection**. This stage consists of several general signs and symptoms, the most prominent of which is persistent swelling of the lymph glands, especially in the neck, armpits, and back of the mouth. Other common signs include fatigue, unexplained weight loss, night sweats, persistent fever, and diarrhea. Many infected individuals have no signs or symptoms.

AIDS is the final stage of HIV infection. People at this stage have badly damaged immune systems. In order for a person to be diagnosed with AIDS, they must have either a CD4 count below 200 cells/mm^3 or have one of the opportunistic infections listed in Table IF4.1. A normal CD4 count can range from 500 cells/mm^3 to 1,000 cells/mm^3. Figure IF4.4 shows the 2010 AIDS diagnosis rates for the states and dependent areas of United States.

> **symptomatic infection**
> The second stage of HIV infection, characterized by HIV antibodies as well as general signs and symptoms such as swollen lymph glands, fatigue, unexplained weight loss, night sweats, persistent fever, and diarrhea.

Although AIDS is classified as a terminal disease, people now live with AIDS for a long time. Newer medication regimens, accompanied by an enthusiastic research agenda, lead some to conclude that AIDS will be considered a chronic disease (like hypertension and diabetes) that can be controlled, if not eradicated.

Testing for HIV

Several types of HIV tests are available. Traditional testing looks for HIV antibodies in either blood, fluid from the cheek, or urine. The most common screening test is called the EIA (enzyme immunoassay), which identifies the presence of HIV antibodies. If antibodies are present, the person is said to be **seropositive**. If no antibodies are present, the person is said to be **seronegative**. However, even though the test results show that HIV antibodies are present, they may be "false positive." Therefore, once the ELISA finding is positive, a more sensitive, and more expensive, test is administered, the Western blot. If the Western blot result confirms the presence of HIV antibodies, the person can be assured that he or she is infected.

> **seropositive**
> The result of a blood test for antibodies to HIV that indicates that such antibodies have been found in the blood.
>
> **seronegative**
> The result of a blood test for antibodies to HIV that indicates no presence of such antibodies.

Some EIA tests use oral fluids and urine to test for HIV antibodies. These oral-fluid tests require a person to place a flat inch-long cotton swab attached to a stick between the gum and cheek for 2 minutes. The swab draws fluid from the mucous membrane, which contains HIV antibodies if the person is infected. This test does

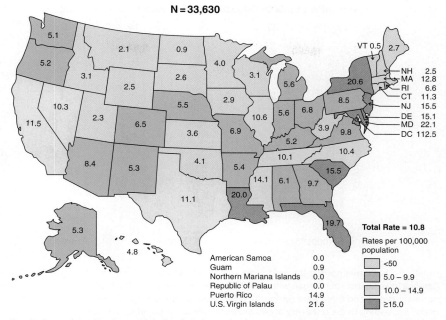

N = 33,630

American Samoa   0.0
Guam   0.9
Northern Mariana Islands   0.0
Republic of Palau   0.0
Puerto Rico   14.9
U.S. Virgin Islands   21.6

Total Rate = 10.8

Rates per 100,000
population

	<50
	5.0 – 9.9
	10.0 – 14.9
	≥15.0

Note: All displayed data have been statistically adjusted to account for reporting delays, but not for incomplete reporting.

FIGURE **IF4.4** Rates of AIDS diagnoses, 2010—United States and dependent areas.
Source: Reproduced from Centers for Disease Control and Prevention. (2012). HIV Surveillance—Epidemiology of HIV Infection (through 2010), Slide 29. Available: http://www.cdc.gov/hiv/topics/surveillance/resources/slides/general/index.htm.

not use saliva. A follow-up confirmatory Western blot uses the same oral-fluid sample.

The sensitivity and accuracy of urine tests for HIV antibodies are less than that of the blood and oral-fluid tests. This EIA antibody test also requires a follow-up confirmatory Western Blot using the same urine sample.

Rapid tests are also available; these are screening procedures that produce results in about 20 minutes. Rapid tests use blood (often from a fingerstick), or oral fluid to look for the presence of antibodies to HIV. As is true for all screening tests, a reactive rapid HIV test result must be confirmed with a follow-up confirmatory test before a final diagnosis of infection is made. These tests have similar accuracy rates as traditional EIA screening tests.

Until 1996, the only way to get tested for HIV was to be tested at a clinic. In 1997, the first home collection kit was approved by the Food and Drug Administration. Today, only two HIV home collection kits are approved and sold legally in the United States (Home Access HIV-1 Test System and Ora-Quick In-Home HIV Test). Although others may advertise and be sold on the Internet, their accuracy cannot be verified. The Home Access kit allows an individual to take a blood sample and send the sample to a laboratory for testing. In July 2012, the Food and Drug Administration approved the first rapid in-home HIV test, OraQuick In-Home HIV Test. The kit tests oral fluid and provides results in 20–40 minutes; there is no need to mail anything. It is approved for sale to individuals 17 years and older. Studies have shown the test to be highly accurate for people who do not have the virus (only 1 false positive result will occur for every 5,000 tests in uninfected individuals). However, the accuracy of this testing mechanism with untrained individuals is lower for individuals who are infected with HIV. There will be 1 false negative result out of every 12 tests performed in HIV-infected individuals (U.S. Food and Drug Administration, 2012b). With both of these tests, a follow-up confirmatory test is needed for any positive results (Centers for Disease Control and Prevention, n.d.).

It should be noted that all of these tests do not directly test for the presence of HIV. Rather, they test for the presence of antibodies produced in response to HIV infection. Thus it is possible that the infection has not yet produced sufficient antibodies to be measured even though the person being tested is infected with HIV. If it is too early for the antibodies to be present in sufficient numbers to be measured, the person can transmit the virus nevertheless.

Total number of new individuals named at each stage of investigation

19   20   24   14   5   8

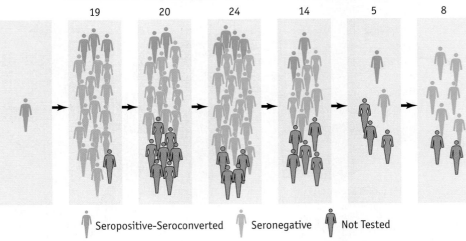

Seropositive-Seroconverted   Seronegative   Not Tested

FIGURE IF4.5 Partner notification programs can be highly productive, as illustrated by results of a South Carolina investigation that began with one HIV-positive man. Of the 19 sexual contacts he named, all but one were tested, and three were seropositive. Those three then named 20 sexual contacts not already identified, leading to the discovery of two more HIV-positive men, who in turn named 24 other previously unidentified contacts, and so forth. When the investigation reached its end point of no new HIV-positive contacts, it had identified a total of 90 persons at risk, tested 68 of them, and found 12 who either were seropositive or seroconverted 6 months after initial testing.

In addition to the tests that detect HIV antibodies, RNA tests are available that look for genetic material of the virus. These tests are used in screening the blood supply and for detection of very early infection cases when antibody tests are unable to detect antibodies to HIV. Because of their high cost, these tests are not commonly used in screening for HIV infection in the United States.

An individual who receives a positive HIV test finding should be given medical and psychological counseling as well as education intended to prevent HIV transmission to others. Additionally, it is important at this time to initiate the process of *partner notification*. Because treatment for HIV is often more successful when initiated early, informing previous partners of their possible infection can potentially help them manage their infection better and also prevent them from unknowingly spreading the infection to others (Figure IF4.5). However, an HIV-infected person may not feel capable of contacting sexual or needle-sharing partners. Many state and local health departments will notify partners without disclosing the name of the infected individual. In fact, some public health programs are utilizing the Internet and other electronic mediums to facilitate this process (National Coalition of STD Directors, 2008).

Treatment of HIV and AIDS

In 1987 the FDA approved **zidovudine** (brand name Retrovir; formerly azidothymidine [AZT]) as the first drug licensed in the United States for the treatment of AIDS patients. Zidovudine is an antiviral drug that slows the replication of HIV in human cells. Studies indicate that zidovudine not only slows the progression of HIV infection when given in early stages, but also prolongs survival and decreases the incidence and severity of opportunistic infections in people living with AIDS.

While somewhat effective by itself, zidovudine is no longer the only antiviral medication to combat HIV infection. There are now six classes of antiretroviral drug therapies (U.S. Department of Health and Human Services, 2011):

1. *Nucleoside/nucleotide reverse transcriptase inhibitors* (for example zidovudine, didanosine, and stavudine): These drugs block the action of reverse transcriptase, thereby preventing HIV RNA from reproducing.

2. *Protease inhibitors* (for example, indinavir, nelfinavir, ritonavir, and saquinavir): These drugs shut down HIV replication by preventing the viral enzyme protease from cutting other viral protein into shorter pieces needed by HIV to make new viral copies for infecting new CD4 cells.

zidovudine
The first drug (brand name Retrovir; also known as AZT) approved by the FDA for the treatment of AIDS. This antiviral drug slows the replication of the AIDS virus, thus slowing the course of the syndrome.

¿? Ethical DIMENSIONS

Should HIV Testing Be Mandatory for Pregnant Women?

If pregnant women are infected with HIV, they can pass on that infection to their babies in utero. Yet, there is a simple way to prevent many of these babies from being born infected. If a pregnant woman receives antiretroviral medications, has an elective cesarean section at 38 weeks of pregnancy, and avoids breastfeeding, the risk of perinatal transmission of HIV drops from 15–25% to less than 2%. For this reason, many physicians and legislators advocate that pregnant women be required to be tested for HIV as part of their routine prenatal care. In that way, the danger to the fetus is identified, and treatment can be administered to the women whose fetuses are at risk.

However, this issue is more complicated than it appears at first glance. For example, if women are required to be HIV tested during prenatal care, many may forgo prenatal care to avoid the test and its possible repercussions. These repercussions may include losing one's job, one's housing, or one's partner. In addition, a woman who lives in a rural area may not be able to find a physician willing to manage her pregnancy and help in the delivery of her child. Avoiding prenatal care places the fetus at risk of being born at low birth weight and/or with a variety of birth defects. Opponents of mandatory testing point out that no other segment of society is required to be HIV tested. Therefore, to require this of pregnant women is to discriminate against these women. There is no disagreement that pregnant women ought to be counseled about the risks and benefits of being tested and that there is a treatment to help prevent their babies from being born infected with HIV even if the mother is infected. But, the choice to be tested for HIV should be the woman's.

Proponents of mandatory HIV testing for pregnant women argue that counseling alone will not persuade enough women to be tested. Too many would choose to avoid testing, and the result would be that too many babies would be born with HIV. To protect the babies, they maintain, women should be required to be tested and their HIV status determined. Only then can pregnant women infected with HIV be administered effective medication, thereby indirectly treating their fetuses. In addition, women who test positive for HIV can be educated about the risk of breastfeeding, another means through which HIV can be transmitted to their babies.

Should the privacy of the mother be protected, or is her privacy less important than the benefits to the fetus? This is not only a policy issue, but also an ethical issue. On which side of this argument do you find yourself?

---

3. *Nonnucleoside reverse transcriptase inhibitors* (for example, delavirdine and nevirapine): These drugs block the reverse transcriptase directly.

4. *Fusion inhibitors* (for example, enfuvirtide): These drugs block HIV from fusing with the CD4 cell.

5. *Integrase strand transfer inhibitors* (for example, raltegravir): These drugs disable integrase, a protein the HIV uses to insert its viral genetic material into the generic material of an infected cell.

6. *CCR5 antagonists* (for example, maraviroc): These types of drug block the entry of HIV into the cells.

In addition to the six classes of antiviral medications, some medications are a combination of two or more anti-HIV drugs from one or more classes of drugs. These medications reduce the number of pills an HIV-infected individual needs to take. Whether taken individually or as a combination pill, the therapy used is called *combination therapy*, or the *AIDS cocktail*. Combination therapy makes sense because it attacks the virus at different steps in the life cycle rather than at one step.

Studies have reported that combination therapy significantly improves the immune system and its ability to fight off infections, which has resulted in a dramatic decrease in opportunistic infections and deaths in both adults and children (Department of Health and Human Services, 2011; Gona et al., 2006; Nesheim et al., 2007).

Early diagnosis is important so individuals can utilize medications that prevent HIV from destroying the immune system. Previously, treatment started when the CD4 count fell to 350 cells/mm^3 or because opportunistic infections began. However, research has shown that it may be easier to maintain higher CD4 counts if HIV treatment is started before the CD4 counts drops that low. Current guidelines recommend antiretroviral treatment if the CD4 count is less than 500 cells/mm^3. Some experts also recommend that HIV-infected individuals with CD4 counts above 500 cells/mm^3 start therapy, while others consider this optional (Department of Health and Human Services, 2011).

Although these medications allow many HIV-infected individuals to live longer and have fewer complications, there are limitations. Some individuals do not tolerate certain drugs well, and the body can develop resistance to some medications, thus new regimens and medication adjustments are often a component of treatment. In addition, toxicity from the medications can affect other body functions.

From a practical standpoint, many of the drugs are expensive. In 2011, the average cost of medications ranged from $300 to $400 per month for some medications to over $3,000 per month for a fusion inhibitor (Berry, 2011b). The total costs for a year average about $20,000 (Gebo et al., 2010). For HIV-infected individuals with low incomes, government assistance may be available through Medicaid and Medicare. In addition, AIDS Drugs Assistance Programs (ADAP), federal- and state-funded programs, provide medication to about one-third of all individuals in the United States receiving HIV treatment (Berry, 2011a). Unfortunately, many states have waiting lists for these programs, and some individuals do not meet program guidelines. In those cases, many pharmaceutical companies also offer co-pay and patient assistance programs to HIV-infected individuals not eligible or not enrolled in other programs (Berry, 2011a). In spite of these programs, the process of obtaining medications and concern about payment for medications can still be challenging for many HIV-infected individuals in the United States. Individuals in other countries often must rely on government programs or pharmaceutical assistance programs for medication. While usage rates of antiretroviral medication are increasing, less than half (47%) of those eligible in middle- and low-income countries (an estimated 14.2 million people) were receiving treatment at the end of 2010 (Joint United Nations Programme on HIV/AIDS, 2011).

■ Prevention of HIV Infection and AIDS

While no cure or vaccine for HIV is currently available, there are both medications and nonmedical strategies for prevention. First, let's review progress towards a vaccine.

HIV Vaccine

At this time, a vaccine for HIV is not available. Historically, vaccines have virtually eliminated spread of infectious diseases such as smallpox, polio, and measles. Because of the success in controlling these other infections, many believe that an HIV vaccine represents the best long-term strategy for ending

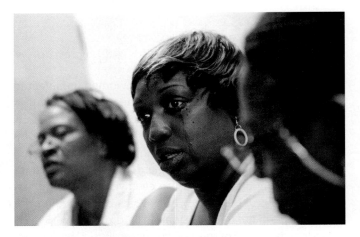

People with HIV must cope not only with the knowledge of their illness but also with society's fear of HIV. Support groups offer emotional support and firsthand advice on coping with the illness.

the HIV pandemic. However, HIV is different from other infectious diseases; the immune system of the human body does not seem capable of effectively preventing the virus from progressing to disease. The most recent vaccine trials have shown moderate success. The "Thai study" tested two different vaccines together, ALVAC-HIV and AIDSVAX, in a primarily low- or moderate-risk group and showed a short-term protective effect against HIV in about one-third of study participants; however, other analyses were not deemed significant (Rerks-Ngarm et al., 2009). Most researchers consider the study's success to be limited. However, given the lack of positive movement toward a vaccine, it provides hope and some direction for future studies. For example, in 2011 another vaccine trial with MSM (at that time the largest ongoing study) increased its participant pool in order to look for the protective changes seen in the Thai study whereas previously the study's primary goal was to determine if the vaccine regimen decreased viral amounts in vaccine recipients who later become infected with HIV (National Institutes of Allergy and Infectious Medicine, 2011).

Pre-Exposure Prophylaxis

While the vaccine efforts have not been successful, studies have demonstrated that the use of antiviral medication before exposure can reduce the risk of becoming infected with HIV. Pre-exposure prophylaxis (PrEP), the daily use of a combined pill of emtricitabine and tenofovir (brand name Truvada) has been shown to decrease the risk of HIV infection in high-risk individuals. Studies have specifically looked at MSM in six different countries (on four continents) and heterosexual men and women in African countries with high rates of HIV. In the MSM study, by taking the pill once a day the risk of HIV infection was reduced by 43.8% on average among men and transgender women who have sex with men and by 72.8% among those with 90% self-reported treatment adherence (Grant et al., 2010). In the heterosexual studies, daily oral doses of Truvada reduced risk 62.6% in one study and 73% in another (Centers for Disease Control and Prevention, 2011a). Daily use of Truvada does have side effects such as nausea, vomiting, and dizziness, but for those truly at risk of HIV because of high-risk sexual practices or because of having an HIV-infected partner, the benefit would likely outweigh those risks. In July 2012, the U.S. Food and Drug Administration approved Truvada as a preventive strategy for healthy people at high risk for acquiring HIV (U.S. Food and Drug Administration, 2012a).

Other Prevention Strategies

In addition to these methods, the best strategy to reduce risk is to refrain from oral, anal, or penile–vaginal sex with an HIV-infected partner and to abstain from sharing needles. This is an important message of HIV and AIDS education efforts—especially for adolescents and young adults who are in a developmental stage at which sexual and drug experimentation is common. Today such experimentation carries the risk of HIV and AIDS.

Abstaining from sexual activity throughout one's life is impractical and undesirable for most people. For those who are uninfected and sexually active, maintaining a mutually faithful monogamous relationship with an uninfected partner prevents the sexual transmission of HIV. Each partner would also need to abstain from sharing needles during drug or steroid use, another high-risk behavior for HIV transmission.

Many people have previously engaged in behaviors that put them "at high risk" of being infected with HIV. People should be considered at risk if they have shared needles or syringes to inject drugs or steroids; are male and have had anal sex (even once) with another male; have had sex with someone they believe may have been infected with HIV; have had another STI; received blood transfusions or blood

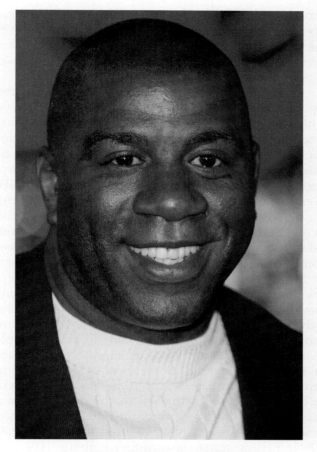

In November 1991, the basketball star Magic Johnson announced that he had acquired HIV infection through unprotected sexual intercourse with an unknown infected woman. Johnson provides living proof of the effectiveness of the AIDS cocktail: The level of HIV in his body has been reduced to an undetectable level.

products between 1978 and 1985; or have had sex with someone who has any of these risk characteristics. In addition, the more sexual partners a person has had, the greater the chances that person will have had contact with an HIV-infected person. The former basketball player Magic Johnson brought this point home to many people when he announced to the world that he was infected with HIV from unprotected

⟨?⟩ Did You Know . . .

Approximately 2.7 million new infections of HIV occurred in 2010, according to the UNAIDS. Of those new infections, 390,000 occurred in children younger than 15 years of age. Furthermore, in 2010 1.8 million deaths occurred worldwide as a result of AIDS. The UNAIDS estimates that an additional 2.5 million deaths have been averted in low- and middle-income countries since 1995 due to antiretroviral therapy being introduced.

sexual intercourse with a woman he could not identify because of his numerous sexual partners over the years. It is important to remember, however, that unprotected sexual intercourse with just one person is risky if that person is infected with HIV.

If an individual decides to engage in sexual activity with a person who is at risk for or is infected with HIV, public health authorities recommend that a condom be used during oral sex on a male, penile–vaginal sex, and anal sex and that latex barriers be used during oral sex on a female. Latex condoms have been shown to be a highly effective barrier to HIV (Centers for Disease Control and Prevention, 2011b).

Yet, even with all the educational efforts and mass attention directed at the issue of condoms and safer sex, studies indicate that many people do not consistently use condoms during penile–vaginal sex. At the time of publication, the largest nationally representative study of sexual and sexual-health behaviors in the United States ever conducted showed that only 1 of 4 acts of vaginal intercourse are condom protected, with a 1 in 3 rate among single people (Sanders et al., 2010). Rates of unprotected anal sex in MSM remain high. Sometimes MSM engage in serosorting—the practice of trying to limit unprotected anal sex to partners with the same HIV status. However, this is not recommended as a safer sex practice, because many MSM are unaware of their HIV-infection status, assumptions about HIV status may not be accurate, some HIV-infected people may not tell their HIV status, and there is still risk for other STIs. For MSM, the most effective way to prevent HIV and other STIs is to avoid anal sex, or when engaging in anal sex, to always use condoms (Centers for Disease Control and Prevention, 2011f). Even if both partners are HIV-infected, engaging in unprotected anal sex poses risk. One individual could be infected with a drug-resistant strain of HIV and transmit that to his partner.

Regarding condom use among adolescents, a 2006–2010 study (Martinez, Copen, & Abma, 2011) showed that 68% of U.S. adolescent females used condoms during their first act of penile–vaginal sex, with less than half (49%) reporting consistent subsequent condom use. The rate for condom use among first time penile–vaginal sex for males was 8 in 10, and consistent condom use among male adolescents was higher than use by females (68%). All of these rates have increased since 2002 (the last time this study was conducted). There were also ethnic differences; black adolescents report the highest rates of consistent condom use, followed by white teens and then Hispanic teens.

Other safer sex strategies are also recommended. If an individual or a sexual partner is at risk for HIV infection, he or she should avoid mouth contact with the penis, vagina, or rectum. Sex with prostitutes should also be avoided, because both male and female prostitutes are often injecting drug users. The possibility of prostitutes having sexual intercourse with high-risk individuals is also great.

Because the current antibody tests for HIV are not 100% accurate, those who are at high risk of HIV infection and those who are known to be infected are asked not to donate blood. Women infected with HIV should strongly consider using birth control to prevent pregnancy, as HIV can be transmitted to the unborn child (see the Ethical Dimensions box on page 643).

Screening tests for HIV are an important preventive tool as an estimated 20% of HIV-infected individuals do not know their status (Centers for Disease Control and Prevention, 2011e). Current recommendations state that healthcare providers screen for HIV in all patients ages 13–64 unless the patient declines the test. The objective is for all individuals to be screened at least once in their life. Individuals at high risk for HIV infection should be screened at least once a year. In addition, HIV testing is recommended for all pregnant women and for any newborn whose mother's HIV status is unknown (Branson et al., 2006). The recommendations include an opt-out standard, meaning that once a patient has been told about the test consent is inferred unless specifically declined. While providers may take this opportunity to counsel about prevention and risky behaviors, counseling is no longer required, because it was seen as a barrier to testing for some individuals. Even for those whose results do not show HIV infection, the testing process can provide a valuable "teachable moment."

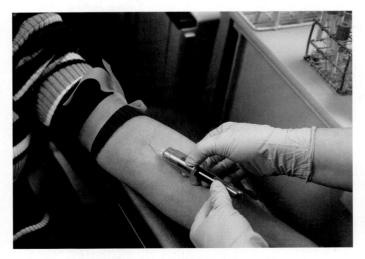

HIV infection is determined by a blood test that looks for antibodies produced in response to HIV. Testing may be accompanied by counseling and education to interpret the results and to discuss ways to prevent infection, or to seek treatment if the test is positive.

Of course, among the ways to prevent the spread of HIV are for those who are infected to let their sexual partners know about their HIV status and to take all the necessary precautions to prevent transmission. Unfortunately, many people do not disclose their status to their partners. Overall rates of disclosure are hard to determine, and study results vary, especially between countries (Arnold et al., 2008; Obermeyer, Baijal, & Pegurri, 2011). A review of U.S. studies showed that 56–81% of individuals disclosed their HIV status to sexual partners, but that rate changed significantly for steady partners (74%) compared to casual partners (25%) (Obermeyer et al., 2011). Given that disclosure can lead to stigmatization and other consequences, it is understandable—though not acceptable—that some HIV infected individuals refrain from informing partners or potential partners. All individuals deserve the right to make informed decisions about the risk of their sexual activities and disclosing an HIV infection, or any other type of chronic STI, allows others that opportunity.

HIV and Young Adults

HIV and AIDS are of particular concern for young adults who have a lot of years left to live. Unfortunately, the HIV infection and AIDS rates for young adults is a growing problem. In 2010, young people aged 13–29 accounted for 35% of all new HIV infections (Centers for Disease Control and Prevention, 2012b). This risk is especially notable for gay, bisexual men, and other MSM and all youth of underserved races and ethnicities. A variety of factors place youth at increased risk, including sexual risk, substance use, and lack of awareness.

Early age at sexual initiation, unprotected sex, and older sex partners are all potential risks for HIV. According to the CDC's 2011 Youth Risk Behavior Survey (YRBS), 47.4% of high school students have had sexual intercourse (YRBS does not specify type of sex), and 6.2% reported first sexual intercourse before the age of 13. Of the 33.7% of students reporting sex during the 3 months before the survey, 39.8% did not use a condom (Centers for Disease Control and Prevention, 2012d). Young people with older sex partners may be at increased risk for HIV because of pressure to not use condoms. CDC data have shown that young gay, bisexual, and other MSM, especially young African American and young Latino MSM, have high rates of new HIV infections. These individuals are less likely to be aware of their HIV infection, and many (approximately 80%) have not received effective HIV interventions or prevention education in the past year. Isolation and lack of support may increase the likelihood of other risk factors, such as risky sexual behaviors (Centers for Disease Control and Prevention, 2011d).

Young people in the United States use alcohol, tobacco, and other drugs at high rates. The CDC's 2011 YRBS found that 21.9% of high school students had consumed five or more drinks of alcohol in a row on at least 1 day during the 30 days before the survey, and 23.1% had used marijuana at least one time during the 30 days before the survey (Centers for Disease Control and Prevention, 2012d). Both casual and chronic substance users are more likely to engage in

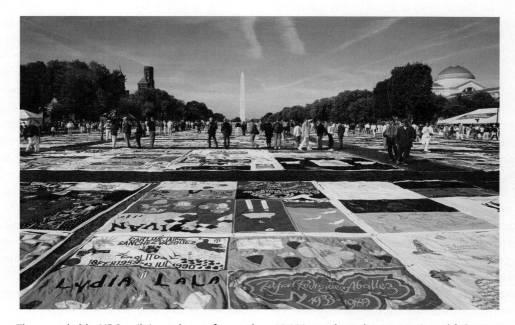

The remarkable AIDS quilt is made up of more than 45,000 panels, each representing a life lost to AIDS. It was created both as a living memorial for those who died and as a brilliant way to help the public visualize the growing toll that AIDS was taking.

high-risk behaviors, such as unprotected sex, when they are under the influence of drugs or alcohol. Runaways, homeless young people, and young persons who have become dependent on drugs are at high risk for HIV infection if they exchange sex for drugs, money, or shelter. There is also a lack of awareness regarding the severity of HIV infection. Research has shown that a large proportion of young people are not concerned about becoming infected with HIV. This lack of awareness can translate into not taking measures that could protect their health (Centers for Disease Control and Prevention, 2011d).

While rates of high-risk sexual behavior among youth have declined from the early 1990s, this decline has stabilized with no significant changes since the early part of the 21st century. For example, although the percentage of students overall who had ever had engaged in sex decreased significantly from 54.1% in 1991 to 47.4% in 2011, the prevalence did not change significantly after 2001 (with a rate of 45.6%). Likewise, the percentage of students who had 4 or more sex partners decreased significantly from 18.7% in 1991 to 14.2% in 2001, but there have been no significant changes since then (including the 2011 rate of 15.3%). Condom use at most recent intercourse follows a similar pattern with a significant increase from the 1991 rate of 46.2% to 63.0% in 2003, but no significant changes since then, including the 2011 rate of 60.2% (Centers for Disease Control and Prevention, 2012c).

Global DIMENSIONS

AIDS in Africa In some areas of Africa, 25% of the population—1 of every 4 people—is infected with HIV. The United Nations reported that at the end of 2010 more than 34 million individuals were HIV-infected and that 68% of those (an estimated 22.9 million) were living in sub-Saharan Africa. Given that this area comprises only 12% of the world's population, the overall effect is devastating (Joint United Nations Programme on HIV/AIDS, 2011).

On the continent, rates of HIV and AIDS range widely between countries. South Africa's epidemic remains the largest in the world, with approximately 5.6 million people living with HIV. Swaziland has the highest adult HIV prevalence in the world at 25.9%. In contrast, the HIV prevalence in West and Central Africa remains comparatively low, with the adult HIV prevalence estimated at 2% or under in 12 countries in 2009.

Although the largest epidemics in sub-Saharan Africa (for example, those in Ethiopia, Nigeria, South Africa, Zambia, and Zimbabwe) have either stabilized or are showing signs of decline, the number of deaths in this area is still high, accounting for 72% (1.3 million) of the total HIV-related deaths in 2009. The increasing availability of antiretroviral treatment has had a profound effect; at the end of 2009, 37% of adults and children eligible for antiretroviral therapy in the region were receiving it, compared with only 2% seven years earlier. However, most people receiving antiretroviral therapy in sub-Saharan Africa start treatment late, which limits the overall impact. In addition, the infrastructure, systems, and staff required to properly monitor treatment retention and loss are becoming increasingly inadequate as the number of people receiving medication increases (Joint United Nations Programme on HIV/AIDS, 2010).

In sub-Saharan Africa, women are disproportionately affected. It is estimated that 40% of all HIV-infected women live in sub-Saharan Africa (Joint United Nations Programme on HIV/AIDS, 2010), which can also affect rates among children. For example, approximately 30% of pregnant women in South Africa are infected with HIV (Health Systems Trust, 2011), and the national transmission rate of HIV from mother to child is approximately 11% (Republic of South Africa, 2010). Not only is the child at risk of contracting the virus prenatally, with the mother (and possibly father) being HIV-infected it is highly likely the child is being born into a family that has already experienced other negative effects of HIV on health, income, productivity, and the ability to care for each other. In South Africa, there are an estimated 1.9 million AIDS orphans, with one or both parents deceased (Joint United Nations Programme on HIV/AIDS, 2010). The HIV/AIDS epidemic is estimated to be responsible for half of the country's orphans (Government of South Africa, 2007) and approximately 70% of the maternal orphans—those who have lost their mother (Budlender et al., 2008).

Theoretically, the rates of HIV infection and death from AIDS should continue to drop as long as there is continued and increased access to antiretroviral medication for those infected or as pre-exposure prophylaxis (PrEP) therapy for those at risk. However, the impact on the family and society of these nations cannot be underestimated.

HIV and College Students

Like adolescents, college students often have the perception that they are not at risk for HIV or other STIs. In reality, some college students are engaging in high-risk behaviors. American College Health Association–National College Health Assessment data from Spring 2011 revealed that 12.4% of male college students and 7.9% of female college students reported having four or more partners in the previous 12 months. For behaviors in the last 30 days, about half of students report engaging in oral (44.9%) or vaginal sex (49.7%) and 5% report engaging in anal sex. Of those engaging in specific behaviors in the previous 30 days, only 5.4% used a condom or latex barrier mostly or always for oral sex, only 51.8% used a condom mostly or always for vaginal sex, and only 31.4% used a condom mostly or always during anal sex. Likewise 16.5% reported having unprotected sex because of alcohol use within the last 12 months (American College Health Association, 2011).

Even more concerning is that individuals who are using condoms may not be doing so correctly. Research has revealed a variety of common condom use errors among adolescents and college students, including inaccurate steps, such as putting the condom on after sex has already started or removing the condom before ending sex; not leaving space at the tip; and placing the condom upside down on the penis and flipping it over (for example Brown et al.,

2008; Crosby et al., 2008; Yarber et al., 2007). Error rates vary, with the highest showing that 93.8% of the adults surveyed reported at least one of nine errors assessed (Topping et al., 2011).

As evidenced by these statistics, too many males and females still engage in unhealthy sexual practices that place them at risk of contracting an STI or becoming infected with HIV. Are college students, who are the most educated people in our society, ready to engage in safer sex? A study of 376 university students concluded that they are not (Dahl, Gorn, & Weinberg, 1997). With the rationale that carrying condoms is the one way to ensure that a condom is available when needed, researchers surveyed college students regarding their likelihood of carrying a condom in different situations (a bar, a concert, a party, and a first date). Part of the study involved the researchers interviewing 346 students (137 females and 209 males) at a university bar known for "fun, cheap beer and ... sex." They offered a five-dollar food coupon for every condom each student possessed. Only 16 students were carrying a condom (less than 5%). What do you think the results of this study would be if conducted today at a bar near your campus?

Why do students not use condoms during sexual activities? A variety of reasons for not using condoms have been identified; these include the belief that condoms reduce pleasure; that their partner would

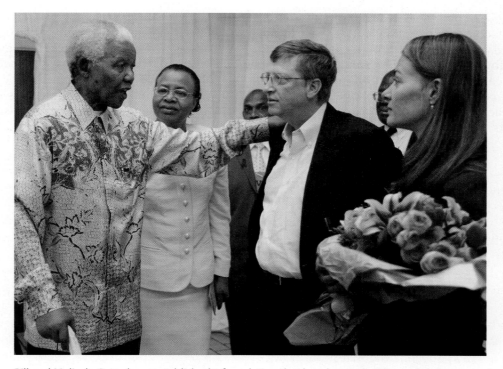

Bill and Melinda Gates have established a foundation that has donated millions of dollars to combat HIV infection and AIDS, especially on the African continent.

Gender
DIMENSIONS

Women and AIDS   AIDS was originally identified as a disease affecting gay men. However, the face of AIDS has changed. Certainly, gay men are still the largest category of those infected with HIV in the United States. Of the new infections in 2010 in the United States, about 21% were among women (Centers for Disease Control and Prevention, 2012b). The global view of HIV is very different; half of all HIV-infected people in the world are women, and more women than men are affected in sub-Saharan Africa (59% of all people living with HIV in that region) and the Caribbean (53%) (Joint United Nations Programme on HIV/AIDS, 2011).

However, in the United States, women need to be aware of their risk. Of the new HIV infections in women in 2010, almost two-thirds (63.5%) occurred in black women. In fact, in 2010 the rate of new HIV infections among black women was almost 20 times that of white women, and more than 4 times the rate among Hispanic/Latina women (Centers for Disease Control and Prevention, 2012b). The lifetime risks show a disproportionate effect on black and Hispanic women. Overall, 1 in 139 women will be diagnosed with HIV infection, but the

rate for black women is 1 in 32. The rate is 1 in 106 for Hispanic/Latina women, 1 in 182 Native Hawaiian/other Pacific Islander women, 1 in 217 American Indian/Alaska Native women, and 1 in 526 for both white and Asian women (Centers for Disease Control and Prevention, 2011c).

Women of color are more likely to contract HIV from a male sexual partner who is infected. Many of these women are also caring for children, which may complicate their treatment. Studies have shown that women infected with HIV are less likely to receive combination therapy and fare more poorly on other access measures than men, often because they have lower incomes, lack transportation, or are too sick to go to the doctor (Kaiser Family Foundation, 2011).

Instituting support groups and community educational campaigns, putting health providers in the community through health clinics and walking of the neighborhoods, and using community health workers to encourage women to seek treatment are ways we can respond to the problem of women and AIDS in the United States.

not approve of condom use; that condoms are not commonly used in their social group; that condoms are embarrassing, hard to discuss, and hard to use; that condoms cause a loss of erection; and that they do not have a condom when sex happens. In addition to these factors, other studies have shown that college students who did not use condoms had high perceptions of invulnerability and low perception of risk associated with their sexual behavior (Thompson et al., 2006). These students also believed they had the ability to identify a partner's HIV status.

With so much at stake in terms of one's health, why do the factors cited seem so insurmountable to many college students and young adults?

Summary

- Acquired immune deficiency syndrome (AIDS) attacks and slowly destroys the immune system, resulting in the development of opportunistic infections such as pneumonia and cancer.

- AIDS is caused by the human immunodeficiency virus (HIV), which is transmitted through the transfer of bodily fluids such as semen, vaginal secretions, and blood. HIV infection is contracted primarily through sexual contact such as penile–vaginal sex, oral sex, or anal sex.

- Although AIDS is still considered a terminal illness, the death rate from this cause has steadily declined since 1996. This decline is predominantly due to new medications that seek to transform AIDS into a manageable chronic illness.

- In the United States most AIDS cases occur among men who have sex with men, although the number of women developing AIDS has increased in recent years. Today, over three-quarters of women who contract HIV infection do so through sexual activity with men.

- There are several tests available to diagnose HIV infection and the eventual development of AIDS. Some screening tests employ blood analysis, whereas others test cheek fluid samples. Two home testing kits have been approved by the FDA for the diagnosis of HIV infection.

- AIDS is treated with one of six classes of antiviral medications: nucleoside reverse transcriptase inhibitors, protease inhibitors, nonnucleoside reverse transcriptase inhibitors, fusion inhibitors, integrase inhibitors, and CCR5 antagonists. Each works on a different aspect of HIV infection, such as preventing HIV from reproducing or preventing HIV from invading the cells.

- Among the safer-sex behaviors to prevent HIV infection are remaining sexually abstinent, being in a sexually monogamous relationship, using a condom or dental dam, and avoiding high-risk behaviors such as anal intercourse.

- College students are particularly vulnerable to HIV infection owing to their relatively frequent sexual activity, their feelings of invulnerability, and the fact that they frequently engage in sexual activities without using a condom.

Discussion Questions

1. Explain the ways HIV is transmitted, the stages of infection, the tests for infection, and how opportunistic diseases occur as a result of AIDS.

2. Which treatments are available for HIV infection? What limits their worldwide availability?

3. List the safer-sex practices that reduce the risk of HIV transmission.

Application Questions

Reread the chapter-opening story and answer the following questions.

1. On June 25, 1998, the Supreme Court ruled that HIV-infected people are protected by a federal ban on discrimination against the disabled—even if they suffer no symptoms of AIDS. If that ruling had been made when Tim was diagnosed with HIV, do you think he might have been more willing to disclose his condition? Why or why not?

2. Regardless of the law, if you were a professor considering granting a graduate assistantship to a student (or an employer making a hiring decision), would the knowledge that the candidate was infected with HIV make a difference? How about if the person were being treated for cancer? Or heart disease? Why should such information make a difference?

3. How would you feel if you knew a fellow classmate or employee were HIV infected?

Critical Thinking Questions

1. Is it fair that the federal government spends a disproportionate share of medical research money on HIV research? Put another way, should federal research money be spent in proportion to the number of people who contract an illness and die of it (such as cancer or heart disease)? Or should the potential threat of a disease becoming more widespread take precedence?

2. You may remember this gender-related issue from another chapter: Men who carry condoms are considered to be "responsible," but women who carry condoms are considered "sluts." Given the need for more condom use to prevent

the spread of STIs and HIV, how can this double standard be overcome?

Critical Thinking Cases

Deciding whether to disclose HIV infection is clearly a troubling decision for anyone to make. But do people have an obligation to disclose that information to protect others?

Consider the case of the two-time double–Olympic diving gold medalist Greg Louganis, who was HIV positive during his second Olympics. Louganis did not disclose his HIV status to Olympic officials. During one dive, Louganis hit the diving board with the back of his head and received a wound that bled. A doctor treated him without knowing of the HIV condition—and thus did not take extra precautions. Also, Olympic competitors are required to supply urine samples to test for illegal substances (such as steroids). Because urine would contain HIV, anyone handling Louganis's sample would have also been at risk unless proper precautions were taken.

Should Louganis have been required to disclose his status before the Olympics? What discrimination may result against an athlete who discloses his or her HIV-infected status? (You may reflect on the problems Magic Johnson faced when he disclosed his status.)

What about typical recreational athletes—people who work out in gyms, play basketball in leagues, fence (saber, epee, or foil), or participate in any recreational activity in which they can be injured accidentally? When do HIV-infected people need to disclose their status?

Exploring Personal Dimensions

Could You Negotiate Safer Sex?

The following items ask you to agree (A) or disagree (D) with the statements presented. Indicate the items about which you are unsure (U) of your response. Compare your responses to those of a friend. Discuss each item about which you said you were unsure of your response. Are there items about which you and a friend disagree? Which changes or adaptations would you or your friend have to make to take on a safer orientation toward sex with a partner?

I believe that . . .

_____ 1. I could use a condom or latex barrier effectively.

_____ 2. I could buy condoms or latex barriers without embarrassment.

_____ 3. If my partner did not want to use a condom or latex barrier during sexual activity, I could convince him or her to do otherwise.

_____ 4. Consumption of alcohol or use of other recreational drugs would in no way affect my determination to use a condom or latex barrier or to convince my partner to respect my wishes.

_____ 5. Having to remember to buy, carry, and use condoms or latex barriers would interfere with sexual spontaneity.

_____ 6. If I suggested using a condom or latex barrier, my partner would think that I must have had many previous sexual partners.

_____ 7. I would feel comfortable insisting on using a condom or latex barrier with a new sexual partner.

_____ 8. I would not feel self-conscious about putting a condom on myself (or on my partner).

_____ 9. I would be able to discuss use of condoms or latex barriers with a partner even before we had any physical intimacy such as touching, caressing, or kissing.

_____10. If I suggested using a condom or latex barrier, my partner would think I did not trust him or her.

_____11. Using a condom during oral, penile–vaginal, or anal sex would interfere with sexual pleasure or sexual functioning.

_____12. Using condoms or latex barriers is an activity primarily for people who have many sexual partners.

_____13. Having to use a condom or latex barrier might subsequently prove to be embarrassing to me or my partner if the mechanics of using one resulted in loss of erection.

_____14. I could tactfully remove and dispose of a condom after sexual intercourse.

_____15. I could convince my partner that use of a condom or latex barrier can be a stimulating part of sexual foreplay.

Suggested Readings

Bartlett, J. G., & Finkbeiner, A. K. *The guide to living with HIV infection: Developed at the Johns Hopkins AIDS Clinic.* Baltimore, MD: Johns Hopkins Press, 2006.

Clark, R. A., Maupin, R. T., & Hayes, J. *A woman's guide to living with HIV infection*, 2nd ed. Baltimore, MD: The Johns Hopkins University Press, 2012.

Gallant, J. E. *100 questions & answers about HIV and AIDS*, 2nd ed. Burlington, MA: Jones & Bartlett Learning, 2012.

Harden, V. A. *AIDS at 30: A history*. Dulles, VA: Potomac Books, 2012.

Piot, P. *No time to lose: A life in pursuit of deadly viruses*. New York: W. W. Norton & Company, 2012.

Skerritt, A. J. *Ashamed to die: Silence, denial, and the AIDS epidemic in the South*. Chicago: Lawrence Hill Books, 2011.

Volberding, P., Greene, W., Lange, J., Gallant, J. E., & Sewankambo, N. (Eds). *Sande's HIV/AIDS medicine: Medical management of AIDS 2012*, 2nd ed. Philadelphia: Saunders, 2012.

Stine, G. *AIDS update 2008*. New York: McGraw-Hill/Dushkin, 2008.

Web Resources

For links to the websites below, visit *go.jblearning.com/dimensions/5e* and click on Resource Links.

AIDS.gov
www.aids.gov

This website has three main objectives: (1) to expand visibility of timely and relevant federal HIV policies, programs, and resources to the American public; (2) to increase use of new media tools to extend the reach of HIV programs to communities at greatest risk; and (3) to increase knowledge about HIV and access to HIV services for people most at-risk for, or living with, HIV. The website includes basic HIV information as well as more complex information regarding strategies for those infected with HIV.

Centers for Disease Control and Prevention: HIV/AIDS
www.cdc.gov/hiv

The Division of HIV/AIDS Prevention of the CDC's National Center for HIV, STD, and TB Prevention maintains this website. It features many differnet resources, including recommendations, guidelines, fact sheets, FAQs, statistics, and materials for prevention and research partners. The CDC also maintains the National Prevention Information Network (CDC NPIN at http://cdcnpin.org/), which features a daily Prevention News Update, reference materials, and referral and distribution services for information on HIV/AIDS, hepatitis, STIs, and tuberculosis.

Henry J. Kaiser Family Foundation: HIV/AIDS
www.kff.org/hivaids/

The Kaiser Family Foundation is dedicated to providing trusted, independent information on the major health issues facing the United States and its people. Its website acts as a clearinghouse of news and information for the health policy community and provides extensive information on both the U.S. and global HIV epidemic, federal actions, and U.S. state HIV/AIDS information.

National Institute of Allergy and Infectious Diseases
www3.niaid.nih.gov

Managed by the federal government, this website presents information pertaining to HIV and AIDS. Links include health and science, research, news and events, the latest news, and research funding.

UNAIDS
www.unaids.org

UNAIDS, the Joint United Nations Programme on HIV/AIDS, works toward achieving universal access to HIV prevention, treatment, care, and support. The website provides country, regional, and global statistics; epidemiological reports; news releases; case studies; and publications on numerous HIV-related topics.

References

AIDS virus gets new name amid feuding, *Medical World News, 27* (1986), 14–15.

American College Health Association. American College Health Association-National College Health Assessment II: Reference Group Executive Summary Spring 2011. Hanover, MD: Author, 2011. Available: http://www.acha-ncha.org/docs/ACHA-NCHA-II_ReferenceGroup_ExecutiveSummary_Spring2011.pdf.

Arnold, E. M., Riceb, E., Flannery, D. & Rotheram-Borus, M. J. HIV disclosure among adults living with HIV. *AIDS Care, 20, no. 1* (2008), 80–82.

Berry, J. It's in the cards: Where to get help to pay for your meds. *Positively Aware* (2011a, March/April), 67–69. Available: http://issuu.com/positivelyaware/docs/2011_march_april_clickable.

Berry, J. The 15th annual HIV drug guide. *Positively Aware* (2011b, March/April), 21–50. Available: http://issuu.com/positivelyaware/docs/2011_march_april_clickable.

Branson, B. M., et al. Revised recommendations for HIV testing of adults, adolescents, and pregnant women in health-care settings. *Morbidity and Mortality Weekly Report, 55*, RR14 (2006), 1–17.

Brown, L. K., DiClemente, R. J., Crosby, R. A., et al. Condom use among high-risk adolescents: Anticipation of partner disapproval and less pleasure associated with not using condoms. *Public Health Reports, 123,* no. 5 (2008), 601–607.

Budlender, D., et al. Developing social policy for children in the context of HIV/AIDS: A South African case study. Children's Institute, University of Cape Town, and the Community Agency for Social Enquiry (2008, December). Available: http://www.ci.org.za/depts/ci/enews/April2009/developing.html.

Centers for Disease Control and Prevention. CDC trial and another major study find PrEP can reduce risk of HIV infection among heterosexuals; CDC assessing data from all heterosexual trials to develop interim guidance for use, 2011a. Available: http://www.cdc.gov/nchhstp/newsroom/PrEPHeterosexuals.html.

Centers for Disease Control and Prevention. Condoms and STDs: Fact sheet for public health personnel, 2011b. Available: http://www.cdc.gov/condomeffectiveness/latex.htm.

Centers for Disease Control and Prevention. HIV among women, 2011c. Available: http://www.cdc.gov/hiv/topics/women/index.htm.

Centers for Disease Control and Prevention. HIV and young men who have sex with men, 2012a. Available: http://www.cdc.gov/HealthyYouth/sexualbehaviors/pdf/hiv_factsheet_ymsm.pdf.

Centers for Disease Control and Prevention. HIV surveillance report, 2010; vol. 22, 2012b. Available: http://www.cdc.gov/hiv/topics/surveillance/resources/reports.

Centers for Disease Control and Prevention. HIV surveillance—United States, 1981–2008. *Morbidity & Mortality Weekly Report, 60,* no. 21 (2011e), 689–693. Available at: http://www.cdc.gov/mmwr/preview/mmwrhtml/mm6021a2.htm?s_cid=mm6021a2_w.

Centers for Disease Control and Prevention. HIV transmission, 2010a. Available: http://www.cdc.gov/hiv/resources/qa/transmission.htm.

Centers for Disease Control and Prevention. National HIV and STD testing resources: Frequently asked questions, n.d. Available: http://www.hivtest.org/faq.aspx#screening.

Centers for Disease Control and Prevention. Serosorting among gay, bisexual and other men who have sex with men, 2011f. Available: http://www.cdc.gov/msmhealth/Serosorting.htm.

Centers for Disease Control and Prevention. Trends in HIV-related risk behaviors among high school students—United States, 1991–2011. *Morbidity and Mortality Weekly Report, 61,* no. 29 (2012c), 556–560. Available: http://www.cdc.gov/mmwr/preview/mmwrhtml/mm6129a4.htm?s_cid=mm6129a4_w.

Centers for Disease Control and Prevention. Youth risk behavior surveillance—United States, 2011. Surveillance summaries, June 8, 2012. *Morbidity and Mortality Weekly Report, 61,* no. SS-4 (2012d). Available: http://www.cdc.gov/mmwr/pdf/ss/ss6104.pdf.

Centers for Disease Control. HIV among youth, 2011d. Available: http://www.cdc.gov/hiv/youth/index.htm.

Crosby, R. A., DiClemente, R. J., Yarber, W. L., Snow, G., & Troutman, A. Young African American men having sex with multiple partners are more likely to use condoms incorrectly: A clinic-based study. *Journal of Men's Health, 2* (2008), 340–343.

Dahl, D. W., Gorn, G. J., & Weinberg, C. B. Condom-carrying behavior among college students. *American Journal of Public Health, 87* (1997), 1059.

Department of Health and Human Services. Guidelines for the use of antiretroviral agents in HIV-1-infected adults and adolescents, 2011. Available: http://aidsinfo.nih.gov/guidelines/html/1/adult-and-adolescent-treatment-guidelines/.

Gebo, K. A., Fleishman, J. A., Conviser, R., Hellinger, J., Hellinger, F. J., Josephs, J. S., et al. Contemporary costs of HIV healthcare in the HAART era. *AIDS 24* (2010), 2705–2715.

Gona, P., Van Dyke, R. B., Williams, P. L., et al. Incidence of opportunistic and other infections in HIV-infected children in the HAART era. *JAMA, 296* (2006), 292–300.

Government of South Africa. HIV and AIDS and STI Strategic Plan for South Africa, 2007–2011, 2007. Available: http://www.info.gov.za/otherdocs/2007/aidsplan2007/index.html.

Grant, R. M. et al., Preexposure chemoprophylaxis for HIV prevention in men who have sex with men. *New England Journal of Medicine, 363* (2010), 2587–2599.

Health Systems Trust. 2010 National Antenatal Sentinel HIV and Syphilis Prevalence Survey in South Africa, 2011. Available: http://www.hst.org.za/publications/2010-national-antenatal-sentinel-hiv-and-syphilis-prevalence-survey-south-africa.

Humar, A., et al., Nucleic acid testing (NAT) of organ donors: Is the 'best' test the right test? A consensus conference report. *American Journal of Transplantation, 10,* no. 4 (2010), 889–899.

Ison, M. G., & Nalesnik, M. A. An update on donor-derived disease transmission in organ transplantation. *American Journal of Transplantation, 11,* no. 6 (2011), 1123–1130

Joint United Nations Programme on HIV/AIDS. Global Report: UNAIDS report on the global AIDS epidemic 2010, 2010. Available: http://www.unaids.org/globalreport/Global_report.htm.

Joint United Nations Programme on HIV/AIDS. UNAIDS World AIDS Day Report, 2011. Available: http://www.unaids.org/en/media/unaids/contentassets/documents/unaidspublication/2011/JC2216_WorldAIDSday_report_2011_en.pdf.

Kaiser Family Foundation. Women and HIV/AIDS in the United States, 2011. Available: http://kff.org/hivaids/upload/6092-09.pdf.

Kuehnert, M. J. CDC: Protect organ transplant patients from unintended disease transmission, 2011. Available: http://blogs.cdc.gov/safehealthcare/?p=1857.

Martinez, G., Copen, C. E., & Abma, J. C. Teenagers in the United States: Sexual activity, contraceptive use, and childbearing, 2006–2010 National Survey of Family Growth. National Center for Health Statistics. *Vital Health Statistics, 23,* no. 31 (2011).

National Coalition of STD Directors. National guidelines for Internet-based STD/HIV prevention—partner services, 2008. Available: http://www.ncsddc.org/sites/default/files/docs/internetpartnerservices.pdf.

National Institutes of Allergy and Infectious Medicine. Bulletin: HVTN 505 HIV vaccine study to expand scope, 2011. Available: http://www.niaid.nih.gov/news/newsreleases/2011/Pages/HVTN505expands.aspx.

Nesheim, S. R., Kapogiannis, B. G., Soe, M. M., et al. Trends in opportunistic infections in the pre- and post-highly active antiretroviral therapy eras among HIV-infected children in the Perinatal AIDS Collaborative Transmission Study, 1986–2004. *Pediatrics, 120* (2007) 100–109.

Obermeyer, C. M., Baijal, P., & Pegurri, E. Facilitating HIV disclosure across diverse settings: A review. *American Journal of Public Health, 101, no. 6* (2011), 1011–1023.

Republic of South Africa. (2010). Country progress report on the declaration of commitment on HIV/AIDS 2010 report. Available: http://data.unaids.org/pub/Report/2010/south-africa_2010_country_progress_report_en.pdf.

Rerks-Ngarm, S. et al., Vaccination with ALVAC and AIDSVAX to prevent HIV-1 infection in Thailand. *New England Journal of Medicine, 361* (2009), 2209–2220.

Sanders, S. A., Reece, M., Herbenick, D., Schick, V., Dodge, B., & Fortenberry, D. Condom use during most recent vaginal intercourse event among a probability sample of adults in the United States. *Journal of Sexual Medicine, 7, s5* (2010), 362–373.

Thompson, S. C., Anderson, K., Freedman, D., & Swan, J. Illusions of safety in a risky world: A study of college students' condom use. *Journal of Applied Social Psychology, 26* (2006), 189–210.

Topping, A. A., Milhausen, R. R., Graham, C. A., Sanders, S. A., Yarber, W. L., & Crosby, R. A. A comparison of condom use errors and problems for heterosexual anal and vaginal intercourse. International *Journal of STD & AIDS, 22, no. 4* (2011), 204–208.

U.S. Census Bureau. *U.S. population projections: National population projections, 2008,* 2008. Available: http://www.census.gov/population/www/projections/summarytables.html.

U.S. Food and Drug Administration. FDA approves first drug for reducing the risk of sexually acquired HIV infection, 2012a. Available: http://www.fda.gov/NewsEvents/Newsroom/PressAnnouncements/ucm312210.htm.

U.S. Food and Drug Administration. First rapid home-use HIV kit approved for self-testing, 2012b. Available: http://www.fda.gov/ForConsumers/ConsumerUpdates/ucm310545.htm.

Yarber, W. L., Graham, C. A., Sanders, S. A., Crosby, R. A., Butler, S. M., & Hartzell, R. M. 'Do you know what you're doing?' College students' experiences with male condoms. *American Journal of Health Education, 38* (2007), 322–331.

Zaidi, I. F., Crepaz, N., Song, R., et al. Epidemiology of HIV/AIDS among Asians and Pacific Islanders in the United States. *AIDS Education and Prevention, 17* (2005), 405–417.

Zou, S., Dorsey, K. A., Notari, E. P., et al. Prevalence, incidence, and residual risk of human immunodeficiency virus and hepatitis C virus infections among United States blood donors since the introduction of nucleic acid testing. *Transfusion, 50* (2010), 1495–1504.

CHAPTER 16

Sexual Dysfunction and Therapy

FEATURES

Gender Dimensions
Sexual Issues for Older Men and Women

Communication Dimensions
Discussing Sexual Dysfunction

Multicultural Dimensions
Sexual Dysfunction and Latino Populations

Global Dimensions
Sexual Disorders Around the World

Ethical Dimensions
Should Surrogates Be Used in Sexual Therapy?

CHAPTER OBJECTIVES

1 Describe the major male and female sexual dysfunctions, including the desire dysfunctions. Evaluate what makes the inability to perform sexually a clinical dysfunction.

2 Identify the multidimensional causes of sexual dysfunction, including the physical, psychological, and sociocultural aspects.

3 Compare and contrast the varied approaches to treating sexual dysfunctions. Explain why many different models of therapy exist.

go.jblearning.com/dimensions5e

Male Sexual Dysfunction
Female Sexual Dysfunction
Treating Sexual Dysfunction

INTRODUCTION

*A*fter he was diagnosed with prostate cancer in 1991, Senator Bob Dole underwent treatment, including surgery. He has since avidly promoted the importance of early detection and encouraged men to speak frankly with their doctors about prostate-related problems.

But it was in May 1998 that Dole made his biggest disclosure: He said on Larry King's talk show that he had been among the men who took part in the trials for the drug Viagra (sildenafil citrate). Viagra is a drug to treat men who have difficulty achieving an erection (erectile dysfunction). In effect, Bob Dole was admitting that he, as do millions of other men, had a sexual dysfunction—specifically, erectile disorder. The next day, Elizabeth Dole, his wife, was asked about the drug during a public appearance. She laughed and said with a beaming smile, "It's a great drug!"

Such public disclosures by celebrities and politicians make taboo topics—such as sexual dysfunctions—the subject of discussion among friends, colleagues, classmates, and even couples. Dole's 1998 public announcement, followed by commercials in March 1999, offered frank and genuine advice: If you have a problem, see a doctor. In the case of erectile disorder, about 80% of problems are physical and can be solved with a prescription or a medical procedure. Other disorders, though, have psychological or sociocultural dimensions at their root.

The Viagra story also touches on the socioeconomic and political dimensions of sexuality. In the 1970s, insurers would not have covered treatments for erectile disorder, because the condition was believed to be psychological. Insurers began coverage as research proved there were physical causes as well. Coverage for Viagra is limited generally to 12 pills per month—the recommended dosage.

When the FDA approved Viagra on March 27, 1998, it was not covered under Medicaid. Thus it was unavailable to those in lower economic brackets. But the political ramifications of denying this wonder drug to the poor caused an uproar. Politicians know that older citizens are more likely to vote. Consequently, many states required Medicaid coverage for Viagra. However, under a law signed by President George W. Bush, as of January 2006, Medicaid no longer covers erectile dysfunction medications, and Medicare stopped coverage as of January 2007, though today some supplemental Medicare drug plans offer it as an added benefit.

Sources: Data from Why is Mrs. Dole smiling? *Washington Post* (May 9, 1998); Postmarketing safety of sildenafil citrate (Viagra), www.fda.gov/cder/consumerinfo/viagra/viagraupdate721.htm; Stark, K. Will insurers pay? Clamor for Viagra could cinch it, *Philadelphia Inquirer* (April 24, 1998).

Sexual Dysfunction

Are you perfect? What seems a silly question has great importance for sexual functioning. Of course, none of us is perfect. And yet, the occasional inability to function sexually (for example, to achieve and maintain an erection or to secrete adequate vaginal lubrication) leads many of us to conclude that something is drastically wrong with us.

This lack of response may be caused by a number of factors that have no bearing at all on your sexual functioning. For example, the ingestion of alcoholic beverages can interfere with sexual response, as can use of drugs such as hypertension medication, narcotics, and barbiturates. In addition, some people have partners with whom it is difficult to respond sexually. For example, your partner may have poor hygiene; he may know so little about sexual physiology that he attempts penile insertion before sufficient vaginal lubrication; or he may touch the scrotum and handle the testicles in a way that causes pain and discomfort. And yet, if the individuals with these sexual partners do not respond as one would expect under more conducive circumstances, they themselves are sometimes accused of having an "abnormality." It might be more accurate to suggest that those who are sexually responsive to dirty, smelly, clumsy sexual partners are the ones experiencing some abnormality.

The media also help to establish unrealistic sexual expectations that, when not met, may lead people to think of themselves as dysfunctional. For example, when movies portray gorgeous specimens of men and women in romantic settings, who seem to have nothing else on their minds but sex, and who are willing and able to engage in any sexual activity that comes to mind, we and our lovers may not measure up. We might conclude something is wrong with us or our love life, although in reality something is wrong with this portrayal. Suffice it to say here that music videos, movies, plays, and advertisements sometimes lead people to decide they are not as sexually adequate as those they see "performing" on satin sheets with unblemished bodies glistening under flattering spotlights.

However, there are people who experience difficulty responding sexually and who wish their sexual responses could be healthier and more sexually satisfying. They may find it difficult to achieve and/or maintain an erection or to relax enough to allow penile penetration. They may ejaculate too soon, or they may experience disturbing pain during coitus. They may wonder why they do not feel sexually aroused enough or do not experience orgasm. Men and women, of all sexual orientations, experience these concerns. They may be young or old, African American or white, well educated or lacking in schooling, and from any socioeconomic group. The one characteristic they have in common, though, is dissatisfaction with their sexual life, and this dissatisfaction often affects other aspects of their relationships.

This chapter explores some of these matters. Specifically, it addresses the types of sexual problems people experience, what causes these problems, and how they can be treated. Notice the difficulty in diagnosing particular sexual dysfunctions (even the experts do not always agree about whether a dysfunction exists) and the varied approaches to treating them once they are identified. This, too, is discussed and its implications explored. We begin with a definition of sexual dysfunction.

sexual dysfunction
A specific, chronic disorder involving sexual performance.

Sexual dysfunction is a chronic inability to respond sexually in a way that one finds satisfying. We do not use the term to describe those situations, common to many people, in which they are temporarily uninterested in sexual activity or unable to respond sexually because of exhaustion, excessive use of alcohol, anger, and so on. The key word in our definition is *chronic*—that is, a consistent long-term inability to respond. It applies both to people who have never had satisfactory sexual relations—lifelong dysfunctions—and to people who have had successful sexual relations at some time but are now having chronic difficulty—acquired dysfunction.

The amount of sexual dysfunction prevalent in society is difficult to determine. As noted earlier, experts may disagree on diagnoses and individuals may not seek treatment. In addition, previous studies focused on rates within married relationships. More recent reports look at individuals' experiences regardless of relationship status and include international studies. The 2004 and 2010 consensus reports estimate that 40–45% of adult women and 20–30% of adult men have at least one sexual dysfunction (Lewis et al, 2010; Lewis et al, 2004). For both men and women, the probability of sexual dysfunction occurring increases directly with age; however, distress about sexual issues seems to decrease with age as well (Connora et al., 2011; Lewis et al., 2010). A study examining U.S. adults between 40 and 80 years old indicated that many individuals experienced sexual problems, but less than 25% sought help for the issue (Laumann et al., 2009). Table 16.1 details the study's findings for particular disorders.

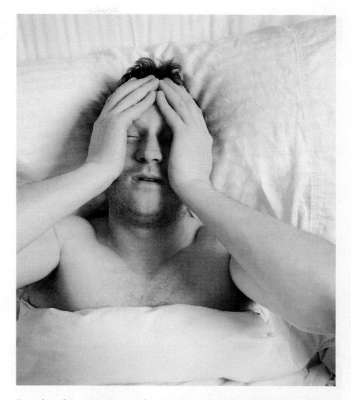

People who experience chronic sexual dysfunction often feel shameful and inadequate. Yet, there are successful treatments for most sexual dysfunctions, whether they are caused by physical or psychological factors.

The underlying cause of any sexual dysfunction may be either organic (physiological) or nonorganic (psychological). Psychological causes, broadly defined, are much more prevalent. More studies are demonstrating that sexual dysfunction may be a result of other medical problems (Berman et al., 2001), and some researchers are concerned that there has been a medicalization of sexual health and sex therapy (Bradley & Fine, 2009; Farrell & Cacchioni, 2012; Marshall, 2012; Tiefer, 2010). *Medicalization* is the process of transforming a personal experience or social situation into one that requires treatment and care by a medical professional. Medicalization may prevent the underlying and causative issues surrounding sexual disorders from being addressed. In 2000, Leonore Tiefer led a group of advocates to reframe ideas about women's sexual dysfunction. Instead of focusing on the physiological processes (often related to Masters and Johnson's sexual response cycle), Tiefer and associates take a more contextual

TABLE 16.1 **Prevalence of Sexual Problems in U.S. Men and Women (ages 40–80)***

Type of Dysfunction	Men (%)	Women (%)
Pain experienced during sex	3.1	12.7
Sex not pleasurable	11.2	19.7
Unable to experience an orgasm	12.4	20.7
Lack of interest in sex	18.1	33.2
Reaching climax too quickly	26.2	N/A
Unable to maintain an erection	22.5	—
Trouble lubricating	—	21.5

*Percentage includes responses of occasional, periodic, and frequent.
Source: Data from Laumann, E. O., Glasser, D. B., Neves, R. C. S., & Moreira, E. for the GSSAB Investigators' Group. A population-based survey of sexual activity, sexual problems and associated help-seeking behavior patterns in mature adults in the United States of America. *International Journal of Impotence Research, 21* (2009), 171–178. doi: 10.1038/ijir.2009.7.

Gender DIMENSIONS

Sexual Issues for Older Men and Women

Contrary to common belief, older people remain sexually active. Still, as with younger men and women, older men engage in sexual activity more often than do older women. In a large scale study[1] of the sexual behavior and health of older Americans, it was found that 84% of men and 62% of women between ages 57 and 64 participated in a sexual activity with a partner at least once during the previous year. Furthermore, although sexual activity declined as respondents got older, 39% of men and 17% of women between ages 75 and 85 still reported engaging in sexual activity with a partner at least once during the previous year.

Older men and women also differed in the sexual problems they experienced. The most prevalent sexual problems experienced by older women were low sexual desire (43%), insufficient vaginal lubrication (39%), and an inability to achieve an orgasm (34%). The most common sexual problems experienced by older men were erectile dysfunction (37%), lack of interest in sex (28%), premature ejaculation (28%), and performance anxiety (27%).

[1]Lindau, S. T., Schumm, L. P., Lauman, E. O., Levinson, W., Muircheartaigh, C. A., & Waite, L. J. A study of sexuality and health among older adults in the United States. *New England Journal of Medicine, 357, no. 8* (2007), 762–774.

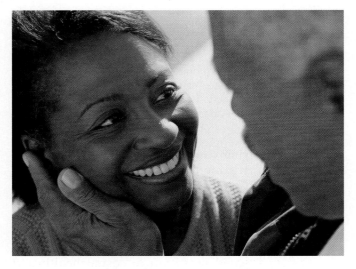

Although the elderly are often perceived as asexual, that is far from the truth. Almost half of adults 60 years of age and older report engaging in sexual activity at least once a month.

approach. The group advocated that women's sexual disorders be framed within four categories: sexual problems resulting from (1) sociocultureal, political, and economic factors; (2) partner and relationship factors; (3) psychological factors; and (4) medical factors (The Working Group on A New View of Women's Sexual Problems, 2000). We applaud the authors' efforts to reconceptualize female sexual dysfunction and to encourage us as sexual health consumers to critically think about labels, context, and the influence of pharmaceutical companies on our lives. As sexuality educators, we also believe students need to be familiar with the existing ideas and terminology about sexual dysfunction and present that

information in this chapter, beginning with sexual dysfunctions experienced by men.

Male Sexual Dysfunctions

Sexual dysfunction in males can be traumatic. In Western culture, gender role expectations dictate that men be experienced and talented in matters of sex. The burden of this expectation is felt most strongly when men have sexual difficulties. In addition to the stress of the sexual dysfunction, they can experience a range of other psychological problems related to self-esteem, feelings of incompetence, and questioning of masculinity.

In addition to the impact on psychological health, the relationship can also be affected. A man may not want to initiate or participate in sexual activity when the results may be failure or a demonstration of ineptness. Only a masochist would allow himself to be placed in such a situation continually and, consequently, his initiation of sexual activity may become sporadic. His partner may perceive this lack of interest as a reflection on his or her attractiveness, as a result of sexual activity outside of the relationship, or some other cause—all of which can affect the relationship as a whole.

However, sexual dysfunction does not have to be exclusively negative. Involvement in sex therapy has been shown to improve ideas about sex and sexual functioning in some aspects. Some studies have shown that even minimal strategies, such as reading materials provided by a sex therapist, can improve sexual functioning (van Lankveld, 2009). Even without therapy, in many cases the sexual dysfunction can be an opportunity for partners to communicate more clearly and openly about their sexual needs and desires. It can also serve as a chance to explore sexual activities that had not been considered previously.

Men experience five main types of sexual dysfunctions: erectile dysfunction, early ejaculation, delayed ejaculation, genital pain, and hypoactive sexual disorders.

Erectile Dysfunction

A man's difficulty in achieving and maintaining an erection used to be called impotence. This term is Latin and means "without power." The word *impotence* is used to connote that a man has lost power—is no longer "manly"—when he cannot achieve or maintain an erection. Furthermore, he has lost power as a lover and has lost his reproductive capacity. Today, the more professional, more sensitive, and more accurate term is **erectile dysfunction**. Men who are unable to achieve or maintain erections may be satisfying lovers; they may be very effective at oral sex or manual masturbation, or other activities.

> **erectile dysfunction**
> The inability of a man to obtain on maintain an erection during sexual activity.

Studies of Western countries estimate that 1 in 5 men will experience erectile dysfunction during their lifetime; however, only a small percentage may experience the issue frequently (Segraves, 2010b). As men age, they are more prone to experience erection problems. A review of epidemiological studies shows rates of 1–10% for individuals younger than 40 years of age, but for those 60–69 years old the rate increases to 20–40%, and for men in their 70s and 80s the rate jumps to 50–100%, depending on the study (Lewis et al, 2010).

> **lifelong erectile dysfunction**
> A condition in which an adult male has never had an erection sufficient to engage in sexual activity.
>
> **acquired erectile dysfunction**
> A condition in which an adult male has previously had an erection sufficient to engage in sexual activity but no longer has.

Men who have never had an erection sufficient to have sexual activity have **lifelong** (or early onset) erectile dysfunction. Men who have previously been able to maintain an erection long enough to have sexual activity but subsequently have an erection problem have **acquired** (late-onset) **erectile dysfunction**. Acquired erectile dysfunction is more prevalent than lifelong, which is extremely rare (Gambescia, Sendak, & Weeks, 2009). Understanding if the condition is generalized (in that it happens in all circumstances) or situational (in that it

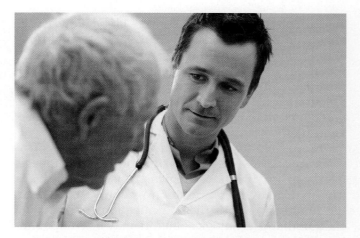

It used to be thought that erectile dysfunction was the result of psychological factors. It is now known that most erectile dysfunctions are the results of physical maladies such as clogged penile arteries.

only happens in some contexts) is also critical. For example, a male who can achieve and maintain an erection during masturbation may not be able to maintain an erection when attempting penetration. This situational disorder would be considered a dysfunction, assuming that it was persistent and caused distress, even though he can maintain an erection in some contexts.

Making a precise diagnosis of erectile dysfunction is not as easy as it might appear. Many men—even college age men—are at times unable to have an erection or lose it before penetration. They may be uninterested in their partner; they may have drunk too much alcohol, which depresses the central nervous system; or they may be using medication that interferes with the erectile reflex. Infrequent erectile difficulties are not cause for alarm. In most cases, the condition needs to be present for 3 to 6 months and occurring 75% of the time for a diagnosis of a dysfunction. Newer definitions also incorporate distress or discomfort about the condition; previously sexual disorders were diagnosed on stringent criteria even if the person was not concerned. Today, incorporating the needs and wants of the individual is an important process in diagnosing a disorder, because some men are not distressed by the condition (Segraves, 2010b). If a condition is persistent and troubling to you or your partner, then you should seek professional help. If it does not bother either of you, then there is no cause for alarm.

The cause of erectile dysfunction can be psychological, physiological, or some combination of psychological and physiological. As men age and experience cardiovascular problems, the likelihood of experiencing erectile dysfunction increases. Although there are a variety of organic causes, approximately

70% of physical causes relate to blood flow issues (Ghanem & Porst, 2006). Neurological conditions and hormonal conditions can also affect erectile functioning (Gambescia, Sendak, & Weeks, 2009). Modifiable physical factors that affect cardiovascular functioning have been linked to erectile dysfunction; these include smoking, poor diet, lack of exercise, and obesity.

Since the advent of Viagra and other medications to address erectile dysfunction, the emphasis has been on the physiological causes. While it is true that many men are able to improve their erectile functioning with these medications, researchers caution that psychological factors may be compounding the issue and that treatment with a combination of physiological and psychological methods is most effective (Althof, 2010; Segraves, 2010b).

Some novel ways to diagnose the causes of erectile dysfunction exist. For example, knowing men normally have erections during their sleep, physicians sometimes place electronic devices around the flaccid penises of men with erection problems while they sleep to determine the presence and frequency of erections (Spark, 2008). If a problem exists during

sleep, the cause is organic. A man who is concerned about an erection problem but who does not yet want to consult a physician or counselor can place a ring of postage stamps around his penis before going to sleep. If the stamps are placed snugly around the flaccid penis and an erection occurs, the ring of stamps will be broken in the morning. Of course, this method is not foolproof, because men may not experience erections during REM (rapid-eye movement) sleep every night.

Early Ejaculation

Early ejaculation, or premature ejaculation, is a common sexual dysfunction in men. It is estimated that 8–30% of men worldwide experience early ejaculation (Lewis et al., 2010). However, as with some of the other dysfunctions, this condition is not easily defined. Years ago, early ejaculation meant the man could not maintain penile insertion without ejaculating within a minimal amount of time (for example, 2

> **early ejaculation**
> Persistent or recurring ejaculation before the person wishes it during partnered sexual activity.

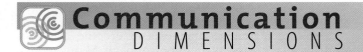

Communication
DIMENSIONS

Discussing Sexual Dysfunction

Two people who love and care for each other can deal with sexual dysfunction together. The key to the resolution of this situation, however, lies in the total relationship, not just the sexual part. Sexual communication is just one form of communication. If the relationship is characterized by ineffective communication in general, assuming that communicating about sex will be different is unrealistic. So, the first step in resolving sexual problems is to develop a relationship of caring, concern, mutual respect, and understanding. For this reason, some sex therapists work with clients to improve their interaction in general and concurrently help them respond to their sexual concerns.

Assuming that the relationship is minimally communicative, the first step is to provide support for each other and the promise of hope: "That's okay, honey; we'll get help and work it out." "It's not that I care any less for you, sweetheart, but something's interfering with my sex-making right now." This form of communication can reduce partners' anxieties that may be interfering with sexual function. Imagine the embarrassment

of experiencing a sexual dysfunction and the resulting pressure during each subsequent sexual encounter. The fear of "failure" and the anticipation of disappointing one's partner can be so frustrating that they can feed on themselves, contributing to, and exacerbating, the sexual problem. Communicating that it is okay, that help can be obtained, that the problem will be faced together, and that there is a commitment to work to make matters better can go a long way in intervening between dysfunctional feelings and resulting dysfunctional sex.

Once counseling starts, the couple needs to continue communicating with each other but now must also begin communicating with the counselor. To be effective, communication with the counselor must be candid. Without candor, the source of the problems may never be uncovered, or at least it will take longer to discover. A commitment is then required to adhere conscientiously to the treatment regimen and remain with it until the problem is resolved.

Certainly, sexual dysfunction puts a strain on both people involved, but caring, supportive lovers can become even closer through facing this problem and overcoming it.

minutes) or could not perform a minimal number of penile thrusts before ejaculating. Masters and Johnson (1970) even proposed a definition that the man's partner had to be satisfied in at least 50% of their coital episodes or it was considered premature. Helen Singer Kaplan (1974) defined premature ejaculation as the man's inability to control his ejaculate voluntarily.

The problems with these definitions were several. The couples in these studies differed in their perception of what was too soon. Some couples were perfectly happy for coitus to last a short period, whereas other couples were dissatisfied with only 2 minutes of insertion or a minimal number of penile thrusts. In addition, Masters and Johnson's definition overlooked the fact that some women do not experience orgasms during coitus and would not achieve orgasm, regardless of the timing of their partner's ejaculation. Kaplan's definition neglected to recognize that men, as a rule, do not possess total voluntary control over ejaculation; this definition would classify most men as sexually dysfunctional.

Newer research considers the desires of the couple in the definition of early ejaculation. For example, one definition divides early ejaculation into a continuum ranging from ejaculation before penile insertion to ejaculation 7 minutes after insertion (Schover et al., 1982). The ejaculate is not classified as early, however, unless the man or his partner considers it to be so. We define early ejaculation as a condition in which the man ejaculates before he wants to or before his partner wants him to during partnered sexual activity.

Unfortunately, the research on early ejaculation focusses on heterosexual men and penile–vaginal sex. Little is known about gay and bisexual men's experiences of early ejaculation or men who engage in other behaviors besides vaginal sex (Segraves, 2010a).

Delayed Ejaculation

For some men, the problem is not ejaculating too soon, but rather being unable to ejaculate at all. This condition is known as **delayed ejaculation**, formerly referred to as retarded ejaculation or ejaculatory incompetence. Delayed ejaculation has a relatively low prevalence—approximately 3% (Perelmen & Rowland, 2006). When a man has never ejaculated after sufficient sexual stimulation and is incapable of doing so, he is classified as having lifelong delayed ejaculation. When he has previously been able to ejaculate but can no longer do so, he is classified as having acquired delayed ejaculation. These men may still be able to maintain an

delayed ejaculation
A condition in which a male is unable to ejaculate or there is marked delay in ejaculation after sufficient sexual stimulation.

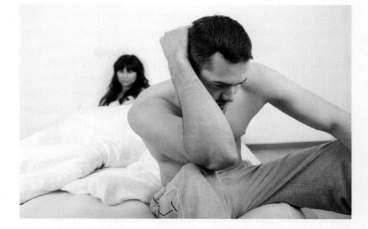

Pain during sex may be caused by infection of the sexual organs or by allergic reactions to spermicidal creams or foams used by their partner.

erection and/or stay sexually aroused. Or they may be able to ejaculate through masturbation. Sometimes, though rarely, this condition can be specific to only one partner or to specific situations.

Another form of delayed ejaculation is called partial ejaculatory incompetence. This condition results in a "half" orgasm—that is, a seepage of semen without true orgasmic sensations. Kaplan (1974) writes of men who, when fatigued or in conflict, "come without realizing they have." This condition appears to be relatively uncommon, even compared to delayed ejaculation.

Delayed ejaculation is a disorder that may have interesting side effects. For example, the ability to maintain penile insertion for long periods without ejaculating may be valued by many men and appreciated by their sexual partners. However, the extreme of being unable to ejaculate at all can result in the partner's questioning her or his own sexual abilities. In this case, the benefit of prolonged insertion quickly dissipates, and frustration and doubt set in. Another side effect is that when the man fakes orgasm to prevent his partner from feeling inadequate, not only does he remain sexually unsatisfied, but deceit, rather than trust and openness, can begin to characterize the relationship as a whole. As with many of the other sexual dysfunctions, treatment must be directed at the relationship as well as at the specific disorder.

Genital–Pelvic Pain

Painful sexual penetration (formerly called dyspareunia) has not been studied extensively in men. Epidemiological studies show prevalence rates ranging from 1–6% (Lewis et al., 2010). During sexual penetration, men may feel pain in the penis, testes, or some other part of the body. Causes of genital pain can be both organic and nonorganic. For example, infections of the penis, foreskin, testes, urethra, or prostate can cause pain. Some men report irritation of the glans caused by an intrauterine device (IUD) string that extends out of the uterus into the vagina.

Other causes of genital pain in men include a foreskin that is too tight and causes pain when an erection develops; smegma (a cheeselike substance secreted by the glans penis) that has not been washed away from the glans penis and causes an infection and/or irritates the glans; and Peyronie's disease, in which fibrous tissue and calcium deposits develop in the area around the cavernous bodies of the penis and may cause pain.

Hypoactive Sexual Desire Disorder in Men

Because of cultural expectations, we often expect men to always want sex. In reality, men may not have a desire for sex. Worldwide 1 in 4 men experience lack of desire or interest in sexual activity (Lewis et al., 2010), though this rate does drop considerably when asked if it is a persistent condition lasting 6 months or more (Brotto, 2010a). This condition, called **male hypoactive sexual desire disorder** (HSDD) (previously called inhibited sexual desire), is characterized by a lack of interest in sexual activity or specific sexual activities, for example, vaginal sex, oral–genital sex, or even sexual fantasizing. As with other conditions, it is considered a dysfunction if the condition causes marked distress or interpersonal difficulty. Without this component it would be extremely difficult to determine a diagnosis. Because each person's interest in sexual activity varies, when is too little interest really too little? When the lack of interest is specific to a sexual partner, is it the partner's fault?

We often compare ourselves—and our relationships—to others. However, when it comes to sexual issues it is important to focus on the context of the relationship. If the degree of interest between two people in a relationship is similar, and the relationship is otherwise healthy, should the couple be concerned? Or should a therapist advise them that they have a problem? Should the therapist attempt to change the couple's degree of interest? What happens when one partner has more interest in a specific activity than the other partner? For example, should an uninterested partner engage in oral sex to satisfy the interest of the partner? Does this situation need to be corrected? These are not easy questions to answer, but they are questions that many individuals struggle with in their relationships.

Male HSDD can have both psychological and organic causes. Low testosterone levels have been weakly associated with male HSDD (although the

> **male hypoactive sexual desire disorder**
> A disorder characterized by a lack of interest in sexual activity or specific sexual activities.

effect seems more prominent in younger men); some medications may also affect desire (Weeks, Hertlein, & Gambescia, 2009). Depression (Brotto, 2010a; Weeks et al., 2009), anxiety, inaccurate beliefs about sex, poor body image, a tendency to fuse sex and affection, and career overload have also been linked with HSDD risk (Weeks et al., 2009). One additional explanation has been proposed by Bancroft and colleagues (2009). Their concept, the dual-control model, postulates that sexual activity is regulated by two competing processes in the brain: the sexual excitation system and the sexual inhibition system. While individuals vary in their predisposition for both sexual excitation and sexual inhibition, most fall in a range that is nonproblematic. However, if those levels are not in normal ranges, arousal disorders or sex addiction (hypersexuality) could develop. For example, individuals with a low predisposition for sexual excitation and/or a high propensity for sexual inhibition could develop an arousal disorder or hyposexuality. Those with a high propensity for excitation and/or low propensity for inhibition may be more likely to engage in high-risk sexual behaviors, like those exhibited with sex addiction (Bancroft et al., 2009).

Female Sexual Dysfunctions

It wasn't too long ago that females were first allowed to express their sexual needs and to be viewed as entitled to sexual satisfaction at the same level as men. However, a double standard is still alive and well. Some men consider women suspect if they initiate sexual activity or are vocal in appreciating it. They are still supposed to be coy, letting the man take the lead, for fear of what might be thought of them if they act too assertively. Given this situation, too many women have adopted a passive attitude toward sexual activity and sometimes have developed shame, guilt, or embarrassment about their sexual behavior. For some women, this has progressed into an inability to function in a sexually healthy and satisfying way. Women may experience sexual dysfunctions in the following areas: sexual interest/arousal disorder in women, female orgasmic disorder, and genital and pelvic pain disorder.

Sexual Interest/Arousal Disorder in Women

While the Masters and Johnson sexual response cycle starts with excitement, the precursors—desire and interest in sex—are critical components. Years ago, in order to be diagnosed with a desire disorder, women had to lack a physical response, such as a lack of vaginal lubrication or vasocongestion. Today, criteria for the disorder include more subjective components of the sexual experience (Brotto, 2010b). For example, women with **sexual interest/arousal disorder** can experience an absence or reduced frequency of interest in sexual activity or even erotic thoughts or fantasies. They may also find themselves initiating sex less often or being unreceptive to a partner's attempts to initiate. Like male HSDD, these can be very subjective ideas of what is normal or what is normal for you as an individual. Women can also be diagnosed with an arousal disorder if there is a lack of sexual pleasure or genital sensations during sexual activity.

> **sexual interest/arousal disorder**
> A sexual dysfunction that causes a woman to experience little or no erotic pleasure through sexual stimulation.

As with other sexual dysfunctions, rates of occurrence are hard to determine. Epidemiological studies show a large range in prevalence rates (17–55%) of women experiencing low levels of desire (Lewis et al., 2010), with most studies typically showing 20–30% of women experiencing arousal issues (Brotto et al., 2010). These rates do increase with age; 10% of those younger than 49 years of age experience arousal difficulties, with the rate increasing to 22% for those 50–65 years of age and again doubling to 47% for those 66–74 years old. Most studies report lubrication difficulties ranging from 8–15%, with some reporting higher rates (21–28%) (Lewis et al., 2010).

Possible causes of sexual arousal disorder can be psychological or organic. However, sexual arousal disorder is more complicated than it appears initially. Experts have recommended considering the sexual partner and environmental conditions when diagnosing sexual arousal disorder (Brotto et al., 2010; Weeks et al., 2009). For example, sexual dysfunction of a male partner, such as erectile dysfunction or early ejaculation, may have a negative impact on a female partner's sexual desire. Women with low arousal report poorer quality relationships, more dissatisfaction with conflict resolution, and less attraction to and emotional closeness with their partners compared with women who do not have low arousal or desire. Relationships that do not include open communication about sexual needs, wishes, and fears also have a negative impact on the woman's desire to engage in sexual activity. Understanding the interactions of all these factors is critical for successful treatment.

Female Orgasmic Disorder

Some women have difficulty experiencing orgasm; women who have a delay or absence of orgasm following normal sexual excitement have a condition called **female orgasmic disorder**. Women who have never had an orgasm are said to have *lifelong*

> **female orgasmic disorder**
> The consistent or frequent inability of a woman to achieve an orgasm.

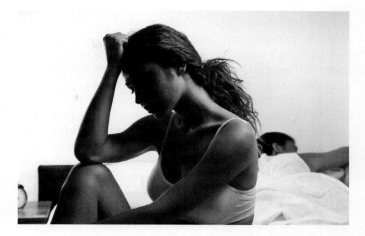

Some women experience pain during intercourse. Possible causes include disorders of the reproductive organs, vaginal infections, or irritation due to the use of some contraceptive products.

orgasmic disorder or *preorgasmia*. Sometimes preorgasmia is referred to as *anorgasmia*. However, anorgasmia implies an inability to achieve orgasm, which is not accurate for many women. Many women simply have not had an orgasm yet—there is no biological cause preventing them from having one (The Trustees of Columbia University, 2012). Those who have experienced an orgasm but are not able to now are said to have *acquired orgasmic disorder*. Some women have orgasms under certain circumstances but not others, for example, while masturbating but not when stimulated by a partner. This condition is referred to as *situational orgasmic disorder*. If a lack of orgasm occurs in all situations, it is considered *generalized orgasmic disorder*.

As with other sexual dysfunctions, there is a lack of quality data with consistent criteria to estimate prevalence rates (Graham, 2010b). Worldwide data regarding the incidence of orgasmic disorder in women varies greatly (Lewis et al., 2010), and few of these studies show the age-related increase that is often associated with other sexual dysfunctions. A U.S. study indicated that in women ages 40–80 about 20% experience the inability to reach orgasm occasionally, periodically, or frequently (Laumann et al., 2009).

Some studies have found associations between orgasmic responsiveness in women and relationship satisfaction (Mah & Binik, 2001), but the absence of orgasm does not mean that a woman cannot have a satisfactory and enjoyable sexual relationship. In reality, some women do not experience distress about the lack of orgasm (Graham, 2010b), and other research has shown that physical aspects of sex (like orgasm) are weak predictors of sexual distress compared to relationship and emotional well-being, which are strong predictors (Bancroft et al., 2003). Each woman places a different level of importance on orgasm, and this is likely related to the level of distress experienced (Bancroft, 2009).

Because many women cannot orgasm through vaginal penetration alone (they require clitoral stimulation), they may consider themselves preorgasmic if they have not explored other activities. Being aware of one's own body becomes critical in understanding stimuli that aid in orgasm. In addition to self-awareness, being in a comfortable and safe relationship that allows honest communication about these issues can facilitate exploration with a partner.

Causes of orgasmic dysfunction seem to be primarily psychological. For women who are preorgasmic, the environment during childhood, such as parental attitudes about sexuality, nudity, and relationships, may affect one's comfort with sexual health issues, body image, communication skills, and other factors. Additionally, stress, levels of fatigue, sexual identity, health, unemployment, and relationship difficulties can all affect orgasmic functioning (McCabe, 2009). Much like arousal disorders, if the woman is partnered, considering the relationship quality is critical. Poor intimacy, affection, and communication have been linked with orgasmic disorder, but it is unclear whether the relationship problems preceded the sexual dysfunction or whether the sexual dysfunction exacerbated relationship challenges (McCabe, 2009).

Genital–Pelvic Pain and Penetration Disorders
Some women experience pain during sexual intercourse or vaginal penetration. Previously, persistent or recurrent pain associated with sexual intercourse was diagnosed as dyspareunia, but this term is being used less as a diagnosis today. Although all women may experience some pain during some particular sexual episodes (due to position, time of cycle, lack of adequate lubrication, etc.), the condition can also be chronic and considered a disorder.

Often the pain manifests itself as a burning feeling or cramping and may occur externally (on the vulva), in the vagina, or elsewhere in the pelvis. Because pain can be different symptomatically, many clinicians and researchers today agree that different syndromes result in dyspareunia. In fact, the pain of dyspareunia can typically be reproduced in nonsexual situations, such as tampon insertion and pelvic exams (Landry & Bergeron, 2009). Two main categories are "superficial" dyspareunia, which includes provoked vestibulodynia (PVD) and vulvovaginal atrophy (VVA), and deep dyspareunia (Binik, 2010). With PVD, women experience pain in the vulva provoked by touch. VVA is a common condition associated with decreased estrogenization of the vaginal tissue. Painful penetration is just one symptom; others include dryness, irritation, soreness, and urinary frequency, urgency, and incontinence. Although VVA can occur at any time in a woman's life cycle, it is more common in the postmenopausal phase (MacBride, Rhodes, & Shuster, 2010). Pain during deep thrust vaginal intercourse is called deep dyspareunia.

Another pain-related condition is when a woman cannot relax the muscles around the entrance to the vagina enough to allow penetration of an object (for example, penis, finger, or speculum) and these muscles involuntarily spasm. Women often report that penetration is almost or completely impossible (Meana, 2009). This condition and diagnosis is called **vaginismus** (see Figure 16.1). There is, however, little research supporting vaginal spasms as a criterion for

> **vaginismus**
> The involuntary contraction of the muscles surrounding the vaginal entrance so that entry of the penis is prevented.

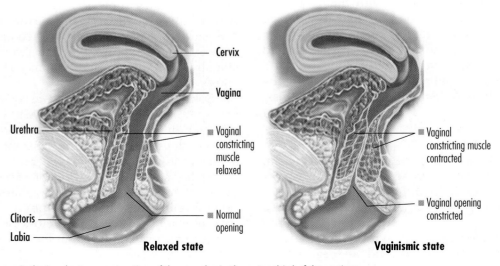

FIGURE **16.1** Vaginismus is the involuntary contraction of the muscles in the outer third of the vagina.

? Did You Know . . .

Testosterone has been used to increase the sex drives of women. In several well-conducted, randomized trials, testosterone delivered in various ways (for example, injections, implants, and patches) resulted in an increase in women's sexual desire, sexual responsiveness, and frequency of sexual intercourse (Heiman, 2006). Yet, as with all medications, there are potential side effects of testosterone use for low sexual desire. Among these side effects are unwanted hair growth and the unanswered question regarding the relationship between testosterone administration and the development of breast cancer (Brotto et al., 2010; Davis et al., 2008), insulin resistance, and metabolic syndrome (Brotto et al., 2010). This medication is currently approved for use in women in Europe, but it has not yet been approved by the FDA in the United States.

diagnosis, and some experts believe that this symptom may be the severe, phobic end of the dyspareunia continuum (Meana & Binik, 1994; Reissing et al., 2004). One aspect of this condition that appears unique is that the fear of penetration can increase to a phobia (Reissing et al., 2004).

Studies examining prevalence rates of pain disorders in women show a range of 14–27% for recent studies (Lewis et al., 2010). The large spectrum of symptoms and conditions that can be included in this category may account for the large range. One concern regarding pain disorders is their potential to lead to other sexual disorders. For example, if a woman anticipates pain during vaginal penetration, this can affect her level of interest and arousal during sexual activity. It is important for any secondary disorders to be considered and treated as well. There is continuing controversy about how to conceptualize and treat these disorders; the uncertainty about best treatment options is complicated by the challenge of dealing with highly distressed patients and the many clinicians who avoid treating these conditions (van Lankveld et al., 2010).

Other Sexual Conditions

Hypersexual Disorder

Hypersexual disorder is often referred to as sex addiction. At the time of this writing, hypersexual activity is a proposed new category for the fifth edition of the *Diagnostic and Statistical Manual* (DSM-V) (Kafka, 2010). Although some believe its inclusion may still be premature (Winters, 2010), many clinicians support and have advocated for its inclusion so that diagnosis and treatment can become more standardized (Turner, 2009).

Sexual Aversion Disorder

Some people have strong feelings of anxiety, fear, or disgust when confronted with a sexual opportunity;

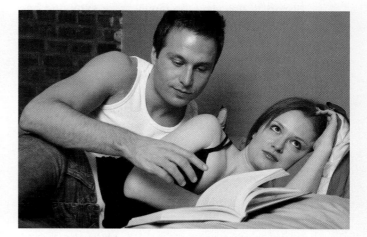

Although people differ in their interest in sexual activity, when one partner experiences lower sexual desire, the other partner may become frustrated and even angry. Understanding and seeking treatment is necessary at this point.

this is called **sexual aversion disorder (SAD)**. The types of sexual stimuli that can produce aversion can range from a specific component (for example, genital secretions) to any sexual stimuli (including kissing, touching, and hugging). Individuals often experience anxiety-like symptoms and may go so far as to avoid sexual behavior (which indicates severe SAD) (Brotto, 2010c). With other phobias (for example, snakes or flying), individuals can often avoid the situation, but with sexual phobias "its avoidance can be profoundly destructive" (Kaplan, 1987) given the role sexuality plays in our lives.

Prevalence of SAD is unknown and difficult to establish given that individuals avoid sexual encounters and usually do not seek out sex therapy services. Some evidence suggests that it is more common

> **sexual aversion disorder (SAD)**
> Disorder characterized by anxiety response when presented with a sexual opportunity.

Multicultural DIMENSIONS

Sexual Dysfunction and Latino Populations

The Hispanic community, as do all subgroups within the United States, has some unique features that need to be considered regarding sexual dysfunction. Many of these features preclude Latinos from seeking professional help for sexual dysfunction. One of these is the language barrier. Not speaking English, or not speaking it well, means that if a sexual dysfunction arises, the person's ability to communicate the condition may prevent him or her from seeking help.

Hispanics also view the family as an extended one, not distinguishing between the nuclear family and the extended family. Cousins, aunts, uncles, and other family members are assumed to be part of the family, and advice is traditionally sought from family members as opposed to people outside the family, such as health professionals. However, matters of sexual function are considered inappropriate for a family discussion and, therefore, often are ignored.

Hispanics also maintain a sense of fatalism. Expressions such as *que sea lo que Dios quiera* ("it's in

God's hands") and *esta enfermedad es una prueba de Dios* ("this illness is a test of God") are examples of this view of health-related problems. Therefore, a sexual dysfunction might be considered a matter for God, not for a sex therapist.

In addition, Latino communities tend to be male dominated, and that condition may interfere with admitting to a sexual dysfunction. In a project to enroll more children in government-sponsored health insurance programs, one of us found that what works for Anglo families does not work for Hispanic families. In Anglo families, it is the mother who is targeted for improving the health of the family's children. In Hispanic families we found it necessary to influence the fathers first. This is because of the concept of *machismo* (in which males are projected as strong, virile, powerful, and in control), which manifests itself in male-dominated families. Given the need to maintain this sense of machismo, Hispanic males may be reluctant to admit a "weakness," especially a sexual dysfunction.

Culturally sensitive approaches are needed in all matters, particularly sexual ones. Sexual dysfunction is no exception.

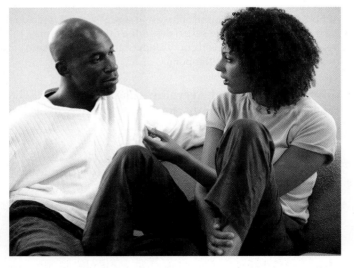

Studies show that males are usually more interested in sexual activity than are women. To resolve these differences, communication is vital for satisfying, long-term sexual relationships to develop.

in women than men, but other evidence suggests that men with SAD may avoid relationships altogether, which limits their distress and subsequent

identification as someone with SAD (Brotto, 2010c). Causes for SAD are unclear; some theorize that the individual had a sexual experience paired with painful or traumatic stimuli. Limited research shows there may be a link with child sexual abuse, but it is not a clear connection.

While sexual aversion disorder (SAD) was specifically listed in the DSM-IV as a sexual disorder, researchers are proposing it be excluded from the DSM-V. The lack of evidence supporting the condition as a distinct diagnosis is the rationale for its exclusion. In addition, experts believe that SAD overlaps with specific phobias in presentation and treatment methodologies, which means that it should be diagnosed as a phobia, not a sexual disorder (Brotto, 2010c).

Dissatisfaction with Sexual Activity Frequency
Not everyone is as interested in sex as his or her partner. A guest speaker in one of our classes characterized this disharmony as only a matter of the mind. To illustrate his point he referred to the way he responds to his spouse's occasional "Leave me alone, I've got a headache" when he is "ready and primed to go." Whereas some men would argue or pout,

he usually says, "Where does your head ache?" and proceeds to massage her head and temples, cheeks and neck gently. After a while he moves to her shoulders and asks, "Does this feel good?" One full body massage later, his spouse's lack of interest has been transformed. Men and women alike can learn to tune into the temporary inhibition, exhaustion, anxiety, or preoccupation that may diminish a partner's sexual interest and learn how that person likes to be treated in such circumstances.

Regardless of the cause, studies have consistently found that men have a greater desire and stronger motivation for sex than do women (Petersen & Hyde, 2010). However, there is some evidence that sexual desire is influenced and expressed differently between men and women. Women's desire may be influenced more by contextual factors and emotional arousal rather than genitals. For example, women are more likely than men to report sexual arousal in response to verbal exchanges and nongenital touching (Fisher, 1999).

If there is a difference in sexual interest between partners, this can have negative impact on other aspects of the relationship. When one person feels he or she is pressuring the other or the other feels pressured, the potential for disagreement is evident. The result may be that both partners feel unloved and guilty. To remedy this problem the couple must maintain effective communication rather than avoid it. In some cases, the assistance of a sex therapist may be warranted.

Sexual Dysfunction and Self-Esteem

Some of us would like to think that sexual functioning is similar to other physical functioning—or that at least it ought to be considered so. If self-worth does not diminish when our digestive functioning goes haywire, why should we think less of ourselves if our sexual functioning is problematic? Well, no matter what we would like to think, sexual functioning is more closely connected to self-esteem than are other body processes. Men and women with sexual dysfunctions often feel less masculine or less feminine because they do not function sexually as they want to. Aside from their desire to function sexually for their own satisfaction, some feel they are depriving their partners of satisfaction. Furthermore, they may fear that their partners will seek other sexual partners and/or leave them, fears that further diminish self-esteem. Not surprisingly, the partners of those struggling with a disorder may also lose some self-esteem. They may feel that the dysfunction is due to their own lack of attractiveness, skill, or attention or that the partner no longer cares for them. Evidence shows that heterosexual women are more likely to experience arousal disorders if their partner is also

suffering from a sexual dysfunction (McCabe & Goldhammer, 2012).

Therapists and counselors have become increasingly sensitive to the matter of self-esteem, of both the person experiencing sexual dysfunction and his or her partner.

■ Causes of Sexual Dysfunction

Sexual dysfunctions can have physical causes, psychological causes, and cultural causes. Many times it is a combination of factors that are influencing the condition. Understanding if the condition is generalized or situational can help an individual or a therapist understand potential underlying causes. Those conditions that are situational have a psychological component. Generalized disorders do not always mean that there is a physical cause, but it increases the likelihood. To prevent and treat sexual problems, these factors need to be understood.

Physical (Organic) Causes

Physical causes can affect many different aspects of sexuality—from desire and cultural to ability to orgasm in both men and women. Natural physical changes that accompany age are one of the prevalent factors affecting sexual functioning. For example, the physical changes accompanying menopause for women also increase the risk of vaginal atrophy, which could cause an increase in painful penetration. As men age, the risk of coronary heart disease and blocked blood vessels increases; this same condition can affect penile arteries, causing erectile dysfunction.

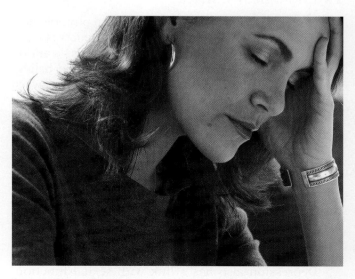

A previous sexual trauma can lead to a sexual dysfunction as this event is recalled during sex.

Extensive research demonstrates that specific medical conditions and health behaviors represent major risk factors for sexual disorders. For men, diabetes, cardiovascular disorders, hypertension, obesity, smoking, lower urinary tract problems, and prostate disorders all have been positively correlated with males experiencing erectile dysfunction (DeRogatis & Burnett, 2008).

For women, chronic illnesses and poor general health status are associated with higher rates of sexual dysfunction. Some specific conditions, such as diabetes, breast cancer, lower urinary tract problems, multiple sclerosis, and clinical depression, are all consistently connected to increased sexual dysfunction (DeRogatis & Burnett, 2008). A U.S. study has also shown that lack of physical activity is associated with a lack of sexual interest for men and women (Laumann et al., 2009).

Surgery for prostate or bladder cancer has demonstrated an impact on erectile dysfunction in men. Similarly, surgical removal of the ovaries affects hormone levels in women, which may cause vaginal atrophy (potentially leading to painful penetration).

Medications can also cause changes in sexual functioning. For example, for both men and women delayed orgasm is the most commonly reported side effect of some antidepressant medications. Approximately 30–60% of those using serotonin reuptake inhibitors (SSRIs) are affected (Graham, 2010a). Medications for a variety of other conditions, such as psychiatric disorders (for example, bipolar) (Nagaraj, Pai, & Rao 2009), hypertension, high cholesterol, heart disease, and allergies, can also affect sexual functioning (Zenilman & Shahmanesh, 2011).

Psychological Causes

Many sexual dysfunctions have no known physiological cause, but rather a psychological basis. Anxiety is a key factor affecting sexual function. Researchers caution against the broad use of the term *anxiety* and believe that clinicians need to consider differences between general anxiety, sexual anxiety, and performance anxiety as possible factors (McCabe et al., 2010). The level of anxiety combined with the setting also needs to be considered. Moderate anxiety in a safe setting may actually facilitate arousal. Imagine the nervousness of a new partner or new activity. However, high levels of anxiety combined with less personal control and a history of chronic anxiety may cause dysfunction. Here, imagine feeling anxious plus being critiqued by your partner; in this situation, one is more likely to experience a disorder (Van Minnen & Kampman, 2000).

Depression also has a link with sexual functioning. The relationship appears reciprocal, because a depressed mood increases the likelihood of sexual dysfunction and sexual dysfunction increases the likelihood of depression. Lower levels of desire caused by antidepressant medication can exacerbate the condition (McCabe et al., 2010).

Many other factors can affect one's sexual functioning. For example, decreased sexual desire can be caused by traumatic experiences, such as child sexual abuse. Other prior experiences, such as problematic attachments, neglectful or critical parents, restrictive upbringing, physical abuse, and violence, increase the risk that one may experience sexual dysfunction (McCabe et al., 2010).

Many times an individual may experience difficulty functioning sexually, but he or she is able to resolve it relatively quickly and without much difficulty. However, some factors prevent improvement of the condition; these include relationship conflict, performance anxiety, guilt, inadequate sexual information or stimulation, loss of sexual chemistry, fear of intimacy, impaired self-image or self-esteem, loss of sexual confidence, restricted foreplay, poor communication, and lack of privacy.

General stress and stress about the sexual experience can also affect sexual functioning. Stress leads to an increase in the hormone epinephrine in the blood, which in turn can interfere with blood flow to the penis or clitoris. Snegroff (1986) studied stressors associated with nonmarital sexual intercourse and found that males differed in some of these stressors and not in others. For males, the following were of most concern:

1. Can I satisfy her?

2. Is my penis the right size?

3. Will I achieve and/or maintain an erection?

4. Will she want a commitment?

5. Will I perform well?

For females, the following were of most concern:

1. Can I satisfy him?

2. Will he like my body?

3. Will he respect me afterward?

4. Does he love/care for me?

5. Will I have an orgasm?

6. Are my breasts large enough?

While this research was conducted almost 30 years ago, the issues are still the same today.

It is quite understandable that psychological factors can cause someone difficulty in functioning in an effective manner sexually. Is it any wonder that someone

Sexual Disorders Around the World

The various perspectives and cultural mores of different countries may contribute to the development of sexual disorders, or at least to a diagnosis of a sexual dysfunction. For example, in China and other countries in which homosexuality is considered immoral, homosexuals, thinking every time they engage in sex they are doing something "dirty" and opposed by their society's expectations, might develop a sexual dysfunction. In Islamic countries in which female genital mutilation is customary, women may have hypoactive sexual disorder. On the island of Inis Beag, off the coast of Ireland, it is considered abnormal for women to experience orgasm. Therefore, women on the island engage in sex but prevent orgasm. Are they

then experiencing orgasmic dysfunction? When men of Inis Beag attempt to ejaculate quickly so as to make sure their partners do not experience orgasm, are they then to be diagnosed with premature ejaculation?

In contrast, countries that have more relaxed sexual mores and accept a wider array of sexual behavior as "normal" tend to cultivate a sexually healthier population. For example, Sweden and Denmark have low rates of sexual dysfunction and teenage pregnancy. In Polynesian countries, known for encouraging sexual exploration at young ages, embarrassment and anxiety associated with sex are almost nonexistent.

Where you grew up and where you live now can have a tremendous effect on your sexual health. What influenced your sexual health? How?

who is self-conscious about his or her body might not function well sexually? Imagine just waiting for a partner to laugh or cringe! Anxiety, guilt, and shame are hardly conducive to healthy sexual functioning.

Cultural Causes

Society also influences sexual functioning. For example, the double standard that judges women as less than moral if they actively seek sexual satisfaction can create shame and guilt that, in turn, interfere with normal sexual functioning. Furthermore, if the double standard is interpreted to mean that the male initiates sex and is more expert at it than a female partner, the pressure to behave in this manner can block the male's normal function. However, if females are taught to expect sexual satisfaction in their relationships comparable to that expected by their male partners, they might unintentionally put the onus for their fulfillment on their partners rather than assume that responsibility for themselves. With the onus placed on them, males may succumb to pressure and be unable to function as usual.

The way we perceive sex is also dependent on what our culture has taught us. Someone once said that sex is so "dirty" it should be saved for someone you love. Thinking of sex as dirty can create negative feelings such as embarrassment and guilt, which can result in sexual dysfunction.

Others (Mayo Foundation for Medical Education and Research, 2011) believe premature ejaculation results from boys' learning by their early teenage years to masturbate. Associated with their masturbatory behavior is guilt that causes them to speed up their orgasm. Having learned to ejaculate rapidly, they have difficulty controlling their ejaculation when they get older.

Religion is also related to sexual function. As one author states: "Rigid adherence to orthodox religious beliefs and practices is a common factor in the backgrounds of men and women with different forms of sexual dysfunction. Strict religious teaching—regardless of the particular religion—often results in negative attitudes toward sexuality. Individuals come to believe that sex is sinful" (Wilson et al., 1996, 241). Of course, not all people who hold such religious beliefs develop a sexual problem, and these beliefs often influence behaviors in a healthy manner.

Another significant cause of sexual dysfunction is related to a lack of information about sexual functioning—for example, not knowing or forgetting that foreplay is necessary to lubricate the vagina before penetration with a penis or a sex toy. Other possible causes are nonsexual problems between sexual partners, ineffective communication (about sex and other matters), and traumatic past sexual experiences (for example, rape). Thus sexual unresponsiveness might, for instance, be caused by an inexperienced, inept, hasty, or insensitive lover; by situational factors, such as thoughts of a sick relative or deep-seated career concerns.

Treating Sexual Dysfunction

In the past few decades many highly effective therapeutic approaches to sexual dysfunction have emerged (although love and concern between partners are still important). Because the effectiveness of the various therapeutic approaches is well publicized, not only do more sufferers seek treatment—a positive step—but more people want to become sex therapists. As might be expected in a field that is emerging, charlatans and quacks, in addition to well-trained professionals, have set up practice. Therefore, anyone experiencing sexual problems would be well advised to investigate the training and experience of a sex therapist carefully before seeking that person's services. To help people select a professional therapist, the American Association of Sex Educators, Counselors, and Therapists (AASECT) has made public its requirements for certifying individuals as sex counselors or sex therapists. AASECT has also published a code of ethics. This code provides guidance for sex counselors and sex therapists, as well as for patients. Counselors and therapists whose behavior is inconsistent with this code may be incompetent and/or unethical.

Generally, sexual therapy for both men and women entails three components, regardless of the number and type of therapists involved: (1) an initial period of abstinence from vaginal sex and/or genital contact to reduce anxiety and facilitate communication; (2) the use of systematic tactile stimulation and exploration to focus on the giving and receiving of pleasure, rather than on the exclusive goal of orgasm; and (3) specific technical suggestions and direction, including sequences and variations on those techniques that facilitate and reinforce success.

Both single individuals and those in relationships may seek therapy for a sexual dysfunction. If in a relationship, the couple may be first seen together by the therapist or therapists. Then they are interviewed separately so they will feel free to discuss matters with the therapist that they might not yet feel comfortable discussing with their partner. Once the nature of the problem is identified, instruction and/or counseling can begin, following the sequence outlined earlier. Usually the couple is at first instructed to abstain from penetrative sex and to learn how to experience pleasure in nongenital touching. Then genital fondling is allowed, and eventually penetrative sex. The touching and sexual activity are private, away from the therapist's office, without the therapist present or in a room with one-way mirrors. Although it is rare, sometimes a *surrogate*, or substitute, partner is used to provide instruction, practice, and feedback for someone with a sexual problem. The use of sexual surrogates is highly controversial, both within the profession and among the public.

Approaches to Sexual Therapy

Several models of sexual therapy have been proposed. Perhaps a good place to begin a discussion of these models is first to consider a stepwise approach to sexual therapy.

The PLISSIT Model
Jack Annon (1976) suggested that relatively minor treatment may be effective for some sexual dysfunctions, whereas more intensive treatment may be required for others. Annon's model of sexual therapy is known as the **PLISSIT** model (an acronym of *P*ermission, *L*imited *I*nformation, *S*pecific *S*uggestion, and *I*ntensive *T*herapy). This model extends from the simplest to the more advanced levels of treatment.

> **PLISSIT**
> A model of sexual therapy that consists of moving through the stages of giving permission, limited information, specific suggestion, and, if that does not work, intensive therapy.

During the permission stage the therapist helps people accept their fantasies and desires and, where appropriate, even gives them permission *not* to engage in sexual intercourse until they are ready to do so. The therapist helps couples not to compare themselves with other couples or with an idealized sexual relationship.

During the limited information stage the therapist provides the factual information that may help the person become more functional sexually. For example, a person may not realize it is natural to fantasize about sexual activity or perceive it as a natural part of one's life. Information can give clients a more realistic perception, thereby removing an impediment to their sexual functioning. Other kinds of information, such as information about penis size and its limited effect on sexual satisfaction, clitoral sensitivity, or proper hygiene, may be all that is needed to help people overcome their sexual dysfunctions.

Specific suggestion is the level of therapy at which the therapist actually recommends activities for the clients. For example, self-stimulation, sensate focus, and the squeeze technique may be suggested. Many of these techniques were developed by Masters and Johnson (1970) but have since been modified by other sexual therapists. These techniques can help the person reduce sexual anxiety, improve communication between partners, or enhance arousal.

¿? Ethical DIMENSIONS

Should Surrogates Be Used in Sexual Therapy?

Early on, some therapists believed that the use of a substitute sexual partner was a vital and necessary component of sexual therapy. This substitute, or surrogate, was an experienced and trained sexual partner who could teach the sexually dysfunctional client effective sexual arousal techniques. Further, the surrogate let the client practice these techniques in a nonthreatening situation, because the surrogate was not a person with whom the client had a relationship or whom the client would ever see again. Advocates of the use of surrogates believed the therapy to be more effective if the client practiced on and received feedback from a real person.

Those opposed to surrogates usually based their arguments on one of two premises—either that sexual activity between people not married to each other is immoral or that the knowledge, skills, and attitudes learned with a surrogate are not readily transferred to one's usual sexual partner. A client's ability to function well with a surrogate does not ensure ability to function well with the usual sexual partner. Those arguing this position believed that sexual dysfunction is a problem between sexual partners and, therefore, needs to be worked out by both partners. Because the couple would have to practice sexually arousing techniques anyhow, why not practice them together from the outset of the therapy? And, finally, some people believed a surrogate was akin to a prostitute. Those employing such a method, therefore, should be subject to criminal prosecution.

Do you think surrogates should be used in sexual therapy? Why or why not?

Intensive therapy may be required when permission, limited information, and specific suggestion are not successful in resolving a sexual problem. Intensive therapy entails a longer-term therapeutic treatment that identifies the deep-seated reasons that interfere with sexual functioning. This therapy has been called *psychosexual therapy* (Kaplan, 1974). Some therapists believe sexual dysfunction is caused by guilt or shame about sex, which leads to sexual anxiety, and the best treatment is intensive therapy to uncover the causes of these feelings.

The Masters and Johnson Model

William Masters and Virginia Johnson advocated a model of sexual therapy with several unique components. First, they believed that sexual problems are relationship problems, and, therefore, therapy works only with couples. Even seemingly healthy partners can learn how to respond and contribute better to their partner's response through sexual therapy. Second, they believed if couples are to be treated, the therapy team should be a couple—that is, a male and a female therapist. They believed that such a team can best appreciate the perspectives and best represent the couple in therapy. In addition, Masters and Johnson felt that clients can better identify with the therapist of the same gender, who may understand them better. Third, clients were medically screened for any potential organic causes of their dysfunction and given a complete psychological evaluation. Finally, treatment at the Masters and Johnson

Myth VS Fact

Myth: Sexual dysfunctions occur because someone either has been sexually abused or raped or has masturbated too often.

Fact: It is true that sexual abuse, such as rape and child abuse, can contribute to the development of a sexual dysfunction. Yet, there are many people who experience those traumatic events and never develop a sexual dysfunction. Regarding masturbation, there is no evidence that the frequency of masturbation is in any way related to the subsequent development of a sexual dysfunction.

Myth: Guys who "can't get it up" are not real men.

Fact: Most cases of erectile dysfunction are caused by physiological problems. To classify these men as less than real men is analogous to characterizing any man who has any physical illness as not a real man. The inability to achieve and maintain an erection is in no way related to manliness.

Myth: Women are not naturally interested in sex, so a woman who cannot be sexually aroused is quite normal.

Fact: Males and females have a natural interest in and capacity for sex. When they do not, they are exhibiting an arousal disorder. If they are upset about this condition, they should seek professional help.

Institute was intensive; couples were seen every day for a 2-week period. Masters and Johnson argued that this intensive interaction between the therapists and the clients is necessary initially to reduce anxiety and help the couple concentrate on overcoming the sexual problem.

There are positives and negatives about the approach Masters and Johnson used. Understanding the possible physical causes of sexual dysfunction is critical to successful treatment; today most sex therapists incorporate treatments affecting psychological and medical aspects, if warranted (Althof, 2010). However, less intensive therapies, such as self-help strategies (van Lankveld, 2009) and sex therapy via the Internet (Althof, 2010), are demonstrating success. In addition, the focus on couples and heterosexuals limits the applicability to single people and gay, lesbian, and bisexual individuals.

Kaplan's Model

Kaplan (1974, 1979, 1983) employs many of the specific techniques of sexual therapy recommended by Masters and Johnson. However, Kaplan believes more intensive therapy is required to uncover the reasons for the sexual anxiety that interferes with normal sexual functioning. Kaplan's triphasic model consists of desire, arousal, and orgasm phases. Desire phase problems are the most difficult to treat because of their association with deep-seated psychological difficulties. Consequently, Kaplan recommends a longer period of sexual therapy to uncover the unconscious rationale for behavior and thought. Kaplan believes that sexual dysfunctions have their roots in multiple causes, some readily accessible and others requiring more intensive therapy to determine them. In addition, Kaplan treats premature ejaculation with the stop–start technique developed by James Semans (1956) rather than the squeeze technique developed by Masters and Johnson. Both the squeeze and the stop–start technique are described later in this chapter.

Other Approaches to Sexual Therapy

There are many other ways in which therapists treat sexual dysfunctions. For example, some behaviorists

(LoPiccolo, 1977; Leiblum & Pervin, 1980) believe most sexual problems are learned and can be unlearned. Behaviorists use positive and negative reinforcement to encourage healthy behaviors and use gradual approaches to problematic sexual behavior. This latter approach is based on the early work of Joseph Wolpe (1958), who argued that one could not be anxious and relaxed at the same time. Consequently, Wolpe taught his clients deep muscle relaxation (for example, meditation) and gradually, over time, introduced more and more components of the anxiety-producing behavior. The sensate focus activity described later in this chapter is an example of Wolpe's desensitization technique.

Barbach (1980, 2000, 2001) organized groups of women to treat sexual dysfunction, in particular, orgasmic dysfunction and sexual unresponsiveness. Barbach's methods include exercises for the woman to do for herself. These exercises are also described later in the chapter.

Ellis and Harper (1975, 1979) developed a therapy model called *rational emotive therapy*. This model is based on the assumption that much of our behavior is a result of our thoughts and interpretations. Sexual problems arise from (irrational) thoughts and interpretations, and these problems can be treated by helping people recognize their irrationality and change these thoughts and interpretations into more rational ones.

Barry McCarthy believes that in the great majority of cases the sexual problem stems from a lack of knowledge, from communication problems, or from psychological difficulties. Consequently he views psychologists, social workers, marriage counselors, and ministers as better suited to working with such patients than physicians. In McCarthy et al.'s (1975) model of sexual therapy, a single therapist sees both sexual partners once a week, sometimes together, sometimes apart. This therapist is not a physician. Because a physical examination is a prerequisite to acceptance in the program, McCarthy considers a physician's skills unnecessary during therapy.

Treating Erectile Dysfunction

Erectile dysfunction can have physiological causes, psychological causes, or a combination of physiological and psychological causes. The first step in treatment is to determine the underlying factors. For disorders influenced by physiological factors, the most common treatment is oral medications, specifically phosphodiesterase 5 (PDE5) inhibitors (Gambescia et al., 2009). We commonly know them as Viagra (sildenafil), Cialis (tadalafil), and Levitra (vardenafil). These medications increase the production of cyclic guanosine monophosphate (cGMP) in

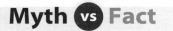

Myth vs Fact

Myth: Treatment for sexual dysfunctions must entail counseling over the long term to be successful.

Fact: Treatments for sexual dysfunctions vary, depending on the nature of the particular dysfunction and the people involved. In many cases, the cause is a physical one, and medications can successfully treat it. In other cases, all that is needed is to educate the couple about effective techniques of sexual arousal. In relatively few cases is long-term counseling necessary.

Myth: Any couple who are not engaging in sexual activities frequently enough, with enough variety, and with orgasm have a sexual dysfunction for which they should seek sexual counseling.

Fact: Some experts believe that, for a sexual dysfunction to exist, one or both of the sexual partners must be dissatisfied with the sexual relationship. If both partners are satisfied, regardless of the nature of their sexual relationship, no sexual dysfunction exists.

the muscle cells by blocking the production of PDE5. cGMP is a chemical produced by the body that allows the arteries in the penis to relax and, as a result, increase blood flow. In terms of toxicity, efficacy, and tolerance, all three medications are similar. However, they differ in how long they last; sildenafil and vardenafil are effective for up to 4 hours, whereas tadalafil can last up to 36 hours.

As with all medications, side effects are possible, as are interactions with other medications. Consequently, consultation with a clinician is required before these medications are taken. It is not wise to order Viagra or other medications over the Internet, because potential medication interactions or health conditions may not be reviewed by a qualified health professional and the pills received may contain no medication or a different medication than that ordered. Common side effects of the PDE5 inhibitors include effects on vision, possible temporary hearing loss, and headache. Because of the possible drop in blood pressure, individuals using organic nitrates or nitric oxide should avoid taking PDE5 medication. Those who have had a recent stroke or myocardial infarction or who have excessively low or high blood pressure or severe liver impairment should also avoid using these medications. One concern with these medications is the risk of priapism, a prolonged erection lasting several hours. If the priapism is caused by the blood being unable to leave the penis, the blood in the penis will lose oxygen and become toxic, which can cause damage or destroy tissues. An untreated priapism can result in erectile dysfunction and disfiguration of the penis (Mayo Foundation for Medical Education and Research, 2010).

It is important to note that PDE5 medications will not increase desire, only the erection. Some therapists are concerned that taking these medications may create unrealistic expectations for a couple about the regularity and duration of sex activity (Rosen et al., 2006). To use a crude analogy, Viagra just cleans the hose of a car—it doesn't fill it with gas. Some wonder about women taking Viagra or other medications; several years ago there was even a *Sex in the City* episode about it. In reality, these medications seem to have little effect on women's sexual functioning when used alone because of the complex etiology of women's arousal (Chivers & Rosen, 2010).

In addition to oral drugs, other treatments may include suppositories, injections, devices, and prostheses. Suppositories containing vasoactive medication are directly inserted into the urethra via an applicator. This is intended to cause an erection, but the effectiveness is low. Alternatively, a vasoactive liquid medication or combination of vasodilators can be injected into the corpus cavernosum of the penis, promoting erection. Injections are safe if used properly, but problems with administration, the required extensive education of patients and their partners, and side effects prevent them from being widely used.

Individuals could also use a vacuum constriction device (VCD), which provides a noninvasive, effective, and safe option for those experiencing erectile dysfunction. The VCD is an acrylic cylinder used with a vacuum pump; the device creates a vacuum that promotes erection. The penis is inserted into the cylinder, and a hand or battery operated pump draws air from the cylinder. The reduced air pressure in the cylinder allows increased blood flow to the penis, causing an erection. Blood is trapped in the penis by a tourniquet or other device around the base of the penis. (It is important to remove the tourniquet after sexual activity or there could be damage to the penis.) Many couples find this method inconvenient, which limits its use. As a last option, penile prostheses are available to those who do not respond to other medical treatments. This option requires invasive and irreversible surgery that may result in scarring and infection and that frequently does not meet patient or partner expectations.

Although oral medications can be successful for 70% of men with erectile dysfunction (Rosen et al., 2004), it is important to consider psychological factors as well. How does one restart a sexual life after an extended period of abstinence? How does one address partner resistance? What happens when the medication addresses the erectile dysfunction but the partner is now identified as having a sexual concern or dysfunction? Even with medication, how does an individual handle lack of confidence, performance anxiety, depression, relationship issues, or unrealistic expectations? It is estimated that 60–70% of those taking PED5s stop treatment (Rosen et al., 2004). However, if strategies address both psychological and physiological issues, success rates are higher (Althof, 2010). Specific counseling strategies and other techniques are described later in this section.

Treating Early Ejaculation

Two techniques are used to help men control early ejaculation. The first is the **squeeze technique**, developed by Masters and Johnson (Figure 16.2), which entails a gentle squeezing of the penis while the man is experiencing full erection. When the man begins to feel the urge to ejaculate,

> **squeeze technique**
> A method of helping men control premature ejaculation whereby the penis is gently squeezed when the man senses ejaculation is imminent.

the partner grasps the penis with the thumb on the underside where the shaft ends and the head begins

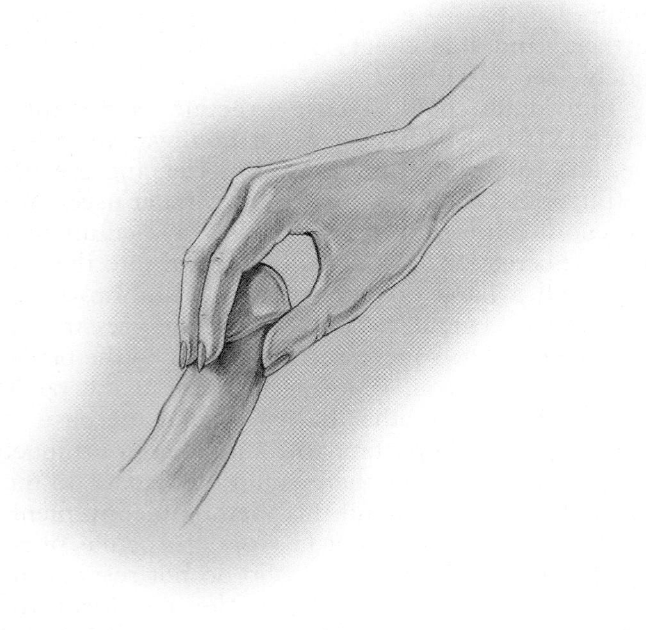

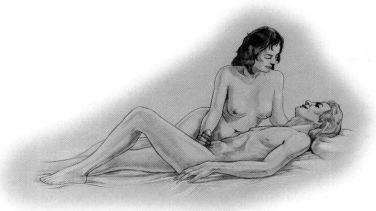

Semans. The man lies on his back and concentrates on his feelings and sensations as his partner stimulates his penis manually (Figure 16.3). When he feels ejaculation approaching, he tells his partner to stop stimulating him. The couple repeats the procedure until the man learns ejaculatory control.

However, other remedies also exist. For example, changing the tempo of thrusting may result in decreased stimulation. Also, changing the angle or depth of penetration may help. Shifting one's thoughts to other events, talking to oneself ("self-talk"), and focusing on the nongenital aspects of the experience can all be of help in controlling ejaculation. The use of a condom can also help because the glans penis is not stimulated directly. Alternatively, some men allow a rapid orgasm, or a small orgasm, knowing that the next one will take longer to arrive. If engaging in penetration, ensuring that there is adequate lubrication may help decrease sensitivity of the glans. Creams designed to decrease sensitivity can be placed on the glans; however, whether the benefit of controlling the ejaculate is worth the price of reduced sensations is a decision that only the man and his partner can make. Finally, some antidepressant medications have been found to control early ejaculation (Betchen, 2009).

Treating Delayed Ejaculation

The therapy for delayed ejaculation includes the technique known as sensate focus (described in the next paragraph), which helps the man focus on his sensual feelings and learn to derive pleasure from sexual behavior. Included in this treatment, in a stepwise fashion, is learning to ejaculate by masturbating alone, by masturbating with his sexual partner present, by asking the partner to masturbate him to

FIGURE 16.2 The squeeze technique. The man signals his partner to squeeze when ejaculation is approaching.

and two fingers on the opposite side. The partner then squeezes for 3 to 4 seconds, after which the urge to ejaculate will have passed. After 15 to 30 seconds, stimulation is provided to full erection once more and the procedure is repeated as necessary. Eventually the man learns to control his ejaculation without his partner's help.

Semans stop–start method
A method of controlling premature ejaculation (developed by James Semans) in which the man tells his partner to stop stimulating him when he feels ejaculation approaching.

The second technique for learning ejaculatory control is called the **Semans stop–start method**, named for its developer, James

FIGURE 16.3 The Semans procedure. The man signals his partner to stop stimulation when he senses that ejaculation is close.

ejaculation, and by asking the partner to masturbate him to the point just short of ejaculation and then inserting the penis into the partner to ejaculate.

Sensate Focus

Sexual therapists treat sexual unresponsiveness in both men and women by teaching the couple a technique termed **sensate focus**. The idea behind this method is to encourage the couple to experience erotic feelings short of penetration so that they will learn to accept sexual pleasuring (both giving and receiving) as part of their lives. The therapist gives the unresponsive partner permission and encouragement to feel nonthreatening sexual feelings, on the assumption that the client has withheld permission from himself or herself (for whatever individual subconscious reason). Eventually the therapy incorporates penetration into the sensate focus program. Figure 16.4 illustrates one of the sensate-focusing positions taught to couples.

> **sensate focus**
> A method of alleviating sexual unresponsiveness by procedures designed to encourage erotic feelings and sexual pleasuring.

Barbach's Technique

Barbach's technique, effective in treating both sexual arousal and orgasmic disorders in women, has been widely disseminated to the general public through Lonnie Barbach's book *For Yourself: The Fulfillment of Female Sexuality* (2000). A woman begins the program by setting aside an hour a day for exploring her body visually (with a mirror) and manually (using body lotion or powder), all the time focusing upon feelings and sensations. Next she is led to do a vulva self-examination and vulva self-stimulation with a body lotion or oil. It is important at this stage that orgasm *not* be the goal of the self-stimulation. Rather the woman is encouraged to become aware of and focus on pleasurable sensations. Eventually the program leads the woman to seek orgasm by using the touching technique she found to be most pleasurable during the self-stimulation stage. The use of a vibrator is recommended for women who still find orgasm elusive after manual stimulation. However, after the woman experiences orgasm with a vibrator, she is encouraged to practice manual stimulation. This transfer is important in helping her to have orgasm with a sexual partner.

Combating Pain Disorders

Pain disorders are treated by a combination of education and practice. The education component entails instruction about the anatomy and physiology of the human sexual response and reproductive systems. Once it is understood that the problem stems from contraction of the muscles of the vagina that prevents penetration, training to control these muscles can begin. The best manner in which to carry out this training appears to be teaching the woman to contract and relax the muscles, becoming conscious of the sensations that accompany both contracted and relaxed vaginal muscles. Next slender rods—first a very narrow one and eventually wider ones—are inserted by the woman into the vagina with relaxed muscles. Once this is mastered (about 1 week), the next step is penetration in a partnered sexual activity with the woman controlling the process. Many times a physical therapist who specializes in pelvic floor dysfunction works with the client to assist with these exercises.

If the pain is a result of insufficient lubrication during penetration, treatment is similar to that used for arousal disorders, such as sensate focus or mindfulness.

Treatment for Hypersexual Disorder

There are limited published treatment models for hypersexuality and few outcome studies assessing treatment (Giugliano, 2009). Many early efforts were

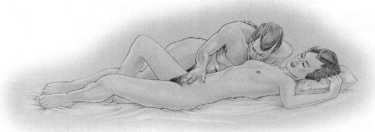

FIGURE 16.4 Sensate focus allows for nondemanding stimulation.

based on modified models of substance addiction treatment, which can include education, spiritual development, behavior strategies, and support groups. Medical treatments tend to focus on diminishing the sex drive and improving control over impulses. Some pharmacological treatments exist as well, but these are not used extensively.

Addressing underlying issues, such as anxieties or childhood issues, is not likely to be effective until the addiction has been addressed and under control (Giugliano, 2009). Therapy may address feelings, insights, and fears as they relate to the addiction. Unlike other addiction plans, it is not realistic for one to abstain from sex; one must learn healthy ways of living with sex as opposed to eliminating it. The clinical literature appears to support an integrative approach as being the most helpful (Woody, 2011).

Treatment for Sexual Aversion Disorder

Treatment for sexual aversion disorder is not well established, and the limited available research focuses on females. The most effective strategy for treatment is related to treatment of anxiety and phobia disorders, specifically, systematic desensitization (Brotto, 2010c). In general, therapists believe that SAD is less responsive to behavioral treatment than arousal disorders, but there have been no studies comparing treatment of the two conditions. Likewise, no longitudinal studies have explored the etiology of SAD, so ideas about treatment are not grounded in research (Brotto 2010c).

Behavior Therapy Model

Joseph Wolpe developed a manner of treating anxiety as the cause of sexual dysfunction. Termed **systematic desensitization**, this model can be applied to people who are anxious about sex. Wolpe reasoned that if people were muscularly relaxed, they could not be anxious at the same time. Consequently, he taught people deep muscle relaxation techniques and then instructed them to think of the anxiety-provoking stimulus. For example, sexually dysfunctional patients might imagine their arms and legs are heavy, warm, and tingly (a relaxation technique called *autogenic training*). Once relaxed, they could imagine the sexual activity about which they feel anxious.

systematic desensitization
A means of overcoming anxiety by approaching the anxiety-provoking stimulus in small steps.

Systematic desensitization also assumes that the gradual introduction of anxiety-provoking stimuli will not produce anxious feelings. Thus this technique involves a fear hierarchy: The initial stimuli are not anxiety provoking, but very gradually more anxiety-provoking stimuli are introduced. For example, the following might be the fear hierarchy of a married woman (Ted's partner) who experiences a genital pain disorder:

1. I go out to a movie with Ted.
2. Ted and I return home and are alone.
3. Ted places his arm around me.
4. Ted nuzzles my neck.
5. Ted fondles my breast.
6. Ted takes my clothes off.
7. Ted removes his clothing.
8. Ted stimulates my clitoris and vagina.
9. Ted inserts his finger into my vagina.
10. Ted inserts his penis into my vagina.

The woman is then asked to imagine the first event in the fear hierarchy without feeling anxious—that is, without an increasing heart rate and rapid, shallow breathing. If she can imagine that event for 30 seconds without feeling anxious, she does deep muscle relaxation for 30 seconds. Then she moves to the next event of the hierarchy. The idea is to take very small steps from something that does not make her anxious to the point at which she is involved in the activity that was the problem (in the example, allowing penile insertion) (Greenberg, 2009).

Behaviorists are concerned with the behavior in question, not the underlying reasons for that behavior. They do not spend a great deal of time analyzing why someone feels or thinks as he or she does. Rather, they begin to manipulate the behavior so it is transformed into the desired behavior. To do this, therapists sometimes employ a technique called *shaping*. Shaping involves rewarding small behaviors along the way to developing the behavior that is the goal of the therapy. For example, if a person becomes anxious on dates and, therefore, refuses to accept a date, the therapist might have the person begin by just speaking to a love interest on the telephone. For doing that, he or she would receive a reward (for example, maybe a pass to a movie theater). To receive a reward the next week, however, the patient needs to spend a few minutes in face-to-face contact with that other person—and so on, until the patient goes out on a date without anxiety.

Self-Care Model

Several of the models and techniques of sexual therapy can be self-administered. For example, couples can employ the stop–start technique or the squeeze technique, and individuals can try systematic desensitization or shaping by themselves. They will thereby save some money and whatever inconvenience is associated with attending therapy. A good first step to solving problems associated with sexual functioning, given that any medical cause has been ruled out, is to employ these self-care techniques (Van Lankveld, 2009). If they are not successful, the person should consider seeking the help of a trained sex counselor or therapist. Often the trained eye can observe something that the untrained cannot.

The Next Era of Sex Therapy

You may have noticed that many of the references in the previous treatment sections were older. These methods are effective and used regularly today, but there are new ideas in sex therapy as well. Althof (2010) identified four innovations in sex therapy: combination of medical and psychological treatment, mindfulness, sex therapy via the Internet, and the reconceptualization of genital pain.

While many psychologists and psychiatrists use medications and therapy to treat mental health disorders (think antidepressants and counseling for depression), there is some resistance within sex therapy regarding the issue. Both medical treatment and counseling strategies have their benefits, but by treating these issues from both perspectives the results are more successful for erectile dysfunction and early ejaculation. Althof (2010) believes that future pharmacological advancements will address female arousal and other disorders, and practitioners and clients need to be open to combining treatment strategies.

Mindfulness is the practice of intentionally being aware of one's thoughts, emotions, and physical sensations without judgment. Brotto and colleagues (Brotto, Sealb, & Rellini, 2012; Brotto, Basson, & Luria, 2008; Brotto, Heiman et al., 2008) have designed studies that incorporate mindfulness techniques for women who have low desire and arousal disorders. Results have shown that for depressed women and survivors of childhood sexual abuse the technique of calming the "busy mind" may be especially helpful in increasing desire and interest in sex.

Sex therapy via the Internet is controversial; benefits of therapy delivery in this mode can include easy accessibility, the removal of constraints related to geographic location and time, and a reduction in embarrassment or humiliation. At the same time, there are concerns related to the subtleties lost in communication without the face-to-face interaction, misinterpretation of written text, and concerns about security and confidentiality of data transmitted via the Internet, as well as professional liability issues.

The few published studies show promise, and further investigation is warranted.

The last innovation identified by Althof (2010) is the reconceptualization of genital pain disorders and treatment. Previously, dyspareunia and vaginismus were considered sexual dysfunctions, but recent studies have advocated for practitioners to focus on the pain and not the function being disturbed (that is, sex). This reconceptualization incorporates pain management techniques as treatment, which has resulted in moderate success for women.

Other Kinds of Therapy

There are other kinds of therapy that treat sexual dysfunction. However, forms of therapy and counseling that are not focused particularly on sexual response can also help people with sexual dysfunctions, especially when conditions are rooted in a more generalized lack of self-acceptance and self-esteem. Also beneficial in some cases is counseling or therapy directed toward improving communication in the nonsexual aspects of a relationship—for example, marriage counseling, family counseling, or crisis counseling for couples.

If you experience any of the sexual dysfunctions described in this chapter, you may want to ask your instructor or student-health service personnel for a referral to a qualified sex therapist. Paying attention to your sexual responsiveness is part of maintaining total well-being. A dysfunction in the sexual aspect of your life requires the same concern and treatment as any other chronic ailment. We are fortunate to live in a time when effective sexual therapy based on sound scientific research is generally available.

Choosing a Sex Therapist

For sex therapy to be effective, the therapist must be qualified. How can you determine this? Someone who claims to be a sex therapist is not necessarily competent in that particular area of expertise. To enhance your chances of choosing a qualified sex therapist, consider the following points:

1. *Does this person have a degree in a recognized profession related to counseling and therapy?* Psychology, marriage and family counseling, pastoral counseling, and social work are examples.

2. *Does this person hold a license or a certification related to counseling and therapy?* Some professions are licensed by the state (psychologists), whereas others are certified by professional organizations (for example, marriage counselors).

3. *Is this person certified by the American Association of Sex Educators, Counselors, and Therapists (AASECT)?* Certification by this professional organization attests to the training specific to sexuality issues the person has had.

4. *Do you know other people who have been helped by this therapist?* Sometimes the best referral is that of someone who has experienced therapy and benefited from it.

To begin choosing a sex therapist, consult local resources. A local hospital might be a good beginning. Perhaps the local medical association can make a referral. The psychology, counseling, social work, or health education department at your university might be able to help, as might your campus health center. Alternatively, you could contact AASECT for a referral in your area.

When first meeting the therapist, or talking with office personnel on the telephone, do not hesitate to inquire about the fee, the therapist's background and qualifications, the licenses and/or certifications the therapist holds, and the usual course of therapy provided for situations such as yours (length of treatment, type of treatment, and so on). Any therapist who objects to your asking these questions should be considered suspect. Reputable therapists should be glad that you are taking such an active interest in obtaining effective treatment. That sort of motivation is critical for a successful outcome.

Exploring the Dimensions of Human Sexuality

Our feelings, attitudes, and beliefs regarding sexuality are influenced by our internal and external environments. Go to go.jblearning.com/dimensions5e to learn more about the biological, psychological, and sociological factors that affect your sexuality.

Case Study

Many of the sexual disorders are multidimensional. In fact, at different times, there can be different causes. Consider an otherwise healthy male who, after getting too little sleep during the week and ingesting too much alcohol, is unable to achieve and maintain an erection with his partner. The dysfunction here is likely physiological. If he understands that alcohol and lack of sleep are to blame, he will probably be fine. However, if he perceives that he "failed" sexually, he may suffer from performance anxiety during his next sexual encounter.

Partners, too, may blame themselves for sexual dysfunction. When partners call into question their attractiveness or sexual ability, their self-esteem may suffer. Further, they may isolate themselves from sexual situations so as not to "cause" failure again.

Both sexuality education and communication can help couples avoid sexual anxiety. The former would help both partners realize why the initial dysfunction occurred. And communication could help both partners' self-esteem, by letting the other person know that he or she is desired.

Biological Factors

- Some sexual dysfunctions, including 80–90% of erectile disorder cases, are of a physiological nature. Age is sometimes a factor, as normal changes in the human body affect sexual desire and arousal.
- Alcohol, drug abuse, and certain medications (for example, for hypertension) can interfere with sexual response.

Sociocultural Factors

- The sexual double standard suggests that men be experienced and talented in sexual matters, leading their partners to sexual bliss. Failure to live up to such expectations can lead to psychological problems.
- Mass media create unrealistic sexual expectations that no real person can meet.
- Relationship problems can lead to some disorders.
- Rigid religious convictions that certain sexual activities are immoral may lead to negative attitudes toward sexuality.

Psychological Factors

- Sexual functioning is closely connected to self-esteem. Men and women with sexual dysfunctions often feel less masculine or feminine because they do not function as well sexually as they wish. Low self-esteem, guilt, or depression can lead to some sexual disorders.
- Gay men, lesbians, and bisexual people seeking treatment for disorders must also confront society's negative attitudes about homosexuality.
- Failure to perform as expected can be devastating psychologically. In turn, such perceived failure could lead to isolation from sexual activities, which would cause further embarrassment. Fear of future sexual inadequacy can create a self-fulfilling prophecy that can result in lowered self-esteem.

Summary

- An individual's sexual desire is not constant; it varies according to situational, emotional, and physical factors. Sexual dysfunction is a *chronic* inability to respond sexually in a way one finds satisfying.

- Lifelong sexual dysfunctions are those in which the person has never been functional in a sexual activity. Acquired sexual dysfunctions are those in which the person was functional at one time but no longer is.

- Male sexual dysfunctions include erectile dysfunction (inability to achieve an erection), early ejaculation (not maintaining penile insertion long enough before ejaculating), delayed ejaculation (inability to ejaculate after sufficient sexual stimulation), male hypoactive sexual desire disorder (low arousal), and genital pain.

- Female sexual dysfunctions include female arousal disorder (not experiencing erotic pleasure from sexual stimulation), orgasmic dysfunction (inability to have an orgasm during sexual activities), and genital pain disorders.

- Both males and females may experience sexual desire dysfunctions, dissatisfaction with sexual frequency, sexual aversion (an irrational fear of sexual activity that leads to avoiding these activities), and hypersexual disorder (recurrent intense sexual fantasies, urges, or behaviors that are difficult to control and cause distress).

- Sexual dysfunctions can have physical causes such as diseases, medications, or blocked blood vessels. They may also be caused by psychological factors such as low self-esteem, guilt and shame, past sexual abuse, or performance anxiety.

- Generally, sexual therapy entails three components: (1) an initial period of abstinence to reduce anxiety and facilitate communication, (2) the use of systematic tactile stimulation and exploration to focus on the giving and receiving of pleasure, and (3) specific technical suggestions and directions that facilitate and reinforce success.

- Among the approaches to treat sexual dysfunctions are the PLISSIT model, teams of cotherapists, the squeeze technique, the stop–start method, sensate focus, surgery, mindfulness, and medication.

Discussion Questions

1. Review the major male and female sexual dysfunctions, including features of diagnosis. What determines what a typical person might consider a sexual problem and what a sexual therapist diagnoses as a sexual dysfunction?

2. List the specific physical, psychological, and sociocultural dimensions that can affect sexual performance. Explain how each could have an effect. (Be specific: Religion is a factor, but state the specific religion. Would it affect all members of that religion or only specific people with a high degree of religious fervor?)

3. Examine the many types of sexual therapy available. Then evaluate which you think would work best for erectile disorder and female arousal disorder. Explain your answer.

Application Questions

Reread the chapter-opening story and answer the following questions.

1. Explain why when a celebrity or a politician discloses a personal problem, it seems easier for the general public to talk about the issue involved. Contrast that with how you might react if a classmate announced in class that he or she had a sexual dysfunction.

2. We know that Elizabeth Dole smiled when asked about Viagra. But if she had been asked about her sex life with Bob before his disclosure, how might she have reacted? Would she have revealed his "dysfunction" (related to prostate-cancer surgery)? If Viagra had not been developed, would either Bob or Elizabeth have realized that there was a dysfunction?

Critical Thinking Questions

1. Masters and Johnson claimed that male and female cotherapists were needed to treat a couple. They reasoned that only a person of the same gender as the client could really understand a sexual problem or dysfunction. Do you agree with Masters and Johnson, or could a couple be successfully treated by one therapist (of either gender)? Explain your answer.

2. The success of the drug Viagra was unprecedented: 36,000 prescriptions in the first week, 3.6 million prescriptions in the first 4 months. Although it is clear that many of the patients had erectile disorders, there is strong anecdotal information to suggest that some men were experimenting with Viagra to improve their sex life. Consider the physical, psychological, and sociocultural dimensions of such experimentation (for example, belief you cannot perform without the pill, the ethics of getting a doctor to write a prescription). Would you take a drug that could possibly improve your sex life, even if it had associated risks?

Critical Thinking Case

Before the 1960s hardly anyone had heard of sexual dysfunction. However, soon after Masters and Johnson's book *Human Sexual Response* was published in 1966, the prevalence of sexual dysfunctions seemed to skyrocket. Some have argued that there are more sexual problems than in previous years because of the greater emphasis people place on sex today. We can now view X-rated movies on the Internet, we can purchase erotic print media at the local bookstore or listen to sexually charged music and lyrics, and we can even observe simulated sex during daytime hours on reality TV or on the Internet. This emphasis on sex, the argument continues, has created unrealistic expectations for people, and when they cannot "perform" as they observe others can, they become dysfunctional.

There is another view, however. Perhaps there was as much sexual dysfunction before 1966 as there is today; however, sex was not a topic for conversation, so problems remained undisclosed. The result was that people were unable to achieve sexual satisfaction.

What is your view? Is there more sexual dysfunction now, or has disclosure of sexual problems increased? Is the situation better today, or was it better before 1966? Is there too much pressure for people to "perform" sexually today?

Exploring Personal Dimensions

What Constitutes Sexual Dysfunction?
Perspectives on what constitutes a sexual dysfunction vary. One important consideration is that if you and your partner are satisfied with your sexual relationship, you probably do not have a disorder.

If you do not participate in any sexual activity, skip this assessment. With that in mind, answer the following statements with one of the following responses:

    a.   Rarely or never

    b.   Sometimes

    c.   Often

    d.   All or most of the time

1. I fantasize about sex.
2. I think about sex.
3. I am able to become aroused.
4. I remain aroused during sexual activities.
5. I enjoy having sex with my partner.
6. I engage in masturbation more than I feel is normal.
7. I worry about my sexual performance.
8. I feel worried about having sexual relations.

Male:

9. I experience pain when I have an erection or ejaculate.
10. I am able to achieve an erection.

Female:

11. I experience pain during vaginal penetration.
12. I have difficulty reaching an orgasm.

This self-assessment is not meant to be scored. Rather, it is intended as a tool to allow you to think critically about sexual performance and dysfunction.

After you have given initial responses to these questions, go back and review them two more times. The first time, consider whether you are satisfied with your initial response. In other words, think about whether you are happy with a particular aspect of your sexuality. Then consider whether your partner may be satisfied with your initial response.

For example, a man with a spinal-cord injury may not be able to achieve an erection. That situation may still be acceptable to both him and his partner, if they have found other satisfying sexual activities in which to engage.

Suggested Readings

Alterowitz, R., & Alterowitz, R. J. *Intimacy with impotence: The couple's guide to better sex after prostate disease.* Philadelphia, PA: Da Capo Press, 2004.

Coady, D., & Fish, N. *Healing painful sex: A woman's guide to confronting, diagnosing, and treating sexual pain.* Berkeley, CA: Seal Press, 2011.

Kleinplatz, P. J. (Ed.). *New directions in sex therapy: Innovations and alternatives,* 2nd ed. New York: Routledge, 2012.

Leiblum, S. (Ed.). *Treating sexual desire disorders: A clinical casebook.* New York: Guilford Press, 2010.

McCarthy, B., & McCarthy, E. *Sexual awareness: Your guide to healthy couple sexuality,* 5th ed. New York: Routledge, 2012.

Metz, M. E., & McCarthy, B. *Coping with erectile dysfunction: How to regain confidence and enjoy great sex.* Oakland, CA: New Harbinger Publications, 2004.

Moynihan, R., & Mintzes, B. *Sex, lies, and pharmaceuticals: How drug companies plan to profit from female sexual dysfunction.* Vancouver: Greystone Books, 2010.

Web Resourcess

For links to the websites below, visit *go.jblearning. com/dimensions5e* and click on Resource Links.

American Urology Association Foundation: Erectile Dysfunction
www.urologyhealth.org/urology/index.cfm?article=60

The educational arm of the American Urology Association, this website provides detailed information on nonsurgical options for treatment of erectile dysfunction. The site includes visuals to assist in understanding the condition. Links to updated pamphlets are provided.

Medline Plus: Sexual Problems in Men and Sexual Problems in Women
www.nlm.nih.gov/medlineplus/sexualproblemsinmen. html and *www.nlm.nih.gov/medlineplus/ sexualproblemsinwomen.html#cat1*

Managed by the National Library of Medicine, these websites provide links to an overview of female and male sexual dysfunctions, diagnosis, symptoms, treatment, prevention and screening, coping, management, clinical trials, and others.

Sexual Advice Association
www.sda.uk.net

A charitable organization in the UK, this website provides information about male and female sexual dysfunctions with links to news and articles and frequently asked questions.

Society for Sex Therapy and Research
www.sstarnet.org

The Society for Sex Therapy and Research (SSTAR) is composed of a broad range of professionals who have clinical or research interests in human sexual concerns. SSTAR's goals are to facilitate communications among clinicians who treat problems of sexual function, sexual identity, and reproductive life, and to provide a forum for exchange of ideas between those interested in research in human sexuality and those whose primary activities are patient care.

References

Althof, S. E. What's new in sex therapy. *Journal of Sexual Medicine,* 7 (2010), 5–13.

Althof, S. E., Leiblum, S. R., Chevret-Measson, M., Hartmann, U., Levine, S. B., McCabe, M., Plaut, M., Rodrigues, O., & Wylie, K. Psychological and interpersonal dimensions of sexual function and dysfunctions. *Journal of Sexual Medicine,* 7 (2010), 327–336.

Annon, J. S. *The behavioral treatment of sexual problems: Brief therapy.* New York: Harper & Row, 1976.

Bancroft, J. *Human sexuality and its problems,* 3rd ed. Edinburgh: Churchill Livingston/Elsevier, 2009.

Bancroft, J., Graham, C. A., Janssen, E., & Sanders, S. A. The dual-control model: Current status and future directions. *Journal of Sex Research,* 46 (2009), 121–142.

Bancroft, J., Loftus, J., & Long, J. S. Distress about sex: A national survey of women in heterosexual relationships. *Archives of Sexual Behavior,* 32 (2003), 193–208.

Barbach, L. *For each other: Sharing sexual intimacy.* New York: New American Library, 2001.

Barbach, L. G. *For yourself: The fulfillment of female sexuality.* New York: Signet, 2000.

Barbach, L. G. *Women discover orgasm: A therapist's guide to a New Testament approach.* New York: Free Press, 1980.

Betchen, S. J. Premature ejaculation: An integrative, intersystems approach for couples. *Journal of Family Psychotherapy, 20* (2009), 241–260.

Binik, Y. The DSM diagnostic criteria for dyspareunia. *Archives of Sexual Behavior, 39, no. 2* (2010), 292–303.

Bradley, P. D., & Fine, R. W. The Medicalization of sex therapy: A call to action for therapists. *Journal of Systemic Therapies, 28, no. 2* (2009), 75–88.

Brotto, L., Basson, R., & Luria, M. A mindfulness-based group psychoeducational intervention targeting sexual arousal disorder in women. *Journal of Sexual Medicine, 5* (2008), 1646–1659.

Brotto, L., Heiman, J., Goff, B., Greer, B., Lentz, G., Swisher, E., Tamimi, H., & Van Blaricom, A. A psychoeducational intervention for sexual dysfunction in women with gynecologic cancer. *Archives of Sexual Behavior, 37* (2008), 317–329.

Brotto, L. A. The DSM diagnostic criteria for hypoactive sexual desire disorder in men. *Journal of Sexual Medicine, 7* (2010a), 2015–2030.

Brotto, L. A. The DSM diagnostic criteria for hypoactive sexual desire disorder in women. *Archives of Sexual Behavior, 39* (2010b), 221–239.

Brotto, L. A. The DSM diagnostic criteria for sexual aversion disorder. *Archives of Sexual Behavior, 39, no. 2* (2010c), 271–277.

Brotto, L. A., Bitzer, J., Laan, E., Leiblum, S., & Luria, M. Women's sexual desire and arousal disorders. *Journal of Sexual Medicine, 7* (2010), 586–614. doi: 10.1111/j.1743-6109.2009.01630.x.

Brotto, L. A., Sealb, B. N., & Rellini, A. Pilot study of a brief cognitive behavioral versus mindfulness-based intervention for women with sexual distress and a history of childhood sexual abuse. *Journal of Sex & Marital Therapy, 38, no. 1* (2012), 1–27.

Chivers, M., & Rosen, R. C. PDE5 inhibitors and female sexual response: Faulty protocols or paradigms? *Journal of Sexual Medicine, 7* (2010), 858–872.

Connora, M. K., Maserejiana, N. N., De Rogatisb, L., Mestonc, C. M., Gerstenbergera, E. P., & Rosena, R. C. Sexual desire, distress, and associated factors in premenopausal women: Preliminary findings from the Hypoactive Sexual Desire Disorder Registry for Women. *Journal of Sex & Marital Therapy, 37, no. 3* (2011), 176–189.

DeRogatis, L. R. & Burnett, A. L. The epidemiology of sexual dysfunctions. *Journal of Sexual Medicine, 5* (2008), 289–300.

Ellis, A., & Harper, R. *A guide to rational living.* North Hollywood, CA: Melvin Powers, Wilshire Book Company, 1975.

Ellis, A., & Harper, R. *A new guide to rational living.* Englewood Cliffs, NJ: Prentice-Hall, 1979.

Farrell, J., & Cacchioni, T. The medicalization of women's sexual pain. *The Journal of Sex Research, 49, 4,* (2012), 328–336. doi: 10.1080/00224499.2012.688227.

Fisher, H. *The first sex: The natural talents of women and how they are changing the world.* New York: Ballantine, 1999.

Gambescia, N., Sendak, S. K., & Weeks, G. The treatment of erectile dysfunction. *Journal of Family Psychotherapy, 20* (2009), 221–240.

Giugliano, J. R., Sexual addiction: diagnostic problems. *International Journal of Mental Health Addiction, 7* (2009), 283–294.

Graham, C. A. The DSM diagnostic criteria for female orgasmic disorder. *Archives of Sexual Behavior, 39* (2010a), 256–270.

Graham, C. A. The DSM diagnostic criteria for female sexual arousal disorder. *Archives of Sexual Behavior, 39* (2010b), 240–255.

Greenberg, J. S. *Comprehensive stress management,* 11th ed. New York: McGraw-Hill Higher Education, 2009.

Heiman, J. R. Treating low sexual desire: New findings for testosterone in women. *New England Journal of Medicine, 359* (2006), 2047–2049.

Kafka, M. P. Hypersexual disorder: A proposed diagnosis for DSM-V. *Archives of Sexual Behavior, 39* (2010), 377–400.

Kaplan, H. S. *Sexual aversion, sexual phobias, and panic disorder.* New York: Brunner-Mazel, 1987.

Kaplan, H. S. *Disorders of sexual desire.* New York: Simon & Schuster, 1979.

Kaplan, H. S. *The evaluation of sexual disorders.* New York: Brunner/Mazel, 1983.

Kaplan, H. S. *The new sex therapy: Active treatment of sexual dysfunction.* New York: Brunner/Mazel, 1974.

Klein, M. *America's war on sex: The attack on law, lust and liberty.* Westport, CT: Praeger, 2006.

Landry, T., & Bergeron, S. How young does vulvo-vaginal pain begin? Prevalence and characteristics of dyspareunia in adolescents. *Journal of Sexual Medicine, 6* (2009), 927–935.

Laumann, E. O., Glasser, D. B., Neves, R. C. S., & Moreira, E. for the GSSAB Investigators' Group. A population-based survey of sexual activity, sexual problems and associated help-seeking behavior patterns in mature adults in the United States of America. *International Journal of Impotence Research, 21* (2009), 171–178.

Leiblum, S. R., & Pervin, L. A. *Principles and practice of sex therapy*. New York: Guilford Press, 1980.

Lewis, R. W., Fugl-Meyer, K. S., Bosch, R., Fugl-Meyer, A. R., Laumann, E. O., Lizza, E., & Martin-Morales, A. Epidemiology/risk factors of sexual dysfunction. *Journal of Sexual Medicine, 1, no. 1* (2004), 35–39.

Lewis, R. W., Fugl-Meyer, K. S., Corona, G., Hayes, R. D., Laumann, E. O., Moreira, E. D., Rellini, A. H., & Segraves, T. Definitions/epidemiology/risk factors for sexual dysfunction. *Journal of Sexual Medicine, 7* (2010), 1598–1607.

LoPiccolo, J. Direct treatment of sexual dysfunction in the couple. In *Handbook of sexology*, Money, J., & Masaph, H., eds. Amsterdam: Elsevier/North-Holland, 1977, 1227–1244.

MacBride, M. B., Rhodes, D. J., & Shuster, L. T. Vulvovaginal atrophy. *Mayo Clinic Proceedings, 85* (2010), 87–94.

Marshall, B. L. Medicalization and the refashioning of age-related limits on sexuality. *The Journal of Sex Research, 49, 4* (2012), 337–343. doi: 10.1080/00224499.2011.644597.

Masters, W. H., & Johnson, V. E. *Human sexual inadequacy*. Boston: Little, Brown, 1970.

Mayo Foundation for Medical Education and Research. Priapism, 2010. Available: http://www.mayoclinic.com/health/priapism/DS00873.

Mayo Foundation for Medical Education and Research. Premature ejaculation: Causes, 2011. Available: http://www.mayoclinic.com/health/premature-ejaculation/DS00578/DSECTION=causes.

McCabe, M. P. Anorgasmia in women, *Journal of Family Psychotherapy, 20* (2009), 177–197.

McCabe, M. P., & Goldhammer, D. L. Demographic and psychological factors related to sexual desire among heterosexual women in a relationship. *Journal of Sex Research, 49* (2012), 78–87.

McCarthy, B. W., Ryan, M., & Johnson, F. A. *Sexual awareness: A practical approach*. San Francisco: Boyd & Fraser, 1975.

Meana, M. Painful intercourse: Dyspareunia and vaginismus *Journal of Family Psychotherapy, 20* (2009), 198–220.

Meana, M., & Binik, Y. M. Painful coitus: A review of female dyspareunia. *Journal of Nervous and Mental Disease, 182* (1994), 264–272.

Nagaraj, A. K. M., Pai, N. B., & Rao, S. A comparative study of sexual dysfunction involving risperidone, quetiapine, and olanzapine. *Indian Journal of Psychiatry, 51* (2009), 265–271.

Perelman, M. A., & Rowland, D. L. Retarded ejaculation. *World Journal of Urology, 24, 6* (2006), 645–652. doi: 10.1007/s00345-006-0127-6.

Petersen, J., & Hyde, J. S. Gender differences in sexuality. In J. C. Chrisler & D. R. McCreary (Eds.), *Handbook of Gender Research in Psychology*. New York: Springer, 2010.

Reissing, E. D., Binik, Y. M., Khalife, S., Cohen, D., & Amsel, R. Vaginal spasm, pain, and behavior: An empirical investigation of the diagnosis of vaginismus. *Archives of Sexual Behavior, 33* (2004), 5–17.

Rosen, R., Janssen, E., Wiegel, M., Bancroft, J., Althof, S., Wincze, J., et al. Psychological and interpersonal correlates in men with erectile dysfunction and their partners. *Journal of Sex & Marital Therapy, 32* (2006), 215–234.

Rosen, R. C., Fisher, W. A., Eardley, I., Niederberger, C., Nadel, A., & Sand, M. The multinational Men's Attitudes to Life Events and Sexuality (MALES) study: I. Prevalence of erectile dysfunction and related health concerns in the general population. *Current Medical Research and Opinion, 20* (2004), 607–617.

Schover, L., Friedman, J., Weiler, S., Heiman, J., & LoPiccolo, J. Multi-axial problem-oriented system for sexual dysfunctions. *Archives of General Psychiatry, 39* (1982), 614–619.

Segraves, R. T. Considerations for an evidence-based definition of premature ejaculation in the DSM-V. *Journal of Sexual Medicine, 7* (2010a), 672–689.

Segraves, R. T. Considerations for diagnostic criteria for erectile dysfunction in DSM V. *Journal of Sexual Medicine, 7* (2010b), 654–671.

Semans, J. Premature ejaculation: A new approach. *Southern Medical Journal, 49* (1956), 353–358.

Snegroff, S. The stressors of non-marital sexual intercourse. *Health Education, 17* (1986), 21–23.

Spark, R. F. Patient information: Sexual problems in men. *UpToDate, 16* (2008), 3. Available: http://www.uptodate. com/patients/content/topic.do?topicKey=~nXT881SoKLFIS 2T&selectedTitle=2~150&source=search_result.

Tiefer, L. Beyond the medical model of women's sexual problems: A campaign to resist the promotion of 'female sexual dysfunction.' *Sexual and Relationship Therapy, 25, no. 2* (2010), 197–205.

The Trustees of Columbia University. What is pre-orgasmic? 2012. Available: http://goaskalice.columbia.edu/ what-pre-orgasmic.

Turner, M. Uncovering and treating sex addiction in couples therapy. *Journal of Family Psychotherapy, 2* (2009), 283–302.

van Lankveld, J. Self-help therapies for sexual dysfunction. *Journal of Sex Research, 46* (2009), 143–155.

van Lankveld, J. J. D. M., Granot, M., Weijmar Schultz, W. C. M., Binik, Y. M., Wesselmann, U., Pukall, C. F., Bohm-Starke, N., & Achtrari, C. Women's sexual pain disorders. *Journal of Sexual Medicine, 7* (2010), 615–631.

Van Minnen, A., & Kampman, M. The interaction between anxiety and sexual functioning: A controlled study of sexual functioning in women with anxiety disorders. *Sexual and Relationship Therapy, 15* (2000), 47–57.

Weeks, G. R., Hertlein, K. M., & Gambescia, N. The Treatment of hypoactive sexual desire disorder. *Journal of Family Psychotherapy, 20* (2009), 129–149.

Wilson, G. T., Nathan, P. E., O'Leary, K. D., & Clark, L. A. *Abnormal psychology: Integrating perspectives.* Needham, MA: Allyn & Bacon, 1996.

Winters, J. Hypersexual disorder: A more cautious approach. *Archives of Sexual Behavior, 39* (2010), 594–596.

Wolpe, J. *Psychotherapy by reciprocal inhibition.* Stanford: Stanford University Press, 1958.

Woody, J. D. Sexual addiction/hypersexuality and the DSM: Update and practice guidance for social workers, *Journal of Social Work Practice in the Addictions, 11, no. 4* (2011), 301–320.

The Working Group on A New View of Women's Sexual Problems. A New View of Women's Sexual Problems, 2000. Available: http://www.newviewcampaign.org/ manifesto5.asp.

Zenilman, J. M., & Shahmanesh, M. *Sexually transmitted infections: Diagnosis, management, and treatment.* Burlington, MA: Jones & Bartlett Learning, 2011.

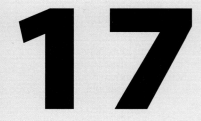

CHAPTER 17

Sexual Consumerism

FEATURES

Communication Dimensions
Feelings About Sexual Themes

Ethical Dimensions
Controlling Cyberspace

Gender Dimensions
Male and Female Use of Autoerotic Materials

Ethical Dimensions
Should Kids Be Sexualized?

Multicultural Dimensions
"Values" of Prostitution in Other Countries?

Multicultural Dimensions
Organizations for Sex Workers

Global Dimensions
International Differences Related to Prostitution

CHAPTER OBJECTIVES

1 Describe the ways in which sexuality is used in the mass media, including advertising, TV, movies, literature, popular music, and on the Internet.

2 Discuss what constitutes sexually explicit materials, the results of research on their effects, and efforts to control their distribution.

3 Describe the different types of sex workers and the economic factors associated with sex work.

go.jblearning.com/dimensions5e

Advertising
Literature
The Control of Sexually Explicit Materials

INTRODUCTION

Not long ago, in a human sexuality class, the conversation turned to the relationship between sexuality and money. Some students were surprised when others became very interested in the topic. They seemed to feel that there was nothing to be gained by continuing the conversation because they did not see a relationship between sexuality and money.

The students interested in the topic persisted. One of the communication majors pointed out that in his classes he learned that messages and products related to sexuality are big business. The saying "You've come a long way, baby" definitely applies to this topic for better or worse, he pointed out. He went on to say that we are all bombarded with sexual themes daily; that you cannot turn on TV, pick up a magazine, or see a billboard without being confronted with sexual topics and themes. This use of sexual content, he indicated, is designed to sell even products that have no relation to sexuality.

Some other students warmed up to the discussion. One student, a psychology major, mentioned that commercialism related to sexuality has taken another form as well. Products specifically related to sexuality are available in large numbers and in great variety. Whether you want to put it in, dangle it about, or place it on, there is a store where you can get whatever "it" is.

Several students started arguing about whether the use of sexual themes to influence consumers is good or bad. One health education major argued that the use of sexual themes to sell products unrelated to sexuality is sexploitation, with the potential for sexism. He said this situation could prompt people to view others as sex objects, and it could interfere with personal relationships and sexual satisfaction as well—because when *one compares one's partner against the commercialized ideal seen in the media, one is likely to be disappointed. This could lead to frustration and a mean-spiritedness that might translate into poor communication, sexual and otherwise.*

Another student, a business major, jumped into the fray and added that the pressure to be like people in the ads—sexy, gorgeous, hunky— may cause people to feel inferior and ashamed of their body. Feelings of inferiority and shame, as we learned earlier, can progress to sexual dysfunction.

Still another student pointed out that appearance may not be the only concern. She expressed concern that as the result of observing the sexual prowess of television and movie stars on-screen, we assume that all of us should be able to affect our partners the same way. If they do not swoon at the very thought of a caress from us, if they do not get light-headed when we place an arm around them, if they do not lick their lips when they see us in a state of semiundress, we may believe that we are ineffective lovers. Thus, because of unrealistic depictions of sexual behavior in the movies and TV, ordinary people like us may fear losing our lovers because we cannot sexually satisfy them.

A nursing major argued that some people value sexual commercialization. Whether because idealized views of sexual activity are exciting, because they have potential for improving sexual relationships by indicating new ways to relate, or because they help to desensitize people to an emotionally charged topic (namely, sexuality), these views are considered a positive trend by many people, he said.

The students' discussion was useful in that it covered most of the points that the instructor wanted to raise before starting the chapter on sexuality and commercial activities. Regardless of our points of view, sexual commercialization is probably here to stay. This chapter considers how sexuality is used in a commercial sense and will help you become a better sexual consumer.

■ Mass Media and the Arts

Advertising

Advertisements in magazines and newspapers that use sexual themes to sell products are abundant. One need only turn at random to any page and more than likely an ad or an article that has some relationship to sex or sexual attractiveness will be evident. In the 1990s, there was a controversy related to ads for condoms.

Because of increasing incidence of HIV/AIDS, many people argued that condom ads were needed to help prevent further spread of disease. Many others argued that there should not be condom ads because they feared such ads would encourage more sexual activity—particularly among adolescents and other unmarried people. Little by little, ads for condoms have become more common, and there have not been increases in sexual activity. In fact, in other countries, where condoms have been openly advertised for years, there are lower rates of STIs, lower rates of unwanted pregnancies, and fewer abortions.

After so much controversy about condom ads, it has been interesting to observe the response to ads for Viagra, Cialis, Levitra, and other products with the sole purpose of enhancing sexual pleasure. These ads are found in newspapers, magazines, on the Internet, and on TV. For some reason, there has not been much controversy about these ads. In some cases, well-known celebrities have talked about how well the products work and how they have helped with their relationships. The presence of these ads seems to have made it more acceptable to talk about sexual behavior in general—even for people in older age groups. This is an excellent example of the impact that advertising can have in certain circumstances.

Most advertising with sexual themes is pretty obvious if you give it a moment's thought, but in the 1970s a book called *Subliminal Seduction*—about subliminal sexual selling—created a furor (Key, 1973). The main premise of the author, Wilson Key, was that many advertisers who used sexual imagery to sell their products intended it to work on the viewer's subconscious, not conscious, awareness. To support his premise Key cited the following kinds of imagery he had found in enlarged photographs taken from magazine ads:

1. Images of people engaged in sexual activity, hidden in the shading of ice cubes in liquor advertisements

2. The word *fuck* or *sex*, written in very small letters, hidden in the ads

3. Pictures that appeared innocent on one side of a magazine page but that made sexual suggestions when held up to the light—for example, a picture of a woman standing on the front of a blank sheet, backed by a picture of a projectile (such as an airplane or cigar) aimed at her vagina

4. Pictures composed to suggest genitals—for instance, of liquor bottles with small round objects on each side (such as oranges or apples) suggesting a penis and two testicles

Some critics have argued that Key went too far and that looking for sexual connotations in ice cubes is in itself perverse. In fact, many feel that Key had no evidence or research to support his ideas. Some marketers today believe that subliminal advertising is a farce. However, research is still done on subliminal exposure. For example, Gillath et al. (2007) looked at the effects of subliminal exposure to sexual

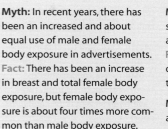

Myth vs Fact

Myth: In recent years, there has been an increased and about equal use of male and female body exposure in advertisements.
Fact: There has been an increase in breast and total female body exposure, but female body exposure is about four times more common than male body exposure.

Myth: Women appear more often than men in television beer commercials.
Fact: Men appear twice as often as women in television beer commercials.

Myth: Television is the main source of information about sexuality for teenagers.
Fact: Friends are the main source of information about sexuality for teenagers.

Myth: Fraudulent sexual aids are not among the top sources of health fraud in the United States.
Fact: According to the Food and Drug Administration, fraudulent sexual aids are among the top 10 sources of health fraud in the United States.

stimuli on men and women. They found that some subliminal exposure to sexual stimuli did not affect the sexual arousal of men, but caused women to have lower sexual arousal. Other subliminal exposure led to more sex-related thoughts in both men and women. So, we are still not certain about the overall influence of subliminal advertising.

Ads crafted to appeal to basic needs are apparently highly effective, even without the kinds of things Key described. For example, some would argue that Paris Hilton washing a car while eating a hamburger is a more recent example of advertising that might be called subliminal advertising and that it appeals to basic needs.

As we shall see in this chapter, we buy many products without fully understanding why. Those selling us these products, though, know that one of the hidden motivations behind our buying habits relates to sexuality. We want to appear sexy, appeal to a potential sexual partner, and feel attractive; knowing this, salespeople use these needs to persuade us to buy products, even though we think we are buying them for reasons totally divorced from sexuality.

Advertisers seem to have made a study of sexual motivation. Some research from as long ago as 1973 suggested that since oral–genital activity had become relatively acceptable and widely practiced (Hunt, 1974), it found its way into product advertising. What better way to sell cigarettes to women, for example, than to associate cigarettes with penises? For years cigarettes have been used as phallic symbols. Beginning in the 1930s, cigarette ads featured only men offering cigarettes to women, employing phallic symbolism. Cigarette ads included words such as *longer, firmer, rounder, more satisfying, better tasting,* and *more pleasing* (not to mention *more fully packed*).

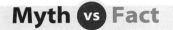

Myth vs Fact

Myth: There are special exercises and/or creams that are helpful in increasing the size of a female's breasts.
Fact: Breast size and shape are the result of glandular influences and cannot be altered by exercise or by application of anything to the breast.

Myth: Prostitution is illegal in most countries around the world.
Fact: In many countries there are no laws against prostitution. In fact, the United Nations adopted a resolution in favor of decriminalization of prostitution.

Myth: It is illegal to release the names of those accused of using prostitutes or the prostitutes themselves publicly until they have been shown to be guilty in a court of law.
Fact: Although some civil liberties groups object, in some states the identities of prostitutes and their customers are made public as soon as they are arrested—before any court action occurs.

Automobile advertisements make obvious use of sexual appeals, along with appeals to such other needs as recognition and esteem. When cars were long and well adorned, they were presented as phallic symbols. *Real* men, the ads suggested, wanted long cars. The tips of automobiles were even ornamented. Today, although car companies sell smaller cars as a rule, their ads still associate the product with sexuality, sometimes by posing pretty, well-endowed, scantily clad, and perfectly proportioned females beside cars. At automobile shows, held in coliseums and arenas throughout the United States, companies employ young female models (again scantily clad) to adorn their displays.

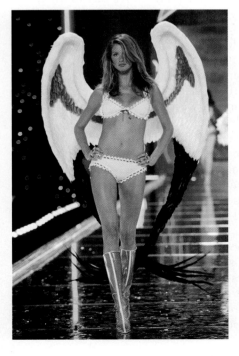

Victoria's Secret became a multi-billion-dollar company by redefining the market for underwear. Here a model shows off the "Angels" line of lingerie at a fashion show. After a single TV ad shown during the 1999 Super Bowl, more than 1 million people inundated the Victoria's Secret website, hoping for a glimpse of more "fashion."

Liquor ads are particularly notable for linking sexual imagery to our aspirations for living well. The people depicted as liquor drinkers are handsome, well dressed, sophisticated, flirtatious, and the object of someone else's unconcealed attention. Readers are supposed to envy the exciting life these attractive people live and, through their choice of liquor purchases, to emulate them.

Whether intended for this purpose or not, advertisements can send sexual messages as well as messages related to gender bias. For example, over a 10-year period there was a significant increase in breast exposure and total female body exposure even though fashion trends did not account for this change. In addition, female body exposure was about four times more common than male body exposure, in part because women were displayed in underwear and bikini swimsuits more often than were men (Plous & Neptune, 1997).

The use of sexual themes to sell products expanded in some interesting ways. For example, in 2001 Abercrombie & Fitch said its summer catalog was sexy in a wholesome sort of way. Critics called it soft porn and joined forces to boycott the trendy youth-oriented retailer. The catalog featured young unclad male and female models to woo younger customers and use sexual themes to popularize the image of the company (Crary, 2001).

Interestingly, in 2005 Abercrombie and Fitch had another related difficulty with its products. The Women & Girls Foundation of Southwest Pennsylvania promoted a national "girlcott" of a new line of Abercrombie and Fitch T-shirts that had "sexist" slogans such as "Who needs brains when you have these," "Blondes are adored, brunettes are ignored," "Give me something to scream about," and "Available for parties." The retailer issued a statement acknowledging that the shirts that were meant to be humorous might be troubling to some. It agreed to stop selling the shirts.

In Europe, Durex, the world's number one condom maker, started a TV and print advertising campaign using humor. In one TV ad a young man walking down the street to meet his date was followed by a boisterous and excited crowd of men dressed in white sperm costumes. The sperm were suddenly trapped, squirming, in a huge condom in the middle of the street. The ad had the tagline "Durex: For a Hundred Million Reasons" (Durex condom maker using "humor" ads to sell condoms in Europe, 2001).

In 2005 another controversy erupted over another type of advertising—store mannequins. Local residents in McLean, Virginia, and Wauwatosa, Wisconsin, were upset about Victoria's Secret scantily clad and provocatively posed mannequins. There were female mannequins on all fours, others intertwined on a bed, and still others in "garters and whatnot, and the only thing missing is a whip," said one resident. Some residents of these communities were very upset, while others failed to see what the fuss was about. A spokesman for Victoria's Secret said: "All we're trying to do is market what we sell. You see bras and underwear. That's lingerie. That's what we sell." In other examples, Diesel's ad campaign celebrated "the world of individual hedonistic pleasure pursuits." One shot featured women with whips. Hipster chain American Apparel had softcore-styled ads including a tight focus on barely covered backsides of women (Barker, 2005).

A different type of controversy arose in 2009 related to Bayer's advertising campaign for its contraceptive Yaz, the most popular birth control pill in the United States. In an agreement with the U.S. Food and Drug Administration (FDA), Bayer launched a $20 million ad campaign to correct previous misleading marketing of Yaz. The FDA believed that Bayer ads had overstated Yaz's ability to treat acne and improve women's moods, while downplaying its health risks. Bayer had to run commercials to set the record straight. In the new ads, an actress said, "You may have seen some Yaz commercials recently that were not clear. The FDA wants us to correct a few points in those ads" ("Unusual" FDA order requiring corrections to Yaz ad campaign, 2009).

Television Advertising and Programming

Kuriansky (1996) provided an interesting historical overview of sexuality and television advertising. Here are some of the highlights:

1. Beer led the way for using sexual themes to sell. One TV ad in the 1950s showed a tired husband growing perky after drinking a beer. He then chased his wife around the room while disrobing.

2. Car spots also pioneered the sexy sell by using sexy models draped over the hood or stroking the wheel suggestively.

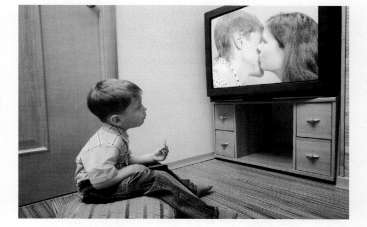

Many sexual themes are used as part of advertising on TV.

3. In 1980 then-15-year-old Brooke Shields panted that nothing came between her and her Calvins. Though some versions of the ad were banned, jeans sales doubled.

4. In the early 1990s a group of female employees sued Stroh's brewery for sexual harassment and named the company's "Swedish Bikini Team" campaign (featuring buxom, blonde, bikini-clad women) as contributing to a "hostile work environment."

5. In 1995 the FBI investigated a Calvin Klein ad featuring an underage teen stripping for a photographer. Many pairs of jeans were sold.

6. Candies hiking boots received more free exposure than paid air time when a furor erupted over the censorship of scenes of a nude couple straddling a chair.

7. What is acceptable on U.S. TV is often tame compared to that in other parts of the world where full frontal nudity is used to sell everything from shock absorbers to sardines. In a Danish TV spot, a newspaper is draped over a man's erect penis as he spies on ladies in the steam room.

(?) Did You Know . . .

Personal ads in newspapers have been around for many years but are much more prevalent now. They can be found on the Internet, in newspapers, in magazines, and on the radio. A radio station that has a phone-dating service will hook you up with people of a similar demographic and music-taste level. Even legitimate regional magazines, like *Boston* magazine,

carry personal ads. Your choice of whom you want may be partially influenced by where he or she advertises. For example, advertising in *Boston* magazine is much more expensive than advertising in the local newspapers, so such ads may attract a more upscale clientele.

8. Cloaking sexuality in romance is one way to prevent controversy. The Taster's Choice soap-opera-like spots follow a handsome neighbor invited in for coffee and whatever else.

9. Humor also relieves the anxiety of sexual suggestion. In another ad, the actress Annie Potts is lifted into a hulk's arms while extolling the virtues of large popcorn kernels.

10. It seems that sexual themes will always sell. The Candies CEO said: "In 30 to 60 seconds, to keep people from going to the refrigerator, you have to astound them. And sex does."

There have also been some interesting events related to the history of sexual themes on TV (Silver, 2011). For example, back in the 1950s, Ricky and Lucy had separate beds and characters couldn't even use the word "pregnant." Two decades later the title character in the *All in the Family* spin-off *Maude* could decide to have an abortion. In the 1970s the network series *Soap* pushed boundaries with an openly gay main character. Still, in 1989 just the sight of two men in the same bed on *Thirtysomething* caused many sponsors to vanish, along with more than a million ad dollars. On the flip side, it was *NYPD Blue's* heterosexual content that aroused the ire of the American Family Association, even before the program hit the air in 1993. The group objected to the show's "steamy sex scenes," and more than 50 ABC affiliates chose not to broadcast the pilot. During its 12-year run the show often flouted authority with its depictions of both male and female bare behinds. In January 2011, a court threw out an FCC fine imposed on ABC for such a shot from an episode that first aired 8 years earlier. Despite ever-changing social mores, nudity on TV can still result in lasting controversies.

Dating shows have become popular in the 21st century. This popularity has shown that people want to observe others in their love and sexual relationships. Not all of the shows are about dating; they may deal with personal relationships in general. All of the shows can make love and romance look phony at best, and vicious at worst. However, large numbers of people seem to enjoy these shows. In 2012 an Internet search listed 54 dating and relationship TV shows (see Table 17.1).

The Kaiser Family Foundation reported that the number of sexual scenes on TV nearly doubled from 1998 to 2005. Approximately 70% of all shows included some sexual content, and these shows

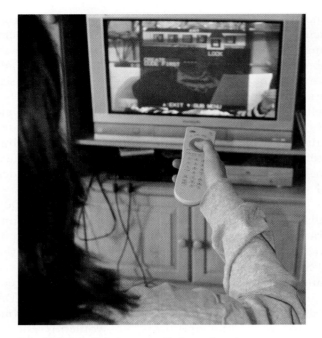

Television is a major source of information about sexuality for people of all ages.

averaged 5 sexual scenes per hour. This compared to 56% and 3.2 scenes per hour in 1998 and 64% and 4.4 scenes per hour in 2002. About 14% of shows with sexual content included reference to sexual risks and responsibilities (such as waiting to have sexual intercourse, using protection, or possible consequences of unprotected sexual activity). This rate was up from 9% in 1998 and about the same as the rate in 2002 (TV sexual scenes nearly double since 1998, 2005).

The Parents' Television Council reported that children watching TV during the first hour of prime time are assaulted by violence, profanity, or sexual content once every 3.5 minutes of noncommercial time. Incidence of sexual content increased by 22.1% from 2002 to 2007. Broadcasters also greatly increased the prevalence of harsh language obscured by bleeps or partial editing such as "f-words" or "s-words" (PTC study: Broadcast TV family hour fare filthier than ever, 2007).

Many people have protested the television industry's portrayal of sexual themes in everyday life. Although objections to the portrayal of explicit sexual activities and the use of sexual language have been raised for some time, today people are beginning to object to the nature and quality of the sexual relationships enacted—stereotypical roles, sexual violence and hostility, incessant teasing, and more physical than emotional display—and to be concerned about the effects of these views of sexuality on socialization of the young.

TABLE 17.1 Dating and Relationship Reality TV Shows

1. Cheaters	28. Meet My Folks
2. The Bachelor	29. My Big Fat Obnoxious Fiance
3. Millionaire Matchmaker	30. #1 Single
4. What Chilli Wants	31. Who Wants to Marry My Dad
5. The Bachelorette	32. Here Come the Newlyweds
6. Blind Date	33. Cupid
7. elimiDATE	34. Chains of Love
8. Daisy of Love	35. Playing it Straight
9. Frank the Entertainer in a Basement Affair	36. Farmer Wants a Wife
10. That's Amore!	37. Mr. Personality
11. Temptation Island	38. Married by America
12. Newlyweds: Nick and Jessica	39. Love Cruise
13. Love Games: Bad Girls Need Love Too	40. Confessions of a Matchmaker
14. Joe Millionaire	41. Dismissed
15. Matched in Manhattan	42. 'Til Death Do Us Part: Carmen and Dave
16. Kept@	43. The Player
17. Dating in the Dark	44. Ex-Wives Club
18. Basketball Wives	45. Anything for Love
19. There's Something About Miriam	46. Bachelorettes in Alaska
20. Average Joe	47. Hooking Up
21. Paradise Hotel	48. Bachelor Pad
22. For Love or Money	49. Shipmates
23. Age of Love	50. Regency House Party
24. Forever Eden	51. Taildaters
25. Momma's Boys	52. G-String Divas
26. Outback Jack	53. Love Is in the Heir
27. The Littlest Groom	54. Star Dates

Source: Data from Yahoo! Directory. Dating and relationships reality TV shows. Available: http://dir.yahoo.com/Entertainment/Television_Shows/Reality_Television/Dating_and_Relationships/?o=a.

A television rating system was adopted in 1997. The ratings system includes age-based symbols like those for movies, such as TV-G, TV-PG, TV-14, and TV-MA, as well as the codes V, S, L, and D to indicate violence, sexual themes, "adult" language, and suggestive dialogue.

Television can be an excellent way to educate people about healthy sexual practices. For instance, the Surgeon General of the United States warned that the spread of HIV and AIDS could be slowed only by sexual abstinence or the use of condoms during coitus. Fortunately, in recent years we have seen an increase in condom ads on television.

Some broadcasters worry that the public disapproves of condom ads, and some worry they would lose sponsors that do not want their ads run alongside condom ads. However, 71% of Americans favor allowing condom ads on TV: 37% support the ads running at any time and 34% support the ads running at certain times, such as after 10 P.M. Even more support exists among adults younger than 50 years of age, of whom 82% say that condom ads should be allowed (Pardun & Forde, 2002/2003).

In early 2011 MTV executives thought they had a new hit drama on their hands called *Skins*. It featured the sexual and drug-fueled exploits of misfit teenagers (Stelter, 2011). Story lines included one boy trying to find a girl with whom his introverted friend could lose his virginity, instances of simulated masturbation, implied sexual assault, and teenagers disrobing and getting into bed together. In one episode a naked 17-year-old was shown from behind as he ran down a street. His erection was a punch line throughout the episode. Some feared that the show might break child pornography laws, because anyone younger than 18 is considered to be a minor. Whatever the reason, MTV cancelled the show in mid-2011. Some thought it was cancelled because it was too controversial; others thought it was simply because the ratings were not high enough. The exact reason was not given.

On cable TV, the fastest-growing segment is adult programming that portrays explicit sexual behavior. As cable availability expands, even more such programming is expected.

Many television programs have been devoted to educating the public about HIV and AIDS, and other programs have focused on such topics as sexual orientation and extramarital sexual activities. Many of these programs follow a talk-show format or are presented as documentaries; however, some sexual topics and issues are dramatized with the intent of entertaining and educating at the same time. For example, one situation comedy depicted a teenager being instructed to use a condom with his girlfriend, and another weekly comedy show depicted an unmarried couple living together and the problems they encountered.

Addressing the media in general, a position statement of the Sexuality Information and Education Council of the United States (SIECUS, 2012) indicates that

> SIECUS believes that the media has a responsibility to present the complexities of human sexuality at all stages of the life cycle in a manner that is medically accurate, sensitive to diversity, and free of exploitation, prejudice, gratuitous sexual violence, and dehumanizing sexual portrayals.

Recommendations for realistic, accurate images concerning sexuality in the media include the following (Edwards, 1996):

1. Dialogue that shows true communication among children, their parents, and trusted adults

2. Situations that show planned mature relationships as opposed to spur-of-the-moment responses to passion

3. Situations in which unprotected sexual encounters have negative repercussions

4. Articulate responsible characters with whom teenagers can identify

Interestingly, teens 15 to 17 years old believe that sexual content on TV influences the behavior of their peers, but not their own. They also report some positive aspects of sexual content on TV. They say they had learned how to say no in an uncomfortable

Communication
DIMENSIONS

Feelings About Sexual Themes

Common communication problems include (1) frame of reference, (2) emotional interference, and (3) physical distractions. Talk with two or three of your classmates about difficulties two people in an intimate relationship might have in these three areas when they are discussing the following topics:

1. Which characters do you think are the sexiest in current television shows? Why?
2. Which ads on TV or in magazines do you find most offensive? Why?
3. What does it take for materials to be considered obscene?
4. Which TV shows and/or movies do you think are most sexually stimulating? Why?
5. If you were a writer for a television series, how would you use sexual themes?

For example, in a discussion about sexy television shows, there could be a difference in which language is considered acceptable or in what might be considered sexy. This could cause emotional interference. Or perhaps one person could not relate to why something is sexually stimulating to another person. Thus one person's frame of reference could cause a problem. Go through each of the five questions with at least two or three other people and see which other possible barriers you can identify. Why do you think these barriers exist? What might be done about them to improve communication?

sexual situation, that they had learned how to communicate with a partner about safer sex, and that they had talked with their parents about a sexuality-related issue because of something they saw on TV (Notes from the research, 2002).

In 2004, Collins et al. conducted a national longitudinal survey of 1,792 adolescents between 12 and 17 years of age. They found that watching sexual themes on TV predicts and may hasten adolescent sexual initiation. They also reported that reducing the amount of sexual content on TV, reducing adolescent exposure to the content, or increasing references to and depictions of possible negative consequences of sexual activity could appreciably delay the initiation of coital and noncoital activities. Alternatively, parents may be able to reduce the effects of sexual content by watching TV with their children and discussing their own beliefs about sexuality and the behaviors portrayed.

Escobar-Chaves et al. (2005) studied the impact of the media on adolescent sexual attitudes and behaviors. In their discussion and in their findings they made many germane points. Among them are:

- Few studies have examined the effects of mass media on adolescent sexual attitudes and behavior.

- Young people report that media messages are an important influence in their lives.

- Two-thirds of youth aged 8 to 18 report having a TV in their bedroom, and more than one-third have their own VCR.

- American adolescents spend an average of 6 to 7 hours per day with some form of media, including TV, videotapes, movies, radio, print media, computers, the Internet, and video games.

- The average teenager spends about 3 hours per day watching TV.

- Much daily TV viewing occurs alone.

- Few parents establish rules about when or what their children may view on TV.

- The overall proportion of programming with sexual content continues to increase.

- Of programs popular with teens, 83% have sexual content, and 20% contain explicit or implicit sexual intercourse. On average, each hour of programs popular with teens contains 6.7 scenes that include sexual topics.

- Most sexual behavior on TV (79%) occurs between people who are not married to each other.

- Negative consequences of sexual activity are rarely portrayed. Very few programs have a primary emphasis on sexual risk and responsibility.

- Watching TV with sexual content has the effect of artificially aging children. Those who watch more than average behave sexually as though they were 9 to 17 months older. The 12-year-olds who watch the most have the sexual behaviors of the 14- and 15-year-olds who watch the least.

- Sexually experienced students are more likely to seek out sexual content on TV than non-sexually experienced youth.

- Adolescents who have just watched an hour of MTV are more likely to report approval of premarital sexual activity than those who have not.

Although a number of researchers have tried, it is difficult to definitively establish the relationship between sexual attitudes and behavior and TV viewing. In various studies it has been reported that those persons who watch more TV initiate sexual intercourse earlier, girls view more sexual content on TV than do boys, younger adolescents view more sexual content on TV than do older adolescents, those who watch more romantic programming are more likely to endorse traditional gender-role beliefs, and college students who are shown sexual TV content and perceive it as realistic are more likely to endorse permissive sexual attitudes and to estimate that more of their female peers are sexually active (Rich, 2008).

Chandra et al. (2008) indicated that teens exposed to high levels of television sexual content are twice as likely to experience a pregnancy in the subsequent 3 years as compared with those with lower levels of exposure. Conversely, Schroeder (2008) pointed out that "We should all raise a skeptical eyebrow whenever any research claims that there's a direct cause–effect relationship between one thing, such as TV viewing, and something as complex as teenage pregnancy." In other words, maybe the same people who are more likely to become pregnant as teenagers are also the same people who want to watch more sexual content on TV—maybe one doesn't cause the other at all.

It remains difficult to legally determine what sexual content is acceptable on TV and what is not, For example, a Supreme Court justice pointed out that when the FCC (Federal Communications Commission) prohibits all "patently offensive" references to sexual behavior, sexual organs, and excretion without giving adequate guidance to what "patently offensive" means, the FCC effectively chills speech because broadcasters have no way of knowing what the FCC will find offensive. This has the effect of promoting wide self-censorship of material that should be completely protected under the First Amendment (Lasar, 2012).

Sexuality and the Movies

Any cursory glance at the entertainment section of your local newspaper will show that movies are often marketed to the public by means of sexual themes—and have been for some time. In *The Blue Angel*, a 1930 film starring Marlene Dietrich (1930 was a time when women's bathing suits were much more than three small patches of flimsy cloth precariously held together by string), images of Marlene's bare thighs in a cabaret outfit made men's heads whirl. In *She Done Him Wrong*, when Mae West invited Cary Grant to "come up and see me some time," men's knees knocked. When Clark Gable (Rhett Butler) carried Vivian Leigh (Scarlett O'Hara) up a flight of stairs to her bedroom in *Gone with the Wind*, women swooned; when Marlon Brando appeared in his ripped undershirt in *A Streetcar Named Desire*, they panted. People's imaginations and perceptions, rather than nudity or sexual activity on film, were integral components of cinematic sexuality during the 1930s, 1940s, and 1950s.

By the 1960s and the 1970s, sexual permissiveness and experimentation had permeated the movies, as well as other segments of society. Movies previously shown as stag films and often called blue movies were elevated to respectable status. With the showing of *I Am Curious (Yellow), Deep Throat, Beyond the Valley of the Dolls, Vixen, The Lickerish Quartet*, and *Behind the Green Door* in movie theaters (in spite of attempts by local communities to ban them), people seemed to be less shocked. Although well-known movie stars had sometimes appeared nude in films in earlier years, a new era began when Marlon Brando appeared in the X-rated *Last Tango in Paris* in the early 1970s. The films of recent years leave little to the imagination and appeal more to the voyeur in us.

To help parents and others make decisions about the appropriateness of a particular movie for themselves or their children, a rating system was developed by the Motion Picture Association of America:

G: Appropriate for the general audience

PG: Appropriate for the general audience; however, parental guidance is advised. There may be brief nudity or some brief moments of sexually explicit language.

PG-13: Parents are advised that some of the material may be inappropriate for younger children.

R: Restricted to people at least 17 years of age or those accompanied by an adult due to sexual content, sexually explicit language, or violence

NC-17: No one under 17 years of age admitted. Extremely sexual in nature, and/or containing explicit sexual language, or extremely violent (but not necessarily pornographic).

In 2004, after parents complained that they wanted to let their kids see R-rated movies but didn't want to sit through the films themselves, a number of theaters in the Midwest started using a parent-approved pass card. To get the card, parents had to accompany their adolescent to the movie theater and sign for the photo ID R-card. Then, the student could get into R-rated films without the parent being

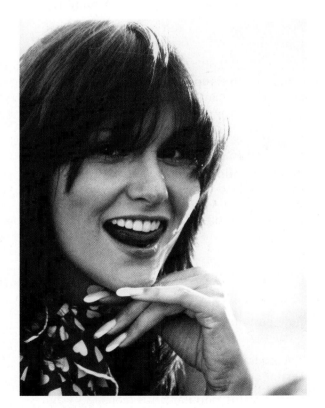

Linda Lovelace, former porn star, openly campaigned against sexually explicit movies. Lovelace was threatened into starring in *Deep Throat* by a physically abusive husband/manager. As were countless other young actresses, Lovelace was led to believe that appearing in adult films would open the door to legitimate film work.

present. This started a debate over convenience versus parental responsibility (Dennis, 2004).

Gunasekera et al. (2005) analyzed the portrayal of sexual themes in the most popular movies of the previous 20 years. Sexual activity, STI prevention, and birth control measures discussed or depicted were recorded. They reviewed 87 movies and found only one suggestion of condom use, which was the only reference to any form of birth control. There were no depictions of important consequences of unprotected sexual behavior such as unwanted pregnancies, HIV, or other STIs. Sexual depictions in popular movies lacked safe sex messages.

Corliss (2005) reported that European films are showing more sexual behavior. It is not pretend sexual behavior, but the real thing. For example, the film *9 Songs* explicitly gives the details of a summer affair. Corliss suggested that the film might better be called *9 Sex Acts*.

As with television and advertising, some people believe that the sexual explicitness of movies is detrimental to society, and others see this trend as positive. The opponents cite the weak commitments of sexual partners as partly responsible for the soaring adultery and divorce rates by setting poor examples of the meaning of intimate relationships. Those in favor of sexual explicitness in movies see this as just one sign of our increased openness about sexuality and the pleasures inherent in sexual behavior. We must make our own decisions about the appropriateness of this trend.

There have been a number of examples of the U.S. federal government's escalating war on indecency (Woellert, 2005). The George W. Bush administration launched a broad assault on sexual content that targeted the entertainment industry from Hollywood production to hotels. The offensive included creation of a Justice Department Obscenity Prosecution Task Force, an FBI anti-porn squad, a crackdown on indecent programming by the Federal Communications Commission, and a wave of indecency legislation. Many in Congress wanted to give regulators more power. However, business has been fighting back. Those selling cell phones, video iPods, and X-rated products could stand to lose a lot of money if the federal government's war on indecency succeeds.

In a different type of regulatory action, the Los Angeles City Council approved a mandate requiring all actors in pornographic films to wear condoms (Medina, 2012). The AIDS Healthcare Foundation had pressed for such legislation for years to help reduce the spread of HIV and to promote the use of condoms. However, the Free Speech Coalition felt that this was an example of government overreaching and intruding into consenting adults' decisions.

A unique aspect of the new mandate was its requirement that the police perform spot checks on any movie set once a permit is issued.

Videos and Video Games

The video rental business has grown by leaps and bounds. Video rental shops can be found in almost every community. These stores stock popular movies soon after they are shown in neighborhood theaters. In addition to these popular movies, often times a separate area houses the X-rated video library, usually out of view so customers are not offended by the movies' enticing packages and children are not exposed to them. Many shelves of the most sexually explicit films are available to rent and to view in the privacy of one's home. However, in recent years these shops have been given lots of competition from online rental sources, companies that handle video rentals through the mail, and various home recorders of TV shows. Some stores have even gone out of business because people have other sources for their videos and video games.

The availability of sexually explicit material has alarmed some people. They consider these X-rated movies to be pure trash with the potential to instigate sexual violence and to stereotype females as sex objects. They argue that these materials are obscene and pornographic and, as such, should be prohibited. However, others view the openness toward sexual expression of various kinds to be healthy. They argue that a couple's sexual relationship can be enhanced by viewing sexually explicit films, learning about new sexual activities, or being implicitly given permission to act out sexual fantasies. The courts have ruled that people have the right to rent sexually explicit videos and rental shop owners have the right to make such videos available. However, pressure from local groups in some communities has convinced shop owners voluntarily to remove the X-rated videos from their stock. In one view, this expression of community standards is considered healthy and the epitome of the democratic process at work. In another view, it is described as the "uptight" majority's dictating sexual mores to the more sexually comfortable minority. As we learned previously, one's view of sexual morality relates to the valuing of one's ethical principles; this is an example of that process at work.

In 1994 the Entertainment Software Rating Board was formed under heat from Congress to crack down on violent video games. It is a self regulating video game industry group. It uses the following rating system:

- EC (Early Childhood—ages 3+) contains no material parents would find inappropriate.

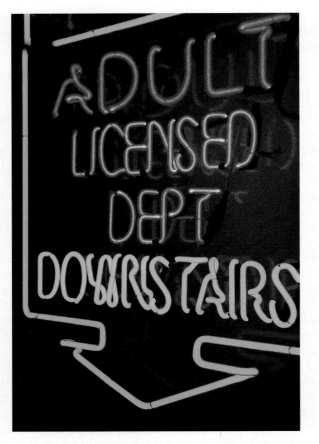

People have various opinions about the legality and availability of sexually explicit materials.

- E (Everyone: ages 6+) contains minimal cartoon, fantasy, or mild violence and/or infrequent use of mild language.

- E10+ (Everyone: ages 10+) contains more cartoon, fantasy, or mild violence, mild profanity, and/or minimally suggestive themes.

- T (Teen: 13+) contains violence, suggestive themes, crude humor, minimal blood, and/or infrequent use of strong language.

- M (Mature: 17+) contains mature sexual themes, more intense violence, and/or strong language.

- AO (Adults Only: 18+) contains graphic depictions of sex and/or violence.

An interesting controversy arose in 2005 related to the series of *Grand Theft Auto* games (Lohr, 2005). In the M-rated game (the top seller one year), the main character seeks bloody vengeance on gang-filled streets, firing automatic weapons and picking up scantily clad women. Family-oriented media watchdog groups became very upset when the PC version had additional scenes in which nude "girlfriends" join

in explicit sex acts. The scenes become "playable" with the help of a freely available download. However, had such sexually explicit content been clearly a part of the retail version, it would have likely earned the game an "adults-only" rating that would have cost millions in lost sales. In an attempt to protect children from "nasty" video games, the Illinois legislature passed a bill making it a crime to sell violent or sexually explicit games to kids under 18. Then-Senator Hillary Clinton worked on a similar bill at the national level.

It seems that a majority of adult videos are rented by females. They are rented most commonly on weekends and are used by married couples after the kids have gone to bed. Common themes of the sexually explicit videos relate to high levels of sexual desire, diverse sexual activity, many sexual partners being readily available, and pleasure as the main purpose of sexual activity. Video rentals and sales represent multibillions of dollars in sales each year. They are a substantial part of the home-video industry's revenue. Some videos have been produced for use by couples in their homes. Sexologists have made videos that provide explicit graphic instruction to help improve sexual relationships.

In 2009, Benedetti observed that video game makers used sexual themes mainly as a means of shocking players and as a means to sell their products. She pointed out that in early 2009 *Afro Samurai* had lots of swordplay, including a scene where players got to slice and dice four topless ninja strippers. In another game, the curvaceous Ayumi, a sword-swinging relic hunter, was dressed in a bum-baring thong and a bikini top. In addition, in a version of *Grand Theft Auto IV*, a man receiving a massage dropped his towel and revealed his flaccid penis for all to see. In these, and many more instances, flesh is used as a tool to sell games.

Ross (2007) pointed out that what is really different about the Internet is that it provides people with the capacity for anonymity in carrying out private cybersex activities. It can serve as a unique site for sexual experimentation. It can also serve as a very important tool for psychological adaptation for gay and lesbian youth.

Literature

As with the content of movies, TV programs, and videos, the public has become desensitized to sexually explicit material in books. However, it was not always this way. For example, in 1928 D. H. Lawrence's *Lady Chatterly's Lover* was published. Because of its sexual explicitness, it was banned in the United States until 1959. James Joyce's *Ulysses*, published in

1934, deals with masturbation, prostitution, adultery, and voyeurism. It was not allowed into the United States for years but is now considered to be a masterpiece.

In the last few decades thousands of books of varying literary quality that openly treat sexual topics have been published. Sometimes they weave themes related to sexuality into a meaningful story, but other times their authors seem to be gratuitously writing about sexual thoughts and activity as much as possible. Many earlier works appear tame compared to what is now available. What was previously considered risque, if not actually immoral or illegal, has now come to be expected in a bestseller.

Sexually arousing material, of course, has existed for centuries. The ancient *Kamasutra* and *The Perfumed Garden*, Chaucer's *Canterbury Tales* and Boccaccio's *Decameron* (both 14th-century works), Li Yu's *Flesh Prayer Mat*, and the *Memoirs of Casanova* are examples of early erotic literature. However, more and more of our popular literature that is not primarily erotic is at least partly concerned with its characters' sexual activities. For example, romance literature relies on fantasy rather than sexual explicitness; its purpose is to tantalize and to nourish sexual fantasies, rather than to tell a good story. Many mass-market paperbacks are romance novels, read by both women and men.

Magazines have made their mark as well. *Esquire: The Magazine for Men* appeared in 1933. Twenty years later *Playboy* appeared on the newsstands. It offered information about sexuality, an open philosophy toward sexuality, and photographs of nude women along with some stimulating stories. Its approach was followed by many other magazines. In the late 1960s other magazines, such as *Penthouse*, *Oui*, and *Hustler*, published pictures of nude males and

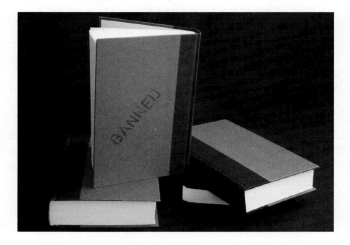

Sexually arousing books and other materials have been available for centuries.

females as well as people engaged in assorted sexual activities. Some even had a classified section allowing people to advertise their sexual services or request sexual partners.

As women asked for a more balanced view, magazines such as *Cosmopolitan* and *Playgirl* began printing photos of nude men and stories with appeal for women. Traditionally, women's magazines have focused on two broad topics: what a woman should do to get a man *(Cosmopolitan)* and what a woman should do once she has the man and his children *(Redbook)*. Other magazines have attempted to include other aspects of women's lives. For example, *Working Woman* and *Savvy* are aimed at women who work outside the home. *Ms.* magazine, the only women's magazine explicitly dedicated to feminism and the facts about women's sexuality, was founded in 1971. It struggled for 20 years to support itself through advertising. It finally gave up on advertising and now relies on its subscription price for revenue. Consequently, its circulation of around 500,000 dropped to 179,000 in the mid–1990s. It currently is around 110,000.

Magazines collectively play a role as communicators on a range of sexual health topics (Sexual health coverage in women's, men's, and teen magazines, 2000). The Kaiser Family Foundation found that 34% of articles in women's magazines, 28% of articles in men's magazines, and 42% of articles in teen magazines focused on sexual health issues. However, the emphasis is different. For example, women's magazines emphasize pregnancy, and especially planned pregnancy, contraception, and abortion. Men's magazines mainly address concerns such as STIs, including HIV and AIDS, and the few male-controlled methods of contraception. Teen magazines focus on the potential adverse outcomes of sexual activity, such as STIs and unintended pregnancy. They also address the difficult decisions many teens face about whether to become sexually active.

Hatton and Trautner (2011) analyzed more than 1,000 images of men and women on *Rolling Stone* covers over a 43–year period. They concluded that representations of both women and men have become more sexualized over time, that women are more frequently sexualized than men, and that the images of women are more intensely sexualized than are those of men. They developed a "scale of sexualization." An image was given points for being sexualized if, for example, the subject's lips were parted or his or her tongue was showing, the subject was only partially clad or naked, or the text describing the subject used explicitly sexual language. The authors said, "We don't necessarily think it's problematic for women to be portrayed as 'sexy,' But we do think it is problematic when nearly all images of women depict them not simply as 'sexy women' but as passive objects for someone else's sexual pleasure."

Adult bookstores specialize in highly sexually arousing books. These stores are adult in the sense that a person must be of legal age to enter. Such establishments also sell sex-illustrated magazines, newspapers, postcards, decks of playing cards, and videotapes. Many communities have attempted to outlaw adult bookstores (through the courts and local government statute) or to limit their location to one part of the community. Nevertheless, all major cities have them, as do many smaller cities and towns. Furthermore, many conventional bookstores, recognizing a market for sexually explicit literature, maintain sections devoted to such books and magazines. As with sexuality in the movies, the cost and benefit of adult bookstores versus the risks of censorship is a topic of heated debate.

In addition to sexually explicit fiction, a how-to publishing business has developed to help people reach their sexual potential. Thus we now have countless books about such topics as using sexual techniques, expressing gay and lesbian sexuality, helping ourselves and our partners to be sensuous women or men, improving our overall sexual relationships, and using sexual aids for pleasure.

Popular Music

The mass phenomenon that may affect more young people than any other is popular music. And in this arena, as in most others, blatant sexuality has become a style. Lyrics (words and grunts), performance (movement and costume), and provocative photos on album covers use sexual suggestion and appeal to our sexual fantasies to sell the music and the entertainer.

Perhaps the epitome of sex in music was Elvis ("The Pelvis") Presley, with his gyrating hips. Aside from his hips, however, Elvis's songs were by today's standards tame. "Heartbreak Hotel," "Love Me Tender," and "Let Me Be Your Teddy Bear," all recorded in the late 1950s, were sexually appealing mainly because of Presley's soft, sultry voice and innuendo, rather than direct sexual language—a far cry from today's popular music and music videos that contain frequent references to relationships, romance, and sexual behavior. Lyrics about sexuality are mixed with lyrics about love, violence, rejection, and loneliness.

Music videos, available on many cable networks, may be influential sources of sexual information for adolescents because they combine visuals of their favorite musicians with music. Many of the visual elements are sexual. Rap music is particularly explicit about both sexuality and violence.

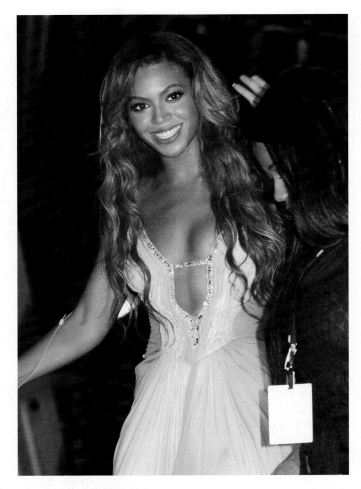

Many entertainers use sexual themes to sell themselves and their products.

Groups of citizens have attempted to ban some of this music from local radio stations and have sometimes been successful. Whether sexually explicit music is harmful (in particular, it is argued, to youths in developmental states) is debatable and depends somewhat on our values.

In 1985 the Recording Industry Association of America (RIAA) reached an agreement with the National Parent-Teacher Association and the Parents Music Resource Center. The agreement specified that music releases containing explicit lyrics, including explicit depictions of violence and sex, be identified so parents can make intelligent listening choices for their children. The Parental Advisory Label on music releases has become a notice to consumers that recordings with the label may contain strong language or depictions of violence, sex, or substance abuse. Parental discretion is then advised. The label is a nonremovable logo that record companies voluntarily place on products to better inform consumers and retailers while also protecting the rights of artists. The decision to label a particular sound recording is

encountering sexual themes; sexual explicitness (and implicitness) is part of our everyday existence. We need to be aware of its presence so that we can better control its effect on our behavior and attitudes. By way of example, knowing that the scantily clad model has no relation to our need to own a new car, we might be better able to ignore the sexual appeal of the ads and purchase a car that is suited to our needs and financial constraints.

Being aware of the uses of sexuality in the marketplace can make you a better consumer, a more enlightened citizen, and a healthier person sexually.

■ Sexually Explicit Materials

Terminology is critical, but somewhat confusing, in relation to sexually explicit materials. You may hear different people use the same terms to describe different things, so it is important to establish definitions. **Pornography** is visual and written material that is used for purposes of sexual arousal. It has been said that pornography, as is beauty, is in the eye of the beholder. Opinions about what it is, its possible uses, and its legal status are extremely varied.

pornography
Visual and written materials used for the purpose of sexual arousal.

Definitions

The legal definition of *obscenity*, established by the Supreme Court in 1973, is that for something to be obscene it must meet all three of the following conditions:

1. The average person, applying contemporary community standards, would find that the work, taken as a whole, appeals to **prurient** interest.

2. The work depicts or describes, in a patently offensive way, sexual conduct specifically defined by the applicable state (or federal) law.

3. The work, taken as a whole, lacks serious literary, artistic, political, or scientific value.

Therefore, although sexually explicit materials are legal in the United States, obscenity is not. Taking the three Supreme Court criteria just listed together, a reasonable definition of **obscenity** is a personal or societal judgment that something

prurient
Characterized by lustful thoughts or wishes.

obscenity
Personal or societal judgment that something is offensive.

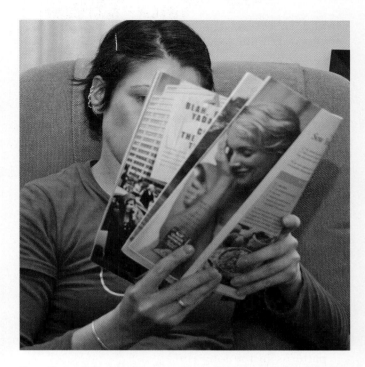

Sexually explicit materials are easily available to people of all ages.

is offensive. Therefore, one person may consider obscene something that another does not.

Another important term is **erotica**, which usually describes sexually oriented material that can be evaluated positively, in contrast to obscenity, which is offensive. Erotica consists of "depictions of sexuality which display mutuality, respect, affection, and a balance of power" (Stock, 1985). Some people will differentiate between pornography and erotica by indicating that pornography provides a degrading or demeaning portrayal of human beings. In contrast, erotica is not degrading or demeaning anyone. Therefore, a person may find pornography to be unacceptable and erotica to be acceptable based upon this differentiation.

erotica
Sexually oriented material that may be artistically produced or motivated.

Effects of Sexually Explicit Materials

Traditionally many people have been opposed to sexually explicit materials. Perhaps this is because they feared that the materials had many undesirable effects, such as causing people to participate in sexual activity they might not otherwise have engaged in, increasing the number of sexual offenses, and corrupting the minds of children. It is difficult to do research in an area where there are so many personal and social variables, but a brief look at research findings about the effects of sexually explicit materials may be helpful.

The report of the Commission on Obscenity and Pornography (1970), sponsored by the federal government, and a review of this report by two researchers at Johns Hopkins University (Money & Athanasiou, 1973) give us some information about the effects of pornography. Although this research summary is almost 50 years old, it still represents a valid summary of the effects of sexually explicit materials. According to these sources, the following appear to be true:

1. There is little, if any, difference in males' and females' sexual responses to sexually explicit materials.

2. People are stimulated only by portrayals of sexual ideas or acts that turn them on. In other words, sexually explicit materials do not seem to plant in people's minds ideas or desires that they do not already have.

3. Exposure to sexually explicit materials does not seem to alter a person's sexual behavior patterns in the long run.

4. Continued exposure to sexually explicit materials tends to lead to indifference and boredom. John Money (1973) believes that stimuli in sexually explicit materials are effective for 2 to 4 hours. After this time a person becomes either more selective or indifferent to the stimuli.

5. Filling out questionnaires on responses to sexually explicit material may be more stimulating than the material itself. (Perhaps this is best explained by human beings' great capacity to fantasize.)

6. Convicted sex offenders have been exposed to fewer sexually explicit and sexuality education materials during their life than nonoffenders. This fact contradicts the common belief that exposure to sexually explicit materials causes people to commit sexual offenses.

The Society for the Scientific Study of Sexuality (What scientists know about pornography, 2007) provides the following summary regarding effects of exposure to sexually explicit material:

- In general, when exposed to nonviolent erotica, men and women show small, short-term increases in the sexual behaviors they already are used to engaging in, but generally they do not add anything new to their sexual repertoire.

- Both men and women are sexually aroused by erotic material, but women report more negative emotional reactions than men, and women seem to be less likely to access sexually explicit materials.

- Findings on the effects of exposure to violent pornography are more mixed. Some researchers have found that exposure to sexually violent materials increases the acceptance of rape myths (beliefs that ascribe responsibility to women who are the victims) and increases men's self-reported likelihood of raping a woman. Other studies have found just the opposite. Still others have found no association between use of sexually explicit media and negative attitudes toward women.

Gender DIMENSIONS

Male and Female Use of Autoerotic Materials

As part of the National Health and Social Life Survey, Laumann and associates (1994) reported on the number of men and women who had used autoerotic materials in the past year. The main activities indicated by the subjects were viewing X-rated movies or videos (23% of the males and 11% of the females), going to a club that has nude or seminude dancers (22% of the males and 4% of the females), and using sexually explicit books or magazines (16% of the males and 4% of the females). Vibrators or dildos were used by 2% of the males and 2% of the females, and other sex toys were used by 1% of the males and 2% of the females.

Forty-one percent of the men and 16% of the women reported using autoerotic materials during the past year.

Interestingly, thinking about sex frequently (defined as "every day" or "several times a day") was reported by 54% of the males and 19% of the females. Thinking about sex infrequently (defined as "a few times a month" to "a few times a week") was reported by 43% of the males and 67% of the females. Thinking about sex never or rarely (defined as "less than once a month") was reported by 4% of the males and 16% of the females.

Source: Data from Laumann, E. O., Gagnon, J. H., Michael, R. T., & Michaels, S. *The social organization of sexuality.* Chicago: University of Chicago Press, 1994.

Rich (2008) summarized research related to the effects of relatively violent pornography on adolescents. Male adolescents were more likely to believe women enjoy forced sexual activity after seeing an excerpt in which a woman was shown as aroused by nonconsenting intercourse. Males who watched films that portrayed violence against females as justifiable and with positive consequences showed increased belief in rape myths and acceptance of violence against women as compared with males who saw films with no sexual violence. Females had the opposite reaction to the same films. Both male and female viewers reported they were more sexually aroused by nonaggressive rather than aggressive sexually explicit materials.

Kingston et al. (2009) looked at pornography's influence on sexually aggressive behavior. They found that pornography use can be a risk factor for sexually aggressive outcomes, principally for men who rate high on other risk factors and who use pornography frequently.

Albright (2008) surveyed more than 15,000 men and women related to pornography. Seventy-five percent of men and 41% of women had intentionally viewed pornography. Women reported more negative consequences, including lowered body image, their partner being critical of their body, increased pressure to perform acts seen in pornographic films, and less actual sexual behavior. Men reported being more critical of their partners' body and less interested in actual sexual behavior.

For years some people have suggested that sexually explicit materials might be stimulating to men, but not to women. Today we know that such materials can be stimulating to both genders, but that there are individual differences in responses. We also know that in most cases exposure to pornography does not influence long-term behaviors or change interests in most sexual behaviors one way or the other.

Watson and Smith (2012) reviewed literature summarizing both negative and neutral-to-positive findings about the effects of sexually explicit materials. They found that despite widespread beliefs that such material causes or contributes to violence, sexual deviance, degradation of women, destruction of relationships, public health concerns, and moral decay, there is little evidence to support such broad claims. When considering the neutral-to-positive impacts of sexually explicit materials, they pointed out that proponents of sexually explicit materials have long held that greater access to information about sexuality/sexual health may diminish anxieties and that encouragement of sexual expression may enhance individual enjoyment and relational connection. Their literature review seems to support these points. Although it is always important to properly prepare and use educational materials, the literature reviewed by Watson and Smith supported the use of sexually explicit material to provide information about sexuality and male and female bodies, to help individuals understand differences in arousal and fantasy, to open lines of communication, and to share thoughts and ideas about sexual topics.

Child Pornography

So far we have considered sexually explicit materials about adults for adults. There is increasing concern about the use of children in pornographic materials and, more recently, about continued eroticization of young children in the print media and on television.

The use of minors in sexually explicit media—**child pornography**—is now prohibited. In the past, many magazine publishers and film producers used their own children in sexually explicit materials they developed. Others advertised in magazines catering to readers of pornography. Still, in spite of the law, magazines and films that depict children in sexually erotic conditions are produced and sold. Given the current societal concern for child abuse (sexual and otherwise) and for missing children, law enforcement agencies have organized to crack down on the kiddie porn industry.

In 1984, the National Center for Missing and Exploited Children was established by the federal

> **child pornography**
> Use of minors in sexually explicit media.

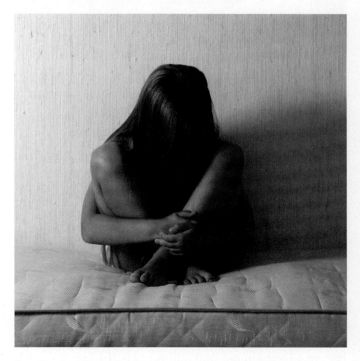

People who might support the availability of sexually explicit materials for adults usually do not condone child pornography.

Ethical
DIMENSIONS

Should Kids Be Sexualized?

There has been a great deal of discussion related to whether to control the routines of high school bands, cheerleaders, and dancers. A Texas legislator sponsored a bill to ban "sexually suggestive" cheerleading in the public schools. A school superintendent in Alabama told bands to clean up their acts. These actions prompted a variety of responses.

On the one hand, one Alabama parent said, "As long as they're not taking any clothes off, I don't see anything wrong with it." A PTA president said, "If we're going to limit our children doing their routines, then take the Dallas Cowgirls off TV."

On the other hand, one band director said, "It is a family show, and high school girls shouldn't be doing college-girl dance routines." A school superintendent said, "It would be much more appealing to have fine sounds produced by the bands than vulgar routines."

Is it ethical for high school bands, cheerleaders, and dancers to be allowed to do suggestive routines? Is it right to have legislation, such as that in Texas, designed to ban "sexually suggestive" cheerleading? Who should decide what is right or wrong related to the possibility of sexualizing students in public schools?

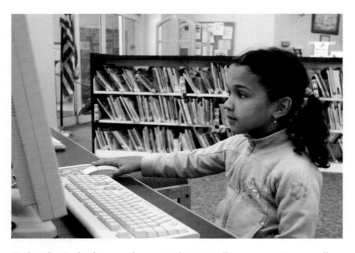

Technological advances have made controlling access to sexually explicit materials very difficult. Debates continue about whether or not it should be controlled at all.

government. In 1997, an Exploited Child Unit was established within this agency to deal with child pornography and other crimes. In 1998, the Cyber-Tipline was launched to have a means of reporting incidents of child sexual exploitation including the possession, manufacture, or distribution of child pornography; online enticement; child prostitution; child sex tourism; extrafamilial child sexual molestation; unsolicited obscene material sent to a child; and misleading domain names, words, or digital images. The CyberTipline (*www.cybertipline.com*) is staffed 24 hours a day, 7 days a week. It received its 200,000th report in 2004, and by April 2009 it had received almost 600,000 reports. In just 1 month in 2011 it received 3,668 reports, and near the end

of 2011 it had received a total of 1,252,274 reports since March 1998. In 2002 a Child Victim Identification Program was established with a dual mission: (1) to help prosecutors get convictions by proving that a real child is depicted in child pornography images (the Supreme Court has ruled that this is required) and (2) to assist law enforcement in locating unidentified child victims.

In 2006, the Sex Offender Registration and Notification Act was passed. It was passed for two reasons: (1) to establish a national database that tracks the location and movements of people convicted of a criminal offense against a victim who is a minor, have been convicted of a sexually violent offense, or are sexually violent predators, and (2) to register and verify the addresses of sex offenders who reside in states without a "minimally sufficient" sex offender registry program. (Today all 50 states have minimally sufficient programs.) Guidelines for this act can be seen at *www.ojp.usdoj.gov/smart/pdfs/final_sornaguidelines.pdf*.

Under federal legislation, child pornography is defined as any visual depiction where a minor is used to engage in sexually explicit conduct, or a technological image is used that is indistinguishable from that of a minor, or it appears that a minor is engaging in sexually explicit conduct. It is a federal crime to knowingly produce, distribute, receive, or possess with intent to distribute, a visual depiction of any kind, including a drawing, cartoon, sculpture, or painting that meets these criteria. A minor is defined as a person younger than the age of 18.

Child pornography exists in multiple formats, including print media, videotape, film, CD-ROM, and DVD. It is transmitted on various platforms within the Internet.

The Control of Sexually Explicit Materials

Should sexually explicit materials be censored and controlled? There are varying opinions. In an attempt to keep sexually explicit materials on the Internet away from the 16 million users younger than 17 years old in the United States, Congress passed the Child Online Protection Act, which forced websites to require a credit card number or some other adult ID. The law made it a crime to knowingly communicate to a minor "for commercial purposes" any online material that is "harmful to minors." Penalties included fines up to $50,000 per day for each violation and up to 6 months in prison. At best, however, the law would make sexually explicit material a bit more difficult for minors to reach. It does not touch areas not on the web, such as email or Usenet newsgroups. It also does not affect noncommercial sites or operations based outside the United States (Head, 2012). This law has been controversial. Some people believe that it is in society's best interest to protect children from sexually explicit materials. Free speech advocates, in contrast, challenge the law on constitutional grounds, arguing it would affect everybody on the web.

In 2009, the long legal drive to shield children from sexually explicit material on the web ended. The Supreme Court struck down the law on free-speech grounds. Judges said parents can protect their children in their own way by installing software filters on their computers.

The Child Pornography and Protection Act was passed in 1996 (High court to hear arguments on child porn amendment, 2001). Since then supporters have claimed that the act was an essential tool to prevent pedophiles from preying on children. Those who disagree have argued that it is so vaguely worded that there is no way to know what is over the line and what is not. Through the years court challenges related to the act have had inconsistent outcomes. For example, one federal district court judge found the law constitutional, and one U.S. court of appeals struck it down. The U.S. Supreme Court struck down the law in 2002 for being overly broad.

A major related event occurred in June 2003 when the U.S. Supreme Court upheld a federal law requiring public library personnel to install pornography filters on all computers providing Internet access as a condition of continuing to receive federal subsidies and grants (Greenhouse, 2003). The law, enacted in 2001, had been blocked by a lower court and never taken effect. Under the law, filters are required for all library users, not just children. The law authorizes, but does not require, librarians to unblock Internet sites at the request of adult users. Many opinions

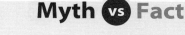

Myth vs Fact

Myth: There is no difference between obscenity and pornography.
Fact: Yes, there is. Obscenity is not protected by the Constitution. It follows the Supreme Court definition, but pornography is material designed to arouse and has no legal or consistent definition.

Myth: Sexually explicit material causes violence against women.
Fact: No reputable research in the United States, Europe, or Asia finds a causal link between pornography and violence.

Myth: Men watch pornography and imitate it or force women to do what they see.
Fact: Violence and intimidation existed for thousands of years before commercial pornography. People do not mimic what they read or view in knee-jerk fashion. Men do not learn coercion from sexual pictures.

Myth: Pornography degrades women.
Fact: Sexism, not sexual behavior, degrades women. Opponents of sexual speech do not understand that it is in everyone's interest to allow a variety of pleasurable materials that enhance well-being and sexual fulfillment.

Myth: Pornography is only for men.
Fact: Half the adult videos in the United States are bought or rented by women alone or women in couples. AIDS and other STIs have made it a public health necessity to encourage sexual fantasy material that offers women and men safe alternatives to unhealthy sexual contact.

exist about the wisdom of this law and how it relates to First Amendment rights to free speech.

Certain segments of the public are very concerned about the increased availability of sexually explicit materials and have organized to combat this trend. They point out that many X-rated movies, CDs, and DVDs are purchased and rented. They talk about the popularity of cable television channels, such as the Playboy Channel, that specialize in sexual broadcasts; they also emphasize the success of such sexually explicit magazines as *Penthouse* and *Playboy*.

The interesting aspect of the organized opposition to sexually explicit materials is that it has united diverse groups. National conservative groups as well as some national feminist groups have joined a loose network of local groups to fight the "Porn War." Among the conservative organizations are the National Federation for Decency, the Citizens for Decency through Law, Morality in Media, the Moral Majority, and the Citizens for Legislation Against Decadence. Among the feminist groups are Women Against Pornography, Feminists Against Pornography, the Pornography Resource Center, and Women Against Violence Against Women.

The objections of these groups to sexually explicit materials are several. Some consider an explicit description or image of sexual acts immoral and irreligious. Others object to women being portrayed as sex objects and believe this view of women will be generalized to "real life." Still others perceive

Myth (vs) Fact

Myth: Women in pornography are exploited or victimized.
Fact: Women are exploited and harassed in all fields, including pornography. Exploitation will stop when it is vigorously prosecuted everywhere it occurs. Some women in pornography say their work gives them independence and a sense of accomplishment; banning it would worsen their lives.

Myth: As an aid to masturbation, pornography is action that is not protected by the First Amendment.
Fact: Pornography may lead to masturbation much as a novel or film may lead to tears or laughter. Feminists for Free Expression does not believe policing masturbation is the proper business of government or well-meaning committees.

Myth: Banning sexual material will protect or help women.
Fact: Historically, censorship has hurt women. It has prevented them from getting information about sexuality and reproduction. The best protection for women's ideas is the constitutional protection of free speech. The answer to bad pornography is good pornography, not no pornography.

that women in sexually explicit materials are treated violently and fear that this type of portrayal might cause more violence toward women. For example, Women Against Pornography (WAP) demanded that sexually explicit materials be prohibited from depicting rape, whipping, or bondage. WAP believed that such depictions lead men to feel superior to women and extend that idea of superiority to nonsexual relationships (such as those in the workplace). Others concentrate predominantly on music and advertising, asserting that commercial degradation of women fosters sexism.

Many groups of women are most vocal in their opinions. However, though not organized, men also suffer from sexploitation. When men are shown performing violent acts on women, they are being taught to be powerful and dominant over the other sex. They are learning that sexual relationships require a measure of forcefulness that in actuality interferes with sexual arousal rather than enhances it. When men learn to treat women as sexual objects, their relationships suffer. Depictions of men and women sharing equally in sexual and loving relationships would teach both sexes that sexual fulfillment is a mutual responsibility; the results would be a decrease of pressure on men to know what to do and how to do it and fewer sexually frustrated women.

The ACLU says that it is no accident that freedom of speech is the first freedom mentioned in the First Amendment. It is not limited to "pure speech"—books, newspapers, leaflets, and rallies. It also protects "symbolic speech"—nonverbal expression whose purpose it is to communicate ideas. It exists precisely to protect the most offensive and controversial speech from government suppression. The best means to counter obnoxious speech is speech. Persuasion, not coercion, is the solution. The ACLU also indicates that the innovation and citizen empowerment inspired by online communications will be lost if civil liberties do not also apply in cyberspace. Furthermore, there are three reasons freedom of expression is essential to a free society: (1) The right to express one's thoughts and to communicate freely with others is the foundation of self-fulfillment. (2) It is vital to the attainment and advancement of knowledge and the search for the truth. (3) It is necessary to our system of self-government and gives the American people a "checking function" against government excess and corruption.

Feminists for Free Expression (FFE) is a leading voice opposing state and national legislation that threatens free speech. This organization defends the right of free expression in court cases, supports the rights of activists whose works have been suppressed or censored, and provides expert speakers. On the topic of sexually explicit materials, FFE published *Feminism and Free Speech: Pornography* to aid in the understanding of pornography, its uses and benefits, and its relation to violence. An overview of its scientific and cross-cultural research is provided in the Myth vs Fact box about pornography on this page. Relatedly, there is more erotica being developed that is not sexist but feminist and gender friendly. It is designed to portray equitable relationships.

The increased easy access to sexually explicit materials has raised an interesting issue: What should we be allowed to watch in public? (Richtel, 2012). For example, is it okay to play explicit materials in the back seat of a car or on buses that could be viewed by others in the vehicle or on the road? Should airlines police what people watch on planes? How about in an Internet cafe or a restaurant? This can be a thorny issue because not everyone agrees on what might be considered offensive. Also, people don't agree on what is acceptable to view in private as opposed to in public settings.

In October 2002 the Museum of Sex opened in New York City. The purpose of the museum is to preserve and present the history, evolution, and cultural significance of human sexuality. Not everyone approves of it. William Donohue, president of the Catholic League for Religions and Civil Rights, denounced the museum for celebrating "smut as sex." He accused the museum of championing or associating with racists, pornographers, and individuals who "exhibit pathological characteristics." On the other side, June Reinisch, a historian adviser to the museum and director emeritus of the Kinsey Institute, characterized it as a serious endeavor, in the sense that it wants to inform and educate as well as to entertain. "Sexuality is a very important part of individual life and to culture," she said. "To not understand it is to be handicapped in your understanding of human relations and culture" (James, 2002). Over a recent 7 year period the Museum of Sex generated 16 exhibitions and 5 virtual installations, each in keeping with its mission of advocating open discourse surrounding sexuality as well as presenting to the public current scholarship unhindered by self-censorship. The museum is committed to addressing a wide range of topics while highlighting material and artifacts from different continents, cultures, time periods, and media.

Finally, the position of the Sexuality Information and Education Council of the United States on sexually explicit materials is as follows:

SIECUS believes that sexually explicit visual, printed, or online materials can be valuable educational or personal aids when sensitively used in a manner appropriate to the viewer's age and developmental level. Such materials can help reduce ignorance and confusion and contribute to a positive concept of sexuality while supporting the sexual rights of all. However, the use of violence, exploitation, or degradation, or the portrayal of children in sexually explicit materials is reprehensible.

SIECUS believes that adults should have the right to access sexually explicit materials for personal use. Legislative and judicial efforts to prevent the production or distribution of sexually explicit materials endanger constitutionally guaranteed freedoms of speech and press, and could be employed to restrict the appropriate professional use of such materials by sexuality educators, therapists, and researchers.

◼ Sex Workers

An important consideration in the study of sexual commercial enterprises is the topic of sex work, or prostitution. The term **prostitution** refers to any situation in which one person pays another for sexual gratification. Sex workers may be males as well as females, but primarily sex workers have been and are females. Women do sex work mainly to make money, but other factors can also motivate them. For example, the lack of education of most sex workers limits their job opportunities. In addition, some women think sex work will be exciting and glamorous, whereas others are motivated to become sex workers because they do not like the discipline and boredom of regular jobs.

prostitution
Participating in sexual activity for pay or profit.

Some women who are drug addicts turn to sex work to support their habit. The background of many sex workers has included emotional deprivation and sexual abuse—even within the family. Some sex workers therefore feel that by providing sexual pleasure they can gain intimacy and attention.

Types of Sex Workers

It is difficult to estimate the number of persons who currently work or have ever worked as sex workers because there are various definitions of prostitution and because sex work is usually illegal. There are many types of sex workers; the major types are call girls, house prostitutes, streetwalkers, massage parlor prostitutes, and bar girls and strippers.

Call Girls
Call girls are at the top of the profession. They do not solicit; rather, their "dates" are arranged by personal referral or by another person. They have regular clients who pay high fees and also pay their bills.

House Prostitutes
House (brothel) prostitutes work in more structured conditions in brothels (houses in which prostitutes work) and serve more men at cheaper rates than call girls would charge. Brothels are legal in some

call girls
Highly paid female sex workers who work by appointment only.

house (brothel) prostitutes
Sex workers who work in brothels.

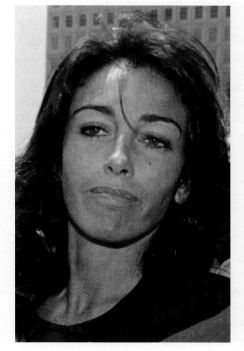

Heidi Fleiss, the so-called Hollywood Madam, ran a high-priced call girl ring in Beverly Hills. She was arrested and convicted on several charges ranging from pandering to tax evasion. However, the case raised ethical questions, because all the call girls were granted immunity and none of the clients was charged. Should prosecutors use government resources to pursue prostitutes' customers?

Did You Know . . .

Did you know that there is a historical connection between Santa Claus and sex workers? In the third century, a rich and good-hearted Turkish man named Nicholas saved poor girls from prostitution by throwing bags of gold coins through their windows or down a chimney. Over the next 700 years, with a little help from Dutch settlers in America and a poet named Clement Clarke Moore, Saint Nicholas was transposed into a merry old gent with a white beard and red suit who spends most of Christmas giving toys to good little girls and boys.

Source: Data from Vrazo, F. Finland town, Rovaniemi, *Birmingham News* (December 18, 1998), 18A.

counties of Nevada but are illegal in all other areas of the United States.

Streetwalkers

Streetwalkers are more independent than house prostitutes but lack the contacts or ability to become call girls. They stand or stroll on streets and approach passing males. Because of their visibility, streetwalkers are the most frequently arrested sex workers.

The ratio of on-street prostitution to off-street prostitution in cities varies with local law, police, and custom. For example, in larger cities experts seem to think that street prostitution is about 10–20% of the prostitution, but in smaller cities (with more limited indoor opportunities), street prostitution might be as much as 50% of the total.

Many women who engage in street sex work experience pregnancies and become mothers. They report that being pregnant or parenting while regularly working the street caused them to feel ashamed of themselves and their work and anxious for their own and their children's safety. Pregnancies and parenting responsibilities also altered their working productivity and practices (Sloss & Harper, 2004).

Massage Parlor Sex Workers

Certainly many **massage parlors** offer only massages, but at others a client can find many "extras." The environment offers an indoor place to work that is safer than the streets, and massage parlor workers may be motivated to earn extra money by providing sexual favors. Fellatio is popular among both customers and masseuses. Many men claim they cannot get their regular partners to participate in fellatio. The masseuses appreciate it because it is efficient: They are trying to earn as much money as they can, so it is useful to be able to service a number of men in a short period.

> **streetwalkers**
> Sex workers who work on the streets.
>
> **massage parlors**
> Places where sex workers can be hired to perform sexual acts under the guise of giving a massage.

Bar Girls and Strippers

Many times **bar girls** and strippers are supposed to act available so men will buy them drinks. This helps the establishment make more on the sale of liquor. Sometimes, however, paid sexual activity is also offered.

> **bar girls**
> Sex workers who are supposed to act available so customers will buy them drinks.

Examples of this type of activity can be found in many countries. For example, an increasing number of Cambodian "beer girls," who sell international beers, wines, and liquors at outdoor eateries and in bars, are also selling sexual activity. If the women refuse a client's offer of sexual activity for money, they may lose a beer sale. Because they depend heavily on commissions, they feel they have to do something to convince the client to buy. To make matters worse, beer girls are less likely than brothel workers to use condoms, and surveys show that as many as one-fifth of them are HIV positive (Increasing number of Cambodian "beer girls" selling sex, 2003).

Japan's sex trade, estimated at $13 billion per year, is one of the nation's fastest-growing industries. Record unemployment has forced many women to work at brothels euphemistically known as fashion, health, soapland, pink salons, or telephone clubs. Only 6% to 25% of sex workers and the public use condoms. HIV has not been widespread in Japan, but the prevalence rate is highest among female sex workers, close to 3%. Because of the lack of HIV and AIDS education, the very low rate of condom use, and the relatively rapid increase in rates of HIV among sex workers, it is feared that HIV and AIDS could become a significant problem in Japan (Kakuchi, 2003).

Kershaw (2004) reported that stripping can be a springboard either to something better or to an abyss of drugs, alcohol, abuse, and prostitution. Sometimes stripping is just a living—the rent. Many dancers say they love what they do, if not for the money then for the attention, or for the power they wield over men who are "stupid enough to pay to see you naked." Most dancers seem to aspire to something else—being an actress, a model, a good mother, or a successful career person. Some make more than $2,000 to $3,000 per week.

There has been greater female attendance at strip clubs in recent years. Some dancers have incorporated female patrons into a sexualized space traditionally designed for men. They have tailored their lap dances for a female patron. In this way, the strip club becomes a potential space for engaging in same-gender eroticism that includes elements of play (Wosick-Correa & Joseph, 2008).

Male Sex Workers

Whereas the majority of sex workers are women, some men also sell sexual services to women or to other men. **Gigolos** provide escort and sexual services for women, and **hustlers** are male sex workers who perform homosexual acts for pay. Male sex workers may be classified as female sex workers are, but the differences are often not obvious.

> **gigolo**
> A man who is paid to provide escort and sexual services, usually for wealthy, middle-aged women.
>
> **hustler**
> A male sex worker who performs homosexual acts for pay.

Percentages of male and female sex workers vary from city to city. Estimates in some larger cities suggest that 20% to 30% of sex workers are male.

In Bangkok, Thailand, a nonprofit group called Swing provides services—including education about condom use—to male sex workers (*Bangkok Post* profiles group providing services for male commercial sex workers, 2005). It is the first organization to focus on Thailand's approximately 4,000 male sex workers. Swing offers English classes, Internet access, and places to nap and shower. The group plans to offer exercise equipment and medical assistance. Although Thai society has become "more tolerant" of female sex workers, it is "less accepting" of male sex workers. People look down on them because they think they are lazy and terrible people. Male sex workers also have experienced stigma in doctors' offices and sometimes avoid being treated for STIs if a doctor or nurse makes them feel uncomfortable. Swing establishes relationships with doctors to make "appropriate referrals" for its clients, and the group plans to have its own in-house physician.

In 2005 Heidi Fleiss, the former "Hollywood Madam," decided to open the "Heidi Stud Farm" in Nevada (Hollywood madam caters for ladies, 2005). She was sure her new service for women would be a hit. She said, "Women make more money these days, they're calling the shots, they're more powerful. And let's face it, it's hard to meet someone."

Pimps

The people who set up sex workers with clients are called **pimps**. Sex workers give the money they earn to their pimps in exchange for affection, concern, and love. Pimps recruit newcomers into sex work, they manage the sex workers' business and provide them counsel, bail them out of jail when necessary, and regulate the streetwalking prostitution enterprise (without a pimp, streetwalking sex workers might be in danger in certain neighborhoods).

> **pimps**
> Individuals who set up female sex workers with clients.

Pitts et al. (2004) sought to answer the question, "Who pays for sex and why?" As compared to those who had not been clients, they found that male clients of sex workers were significantly older, less likely to have been educated beyond high school, less likely to report having a regular partner in the past 6 months, and more likely to report that their most recent sexual encounter was with a casual partner.

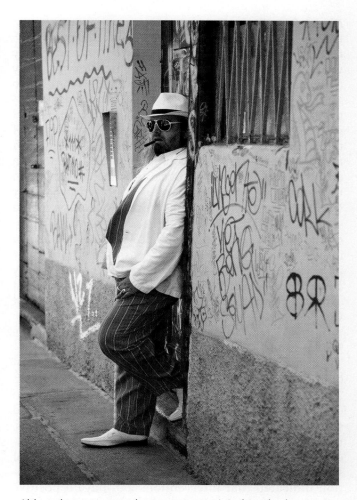

Although most sex workers are women, it is thought that as many as 20% to 30% of sex workers are men.

Clients said their major reasons for paying for sexual activity were to satisfy their sexual needs (44%), followed by the belief that paying for sexual activity was less trouble (36%), and that it would be entertaining (36%).

Little is known about the magnitude of prostitution or changes in its incidence. Because prostitution is an illegal (except in rural Nevada) and socially stigmatized profession in the United States, the amount of reliable information is very limited. Smith (2003) summarized existing studies indicating that between 1.6% to 2% of U.S. women had ever had sexual activity in exchange for money or drugs. He also indicated that 0.6% of U.S. men had a prostitute for a sex partner during the last year, 5.9% within the past 5 years, and 16.3% at some point in the past. Sexual activity with prostitutes does not consistently vary by education or age. It is higher among those living in metropolitan areas, African Americans, those with lower incomes, veterans (probably when in military service), those who attend church less frequently, and those who have gone through a divorce.

Phone Sex Workers

Female employees of a phone sex company were interviewed to find out who they are and why they work at a job they often can't mention publicly (Rich, 2004). The women ranged in age from 21 to 45 and came from a variety of educational backgrounds. Many felt they held an important social role. While some lost respect for men as a result of their job, others believed that by taking callers with rape fantasies, they kept potentially violent men from enacting real-life crimes. Because some callers claim to be virgins, some employees reported that they were educating men about female sexuality. Some workers cited that they liked the casual environment, or the chance to have fun before settling down in a more serious career. The main reason they took their jobs was money. They made more than most felt they could earn elsewhere. They said the income came at a price, however, because they could not be honest with people about what they do to make money.

Public Health Perspective

The issue of commercial sex work causes a lot of debate among public health professionals (Kempner, 2005). Historically, public health professionals focused on sex workers as disease vectors—those who could spread STIs to the wider population. Interventions, therefore, focused not on the health of the sex workers but rather on their role in shaping the health of society. More recently, the World Health Organization indicated that interventions can have a positive impact on both the spread of disease and the lives of those involved in sex work. Paying more attention to the health of sex workers involves adopting a nonjudgmental attitude, respecting sex workers' human rights, involving sex workers in program development, and recognizing that sex workers are part of the solution. This kind of model can be controversial because it seeks to improve conditions and health without necessarily eliminating potentially harmful behavior or behavior that some people would feel is wrong or immoral.

Sexual Slavery

Human rights groups estimate that between 12.3 million and 27 million people are enslaved in forced or bonded labor, child labor, sexual servitude, and involuntary servitude at any given time. Human trafficking is estimated to generate $9.5 billion in annual revenue. Although there are many different kinds of trafficking, women and girls make up the majority of human victims (66% and 13%, respectively). Sex trafficking appears to be growing in scope and magnitude. It is estimated that only about 5% of trafficking cases are ever reported. Those most vulnerable to trafficking include impoverished and drug-addicted women and runaway girls. Children as young as 1 and 2 years old have been found in brothels. Organized crime is largely responsible for the proliferation of human trafficking. Women and girls are lured with promises of love, marriage, educational opportunities, and a better life. Sex trafficking of women and girls has astronomical costs, both to the women and girls who are its primary victims, and to society as a whole (The new face of slavery, 2010).

Girls are lured from other countries to the United States. They are promised restaurant jobs, modeling jobs, and other opportunities. But then people who traffic in sex slaves seize their passports. They tell the girls that they owe a large sum of money to pay for their trip and other expenses. Of course, the girls don't have the money so they are forced to work in brothels. Some of the girls are baited by promises of legitimate jobs and a better life in America, many are abducted, and others have been bought from or abandoned by their impoverished families. Some women are sold four or five times to different people like a piece of property (Vitagliano, 2004).

In 2005, *48 Hours*, a CBS News presentation, did a special on sex slavery (Rescued from sex slavery, 2005). Reporters traveled to Romania with hidden cameras to find out if it was really possible to purchase a sex slave. In a very short time, they learned about girls who were for sale as slaves. One contact

? Did You Know . . .

Even obtaining the services of a sex worker has changed with the advent of the Internet. For example, you can search under "prostitutes" and "[name of city]" and get a listing of the best spots to find a sex worker. Local police monitor such sites as well. Also, you can link up with an "escort" service via the Internet, ordering online.

told them that, "You can buy 10 girls in one night if you want to." The contact helped them meet with a sex trafficker. The woman brought out a young girl who was for sale. She had the girl undress to show that she didn't have any marks or skin disease. After some haggling, Peter Van Sant, the CBS newsman, bought the girl for $1,800. Later, the girl told the newsman it was the first time she had been outside for over a year. She said her owners brutally beat her, and that she was fed like a dog. She had become a sex slave after her mother abandoned her in an orphanage. The *48 Hours* crew brought the girl to a shelter where she started a new life. They had demonstrated how easy it was to buy a sex slave.

The Trafficking Victims Protection Act of 2000 and its reauthorizations in 2003, 2005, and 2008 define a human trafficking victim as a person induced to perform labor or a commercial sex act through force, fraud, or coercion. The act was put in place to combat international trafficking in persons, to combat trafficking in persons in the United States, and to provide funding to assist with these efforts. In its first 21 months of operation (January 2007 to September 2008), the Human Trafficking Reporting System recorded information on more than 1,200 alleged incidents of human trafficking in the United States. Most (83%) of the incidents involved sex trafficking. About one-third of the 1,200 incidents involved children (More than 1,200 alleged incidents of human trafficking reported in the U.S., 2009).

Even though the Trafficking Victims Protection Act enables the federal government to distribute funding for victims of severe forms of trafficking, there has been controversy about use of the money. In 2009, the ACLU filed a lawsuit against the U.S. Department of Health and Human Services alleging that the agency was allowing a Roman Catholic organization to limit grant money to organizations that do not provide access to contraception and abortion services for human trafficking victims. The ACLU said the restrictions present serious health risks because sex trafficking victims have a higher incidence of HIV and other STIs. It further said that the organization was misusing taxpayer money and attempting to impose its religious beliefs on trafficking victims (ACLU sues HHS over religious

restrictions on funds for programs serving sex trafficking victims, 2009).

The U.S. Department of State has an Office to Monitor and Combat Trafficking in Persons. Annually, it publishes a *Trafficking in Persons Report*. Organizations that work on the issue of sex slavery include the International Justice Mission (*www.ijm.org*) and Free the Slaves (*http://freetheslaves.net*).

Opinions About Sex Work

The subject of sex workers produces strong emotional reactions in many people. For example, some people believe sex workers should have the right to do their work. Others believe that this practice maintains a world where women are subordinate and sex workers reinforce broad patterns of discrimination. From an economic perspective, it has been argued that sex work helps many women escape poverty and hunger. They get paid much more than they could earn by doing anything else, so they can better help their families. Also, legalizing sex work would make it easier for sex workers to organize into unions as other workers have, which could help improve their working conditions, raise the status of their profession, and promote respect for their human rights.

Of course many people would argue against sex work on moral grounds. Perhaps they feel that sexual activity should be restricted to marital relations or that it is immoral for sex workers to participate in sexual activity with many different people.

In contrast to those who organize against sex work, the North American Task Force on Prostitution (NTFP) was founded in 1979 to act as an umbrella organization for prostitutes and prostitutes' rights organizations. It is a network of sex workers and their supporters that advocates for the rights of sex workers to organize on their own behalf, work safely and without legal repression, travel without legal restrictions, have families and raise children, and enjoy the same rights, responsibilities, and privileges as other people. The goals of the NTFP are to (1) repeal the existing prostitution laws; (2) ensure the right of prostitutes and other sex workers to bargain with their employers, when they work for

Multicultural DIMENSIONS

"Values" of Prostitution in Other Countries?

In Russia, tens of thousands of female college students work as prostitutes or carry on exclusive relationships with so-called sponsors to pay for college. The Russian Internet is replete with websites that offer free search engines that match potential clients with students. Most sites provide the woman's age, body measurements, types of sex she practices, corresponding costs, and even reviews by former clients. One girl used to work as an elementary teacher earning the equivalent of $60 per month. Now she works as a prostitute and earns the equivalent of $200 to $300

for a night of sexual activities. Of course, the women have expenses such as paying for a madam (agent) and use of an apartment or other appropriate facility. When asked how her parents feel about her work, one student said, "We tell them we work as waitresses. They don't ask any questions" (MacWilliams, 2002).

In some situations, prostitutes are very concerned about their rights. For example, in Paris hundreds of prostitutes wearing white masks with tears painted on them rallied in front of the French Senate to protest a high-profile government crackdown on their livelihood (French prostitutes protest crackdown, 2002).

---

third parties, to improve their working conditions; (3) inform the public about a wide range of issues related to prostitution and other forms of sex work; (4) promote the development of support services for sex workers, including HIV, AIDS, and STIs and violence-prevention projects, as well as health and social support services for sex workers (including supportive programs to deal with STIs, violence, and substance abuse), legal assistance projects, and job retraining and other programs to assist prostitutes who wish to change their occupation; and (5) end the public stigma associated with sex work.

There are other examples of giving a louder voice to a business that has thrived in silence. In Huntsville, Alabama, a chapter of the Sex Workers Outreach Project was formed. It is part of a national movement to demand greater acceptance and protection for sex workers. In San Francisco there is a Center for Sex and Culture where prostitutes met to plot their next political move after losing a ballot initiative that would have eased police enforcement of prostitution laws. In New York there is a magazine for people in the sex industry. On the Internet, prostitutes have found ways to find one another, form online communities, and connect with groups in other communities. The ultimate goal for some in the movement is decriminalization of prostitution. They say there are safe ways to work—that sex work is only a risk when it is illegal. They also argue that prostitution is a viable source of income for many people, and that sexual activity between adults for money should be treated as any other form of legal labor. However, some former prostitutes oppose this movement because they see the business as inherently exploitative and degrading.

In 2005 the United Kingdom Royal College of Nursing called on the British government to decriminalize prostitution in an attempt to limit associated negative health consequences (Prostitutes are people too, 2005). It was pointed out that prostitutes face many occupational hazards such as STIs, physical violence, psychological disorders, and a lifestyle associated with substance abuse. Compounding the situation is a propensity for them to be excluded from routine preventive and therapeutic health care. It was further indicated that prostitutes, be they men or women, are real people and suffer real illness and experience real pain from circumstances forced on them. They need medical care and treatment with the same respect afforded to other members of the community. The conclusion was that decriminalization of prostitution would be a fundamental step to help these often vulnerable people.

Controlling Sex Work

Some officials have tried various ways to manage sex work. For example, San Francisco took a laissez-faire approach. As a result, sex work is highly visible in tourist sections in the form of massage parlors, escort services, bar sex workers, hotel sex workers, and call girls (or boys). The major benefit of this approach has been to restrict sex work to nonresidential parts of the city. The control model—whereby certain neighborhoods strictly enforce laws against sex work—has been employed in North Dallas; the results have been reductions in crime and in visibility of sex workers. The regulation model—whereby sex work is legalized and subject to certain regulations—has been tried in rural Nevada, where it has resulted

Multicultural DIMENSIONS

Organizations for Sex Workers

One organization for sex workers is Call Off Your Tired Ethics (COYOTE), which was founded in 1973. It works for the rights of all sex workers of all genders and persuasions. COYOTE supports programs to assist sex workers if they choose to change their occupation, works to prevent the scapegoating of sex workers for AIDS and other STIs, and educates sex workers, their clients, and the general public about safer sex.

Prostitutes of New York (PONY) is a support and advocacy group for all people in the sex industry. PONY advocates the decriminalization of prostitution and calls for an end to illegal police activity in the enforcement of existing laws. It provides legal and health referrals to sex workers and encourages members to recommend doctors, therapists, and other professionals who provide high-quality service to sex workers. PONY encourages all people who sell sex or profit from sex to learn about the diversity of their industry, to promote professional standards in their sector, and to learn more about the history of the world's oldest profession (and its allied industries).

There are similar groups in other countries. One example is the Prostitutes Collective of Victoria (PCV) (Australia), which is a community-based organization developed to include and represent sex-industry workers' concerns about the issue of prostitution as a part of a worldwide prostitutes' rights movement. It works for basic human rights and occupational health and safety rights for all prostitution workers.

The Network of Sex Work Projects (NSWP) was formed in 1991. It consists of sex workers and organizations that provide services to sex workers in more than 40 countries. The NSWP focuses on issues similar to those of interest to the other groups and aims to facilitate opportunities for the voices of sex workers to be heard in relevant international forums.

---

in a minimal amount of crime and where, for the most part, sex work is limited to controlled brothels. Finally, there is the zoning model—whereby sex work is tolerated but not legal only in certain parts of the city. With this model, sex workers are supposedly visible only in a certain part of the city, and crime associated with sex work is limited to that area. None of these approaches has been totally successful, and each has advantages and disadvantages.

Another method of trying to control sex work has been making public the identities of sex workers and their customers. For example, in 1997 "John TV" started in Kansas City. Every Wednesday morning viewers of the local government cable TV channel saw the names, photographs, dates of birth, and addresses of people—mostly men—who were arrested for visiting sex workers. Above each picture was this disclaimer: "This person is innocent until found guilty by a court." The ACLU objected to this practice because it targeted people before they were convicted of a crime and used a government-controlled medium to deliver its message of humiliation.

"John TV" has been used in other places as well. In Oklahoma, its goals include to expose and identify those who have preyed upon women lost to drug addiction and street prostitution, use those caught and published as an example to dissuade others, and to forward the ideology of decriminalization of 100% private, consensual and nonorganized prostitution so that the community's limited resources can be focused on street, forced, and organized prostitution and trafficking. More detail is available about John TV at *http://johntv.com*.

Another method of controlling sex workers involves organizations that provide help and support for sex workers who desire to change their life and stop being sex workers. One such organization is the Council for Prostitution Alternatives in Portland, Oregon. Its goal is to help women who want to leave the sex industry find alternatives to lives in prostitution. A number of services are provided, including education, health care, referrals to services when needed, legal assistance, mentoring, and hospitality. More information can be found at *www.prostitutionalternatives.org*. Children of the Night is a similar organization located in San Francisco.

A different approach to controlling sex work came about in 1996 when the Lusty Lady Theater in San Francisco became the first women-managed strip club in the United States to unionize. This resulted in elimination of racist hiring practices and the practice of customers being allowed to videotape dancers without their consent via one-way mirrors. It also resulted in having consistent disciplinary policies, better health benefits, and better job security (Brooks, 2005).

Global DIMENSIONS

International Differences Related to Prostitution

From a selection of 100 countries inclusive of major religions, geographical regions, and policies towards prostitution, prostitution is legal in 50 of the countries, of limited legality in 11 of the countries, and illegal in 39 of the countries. Countries where prostitution is legal include Argentina, Austria, Belgium, Brazil, Canada, Chile, Denmark, Ecuador, Finland, Greece, Germany, Hungary, Ireland, Israel, Italy, Mexico, the Netherlands, New Zealand, Poland, Portugal, Switzerland, Turkey, and the United Kingdom. Countries where prostitution is illegal include Afghanistan, the Bahamas, China, Cuba, Egypt, Haiti, Iran, Jamaica, Kenya, North and South Korea, Liberia, the Philippines, Romania, South Africa, Thailand, Uganda, and the United

Arab Emirates. Countries with limited legality include Australia, Bulgaria, Iceland, India, Japan, Norway, Spain, Sweden, and the United States.

The percentage of men who have paid for sexual activity at least once varies quite a bit among countries. For example, in the United States estimates are between 15% and 20%. At the higher end are Cambodia (59–80%), Thailand (75%), Italy (17–45%), Spain (27–39%), and Japan (37%). At the lower end are Australia (16%), Sweden (8–14%), Finland (10–13%), Norway (13%), and the United Kingdom (7–9%).

Source: Data from Prostitution. ProCon.org, 2012. Available: http://prostitution.procon.org/view.resource.php?resourceID=000772 and http://prostitution.procon.org/view.resource.php?resourceID=004119.

The federal government has tried another way to control sex work. Since 2003 all foreign nongovernmental organizations seeking U.S. global HIV/AIDS funds have been required to pledge their opposition to prostitution and sex trafficking to be eligible to partner with the U.S. government in combating HIV/AIDS in the developing world. In 2005 the rule was extended to American organizations as well (U.S. requirement that AIDS groups sign pledge against commercial sex work "harms" AIDS work, 2005).

Ditmore (2005) pointed out that many agencies are severely restricted by the policy. For example, some projects advocate the empowerment of sex workers to help them develop better lives. Other projects assist trafficked persons and sex workers in various ways. Some help sex workers to obtain high school diplomas so they can get other employment. As one project administrator said: "How can we ask prostitutes to take a position against themselves?" As a result of the governmental policy, those in a number of worthwhile projects decided to turn down the money. This meant they could not help as many people.

Arguments about the pros and cons of controlling sex work and its safety will probably continue for many years to come. Schmidt (2011) summarized the research and the beliefs of other researchers. He pointed out that some research indicates that Nevada's legal model is a better solution than criminalization. Women working in Nevada brothels do so under the protection of other brothel employees in rooms equipped with intercoms and panic

buttons. It seems that women in Nevada brothels are far safer than those engaged in street prostitution or, for that matter, many women in the ordinary dating scene. Some researchers found no evidence "that selling sex is harmful to women." Other researchers, however, feel that women in Nevada's legal brothels are vulnerable to violence, STIs, and a host of other ailments; that some women were placed in the brothels by their pimps as punishment for not earning more money elsewhere; that some women appear to have been trafficked into Nevada's brothels; and that many working in them appear to be brainwashed.

The Law and Prostitution

Should prostitution be legal? This question has been argued for many years. Some people believe there are potential benefits of legalizing prostitution, such as increased human rights protection and health precautions. They argue that prostitution always has been and always will be. Legalization would increase condom use and, in turn, lead to a reduction of HIV and AIDS and other STIs. They feel prostitutes have the right to choose the way they earn their income; therefore, how can society stand in the way of someone's earning a good living?

Opponents of prostitution argue that most prostitutes are forced into sexual slavery. They suggest that legalization would give rise to a black market that would be frightening and abusive. For some opponents to prostitution, the issue is a moral one because prostitution gives rise to dehumanizing, unsafe, illegal activities. It is morally reprehensible, they say, for prostitutes to be treated as too many are treated. They conclude that the abuses and potential threat for ongoing abuse far outweigh any potential benefits of legalization. And the argument continues (Should prostitution be legal?, 2003).

Agustin (2008) has pointed out that a large number of those who would be governed by legislation on commercial sexual activity don't identify with such legislation or consider it useful to their lives. Even in those places in the world where sex workers can legally register and operate within the law, many do not bother to do so because they fail to see any benefit. Few sex workers join trade unions or interest groups where they exist.

Is prostitution safer when it is legal? This question was debated by eight experts in 2012 (Is prostitution safer when it's legal?, 2012). The main points raised included:

1. Labor laws, not criminal laws, are the answer. Prostitutes should be allowed to protect themselves, organize, and advocate.

2. Legality leads to more trafficking. The presence of an adult sex industry increases the rates of child sexual exploitation and trafficking. The argument that legalizing prostitution makes it safer hasn't been borne out in countries implementing legalization.

3. Prostitution should not be illegal, but the buying of sexual activity should be criminalized. (The customers should be prosecuted, but not the prostitutes.)

4. The legalization of prostitution would likely make things a little better for those women who have few options to begin with. If options are not good, the focus should be on education, skills training, and job creation.

5. In legal brothels, employees report that they feel safe, are free to come and go, and are bound only by their contract. The police, employers, and coworkers are there to protect them. Legality brings protection and better care.

6. The way to address oppression is to end it—not legalize, regulate, or make it more tolerable. Prostitution teaches people that other people can be rendered into sexual commodities that can be bought or sold for sexual use and abuse.

7. Legal brothels can be coercive. Some have been like prisons or detention camps.

Child Prostitution

A particularly disturbing feature of sex work is the presence of minors selling sexual activity. Child prostitution has become more common in recent years. In some instances, children are forced by adults to perform sexual acts. In other instances, the minors may appear to be selling sexual activity by choice—though many would argue that it is not really voluntary.

Cultures exist around the world in which children, as belongings, are property to be bought and sold. In some developing countries, boys outnumber girls on the streets because girls are often put into brothels. These children are prostituted, or even sold, to prevent themselves and their families from starving. The customers who purchase the children or their services are adults who are commonly pedophiles or sadists.

In some instances there can be links between child prostitution and child pornography. For example, costumed children might act out a customer's fantasy in special surroundings while filming is done. The acting might be done as part of a story, such as an abduction of a virgin or a "schoolgirl tease," or the action might simply be rape and torture. There is money to be made from the prostitution activities and the selling of videos.

In the United States a large number of adolescent sex workers are runaways who are looking for

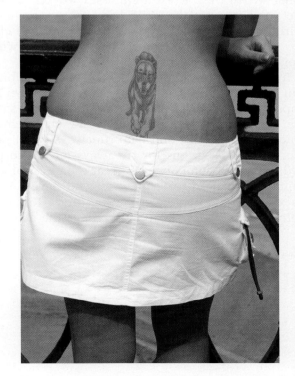

To survive on the streets, adolescents who have run away from home often sell drugs or their bodies.

companionship, friendship, love, and approval, as well as a way of supporting themselves financially. Unfortunately, many of them are ideal targets for gangs, drug pushers, and pimps. To survive on the streets, runaways often sell drugs or their bodies, and a large number turn to other types of crime to support themselves.

It is estimated that between 300,000 and 400,000 girls and boys, aged 9–17 years, trade their bodies to pay for food, shelter, clothing, and other basic needs to survive on America's streets (Uhlman, 2001). Some U.S. children engage in commercial sexual activity while living at home and generally find customers among their peers. Those children at highest risk for commercial sexual exploitation are those who run away or are thrown out by their relatives. Fewer than 25% are members of impoverished families. A significant number of their customers are married men, many with children of their own. Other children at higher risk to become victims of commercial sexual activity include female gang members who get involved to raise money for the gang; foreign children; and teenagers living along the Canadian or Mexican borders who cross into those countries specifically to solicit sexual activity.

The fact that runaways make up a significant percentage of adolescent sex workers creates a particularly difficult problem for law enforcement personnel. When they arrest a child sex worker, it does little good to send the child back to a poor home environment. In fact, there have been reports of children setting up their own prostitution rings, while living at home, to earn spending money.

In response to childhood sex work, law enforcement personnel have attempted to crack down on pimps of adolescent sex workers and at the same time better coordinate with other law enforcement agencies to recognize and help runaways when possible. Service programs for runaways have incorporated a medical component to treat the physical and mental health needs of runaways who have turned to sex work (and of other runaways, too). Runaway shelters provide services to help reduce the need for runaways to turn to sex work. Such services include medical services, crisis intervention services, individual and group counseling, vocational training and job placement, legal services, independent living skills training, and support and friendship. The hope is that the many shelters and service centers around the United States will help convince young people that they need not turn to pimps and sex work to meet their needs.

Thousands of British university students have turned to sex work to cover their college expenses. They work as strippers, lap dancers, escorts, and pornographic movie actors. One student said she cannot find another job that fits in with her academic obligations. Another said that taking his clothes off is easier than waiting on tables and he makes 10 times more. In Leeds, 60% of the city's sex workers are university students. One madam opened a brothel close to the University of Leeds to make it easier for students to commute to work (Birchard, 2001).

A survey of 56 county social service providers showed that the exploitation of children for money, whether it is pornography or prostitution, is an often unseen but very real problem (Invisibility, 2011). For example, 87% of the respondents said children who are sexually exploited are working for a pimp or are being pimped by a parent, many of the pimps are members of the child's family, an equal number of blacks and whites were involved, and a little over half of the young people were homeless. The vast majority of those surveyed said there were no programs in place designed to specifically help the young people.

Research about all forms of sex work has changed more in recent years than at any time in the past. We now know more about the extent of sex work and its changing nature worldwide, but particularly in the West. We also have a better grasp of the reasons why some people enter the sex industry. With the growth of sex-worker organizations, there is greater access to research subjects. The existence of a pool of volunteers willing to contribute to both their own research projects and those of others has the potential of adding greatly to our knowledge about this area of human sexual behavior.

Our feeling, attitudes, and beliefs regarding sexuality are influenced by our internal and external environments. Go to go.jblearning.com/dimensions5e *to learn more about the biological, psychological, and sociological factors that affect your sexuality.*

Case Study

Marketing of sexual products and use of sexual imagery to market nonsexual products are multibillion-dollar businesses. The alluring imagery may draw attention to the product but does not necessarily result in a sale unless the product is sexually related, such as a product to enhance one's appearance.

As marketers attempt to target certain groups (typically younger populations) with sexual imagery, they need to be aware that other people may find their ads offensive.

Marketing of sexually explicit materials to consumers in conditions of privacy (i.e., at home) has driven the markets for DVDs and the Internet.

But marketers also face legal challenges to distributing sexually explicit material. Because "community standards" are used to judge whether material is obscene, a website operator in one state can be charged with obscenity under the community standards of a person in another state who downloads the materials.

Marketing of any sexually explicit material involving children is prosecuted harshly. Even just downloading such material is a violation of the law.

Biological Factors

- Prostitutes in general have a much higher rate of HIV infection. About one-third of New York City streetwalkers are infected with HIV.
- No externally used products can enlarge the penis or breasts.

Sociocultural Factors

- Fraudulent sexual aids are among the top 10 sources of health fraud in the United States.
- Prostitution is outlawed in every U.S. state except Nevada (and even there it is legal in only a few counties).
- Many countries allow prostitution. South Korea issues identification cards to prostitutes that serve as hotel passes. South Korea and Thailand consider prostitution of young girls to be a tourist attraction.
- Some countries, such as Iran and China, have attempted to ban distribution of sexually explicit materials. Laws govern distribution and possession of sexually explicit photos of children.
- Media often fail to depict safer sexual practices in books, articles, TV shows, and movies.
- Sexually explicit materials helped create and expand the market for home videos and the Internet.

Psychological Factors

- Media images may negatively impact body image and self-esteem.
- Many ads use sexual imagery to attract attention and stimulate senses.

Summary

- There are countless advertisements in magazines, in newspapers, and on TV that use sexual themes to sell products. Advertisers seem to have made a careful study of sexual motivation.

- The sexual content of TV programs has increased immensely in the past few decades. TV can be an excellent way to educate people about healthy sexual practices, but it is rarely used that way.

- The sexuality content of movies has also increased greatly in the past few decades. Some people believe the sexual explicitness is detrimental to society, whereas others see this trend as positive.

- The availability of sexual material in DVDs and video games continues to increase. Businesses related to these products have grown by leaps and bounds.

- The mass phenomenon that may affect more young people than any other is popular music. Blatant sexual themes in music are very common today.

- Sexual content available on the Internet has raised many interesting issues. Among them is whether and how to apply censorship, whether and how to control access to the Internet for children, and how to deal with sexual predators on the Internet.

- Sexually explicit materials have been around for centuries and have often spawned controversy. Some people believe it is necessary to strictly control such materials, but others feel they are not harmful if used by adults. Most agree that child pornography should be prohibited.

- There are many types of sex workers, including call girls, house prostitutes, streetwalkers, massage parlor sex workers, bar girls, gigolos, hustlers, and pimps. In addition, in more recent years new types have emerged—phone and Internet sex workers, sex shop operators, and owners of stores that sell toys and devices related to sexuality.

- Sexual slavery has become a huge international problem. Millions of people around the world are trapped in virtual prisons on farms, in sweatshops, or in brothels.

Discussion Questions

1. Analyze the value of sexuality in selling products. Discuss sexually oriented ads, including the ways sex helps sell products (bikini-clad calendars, sexually explicit rap music, "dirty" classic literature, and so on).

2. Create a legal standard for distributing sexually explicit materials. Include in the standard what constitutes art, child pornography, literature, and the like.

3. Compare and contrast the varied types of sex workers. Then describe efforts to control sex work.

Application Questions

Reread the chapter-opening story and answer the following questions.

1. Of the students who had opinions about sexual consumerism, with whom do you agree? Explain your answer, citing contemporary examples.

2. In what ways do actor portrayals of sexuality—or models with "perfect" bodies—make us feel inferior? Could those same images be said to promote erotic feelings and thus have value?

3. Does the use of naked flesh make ads sexier? Or have ads from the past, albeit with less flesh, been just as sexually oriented?

Critical Thinking Questions

1. When planning an ad campaign, a marketer needs to think about all audiences who will view the ad. Consider the anecdotal story that has appeared in various advertising publications about the former first lady Nancy Reagan and her daughter, Patty Davis: During the early 1990s, the two women were waiting in a hotel lobby when the conversation turned to sexual consumerism. Mrs. Reagan, showing her daughter a perfume ad in a magazine, said that she did not like having to look at a nearly naked man in the ad. Her daughter replied, "Well, I sure do!" They both laughed.

   Clearly, the marketer was targeting the demographics of Reagan's daughter. But should a marketer have to be concerned about offending people in other demographics—older and more conservative people as well as minors? Describe the steps a marketer should have to take before placing ads.

2. Although it is billed as the "world's oldest profession," prostitution is not legal in the United States except in a few counties in Nevada. Should prostitution be legalized? Consider the social, legal (including tax ramifications), health, moral, and other dimensions of sexuality of both clients and prostitutes in your answer.

3. Former stars of sexually explicit films, such as Linda Lovelace and Traci Lords, described the world of porn films as one of physical abuse (actual and threatened) and drugs. If an actress participated in explicit sexual activity under such coercion, does that constitute rape? Should distribution of such movies be illegal?

4. Distribution of photos of naked minors is illegal. But prominent "art" photographers often take photos of naked minors, and such photos are distributed in photo anthologies through major bookstore chains. How is it possible to differentiate between art and child pornography?

5. China, Iran, and other countries limit Internet access for their citizens. Two major concerns are antigovernment rhetoric and sexually explicit material. Given the ease with which minors can access sexually explicit material, should the U.S. government restrict the Internet access of U.S. citizens? Should the Internet be regulated?

Critical Thinking Cases

In parts of Japan, December 24 is the "hottest" night of the year. Societal pressure is strong for every unmarried person to have a date on Christmas Eve and for that date to include an overnight stay. In this respect December 24 is not dissimilar to prom night here in America. Just about every major hotel in Tokyo is sold out for that night months in advance. The Japanese describe Christmas Eve as a night to make love and refer to it as "H-Day" (for "hormone," the Japanese euphemism for sex).

This evening is quite expensive for young Japanese, as the cost typically exceeds $1,000. Men are expected to buy their date a present ($215), take her to Tokyo Disneyland ($100), provide dinner at a fancy restaurant ($385), take a room at a nice hotel (between $350 and $650), have breakfast the next morning ($35), and rent a limousine ($150)—all of this in a country less than 1% Christian and where December 25 is a normal working day.

1. Discuss H-Day in terms of the dimensions of sexuality. Include safer-sex practices, the psychological implications of engaging in sexual activity with someone because of societal pressure, religion, culture, and other factors.

2. Which cultural factors would prevent H-Day from being accepted in the United States? (Assume that the date would be changed from December 24.)

Exploring Personal Dimensions

Are You a Good Sexual Consumer?

Answer the following statements with one of the following responses. When you are finished, total your points and find out how good a sexual consumer you are.

1. Rarely or never
2. Sometimes
3. Often
4. All or most of the time

_____ 1. I make sure the date on any product (such as condoms or oral contraceptives) has not expired.

_____ 2. I am not influenced by sexually alluring images to purchase products.

_____ 3. I am aware of whether any sexually explicit material I view involves minors.

_____ 4. I make sure that any sexually explicit material I view is kept away from minors.

_____ 5. I understand that sharing sexual aids (or toys) with others is a high-risk activity, capable of transmitting STIs and AIDS.

_____ 6. I am aware that sexual contact with sex workers or former sex workers is a high-risk activity because of the potential for STI and/or HIV transmission.

_____ 7. I believe that aphrodisiacs offer no sexual help physiologically, and I consider their side effects before using them.

_____ 8. I evaluate "research" claims made by marketers before buying a product.

_____ 9. I consider the source of sexual health information before purchasing any product.

_____10. I have sought recommendations from friends for whom to consult in case of sexually related healthcare needs.

_____11. I have regular exams by a physician.

_____12. I understand that certain prescription drugs (such as antibiotics) can affect the effectiveness of oral contraceptives.

_____13. I read labels of health products and follow directions.

_____14. I do a monthly breast or testicular self-exam.

_____15. When friends state a sexual myth as though it were a fact, I use knowledge from this course to correct them tactfully.

Scoring

0–15   Your sexual consumer skills are weak.

16–30   Your sexual consumer skills are below what they should be.

31–45   Your sexual consumer skills are good but can stand improvement.

Suggested Readings

Brennan, B. Competing claims of victimhood? Foreign and domestic victims of trafficking in the United States. *Sexuality Research & Social Policy, 5, no. 4* (December 2008), 45–61.

Herbenick, D., & Reece, M. Sex education in adult retail stores: Positioning consumers' questions as teachable moments. *American Journal of Sexuality Education, 2, no. 1* (2006), 57–75.

Johansson, T., & Hammaren, N. Hegemonic masculinity and pornography: Young people's attitudes toward and relations to pornography. *Journal of Men's Studies, 15, no. 1* (January 2007), 57–70.

Brief history: Sex on TV. *Time 177, no. 5* (February 7, 2011), 19.

Brown, J. D., Keller, S., & Stern, S. Sex, sexuality, sexting, and sex ed: Adolescents and the media. *The Prevention Researcher 16, no. 4* (November, 2009), 12–16.

The national report on domestic minor sex trafficking: America's prostituted children, May 2009. Available: www.sharedjope.org.

Soderlund, G., Journalist or panderer? Framing underage webcam sites. *Sexuality Research & Social Policy, 5, no. 4* (December 2008), 62–72.

Teens talk About TV, sex, and real life, (2012). Available: www.k4health.org/es/popline/teens-talk-about-tv-sex-and-real-life

Web Resources

For links to the websites below, visit *go.jblearning.com/dimensions5e* and click on Resource Links.

The Dove Foundation
www.dove.org

The Dove Foundation supports efforts to move Hollywood in a more family-friendly direction. It provides film reviews for consideration by consumers.

The Free Speech Museum
www.spectacle.org/musm.html

The Free Speech Museum is intended to serve as a permanent Internet resource on the freedom of speech. It is very concerned that many current efforts are designed to cut down or eliminate free speech.

Good Vibrations
www.goodvibes.com

Good Vibrations considers itself the place to go for sex toys, sex education, erotic and informative books, adult DVDs, and more.

National Coalition for the Protection of Children and Families
www.nationalcoalition.org

The Coalition's mission is to move the people of God to embrace, live out, preserve, and advance the biblical truth of sexuality. It wants to educate the Christian community on sexual ethics according to a biblical worldview, encourage and challenge Christians to live sexually pure lives, engage Christians in public policy relative to sexual ethics, and embrace those harmed by pornography and help restore them to sexual wholeness.

Prostitution Research and Education
www.prostitutionresearch.com

The purpose of Prostitution Research and Education is to abolish prostitution and advocate for alternatives to prostitution—including emotional and physical health care for women in prostitution. PRE seeks to give voice to those who are among the world's most disenfranchised groups: prostituted/trafficked women and children. Its goal is to empower this constituency by documenting their perspectives through research, public education, and arts projects.

Veronica's Voice
www.veronicasvoice.org

This organization encourages prostitutes to choose lifestyle changes that lead to recovery of their minds, bodies, and spirits. It is targeted to help women make the choice to leave prostitution, drug addiction, and a life of violence, transitioning into new lives free from abuse. Survivors of the sex industry direct the program.

References

ACLU sues HHS over religious restrictions on funds for programs serving sex trafficking victims. *Daily Women's Health Report* (January 13, 2009). National Partnership for Women and Families. Available: http://nationalpartnership.org/.

Agustin, L. Sex and the limits of enlightenment: The irrationality of legal regimes to control prostitution. *Sexuality Research & Social Policy, 5, 4* (December 2008), 73–85.

Albright, J. M. Sex in America online: An exploration of sex, marital status, and sexual identity in Internet sex seeking and its impacts. *Journal of Sex Research, 45, 2* (April–June 2008), 175–186.

Bangkok Post profiles group providing services for male commercial sex workers. *Kaiser Daily HIV/AIDS Report* (January 5, 2005). Available: http://www.kaisernetwork.org.

Barker, O. Victoria's Secret tones down suggestive displays. *USA Today* (October 10, 2005), p. 1D.

Benedetti, W. The naked truth: Junk and jubblies sell games. *MSNBC.com*, February 27, 2009. Available: http://www.msnbc.msn.com/id/29417313/.

Birchard, K. Sex, please, we're British: Many students strip to pay bills, BBC reports. *Chronicle of Higher Education*, Today's News (May 2, 2001). Available: http://chronicle.com/daily/2001/05/2001050205n.htm.

Brooks, S. Exotic dancing and unionizing: The challenges of feminist and antiracist organizing at the Lusty Lady Theater. *SIECUS Report 33, 2* (Spring 2005), 12–15.

Chandra, A., Martino, S. C., Collins, R. L., Elliott, M. N., Berry, S. H., Kanouse, D. E., & Miu, A. Does watching sex on television predict teen pregnancy? Findings from a national longitudinal survey of youth. *Pediatrics, 122, 5* (November 2008), 1047–1054.

Collins, D., Elliott, M., Berry, S., Kanouse, D., Kunkel, D., Hunter, S., & Miu, A. Watching sex on television predicts adolescent initiation of sexual behavior. *Pediatrics, 114, 3* (September 2004), e280–e289.

Commission on Obscenity and Pornography. *The report of the Commission on Obscenity and Pornography*. New York: Bantam, 1970.

Corliss, R. Sex, sex and rock 'n' roll. *Time, 166, 5* (August 1, 2005), 83.

Crary, D. Abercrombie & Fitch's racy catalog draws odd coalition to call for boycott. *The Birmingham News* (June 22, 2001), 7C.

Daneback, K, Cooper, A., & Mansson, S. An Internet study of cybersex participants. *Archives of Sexual Behavior, 34, 3* (June 2005), 321–328.

Dennis, J. Theater's pass cards let teens see films rated R. *The Birmingham News* (June 9, 2004), 1G.

Ditmore, M. New U.S. funding policies on trafficking affect sex work and HIV-prevention efforts worldwide. *SIECUS Report 33, 2* (Spring 2005), 26–29.

Durex condom maker using "humor" ads to sell condoms in Europe. *Kaiser Network Daily HIV/AIDS Report*. Henry J. Kaiser Family Foundation. Available: http://www.kaisernetwork.org.

Edwards, M. We have a responsibility to dialogue with the media. *SIECUS Report, 24, 5* (June/July 1996), 5.

Escobar-Chaves, S., Tortolero, S., Markham, C., Low, B., Eitel, P., & Thickstun, P. Impact of the media on adolescent sexual attitudes and behaviors. *Pediatrics, 116, 1* (July 2005), 303–326.

Fisher, C., Herbenick, D., Reece, M., Dodge, B., & Fischtein, D. exploring sexuality education opportunities at in-home sex-toy parties in the United States. *Sex Education, 10, no 2* (May 2010), 131–144.

French prostitutes protest crackdown. *The Birmingham News* (November 6, 2002), 9A.

Gillath, O., Mikulincer, M., Birnbaum, G. E., & Shaver, P. R. Does subliminal exposure to sexual stimuli have the same effects on men and women? *Journal of Sex Research, 44, 2* (April 2007), 111–121.

Goodwill ambassador and former "Spice Girl" Geri Halliwell to launch British sex education web site. *Kaiser Daily Reproductive Health Report* (October 25, 2001). Available: http://www.kaisernetwork.org.

Greenhouse, L. Justices back law to make libraries use Internet filters. *The New York Times* (June 24, 2003). Available: http://www.nytimes.com.

Gunasekera, H., Chapman, S., & Campbell, S. Sex and drugs in popular movies: An analysis of the top 200 films. *Journal of the Royal Society of Medicine, 98* (2005), 464–470.

Hall, P. C., West, J. H., & Hill, S. Sexualization in lyrics of popular music from 1959 to 2009: Implications for sexuality education. *Sexuality & Culture*. DOI: 10.1007/s12119-011-9103-4.

Hatton, E., & Trautner, M. N. Equal opportunity objectification? The sexualization of men and women on the cover of *Rolling Stone. Sexuality and Culture, 15, 3* (September 2011), 256–278.

Head, T. The Child Online Protection Act (COPA) of 1998. About .com Civil Liberties, 2012. Available: http://civilliberty.about.com/od/freespeech/p/copa1998.htm.

High court to hear arguments on child porn amendment. *The Birmingham News* (October 28, 2001), 20A.

Hollywood madam caters for ladies. *BBC News* (November 11, 2005).

How popular is Danni Ashe compared to other stars? (2003). Available: http://www.billiondownloadwoman.com/pop.html.

Hunt, M. *Sexual behavior in the 1970s*. Chicago: Playboy Press, 1974.

Increasing number of Cambodian "beer girls" selling sex. *Kaiser Daily HIV/AIDS Report* (January 15, 2003). Available: www.kaisernetwork.org/daily_reports.

Invisibility. Youth and Family Services Network, 2011. Available: http://media.al.com/spotnews/other/Invisibility.final.revised%281%29.pdf.

Is prostitution safer when it's legal? *The New York Times* (April 19, 2012). Available: http://www.nytimes.com/roomfordebate/2012/04/19/is-legalized-prostitution-safer.

James, M. S. Museum of Sex to debut in New York (2002). Available: http://www.ABCnews.com.

Jesdanun, A. Internet porn district clears hurdle with initial approval of .xxx domain. *The Birmingham News* (June 13, 2005), 9C.

Kakuchi, S. Japan only now confronting rising HIV rate—women in sex trade most at risk. *San Francisco Chronicle* (March 17, 2003), A8.

Kempner, M. E. Sex workers: A glimpse into public health perspectives. *SIECUS Report, 33, 2* (Spring 2005), 2.

Kershaw, S. A life as a Live! Nude! Girl! has a few strings attached. *The New York Times* (June 2, 2004).

Key, W. B. *Subliminal seduction*. Englewood Cliffs, NJ: Prentice Hall, 1973.

Kingston, D. A., Malamuth, N. M., Federoff, P., & Marshall, W. L. The importance of individual differences in pornography use: Theoretical perspectives and implications for treating sexual offenders. *Journal of Sex Research, 46, 2 & 3* (March 2009), 216–232.

Kuchment, A., & Springen, K. The tangled web of porn in the office. *Newsweek* (December 8, 2008), 14.

Kuriansky, J. Sexuality and television advertising: An historical perspective. *SIECUS Report, 24, 5* (June/July 1996), 13.

Lasar, M. Supreme Court justice: Broadcast TV on "borrowed time," so why worry about indecency? *Law and Disorder*, January 11, 2012. Available: http://arstechnica.com/tech-policy/news/2012/01/supreme-court-justice-broadcast-tv-living-on-borrowed-time-so-why-worry-about-indecency-rules.ars?comments=1#comments-bar.

Lohr, S. In video game, a download unlocks hidden sex scenes. *The New York Times* (July 11, 2005).

MacWilliams, B. Turning tricks for tuition. *Chronicle of Higher Education, 49, 11* (November 8, 2002), A48.

McClain, D. L. Sex and chess: Is she a queen or a pawn? *The New York Times* (November 27, 2005).

Medina, J. Los Angeles mandates use of condoms for sex films. *The New York Times* (January 17, 2012). Available: http://www.nytimes.com/2012/01/18/us/los-angeles-makes-condoms-mandatory-for-adult-film-actors.html.

Money, J. Pornography in the home. In *Contemporary sexual behavior*, Zubin, J., & Money, J., eds. Baltimore: Johns Hopkins Press, 1973.

Money, J., & Athanasiou, R. Pornography: Review and bibliographic annotations. *American Journal of Obstetrics and Gynecology, 115* (January 1973), 130–146.

More than 1,200 alleged incidents of human trafficking reported in the U.S. U.S. Department of Justice, January 15, 2009. Available: http://www.ojp.usdoj.gov/bjs/pub/press/cshti08pr.htm.

Navarro, M. Women tailor sex industry to their eyes. *The New York Times* (February 20, 2004).

The new face of slavery. Soroptimist International, November, 2010. Available: http://www.soroptimist.org/whitepapers/WhitePaperDocs/WPNewFaceSlavery.pdf.

Notes from the research. *SIECUS Development* (Summer/Fall 2002), 2.

Padgett, P. M. Personal safety and sexual safety for women using online personal ads. *Sexuality Research & Social Policy, 4, 2* (June 2007), 27–37.

Pardun, C. J., & Forde, K. R. Sex in the media: Do condom ads have a chance? *SIECUS Report, 31, 2* (December 2002/January 2003), 22–23.

Parental advisory. The Recording Industry of America, 2003. Available: http://www.riaa.com/issues/parents/advisory.asp.

Pastor's column hits the growth of porn. *The Birmingham Post Herald* (September 1, 2001), D9.

Pitts, M., Smith, A., Grierson, J., O'Brien, M., & Mission, S. Who pays for sex and why? An analysis of social and motivational factors associated with male clients of sex workers. *Archives of Sexual Behavior, 33, 4* (Aug. 2004), 353–358.

Plous, S., & Neptune, D. Racial and gender biases in magazines and advertising. *Psychology of Women Quarterly, 21, 4* (December 1997), 627–644.

Prostitutes are people too. *Lancet Online, 365* (May 7, 2005), 1618.

PTC study: Broadcast TV family hour fare filthier than ever. Parents' Television Council, September 5, 2007. Available: http://parentstv.org.

Rescued from sex slavery. *CBS News, 48 Hours* (July 22, 2005).

Rich, G. Midnight callers. *Psychology Today Here to Help*, 2004. Available: http://www.psychologytoday.com/articles/pto-19990701-000010.html.

Rich, M. *The influence of entertainment media on sexual attitudes and behavior: Managing the media monster*. Washington, DC: National Campaign to Prevent Teen and Unplanned Pregnancy, 2008.

Richtel, M. He's watching that, in public? Pornography takes next seat. *The New York Times* (July 21, 2012). Available: http://www.nytimes.com/2012/07/21/us/tablets-and-phones-lead-to-more-pornography-in-public.html?pagewanted=all.

Rimm, M. Marketing pornography on the information superhighway. *Georgetown Law Journal* (1998).

Rolfe, D. Wal-Mart sells "sanitized" music, film—censorship or public service? The Dove Foundation, 2005. Available: http://www.dove.org.

Ross, M. W. Situating sexuality electronically: The Internet and sexual expression. *Sexuality Research & Public Policy, 4, 2* (June 2007), 1–4.

Schmidt, P. Scholars of legal brothels offer a new take on the "oldest profession." *Chronicle of Higher Education 58, 5* (September 23, 2011), A14–A15.

Schroeder, E. Blaming TV for teen pregnancy is a convenient excuse. *New York Daily News* (November 28, 2008). Available: http://www.nydailynews.com/opinion/blaming-tv-teen-pregnancy-a-convenient-excuse-article-1.339238.

Sex and Tech. Washington, DC: National Campaign to Prevent Teen and Unplanned Pregnancy, 2008. Available: http://www.thenationalcampaign.org/sextech/PDF/SexTech_Summary.pdf.

Sexual health coverage in women's, men's, and teen magazines. Henry J. Kaiser Family Foundation (2000). Available: http://www.kff.org.

Should prostitution be legal? In *Taking sides: Issues in family and personal relationships*, Schroeder, E., ed. Guilford, CT: McGraw-Hill/Dushkin, 2003.

Silver, A. Brief history—sex on TV. *Time, 177, 5* (February 7, 2011), 19.

Sloss, C., & Harper, G. When street sex workers are mothers. *Archives of Sexual Behavior, 33, 4* (August 2004), 329–341.

Small operators can make a real killing on the Web. *USA Today* (August 20, 1997), 1.

Smith, T. W. *American sexual behavior: Trends, socio-demographic differences, and risk behavior*. Chicago: National Opinion Research Center, 2003.

Soderlund, G. Journalist or panderer? Framing underage webcam sites. *Sexuality Research & Social Policy, 5, 4* (December 2008), 62–72.

Stelter, B. A racy show with teenagers steps back from a boundary. *The New York Times,* (January 19, 2011). Available: http://www.nytimes.com/2011/01/20/business/media/20mtv.html.

Stock, W. The effect of pornography on women. Paper presented at a hearing of the Attorney General's Commission on Pornography. Houston, September 11–12, 1985.

Summers, N. Podcasting: Talking dirty on your iPod. *Newsweek Periscope* (August 1, 2005). Available: http://msnbc.msn.com/id/8681666/site/newsweek/?rf=technorati.

Teen girls help FBI nab cyber stalkers. *ABC News,* June 28, 2005. Available: http://abcnews.go.com/WNT/print?id=889662

TV sexual scenes nearly double since 1998. Kaiser Family Foundation, *Kaiser Daily Women's Health Policy* (November 10, 2005). Available: http://kaisernetwork.org.

U.S. Department of Justice. Attorney Holder announces results of international child pornography investigation at Operation Delego press conference, August 3, 2011. Available: http://www.justice.gov/iso/opa/ag/speeches/2011/ag-speech-110803.html.

U.S. Requirement that AIDS groups sign pledge against commercial sex work "harms" AIDS work. *Daily HIV/AIDS Report,* Kaiser Family Foundation, 2005. Available: http://www.kaisernetwork.org/daily_reports/rep_index.cfm?hint=1&DR_ID=32372

Uhlman, M. Many children trade sex to survive, study says. *The Birmingham News* (September 11, 2001), 1A.

"Unusual" FDA order requiring corrections to Yaz ad campaign. National Partnership for Women & Families, *Daily Women's Health Policy Report* (February 11, 2009).

Vitagliano, E. Malevolent bargains. *American Family Association Journal* (April 2004).

Watson, M. A., & Smith, R. Positive porn: Educational, medical, and clinical uses. *American Journal of Sexuality Education, 7, 2,* (2012), 122–145.

What scientists know about pornography. Allentown, PA: Society for the Scientific Study of Sexuality, 2007.

Woellert, L. An all-out assault on sexual content. *BusinessWeek* (November 21, 2005), 118.

Wong, N. C. Study: 1 in 5 kids pressed for sex online. *The Birmingham News* (June 21, 2001), 7A.

Wosick-Correa, K. R., & Joseph, L. J. Sexy ladies sexing ladies: Women as consumers in strip clubs. *Journal of Sex Research, 45, 3* (July 2008), 201–216.

CHAPTER 18

Sexual Ethics, Morality, and the Law

CHAPTER OBJECTIVES

1 Define *ethics, morals, ethical principles, ethical dilemmas, values,* and the five ethical principles that serve as a basis for deciding whether a decision is moral.

2 State the ethical considerations of such sexually related topics as sexually transmitted infections, sexual activity between unmarried partners, sodomy, contraception, abortion, amniocentesis, fetal tissue implantation, prostitution, in vitro fertilization, genetic engineering, and sexual responsibility to a partner.

3 Identify the rationale for laws pertaining to homosexuality, obscenity and pornography, rape, statutory rape, marriage, polygamy, adultery, and divorce.

go.jblearning.com/dimensions5e

Commonly Accepted Ethical Principles
Genetic Engineering

INTRODUCTION

Wendy Weaver was a well-respected high school philosophy teacher and girls' volleyball coach in the Nebo, Utah, school district (Associated Press, 1998). Concerned about her student athletes, in the summer of 1997 she telephoned each one to ask about her summer camp schedule. That is when it happened. A student asked, "Are you gay?" Weaver answered that she was, eliciting a response from the student that she would not play on Weaver's volleyball team in the fall. When school district officials heard what Wendy Weaver disclosed to the student, they immediately fired her from her coaching responsibilities and instructed her not to speak of her sexual orientation to either students or school staff, in or outside school.

The Nebo school district officials believed they were right to protect young people in their school from what they perceived to be disclosure of immoral behavior. They believed that homosexuality was wrong and that it was sinful.

Wendy Weaver, however, believed that she had a moral right to express her sexuality in any way she sought, as long as she did not impose it on her students. After all, she argued, heterosexual teachers are not forbidden to disclose their sexual orientation. Therefore, she asserted that it was wrong—immoral—to forbid her to do so.

Eventually a judge determined the legal issues involved in this case. In November 1997, U.S. District Court Judge Bruce Jenkins ruled that Wendy Weaver's rights of free speech, equal protection under the law, and due process were violated. He ordered that the gag order be lifted and that Wendy Weaver be reinstated as coach of the girls' volleyball team. In his ruling Judge Jenkins stated, "Although the Constitution cannot control prejudices, neither this court nor any other court should, directly or indirectly, legitimize them."

This case includes issues of morality, ethics, and law. The school officials believed that they were acting morally by protecting young people from a teacher they thought might inappropriately affect their sexual orientation. Wendy believed she was acting morally when she answered the team member honestly and when she asserted her constitutional rights. And the judge believed he was acting morally when he applied a law designed to prevent prejudice from depriving a person of her rights in a democratic society. Certainly everyone could not be right; nor could everyone be wrong. Certainly, everyone was not purposefully acting immorally. We shall see in this chapter how complex issues of morality really are and how a systematic approach can manage some of this complexity when these issues relate to matters of sexuality. Furthermore, we shall see how the law is used to codify societal consensus about morality and how it is applied to express societal mores.

Many ethical dilemmas relate to sexuality. For example, whether women should use intrauterine devices (IUDs) as a means of contraception that may prevent fertilized ova from successfully implanting on the uterus's endometrial lining involves the moral question of when life begins. Whether fetal tissue or stem cells—that is, from aborted fetuses—should be made available as a treatment for such conditions as Parkinson's disease concerns the moral issue of the sanctity of the human body.

These and other questions of sexual morality are pervasive. They affect every one of us, if not directly and daily, then certainly as members of a society wrestling with their resolutions. They are also emotionally charged. This point should not go unnoticed. When issues evoke emotional reactions—as sexual issues tend to do—these emotions too often interfere with a rational investigation. Consequently, people argue their own viewpoints while ignoring other perspectives, and that method of argument is not conducive to learning.

This chapter serves to explore the morality and ethics of particular sexually related behaviors or decisions in a unified, systematic manner. In addition, it highlights the importance of considering the ethics and morality of all sexual matters.

Talking about sexual morality is not easy. Whose morality should we focus on? Which morals, if any, should we advocate? How can we prevent offending people whose morals differ from ours? It would be arrogant for us to insist that everyone adopt a single set of sexual morals, and it would be particularly

The story of Wendy Weaver illustrates the multidimensional facets of ethics, morality, and the law.

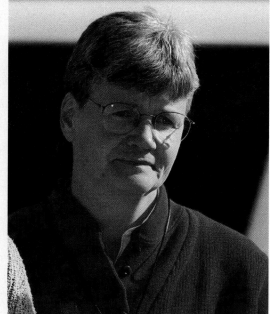

impertinent to suggest that our own morals be the ones adopted. Therefore, in this chapter, rather than advocating a particular set of morals or ethical principles, we describe the process of moral reasoning. We sketch our society's moral stance on STIs, contraception, in vitro fertilization, rape, prostitution, and so on, and describe the background and enforcement of some laws. Along the way we acknowledge some of the religious, philosophical, cultural, family-related, and experiential reasons for the differences in sexual morality among individuals and among societies.

■ Ethics: The Basis for Making Decisions

To begin investigating sexual morality, we need to distinguish between the terms *ethics* and *moral*. **Ethics** refers to a *system* by which we determine whether some action is moral or immoral. An action is **moral** if it is judged to be *good* or *right;* it is **immoral** if it is judged to be *bad* or *wrong*. To guide the decision of whether an action is moral or immoral, the system of ethics employs **ethical principles**. These ethical principles provide answers to abstract questions—they are general guidelines, not meant for individual cases. With regard to abortion, for example, ethicists would be more concerned with the general question of when life begins or with a woman's right to control her own reproductive capacity than with whether abortion is appropriate in a particular case. Decisions about what is moral are determined by many different experiences and influences. Religious beliefs and values, social mores, humanistic views, education, culture, and friends and family are but a few of these influences.

When a set of ethical principles is available and accepted by a society, the people of that society know how they are

ethics
A system that uses ethical principles to make decisions about morality.

moral
What is judged to be right according to a system of ethics.

immoral
What is judged to be wrong according to a system of ethics.

ethical principles
Guides by which we can judge an action or decision as moral or immoral.

expected to behave. Professional societies attempt to develop guiding principles—or *codes of ethics*—to govern their members' behaviors. The code of ethics developed by the American Association of Sex Educators, Counselors, and Therapists, for example, sets guidelines for its members.

Ethical Principles

Table 18.1 introduces five examples of ethical principles that can be used to make moral decisions. As will be discussed, though, these kinds of principles may be in opposition to one another in any given situation.

Nonmaleficence

Is it moral to convince someone else to engage in sexual intercourse in spite of his or her reluctance? One ethical principle that speaks to this issue is maleficence—the act of committing harm or evil. The principle of *nonmaleficence* is that whatever is moral—right or good—can be determined by asking whether it does any harm. If it does harm, it is not moral. Does coercing someone to engage in sex do physical, psychological, or spiritual harm? If so, that behavior is immoral.

TABLE 18.1 Selected Ethical Principles

1. Nonmaleficence	Whatever else, do no harm. This includes preventing harm, not inflicting harm, and removing harm when it is present.
2. Beneficence	Not only should one not do harm, but one is also obligated to do good.
3. Autonomy/liberty	People should be free to decide their own course of action as long as they do not harm others.
4. Justice/fairness	Each person should be treated fairly.
5. Social utility	The greatest good for the greatest number should be considered. What is best for society may outweigh what is best for the individual.

Source: Created by Jerrold Greenberg.

Ethical
DIMENSIONS

Extramarital Sex   Actually making a decision regarding sexual morality may help you comprehend the rather abstract material to come. Therefore, we quote here an argument that adultery, or extramarital relationships, can be moral and ask you to react to it. (Bear in mind that although this argument describes only men, women have extramarital affairs.)

Albert Ellis, a prominent psychologist, wrote that there is a healthy adulterer. Although Ellis's argument was presented a number of years ago, it is as applicable today as it was then. Ellis wrote (1977, 374–375):

1. The healthy adulterer is nondemanding and noncompulsive. He prefers but he does not need extramarital affairs. He believes that he can live better with than without them, and therefore he tries to have them from time to time. But he is also able to have a happy general and marital life if no such affairs are practicable.

2. The undisturbed adulterer usually manages to carry on his extramarital affairs without unduly disturbing his marriage and family relationships nor his general existence. He is sufficiently discreet about his adultery, on the one hand, and appropriately frank and honest about it with his close associates, on the other hand, so that most people he intimately knows are able to tolerate his affairs and not get too upset about them.

3. He fully accepts his own extramarital desires and acts and never condemns himself or punishes himself because of them, even though he may sometimes decide that they are unwise and may make specific attempts to bring them to a halt.

4. He faces his specific problems with his wife and family as well as his general life difficulties and does not use his adulterous relationships as a means of avoiding any of his serious problems.

5. He is usually tolerant of himself when he acts poorly or makes errors; he is minimally hostile when his wife and family members behave in a less than desirable manner; and he fully accepts the fact that the world is rough and life is often grim, but that there is no reason why it must be otherwise and that he can live happily even when conditions around him are not great. Consequently, he does not drive himself to adultery because of self-deprecation, self-pity, or hostility to others.

6. He is sexually adequate with his spouse as well as with others and therefore has extramarital affairs out of sex interest rather than for sex therapy.

Although the adulterer who lives up to these criteria may have still other emotional disturbances and may be having extramarital affairs for various neurotic reasons, Ellis argues that there is also a good chance that this is not true.

Do you believe there is such a thing as a healthy adulterer?

Beneficence

For some ethicists, doing no harm is not enough. For an action to be moral, it has to do good. That is what is meant by the ethical principle of *beneficence*. School officials who banned Wendy Weaver from coaching volleyball thought they were doing good for the students in that school. Therefore, they thought they were acting morally. Those who opposed the ban believed they were doing good by upholding the right of people to acknowledge their sexuality in an appropriate and honest manner, regardless of their particular sexual orientation. Therefore, they thought they were acting morally. We will soon discuss how these contradictions can be resolved.

Autonomy/Liberty

The ethical principle of *autonomy* or *liberty* requires people be free to decide an issue for themselves before that decision can qualify as moral. That does

not mean that every decision made freely is a moral one, only that any decision made under coercion is immoral. Was the decision to bar Wendy Weaver made freely by school officials, or was it coerced by a small group of vocal parents? Was Weaver allowed to decide freely whether she would discuss her sexual orientation, as could heterosexuals teaching in that school, or was she being coerced by school officials? The way you answer these questions will help you determine which actions you think were moral in this case.

Justice/Fairness

Some ethicists believe that for an action to be moral, it must treat people fairly. They term this ethical principle *justice* or *fairness*. That does not mean that people must be treated equally. For example, our culture has determined that homosexuals and heterosexuals may be treated differently by different segments of society. That is, in private clubs or homes, or in certain churches or synagogues, gays may be excluded. However, our society has determined that excluding gays from public facilities is not just or fair—it is immoral—and has codified that decision by making a law defining that behavior illegal/unconstitutional.

Social Utility

Sometimes there is a clash between individual rights and the rights of a large group of people. In these instances, some ethicists use the ethical principle of *social utility* to determine the morality of various actions being contemplated. Social utility defines the moral decision as the one that is best for society (or the large group) rather than what is best for the individual (or the small group). School officials in Nebo, Utah, determined that removing Wendy Weaver from coaching was the greater good for the greater number of people (the students). Whether they were aware of it or not, they were using social utility to justify their decision. Of course, others might argue that the greater number of people in this instance ought to have been the gay community throughout the United States whose rights have been violated for far too long.

Ethical Dilemmas

We often experience situations in which one ethical principle clashes with another. We call these clashes **ethical dilemmas**. For example, consider again the question of adultery. Suppose you held the following ethical principles: Marriage should be a sexually monogamous relationship and people have a right to a satisfying, fulfilling sexual life. Obviously if you were in a marriage in which you were sexually unfulfilled for some reason, these two ethical principles would conflict. In such a situation which principle would be operative? Which one would take precedence over the other? Sometimes religion or culture provides answers to ethical dilemmas. For instance, in Islamic countries adultery is opposed by tradition and the law; such a society has resolved our ethical dilemma—at least officially—by placing the higher value on fidelity within marriage. Where there are no such prohibitions, individuals must rank their own values to make a choice.

The existence of such dilemmas has led to the development of situation ethics, in contrast to rule ethics. **Rule ethics** are exhaustive principles intended to guide people in their moral decision making in

> **ethical dilemma**
> When two or more ethical principles work in opposing fashion in a particular situation, resulting in bewilderment regarding what is moral and what is immoral.

all situations. These principles are explicit, specific, and all-encompassing. People who hold to the letter of the law and proponents of religious dogmas are rule ethicists. **Situation ethics**, in contrast, are based on the premise that all situations are unique, and therefore no one set of rules is applicable in all cases. Consequently a situation ethicist faced with a moral decision carefully reviews, analyzes, and evaluates each specific situation to determine which principles are applicable; a rule ethicist applies a given principle, regardless of the specific circumstances. As an example, a rule ethicist believes abortion is wrong in all cases. A situation ethicist may also believe abortion is wrong but may also believe it is moral in the case of a 12-year-old rape victim who becomes pregnant.

> **rule ethics**
> Guiding principles used in all situations to arrive at moral decisions, which are considered applicable to all situations.
>
> **situation ethics**
> A belief that no one set of rules can apply to all situations and each specific situation must be analyzed to determine which ethical principles are applicable.

Trying to decide which viewpoint—rule ethics or situation ethics—is correct is itself an ethical dilemma. When we narrow our focus to sexual behavior, we can see that the rule/situation dichotomy has relevance. Are there general rules to guide sexual behavior, or does each situation require its own set of rules? Which rules, if any, will guide your behavior? Given your intuitive responses to the questions we raise in this chapter, see whether you consider yourself a rule or situation ethicist

■ Moral Decision Making and Sexual Behavior

What influences the decisions we make about sexuality? Such factors as our knowledge or lack of knowledge; our sense of who we are; our ideals regarding fidelity and responsibility; our desire to express affection, passion, and delight; the emotional excitement we experience while facing the decision; and external cultural influences such as the double standard are all involved. The questions one asks in making moral decisions about sexuality or any other area of life are, What is *right*? What is *good*? What is *wrong*? What is *bad*? If it is right or good, it is moral! If it is wrong or bad, it is immoral! Thus morals relate to concrete decisions in particular situations.

To determine whether an action or decision is moral or immoral, we use our system of ethics. This system of ethics involves our ethical principles, which are guides by which we can judge an action or decision

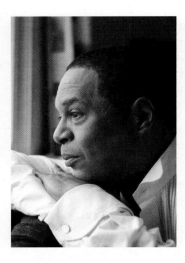

Deciding whether a rule should be applied to a particular ethical issue, or whether the situation is unique and requires a unique decision, is a dilemma faced by ethicists.

as moral or immoral. If the decision is inconsistent with our ethical principles, it is immoral; if it is consistent with them, it is moral.

Ethical principles specific to sexual matters include the following:

1. Sexual behavior should not be forced on anyone.

2. Sexual behavior between consenting adults is acceptable.

3. Fidelity (faithfulness) in marriage is a must.

4. Marriage partners and loved ones must be responsive to each other's needs (Bruess & Greenberg, 2009).

Unfortunately, most situations are not so cut and dried. Applying ethical principles is often a complex matter because they provide only guidance, not ready-made answers. If our principles are in conflict, we must examine our personal values to rank conflicting ethical principles in order of importance. By personal *values* we mean the worth or importance we assign to our ethical principles. If we personally value our commitment to a monogamous relationship more than we value sexual fulfillment, for example, then we resolve a conflict between the two by choosing not to have extramarital relationships. If we value sexual fulfillment more highly, then we resolve the same conflict differently.

To summarize, then, we decide the morality of an action or decision after identifying and ranking ethical principles in order of our personal values. Most people learn that the many moral decisions they make about sexual behavior are ultimately based on their personal values.

Our intention is to help you explore your own values and ethical principles so you may apply them in specific situations, and thereby act morally.

Commonly Accepted Ethical Principles

This discussion is not intended to convey the notion that *anything goes*. Although we value and recognize the need for diversity, as a society we have reached agreement on a set of ethical principles. For example,

we have societal consensus that caring, respect, honesty, responsibility, and trust ought to guide our decisions regarding morality. In fact, a whole educational movement that seeks to convey these principles to school-aged children and youth has sprouted. That movement is called *character education*. Its objectives are consistent with the societal consensus regarding ethical principles described: respect for the rights of all people regardless of their race, religion, gender, age, and sexual orientation; understanding, sympathy, concern, and compassion for others; and personal integrity and honesty. These are principles to which all citizens should adhere, and to emphasize their importance, society has passed laws specifying sanctions for acting contrary to them. For example, we have laws against discrimination by gender, race, ethnicity, and sexual orientation. And we have laws punishing those who sexually abuse others. If someone lies to a sexual partner about his or her HIV status and infects that partner, we have laws to punish that behavior. If someone takes advantage of someone else by engaging in coitus with that person while he or she is incapable of deciding freely to participate (for example, if intoxicated or mentally impaired), we have laws punishing that behavior. And if someone fires someone else from a job solely because of that person's sexual orientation, we have laws to punish that behavior (as the school officials who fired Wendy Weaver found out).

In matters of sexuality and sexual morality, it is important to keep these consensually agreed-on ethical principles in the forefront. Certainly we, as the writers of this chapter, value diversity and recognize the influence of different experiences and values as they play out in various ethical dilemmas. Still, these consensually accepted ethical principles are ones to which we are committed. The problem arises when behaving consistently with one or more of these principles means violating one or more of the others. This is what we earlier described as an

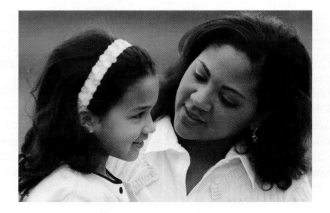

Although people may value ethical principles differently, there is agreement on a set of common principles such as caring, respect, and honesty.

ethical dilemma. Ethical dilemmas apply to human sexuality, as we shall now see.

Government Control and Regulation

As will be evident in the rest of this chapter, each sexual ethical issue can be controlled or regulated by government. The broader issue, then, is how much control should we expect the government to exert through regulation, and how much should individuals be allowed to decide these issues for themselves. Laws are a reflection of moral judgments. For example, we judge stealing from another to be immoral so we pass laws penalizing those who steal. Because many sexual ethical issues are controversial, passing regulations or laws to control sexual behavior can be problematic. Whose morals should be the basis for law? How will the minority view of morality be protected? These are important, but not easily answered, questions. The government has an obligation to pass laws to regulate behaviors believed to be harmful— that is, to protect the health of Americans. Where should the line between individual freedoms and governmental protections be drawn?

To resolve many of these sexual ethical issues raised by government regulations, as manifested in laws, these laws are juxtaposed against constitutional protections. The U.S. Constitution is the arbiter of issues that divide the populace. It offers guidance to lawmakers and others to help them protect the public without infringing on their rights. As you will soon see, it is not unusual for the government to pass laws pertaining to sexual behavior (for example, sodomy) or other sexually related issues (such as abortion), only to have these laws challenged, and sometimes overturned, by the U.S. Supreme Court.

Sexually Transmitted Infections

To treat sexually transmitted infections (STIs) effectively on a large scale, health care workers often ask their patients to identify their sexual contacts. The purpose is to inform these contacts that they have been exposed to a disease and encourage them to seek treatment. Generally the carrier is inclined, at least fleetingly, to protect the anonymity of his or her sexual contacts (and perhaps his or her own identity and reputation). One of the ethical principles commonly underlying such a reaction is probably, *One should not discuss other people's private sexual behavior.* However, a competing ethical principle might be, *People should not intentionally harm the health of others.* Most individuals would probably value the second principle over the first and would therefore identify their sexual contacts. Observers who also value health over confidentiality would judge this decision

to be moral. If the infected person is married and has contracted the disease through nonconsensual extramarital activity, the principle of not harming others becomes harder to apply. In this situation the patient would have to decide whether the health of the marriage partner was more valuable than potential damage to the marital relationship and the family and whether the couple had an agreement regarding fidelity that had been breached.

An important ethical issue raised by the HIV and AIDS epidemic is whether to require pregnant women to be tested for HIV. With modern medications and medical regimens, approximately two-thirds of HIV and AIDS can be prevented in babies born to infected mothers. Consequently, using the ethical principle of beneficence, some medical experts argue that all pregnant women should be required to be tested for HIV, thereby identifying mothers who ought to be treated before their babies' births and newborns who ought to be treated as soon after birth as possible. However, others argue that requiring all pregnant women to be tested would actually harm newborns (maleficence). They believe that if pregnant women are required to be tested they will refrain from identifying themselves as pregnant, thereby depriving their babies of the prenatal care that can prevent all kinds of health problems, not just HIV and AIDS. This would, in turn, increase the infant mortality rate, which is already too high, especially in low-socioeconomic-status populations. Therefore, opponents of mandatory pregnancy testing for HIV believe testing ought to be voluntary (autonomy/liberty) with educational campaigns to communicate the advantages of being tested.

There are other ethical issues related to HIV and AIDS. For example, should research funds be used for treating AIDS patients or for finding a cure or for developing a vaccine? What is the appropriate balance in this funding? Are funds best used for education about HIV and AIDS to prevent the greatest possible number of cases?

These questions are more than issues for academic consideration: Decisions are being made on a regular basis by research institutes, the government, and insurance companies. Are these decisions being made ethically? Are they moral decisions? Your answers to these questions depend on the way you value your ethical principles. Although no one answer will meet with everyone's approval, society adopts a consensus view of morality as a matter of necessity. That is, *something* must be decided, even if the decision is to ignore the situation. Further, because we are citizens in a society that allows for our input, we are contributing to this ethical exercise by our votes, letters, and attitudes (as determined by opinion polls).

Sexual Activity Between Unmarried Partners

Whether to participate in sexual activity without being married is another common moral decision. Those who decide that such behavior is immoral might value the following ethical principle: *Marriage is a unique relationship blessed by God and allowing for a total expression of love.* Those who consider sexual intercourse to be moral in any circumstance, unless one participant is harmed in some way, might value another principle more, such as *You should experience life fully.* However, decisions regarding premarital or nonmarital sexual behavior are usually more complicated than a choice between two principles. Situation ethicists pondering the morality of premarital sex in a given situation might ask the following questions:

1. How old are the people involved? Seventeen? Forty-five?

2. What do the people feel for each other?

3. Is their intention to marry or enter into a union? Soon?

4. What are their religious beliefs?

5. In which society (country, culture) do they live?

In your own situation, which special considerations are or were relevant to your decisions about the morality of your sexual behavior?

Sodomy

It is impossible to define the term **sodomy** because states lump together those sexual activities they consider immoral and codify their views by passing laws that make these sexual behaviors illegal. Usually sodomy laws refer to such sexual activities as anal intercourse, oral–genital sexual behavior, homosexual activities, and any sexual behavior with animals. In earlier years, some states defined *sodomy* as any sexual activity of anyone other than a married couple. In fact, as late as 1990, a bill was proposed by a Washington state legislator that would allow the state to prosecute anyone younger than 18 years old who was "necking" or "petting." The proposed penalty was a maximal sentence of 90 days in jail and a $5,000 fine.

sodomy
A term that specifically refers to anal intercourse, but is often used to refer to almost any sexual behavior someone might not consider normal.

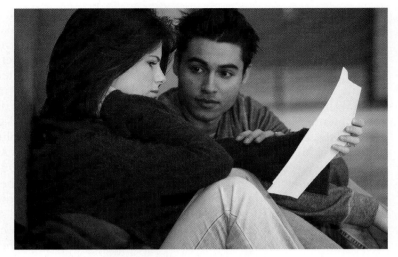

One ethical dilemma is whether sexual intercourse between unmarried partners is moral. Should the age of the partners matter? Should the quality of the relationship matter? What other factors do you think need to be considered when deciding on the morality of coitus between unmarried partners?

Most sodomy laws were applied primarily against homosexuals. The penalties varied from state to state, ranging from a $200 fine to 20 years of imprisonment. Violators of sodomy laws have been imprisoned, lost their jobs and homes, lost custody of their children, and even been beaten and killed. One test of the constitutionality of sodomy laws occurred in 1986. In the *Bowers v. Hardwick* case, an Atlanta man was arrested after police officers entered his home at the request of his roommate regarding another matter and found him in bed with another man. When this case finally reached the U.S. Supreme Court, the Court upheld Georgia's sodomy law in spite of recognizing that the Constitution creates "zones of privacy." Dissenting from this decision was Justice Harry A. Blackmun, who wrote that the Court mistakenly refused to recognize "the fundamental interest all individuals have in controlling the nature of their intimate associations with others." However, on June 26, 2003, in a landmark ruling on sexuality and privacy, the U.S. Supreme Court overturned *Bowers v. Hardwick*. In *Lawrence v. Texas*, the Court found that *Bowers* "was not correct when it was decided, is not correct today, and is hereby overruled." Further, the *Lawrence* decision states, "When homosexual conduct is made criminal by the law of the State, that declaration in and of itself is an invitation to subject homosexual persons to discrimination both in the public and private spheres... Its continuance as precedent demeans the lives of homosexual persons."

Contraception

People who oppose so-called artificial methods of contraception for religious reasons are usually guided by the ethic, *All life is sacred*. They argue that prevention of a conception that would occur without interference is interference with God's creation of life. Proponents of modern birth control, in contrast, are often guided by the ethic, *Every child deserves to be wanted and loved*. They argue that when unwanted children are born, the quality of life diminishes for the parents and the society, and the children themselves often have difficult lives as well.

In 1914 Margaret Sanger began publishing her newspaper, *The Woman Rebel*, in which she argued that women should be free to choose whether to bear children. Sanger had witnessed the death of a young woman who tried to perform an abortion on herself and cited this incident as her motivation for working for a woman's right to control her fertility.

For some people, certain types of fertility-control methods are acceptable and others are not. For example, methods that prevent a fertilized egg from implanting on the endometrial lining of the uterus might be unacceptable to people who believe life begins at conception. For others, any action taken before birth is acceptable because they believe that birth is when human life begins.

Then there is the issue pertaining to who should be responsible for contraception. Some people wonder why most methods of contraception are designed to be used by women. Accompanying these methods of contraception are potential side effects that can have significant health implications. Why aren't men subjected to the same risks, some wonder

Gender DIMENSIONS

The "Umbrelly" (A Little Humor)

Critics of research on contraceptive technology argue that research is immoral—that is, sexist. It focuses on female techniques, largely ignoring male methods of contraception. Others argue it is the characteristics and complexities of the male reproductive system that make the development of effective male contraception difficult. In an attempt to have males develop a greater appreciation for how the critics view the morality of contraceptive research, the following facetious description of a new male contraceptive was written:

The newest development in male contraception was unveiled recently at the American Women's Surgical Symposium held at the Ann Arbor Medical Center. Dr. Sophia Merkin, of the Merkin Clinic, announced the preliminary findings of a study conducted on 763 unsuspecting male grad students at a large Midwest university. In her report Dr. Merkin stated that the new contraceptive—the IPD—was a breakthrough in male contraception. It will be marketed under the trade name "Umbrelly."

The IPD (intrapenal device) resembles a tiny folded umbrella that is inserted through the head of the penis and pushed into the scrotum with a plunger-like instrument. Occasionally there is perforation of the scrotum but this is disregarded, since it is known that the male has few nerve endings in this area of his body. The underside of the umbrella contains a spermicidal jelly, hence "Umbrelly."

Experiments on a thousand white whales from the Continental Shelf (whose sexual apparatus is said to be closest to man's) proved the Umbrelly to be 100% effective in preventing production of sperm and eminently satisfactory to the female whale, since it doesn't interfere with her rutting pleasure.

Dr. Merkin declared the Umbrelly to be statistically safe for the human male. She reported that of the 763 grad students tested with the device, only two died of scrotal infection, only 20 experienced swelling of the tissues, three developed cancer of the testicles, and 13 were too depressed to have an erection. She stated that common complaints ranged from cramping and bleeding to acute abdominal pain. She emphasized that these symptoms were merely indications that the man's body had not yet adjusted to the device. Hopefully the symptoms would disappear within a year.

One complication caused by the IPD and briefly mentioned by Dr. Merkin was the incidence of massive scrotal infection necessitating the surgical removal of the testicles. "But this is a rare case," said Merkin, "too rare to be statistically important." She and the other distinguished members of the Women's College of Surgeons agreed that the benefits far outweighed the risk to any individual man.

Source: Unknown.

(see Gender Dimensions). Is it moral to subject women to health risks disproportionate to the risk expected of men so as to prevent conception?

Lastly, different cultural groups view the morality of contraception differently. Some countries' health insurance plans will not reimburse its subscribers for contraceptive devices or pills. In other countries, contraceptive services are part of reimbursable expenses. Countries with large Hispanic populations, such as in Latin America, with a strong belief in Catholicism, may not be as accepting of contraception as non-Catholics. Once again, morality is influenced by many variables and, therefore, what one person determines to be moral, another may determine to be immoral.

Emergency Contraception

A more recent contraceptive development pertains to *emergency contraception*. This is the use of oral contraceptives after unprotected sexual intercourse has occurred and there is a fear of pregnancy. For example, emergency contraception can be used in the case of rape or condom failure to prevent conception. The oral contraceptives must be taken within 72 hours of intercourse.

One of the issues debated was whether to allow women access to emergency contraception without a physician's prescription. An expert Food and Drug Administration (FDA) panel recommended the FDA approve emergency contraception to be disbursed by pharmacists. The FDA asked the panel to gather more information and did not follow through on its recommendation. Some accused the FDA of bowing to political pressure from social conservatives (Kaufman, 2005). They argued that making emergency contraception available through pharmacists would make emergency contraception more effective. Their reasoning was that since it has to be used within 72 hours of coitus, why jeopardize that time frame by requiring a physician be contacted and a prescription be written. Further, they argued, studies have shown emergency contraception to be safe and effective.

Others, though, considered emergency contraception to be an abortion pill. That is, it prevents a fertilized egg from developing into a fetus and, eventually, a baby. They were opposed to any action that interfered with a pregnancy. They also believed that with emergency contraception available as a back-up, people (in particular, youth) might engage in riskier sexual behavior. Studies, however, have found this fear to be unfounded (Kaufman, 2005). Whether and how emergency contraception should be available elicits more debate. As a responsible citizen, you should keep abreast of this debate and let your elected representatives know your views.

Abortion

Is induced, or voluntary, abortion simply a method of fertility control and as such the right of every woman, or is it taking of life that has a right to exist? Can it be both? If so, how can the dilemma be resolved? Some people seek to solve the problem by looking for evidence—or a definition—of when life begins. Does it begin at conception or does it begin when a fetus is capable of living outside the mother (at birth, or shortly before)? Others seek to solve it by asking who controls a woman's reproductive capacity. One must decide whether preserving the life and quality of life of the living is more or less important than maintaining the existence or viability of the unborn. This ethical dilemma is one of the most divisive issues in modern society. Laws are no sooner made than they are challenged. Some of these laws seek to limit abortions or encourage women to reconsider before deciding to abort. For example, some states require a waiting period before abortions can be done. Other states are seeking to require women to view sonograms of the fetus, obtain parental consent if a minor, or prohibit government funds from supporting organizations (such as Planned Parenthood) that support a woman's right to abort. What is your view of the morality of these legal strategies? The morality of abortion is a subject of ongoing debate in many arenas of modern life—from the purely personal to the political.

Amniocentesis

Amniocentesis involves withdrawing, via a needle inserted into the uterus through the abdominal wall, a small amount of amniotic fluid surrounding the fetus. The procedure is recommended for women whose risk of producing babies with birth defects is greater than average (for example, women older than 35 years or women who have previously given birth to babies with birth defects). The moral question arises because if the test shows that the fetus will be deformed, mentally retarded, or seriously ill, the parents can choose to have an abortion rather than let the pregnancy run its course. Is it moral to take the risk (for example, of miscarriage) of having the test at all? Other issues are raised as well. For example, the sex of the fetus can be determined through amniocentesis. Is abortion moral when parents who have, say, four sons discover that their unborn child is a boy? Should the genes of an unborn baby be manipulated to conform with the parents'—or society's—idea of a superior human being? How much genetic manipulation is consistent with our ethical principles and values? As science becomes more sophisticated in this area, new ethical dilemmas arise.

Fetal Tissue Implantation

Parkinson's disease patients suffer tremors, muscular rigidity, and loss of balance as a result of a lack of the brain neurotransmitter dopamine. Research has discovered that fetal brain tissue, if implanted within the brain of Parkinson's patients, can produce enough dopamine to relieve many of the symptoms. However, the potential for abuse of this knowledge has prompted many groups and individuals to oppose the use of fetal tissue for implantation, or even for research purposes. One of the concerns is that a woman will become pregnant with the intention to abort the fetus and use its brain tissue for a family member suffering from Parkinson's disease. Others argue that using human tissue in this manner defiles the sanctity of the human body.

Yet there are those who strongly support the use of fetal tissue to relieve Parkinson's and other diseases. They point to the socially acceptable practice of donating and transplanting organs such as hearts, livers, kidneys, lungs, and corneas.

In 1988, the federal government banned the use of federal funds for research involving aborted fetal tissue implantation. Believing this policy deprives certain patients from receiving adequate care, the American College of Obstetrics and Gynecology and the American Fertility Society in February 1991 established a private advisory body to guide scientists conducting fetal tissue and fertility research. This board, the National Advisory Board on Ethics in Reproduction, sets uniform standards, reviews proposed projects, advises researchers, and serves as a clearinghouse of information.

By 1993, the federal government's ban on research with fetal tissue implantation was lifted. Since then the National Institutes of Health (NIH) has awarded

Global DIMENSIONS

Marital Age Around the World

It is not surprising that different countries with different cultures have different views of ethical issues. One of these issues is age at marriage. In the United States, it is believed to be immoral for a 13-year-old girl to marry, especially an older man. We even maintain legislation defining this as a violation of law. However, in other countries, the morality of early marriage, even to an older man, is not called into question. In developing countries, more than 60 million women aged 20–24 were married/in union before the age of 18. More than 31 million of them live in South Asia. In countries such as Bangladesh, Central African Republic, Chad, Guinea, Mali, and Niger, more than 60% of women entered into marriage or into a union before their eighteenth birthdays. Girls living in the poorest 20% of households are more likely to get married at an early age than those living in the wealthiest 20%. For example, in Peru, 45% of women were married by age 18 among the poorest 20% of the population, compared to 5% among the richest 20%. Women with primary education were significantly less likely to be married as children than those who received no education. In Zimbabwe, 48% of women who had attended primary school had been married by the age of 18, compared to 87% of those who had not attended school.

Parents choose to marry off their daughters early for a number of reasons. Poor families may regard a young girl as an economic burden and her marriage as a necessary survival strategy for her family. They may think that child marriage offers protection for their daughter from the dangers of sexual assault or, more generally, offers the care of a male guardian. Child marriage may also be seen as a strategy to avoid girls becoming pregnant outside of marriage. Gender discrimination can also underpin child marriage. Girls may be married young to ensure obedience and subservience within their husband's household and to maximize their childbearing.

UNICEF argues that child marriage can have serious harmful consequences for children, including *denial of education* (once married, girls tend not to go to school), *health problems* (including premature pregnancies, higher rates of maternal and infant mortality, and STIs, including HIV/AIDS), and *abuse* (a practice common in child marriages; children who refuse to marry or who choose a marriage partner against the wishes of their parents are often punished or even killed by their families in so-called honor killings).

Sources: Data from UNICEF. Child protection from violence, exploitation and abuse: Child marriage. 2009. Available: http://www.unicef.org/protection/index_earlymarriage.html. UNICEF. *The state of the world's children 2009: Maternal and newborn health.* New York: UNICEF, 2009. Available: http://www.unicef.org/sowc09/docs/SOWC09 Figure-2.4-EN.pdf.

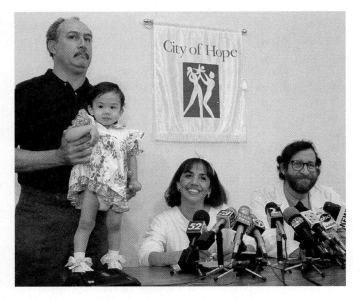

In 1990, Mary and Abe Ayala were told that the only chance to save their 17-year-old daughter Anissa from dying of leukemia was for her to have bone marrow transplantation. With no matching donors, the Ayalas decided to have another child (Marissa Eve) to use his or her bone marrow. Did the Ayalas act in a moral way? Did their physicians? What would you have done faced with such a dilemma?

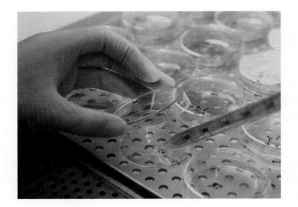

Stem cell research has the potential to result in cures for debilitating diseases, but it is fraught with moral potholes. What do you think the policy ought to be regarding stem cell research and the appropriate source of stem cells?

millions of dollars in grants for research involving the study, analysis, and use of human fetal tissue. Today research continues on the potential of fetal tissue in treatment of not only Parkinson's disease but also Alzheimer's disease, Huntington's disease, diabetes, multiple sclerosis, epilepsy, blindness, leukemia, hemophilia, sickle cell anemia, spinal-cord injuries, deficiencies of the immune system, birth defects, and pain (Kenney, Reinholtz, & Angellini, 1997). Supporting this research are the Alzheimer's Association, the Epilepsy Foundation of America, the Cystic Fibrosis Foundation, the Parkinson's Disease Foundation, and the Society for Pediatric Research.

Part of the remaining ethical issues regarding the use of human fetal tissue pertains to the finding that tissue from miscarriages and ectopic pregnancies appears rarely to be suitable for transplantation. However, tissue from induced abortions is effective when transplanted. Researchers argue that legal barriers to harvesting tissue from induced abortions stand in the way of building up the supply of usable fetal tissue.

Stem Cell Research

Stem cells are cells that can be found in embryos, fetuses, and adults. In adults, stem cells are specialized and can evolve into more cells of their own kind. In embryos, however, stem cells have the capacity to evolve into many different types of tissues and organs, depending on a complex of biological instructions. However, scientists think that tissues derived from embryonic and adult stem cells may differ in the likelihood of being rejected after transplantation. It is not yet known whether tissues derived from embryonic stem cells will cause transplant rejection, because the first-phase clinical trials involving embryonic stem cells have only recently been approved by the U.S. Food and Drug Administration (FDA). However, adult stem cells, and tissues derived from them, are currently thought to be less likely to initiate rejection after transplantation. This is because a patient's own cells could be expanded in culture, coaxed into assuming a specific cell type (differentiation), and then reintroduced into the patient. The use of adult stem cells and tissues derived from the patient's own adult stem cells would mean that the cells are less likely to be rejected by the immune system. This represents a significant advantage, because immune rejection can be circumvented only by continuous administration of immunosuppressive drugs, and the drugs themselves may cause deleterious side effects (National Institutes of Health Resource for Stem Cell Research, 2011).

Embryonic stem cells are taken from embryos at the blastocyst stage of development (4 or 5 days after conception) when they are, in essence, a "blank page." Scientists are working on ways of instructing stem cells to develop into specific tissue—for example, into insulin-producing pancreatic cells for implantation in diabetics.

The moral debate about stem cells involves a number of complex issues. For example, is it moral to use stem cells from aborted fetuses? Will this practice encourage more abortions? Is it moral to use stem cells from embryos created specifically for

(?) Did You Know ...

Fetal brain tissue is not the only type of fetal cell that has potential for medical use. Early in development, the fetus's blood cells are produced by stem cells in the liver. Eventually these blood cells move into the fetus's bones and become bone marrow. Therefore, injecting fetal liver cells intravenously into patients is, in effect, giving them immune system transplantation.

Fetal liver transplants hold promise for such conditions as certain leukemias, sickle cell anemia, aplastic anemia, AIDS, and severe combined immunodeficiency disease.

Diabetics have also been given fetal insulin-producing pancreas cells, and fetal brain tissue's potential to aid in the treatment of Alzheimer's disease is very real.

their stem cells? Is this the destruction of one human life to benefit another human life? Should scientific research, and consequently money that is devoted to scientific research, be concentrated on developing techniques for using adult stem cells rather than on embryonic stem cells? What should be the government's role in regulating and/or supporting stem cell research? Given the potential for stem cells to contribute to cures and/or treatments for Parkinson's disease, Alzheimer's disease, diabetes, heart disease, and arthritis, among others, should scientific research be entailed by governmental restrictions? Is that moral?

In 2001, President George W. Bush approved a regulation that would provide government funding for limited stem cell research. Bush, a conservative politician, tried to walk the fine line between what he believed to be morally justified and the potential for the enhancement of a large number of American lives—another moral consideration. He decided that, on the one hand, stem cell research had a great deal of potential to cure diseases that affect large numbers of Americans. On the other hand, he believed that developing "human life" (embryos) to harvest their stem cells was immoral. Consequently, Bush decided that the government would provide funding for scientific research that used only adult stem cells or embryonic stem cells that had already been harvested. Bush estimated that there were about 60 of those groups of embryonic stem cells around the world. Staunch conservatives viewed this decision as immoral because it did not make a statement about the sanctity of life and allowed "immorally produced" embryonic stem cells to be used for research purposes. Scientists considered this decision immoral because it limited research to a small number of embryonic stem cells that were thought to be too homogenous to produce wide-scale cures (for example, many of these existing colonies of embryonic stem cells were obtained from white populations). Furthermore, scientists argued, adult stem cells do not have the capacity to develop into a range of tissue as do embryonic stem cells but

are, instead, tissue specific. That limits their potential for a scientific breakthrough.

When Americans were surveyed, a majority supported stem cell research (Stem cell research, 2005). When asked if they favored or opposed stem cell research using embryonic stem cells, 58% were either strongly or somewhat in favor, 29% were either strongly or somewhat opposed, and 13% had no opinion. Of those opposed to the use of embryonic stem cells for research, 57% were opposed on religious grounds. Furthermore, 78% stated they thought the United States should be the global leader in medical and scientific research, in general. However, this is not the case when it comes to stem cell research. Whereas the federal government has restricted funding, several other countries have proceeded vigorously in stem cell research. They believe that, aside from developing techniques to cure many of the diseases plaguing humankind today, embryonic stem cell research is both moral and has tremendous economic potential for these countries' economies.

In 2009, bringing a different perspective to this issue, President Barack Obama lifted the restriction on federal funding of human embryonic stem cell research.

If you were the person deciding the role government ought to play in stem cell research, what would you decide? Which moral justifications would you offer to support that decision?

Prostitution

Prostitution is the selling of sexual gratification. Examples of prostitution were recorded even in ancient times, so contemporary society can take neither credit nor blame for inventing this trade—only for the way in which it treats it.

People who consider prostitution immoral often argue that it degrades sexual intercourse, which is sanctified within marriage as an expression of love, into a mere animalistic act. Centuries ago Christianity adopted the Persian view, that the demands of the spirit and flesh were in conflict with each other, rather than the Greek view, which saw no conflict and allowed for prostitution (so long as the prostitutes were male). Nevertheless making some allowances for the flesh, Christianity developed incentives for marriage and deemed sexual intercourse within marriage appropriate and outside it sinful. Our culture has largely adhered to this view of who is a legitimate and morally acceptable sexual partner. To make a judgment about prostitution, a person must decide whether the desire for sexual services and sexual outlets is more important than the principle that coitus outside marriage is immoral.

In Vitro Fertilization

In 1980 the first "test-tube" baby clinic in the United States was approved by the state of Virginia. Located at the Norfolk General Hospital in Norfolk, Virginia, this clinic offers its services to couples who wish to conceive but are infertile as a result of blocked, missing, or damaged fallopian tubes of women. (It does not treat male infertility.) The clinic, officially named the In Vitro Clinic (for **in vitro fertilization**), had a waiting list of from 1 to 2 years just 1 week after gaining state approval.

in vitro fertilization
The creation of a pregnancy in a laboratory by uniting the sperm and egg outside the womb; sometimes termed the "test-tube" baby technique.

There are some who believe using in vitro fertilization to produce babies is immoral. For example, in March 1987 the Catholic Congregation for the Doctrine of the Faith issued "Instruction on Respect for Human Life in Its Origin and on the Dignity of Procreation," a document that defined generation of human life outside the body as "morally illicit." In addition to in vitro fertilization, other biomedical breakthroughs were condemned as immoral. Among these were genetic engineering, surrogate motherhood, cloning, and manipulations to produce human beings according to sex or other predetermined qualities. According to the document, the only approved method of human procreation is "the act of conjugal love."

Other ethical issues pertain to in vitro fertilization. For example, what will be its effect on the population of the world? Will it produce too many people for the available resources? What would that mean for the quality of life of the world's population? What should be done if the fetus develops defectively once it has been implanted in the uterus? When choosing to have a baby by artificial means, should parents be allowed to select the baby's sex, eye color, intelligence, and so on? These issues need societal attention; we as citizens need to inform our representatives of our judgments regarding what is moral and immoral relative to in vitro fertilization.

Genetic Engineering

In vitro fertilization evokes images of genetic manipulation in the minds of some people. Of course, that is not its intent. However, as science progresses and reproductive technology develops new ways to manage and enhance reproduction, fears of Huxley's *Brave New World* emerge. There are hundreds of biotechnology companies devoted to identifying genes and their functions with the hope of obtaining patents for these genes and the ways in which they can be put to use. It is envisioned that these genes will lead to designer medicines, engineered foods, and eventually custom-made kids (Achenbach, 1998), and the companies that own these patents will make a lot of money. Even the U.S. government staked out a claim to this research by funding the largest scientific project, the Human Genome Project. The $3 billion Human Genome Project, in collaboration with the private firm Celera Genomics, decoded the entire human genetic code in 2003.

All this research raises the possibility that a new generation will be genetically manipulated so that parents will be able to select the color of their babies' eyes, height, athletic and intellectual abilities, and artistic talents. However, some experts are concerned about this possibility. Jeremy Rifkin, the eminent futurist, argues that in a few generations babies will be "engineered." The biologist Lee Silver believes that the human race will be divided into two distinct species, the "Naturals" and the "GenRich" (Achenbach, 1998).

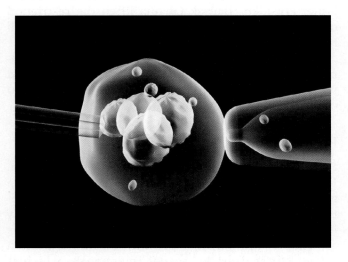

What is the appropriate and/or moral use of reproductive technologies such as in vitro fertilization? Should reproduction remain a natural phenomenon, or should medical advancements and techniques be used to enhance conception?

However, there are other experts who disagree. They argue that although a sheep (Dolly) has been cloned, researchers are a long way from being able to clone humans. And, even if that were possible, scientists are too ethical to do that. However, it is disconcerting that there are groups of scientists who are attempting to clone a human as of the time of this writing. Finally, experts who do not see a *Brave New World* on the horizon expect that as we approach new and more sophisticated reproductive technological advancements, ethicists, clergy, philosophers, politicians, and others, will intervene to develop gene-technology protocols that are acceptable to our societal values and mores.

Whether we will have "designer babies" is still an open question. As citizens in a democratic society we need to keep abreast of the latest developments in this area, because the very nature of the human race may be at issue. The uses of this new technology may be as much a function of the will of the people as it is the interests of the scientists, and, if so, every person has a responsibility to become involved in some way.

The issue of bioethics is recognized throughout the world. The United Nations (UN) Commission on Human Rights adopted the first international guidelines on bioethics and the human genome. The "Universal Declaration on the Human Genome and Human Rights," cosponsored by 86 countries, sets standards for people researching and using genetic information and techniques. Although it specifically recognizes the rights to freedom of research and freedom of thought, it states that "practices which are contrary to human dignity, such as reproductive cloning of human beings, shall not be permitted." The United States is one of the countries that support the UN declaration.

Sexual Responsibility to a Partner

The last sexual ethical dilemma we discuss is, What degree of responsibility do we have, sexually, with respect to others? Should our sexual behavior achieve our own ends, regardless of the desires of our sexual partners? Conversely, are we under an obligation to subjugate our own sexual needs to the needs of our sexual partners? Given that two individuals are involved, just what is moral sexual behavior?

The issue of sexual responsibility, as are all the issues discussed so far, is complex. Certainly we are all responsible for ourselves and our own behavior, but when we take care of ourselves by involving someone else, the issue becomes clouded. As an example imagine that a typical couple, Paul and Paula, love each other and are engaged to be married. Paula wants to share coitus with Paul, but Paul considers sexual intercourse outside marriage immoral. Should Paula

attempt to convince Paul that they should have intercourse? Would it be reasonable for her to threaten to date someone else if he refuses? Should Paul relegate his beliefs to second place and give in to Paula? What is their responsibility to themselves? To each other? To their future? To their relationship? These questions are not easy to answer. However, when sexual behavior involves someone else, there is always potential for manipulation or coercion. The moral nature of such behavior should be explored.

Even when a decision is the individual's alone, ethical dilemmas may arise. For example, should sexually active people use some means of contraception, even if their partners do not care? If not, are they behaving responsibly? What if one's religion opposes the use of contraception but one is sexually active and unwilling to risk pregnancy? As with all the issues we have explored, the means of resolving these questions is to rank the conflicting ethical principles according to our personal values.

■ Laws Regulating Sexual Behavior

Laws formalize moral decisions for a society. Our laws regarding sexual behavior developed from a general acceptance of specific ethical principles, values, and judgments about behaviors such as those we have explored. They have their roots in experience, in religious dogma, and in economics and politics.

Consensus—or general agreement—about which sexual actions should be considered permissible has not always been easily achieved. Indeed, communities have sometimes had to devise ingenious compromises to keep peace among their various moral factions. Consider, for example, the "Combat Zone" in Boston, Massachusetts. To meet the needs of people who frequented bars featuring topless dancers, attended X-rated movies, and so forth, but also to protect citizens opposed to such activities from exposure to them, the municipal government restricted the bars and theaters in question to a specific part of the city, nicknamed the "Combat Zone." The Combat Zone has subsequently been abolished. For similar reasons, some European countries have established red-light districts, in an attempt to limit prostitution to a single section of town.

However, even when consensus is achieved and codified into city, state, or federal law, it is by no means stable. State laws prohibiting prostitution, which were widely acceptable when they were enacted, are periodically under attack and may well someday be modified or rejected. Supreme Court rulings on abortion and on pornography have not settled those issues. Changes occur—albeit slowly—when there is a conflict between existing law and new

Myth 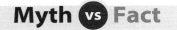 Fact

Myth: Morality is morality. What is right is right, and what is wrong is wrong.

Fact: Most people agree that what is moral in one society may not be moral in another. Furthermore, what is considered moral in one situation may not be considered moral in another situation.

Myth: There is no systematic way in which to resolve ethical and moral issues. It is mostly a matter of intuition and subjective judgment.

Fact: Ethics is a system that uses ethical principles to determine the morality of a situation or decision. Ethical principles are valued according to many factors, including experience, religious teachings, cultural background, education, and family values.

Myth: In our diverse society, there are no commonly accepted ethical principles. Different groups have different values and different views of morality.

Fact: Although it is true that in a country with many different cultural groups living together there are many different views of morality, there are some ethical principles that we can all agree on. These include caring, respect for others, honesty, responsibility, and trustworthiness.

Myth: There are some situations about which there is no disagreement regarding morality. For example, there is no disagreement about HIV and AIDS, because AIDS is such a serious and deadly disease.

Fact: HIV and AIDS provide a good example of how complex moral decisions can be. For example, there is disagreement regarding whether condom advertisements should be allowed on television and whether needle-distribution programs for intravenous drug users should be developed.

morality. An illegal activity might begin to be seen as moral; a legal act, as immoral.

We will see in this discussion that sexual laws develop through a societal consensus of the valuing of ethical principles. The process of devising such laws involves identifying ethical principles, valuing them to define moral behavior, and then encoding laws to enforce that behavior (or prohibit it if defined as immoral). Because our values may change over time, however, we periodically reassess and change our laws governing sexual behavior.

Obscenity and Pornography

Some issues continue to be debated even in the face of definitive opinions from the Supreme Court. An example involves the definitions of **obscenity** and **pornography**. The Comstock Act of 1873, the first major law concerning obscenity in the United States, prohibited the mailing of

obscenity
Something offensive to modesty or decency; often sexually related.

pornography
Sexually arousing music, art, literature, or films; a determination that may vary from individual to individual and from community to community.

obscene or lewd material. The interpretation of what was obscene or lewd was left to the Postal Service. In 1957 the Supreme Court attempted to clarify the issue by ruling that sexuality-related material and obscene material were not one and the same. Rather, sexual material was ruled obscene (and therefore outside the protection of the First Amendment) only when sexual behavior was presented in a lewd and lascivious manner. But how was it to be determined whether some particular material was lewd or lascivious? The Supreme Court stated that the standard to be applied was whether the average person would judge it as such.

Further rulings between 1957 and 1968 (55 separate legal opinions in 13 obscenity cases) attempted to define obscenity more explicitly. As a result, the phrase "utterly without redeeming social value" was added to the definition. In 1973 the Court rejected its own "utterly without redeeming social value" criterion and defined the standards of obscenity that are currently in effect:

1. Whether the average person applying contemporary community standards would find that the work, taken as a whole, appeals to the prurient (lustful) interests

2. Whether the work depicts or describes, in a patently offensive way, sexual conduct specified by state law

3. Whether the work, taken as a whole, lacks serious literary, artistic, political, or scientific value

Despite the history of legal activity, a consensus in the society as to the definition of obscenity has yet to be reached. With the advent of the Internet and the access it provides to sexually explicit material, the problem is exacerbated.

Rape

Although there is considerable debate about the psychological, sociological, and cultural causes of rape, the chief legal issue involves achieving consensus on a set of standards for enforcing the laws against rape. The legal definition of forcible rape is sexual intercourse against one's will, but because anyone might accuse another of rape, society has had to define acceptable evidence. Until recently a prosecutor had to prove that semen was present—on the woman's body or clothing—to gain a conviction of rape. However, many female victims do not have a medical exam after rape; others bathe or shower before being examined; and in many cases of true rape, the rapist fails to ejaculate. Because many rapists have been pronounced innocent because of a lack of such evidence, the presence of semen is no longer

Communication DIMENSIONS

The Morality of Requesting a Variety of Sexual Behaviors

In some sexual relationships, one partner desires more variety in sexual activities than the other. For example, one partner may prefer anal sexual intercourse, and the other may object. Or one partner may be extremely excited by oral–genital sex, and the other may be turned off by it. One person may think of certain sexual activities as immoral, another as exciting. Too often, these conflicts result in anger and resentment, thereby interfering with other aspects of the relationship, not merely the sexual part. Consequently, partners should discuss differing sexual desires and resolve these issues. Fortunately, there are ways to do just that.

To begin, each person's thoughts and feelings should be expressed. A comment like "That's sick!" short-circuits any meaningful communication. The initial part of the conversation should be devoted to understanding the viewpoint of the other person, and that requires listening. There is time to express an opposing point of view, but not until one person has had the chance to be understood. Once one person has expressed his or her viewpoint, the other should. Refrain from arguing or disagreeing at this point. Merely listen.

Once both points of view have been aired, points of agreement should be identified. For example, both partners might agree that sex is a normal and desirable part of their relationship; that variety of sexual behaviors enhances the sexual relationship and thereby positively influences other aspects of their life together; that each cares about the other's feelings and sexual satisfaction; and that they want to make each other happy.

The part of communication regarding conflicts of ethics and morality that is most difficult is finding a compromise with which both persons are satisfied. Identifying areas of agreement provides a starting point in this process. Perhaps one partner is willing to try a particular sexual activity because he or she has identified a concern for making the other person happy. Perhaps the other is willing to forgo a particular sexual activity because it will make the other unhappy. The goal is to maintain the relationship as a stimulating one, not to engage in specific behaviors. The original focus on the behaviors is what is "wanted," whereas the real issue is the "need" for excitement and stimulation. That need can be met in ways that satisfy both partners with a little ingenuity and creativity.

Remember, though, no one should be forced, coerced, or manipulated to behave in any way that he or she considers immoral. That will result only in guilt, shame, or embarrassment and will not be healthy for the person or the relationship. If your partner is trying to manipulate you, the relationship is probably not worth saving.

---

considered the sole evidence of forcible rape; bruises, the presence of a weapon, and even threats of force may now be accepted.

Defense attorneys have often focused on the victims, attempting to show that they were promiscuous and thus responsible for provoking sexual attacks. New laws reflect society's growing concern with protecting victims from unfair questioning, as well as with ensuring conviction when rape has actually occurred. These laws now prohibit questions regarding the victim's sexual experience during a rape trial. Thus the focus of the trial is on determining the guilt or innocence of the accused, not on the moral character of the victim.

Statutory Rape

Statutory rape is placed in a different legal category from forcible rape, and a situation ethicist might also

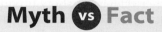

Myth: As long as two adults agree, any sexual activity in which they engage is legal, as long as it is done in private.
Fact: Not long ago, most states had sodomy laws that made certain sexual activities illegal even though they were consensual and performed by adults. These laws have since been declared unconstitutional.

put it in a different moral category. Statutory rape is sexual intercourse with a person below the legal age of consent, which varies from state to state. The statute is designed to protect children considered too immature to make sexual decisions for themselves. Even if boys or girls willingly participate in sexual intercourse, their consent is ignored for legal purposes. And even if they appear to be of age or lie about their age, the laws still apply, with few exceptions. In some states the exception is that a child proved to be sexually promiscuous or a prostitute may be considered an adult.

Adultery

Adultery, or extramarital intercourse, is quite prevalent in the United States. Kinsey reported back in 1948 that more than one-third of the men in his study reported extramarital coitus; in 1953 he reported that half of the men and 26% of the women he studied had extramarital sexual intercourse by age 40 years. Many suspect that the incidence of extramarital coitus has increased since Kinsey's studies. However, Hicks and Leitenberg (2001) report that men are engaging in fewer instances of extramarital sexual intercourse. They report the incidence for men at 28%, similar to women (29%). Other researchers have found the prevalence of adultery to be even lower, between 20% and 25% (Smith, 2006; Atkins, Baucom, & Jacobson, 2001). Even so, our concept of morality vis-à-vis marriage still leads us to sustain the laws against it. Adultery is frequently a legal ground for divorce. When adultery is the basis of divorce and custody of children is challenged in court, the adulterous partner often loses custody.

Polygamy

Two popular television programs have recently brought the practice of polygamy to the forefront. *Sister Wives*, a reality show broadcast on the TLC network, documented the life of a polygamist family living in Lehi, Utah. The family consisted of a husband living with his 4 wives and their 16 children. *Big Love*, another television show broadcast on HBO, was about a fictional fundamentalist Mormon family in Utah that also practiced polygamy.

Polygamy is when one man is married to more than one woman at the same time. The women know each other and are aware they are sharing one husband. Polygamy has been practiced in the United States over a long period of time, although currently it is illegal. Many Native American tribes practiced polygamy, as did some Scottish, Irish, and Welsh settlers. Some polygamous marriages also occurred in the southern United States shortly after the Civil War. Today, the most prominent polygamous group is the Fundamentalist Church of Jesus Christ of Latter-Day Saints (FLDS), a sect of the Mormon Church. FLDS

> **polygamy**
> When one man is married to more than one woman.

members practice polygamy in arranged marriages that often, though not always, involve young girls with older men. FLDS members can be found primarily in Hildale, Utah, and Colorado City, Arizona. Other FLDS communities exist in Canada, Texas, and other areas of western North America.

In 2001, Tom Green, a fundamentalist Mormon, was convicted and sentenced to 5 years in prison for polygamy. He had 5 wives and 30 children. Despite the fact that the Mormon Church and the state of Utah are formally against the practice of polygamy, as well as further charges that one of Green's wives was actually only 13 years old when he first had intercourse with her, Green argued he was being singled out among an estimated 30,000 polygamists in the United States. Another publicized case occurred in 2008. Texas officials took 436 children into temporary legal custody after a 16-year-old girl called authorities claiming that she had been beaten and forced to become a wife of an adult man. The raid occurred at the YFZ Ranch, which is owned by the FLDS. The children ranged in age from infants to teenagers, including teenage mothers and pregnant teens.

Should men be able to decide how many wives they wish to have at one time? For that matter, should women also be able to decide to have more than one husband at the same time (autonomy/liberty)? Or is there a societal interest in preserving the current legal standard of one husband being married to only one wife at the same time (social utility)? Does polygamy do harm to those involved; husbands, wives, and children (nonmaleficence)? Do you believe the law should be changed, or vigorously enforced?

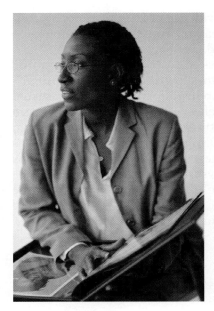

Although it is illegal for a typical person to photograph and publish nude photos of minors, many "artists" seem to have few problems getting away with it. Many bookstores sell photo albums that contain full nudity of clearly underage boys and girls, without prosecution. Is it possible to distinguish ethically or legally between nude photos of minors that are taken for the purpose of arousal from those that are taken as "art"?

Divorce

Laws involving divorce have been reformed over the years. Originally marriage and divorce laws in the United States were based on Judeo-Christian ethical principles involving the sanctity of the family and of parenthood. These laws reinforced the idea that the family was an economic necessity, both for the individual and for the society. Consequently divorce was granted by law only if misbehavior was proved in court. In other words, one of the marriage partners had to be at fault by being adulterous, mentally or physically cruel, and so on. When the number of divorces increased, and it became a common belief that people wishing to be free of each other should not be forced to remain married, many states adopted **no-fault divorce**. No-fault divorce statutes allow courts to dissolve marriages when no fault is cited and both partners agree to end the marriage.

Some people argue that no-fault divorce laws have led to more divorces (a bad thing); others say they have led to happier people (a good thing). Another way of looking at the prevalence of divorce—regardless of fault—is to argue that we should make marriage laws stricter, rather than making

Polygamist Tom Green with his "family."

divorce laws looser. People would then have to work harder to get married, and those without a strong commitment to each other would be unlikely to follow through.

Alimony is money that a judge orders the partner who earns more to pay on the granting of a divorce to the partner who earns less or no money. As are other matters related to divorce, alimony is being reevaluated. Previously alimony was handled as punishment for divorce, and the husband was forced to make payments to his wife. Today judges are more likely to assess the particular circumstances in a case and award alimony to either the man or the woman, on the basis of their respective resources and contributions to the marriage.

no-fault divorce
The granting of divorce without either partner's proving the other was the cause of the marriage's failure.

alimony
Money a divorced person is instructed by the courts to pay regularly to his or her ex-spouse.

Exploring the Dimensions of Human Sexuality

Our feelings, attitudes, and beliefs regarding sexuality are influenced by our internal and external environments. Go to go.jblearning.com/dimensions5e *to learn more about the biological, psychological, and sociological factors that affect your sexuality.*

Case Study

At the center of many ethical and moral dilemmas are cultural underpinnings—especially religious and political beliefs.

However, sometimes those cultural underpinnings clash. Consider the woman who unexpectedly finds herself pregnant. Raised as a member of the Roman Catholic religion—with its antiabortion doctrine—the woman has also been raised as a feminist, with a pro-choice doctrine. Further, consider the rights of her partner, who may have a different set of sociocultural doctrines to rely on for making moral decisions.

On a more personal level, it is important to make moral decisions regarding sexual relationships before becoming sexually involved. During a state of sexual arousal and response, it is often hard to put moral feelings ahead of intense physiological feelings.

States may pass specific laws dealing with sexuality; however, such laws must not conflict with federal laws and may be challenged for their constitutionality.

Biological Factors
- Alcohol and drugs can blur decision-making ability.

Sociocultural Factors
- Religions often establish codes of ethics, which state for members beliefs on matters including abortion, premarital sexual activity, extramarital sexual activity, same-gender sexual relations, and nonintercourse sexual activities.
- Political beliefs often suggest ethical standards. Although there are exceptions, in general, Democrats and feminists generally take a pro-choice stance (not always), and Republicans and fundamentalist Christians take an antiabortion stance. Laws in the United States ban discrimination based on race, religion, gender, age, and sexual orientation for public organizations, but private organizations can still discriminate. In many Islamic countries, adultery is illegal—even punishable by death. Gender selection through female infanticide or amniocentesis coupled with abortion is tolerated in some countries.

Psychological Factors
- During the state of sexual arousal and response, it is often hard to make moral judgments that conflict with intense physiological feelings.

Summary

- Ethics is a system on which we base our moral decisions. Ethical principles provide guidelines for abstract questions, not solutions to individual cases.

- When ethical principles clash, we have an ethical dilemma. Ethical dilemmas are resolved by placing a value on the competing ethical principles, with the principle carrying the highest value being the one that guides the decision.

- Rule ethics uses ethical principles to guide decisions in all situations. Situation ethics is based on the premise that all situations are unique and, therefore, there are no ethical principles that can be used the same way to guide all moral decision.

- If a decision or action is moral, it is *good* or *right*. If a decision is immoral, it is *bad* or *wrong*.

- Laws represent the encoding of generally accepted societal views of morality. Laws regarding sexual behavior develop from a general consensus of specific ethical principles, values, and judgments about behavior. When laws are not representative of societal views of morality, they are not followed and often need to be changed.

- Sexual morality is a consideration in such sexually related areas as sexually transmitted infections, sexual activity among unmarried persons, emergency contraception, abortion, amniocentesis, fetal tissue implantation, stem cell research, prostitution, in vitro fertilization, genetic engineering, and sexual responsibility to a partner.

- Among laws pertaining to sexual behavior are those regarding obscenity and pornography, rape, statutory rape, marriage, polygamy, adultery, and divorce.

Discussion Questions

1. Differentiate between ethics and morals. Apply the ethical principles of nonmaleficence, beneficence, autonomy/liberty, justice/fairness, and social utility to issues in human sexuality.

2. Discuss commonly accepted ethical principles and ways they can be applied in situations involving sexual behavior.

3. Which types of sexual behavior are regulated by laws? What is the basis of those laws?

Application Questions

Reread the chapter-opening story and answer the following questions.

1. Consider the ethical principles of nonmaleficence, beneficence, autonomy/liberty, justice/fairness, and social utility as they relate to the opening story. Which of the ethical principles did Wendy Weaver and the Nebo school district follow? Then explain how the case might have been affected if Weaver and the school district had followed other principles.

2. Was it ethical for Weaver to disclose her sexual orientation to a minor student? Should Weaver have considered the student's possible religious (70% of Utah residents are Mormon) objections to homosexuality before answering?

Critical Thinking Questions

1. Is practicing safer sex an ethical issue or a legal issue? For example, is it unethical not to have STI and HIV tests before starting a new relationship? Can this become a legal issue?

2. An unmarried woman who has been in a steady sexual relationship for 5 months discovers she is pregnant. Is it ethical, moral, or legal for the male to decide whether the female should have the child and keep it, give the child up for adoption, or have an abortion? What if the couple breaks up before she finds out she is pregnant? What rights, if any, does the man have in relation to the baby he helped create?

3. The ethics and morality of creating (or re-creating) life sometimes reflect technological innovations of the times. As the age of electricity dawned in the 1800s, Mary Shelley's *Frankenstein* (1818) provoked ethical and moral concerns about the use of electricity. Today, the use of electricity in the defibrillator to save a heart attack patient is accepted as ethical, moral, and legal. In fact, it would be considered unethical, immoral, and illegal not to use a defibrillator when a life could be saved. During our current age of genetic research (beginning with the 1950s discovery of DNA), Michael Crichton's *Jurassic Park* provoked similar concerns about the misuse of genetic engineering. However, even as you read this question, new technological applications are being devised that can and will save lives. Do you think people in 200 years will look back at *Jurassic Park* and wonder why we feared genetic research?

Critical Thinking Case

The ability to select the gender of a child has for years been the source of ethical debate. In some countries, cultures approve of female infanticide or amniocentesis coupled with abortion. However, the cultural morals of the United States do not favor such methods.

Would the current U.S. culture accept a scientifically based method of gender selection? The Genetics and IVF Institute (Fairfax, Virginia) announced in September 1998 that it had found a way to separate male and female sperm cells. Using specialized technology, its personnel are able to sort out 85% of X-bearing sperm (females) and 65% of Y-bearing sperm (males). Using artificial insemination, the Institute can give parents potential for gender selection, in proportion to the sperm-sorting abilities.

The technique has been used for some time on animals, which are easier to sort by gender. Testing with humans began in 1998. Human applications include preventing the birth of children with rare genetic sex-linked diseases (such as X-linked hydrocephalus) or "balancing" families with an opposite-sex sibling. The Institute is not planning to market the sorting procedure to first-time parents who simply have a dream of a specific-gender child.

Do you think that sperm-sorting technology is ethically acceptable in the case of raising farm animals? How about in the name of protecting endangered species from extinction?

As far as human applications are concerned, do you find it ethical to use sperm sorting to prevent the birth of a child who has a genetic sex-linked disease? How about to have an additional child to provide needed bone marrow for transplantion to a current child? Finally, is it ethical to use sperm sorting to have a third or fourth child of the opposite gender?

Exploring Personal Dimensions

Determining Your Ethical Compass
Several ethical dilemmas are presented in this activity to help you determine which ethical principles you use to guide your behavior and your view of morality. Choose the one option for each dilemma that best represents your views, even though you might agree with more than one.

1. Juan and Maria decide to live together and share a sexual relationship. They are thinking that they may marry in the future, but not anytime soon.

   a. Juan and Maria should not move in together because we know that when men and women live together, they are not equals. Women tend to take on more of the household chores than men.

   b. Juan and Maria should be free to decide what is best for them.

   c. Juan and Maria should not live together because Maria will suffer if she does not eventually marry Juan. She will be perceived as immoral by her family and her community.

   d. No good will come of Juan and Maria's living together. In fact, it might harm society by encouraging sexual relations between people who are not married to each other.

2. Evan and Rhonda place their 2-year-old son in child care so they can both work outside the home.

   a. This is unfair because Evan and Rhonda are placing their interests above the welfare of their son.

   b. Each couple should be able to decide what is best for their family unit.

   c. Without the direct and extensive contact with one of his parents, Evan and Rhonda's son will not grow and develop to his potential.

   d. Society will suffer if this becomes a common practice because of the emotional cost and health effects that the community will eventually have to absorb.

3. Although Kevin and Latisha have a sexual relationship, Kevin has not disclosed to Latisha that he has herpes. Kevin argues that their relationship is not "serious" and, therefore, he should not have to divulge his STI to Latisha. Furthermore, Kevin states, he refrains from having intercourse with Latisha when he has noticeable sores.

   a. Because Kevin knows about his STI and Latisha does not, Kevin is treating Latisha unfairly. He has more information than she, and that is not right.

   b. Kevin has a right to decide to whom information about his health is released, as well as the nature of that information.

   c. Lacking knowledge of Kevin's herpes, Latisha is likely to engage in behavior that can cause her harm.

   d. If Kevin continues to withhold information about his health and infects other sexual partners, society will suffer, health premiums will be raised for the rest of us, and hospital and medical staff resources may have to be redirected from other health issues.

4. Frankie and Lynn had been married for 10 years when Frankie began a sexual relationship with his coworker Flo.

a. It is not fair that Frankie engages in sex outside his marriage whereas Lynn refrains because of her vows of fidelity. If Frankie engages in extramarital sex, why should Lynn not have affairs as well?

b. Frankie may have many reasons for deciding to have a sexual relationship with Flo. He is an adult and should be free to decide whether the risk outweighs the benefits he derives from the relationship with Flo.

c. If Lynn ever found out she would be devastated, and their marriage might end. If they have children, even more harm would be done.

d. Society cannot allow extramarital affairs to be unpunished; otherwise, we would have chaos, unstable families, and dysfunctional children growing into dysfunctional adults.

5. Rose and Amber are lovers who are often seen by their neighbors holding hands as they enter their apartment building. Several of the more conservative tenants have complained about being "confronted by two lesbians flaunting their relationship to everyone else."

a. It is not fair that heterosexual tenants can hold hands but gay couples are expected to refrain from doing so.

b. Rose and Amber should be able to do whatever they choose. It is a free world. The other residents are free to look away.

c. Raising this issue with Rose and Amber might make them self-conscious and lead to their questioning whether they are welcome in that apartment building. Furthermore, the strain of this confrontation might lead to stress that could harm their health.

d. It is harmful to young children, who are impressionable and in the process of developing their own sexual orientation, to see outwardly gay couples' being accepted by society. For the good of the total society, gay couples should be more discreet.

If you found yourself selecting choice (a) more often than the other choices, you are predominantly guided by the ethical principle of *justice*, believing people ought to be treated fairly. If you selected choice (b) over the others, you are guided by *autonomy*, believing people ought to be free to make their own choices without interference from others. However, if you selected choice (c) most often, you are guided by the ethical principle of *nonmaleficence*, believing no harm ought to be done, and, when it is, the decision is immoral. And, if you found yourself most often selecting choice (d), you are guided by *social utility*, believing a decision needs to be considered in terms of the benefit or harm to society.

Suggested Readings

Ali, K. *Sexual ethics and islam: Feminist reflections on Qur'an, hadith, and jurisprudence*. London, UK: Oneworld, 2006.

Arthur, J. *Morality and moral controversies: Readings in moral, social and political philosophy*, 8th Ed. Saddle River, NJ: Prentice Hall, 2008.

Blackburn, S. *Being good: A short introduction to ethics*. Oxford, UK: Oxford University Press, 2003.

Gert, B. *Common morality: Deciding what to do*. Oxford, UK: Oxford University Press, 2004.

Greenberg, J. *The code of ethics for the health education profession: A case study book*. Boston: Jones and Bartlett, 2001.

Hollinger, D. P. *The meaning of sex*: Christian *ethics and the moral life*. Grand Rapids, MI: Baker Academic, 2009.

Ingram, P. *The signifying body: Toward an ethics of sexual and racial difference*. Albany, NY: State University of New York Press, 2009.

Mappes, T. A., & Zembaty, J. *Social ethics: Morality and social policy*. New York: McGraw-Hill Humanities, 2006.

Martin, M. W. *Everyday morality: An introduction to applied ethics*. Florence, KY: Wadsworth, 2006.

Piderit, J. *Sexual morality: A natural law approach to intimate relationships*. Cary, NC: Oxford University Press, 2011.

Teutsch, D. A. *Family and sexual ethics (guide to Jewish practice)*. Wyncote, PA: Reconstructionist Rabbinical College Press, 2010.

Twomey, V. *Moral theology after Humanae Vitae: Fundamental issues in moral theory and sexual ethics*. Dublin, Ireland: Four Courts, 2010.

Web Resources

For links to the websites below, visit *go.jblearning.com/dimensions5e* and click on Resource Links.

The Feminist Sexual Ethics Project
www.brandeis.edu/projects/fse

Explores sexual ethics within Judaism, Christianity, and Islam, and presents how the toleration of slavery in the early teachings of these religions affects the lives of women today. Among the links are those dealing with Jewish sexual ethics, Christian sexual ethics, and Muslim sexual ethics.

United Nations High Commissioner for Human Rights (UNHCHR)

www.ohchr.org/EN/Pages/WelcomePage.aspx

The Office of the High Commissioner for Human Rights (OHCHR) is a department of the United Nations Secretariat. It is mandated to promote and protect the enjoyment and full realization, by all people, of all rights established in the Charter of the United Nations and in international human rights laws and treaties. The mandate includes preventing human rights violations, securing respect for all human rights, promoting international cooperation to protect human rights, coordinating related activities throughout the United Nations, and strengthening and streamlining the United Nations system in the field of human rights. Among these rights are those that pertain to sexual issues— for example, female clitoral mutilation.

Sexual Ethics in Psychology

www.rotten.com/library/sex/sexual-ethics-in-psychology

Presents case studies to discuss the American Psychological Association's code of ethics that governs the interaction between therapists and patients. The sexual interaction between clinician and patient is emphasized.

Human Rights Campaign

www.hrc.org

The Human Rights Campaign is America's largest civil rights organization working to achieve gay, lesbian, bisexual, and transgender (GLBT) equality. HRC seeks to improve the lives of GLBT Americans by advocating for equal rights and benefits in the workplace, ensuring families are treated equally under the law, and increasing public support among all Americans through innovative advocacy, education, and outreach programs. The website includes links to legislation, laws, work life, religion and faith, employment opportunities, and other subjects.

Sexual Ethics in Islam and in the Western World

www.al-islam.org/sexualethics/

Offers chapters from a book describing sexual ethics as it relates to Islam. Chapters explore traditional sexual ethics, sexual ethics as conceived by modern thinkers; proposed new sexual freedom; a critical examination of the theoretical basis of the proposed new sexual freedom; the basic need for humane conditioning of natural instincts and desires; and love, sexual discipline, and chastity.

References

Achenbach, J. Splice of life. *The Washington Post Magazine* (November 29, 1998), 12–19, 27–30.

Associated Press. Lesbian can resume coaching, judge rules. *Washington Post* (November 27, 1998), A12.

Atkins, D. C., Baucom, D. H., & Jacobson, N. S. Understanding infidelity: Correlates in a national random sample. *Journal of Family Psychology*, 15 (2001), 735–749.

Catholic Church. *Encyclical of Pope Paul VI, humanae vitae, on the regulation of birth, and Pope Paul VI's credo of the people of God.* Glen Rock, NJ: Paulist Press, 1968.

Ellis, A. Healthy and disturbed reasons for having extramarital relations, in *Encounter with family realities*, Powers, E. A. & Lees, M.-W., eds. St. Paul, MN: West, 1977, 374–375.

Hicks, T., & Leitenberg, H. Sexual fantasies about one's partner versus someone else: Gender differences in incidence and frequency. *Journal of Sex Research*, 38 (2001), 43–50.

Kaufman, M. Morning-after pill study contradicts claim by foes: Easy access did not lead to riskier behavior. *Washington Post* (January 5, 2005), p. A09.

Kenney, J. W., Reinholtz, C., & Angellini, P. J. Ethnic differences in childhood and adolescent sexual abuse and teenage pregnancy. *Journal of Adolescent Health 21, 1* (1997), 3–10.

National Institutes of Health Resource for Stem Cell Research. Stem cell information: Stem cell basics. 2011. Available: http://stemcells.nih.gov/info/basics5asp.

Smith, T. W. American sexual behavior: Trends, socio-demographic differences, and risk behavior. GSS Topical Report no. 25. Chicago, IL: National Opinion Research Center, University of Chicago; 2006.

Stem cell research: What Americans think. *Parade* (July 10, 2005), p. 5.

Epilogue: Taking Responsibility for Your Sexual Health

THE SEXUAL FUTURE

It was a morning of unmatched brilliance; the sun shone brightly, the robins were singing, and the spring air was morning fresh. It was a typical morning in the year 2099 for Todd and his housemates Keri, Karen, and Jerry.

Excuse me. I am being impolite. I forgot that you were from another time. I should have introduced you to our way of life before mentioning my friends. Of course we have made lots of technological advances, as you will soon see. But given what was going on in your day, you could probably see that coming, even if you could not foresee the form. Beyond that, however, we have changed our attitudes and values, our ways of doing work, and our social, sexual, and family relationships. For example, in 2099 we are altogether more respectful of individual differences than you were in your time. Questions of morality do not dominate our way of life as they did yours, and much ignorance has been dispelled. Is it a good or bad time, you ask? Let me describe our ways to you and you can answer for yourself.

Keri, Karen, Jerry, and Todd range in age from 21 to 41 years, but they are not rushing off to work today. In fact they never rush off to work, because they all work at home. Most people do. It is the computer and all the other technological and communication advances, you see. Of course, as you did in the early part of this century, we all have computers, smartphones, and tablets at home, and we use them for work and play, as well as for banking, shopping, and communicating with one another over long and short distances. We play games on them and can program our devices to play music for us. Our physicians even use them to diagnose illnesses and prescribe medication. (Wait until you hear about the medication we have!) Anyway, why do you think the morning air is so fresh? No cars to pollute it! In fact, there is very little transportation as you knew it. We have little need to go anywhere. Our computers meet most of our needs. Life really is easy.

Family life, as you can imagine, is also quite different from home life as you knew it. Long ago we realized that marriage was archaic—it just did not make sense in a rapidly changing society to expect two people to live together forever. People change as the society changes, but not all marriage partners change at the same pace. Once we understood this, we changed our laws to allow for a number of different marriage styles. The styles are not really new, but the legal and social ease of choosing and changing *is*. For example, we have repeating monogamous marriages

(RMMs), wherein one maintains only one partner at a time but, when the marriage becomes stale, one can dissolve the marriage easily and marry another partner. Some people marry 10 or more times in this manner. Polygamy (one person married to several people at the same time) is also common, as are multiple marriage partners (MMPs). MMPs allow several males to share several female marriage partners, and vice versa.

In spite of all our attempts to adapt marriage to our society, however, most people never marry. Rather they establish informal arrangements of convenience. Some live together, some raise children together (their own or those of others), and some just share particular events together. I, for example, have an informal arrangement with Betty for sexual play, with Tina for computer game play, and with Tasha for sharing of thoughts and important feelings.

By the way, we laugh when we hear stories of your struggle with sexual equality. In 2099 we cannot imagine that males would be treated differently from females. I guess our attitude evolves partly because the need for physical strength continued to decrease, just as it was in your day, and that eliminated the male's biological advantage. You see, robots do all our strenuous work, and competitive sports (other than computer games) have long since been outlawed. They were thought to contribute to warlike attitudes that, with the existence of weapons that could destroy the world, were deemed intolerable. But really that only partly explains our sexual equality. We realize that people who are discriminated against eventually revolt. It is only a matter of time—treat a group unfairly and it eventually rebels, disturbing the peace. Furthermore, our scientists have discovered treatments that allow everyone, male and female, to feel however they wish and to acquire almost any trait they want or need. Because people can change themselves nearly at will, how could we believe any one or any group to be inferior?

Scientists have made other important advances, too. Most diseases are curable now—your dreaded cancer and heart diseases among them. But perhaps the single most significant advance has been the discovery of K25W. Added to our water supply by our leaders (all of whom are scientists rather than politicians), K25W is a chemical that prepares the mind to receive and accept subliminal messages.

What are subliminal messages, you ask? Just a little trick of the media trade. The subliminal messages are verbal messages delivered so quickly and at such a low volume that those who receive them are not even aware that messages have been conveyed. Subliminal messages can be visual, too, images relayed so quickly along with other broadcast material that viewers remain unaware of them. Your society experimented with a crude form of subliminal messages when, for instance, voices were hidden beneath the pleasant music that department store customers heard while shopping reminding customers to be polite and not to shoplift. But you did not have K25W in your water! We use subliminal messages to plant many ideas, one of which is sexual equality, in the minds of our citizens.

The one problem we are still wrestling with is how to solve the discontent of our elderly. Having eradicated many of the diseases that plagued you, plus eliminating traffic accidents, we have lengthened the life span of most people, and so the size of our elderly population has grown enormously. By the way, we do not think of 70-year-olds as elderly; people live now to the ages of 120, 130, even 140 years. Mind you, our old people are quite happy (remember K25W) and able to care for themselves (remember our medications). Still, they tell stories of their past, and young people wonder whether our society is really better than the one the old folks recall. There is much ambivalence in those recollections. The old ones speak of illness, on the one hand, and the joy of life, on the other hand; of cruelty and war, on the one hand, and the Peace Corps, on the other hand; of nursing homes, on the one hand, and growing old with families to care for you, on the other hand. No small wonder the younger ones are confused. But our scientists are working on this issue even as we speak. Before long it will be clear to all that our new society is developing in the right direction. After all, do we not live longer? Have we not eliminated sexual bias? Can we not take a pill and acquire just about any trait we want?

Well, that gives you a quick overview of some major areas of our life. Now let me tell you about my friends to show you examples of how some personal relationships work.

Todd is an Edibilist. His job relates to developing new strains of foods and nutrients. Because many of our citizens live to be 130 years old, world population has skyrocketed, and all the life-sustaining resources (food, energy, oxygen) are at a premium. Todd is married to Jerry (homosexual marriage is not uncommon among us, because people do not marry primarily to have babies). His recreational needs are met by Keri and his intellectual needs by Karen. Jerry is also Karen's sexual mate. As a matter of fact, they had a scare recently. No, not an unwanted pregnancy. That is no longer a problem. We have an enormous range of effective contraceptives (male contraceptives that prevent sperm development or immobilize sperm and female contraceptives are taken only once a year). Furthermore, someone who misuses reproductive privileges—by becoming pregnant without written

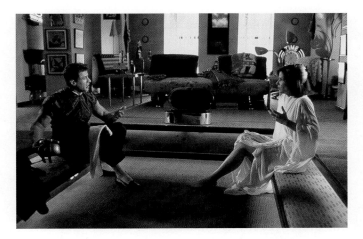

In *Demolition Man*, Sylvester Stallone plays a rogue cop put into cryogenic captivity and awakened in the year 2032. He is understandably perplexed by this strange new world, but when Sandra Bullock asks him to have sex and he realizes it involves a virtual reality helmet and no touching, he is outraged! What are the missing dimensions of sexuality in this scenario?

approval from the Population and Parenthood Screening Bureau—is liable to be sterilized by court order. As you can imagine, population control is a major concern, and reproductive control is therefore a governmental issue. At least we have no need for abortions!

No, Jerry and Karen's problem pertained not to pregnancy but to sexual dysfunction. We have eliminated the kinds of sexual dysfunction you were familiar with. Pills are available that eliminate inhibitions to sexual response. They can also lubricate vaginas, make penises erect, and even increase sexual desire. Jerry and Karen's problem arose when she popped a "desire" pill and Jerry did not want to take his. As yet it is not a matter of policy to add these chemicals to the water supply, as we do with K25W, to make people's sexual desires compatible. The controversy is ongoing as to whether controlling sexual desire should be left to individual discretion. At present the *dysfunction of the sexual union*, the term for our form of sexual dysfunction, is subject to the whims of the sexual partners. Opponents of adding desire chemicals to the water supply suggest that if one person drank a glass of water, felt a rush of desire, and could not find his or her partner, hysteria, frustration, violence, or a change of partner could ensue. Well, Jerry finally took his "desire" pill and the dysfunction was eliminated. It is my guess that if this incompatibility recurs, they will be looking for new mates.

Speaking of new mates, Keri is presently looking for one. Her old mate is raising her child and Keri would like a new mate with a drastically different endowment than the last. Keri's child was a dream come true, but only after some medical intervention. The Population and Parenthood Screening Bureau tested Keri both physiologically and psychologically to determine her qualifications for parenthood and approved her application. She chose John as the father because of his blond hair, blue eyes, impressive height, and high intelligence. Several months after conception, the amniotic fluid tests revealed that the fetus was male and had brown eyes and a cleft palate—not at all like John. You can imagine how quickly Keri ordered a genetic manipulation (GM)! When her daughter was born with blue eyes and devoid of any defects, Keri was elated and decided to keep her.

Keri's friend Josie is an interesting case. In fact, her situation would make a good riddle for you: How can someone be both the biological mother and the biological father of the same child? Well, Josie was not always Josie; she was once Joseph! Joseph was born a male and as a young adult deposited sperm in one of our neighborhood sperm banks. Joseph then decided that his maleness was unsuited to his disposition (unfortunately, his mother had not ordered a GM but had let nature take its course), and he had a sex-change operation. Joseph's male genitals were surgically removed and replaced with two ovaries, two fallopian tubes, a uterus, and a vagina. Once recuperated, Joseph, now Josie, used the deposited sperm to fertilize the ovum during her ovulation period. Hence when the baby was born, its mother and father were one and the same.

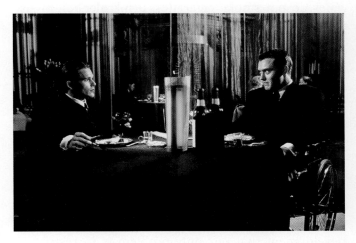

How important our genetic makeup may be in the future is explored in the film *Gattaca*. Ethan Hawke plays a young man labeled an "invalid" because his parents decided not to undergo genetic engineering while he was in the womb. Barred from well-paying or respectable jobs, Ethan must take on the identity of a "valid" and risk his life to pursue his dreams. What possible effects do you think genetic engineering may have on sociocultural dimensions of sexuality?

But enough of unusual stories. Josie's situation is unique. Keri's case is more common. Perhaps she can soon choose another accurately genetically analyzed mate to make the kind of child she wants. If not, the GM people should be able to help, although, because they are in such demand, we encourage our citizens to do their genetic planning as much beforehand as possible (even though, as Keri's case indicates, this may result in something short of perfection).

By the way, the birthing process has changed much since your time. In 2099 women neither experience pain nor use unnatural chemicals during the delivery of babies. Instead we use endorphins. These substances were discovered more than a century ago but were not put to much use right away. Maybe you remember that endorphins are chemicals naturally produced by the human body that decrease pain and are related to relaxation. Since their discovery in the human brain, we have learned how to produce them synthetically. We administer these synthetic endorphins during childbirth (which, by the way, occurs in people's homes rather than in birthing factories—hospitals, I think you called them). Thus the birth of a baby involves nothing but joy—more joy than we have been able to develop with our medications.

For women too busy to carry the unborn for the 6 months required (we sped up the gestation process for convenience), surrogate mothers are available to do the job. A surrogate receives the fertilized ovum in her uterus and goes through the birth process as usual. The baby is then presented to the original parents and the surrogate is paid according to the birth weight and health of the baby (consequently surrogates do not smoke cigarettes, drink alcohol, or use drugs, and they monitor their nutrition carefully). Other options are available for parents of lesser financial means—animal uteruses serve as surrogate fetal development sites, as does the womb simulator (a machine in which a fetal development is maintained). These options allow the original mother to continue her usual routine unimpeded by pregnancy. However, the price she pays for this convenience is losing the joy of birthing. Moreover, a certain detachment often characterizes the mother–child relationship in such cases.

As you could probably guess, infertility does not exist today. We have so many ways of fertilizing ova and so many ways of organizing embryo and fetal development that our only problem is in restricting birth to a number that does not draw too heavily upon our society's resources.

Before you leave us, take with you the knowledge that sexual infections need not exist—it does not for us. As you can gather, I am sure, we are quite active sexually. And yet we managed to eliminate sexually

transmitted infections by the year 2047. We finally found the link among all the causative agents of STIs, including AIDS. We termed this link the *Syphgon factor*, after syphilis and gonorrhea, although a more appropriate name might be *basic biological matter–thwarting factor*. Soon after the link was found, a vaccine was developed to immunize people against STIs. Originally injected into the bloodstream, this chemical is now in pill form and is designed to dissolve under the tongue. Regarding cancer—breast, uterine, vaginal, testicular, and others—we have been able to teach people, using no medication, to control the flow of T lymphocytes to the cancerous area, thereby eliminating the cancer. Of course, to allow the technique to work, early detection is imperative; the required monthly screening (consisting only of passing through a sensitive doorway similar to that used by your generation to screen airline passengers) serves this purpose. Cancer has virtually been eliminated.

What? You want to know how we arrive at ethical and moral decisions? I am afraid you can only get into trouble asking these questions. Do you not remember the trouble they caused in your time? We leave ethical issues to our leaders. You ask why our leaders are scientists and not ethicists, philosophers, clergy, psychologists, or sociologists? Well, would you have nonscientists leading this highly technical society? We have to trust our leaders to do what is best for us.

To be honest, though, the questions you ask trouble me, too. For us, however, the opportunity to make some other choices has passed. Our society is what it is. It is, you might say, a snowball rolling downhill picking up more and more snow. But take a look at your time. Are not the seeds of our society already planted? Perhaps you still have the chance to nurture the humanizing aspects of your society and to prevent its dehumanizing aspects from developing and taking over your future.

■ Commentary

Interestingly, the scenario you just read was written in the mid-1980s to promote discussion about the future and dimensions of sexuality (Greenberg & Bruess, 1986). As we reread this in preparation for its inclusion in this book, it struck us just how on target our predictions were. It made us think that we should be advising people on which stocks to invest in. Let us take a closer look at the future we projected two decades ago, at the characteristics of that future that already have come to pass and those that have not.

Social Dimensions

We described the year 2099 as one in which fewer people left their home and family to travel to work. Rather, they worked from home with the help of new technologies. We do not have to wait for 2099 for that to occur; it is already happening today. With the advent of the computer, smartphones, tablets, and telecommunications capabilities, more people are "telecommuting" than ever before. As in the scenario, more and more people are shopping, banking, and communicating from home. If you want a book, you need only go to the website of Amazon.com or Barnes and Noble. If you want to switch money from one bank account to another, you can hit a few keys on your home computer or a few numbers on your smartphone and the transfer is completed. And, if you want to communicate with someone, you can do so by email, instant messaging, or iPhones and Blackberrys. The result should be more time for the family and for people about whom we care. However, this does not seem to be a social benefit we have as yet derived from technological advances. Too many people spend too much time at their computers or on their smartphones, checking out Internet sites, receiving and sending email messages, or playing computer games.

Physical Dimensions

We also guessed right about the ability of physicians to use computers to treat patients better. Today, physicians can call on experts from afar, using computers and telecommunications to read X rays, computed tomography (CT) scans, and magnetic resonance imaging (MRI) results and make a diagnosis that a local physician may be incapable of making. Robots are even conducting surgeries managed from afar. This technology has tremendous potential for the diagnosis and treatment of sexually transmitted infections and other sexual illnesses.

In 2099, sexual dysfunction is not one of those matters about which citizens are concerned; they have a "desire pill." In a way, this is not much different from today's Viagra and Cialis and other drugs that treat sexual dysfunctions. In addition, microsurgical techniques are available to alleviate some sexual dysfunctional problems.

However, in 2099 the reason the "desire pill" is not added to the water supply is that a person who took a drink and experienced sexual desire might form a "sexual union" with a stranger who happened to be nearby and available. Today, we have a different variable serving as a barrier to "haphazard" sexual unions: HIV and AIDS. The fear of contracting

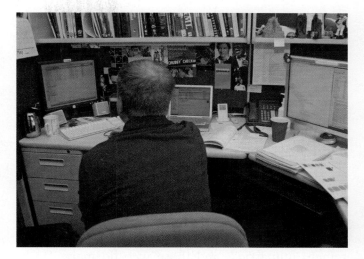

Many people telecommute, working from their homes with new technology. With decreased human contact, will our society change? For the better or for the worse?

HIV has led to a decrease in casual sex and an increase in condom use when sexual activity does take place. Still, research to develop an HIV and AIDS vaccine, if successful, might once again lead to a more cavalier attitude toward sex and a reemergence of the sexually free attitude of the 1960s. And yet, many Americans and others around the world are not waiting for a vaccine. Too many refuse to adopt responsible sexual behavior and engage in safer-sex practices.

Marital Dimensions

In the year 2099, there is a new form of marriage—repeating monogamous marriage (RMM). Today, with the divorce and remarriage rates as they are, we have a de facto RMM system. We have even developed a name for the convoluted family structure possible when remarriage occurs (possibly several times for

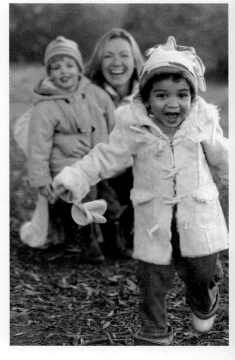

Blended families, as well as the large number of international adoptions, are having a dramatic effect on the families in the 21st century.

the same parent): *blended families*. However, we have not institutionalized polygamy as was described in the scenario. We still believe in the fidelity of one marital partner to the other, although some might argue that the prevalence of extramarital sex provides evidence of a trend in the opposite direction. And today, as in the scenario, it is common for people to live together and not be married to each other. Young couples move in together to determine whether a long-term relationship is feasible for them. Gays live together as unmarried, in the eyes of the law at least, because legislators in many states have proscribed gay marriage. And elders cohabit because our society reinforces that arrangement through our tax codes and social welfare programs. Many Americans choose to remain unmarried, and those who do marry do so at a later age.

Gender Dimensions

We have discussed gender dimensions of sexuality throughout this book, and in 2099 attention is paid to this issue as well: Gender equality is a reality. In present-day society we have made great strides toward gender equality. It is no longer unusual for a female to be a physician or a lawyer. It is no longer unusual for a male to assume such household chores as cooking, cleaning, and child rearing. And yet, women are still paid less than men even when they do the same job; also, although men do more household chores when they and their spouses work full-time outside the home, women still assume a disproportionate share. And female genital mutilation is still practiced in many parts of the world. We have yet to discover a way to remedy the disparity in the way we treat our females and males in a manner that is best for women, men, children, and the rest of society, as they did in 2099 with the magical K25W. Still, we are headed in the right direction; the trend is toward greater gender equality and fairness. We hope that we will not have to wait until 2099 to see their full development.

Pregnancy and Childbearing Dimensions

In 2099, there are no unintended pregnancies. That is certainly not where we are today. More than half of all pregnancies in the United States are unintended, and our teenage pregnancy rate is one of the highest among developed countries. As in 2099, we have a wide range of effective contraceptives. The difference is that too few Americans use them or use them irregularly or incorrectly. That leads to a greater number

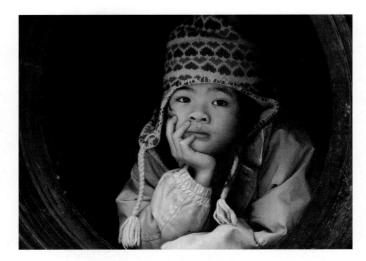

Some countries value male babies for their ability to support the family. This has resulted in infanticide in the form of female babies being aborted. How do you imagine females feel in such societies?

of unwanted births, abortions, and adoptions than would otherwise be the case.

Perhaps our descendants in 2099 have the right idea with the Population and Parenthood Screening Bureau. Today, we have too many children who are abused and neglected. We have too many children who are taken from their birth parents and placed in foster care with the intent of having them adopted, although many never do get a stable family and remain in the foster care system until they become of emancipated age. Perhaps we need to pay as much attention to enhancing parenting skills as our descendants do in 2099.

One area in which we do not have to wait for 2099 is that of genetic manipulation. With medical scientific advances, it is possible to perform surgery on fetuses in the womb to remedy structural abnormalities. Soon we will be able to apply different genes to influence eye color, intelligence, or other traits. Researchers have already isolated stem cells from embryonic tissue that can eventually be used to grow human replacement parts for transplantation. People wonder, if Dolly the sheep has been cloned, will humans eventually be cloned? The ethical implications of rapidly developing scientific advances have outstripped our society's ability to develop laws that will assure that technology will be used to enhance our culture rather than diminish it.

Want a boy baby? No need to engage in abortion or infanticide, as in some countries. Just use sperm-separation techniques to improve the odds. No, this is not part of the 2099 scenario. This is occurring today. Want a child who is likely to be an athlete or a musician? Just be selective at the sperm bank, careful to choose sperm from a male who has the characteristics you want for your child. No, this is not part of the 2099 scenario. This is occurring today. The future is here!

■ Tonow

As the 21st-century narrator of our story implies, being aware of present trends and considering what personal and social agreements about sexuality may be like in the future can be fun, but it can also be a responsibility.

As our society evolves, we must not lose sight of our heritage and what we have learned from it. To that knowledge we must add new information—information filtered through ethical and moral awareness and values. As citizens of today and of the future, we can ill afford to shirk our responsibility to help shape our sexual society.

The physician Bernie Siegel worked with cancer patients—"cancer survivors," he called them. Knowing they probably had little time left to live, he helped them live "well" during the time left to them. This is a lesson that all of us could profit by learning. Siegel was fond of speaking of today, tomorrow, and "tonow." Using Siegel's terminology, many sexual futuristic issues are actually occurring tonow.

A woman is judged guilty of a criminal act and is considered to be a poor mother, so a judge prevents her from having other children. He offers her a choice of going to jail or having a contraceptive implant (Norplant) surgically placed on her arm. Tonow.

A society experiments on itself. Its children grow up with the majority of their mothers working full-time outside the home. In many cases, a male figure is absent from the home because of desertion, death, or divorce. What will the effects be? Tonow.

A country changes dramatically. What were once "minorities," when grouped together, become the majority. In many areas of the United States, Hispanic, Asian American, and African American populations have increased in numbers and in percentage of population. What will be the effects on sexuality? On attitudes toward sexual issues? On views of censorship, morality, abortion, and family life? Many believe the country will profit from this diversity. Will it? Tonow.

As people wrestle with a threat to their very lives, AIDS stalks all segments of the population. During the sexual revolution individuals fought for the right of free sexual expression; however, in this day there can be heavy consequences for such behavior. Will behavior change? How many deaths will occur before that happens? Will relationships ever be the same? Tonow.

It is our hope that this book helps to prepare you for your sexual tonow and your sexual tomorrow. Most likely your instructor hopes your sexuality course will have the same effect. No one can predict the future, but we can anticipate trends and prepare for them. How will you prepare? When will you start?

Discussion Questions

1. Vaccines were one of the greatest wonders of the 20th century and eradicated several major diseases. However, a small percentage of people contract the disease through the vaccine and are left disabled or dead. Would you be willing to take such a risk to be vaccinated for STIs or HIV? Would you subject your infant children to such vaccines to protect their future? Explain why or why not.

2. Over the time you have taken this course, you have undoubtedly heard news stories about current research that could affect your future sexuality. Relate some of the more interesting research projects, and discuss whether they are feasible, given the biological, psychological, and sociocultural dimensions of sexuality.

Application Questions

Reread the chapter-opening scenario and answer the following questions.

1. Would you prefer to live in your current world or in the world of 2099 described in the scenario? Explain your answer.

2. Allowing government control over subliminal messages (and lacing the drinking water with K25W) would give the government complete control of the population. How could government be regulated so that only positive messages (for example, gender equality) would be conveyed? What if the government decided to convey messages like "Don't vote for the opposing political party"—or worse?

Critical Thinking Questions

1. As our society continues to accept the ideal of diversity, we seem less and less likely to unify as a nation on any issue—especially sex! Consider the use of stem cells in the United States. Which sociocultural groups are likely to be in favor of their use? Which groups would be against it? Under which circumstances do you think the federal government should approve the use of embryonic stem cells?

2. Aldous Huxley, in *Brave New World*, portrayed a government that kept control of its people by granting them unrestrained sexual pleasures. George Orwell, in *1984*, took the opposite position: The government keeps control by discouraging sexual contact among spouses and forbidding it among nonmarried people.

Compare and contrast these methods given what you know about the many dimensions of human sexuality.

Critical Thinking Cases

What Is "Quality of Life"?

The year 2099 seems to have some attractive features. Diseases are curable. Computers do a lot of the work, and the remainder can often be done at home. Cars do not pollute air. People live longer and establish numerous relationships—each designed to meet a specific need.

And yet some of the citizens in the year 2099 seem disenchanted. Their marriages often do not last very long. They cannot have children whenever they want. They cannot engage in competitive sports. Their mind is manipulated as a result of K25W in their water supply.

Given these and the other conditions we have described, would you want to live in the year 2099? Why or why not?

What in life is important to you aside from *how long you live?*

What is present and what is absent in 2099 that you need to be happy sexually?

Exploring Personal Dimensions

The form below might be used in our fictional story set in 2099. In our story, those individuals wishing to conceive may have to answer questions very much like those in the form. Their answers determine whether they are given permission to have a child, as well as specifying the gender and appearance of the child. As you read through this form, consider whether it is ethical to ask such questions of potential parents. What would be the effects on the sociocultural dimensions of sexuality of applying such rules to parenting?

POPULATION AND PARENTHOOD SCREENING BUREAU

Parenthood Application

Name: _____

Mate's Name: _____

Address: _____

Computer Access Number: _____

Answer all of the following questions:

1. How long have you been mating? _____

2. List all illnesses/diseases experienced within the last year by the female mate: _____
_____
_____

3. List all illnesses/diseases experienced within the last year by the male mate: _____
_____
_____

4. On the breakup of your relationship, what do you plan for your child?
_____
_____
_____

5. What time is best for you to be interviewed by our psychological team?
_____
_____
_____
_____

6. List those traits you want ensured in your child:
   a. Sex: _____

   b. Eye color: _____

   c. Hair color: _____

   d. Intelligence quotient: _____

   e. Height: _____

   f. Special abilities (for example, athletic, mathematical, artistic):
   _____
   _____

7. Which method of birth control do you employ?
_____

8. Do you have any other children? _____

9. Which method of birthing do you plan?

10. How will your child be cared for during the workday? _____
_____
_____

11. List any parenting training you and your mate have received: _____
_____
_____

12. Will you agree to amniotic fluid screening during the pregnancy?
_____
_____

Special Note: Be aware that approval will not be granted to individuals who already have a child, who are untrained for parenthood, who do not agree to amniotic fluid screening, who have not planned for the daily care of their child-to-be, or who have not prepared for the breakup of their relationship.

Reference

Greenberg, J. S., Bruess, C. E., & Mullen, K. D. *Sexuality: Insights and issues*. Madison, WI: WCB Brown & Benchmark, 1986.

Glossary

69 Two partners' simultaneous stimulation of each other's genitalia orally. The numerals 6 and 9 visually describe the body positions.

abortifacient A medical method that causes an embryo or fetus to die.

abortion Purposeful termination of a pregnancy.

abstinence Avoidance of any type of sexual intercourse.

acquaintance rape Rape by a friend, acquaintance, or date; also known as *date rape*.

acquired erectile dysfunction A condition in which an adult male has previously had an erection sufficient to engage in sexual intercourse but no longer has.

acquired immune deficiency syndrome (AIDS) A syndrome caused by the human immunodeficiency virus (HIV), characterized by a depressed immune system and the presence of one or more opportunistic diseases.

active listening Paraphrasing what someone has said to demonstrate interest and understanding.

adipose Pertaining to fat tissue in the body.

afterbirth The delivery of the placenta.

aggressiveness Standing up for one's basic rights, but at the expense of someone else's basic rights.

alimony Money a divorced person is instructed by the courts to pay regularly to his or her ex-spouse.

amenorrhea The absence of menstruation in a woman who should be menstruating.

amniocentesis Withdrawal by syringe of amniotic fluid to determine the presence of fetal abnormalities.

amniotic fluid The fluid inside the amniotic sac in which the fetus floats; it acts as a shock absorber, maintains the fetus at a constant temperature, and serves as a nutrient.

amniotic sac A fluid-filled membrane that surrounds the developing infant in the uterus.

ampulla The enlarged portion of the vas deferens where sperm are provided nutrients from the seminal vesicles; also, the part of the fallopian tube of women containing the cilia.

anal intercourse Insertion of the penis into the anus.

analgesics Substances that decrease pain locally, such as topical creams.

analingus Licking of the anus.

androgens Male sex hormones.

androgynous Exhibiting a combination of masculine and feminine traits as defined by the society.

anesthetics Substances that elicit unconsciousness and thereby relieve pain.

annular Type of hymen that surrounds the vaginal opening.

anorexia nervosa A condition in which the individual severely limits caloric intake.

antiandrogen drugs Chemicals that reduce the sex drive by lowering the testosterone level in the bloodstream.

antibodies A class of proteins secreted by the immune system that bonds with antigens. Antibodies fight off disease-causing organisms.

areola The darkened part of the breast immediately surrounding the nipple.

arousal phase The second stage of Kaplan's model of sexual response, which consists of physiological arousal and changes and, possibly, orgasm.

asphyxiophilia Desire for a state of oxygen deficiency to enhance sexual excitement.

assertiveness Standing up for one's basic rights without violating anyone else's rights.

aversion therapy Pairing an undesirable sexual behavior with a painful response.

bar girls Sex workers who are supposed to act available so customers will buy them drinks.

Barbach's technique A method of treating orgasmic dysfunction and sexual unresponsiveness developed by Lonnie Barbach that focuses on awareness of feelings and sensations through self-exploration and stimulation.

Bartholin's glands Small glands located within the labia minora that secrete a few drops of fluid during sexual arousal.

basal body temperature A woman's body temperature immediately upon waking.

basal body thermometer A special thermometer used to measure changes in basal body temperature.

behavior therapy Applying learning principles to help people change behavior.

bestiality Sexual contact with animals—also called *zoophilia*.

binge-eating disorder (BED) Eating disorder characterized by recurrent binge eating but not by inappropriate weight-control measures.

biopsy (open biopsy) Usually referred to as an open biopsy, a minor surgical procedure during which tissue of a tumor is removed and examined for presence of cancer.

birthing room A homelike birth setting now available in some hospitals.

bisexual One whose erotic, romantic, and affectional attraction is toward both genders.

blended orgasm An orgasm in a female in which there are contractions of the muscles in the outer third of the vagina as well as breath holding; a combination of the vulval and uterine orgasms.

bloody show The expelling of the mucus plug (often streaked with blood) that has closed off the cervix during pregnancy.

body composition The percentage of fat versus lean tissue.

body image The mental image we have of our own physical appearance

body mass index (BMI) Weight in kilograms divided by the square of the height in meters.

bondage perversion Getting sexual pleasure from being bound, tied up, or otherwise restricted.

bonding A process of developing a close physical and psychological relationship with one's caregiver. A sense of close emotional attachment.

Braxton-Hicks contractions Weak and slow uterine contractions that occur during the last few months of pregnancy.

breast abscess Infection of the breast characterized by redness, swelling, and a painful or tender mass.

breast budding First stage of breast development in females, whereby breast tissue elevates as a small mound.

breast cancer The second most common type of cancer in women.

breast self-examination (BSE) A periodic self-care procedure that involves feeling the breast for any abnormalities. The test is performed once every menstrual cycle or every month after menopause.

breech delivery A delivery in which the infant is born with another body part first, rather than head first. This form of delivery can be hazardous for both mother and infant.

bulbocavernosus muscle A muscle that encircles and supports the vagina.

bulimia nervosa A condition in which the individual periodically binges and purges, with an obsessive fear of becoming fat.

bypassing When misunderstandings result from missed meanings.

calendar method Charting of the length of a woman's periods for several months to determine the days she is most likely to be fertile.

call girls Highly paid female sex workers who work by appointment only.

candidiasis A common form of vaginitis, sometimes called a yeast infection, which is caused by the fungus *Candida albicans*.

carcinoma A type of cancer emanating from epithelial cells.

case study In-depth study of individual(s) or small groups.

causation A relationship in which one event causes another event to occur.

cerebral cortex The part of the brain called the gray matter that controls higher-order functioning such as language and judgment.

cervical cap Shallow rubber cap, smaller than a diaphragm, that covers the cervix to prevent sperm from entering the uterus.

cervical secretions Normal fluids from the cervix that change consistency during the month.

cervix The mouth of the uterus, through which the vagina extends.

cesarean section (C-section) Surgical intervention to deliver the fetus, placenta, and membranes through an incision in the walls of the abdomen and uterus.

chancre A painless lesion that is symptomatic of the primary stage of syphilis and appears at the site of contact.

change-of-life baby A baby born to a menopausal woman who, in spite of not menstruating regularly, ovulated.

chemotherapy Use of chemicals (medication) to treat disease may be oral, intravenous, intramuscular, or topical.

child pornography Use of minors in sexually explicit media.

child sexual abuse Any sexual abuse involving fondling, erotic kissing, oral sexual activity, or genital penetration between an adult and a child, including pedophilia and incest.

chlamydia A term that encompasses several major diseases caused by *Chlamydia trachomatis*, including genitourinary tract infection, a type of conjunctivitis in newborns, a type of pneumonia in infants, lymphogranuloma venereum, and trachoma.

Chlamydia trachomatis An intracellular parasite that causes chlamydial infections.

chloasma A yellow to brown patch of skin pigmentation that may appear on the faces of pregnant white women; sometimes referred to as the "mask of pregnancy."

chorionic villi sampling (CVS) A technique for prenatal detection of genetic defects that involves removal of some of the villi growing on the outer surface of the chorion and examining their chromosomes.

cilia Hairlike structures that guide objects, such as ova, moving past them.

circumcision The surgical removal of the foreskin covering the glans penis.

clinical breast exam A breast examination conducted by a physician to detect any abnormalities.

clitoral hood The skin covering the clitoris.

clitoridectomy Surgical removal of the clitoris.

clitoris The structure located at the upper part of the labia minora that is homologous to the penis and is very sensitive to stimulation.

cognitive development Explains the ability to think concretely or abstractly.

cohabitation Situation in which people who live together and share a sexual relationship are not married.

coitus interruptus The Latin term for *withdrawal*, which means "interrupted intercourse."

colostrum The yellow fluid secreted by the breasts just before and after childbirth until milk production begins.

colposcopy An examination of the vagina and cervix using an instrument—a colposcope—to detect abnormal tissue growth.

combined pill (COC) Oral contraceptive containing estrogen and progestin.

come out Accept and make homosexual orientation public.

common-law marriage The recognition by some states that heterosexual couples who have lived together for a specified period and have represented themselves as married are in fact legally married.

conception The union of the sperm and ovum; also called *fertilization*.

conceptual identity Who am I in my world?

conceptus The fertilized ovum; the product of conception.

condom A sheath that covers the penis.

conformity with peers Desire to be like everyone else.

consensual In this context, a married person's engaging in extramarital sexual activity with the knowledge and permission of the spouse.

contraception Means of preventing pregnancy in spite of sexual intercourse.

contraction The shortening or tension of uterine muscles during labor.

control group In an experiment, the group not subjected to a particular event or condition.

coprophilia Sexual pleasure associated with feces.

coronal ridge (corona) The raised ridge where the glans penis ends and the penile shaft begins.

corpora cavernosa A cavernous structure located within the clitoris and the penis that fills with blood during sexual excitement, causing erection.

corpus The upper two-thirds of the uterus.

corpus luteum A yellowish structure that develops in the Graafian follicle at the discharge of an ovum and that produces progesterone and estrogen.

corpus spongiosum A spongy body in the penis that contains a network of blood vessels and nerves.

correlation A relationship between two events; a statistical measure that shows how variables are naturally related to each other.

cosmetic surgery Surgery done for the sole purpose of improving the appearance.

Cowper's glands Two pea-sized glands adjacent to the urethra that secrete a lubricating fluid before ejaculation.

cribriform Type of hymen that creates a sievelike covering for the vaginal opening.

critical thinking Thinking that avoids blind acceptance of conclusions or arguments and closely examines all assumptions.

crowning The presentation of the baby's head at the vaginal opening.

cunnilingus The stimulation of the female genitalia by the mouth, lips, and/or tongue of the sexual partner.

cystic mastitis Known also as fibrocystic disease, a condition characterized by fluid-filled lesions (cysts) that are tender and believed to be related to estrogen activity.

date-rape drugs Sedative hypnotic drugs used to incapacitate victims who are then sexually molested or raped.

decoding Translating the message from its symbol form into meaning.

delivery The stage of childbirth characterized by the expulsion of the infant and the placenta.

Depo-Provera (DPMA) An injectable progestin-only contraceptive.

dermoid cyst A type of benign ovarian cyst commonly found in young women.

desire phase The first stage of the sexual response cycle, as described in Helen Singer Kaplan's model, which consists of psychologically becoming interested in sex before any physical changes occur.

diaphragm Shallow rubber cap that covers the cervix and prevents sperm from entering the uterus.

digital rectal examination (DRE) A rectal examination whereby a physician inserts a finger into the rectum of a male patient to check for any abnormalities of the prostate.

dilation In childbirth, the gradual opening of the cervix during labor.

dilation and evacuation (D&E) Surgical procedure that involves dilating the cervix, scraping the walls of the uterus, and removing the endometrial lining with suction.

dildos Artificial penises.

douche Cleansing of the vagina by inserting a nozzle that secretes a recommended cleansing substance, a controversial procedure.

duration How long something occurs or has occurred.

dysmenorrhea Painful menstruation.

early adolescence First stage of adolescence, defined by pubertal changes—usually ages 9–13 years for females and ages 11–15 years for males.

early ejaculation Persistent or recurring ejaculation before the person wishes it during partnered sexual activity.

eclampsia Pregnancy-induced hypertension accompanied by swelling of the face, neck, and upper extremities, plus convulsions or coma, which may be fat.

ectopic pregnancy The attachment and development of the zygote in a location other than in the uterus.

ejaculation The ejection of semen from the penis during orgasm.

Electra complex Freud's theory that 3- to 5-year-old girls want to take their father away from their mother.

electronic fetal monitoring A technique used during labor whereby a physician places an electrode on the woman's abdomen to monitor the fetal heart rate for signs of fetal distress.

embryo The developing fetus during the 2 months after conception.

embryonic stage The stage of prenatal development that includes the first 8 weeks of pregnancy.

emergency contraception The use of oral contraceptives or insertion of an IUD after unprotected sex has occurred at midcycle.

encoding Converting an idea into words or gestures to convey meaning.

endocrine glands Glands that secrete their products into the bloodstream.

endometriosis The growth of the endometrium uterine lining at a location other than in the uterus.

endometrium The innermost layer of the uterus, to which the fertilized egg attaches and by which it is nourished as it develops before birth, which is partly discharged (if pregnancy does not occur) with the menstrual flow.

epididymis The location where sperm are stored in the testes and where nutrients are provided to help the sperm develop.

episiotomy Incision between the vulva and anus to enlarge the vaginal opening at the time of birth.

erectile dysfunction The inability of a man to obtain or maintain an erection during sexual activity.

erection The extension of the penis and its engorgement with blood when the male is sexually stimulated.

erotica Sexually oriented material that may be artistically produced or motivated.

essentialism Belief that once the cultural and historical aspects are taken away, the essence of sexuality is biological.

estrogen A hormone produced by the ovaries whose level in the blood helps control the menstrual cycle.

ethical dilemma When two or more ethical principles work in opposing fashion in a particular situation, resulting in bewilderment regarding what is moral and what is immoral.

ethical principles Guides by which we can judge an action or decision as moral or immoral.

ethics A system that uses ethical principles to make decisions about morality.

ethnicity The degree of identification an individual feels with a particular ethnic group.

excitement phase The second stage of Kaplan's model of sexual response, which consists of physiological arousal and changes and, possibly, orgasm.

exhibitionism Achievement of sexual gratification by exhibiting the genitals to observers.

expected date of confinement (EDC) Due date for normal pregnancy that is usually estimated by Nägele's rule.

experiment Observation of behavior (or effects) under controlled conditions.

experimental group In an experiment, the group subjected to a particular event or condition.

external urethral sphincter The valve that closes during the emission stage, resulting in a buildup of semen, and that opens during the ejaculation stage, allowing semen to be expelled.

fallopian tubes (oviduct) The routes through which eggs leave the ovaries on their way to the uterus, in which fertilization normally occurs.

feedback When the receiver responds verbally or nonverbally.

fellatio Oral contact with a male's penis.

female condom A polyurethane or synthetic rubber sheath with flexible inner and outer rings worn inside the vagina.

female orgasmic disorder The consistent or frequent inability of a woman to achieve an orgasm.

femininity Those qualities characteristic of and suitable for girls and women according to the rules and expectations of a society.

fertility-awareness methods Methods used to determine fertile days.

fertility-awareness-combined methods Calculation of a woman's fertile times and use of a barrier or withdrawal on fertile days.

fetal alcohol spectrum disorders (FASD) The full spectrum of birth defects that are caused by prenatal alcohol exposure.

fetal alcohol syndrome (FAS) Impaired psychological and physical characteristics common in infants born to alcoholic women.

fetal stage Period from the ninth week of pregnancy to birth.

fetishism Paraphilia in which an inanimate object elicits sexual arousal.

fetus The developing child from the ninth week after conception until birth.

fibroadenoma A benign (noncancerous) tumor that is firm, round, and somewhat movable.

fimbriae The fingerlike ends of the fallopian tubes that catch the ova when they are discharged from the ovaries.

flaccid The relaxed, unerect state of the penis.

flooding Experiencing something so frequently that you no longer are aroused by it. This is a technique used to become more comfortable with sexual terminology.

focus group A form of research where a group of 6 to 10 people are asked about a topic and then discuss related issues.

follicle-stimulating hormone (FSH) A hormone, secreted by the anterior portion of the pituitary gland, that "instructs" the ovaries to prepare an egg to be released from a follicle.

follicular phase The part of the menstrual cycle during which menstruation occurs and the pituitary increases the production of FSH so the follicles mature: a combination of the menstrual and proliferative phases.

foreplay Physical contact preceding sexual intercourse.

foreskin (prepuce) The covering of the glans penis, which is removed during circumcision.

frequency How often something occurs or has occurred.

frottage Obtaining of sexual pleasure from rubbing or pressing against another person.

functional cyst An ovarian cyst that occurs on the follicle or corpus luteum, usually caused by the failure of the follicle to rupture and release an egg.

functional identity What adult roles will I play in the world?

fundus The upper end of the uterus, closest to the opening of the fallopian tubes.

gay Male or female homosexual. (*Gay* used alone probably refers to a male, though it is acceptable to refer to a *gay female*.)

gender constancy The concept that people's gender does not change—even if they change their dress or behavior.

gender dysphoria Feeling trapped in the body of the "wrong" sex.

gender identity The awareness and acceptance of one's gender.

gender role Complex groups of ways males and females are expected to behave in a given culture.

gender-role stereotyping Expectation that individuals will behave in certain ways because they are male or female.

gender schema A grouping of mental representations about male and female physical qualities, behaviors, and personality traits.

gender stereotypes Beliefs about how each gender should behave, which may be over-generalized or rigidly held.

gender typing The process whereby children develop behavior that is appropriate to their gender.

generalization The ability to conclude that the same results would be obtained outside the study.

genital herpes An STI characterized by tiny fluid-filled blisters that appear on the genitals and in the genital tract.

gigolo A man who is paid to provide escort and sexual services, usually for wealthy, middle-aged women.

glans penis The head of the penis.

gonadotropins Sexual hormones secreted by the pituitary that stimulate the gonads to produce their hormones.

gonads The male testes and the female ovaries, which produce gonadotropin hormones responsible for the development of secondary sexual characteristics.

gonorrhea An STI that commonly starts with inflammation of the mucous membrane lining of the openings of the body (e.g., mouth, vagina).

Graafian follicle A part of the ovary from which a mature egg ruptures, allowing the corpus luteum to develop in the location where the egg was released.

Grafenberg spot (G spot) An area located along the anterior wall of the vagina, several inches into the vaginal canal, that when stimulated in some women may result in sexual excitement and/or orgasm.

gynecologist A physician specializing in women's reproductive health.

gynecomastia Glandular tissue development in the breasts of boys.

herpes simplex virus (HSV) The virus that causes oral and genital herpes infections.

heterosexist An attitude that reinforces heterosexuality as the privileged and powerful norm.

heterosexual One whose primary erotic, romantic, and affectional attraction is toward members of the other gender.

homologous Organs that differ but that developed from the same tissue—for example, the glans penis and clitoris.

homophobia An irrational fear of homosexuality.

homosexual One whose primary erotic, romantic, and affectional attraction is toward members of one's own gender.

hormone A chemical substance secreted by a ductless gland, which is carried to an organ or tissue where it has a specific effect.

hormone therapy Form of treatment for cancer that uses hormones to combat cancer cell growth.

hot flashes Intermittent sensations of heat reported by menopausal women, possibly caused by decreased estrogen production.

house (brothel) prostitutes Sex workers who work in brothels.

human chorionic gonadotropin (HCG) A hormone secreted by the placenta whose presence in a woman's urine is the most common medical method of determining pregnancy.

human immunodeficiency virus (HIV) A retrovirus that causes AIDS.

human papillomavirus (HPV) A persistent STI caused by any of a group of viruses associated with the development of cervical cancer and/or genital warts.

human sexuality A part of your total personality. It involves the interrelationship of biological, psychological, and sociocultural dimensions.

hustler A male sex worker who performs homosexual acts for pay.

hymen A thin connective tissue covering the opening of the vagina.

hyperthyroidism Excessive functional activity of the thyroid gland.

hyperventilation Deep and rapid breathing that occurs during sexual excitation.

hypogonadism Decreased activity of the gonads that may result in retardation of growth and sexual development.

hypothalamus A structure in the brain that controls the pituitary gland and is directly connected by nerve pathways to various organs of the body.

hypothesis Tentative proposal or an educated guess about the results of a research study.

hypothyroidism A deficiency of thyroid activity.

"I" statement Statement that begins with an "I" to express personal feelings.

imaginary audience Belief in early adolescence that other people are looking at you as if you are onstage.

immoral What is judged to be wrong according to a system of ethics.

incest Sexual behavior between relatives who are too closely related to be married.

infants Babies from birth to 1 year old.

infertility The inability to reproduce.

informed consent Document required to participate in a research study after the purposes, risks, and benefits of the study have been explained.

internal urethral sphincter The valve that prevents urine from entering the urethra and sperm from entering the bladder during ejaculation.

interstitial cells The cells (sometimes called Leydig's cells) between the seminiferous tubules, where testosterone is produced.

interstitial-cell-stimulating hormone (ICSH) A hormone, secreted by the anterior portion of the pituitary gland in males, that stimulates the production of sperm.

interview Oral research method designed to gather information.

intrauterine device (IUD) Synthetic device that is inserted into the uterus to prevent the sperm from fertilizing the ovum.

intrauterine insemination Introduction of semen into the uterus by noncoital means.

intrauterine system (IUS) Synthetic device placed in the uterus that releases a continuous amount of hormone (levonorgestrel) to prevent ovulation, fertilization, or implantation.

introitus The vaginal entrance.

invasive cervical cancer Cancer that has invaded a wide area of cervical tissue.

in vitro fertilization The creation of a pregnancy in a laboratory by uniting the sperm and egg outside the womb; sometimes termed the "test-tube" baby technique.

Kamasutra Ancient sex manual from India.

Kegel exercises Exercises to help women develop greater control of muscles supporting the genitalia.

klismaphilia Sexual arousal produced by the use of enemas.

labia majora Two large folds of skin whose main function is to protect the external genitalia and the opening of the vestibule (defined later).

labia minora Two folds of skin lying inside the labia majora, which contain numerous blood vessels and nerve receptors.

labor The process of expelling a child by uterine contractions, dilation of the cervix, and bearing-down pressure.

lactation Production of breast milk.

lactobacilli Bacteria in the vagina that aid in keeping it healthy; also called *Doderlein bacilli*.

lactogen A hormone that stimulates the production of milk, the principal one being prolactin.

Lamaze method An approach to childbirth in which exercise and breath control are central to reducing anxiety and discomfort.

laparoscopy Female sterilization procedure that involves inserting a narrow viewing instrument—a laparoscope—through an incision in the abdomen and then performing ligation or applying clips or rings to block the fallopian tubes.

late adolescence Period of transition to adulthood, beginning usually at age 16 years for females and age 17 years for males.

late luteal phase dysphoric disorder (LLPDD) A type of premenstrual syndrome in which mental and emotional symptoms occur the week before menstruation. This is the name given to that condition by the American Psychiatric Association.

latency period Outdated Freudian theory that children aged 6–12 years old have no sexual feelings or interest.

latent genital herpes The stage of genital herpes characterized by inactivity of the herpesvirus, during which an infected individual is asymptomatic and transmission of the virus is rare.

latent syphilis A stage of syphilis that may last for years: early latent (about 1 to 4 years in duration) and late latent (may last for years); it may be symptom free or cause degenerative complications.

latex A synthetic rubber.

lesbian Female homosexual.

letdown The tingling sensation in the breasts when milk is forced out about 30 to 60 seconds after the infant begins to suckle.

libido Sexual desire, or drive.

lifelong erectile dysfunction A condition in which an adult male has never had an erection sufficient to engage in sexual intercourse.

ligation The tying of the fallopian tubes to prevent the sperm–egg union.

limbic system The part of the brain referred to as the "seat of emotions," which produces emotions in response to physical and psychological signals.

liposuction A technique for removing adipose tissue with a suction-pump device.

locus of control Refers to an individual's perception of the main causes of events in life. More simply, is life's destiny controlled by the self (*internal locus*) or by external forces such as fate or other people (*external locus*)?

lumpectomy Removal of a lesion, benign or malignant.

luteal phase The same phase of the menstrual cycle as the secretory phase, which includes ovulation and the production of LH from the corpus luteum.

luteinizing hormone (LH) A hormone, secreted by the anterior portion of the pituitary gland, that stimulates ovulation.

male climacteric Sometimes termed the "male menopause," which occurs at about the same age that women experience menopause, when men experience slightly decreased testosterone production and begin to question the directions in which their lives are headed.

mammary glands Milk-secreting glands located in the female breast.

mammography An X ray of the breasts to detect any abnormality before it is visible or palpable.

manual vacuum aspiration (MVA) A variation of vacuum aspiration that uses nonelectric suction instruments and can be used from detection of pregnancy through 12 weeks.

masculinity Those qualities characteristic of and suitable for boys and men according to the rules and expectations of a society.

massage parlors Places where sex workers can be hired to perform sexual acts under the guise of giving a massage.

masturbation Self-stimulation of the genitals.

meatus The opening of the urethra in the head of the penis, where both seminal fluid and urine are passed.

medical abortion A procedure that uses drugs to induce abortion.

menarche The time when a female begins her first menstrual cycle, usually at 8 to 16 years of age.

menopause The time when a woman's menstrual cycle ceases, usually between 40 and 55 years of age.

menstrual phase The part of the menstrual cycle during which the endometrial lining is sloughed off as the menstrual flow.

menstruation The cyclical emission of the blood-enriched endometrium when pregnancy does not occur.

metastasis Spread of cancer from a primary site to other parts of the body.

methotrexate A drug that blocks the hormone progesterone, which is needed to maintain a pregnancy.

middle adolescence The typical "teenage years," usually ages 13–16 years for females and ages 14–17 years for males.

midlife crisis A time of life, usually between 40 and 50 years of age, during which men question the path their lives have taken and make plans for changing their goals.

midwifery The practice by nonphysicians of assisting in the process of pregnancy and childbirth. Lay midwives are not trained healthcare professionals; nurse midwives are registered nurses who have received advanced training and often certification in the techniques of the birthing process.

mifepristone A drug that blocks the hormone progesterone, which is needed to maintain a pregnancy.

minilaparotomy Female sterilization procedure that involves a small incision in the abdomen through which the fallopian tubes are pulled so they can be blocked.

minipill (POP) A progestin-only pill.

misoprostol A prostaglandin that causes uterine contractions.

mons pubis (mons veneris, mount of Venus) The rounded, soft area above the vaginal opening that becomes covered with hair at puberty.

moral What is judged to be right according to a system of ethics.

morning sickness The condition of nausea and vomiting that is common in early pregnancy; thought to be caused by hormonal changes.

motility The ability to move spontaneously, which is required for fertilization.

multiple orgasms Orgasms that occur without the need for a refractory, or recovery, period.

muscle dysmorphia A disorder whereby a bodybuilder in top shape considers himself or herself to be puny.

myometrium The middle layer of the uterus, consisting of smooth muscle that aids in the pushing of the newborn through the cervix.

myotonia Muscle tension occurring during sexual arousal.

natural childbirth Drug-free childbirth; sometimes called *prepared childbirth*.

natural family planning (NFP) Calculation of a woman's fertile times and abstention from penile–vaginal sex on fertile days.

necrophilia Sexual relations with a dead person.

needle biopsy Insertion of a needle into a lump in a breast to see whether fluid (which indicates a cyst rather than a tumor) can be removed.

Neisseria gonorrhoeae The bacterium that causes gonorrhea; also known as *gonococcus*. Street names include "clap" and "drip."

no-fault divorce The granting of divorce without either partner's proving the other was the cause of the marriage's failure.

nonassertiveness Giving up one's basic rights so others may achieve theirs.

nonconsensual In this context, a married person's engaging in sexual intercourse without the consent of the spouse.

nongonococcal urethritis (NGU) Inflammation of the urethra caused by *Chlamydia trachomatis*, and *Ureaplasma urealyticum, Mycoplasma hominis, Trichomonas vaginalis*, herpes simplex virus, and unknown organisms.

Nonoxynol 9 (N-9) The major spermicidal ingredient in U.S.-made products.

nuclear family A father and mother and their children.

nymphomania An excessive, insatiable sexual drive in women.

objectivity Being sure the results are the same no matter who asks the questions or records the answers.

obscenity Personal or societal judgment that something is offensive. Something offensive to modesty or decency; often sexually related.

observation Watching subjects in a particular setting.

obstetrical analgesia A nondrug pain reliever used in delivery (e.g., hypnosis).

obstetrician A physician who specializes in the care of pregnant women and the process of childbirth. Because these physicians are also gynecologists, they are often referred to as obstetrician–gynecologists or OB–GYNs.

Oedipus complex A development stage in which the boy wants to possess his mother sexually and sees the father as a rival (similar to the female *Electra complex*).

open marriage A marriage in which partners allow each other to have intimate and emotional relationships with others.

opportunistic diseases A major manifestation of AIDS, diseases that occur in the presence of a suppressed immune system.

oral contraceptive (OC) A daily pill taken to prevent pregnancy.

orgasm The peak release of sexual tension, accompanied by sensory pleasure and involuntary rhythmic muscular contractions; ejaculation in the male.

orgasmic platform The narrowing of the outer third of the vagina during orgasm caused by contractions of the muscles in that area.

orgasmic reconditioning Increasing sexual arousal to socially appropriate stimuli.

os The opening to the uterus.

osteoporosis A condition of weakened bones resulting from decalcification (loss of calcium) of bone that increases in the absence of estrogen and is of particular concern in postmenopausal women.

ovarian cancer Cancer of the ovaries that causes more cancer deaths than any other cancer of the female reproductive system.

ovary A structure of the female genitalia that houses ova before their maturation and discharge and that produces estrogen and progesterone.

Ovist Adherent to the 17th-century belief that the preformed baby was contained within the female body and that the male's sperm simply activated its development.

ovulation The part of the menstrual cycle when the ovum is discharged from the ovary.

ovulation methods Observation of signs of ovulation to calculate fertile days.

oxytocin A pituitary hormone that stimulates the breasts to eject milk so that breastfeeding may occur after childbirth.

Pap smear A test of the tissue of the cervix for cervical cancer (named after its founder, Dr. Papanicolaou).

paracervical block An anesthetic used during childbirth that blocks pain sensations in the pelvic area, in which injections are given at positions around the cervix.

paraphilia Literally meaning "love (*philia*) beyond the usual (*para*)," this term refers to various sexual behaviors previously referred to as deviant.

partialism Paraphilia in which sexual arousal is associated with a particular body part.

parturition The process of giving birth.

pediculosis lice Also known as crabs, of three common types: *Pediculus corporis*, a body louse; *Pediculus capitis*, a head louse; and *Pediculus pubis*, a pubic louse.

pedophilia Sexual behavior in which a child is the sexual object.

peer marriage Relationship in which partners have equal status.

pelvic inflammatory disease (PID) Infection of the reproductive organs, particularly the uterus, fallopian tubes, and pelvic cavity.

penetrative behaviors Any behavior whereby penetration occurs—for example, penile–vaginal sex, oral sex, or anal sex.

penile strain gauge A wire or cuff placed around the penis to measure physiological changes over time.

penis Structure of the male external genitalia consisting of the root, shaft, and glans; also contains the urethra, through which urine is excreted.

perfect use The ability of a method of contraception to prevent pregnancy as measured by consistent and correct use.

perimenopause (climacteric) The period just before menopause when the production of estrogen and progesterone is decreasing, usually a 5- to 10-year period.

perimetrium The outermost layer of the uterus, sometimes termed the *serosa*, a very elastic layer that allows the uterus to accommodate a growing embryo and fetus.

pheromones Substances that when secreted have a specific scent found to be sexually arousing.

phimosis Condition resulting when penile erection causes pain because the foreskin is too tight.

pimps Individuals who set up female sex workers with clients.

pituitary The "master gland," an endocrine gland located at the base of the brain that stimulates the other endocrine glands to produce their hormones.

placenta An organ of interchange between mother and fetus; oxygen, nutrients, and waste are exchanged through its cells.

plethysmograph A laboratory measuring device that charts physiological changes over time.

PLISSIT A model of sexual therapy that consists of moving through the stages of giving permission, limited information, specific suggestion, and, if that does not work, intensive therapy.

polygamy When one man is married to more than one woman.

polyurethane A type of plastic.

population The group being studied in a research project.

pornography Visual and written materials used for the purpose of sexual arousal.

precocious puberty Pubertal development before the age of 7 years.

preeclampsia Pregnancy-induced hypertension; symptoms include swelling of the face, neck, and upper extremities; and excess levels of protein in the urine.

premature Type of birth in which an infant is born before the complete term of gestation but late enough in the pregnancy that it has a chance to survive.

premenstrual syndrome (PMS) Marked mood fluctuation during the week before menstruation, accompanied by physical symptoms.

prenatal care Care given to an expectant mother before the birth of her child that typically consists of monitoring fetal development, screening for high-risk pregnancy, and providing education for pregnancy and childbirth.

primary amenorrhea A condition in which a woman of age 18 years or older has never menstruated.

primary dysmenorrhea Painful menstruation, the cause of which is unknown.

primary genital herpes The first stage of a genital herpes infection; it begins with infection by the herpesvirus and the formation of antibodies. Common symptoms include painful lesions in or around the genital area, a sluggish feeling, fever, and possibly swollen lymph nodes.

primary syphilis The first stage of syphilis most generally manifested by the appearance of a painless lesion called a *chancre*.

procreation Sexual intercourse for the purpose of reproduction.

prodrome Itching, tingling, or burning sensations that occur where a herpes lesion will appear.

progesterone A hormone secreted by the corpus luteum signaling the endometrium to develop in preparation for a zygote.

prolactin A pituitary hormone that stimulates the production of milk from the mammary glands.

proliferative phase The first part of the menstrual cycle, during which FSH production is increased and the follicles are maturing.

prostaglandins Hormonelike substances produced by body tissue that may cause dysmenorrhea.

prostate gland A structure of the male internal genitalia that secretes a fluid into the semen before ejaculation to aid sperm motility and prolong sperm life.

prostatitis Infection of the prostate gland.

prostitution Participating in sexual activity for pay or profit.

prurient Characterized by lustful thoughts or wishes.

psychosexual development The blending of sexual aspects of one's development with other psychological factors.

pubic lice A parasite, commonly referred to as crabs, a louse that grips the pubic hair and feeds on tiny blood vessels of the skin.

pubococcygeal muscle A muscle that encircles the vagina and supports it.

questionnaire Written instrument designed to gather information.

quickening Movements of the fetus felt by the mother; usually occurs about the fourth month of pregnancy.

radiation therapy A form of treatment for cancer that uses carefully directed radiation to destroy cancer cells.

random sample A sample that represents the larger population and that is chosen without bias, so that every member of the larger population had an equal chance to be selected.

rape Forcible sexual intercourse with a person who does not give consent.

rape trauma syndrome A two-phase reaction to rape. An acute phase involves intense emotional responses for several weeks. The long-term phase may last several years and involves reorganization and establishment of control.

recurrent genital herpes The fourth stage of a genital herpes infection, which is characterized by a reactivation of the virus and the appearance of blisters on the skin. Not all people with herpes have recurrences.

refractory (recovery) period The time needed by males for recovery between orgasms.

releasing factors Chemicals released from the hypothalamus that affect the function of various body parts.

resolution phase A stage of the sexual response cycle consisting of a return to the prearoused state.

reticular activating system (RAS) A network of nerves that connect the cortex and the subcortex—the connection between mind and body.

retroviruses A group of viruses consisting of ribonucleic acid (RNA) surrounded by a protein coat that can convert their RNA into deoxyribonucleic acid (DNA) once they have invaded a living cell, allowing them to take over the cell and reproduce themselves.

Rh factor The presence of Rh agglutinogens (antigens) in the blood, which indicates that a person is Rh positive, whereas its absence designates the person as Rh negative.

rhinoplasty Surgery done to change the shape of the nose.

rule ethics Guiding principles used in all situations to arrive at moral decisions, which are considered applicable to all situations.

saddle (epidural) block An anesthetic used during childbirth that blocks pain sensations in the buttocks, perineum, and inner thigh.

same-gender marriage A marriage between two people who perceive themselves to be of the same gender.

sample A segment of the larger population.

satyriasis An excessive, insatiable sexual drive in men— also called *Don Juanism*.

scabies Skin irritation caused by a tiny mite that is transferred from one person to another by close contact, sexual or otherwise.

scientific method Research conducted in an atmosphere free from bias.

scrotum (scrotal sac) A sac of skin that contains the testes and spermatic cords.

secondary amenorrhea A condition in which a woman has ceased menstruating after menarche.

secondary dysmenorrhea Painful menstruation caused by some identifiable condition such as endometriosis.

secondary sexual characteristics Changes occurring during adolescence—such as growth of pubic hair, breast development, and testes and penile development.

secondary syphilis The second stage of syphilis, often characterized by a rash.

secretory phase The second part of the menstrual cycle, during which ovulation occurs and the production of LH stimulates the development of the corpus luteum.

self-esteem Sense of personal worth.

self-report data The respondents' descriptions of something.

Semans stop–start method A method of controlling premature ejaculation (developed by James Semans) in which the man tells his partner to stop stimulating him when he feels ejaculation approaching.

semen The male ejaculate, which contains sperm and other secretions.

semenarche First ejaculation of semen for boys.

seminal vesicles Two sacs of the male internal genitalia that secrete nutrients to nourish sperm.

seminiferous tubules The structures located within the testes that actually produce the sperm.

sensate focus A method of alleviating sexual unresponsiveness by procedures designed to encourage erotic feelings and sexual pleasuring.

septate Type of hymen that bridges the vaginal opening.

seronegative The result of a blood test for antibodies to HIV that indicates no presence of such antibodies.

seropositive The result of a blood test for antibodies to HIV that indicates that such antibodies have been found in the blood.

sexism The prejudgment that because of gender a person will possess negative traits.

sexology The study of sexuality.

sexual cognition Attitudes, expectations, beliefs, and values framing one's sexual experiences.

sexual dysfunction A specific, chronic disorder involving sexual performance.

sexual fantasies Thoughts, images, and daydreams of a sexual nature.

sexual harassment Unwelcome verbal, physical, or sexual conduct that has the effect of creating an intimidating, hostile, or offensive environment.

sexual identity Inner sense of oneself as a sexual being, including one's identification in terms of gender and sexual orientation.

sexual interest arousal disorder A sexual dysfunction that causes a woman to experience little or no erotic pleasure through sexual stimulation.

sexual masochism Sexual gratification that results from experiencing pain.

sexual orientation One's erotic, romantic, and affectional attraction to the same gender, to the opposite gender, or to both.

sexual preference Term formerly used to describe sexual orientation that is now outdated, because sexual orientation is no longer commonly considered to be a conscious individual preference or choice, but to be formed by a complicated network of factors.

sexual response cycle The sequence of physiological and psychological reactions as a result of sexual arousal.

sexual sadism Sexual gratification that results from inflicting pain on another person.

sexual self-concept Who am I as a sexual being?

sexually healthy relationship Consensual, non-exploitative, honest, mutually pleasurable, safe and protected from unwanted pregnancy, STIs, and other harm (National Guidelines Task Force, 2004).

sexually related diseases (SRDs) Diseases of the reproductive system that can occur in either sexually active or sexually inactive individuals.

sexually transmitted infections (STIs) Infections that are primarily contracted through sexual contact.

silent infection A stage of HIV infection characterized by no symptoms other than the presence of HIV antibodies.

single-parent family For whatever reason, only one parent who is living with a child or children.

situation ethics A belief that no one set of rules can apply to all situations and each specific situation must be analyzed to determine which ethical principles are applicable.

situational homosexuality Homosexual behavior limited to circumstances in which members of the same gender are deprived of contact with the other gender.

Skene's glands Glands located along the walls of the vagina that are thought to be analogous to the male prostate gland and the site from which some women eject a fluid during orgasm.

smegma A cheeselike substance secreted by the glans penis that must be removed from below the foreskin of uncircumcised males to prevent irritation and/or infection.

social cognition Ability to see a situation from another person's point of view.

social constructionism The belief that sexual identities are acquired from and influenced and modified by an ever-changing social environment.

social training Improving a person's social skills.

socialization The process of guiding people into socially acceptable behavior by providing information, rewards, and punishments.

sodomy A term that specifically refers to anal intercourse, but is often used to refer to almost any sexual behavior someone might not consider normal.

sonogram A diagnostic picture revealing the fetal outline. In ultrasonography, sound waves are bounced off the fetus. With a scanner, the image is then projected onto a computer screen, revealing whether certain defects are present.

speculum A metal (or plastic) instrument that is inserted into the vagina to hold the walls apart, allowing for medical examination.

spermatic cord The cord from which the testicle is suspended that contains the vas deferens, blood vessels, nerves, and muscle fibers.

spermatocytes Cells that develop through several stages to form sperm.

spermatogenesis The manufacturing of sperm in the seminiferous tubules.

spermatorrhea (wet dreams, or nocturnal emissions) Emission of semen during sleep.

spermatozoa (sperm) The mature male sperm cell.

spermicide Chemical detergent compound that immobilizes or kills sperm on contact; as a barrier, prevents sperm from entering the uterus through the cervical os.

spirochete A spiral-shaped bacterium, one of which, *Treponema pallidum*, causes syphilis.

spontaneous abortion (miscarriage) The natural termination of a pregnancy.

squeeze technique A method of helping men control premature ejaculation whereby the penis is gently squeezed when the man senses ejaculation is imminent.

statistical significance The likelihood that a study's results are due to the relationship uncovered between the study's variable as opposed to chance.

statutory rape Intercourse with a person younger than the legal age of consent.

Stein–Leventhal syndrome Reproductive malfunction in women; a syndrome of endocrine origin that involves ovarian cysts, amenorrhea, and infertility.

stepfamily A family with children that is formed as a result of remarriage.

stereotyping The expectation that individuals will exhibit certain characteristics or behaviors.

sterilization A procedure that makes a person biologically incapable of reproducing.

steroids Synthetic versions of the male hormone testosterone that promote tissue growth.

stranger rape Rape of a person by an unknown person.

streetwalkers Sex workers who work on the streets.

survey Research in which people complete questionnaires or are personally interviewed.

swinging Swapping of mates for sexual activities.

symptomatic infection The second stage of HIV infection, characterized by HIV antibodies as well as general signs and symptoms such as swollen lymph glands, fatigue, unexplained weight loss, night sweats, persistent fever, and diarrhea.

symptothermal method A combination of natural family planning methods, in which both temperature and signs of ovulation are observed and charted.

syphilis An STI caused by the spirochete *Treponema pallidum*.

systematic desensitization A means of overcoming anxiety by approaching the anxiety-provoking stimulus in small steps.

tachycardia An increase in heart rate that occurs during sexual activity.

Tanner scale Scale developed by Dr. John Tanner for measuring pubertal development in boys and girls.

teratology The study of causative factors of birth defects.

testes Male gonads contained within the scrotal sacs that produce sperm cells and the male sex hormone testosterone. Singular form: testicle.

testicular cancer Cancer of the testicles; the most common form of cancer in men aged 29 to 35 years.

testosterone The male sex hormone produced in the testes that is responsible for the development of male secondary sexual characteristics.

thriving Normal physical and psychological pattern of weight gain, neuromuscular development and other developmental attributes of infants.

toxemias of pregnancy Hypertensive conditions, subdivided into preeclampsia and eclampsia.

toxic shock syndrome (TSS) A syndrome caused by *Staphylococcus aureus* bacteria in which symptoms include high fever, nausea, vomiting, diarrhea, and a drop in blood pressure; a potentially fatal syndrome that has been linked with the use of superabsorbent tampons.

transgender A general term used when one's identity does not match one's physical/genetic sex. It includes such diverse categories as transsexualism and transvestism.

transsexual A person whose gender identity does not match her or his biological sex; also a person who wishes to have, or has had, his or her gender surgically altered to conform to his or her gender identity.

transudation The process of vaginal lubrication resulting from engorgement of blood that creates pressure that forces moisture to seep from the spaces between the cells.

transvestite A person who achieves sexual satisfaction from wearing clothes usually worn by the other gender.

tribadism Rubbing genitals against someone's body or genital area.

trichomoniasis (trick) A type of vaginitis that can be an STI or an SRD. Symptoms include a foul-smelling, foamy white or yellow-green discharge that irritates the vagina and vulva. Urethritis may also be present.

troilism Having sexual relations with another person while a third person watches.

true labor Characterized by regularly spaced contractions of the uterus, thinning and dilation of the cervix, and a descending of the presenting part of the fetus into the vagina.

tummy tuck Extensive surgical procedure that removes excess skin and fat from the abdomen.

typical use The ability of a method of contraception to prevent pregnancy as actually used at home by people not being monitored.

umbilical cord The lifeline between mother and fetus, which contains two arteries and one vein. Food, oxygen, and chemicals are transported to the child through the arteries, and waste is returned to the mother through the vein.

urethra The tube through which the bladder empties urine outside the body and through which the male ejaculate exits.

urine The body-waste product stored in the bladder and eliminated through the urethra.

urophilia Sexual pleasure associated with urine.

uterine orgasm An orgasm in a female that can occur only in the presence of penile penetration and that involves a woman's holding her breath just before orgasm and then exhaling when the climax occurs.

uterus A pear-shaped hollow structure of the female genitalia in which the embryo and fetus develop before birth.

vacuum aspiration Surgical procedure that uses a suction tube to evacuate the contents of the uterus, which can be used through the first weeks of the second trimester.

vagina A hollow, tunnellike structure of the female internal genitalia whose reproductive functions are to receive the penis and its ejaculate, serve as a route of exit for the newborn, and provide an exit for menstrual flow.

vaginal plethysmography Insertion of a probe into a woman's vagina to measure changes in blood volume.

vaginismus The involuntary contraction of the muscles surrounding the vaginal entrance so that entry of the penis is prevented.

validity, validation Demonstration that tests measure what they are designed to measure.

values Those beliefs to which we attach the most worth.

variable A measurable event that varies or is subject to change.

vas deferens The duct, through which sperm stored in the epididymis is passed, that is cut or blocked during vasectomy.

vasa efferentia The duct through which sperm produced in the seminiferous tubules travel to the epididymis.

vasectomy Cutting or cauterizing of the vas deferens to prevent sperm from being ejaculated; a means of sterilization.

vasocongestion Increased blood flow to an area of the body; which occurs in the pelvic area during sexual arousal.

vasovasectomy Reversal of a vasectomy, so that sperm can be ejaculated.

vestibule The area containing the vaginal and urethral openings.

viral shedding HSV is excreted from the body even though an infected individual experiences no signs or symptoms.

volunteer bias Characteristics of volunteers that are likely to influence research results.

voyeurism Obtaining of pleasure from watching people who are undressing or engaging in sexual behavior.

vulva The female external genitalia.

vulval orgasm An orgasm in a female that includes the contractions of the orgasmic platform, which is not sexually satisfying and, as a result, allows another orgasm to occur almost immediately.

withdrawal Removing the penis from the vagina before ejaculation.

zidovudine The first drug (brand name Retrovir; also known as AZT) approved by the FDA for the treatment of AIDS. This antiviral drug slows the replication of the AIDS virus, thus slowing the course of the syndrome.

zoophilia Sexual contact with animals—also called *bestiality*.

zygote A fertilized egg.

Index

Implants, 205
Impotence, 661
Incest, 574–576
Indecent exposure, 533
India, gender equity promoting
    programs in, 309
Induced abortions, 276
Infanticide, 291
Infants
    conjunctivitis and pneumonia,
        602, 603
    defined, 409
    genital touching, 410–411
    mortality, 258
    sexual development and, 408–412
    touch, role of, 410
Infertility
    causes of, 261–262
    defined, 260
    surrogate mothers, 261
    testing and treatment for, 262–264
Infibulation, 99
Informed consent, 38
Inguinal hernia, 260
Injectables, 205
Integrase strand transfer
        inhibitors, 643
Integrated theories, sexual orientation
        and, 379
Internal urethral sphincter, 162
Internet
    cyber relationships, 456
    cybersex addiction, 543
    dating, 459
    infidelity, 472
    pedophilia, 569
    sex and the, 703–707
    sex therapy and, 679
    sexual abuse using the, 433, 437
    sexual harassment on the, 583
    sexual information on the, 39–40
Interstitial cells, 144
Interstitial-cell-stimulating hormone
        (ICSH), 108
Interviews, 34
Intimate-partner violence, 8,
        577–581
Intracytoplasmic sperm injection
        (ICSI), 264
Intrauterine devices (IUDs), 16
    advantages and disadvantages, 207
    defined, 206
    effectiveness of, 206–207
    emergency contraception, 203, 206
    how it works, 206
    reversibility, 207
    STIs and, 207
Intrauterine insemination
        (IUI), 263
Intrauterine systems (IUSs), 206
Introitus, 101
Invasive cervical cancer, 124–125
In vitro fertilization (IVF),
        263–264, 746
Islamic influence, 11
"I" statements, 85

J

Jefferson, T., 464
John Paul II, 505
Johnson, M., 645–646

Johnson, V., 5, 13, 35, 44–46, 102,
        161–166, 172, 483–484, 521, 663,
        673–674, 675
Johnson & Johnson, 203
Justice/fairness, 735, 736–737

K

Kaiser Family Foundation, 49–50, 52,
        694, 701
Kamasutra, 103, 138, 701
Kanka, M., 574
Kaplan, H.S., 102, 166–167, 663, 674
Kaplan's triphasic model, 166–167
Kegel exercises
    female, 101–102
    male, 139–140
Kennedy, E., 609
Kennedy, J.F., 491
Kenya, gender equity promoting
        programs in, 309
Ketamine hydrochloride, 561
Key, W., 691
King, J.L., 386
Kinsey, A.C., 13, 43–44, 371, 372
Kinsey Institute for Research in
        Sex, Gender, and Reproduction,
        44, 49
Kinsey sexual orientation continuum,
        44, 371
Kissing, 512
Klinefelter's syndrome, 260
Klismaphilia, 540
Koch, E., 393
Kushner, R., 123

L

Labia majora, 98
Labia minora, 98
Labor
    See also Childbirth
    defined, 248
    stages, 249–250
Lactation, 256
Lactobacilli, 620
Lactogen, 256
Lamaze, F., 252
Lamaze method, 253
Lambskin condoms, 189
Laparoscopy, 213
Laparotomy, 116
Late adolescence, 424, 425–426
Late luteal phase dysphoric disorder
        (LLPDD), 114
Latency period, 415
Latent stage of genital herpes, 615
Latent syphilis, 610
Latex condoms, 189
Law, B., 572–573
Laws regulating sexual behavior, 747
    abortion and court decisions,
        278–279
    adultery, 750
    divorce, 751
    myths versus facts, 749
    obscenity and pornography, 748
    polygamy, 750
    rape, 748–750
L-dopa, 170
Learned behavior theory, 378–379
Learning assertiveness, 82–83
Leonardo da Vinci, 21

Lesbian
    See also Homosexuality
    defined, 371
    sexual activities, 521–522
Lesbian, gay, bisexual, and transgender
        (LGBT), 380–383, 388
Letdown, 256
Liberty, 735, 736
Libido, 145, 160
Life expectancy, gender
        differences, 310
Lifelong erectile dysfunction, 661
Ligation, 213
Limbic system, 158–159
Liposuction, 360
Listening
    active, 85, 86
    importance of, 83–85
    reflective, 86
Literature, sex and, 700–702
Liu, D., 44
Lochia, 255
Locus of control, 416
Love
    attraction, what causes, 453–454
    characteristics of romantic, 450–452
    hormonal and chemical aspects
        of, 452
    problems, 452–453
    Sternberg's triangular theory of love,
        450
    theories about, 448–449
    types of, 449–450
LUMA Cervical Imaging System, 125
Lumpectomy, 121
Lunelle, 205
Luteal phase, 111
Luteinizing hormone (LH), 108,
        109–111

M

Magazines, sex and, 701
Magnetic resonance imaging (MRI),
        breast, 121
Male climacteric, 483
Male condoms. *See* Condoms, male
Male genital mutilation, 142
Male hypoactive sexual desire disorder
        (HSDD), 664
Male reproductive system
    circumcision, 140–142
    diseases, self-care and prevention,
        146–151
    external genitals, 138–143
    hormones, 145–146
    internal genitals, 143–145
    myths versus facts, 143
    organs, diagrams of, 138, 139
    organs, functions of, 145
    penis, 138–142
Males
    puberty in, 417–418
    rape of, 563–565
    sexual dysfunctions, 660–664
    sex workers, 717
Male sterilization, 211–212
Maltz, W., 17
Mammary dysplasia, 123
Mammary glands, 106–107
Mammography, 119, 121, 122
Mansfield, B., 704–705

Photo Credits

© Science Photo Library/Alamy; **top (b)** © Jacqueline Shaw/ShutterStock, Inc.; **(bottom right)** © Stephen Coburn/ShutterStock, Inc.; **page 241** © Photos.com; **page 242** © Pixtal/SuperStock; **page 244** © LiquidLibrary; **page 251 (upper left)** © Photos.com; **(upper right)** © Bubbles Photolibrary/Alamy Images; **(lower left)** © Francois Etienne du Plessis/ShutterStock, Inc.; **(lower right)** © Photos.com; **page 252** © Bill Crump/Brand X Pictures/Alamy Images; **page 254** © Francois Etienne du Plessis/ShutterStock, Inc.; **page 256** © Kari Weatherly/Photodisc/Getty Images; **page 262** © Jiang JingJie/ShutterStock, Inc.

Unexpected Pregnancy Outcomes
page 279 (top) © Reuters/Larry Downing /Landov; **(bottom)** © ZUMA Wire Service/Alamy; **page 294** © Varina Hinkle/ShutterStock, Inc.

Chapter 9
page 305 © pryzmat/ShutterStock, Inc.; **page 307** © Anita Patterson Peppers/ShutterStock, Inc.; **page 308** © David Buffington/Photodisc/Getty Images; **page 310** © LiquidLibrary; **page 311** © Jim Ruymen/UPI/Landov; **page 313** © Photos.com; **page 314** © Jennifer Hogan/ Dreamstime.com; **page 318** © Dan Thomas Brostrom/ ShutterStock, Inc.; **page 320** © AP Photos; **page 322** © Photos.com; **page 324** © David Gray/Reuters/Corbis; **page 327** © Thinkstock LLC; **page 328** © Stephen Coburn/ ShutterStock, Inc.; **page 329** © Bartomeu Amengual/ age fotostock; **page 330** Courtesy of Library of Congress, Prints & Photographs Division, [reproduction number LC-USZ62-25812]; **page 332** © Jeff Greenberg/PhotoEdit, Inc.; **page 333** © Photo Works/ShutterStock, Inc.

Body Image
page 344 (top) © Gabi Moisa/ShutterStock, Inc.; **(bottom)** © Kzenon/ShutterStock, Inc.; **page 345** © Patricia Malina/ShutterStock, Inc.; **page 348** © Bjorn Svensson/Alamy Images; **page 350** © Michael Germana/ SSI Photo/Landov; **page 351** © Reuters/Eriko Sugita/ Landov; **page 352** © Photodisc; **page 355** © Photodisc; **page 356 (left)** © AP Photos; **(right)** © Kelley Chin, The Kansas City Star/AP Photos; **page 357** © Banana Stock/ age fotostock **page 358** © Patrick Tuohy/ShutterStock, Inc.; **page 359** © A. Ramey/PhotoEdit; **page 360** © Noel Hines/Landov; **page 362** © Reuters/Alex Grimm/Landov

Chapter 10
page 373 © Photos.com; **page 375** © Photos.com; **page 376** © Paige Falk/ShutterStock, Inc.; **page 378** © Liang Wen You/ShutterStock, Inc.; **page 380** © Joe Gough/ ShutterStock, Inc.; **page 385 (top)** © kzenon/iStockphoto. com; **(bottom)** © LiquidLibrary; **page 390** © Kevin Dietsch/UPI/Landov; **page 391** © Scott Anderson, Racine Journal Times/AP Photos; **page 392** The Kobal Collection at Art Resource, NY; **page 394** © EdStock/iStockphoto. com; **page 396** © BananaStock/Thinkstock

Chapter 11
page 408 © Thinkstock LLC/Jupiterimages; **page 412** © LiquidLibrary; **page 413 (left)** © Andrey Stratilatov/ ShutterStock, Inc.; **(right)** © WizData, Inc./ShutterStock, Inc.; **page 414** © Jones and Bartlett Publishers. Photographed by Kimberly Potvin and Christine McKeen.; **page 415** © Dennis MacDonald/age fotostock; **page 416** © Reuters/Family Communications/Landov; **page 419 (left)** © Photos.com; **(right)** © Mark E. Stout/ ShutterStock, Inc.; **page 421** © Jason Stitt/ShutterStock, Inc.; **page 427** © Stephen Coburn/ShutterStock, Inc.; **page 438** © Richard Hutchings/Photo Researchers, Inc.

Chapter 12
page 449 © digitalskillet/ShutterStock, Inc.; **page 451** © Photos.com; **page 453** © Photos.com; **page 455** © Photos.com; **page 456** © Directphoto.org/Alamy Images; **page 458** © AbleStock; **page 461** © Photos. com; **page 462** © PhotoCreate/ShutterStock, Inc.; **page 463** © WizData, Inc./ShutterStock, Inc.; **page 465** © Photos.com; **page 466** © WizData, Inc./ShutterStock, Inc.; **page 468** © Photos.com; **page 469** © Photos. com; **page 471** © Graca Victoria/ShutterStock, Inc.; **page 473** © Suzanne Tucker/ShutterStock, Inc.; **page 475** © Dhannte/ShutterStock, Inc.; **page 476** © Ami Beyer/ ShutterStock, Inc.; **page 477** © Photos.com; **page 478** © Sylvia Cordaiy Photo Library Ltd./Alamy Images; **page 479** © Sandy Schaeffer/MAI/Landov; **page 481 (left)** © Zdenka Micka/ShutterStock, Inc.; **(right)** © Diane Critelli/ShutterStock, Inc.; **page 482** © Simone van den Berg/ShutterStock, Inc.; **page 484** © bikeriderlondon/ ShutterStock, Inc.; **page 486** © ejwhite/iStockphoto.com; **page 487** © Photodisc/Getty Images; **page 488** © Photos. com; **page 490** © Mark Richards/PhotoEdit

Chapter 13
page 505 Courtesy of AIDS Action Committee of Massachusetts, Inc.; **page 511** © Photos.com; **page 512** © Gertjan Hooijer/ShutterStock, Inc.

Alternative Sexual Behavior
page 533 © Jones and Bartlett Publishers. Photographed by Christine McKeen.; **page 534** © Darren Baker/ ShutterStock, Inc.; **page 536** © Karen Struthers/ ShutterStock, Inc.; **page 537** © Rusian/ShutterStock, Inc.; **page 538** © Figaro Magahn/Photo Researchers, Inc.; **page 543** © Vlad Mereuta/ShutterStock, Inc.

Chapter 14
page 551 Courtesy of Men Can Stop Rape – www. mencanstoprape.org; **page 555 (left)** The Kobal Collection at Art Resource, NY; **(right)** © Tim Harman/ ShutterStock, Inc.; **page 556** © Luba V. Nel/ShutterStock, Inc.; **page 558** © www.imagesource.com/Jupiterimages; **page 560** Courtesy of DEA/U.S. Department of Justice.; **page 561** © Joseph/ShutterStock, Inc.; **page 563** © Charles Rex Arbogast/AP Photos; **page 564** © Hader

Glang/ShutterStock, Inc.; **page 572** © Goldenkb/ Dreamstime.com; **page 575** © franckreporter/iStockphoto. com; **page 577** The Kobal Collection at Art Resource, NY; **page 578** Courtesy The National Coalition Against Domestic Violence; www.ncadv.org; **page 582** © Andres Rodriguez/ShutterStock, Inc.; **page 583** © Louis Lanzano/ AP Photos; **page 585** © Jaimie Duplass/ShutterStock, Inc.; **page 589** © Rena Schild/ShutterStock, Inc.

Chapter 15
page 605 (top) Courtesy of CDC/Joe Miller.; **(bottom)** © Mediscan/Visuals Unlimited; **page 606** Courtesy of CDC/ Dr. Norman Jacobs.; **page 607** Courtesy of CDC.; **page 609** Courtesy of CDC.; **page 610 (top)** Courtesy of CDC/Bill Schwartz.; **(bottom)** Courtesy of CDC/ J. Pledger, BSS/VD.; **page 612 (left)** Courtesy of CDC/ Susan Lindsley.; **(right)** Courtesy of CDC/Joe Millar.; **page 614** Courtesy of CDC/Dr. Herrmann.; **page 615** Courtesy of CDC/ Susan Lindsley.; **page 616** Courtesy of CDC/Dr. N.J. Flumara/Dr. Gavin Hart.; **page 618 (left)** Courtesy of National Cancer Institute; **(right)** Courtesy of Tom Watanabe/U.S. Navy; **page 619** Courtesy of CDC.; **page 620** © Ken Greer/Visuals Unlimited; **page 621** Courtesy of WHO/CDC.; **page 622** Courtesy of CDC/ Susan Lindsley.; **page 624** © Elena Ray/ShutterStock, Inc.; **page 625** © Jones and Bartlett Publishers. Photographed by Kimberly Potvin.

HIV and AIDS
page 637 © Timothy E. Goodwin/ShutterStock, Inc.; **page 639** © rlw/Roger L. Wollenberg/UPI/Landov; **page 644** © Fort Worth Star-Telegram/MCT/Landov; **page 645** © Landov; **page 646** © LiquidLibrary; **page 647** © Hisham Ibrahim/Corbis; **page 649** © Reuters/Jeff Christensen/Landov

Chapter 16
page 659 © gollykim/iStockphoto.com; **page 660** © Ryan McVay/Photodisc/Getty Images; **page 661** © Yuri_Arcurs/ iStockphoto.com; **page 663** © Andrey_Popov/Shutter-Stock, Inc.; **page 665** © -ilkeryuksel-/iStockphoto.com;

page 667 © JJJ/ShutterStock, Inc.; **page 668** © Creatas; **page 669** © Photos.com

Chapter 17
page 692 © Reuters/Mike Segar/Landov; **page 693** © Andrey Burmakin/ShutterStock, Inc.; **page 694** © Jones and Bartlett Publishers. Photographed by Christine McKeen.; **page 698** The Kobal Collection at Art Resource, NY; **page 700** © Jacqueline Abromeit/ ShutterStock, Inc.; **page 701** © Jones and Bartlett Publishers. Photographed by Christine McKeen.; **page 702** © TOSP Photo/ShutterStock, Inc.; **page 704** Courtesy of www.persiankitty.com; **page 707 (left)** © Jones and Bartlett Publishers. Photographed by Kimberly Potvin.; **(right)** © Ismael Montero Verdu/ ShutterStock, Inc.; **page 709** © Jones and Bartlett Publishers. Photographed by Kimberly Potvin.; **page 711** © Natalja/ShutterStock, Inc.; **page 712** © Rob Marmion/ShutterStock, Inc.; **page 715** © Reuters/Sam Mircovich/Landov; **page 717** © maxphotography/iStockphoto.com; **page 723** © Kuzma/ShutterStock, Inc.

Chapter 18
page 734 © AP Photo/The Daily Herald, Brian Winter; **page 738 (top left)** © Matthew Gough/ShutterStock, Inc.; **(bottom right)** © Rob Marmion/ShutterStock, Inc.; **page 740** © Photos.com; **page 744 (left)** © Julie Markes/AP Photos; **(right)** Courtesy of National Cancer Institute/Linda Bartlett.; **page 746** © Antonio Petrone/ ShutterStock, Inc.; **page 750** © Dynamic Graphics/ Jupiterimages; **page 751** © Associated Press, Tom Green Defense Team/AP Photos

Epilogue
page 759 (upper left) The Kobal Collection at Art Resource, NY; **(lower right)** The Kobal Collection at Art Resource, NY; **page 761 (top)** © Jones and Bartlett Publishers. Photographed by Christine McKeen.; **(bottom)** © Darren Baker/ShutterStock, Inc.; **page 762** © jean schweitzer/ShutterStock, Inc.